Supplement to Circulation • Volume 102 • Number 8 • August 22, 20?~

Guidelines 2000 for Cardiopulmonary R
and Emergency Cardiovascular Care

INTERNATIONAL CONSENSUS ON SCIENCE

CIRCULATION (ISSN 0009-7322) is published weekly except combined the first two weeks in January and the last two weeks in December by Lippincott Williams & Wilkins at 12107 Insurance Way, Hagerstown, MD 21740. Business offices are located at 227 East Washington Square, Philadelphia, PA 19106-3780. Production offices are located at 351 West Camden Street, Baltimore, MD 21201-2436. Individuals may subscribe for their personal use at the following rates: $177 for members of an American Heart Association scientific council and $236 for nonmembers; international: $314 for members of an American Heart Association scientific council and $418 for nonmembers. Periodicals postage paid at Hagerstown, MD, and additional mailing offices. POSTMASTER: Send address changes to CIRCULATION, American Heart Association, Lippincott Williams & Wilkins, 12107 Insurance Way, Hagerstown, MD 21740.

Editorials

Guidelines 2000 for Cardiopulmonary Resuscitation and Emergency Cardiovascular Care

An International Consensus on Science

The American Heart Association in Collaboration With the International Liaison Committee on Resuscitation (ILCOR)

ILCOR Member Organizations
American Heart Association (AHA)
Australian Resuscitation Council (ARC)
European Resuscitation Council (ERC)
Heart and Stroke Foundation of Canada (HSFC)
InterAmerican Heart Foundation (CLAR)
New Zealand Resuscitation Council (NZRC)
Resuscitation Council of Southern Africa (RCSA)

International Editorial Board

Richard O. Cummins, MD, MPH,
    MSc—AHA
Mary Fran Hazinski, RN, MSN—AHA
Peter J.F. Baskett, MD—ERC
Douglas Chamberlain, MD—ERC
Leo L. Bossaert, MD—ERC
Vic Callanan, MD—ARC
Pierre Carli, MD—ERC
Marc Gay, MD—HSFC
Anthony J. Handley, MD—ERC
Ian Jacobs, MD—ARC
Richard E. Kerber, MD—-AHA
Walter G.J. Kloeck, MD, BCh—RCSA
Pip Mason, RN—NZRC
William H. Montgomery, MD—AHA
Peter T. Morley, MD—ARC
Martin H. Osmond, MDCM—HSFC
Colin Robertson, MD—ERC
Michael Shuster, MD—HSFC
Petter A. Steen, MD—ERC
James Tibballs, MD—ARC
Sergio Timerman, MD—CLAR
David A. Zideman, MD—ERC

Emergency Cardiovascular Care Committee (1999–2000)

Richard E. Kerber, MD
*Chair, Emergency Cardiovascular Care
    Committee*
Cardiology Division
University of Iowa
Iowa City, IA

Peter J. Kudenchuk, MD
*Vice Chair, Emergency Cardiovascular Care
    Committee*
University of Washington Medical Center
Seattle, WA

Robert A. Berg, MD
*Chair, Subcommittee on Pediatric
    Resuscitation*
Pediatric Critical Care
University of Arizona
Tucson, AZ

Richard O. Cummins, MD, MPH, MSc
*Past Chair, Emergency Cardiovascular Care
    Committee*
University of Washington Medical Center
Seattle, WA

Mary Fry Davis, RN, MN, MEd
Member at Large
Benefits Healthcare
Great Falls, MT

Mary Fran Hazinski, RN, MSN
*Immediate Past Chair, Emergency
    Cardiovascular Care Committee*
Vanderbilt University Medical Center
Nashville, TN

Louis Gonzales, BS, NREMT-P
Member at Large
Department of EMS Technology
Temple College
Temple, TX

Ahamed H. Idris, MD
Chair, Subcommittee on Basic Life Support
Division of Emergency Medicine
University of Florida
Gainesville, FL

Karl B. Kern, MD
*Chair, Subcommittee on Advanced
    Cardiovascular Life Support*
Section of Cardiology
University of Arizona
Tucson, AZ

Rashmi U. Kothari, MD
Member at Large
Borgess Research Institute
Kalamazoo, MI

Mark E. Swanson, MD
*Chair, Subcommittee on Program
    Administration*
The Nemours Children's Clinic
Orlando, FL

Science Product Development Panel (1999–2000)

Mary Fran Hazinski, RN, MSN
Senior Science Editor

Vanderbilt University Medical Center
Nashville, TN

Richard O. Cummins, MD, MPH, MSc
Senior Science Editor
University of Washington Medical Center
Seattle, WA

Tom P. Aufderheide, MD
BLS Editor
Department of Emergency Medicine
Medical College of Wisconsin
Milwaukee, WI

Lance B. Becker, MD
*Conference Coordinator, Evidence
    Evaluation Conference*
University of Chicago Hospital
Chicago, IL

John Field, MD
ACLS Editor
Pennsylvania State University
College of Medicine
Hershey, PA

Vinay M. Nadkarni, MD
Pediatric Resuscitation Editor
A.I. duPont Hospital for Children
Wilmington, DE

Arthur B. Sanders, MD, MHA
*Conference Coordinator, Guidelines 2000
    Conference*
Department of Emergency Medicine
University of Arizona
Tucson, AZ

Edward R. Stapleton, EMT-P
BLS Editor
Prehospital Care and Education
State University of New York at Stony
    Brook
University Hospital
Stony Brook, NY

Arno Zaritsky, MD
Pediatric Resuscitation Editor
The Children's Hospital of King's Daughters
Division of Critical Care
Norfolk, VA

Financial Support

Laerdal Medical Corporation
Agilent Technologies
Survivalink Corporation
Wyeth-Ayerst Pharmaceuticals
Zoll Medical Corporation

Contributors

Dianne L. Atkins, MD
Tom P. Aufderheide, MD
Charles F. Babbs, MD, PhD
Thomas A. Barnes, EdD, RRT
Robert A. Berg, MD
John E. Billi, MD
Paul Berlin, MS, NREMT-P
Leo L. Bossaert, MD
Barry Brenner, MD, PhD
Vic Callanan, MD
Douglas Chamberlain, MD
Leon Chameides, MD
Richard O. Cummins, MD, MPH, MSc
Mary E. Fallat, MD
John Field, MD
Michael J. Gerardi, MD
Louis Gonzales, BS, NREMT-P
Henry R. Halperin, MD, MA
Anthony J. Handley, MD
Mary Fran Hazinski, RN, MSN
Mark C. Henry, MD
Robert W. Hickey, MD
Ahamed H. Idris, MD
Lenworth M. Jacobs, MD, MPH
Richard E. Kerber, MD
Karl B. Kern, MD
Walter G.J. Kloeck, MD, BCh
Rashmi U. Kothari, MD
Peter J. Kudenchuk, MD
Karl H. Lindner, MD
Keith G. Lurie, MD
Thomas G. Martin, MD, MPH
David G.C. McCann, MD
William H. Montgomery, MD
Peter T. Morley, MD
Vinay M. Nadkarni, MD
Graham Nichol, MD, MPH
Susan Niermeyer, MD
Jerry Nolan, MD
Deems Okamoto, MD
Joseph P. Ornato, MD
Martin H. Osmond, MDCM
Charles W. Otto, MD
Michael Parr, MD
Mary Ann Peberdy, MD
Paul E. Pepe, MD, MPH
Barbara Phillips, MD
Gail E. Rasmussen, MD
Robb S. Rehberg, MS, ATC, NREMT
Amelia Gorete Reis, MD

Flavio Ribichini, MD
Colin Robertson, MD
Mitchell P. Ross, MD
Peter Safar, MD
Ricardo A. Samson, MD
Arthur B. Sanders, MD, MHA
Michael R. Sayre, MD
Charles L. Schleien, MD
L.R. Scherer III, MD
Donna L. Seger, MD
Michael Shuster, MD
Michael J. Silka, MD
Adam Singer, MD
Edward R. Stapleton, EMT-P
Petter A. Steen, MD
Fritz R. Sterz, MD
Lark Stewart, MS, NREMT
Ian Stiell, MD, MSc
Mark E. Swanson, MD
Wanchun Tang, MD
Thomas E. Terndrup, MD
James Tibballs, MD
Sergio Timerman, MD
Francisco de la Torre, MD
Patrick Van Reempts, MD, PhD
Max Harry Weil, MD, PhD
Volker Wenzel, MD
Roger D. White, MD
Arno Zaritsky, MD
David A. Zideman, MD

AAP, AHA, and ILCOR Neonatal Resuscitation Contributors and Reviewers

Susan Niermeyer, MD
John Kattwinkel, MD
Vinay M. Nadkarni, MD
Robert A. Berg, MD
David Boyle, MD
Robert Boyle, MD
David Burchfield, MD
Waldemar Carlo, MD
Leon Chameides, MD
Susan E. Denson, MD
Michael J. Gerardi, MD
Alistair Gunn, MD
Walter G.J. Kloeck, MD, BCh
Anthony Milner, MD
Barbara Nightengale, CNNP
Martin H. Osmond, MDCM
Jeffrey Perlman, MD
Barbara Phillips, MD
Gail Rasmussen, MD
Ola Didrick Saugstad, MD
Alfonso Solimano, MD
Michael Speer, MD
James Tibballs, MD

Suzanne Toce, MD
Patrick Van Reempts, MD, PhD
Thomas Wiswell, MD
Arno Zaritsky, MD
David A. Zideman, MD
Jelka Zupan,MD

Collaborating Organizations

American Academy of Pediatrics (AAP)
American Association for Respiratory Care
American Association of Critical-Care
    Nurses
American College of Cardiology
American College of Emergency Physicians
American College of Surgeons
American Heart Association:
    Cardiopulmonary and Critical Care
    Council
American Heart Association: Council on
    Cardiovascular Nursing
American Medical Association
American Safety and Health Institute
American Society of Anesthesiologists
Association of Black Cardiologists, Inc.
Australian Resuscitation Council
Centers for Disease Control and Prevention:
    Cardiovascular Health Branch, National
    Center for Chronic Disease Prevention
    and Health Promotion
Emergency Room Nurses Association
EMP International, Inc.
European Resuscitation Council
Health Resource Service Administration:
    Maternal Child Healthcare Bureau,
    Emergency Medical Services for Children
    Program
Heart Association of Thailand
Heart and Stroke Foundation of Canada
InterAmerican Heart Foundation: Emergency
    Cardiovascular Care Committee
International Liaison Committee on
    Resuscitation (ILCOR)
Japan Resuscitation Council
National Association of EMS Educators
National Association of EMS Physicians
National Association of EMT's
National Heart, Lung, and Blood Institute:
    Heart Research Program
National Institute of Neurological Disorders
    and Stroke
National Registry of Emergency Medical
    Technicians
National Resuscitation Council of Taiwan
National Safety Council
New Zealand Resuscitation Council
Resuscitation Council of Southern Africa
Saudi Heart Association
Society for Academic Emergency Medicine
Society of Critical Care Medicine

Acknowledgments

The editors and contributors gratefully acknowledge the extraordinary dedication of the AHA staff who made this publication possible, in particular Jackie Haigney, Mary Ann McNeely, F.G. Stoddard, and Starr Wheelan.

Part 1: Introduction to the International Guidelines 2000 for CPR and ECC

A Consensus on Science

International Guidelines

This publication presents the conclusions of the International Guidelines 2000 Conference on Cardiopulmonary Resuscitation (CPR) and Emergency Cardiovascular Care (ECC). We have achieved a long-term goal: to create valid, widely accepted international resuscitation guidelines based on international science and produced by international resuscitation experts. The Guidelines 2000 Conference was more than an update of previous recommendations for CPR and ECC published by the AHA (in 1974,[1] 1980,[2] 1986,[3] and 1992[4]) and similar recommendations published by the European Resuscitation Council (in 1992,[5] 1996,[6] and 1998[7]). The Guidelines 2000 Conference was the world's first international conference assembled specifically to produce international resuscitation guidelines.

At all stages of planning, coordination, and implementation, conference planners sought and achieved active involvement of individuals and councils outside the United States.

Important new recommendations were developed either at the 2000 conference or during the post-conference period of writing, review, and rewriting. Positive new additions had to pass our rigorous evidence-based review. Revisions of or deletions from existing guidelines occurred for any of 3 reasons: (1) lack of evidence to confirm effectiveness, (2) additional evidence to suggest harm or ineffectiveness, or (3) evidence that superior therapies have become available.

We have also produced the *International Consensus on Science: Proceedings of the 2000 Guidelines Conference on CPR and ECC*. The proceedings are detailed articles that recount the discussions and debates at the 2 conferences.

The International Guidelines 2000 represent a consensus of experts from a variety of countries, cultures, and disciplines. The conference experts, participants, and resuscitation councils do not dictate or impose these recommendations on any person, Emergency Medical Services (EMS) system, hospital, healthcare facility, community, state, country, or resuscitation council. The majority of the therapeutic interventions in the guidelines are "acts of medical practice." Most resuscitation personnel in the conference countries can use these interventions on a human being **only** when authorized by the "proper" local, state, or national agencies. Enforcement, authorization, and certification are medicolegal concepts with no role to play in the science-based International Guidelines 2000.

The recommendations of the Guidelines 2000 Conference confirm safety and effectiveness for many approaches, acknowledge ineffectiveness for others, and introduce new treatments that have survived intensive evidence-based evaluation. These new recommendations do not imply that care using past guidelines is either unsafe or ineffective. The conference participants consider these new guidelines to be the most effective and easily teachable guidelines that current knowledge, research, and experience can provide.

Historical Perspective

During the 40 years since the introduction of modern CPR and ECC there have been many advances in ECC for cardiac arrest victims. These interventions have restored the lives of many people when breathing has ceased and the heart has stopped. For those with preserved neurological function and treatable cardiopulmonary disease, a lengthy, vigorous, and high-quality life may often follow.

Until 1960 successful resuscitation was limited to victims of respiratory arrest. Emergency thoracotomy with "open-chest heart massage" was sometimes successful when proper personnel and equipment were readily available.[8] Termination of ventricular fibrillation by externally applied electricity was first described in 1956.[9] The ability of defibrillators to reverse a fatal arrhythmia was a dramatic achievement. Defibrillators challenged the medical community to develop ways to get the defibrillator to the patient's fibrillating heart as fast as possible while simultaneously sustaining ventilation and circulation. These challenges will continue into the next millenium.

In the 1950s Safar et al[10] and Elam et al[11] "rediscovered" mouth-to-mouth ventilation by reading how midwives used the technique to resuscitate newly born infants. In 1958 Safar et al confirmed the effectiveness of the mouth-to-mouth ventilation technique of Elam et al. In 1960 Kouwenhoven et al[12] observed that forceful chest compressions produced respectable arterial pulses. In a series consisting chiefly of anesthesia-induced cardiac arrests they confirmed that chest compressions alone could sustain life while awaiting more definitive care. The critical steps of modern CPR—"closed-chest" compressions and "mouth-to-mouth" ventilations—had arrived.[12]

Over the next several years, through casual conversations, Safar and Kouwenhoven saw the rationale for combining closed-chest compressions with mouth-to-mouth ventilations. Soon Safar confirmed the combined technique, now known as basic CPR. The simplicity of this technique has led to its

Circulation. **2000;102(suppl I):I-1–I-11.**
© 2000 American Heart Association, Inc.

Circulation is available at http://www.circulationaha.org

TABLE 1.   Milestones on the Way to International Guidelines 2000—The First International Conference on Guidelines for CPR and ECC

1966—First Conference on CPR: National Academy of Sciences, National Research Council	Recommended training medical, allied health, and other professional personnel in external chest compressions according to American Heart Association standards.[13,14]
1973—Second National Conference on CPR: American Heart Association, National Academy of Sciences, National Research Council	Recommended that CPR training programs be extended to the general public.
1979—Third National Conference on CPR: American Heart Association	Developed ACLS; recommendations for training, testing, and supervising medical and allied health personnel.
1983—First National Conference on Pediatric Resuscitation: American Academy of Pediatrics, American Heart Association	Developed guidelines for pediatric BLS and ALS, with separate guidelines for neonatal ALS.
1985—Fourth National Conference on CPR and ECC: American Heart Association, American Academy of Pediatrics	Reviewed experimental and clinical research published since the 1979 conference.
1992—Fifth National Conference on CPR and ECC: American Heart Association plus collaborating Councils. First meeting of ILCOR	Reviewed developments over the previous 7 years. These required review and resolution of disputes and disagreements. ILCOR founded; began 2 meetings a year until 2000.
2000—The First International Guidelines Conference on CPR and ECC: International Collaboration of AHA, ERC, HSFC, RCSA, ARC, CLAR, and others	First conference that was international in planning, topics, experts, writing, review, and publication. First to be evidence-based; used new class of recommendations.

ARC indicates Australian Resuscitation Council; CLAR, Resuscitation Councils of Latin America; ERC, European Resuscitation Council; HSFC, Heart and Stroke Foundation of Canada; RCSA, Resuscitation Councils of Southern Africa.

widespread dissemination: "All that is needed is 2 hands." The technique gives hope for reducing the nearly 1000 sudden deaths (on average) that occur each day, both in the United States and also in the whole of Europe, before patients reach the hospital.

Achievements and Recommendations from Previous Guideline Conferences

The Guidelines 2000 Conference must not be considered an American conference or an AHA conference. The most valid descriptive term is *international*. This conference, planned and organized by a liaison of the world's major resuscitation councils, embraced a wide range of topics and issues. Each previous conference also established important milestones (Table 1).

Beginning with the original 1966 conference of the National Academy of Sciences–National Research Council, every AHA conference has invited numerous international experts as well as delegates from international resuscitation councils. International intellectual exchange was pervasive, and all perspectives benefited from the exchange. Whether we think of ourselves as AHA delegates or European Resuscitation Council delegates matters nothing. We are now the World's Resuscitation Council; we hold a sobering responsibility to rise above national pride and self-interest and work together to achieve our simple goal—to reduce morbidity and mortality from cardiovascular and cardiopulmonary disease. Table 1 summarizes the important work that paved the way for modern CPR and ECC. The scientists, clinicians, experts, leaders, managers, and instructors who planned, developed, and conducted these conferences deserve our thanks and gratitude. We are in debt to their creativity, industry, and hard work.

Scientific Advances: ILCOR, Stroke, Acute Coronary Syndromes, and Public Access Defibrillation

Resuscitation is an active and exciting area of research. By 1997 ECC leaders recognized the need to incorporate new scientific advances into international guidelines in a timely fashion. The member councils of the International Liaison Committee on Resuscitation (ILCOR) provided strong support for this idea. As an international "council of councils," ILCOR embarked on a 2-year plan to develop a series of "advisory statements." These statements pursued 2 objectives: to identify all differences and inconsistencies among existing guideline publications and to conduct evidence-based review of resuscitation topics and advise the liaison councils on topics to revise, delete, or insert. ILCOR has published these advisory statements in *Circulation* and *Resuscitation*.

Rapid change occurred in the management of acute ischemic stroke and acute coronary syndromes between 1992 and 1997. In collaboration with other societies, a Stroke Task Force plus an Acute Coronary Syndrome Working Group developed interim guidelines. These guidelines have appeared in the 1995, 1997, 1999, and 2000 ECC handbooks.

New guidelines for the lay-responder's use of automated external defibrillators (AEDs) were developed following 2 national conferences on public access defibrillation (PAD).[15] This led directly to the development of the Heartsaver AED program, which provides a 3- to 4-hour course in both CPR and the use of an AED. The course is addressed to lay rescuers and first responders in the community.[16]

2000—The First International Conference on Guidelines for CPR and ECC

The objectives of the Guidelines 2000 Conference were to

1. Fulfill the 1992 goal of producing the first (a) international guidelines (b) supported by international science and (c) developed by international collaboration. A related goal was to have >50% of the conference participants affiliated with non-US organizations.
2. Establish ILCOR as the committee responsible for coordinating the international science review and communicating the international science conclusions via the recurring ILCOR advisory statements.

3. Confirm our strong commitment to these goals by requiring numerical equality—AHA versus non-US councils—on all guideline panels, topic discussions, summary presentations, moderator positions, panel experts, writers, summary presenters, and members of editorial boards.
4. Draft a consensus document that explained evidence-based guidelines development and evaluate the success or failure of evidence-based guidelines development. The draft consensus document was evaluated formally multiple times with appropriate revisions and modifications after each evaluation:
   • Mini-Evidence Evaluation Conference, March 1999
   • 2000 Evidence Evaluation Conference, September 1999
   • Guidelines 2000 Conference, February 2000
5. Review and revise recommendations from past conferences, based on scientific evidence that had accumulated since the previous guidelines. Develop guidelines for first aid at home and at the work site.
6. Review and recommend changes in the methods recommended for teaching the knowledge and skills of ECC, basic life support (BLS), pediatric advanced life support (PALS), and advanced cardiovascular life support (ACLS) in education and evaluation.

Evidence-Based Resuscitation Guidelines

Conference participants used evidence-based criteria to identify, evaluate, and appraise scientific publications and to propose needed changes. We supplied all experts, panel members, and attendees with a Worksheet for Proposed Evidence-Based Guidelines with step-by-step directions (these materials are available on the AHA website at http://www.americanheart.org/ECC/index.html). To increase the validity of the results obtained by this evidence-based approach, conference leaders requested help from topic experts, panel members, and members of the ECC Committee and the International Editorial Board. These reviews checked all changes and new interventions, not just for scientific accuracy, but also for possible future effects on *safety*, *cost*, *effectiveness*, and *teachability*.

All resuscitation councils and experts that participated in the Guidelines 2000 Conference applied the tools and principles of evidence-based medicine on all proposed guidelines:

1. Search for evidence: yield is a series of individual studies/publications
2. Determine the *level* of each piece of evidence (a single study's methodology) (see Table 2)
3. Critically *appraise* the quality of each article
4. Integrate all the acceptable evidence into a final *class of recommendation*.

Tables 2, 3, and 4 define the steps and terms used for this process.

The Effectiveness of ECC

Emergency Cardiovascular Care Defined

ECC includes all responses necessary to deal with sudden and often life-threatening events affecting the cardiovascular, cerebrovascular, and pulmonary systems. ECC specifically includes

1. Recognition of early warning signs of heart attack and stroke, efforts to prevent complications, reassurance of the victim, and prompt availability of monitoring equipment
2. Provision of immediate BLS at the scene when needed
3. Provision of ACLS at the scene as quickly as possible to defibrillate if necessary and stabilize the victim before transportation
4. Transfer of the stabilized victim to a hospital where definitive cardiac care can be provided

The most important link in the ECC system in the community is the layperson. Successful ECC depends on laypersons' understanding of the importance of early activation of the EMS system, their willingness and ability to initiate effective CPR promptly, and their training in and safe use of AEDs. Accordingly, providing lifesaving BLS at this level can be considered primarily a public, community responsibility.

ACLS includes the use of adjunctive equipment in supporting ventilation, the establishment of intravenous access, the administration of drugs, cardiac monitoring, defibrillation or other control of arrhythmias, and care after resuscitation. In virtually every EMS system in the world a medical physician must be involved to supervise and direct ACLS efforts (1) in person at the scene, (2) by direct voice communication, or (3) by the widely used mechanism of "standing orders." These are a set of written, condition-specific orders that instruct the nonphysician responders.

The Chain of Survival

The highest potential survival rate from cardiac arrest can be achieved only when the following sequence of events occurs as rapidly as possible: (1) recognition of early warning signs, (2) activation of the EMS system, (3) basic CPR, (4) defibrillation, (5) management of the airway and ventilation, and (6) intravenous administration of medications.[17] These events are indispensable for any success of the ECC endeavor. They have been likened to links in a chain. If any link is weak or missing, the chance of survival is lessened, and the EMS system is condemned to poor results. The links in the adult Chain of Survival are (1) early access, (2) early CPR, (3) early defibrillation, and (4) early ACLS.

Effectiveness of the Chain of Survival

Cost-effectiveness studies relate money expended to lives saved.[18–24] ECC-CPR leaders have asked questions about the proven effectiveness of the Chain of Survival and the separate links in the Chain. Is there a positive balance between the outcomes from adding new drugs or medical devices and the costs to obtain the new interventions?[25,26]

Our Most Effective Intervention: Defibrillation

Defibrillation, as an intervention, can be analyzed as a balance between costs expended and the clinical outcome. One study examined how many person-years of life would be added to a community if firefighters not currently providing any emergency medical care were trained to do CPR and defibrillation.[21] Another model estimated how many years of *quality-adjusted* person-years of life would be gained by decreasing time to defibrillation by 1 minute with a new PAD program.[22] If PAD is implemented with lay responders, the

TABLE 2. Levels of Evidence

Evidence Level	Definition
1. Positive RCTs ($P<0.05$)	A prospective RCT. Conclusions: new treatment significantly better (or worse) than control treatment.
2. Neutral RCTs (NS)	An RCT. Conclusions: new treatment no better than control treatment.
3. Prospective, nonrandom	Nonrandomized, *prospective* observational study of a group that uses new treatment; *must* have a control group for comparisons.
4. Retrospective, nonrandom	Nonrandomized, *retrospective* observational study; 1 group used new treatment; must have a control group for comparisons.
5. Case series	Series of patients received new treatment in past or will receive in future; watch to see what outcomes occur; no control group.
6. Animal studies (A and B)	Studies using animals or mechanical models; A-level animal studies are higher quality than B-level studies.
7. Extrapolations	Reasonable extrapolations from existing data or data gathered for other purposes; quasi-experimental designs.
8. Rational conjecture, common sense	Fits with common sense; has face validity; applies to many non–evidence-based guidelines that "made sense." No evidence of harm.

RCT indicates randomized, controlled trial.

program costs 1.5 times more per added quality-adjusted life-year than if implemented with police.

Decision analysis was used recently to assess the effectiveness of decreasing time to defibrillation by adding an early defibrillation program to the gaming casinos of Las Vegas, Nevada (USA). The program enrolled casino security guards and trained and equipped them to respond within 2 to 4 minutes to any arrest in the facility.[23] This early defibrillation program published the lowest cost per year of added life of any published out-of-hospital care program.

Decreasing time to defibrillation appears most cost-effective when a low-intensity intervention is used, such as police or lay responder defibrillation. Currently adding more professional responders to an existing EMS system to decrease the collapse-to-first-shock interval is economically unattractive.

Advanced Life Support

Studies that have evaluated the cost of ACLS for out-of-hospital sudden cardiac arrest have been severely limited. The best methodology, using the most comprehensive costing methods, confirmed the value of decreasing time to defibrillation by implementing early defibrillation in gaming establishments.

TABLE 3. Steps to Follow for Evidence Integration

Integrate all evidence following these steps:

1. Determine **level of evidence** based on methodology (as in Table 2)

2. Perform **critical appraisal** *(poor to excellent)*

3. Integrate all evidence into a final **class of recommendation** (see Table 4). Experts must distill many articles, at different evidence levels, at different quality levels, into one class of recommendation. Steps used include

   Consensus discussions by experts, plus

   1999 Evidence Evaluation Conference discussions, plus

   Guidelines 2000 Conference input, plus

   Final editorial review by *International Editorial Board, Science Product Development Panel, ECC Committees and Subcommittees*

The goal of CPR-ECC programs is to increase the number of lives saved by prevention, risk factor modification, and emergency intervention at comparatively little cost.[27] Improving the efficacy of emergency cardiovascular intervention for victims of cardiopulmonary arrest requires aggressive implementation strategies.

Cardiopulmonary-Cerebral Resuscitation

Although the importance of CPR and BLS is undisputed, the efficacy of CPR in prolonged arrest is modest at best. When CPR and defibrillation are delayed or when definitive care is not closely followed, the Chain of Survival is broken. The cerebral cortex, the tissue most susceptible to hypoxia, is irreversibly damaged, resulting in death or severe neurological damage. The need to preserve cerebral viability must be stressed both in research endeavors and in practical interventions. The term *cardiopulmonary-cerebral resuscitation* has been used to further emphasize this need.[28,29]

The initial hope for closed-chest CPR was that circulation and oxygenation could maintain viability long enough to bring the defibrillator to the victim's aid.[12] BLS is often successful if defibrillation (and other modes of definitive care) occurs sooner than 8 to 10 minutes after collapse.[30–32] If restoration of spontaneous circulation occurs after the 8- to 10-minute limit, the frequency of significant, permanent neurological damage becomes unacceptably high. Responding and shocking as fast as possible, seldom exceeding 8 to 10 minutes, is a central objective of all EMS systems. In many communities it rarely happens.

The Hope of Public Access Defibrillation

By the mid and late 1990s great optimism arose because of reports of success from early PAD-like programs. PAD programs stay within the limit of 8 to 10 minutes, and can even decrease the response interval to as little as 3 to 5 minutes.[33–40] These and other preliminary data from PAD programs confirm epidemiological observations that every minute increment from the time of collapse to defibrillation will result in a substantial decrease in survival. This objective

TABLE 4.   Classes of Recommendations 2000: Classification of Therapeutic Interventions in CPR and ECC

1. Search for Evidence: Locates the Following	2. Consensus Review by Experts: Intervention Is Placed in Following Class	3. Interpretation of This Class of Recommendation When Used Clinically
Minimum evidence required for a Class I recommendation • Level of evidence: 1 or more RCTs • Critical assessment: *excellent* • Results: homogeneous, consistently positive, and robust	*Class I: Excellent* *Definitely recommended* Supported by ***excellent*** evidence Proven efficacy and effectiveness	**Class I** interventions are always acceptable, proven safe, and definitely useful.
Minimum evidence required for a Class IIa recommendation • Level of evidence: higher • Number of studies: multiple • Critical assessment: *good to very good* • Weight of evidence/expert opinion: more strongly in favor of intervention than Class IIb • More long-term outcomes measured than Class IIb • Results: positive in majority of studies • Observed magnitude of benefit: higher than Class IIb • Results: positive in majority of studies • Observed magnitude of benefit: higher than Class IIb	*Class IIa: Good to very good* *Acceptable and useful* ***Good/very good*** evidence provides support Note*: "Contextual" factors: In addition to level of evidence, these additional factors are considered in making final class of recommendation. Contextual factors include small magnitude of benefit, high cost, educational and training challenges, large difficulties in implementation, and impractical, unfavorable cost-benefit ratios.	**Class IIa** interventions are acceptable, safe, and useful. • Considered standard of care: reasonably prudent physicians can choose • Considered ***intervention of choice*** by majority of experts • Often receive AHA support in training programs, teaching materials, etc *"Contextual" or "mismatch" factors may render an intervention Class IIa in one context and Class IIb in another (see Note*).*
Minimum evidence required for a Class IIb recommendation • Level of evidence: lower/intermediate • Number of studies: few • Critical assessment: *fair or poor* • Weight of evidence/expert opinion: less in favor of usefulness/efficacy • Outcomes measured: immediate, intermediate, or surrogate • Results: generally, not always, positive	*Class IIb: Fair to good* *Acceptable and useful* ***Fair to good*** evidence provides support. Note: Contextual/mismatch factors should not be used to avoid the trouble and expense of adopting new but clinically beneficial interventions.	**Class IIb** interventions are acceptable, safe, and useful. • Considered within "standard of care": reasonably prudent physicians can choose • Considered *optional* or *alternative interventions* by majority of experts
Evidence found but available studies have one or more shortcomings • Promising but low level • Fail to address relevant clinical outcomes • Are inconsistent, noncompelling, or report contradictory results • May be high level but report conflicting results	*Class Indeterminate* *Preliminary research stage* Available evidence insufficient to support a final class decision Results promising but need additional confirmation Evidence: no harm, but no benefit No recommendation until further evidence is available.	Note: Interventions classed **Indeterminate** can still be recommended for use, but reviewers must acknowledge that research quantity/quality fall short of supporting a final class decision. Do not use *Indeterminate* to resolve debates among experts, especially when evidence is available but experts disagree on interpretation. *Indeterminate* is limited to promising interventions.
Positive evidence completely absent *or* **Evidence strongly suggests or confirms harm**	*Class III: Unacceptable, no documented benefit, may be harmful* *Not acceptable, not useful, may be harmful*	Interventions are designated as Class III when evidence of benefit is completely lacking or studies suggest or confirm harm.

RCT indicates randomized, controlled trial.

of earlier defibrillation has been attained in multiple PAD venues, including police, first responders, airports, and commercial airline flights. These researchers also reported substantial increases in the frequency of neurologically intact survivors.

With reported survival rates of up to 49%, PAD has the potential to be the single greatest advance in the treatment of prehospital sudden cardiac death since the invention of CPR.

The Preventive Cardiology–CPR Paradox

Fully 50% of men and women in western society with serious coronary artery disease (CAD) experience their first signs of the disease in a dramatic way—sudden cardiac arrest. This statement may apply to women as well, but no study has examined this issue in women. The first sign of progressive narrowing of the coronary arteries from the decades-long buildup of intra-arterial plaque can be a rapid sequence of sudden plaque rupture or erosion, platelet adhesion, and an occluding thrombus. The arterial obstruction leads to severe ischemia, an irritable myocardium, and sudden generation of ventricular fibrillation, collapse, and death. Whether a victim lives or dies at this point depends on whether the collapse is witnessed; whether the people who respond are trained in CPR, resuscitation, and defibrillation; and whether they work within an emergency response system that can bring about early arrival of BLS and ACLS resources.

The "Risk Factors Modification and Prevention Message" for Preventive Cardiology.

The following statements are modified from the 1992 *Guidelines for CPR and ECC*, pages 2175–2176.

1. Cardiac arrest and MI are, in the vast majority of cases, end points in the evolution of atherosclerotic arterial disease over a period of decades.
2. The rate of progression of atherosclerosis is the primary determinant of the age at which MI and sudden death occur.
3. The rate of progression can be significantly influenced by specific conditions and behaviors referred to as *risk factors*.
4. Control or elimination of risk factors can be achieved by establishing positive health attitudes and behaviors in the young.
5. Modification of cardiovascular risk factors in adults, even in those who have had an MI, can alter the rate of progression of arterial disease and reduce the incidence of major end points, ie, sudden death, MI, and stroke.
6. Effective strategies to delay death due to cardiovascular disease include primary, secondary, and tertiary prevention and therapy.
7. Significant modifications in risk factors can occur by exercise; cessation of smoking; dietary modification; treatment and control of hypertension; and use of statin agents, anticoagulants, antiplatelet agents, angiotensin-converting enzyme inhibitors, as well as aspirin and β-blockers.
8. Effective strategies to delay death after successful treatment of sudden cardiac arrest include use of amiodarone or implantable cardioverter-defibrillators.

The perspective of preventive cardiology is to point out the strange paradox of investing so much time and so many resources into an EMS response when such a death would have been so easy to prevent or at least delay through the principles of preventive cardiology.

The sidebar reprints statements endorsed by the 1992 Guidelines Conference. The elimination of most of this material from lay and healthcare provider CPR training implies no disagreement with these concepts and recommendations. Neither does this imply rejection of the concept that prevention is the best way to reduce the heavy toll of premature morbidity and mortality from heart disease and stroke.

The goals of teaching the community to function as a prevention intervention and as the ultimate coronary care unit are as follows:

1. Adoption of healthy heart living at the earliest age possible, focusing on diet and preventive screening before any development of a disease process (primary prevention)
2. Recognition and reduction of reversible risk factors among the population free of clinical manifestations of CAD, especially among the young (secondary prevention)
3. Recognition and reduction of reversible risk factors among the population in which disease is progressing and clinical manifestations of CAD are beginning (tertiary prevention)
4. A lay public able to recognize the symptoms of a possible MI and educated to seek prompt entry of the victim into the EMS system
5. A lay public educated in the importance of early BLS and ACLS and eager to support an effective EMS system in the community
6. A lay public able to support the life of the cardiac arrest victim until ACLS becomes available

Final Comments: Have We Achieved "International Guidelines" at the Guidelines 2000 Conference on CPR and ECC?

The authors named the *International Guidelines 2000 Conference* appropriately. Participants from outside the United States comprised 40% of the total number of people attending. Planning for the new international guidelines included concerted efforts to have international representation at all stages. The Conference did achieve equality in terms of the important roles of primary reviewers and writers, topic experts, and panel moderators. At least 1 US scientist and 1 non-US scientist evaluated each topic.

During the *Guidelines 2000 Conference* the ECC Committee delegated final review of the guidelines to the existing *AHA Scientific Product Development Panel*. This Panel comprises the chairs of the ECC subcommittees, the panel of Science Editors (1 or 2 for each subcommittee), and the 2 Senior Science Editors. The ILCOR and other international delegates appointed an International Editorial Board.

Resource staff posted drafts of the guidelines on a secure website accessible to the 2 editorial groups for review and comment. Most scientific issues had been resolved by the end of the conference.

Some issues did arise as a product of the international nature of this process. Most occurred during the months of postconference writing and review. The scientific infrastructure, the debates and discussions, and the final recommendations were close to identical for all of the participating organizations. Some differences, however, remained. Thematically these issues grew out of preexisting international differences in law, ethics, system management, and local regulations. Scientific issues were virtually nonexistent.

Resuscitation councils must confront geographic and economic differences in the availability of medical devices and pharmacological agents. Each resuscitation council struggles with international differences in instructional methods, teaching aids, and training networks. The world's resuscitation councils must develop organized plans to support instruction in the new guidelines to citizen responders, BLS providers, and advanced healthcare professionals.

The worldwide distribution of these guidelines will be enhanced by publication in an official journal of the AHA, *Circulation,* and the official journal of the European Resuscitation Council, *Resuscitation. Circulation* and *Resuscitation* will publish the International Guidelines 2000 as a statement that strongly merits the description "international." Publication of the guidelines is the product of these councils:

- American Heart Association
- Australian Resuscitation Council
- European Resuscitation Council
- Heart and Stroke Foundation of Canada
- New Zealand Resuscitation Council
- Resuscitation Councils of Latin America
- Resuscitation Councils of Southern Africa

Appendix: Educational and Training Issues in ECC and CPR—Experiences and Plans of the AHA

Editors' Note: Throughout the process of writing the International Guidelines 2000 the Senior Science Editors and the Editorial Board have attempted to create a work that is *geopolitically neutral.* Guidelines dominated by the perspectives of 1 country or 1 resuscitation council would be unacceptable.

This Appendix breaches this objective of geopolitical neutrality. This discussion of educational and training issues depicts the experiences of the AHA. In addition to being actively involved in resuscitation research, the AHA is responsible for an immense infrastructure supporting resuscitation training and education across the United States. The experiences of the AHA have accumulated for more than a quarter century. We have learned from both our mistakes and our successes. We share these experiences with you with the hope that they will facilitate development and improvement of ECC programs in your community. —R.O.C. and M.F.H.

Long-Term View of CPR Training

Training in CPR has been recommended for healthcare professionals for more than 3 decades[13,14] and for the lay public since 1974.[1] These recommendations have resulted in the development of a wide variety of BLS programs sponsored by ECC organizations around the world. In most programs BLS instructors are trained by the sponsoring organization to deliver information, to teach skills, and to evaluate the knowledge and skills of those they teach.[41-43] This type of training relies on a traditional course format of lecture, skills demonstrations, skills practice, and evaluation using detailed skills performance checklists. In essence such courses are "instructor centered" because the instructor is free to organize the course as he or she desires, including deciding how much time to devote to lectures, demonstrations, and practice; how to communicate the information; and how to evaluate the knowledge and performance of each student. Courses cover numerous topics, including anatomy and physiology, recognition of heart attack and stroke, actions to increase survival, risk factors for heart disease and stroke, lifestyle behaviors, recognition of foreign-body airway obstruction (FBAO), and the skills of rescue breathing, CPR, and relief of FBAO. This material is typically covered in a 4- to 8-hour course.[44] The amount of time for each specific unit of the course often is not defined, which allows the instructor to choose which units should be emphasized and how information should be distributed.

Numerous studies have evaluated this type of program for instructor performance,[45] postcourse skills performance,[46] and retention 3 months, 6 months, and 1 year after training.[47-51] Most studies have documented poor postcourse performance and poor retention of core BLS skills. This educational failure has been attributed to multiple factors, including insufficient practice time, the complexity and large amount of information covered, and numerous other factors across the educational spectrum. One study showed that instructors tend to spend too much time lecturing and allow too little time for practice. In addition, instructors provided poor feedback and correction of skills and did not follow the prescribed curriculum.[45] The quality and accuracy of skills evaluation by instructors has also been questioned. Studies have noted poor interinstructor reliability during skills evaluation even when standardized checklists were used.[52,53] Use of manikins with tape readouts in conjunction with instructor observation and computerized feedback with instructor observation have been shown to be the most objective and accurate forms of evaluation, but these methods were criticized as a cause of "strict constructionist" behavior in the classroom. Instructors tended to expect an unrealistic skill level during evaluation, which in turn led to excessive criticism and negative feedback to students. Beginning in the early 1990s, instructors and trainers started to reshape CPR training by developing simpler skills checklists and equipment manufacturers simplified the design of manikins.

In addition, studies have shown that participants are frequently reluctant to perform CPR even after they are trained.[54] This reluctance is related to such concerns as anxiety, guilt, fear of imperfect performance, responsibility, and infection. These issues must be addressed during the CPR course to alleviate participants' concerns.

Numerous innovative instructional methods have been used to improve performance. These include overtraining,[55] simplification of course content, videotaped instruction for initial learning and reinforcement,[56-58] videotaped self-instruction with manikins,[59-61] use of "practice-after-watching" videotapes with instructor support,[16] and use of audio prompts.[62-64]

Simplification

There is now widespread consensus that BLS training needs to be simplified so that students can focus on learning the essential skills of CPR. Skills performance sheets have been revised to reduce the number of critical steps needed to successfully perform CPR. The complexity of the sequences and the precision required to perform them contribute to widespread learning difficulties. No evidence supports rigorous training requirements as a way to improve outcomes. Simplification of the educational content of materials will improve learning and retention in both basic and advanced ECC programs. A comparison of video self-instruction and traditional CPR training revealed that students who watched a 34-minute video focusing on a single task (1-rescuer adult CPR) retained more information and skills than students taught in a 4-hour course covering numerous topics.[59] Audio prompts and home learning systems have also been used successfully to simplify CPR education.[63,64]

In 1 study, reducing the number of steps in CPR from 8 steps to 4 resulted in superior skills retention. Shorter, objective-focused ACLS courses do a better job at teaching core skills and improving retention than long courses do.[65] Peer training provides a mechanism for training large numbers of people in a cost-effective manner. Simplification of the design of peer-training courses has significantly improved learning and retention.[66]

Use of core objectives to determine the essential content of a course may be a helpful method for focusing on the essential information needed for a target audience. Table 5 describes the core objectives of BLS and thus the core content of BLS courses defined in a recent consensus process.

Future research should focus on controlled trials of simplified action sequences and skills in ECC courses. Outcome studies should be performed to verify proficiency when new, simpler sequences and skills are used, and clinical studies should be conducted if there are significant changes in resuscitation sequences or procedures.

Targeting Populations for CPR Education

Target: Family Members of High-Risk Cardiac Patients

Past CPR guidelines recommended aiming courses at relatives and close friends of persons at risk.[67] The International Guidelines 2000 also recommend that the public be taught both adult and pediatric BLS on the basis of individual need for CPR training. In particular, pediatric BLS training is recommended for caretakers of children, including parents, teachers, baby sitters, daycare workers, and in some cases siblings.

Scientific evaluations support establishment of priority groups to guide CPR education, training, practice, and research. Several studies[68–70] have shown that family members of high-risk populations benefit from learning CPR. Research confirms that tailoring CPR education to family members results in positive attitudes toward learning and implementing CPR.[68,70,71] Many family members of high-risk patients learn CPR successfully without deleterious psychosocial consequences,[69] yet they are less likely to seek CPR training and least likely actually to receive CPR training. We must continue to aim CPR courses at family members of high-risk patients.

On the basis of evidence presented at the international Guidelines 2000 Conference, we recommend that strong recruitment efforts be directed at

- Families and caregivers of infants and children at risk for life-threatening events
- Families and caregivers of adults at risk for sudden cardiac events, especially elderly couples

After thorough discussion this was made a Class IIa recommendation.

Additional studies are needed (1) to determine which individual characteristics of courses lead to increased participation in CPR training, (2) to describe the factors that prevent healthcare professionals from recommending CPR training to families of at-risk patients, and (3) to identify the CPR training methods that are most attractive to families and caretakers of at-risk patients.

A New Era? Video-Mediated Instruction

Video self-instruction, like many other learning methods, is effective in teaching the initial cognitive and psychomotor skills of CPR. Unfortunately most people who learn CPR by this method do not retain their skills for long. Even those who care for high-risk patients tend to forget what they have learned,[72,73] probably because they do not practice their skills. Only highly motivated family members use video self-instruction or other materials to practice, review, and maintain their knowledge and skills.[72] The less educated, males, and elderly learn CPR poorly without instructor training and support. Studies[72,73] of these groups show that instructor-led CPR training is more effective in terms of CPR knowledge and skills than video self-instruction. Participants at the international Guidelines 2000 Conference agreed that the evidence supports the following conclusions:

Validated learning systems are effective methods for conveying initial CPR skills but only for motivated families and caretakers (Class IIb).

Video self-instruction without manikins or instructor feedback fails to yield an adequate level of BLS skills after initial training (Class Indeterminate; not recommended).

Summary: Innovative Teaching Featuring Video-Based Instruction for Healthcare Professionals and the General Public

Any reference to video-based instruction and learning must be placed in context with the ways in which videotapes are used in modern CPR training.

Passive Watching

The passive watching technique conveys information only. The video gives an overview of knowledge and skills and may be

---

TABLE 5. Core Objectives of BLS Training

Immediately after a BLS course (initial skill acquisition) and any time <1 year after training (remote skill retention), the BLS provider who encounters an unresponsive person should be able to

1. Recognize unresponsiveness or other emergency situations when resuscitation is appropriate (eg, the victim does not have a "do not attempt resuscitation" order)

2. Phone the EMS number at the appropriate time within the BLS sequence

3. Provide an open airway using the head tilt–chin lift or jaw-thrust technique

4. Provide effective rescuer ventilations (breathing) that make the chest rise using the mouth-to-mouth, mouth-to-mask, or mouth-to–barrier device technique

5. Recognize and relieve FBAO in *conscious* victim as a part of the core breathing step (lay providers are not required to perform this step in unconscious victims)

6. Provide proper chest compressions sufficient to generate a palpable carotid pulse

7. Perform all skills in a manner that is safe for the rescuer, victim, and bystanders

If use of an AED is taught as part of the course, an additional core objective is to

8. Use an AED safely, correctly, and in the appropriate sequence

---

motivational. We do not know how much of the information is actually learned, but students reportedly "feel more comfortable" after passively watching a video.

Learn or Practice While Watching

In this technique the student watches the instructor on a monitor and attempts to follow the actions demonstrated by the instructor. This technique was used in the pioneering studies of Brennan, Braslow, Kaye, Todd, and others. Researchers have evaluated this technique more than any other video-based technique using the highest level of methodology. This technique does not require the presence of an on-site instructor but does require personal manikins for each student.

Learn or Practice After Watching

In this technique students watch a video with an instructor demonstrating brief but critical actions (eg, head tilt–chin lift). The on-site instructor pauses the video after each action and closely observes the students as they perform the actions demonstrated by the video instructor. This sequence of "watch then practice" is repeated until all students learn the particular action. On-site instructors and manikins for each student are required. This technique can lead to standardized CPR education if the same videotape is used across the country. Such courses are so tightly scripted that instructor flexibility is markedly restricted. Nevertheless this approach is popular among instructors because their role is important and demanding.

The traditional CPR training model that allows maximum instructor flexibility has resulted in transmission of inconsistent information and insufficient practice time for students, resulting in poor outcomes at the end of training.[46–51,59] Rather than prohibit instructor flexibility, the AHA ECC Committee aims to improve the consistency of information presented and maximize skill practice time by incorporating more video-based experiences and extra time for hands-on practice.

Past attempts at video-based training without manikin practice (passive watching model) resulted in poor initial and long-term outcomes.[58] Passive watching combined with review of written materials is a somewhat successful model for renewal courses.[56] In 1 study investigators mailed videotapes to laypersons in a county-wide area to determine whether a free 10-minute lesson in CPR would result in an increase in the percentage of arrests in which a witness or bystander started CPR. Under the actual arrest situations in this study, the investigators could detect no effect of the videotape.[57]

The same investigators attempted to provide CPR instruction through public service announcements delivered in the early morning hours. This initiative did result in a statistically significant increase in performance of bystander CPR.[74] Recently Braslow and Todd[59–61] showed that video self-instruction could teach adequate adult 1-rescuer CPR skills in 30 minutes. This contrasted with the 4 hours required in the traditional CPR course. The study noted that less hands-on practice time occurred during the traditional 4-hour course than during the 30-minute video-based course.

Video instruction was initially incorporated into AHA courses during pilot studies conducted by Edward Stapleton and Tom Aufderheide of the Heartsaver AED Course. The Heartsaver AED Course teaches 1-rescuer adult CPR, use of the pocket mask, and use of an AED.[16] All of these skills are taught and learned using the practice after watching technique.

Video-based instruction has many advantages: consistency of content, less time required for skills demonstration, more time for skill practice, and a shift from a teacher-centered to a student-centered classroom environment. Video also has the potential to motivate students by presenting real-life cases. Video is a visually stimulating educational tool. Practice after watching video-based instruction with instructor feedback is a validated primary learning strategy for training of lay rescuers (Class IIa).

Audio devices that talk the rescuer through the steps of CPR in the classroom have also been used to enhance performance during CPR instruction.[63,64] These devices can enhance learning for individuals who cannot be reached by traditional lecture methods. Audio prompting devices facilitate consistent repetitive practice, which results in improved initial acquisition and retention of skills. Use of audio prompting devices is recommended (Class IIb).

CPR in the Schools

Several studies in the 1990s led to rediscovery of the value of teaching CPR in schools. In 1998 the AHA began a large-scale evaluation of CPR in schools in the United States. Experts at the international Guidelines 2000 Conference strongly recommended development of in-school CPR programs as a *primary educational strategy* to ensure widespread learning of CPR and other BLS skills. Because 70% to 80% of cardiac arrests occur at home,[3] widespread training of a national population is needed to increase the likelihood of CPR being performed before the arrival of EMS personnel.

PAD programs that provide AEDs for individual homes are not expected to provide much benefit because of the small population that would be served and the cost of AEDs.[15] CPR is a critical action that can be performed in the home, where adolescents are often present. In addition, the major causes of death in school-aged children are unintentional injury, drowning, suffocation, and other conditions treatable with BLS. In 1998 the AHA trained 2.4 million lay rescuers in adult and pediatric CPR,[75] approximately 0.9% of the US population. Evidence gathered about CPR in schools included findings of 7 studies (level of evidence 3). All 7 studies support this guideline and present no opposing evidence. These studies have consistently demonstrated the effectiveness of school-based curriculums in ensuring both knowledge and skills retention consistent with outcomes among adult populations.[76–81]

Teaching CPR in schools is a powerful educational strategy. Research is needed to identify the best content, process, and structure of the curricula. Such a program will ensure widespread dissemination of CPR and other BLS skills to citizens around the world. The evidence for these recommendations does not include evidence from prospective, randomized clinical trials. Therefore, the concept of CPR in midlevel schools does not yet merit a Class I recommendation.

TABLE 6.   Course Elements Versus Allowed Variability

Element of Course	Variability
Course format and style	High, based on participants' needs
Course objectives (knowledge and skills to learn)	Constant
Evaluation methods and tools (checklists, written evaluations)	Constant

For maximum benefit to the participants, all evaluation instruments (eg, checklists of actions) should be shared with participants throughout the learning process, including *before the course* (to facilitate preparation), *during the course* (to provide real-time feedback and direct efforts for improvement), and *after the course* (to refresh memory and to stimulate practice).

Evaluation: A Process to Improve Learning

Evaluation in ECC courses is critical for both instructors and students. Evaluation helps achieve the overall course goal of having each participant acquire the skills and knowledge needed for his or her role in a potentially life-threatening situation. Teachers must teach effectively and students must learn effectively. Evaluation provides the tools by which instructors and students measure their success and plan for improvement. Evaluation of ECC courses has multiple overlapping purposes:

1. To help students identify areas in which they require more learning and review
2. To help instructors identify students who need additional help and the areas in which they need help
3. To help instructors identify topics or skills in which they can improve their organization, use of time, teaching techniques, or understanding
4. To help the course director identify areas of the course that require revision and assess the overall success of the course
5. To support efforts to improve the quality of the course within and across community training programs and larger training networks
6. To support consistency in course objectives and outcomes across community training programs and larger training networks
7. To provide participants with additional motivation to study and review

Variability in Students Versus Variability in Courses

Persons who participate in ECC courses have different needs, skills, experiences, motivation, and learning styles. This diversity requires flexibility in presentation and format that must be balanced against the need for predictable educational outcomes. Course objectives, however, must remain consistent across the training network. Uniform course objectives can be maintained by use of standardized evaluation instruments. Table 6 lists the elements of ECC courses, areas in which variability is allowable, and the level of variability that is allowable.

References

1. Standards for cardiopulmonary resuscitation (CPR) and emergency cardiac care (ECC). *JAMA*. 1974;227:833–868.
2. Standards and guidelines for cardiopulmonary resuscitation (CPR) and emergency cardiac care (ECC). *JAMA*. 1980;244:453–509.
3. Standards and guidelines for Cardiopulmonary Resuscitation (CPR), and Emergency Cardiac Care (ECC). National Academy of Sciences–National Research Council. *JAMA*. 1986;255:2905–2989.
4. American Heart Association. Guidelines for Cardiopulmonary Resuscitation Emergency Cardiac Care. *JAMA*. 1992;268:2212–2302.
5. Guidelines for advanced life support: a statement by the Advanced Life Support Working Party of the European Resuscitation Council, 1992. *Resuscitation*. 1992;24:111–121.

6. Guidelines for the basic and advanced management of the airway and ventilation during resuscitation. *Resuscitation*. 1996;31:187–230.

7. Bossaert L. *European Resuscitation Council Guidelines for Resuscitation*. Amsterdam, Netherlands: Elsevier; 1998.

8. Stephenson HE, Corsan Reed L, Hinton JW. Some common denominators in 1200 cases of cardiac arrest. *Ann Surg*. 1953;137:731–744.

9. Zoll PM, Linenthal AJ, Gibson W, Paul MH, Normal LR. Termination of ventricular fibrillation in man by externally applied electric countershock. *N Engl J Med*. 1956;254:727–732.

10. Safar P, Escarraga LA, Elam JO. A comparison of the mouth-to-mouth and mouth-to-airway methods of artificial respiration with the chest-pressure arm-lift methods. *N Engl J Med*. 1958;258:671–677.

11. Elam JO, Greene DG, Brown ES, Clements JA. Oxygen and carbon dioxide exchange and energy cost of expired air resuscitation. *JAMA*. 1958;167:328–341.

12. Kouwenhoven W, Jude JR, Knickerbocker GG. Closed-chest cardiac massage. 1960;173:1064–1067.

13. Cardiopulmonary resuscitation: statement by the Ad Hoc Committee on Cardiopulmonary Resuscitation of the Division of Medical Sciences, National Academy of Sciences, National Research Council. *JAMA*. 1966;198:372–379.

14. Cardiopulmonary Resuscitation. Conference Proceedings, May 23, 1966. Washington, DC: National Academy of Sciences, National Research Council; 1967.

15. Weisfeldt ML, Kerber RE, McGoldrick RP, Moss AJ, Nichol G, Ornato JP, Palmer DG, Riegel B, Smith SC Jr. Public access defibrillation: a statement for healthcare professionals from the American Heart Association Task Force on Automatic External Defibrillation. *Circulation*. 1995;92:2763.

16. Aufderheide T, Stapleton ER, Hazinski MF, Cummins RO. *Heartsaver AED for the Lay Rescuer and First Responder*. Dallas, Tex: American Heart Association; 1998.

17. Cummins RO, Ornato JP, Thies WH, Pepe PE. Improving survival from sudden cardiac arrest: the "chain of survival" concept: a statement for health professionals from the Advanced Cardiac Life Support Subcommittee and the Emergency Cardiac Care Committee, American Heart Association. *Circulation*. 1991;83:1832–1847.

18. Hallstrom A, Eisenberg MS, Bergner L. Modeling the effectiveness and cost-effectiveness of an emergency service system. *Soc Sci Med*. 1981;15C:13–17.

19. Urban N, Bergner L, Eisenberg MS. The costs of a suburban paramedic program in reducing deaths due to cardiac arrest. *Med Care*. 1981;19:379–392.

20. Ornato JP, Craren EJ, Nelson N, Smith HD. The economic impact of cardiopulmonary resuscitation and emergency cardiac care programs. *Cardiovasc Rev Rep*. 1983;4:1083–1085.

21. Nichol G, Laupacis A, Stiell I, O'Rourke K, Anis A, Bolley H, et al. A cost-effectiveness analysis of potential improvements to emergency medical services for victims of out-of-hospital cardiac arrest. *Ann Emerg Med*. 1996;27:711–720.

22. Nichol G, Hallstrom AP, Ornato JP, Riegel B, Stiell IG, Valenzuela T, Wells GA, White RD, Weisfeldt ML. Potential cost-effectiveness of public access defibrillation in the United States. *Circulation*. 1998;97:1315–1320.

23. Nichol G, Stiell IG, Laupacis A, Pham B, De Maio VJ, Wells GA. A cumulative meta-analysis of the effectiveness of defibrillator-capable emergency medical services for victims of out-of-hospital cardiac arrest. *Ann Emerg Med*. 1999;34:517–525.

24. Valenzuela T, Criss EA, Spaite D. Cost-effectiveness analysis of paramedic emergency medical services in the treatment of prehospital cardiopulmonary arrest. *Ann Emerg Med*. 1990;19:1407–1411.

25. Gold MR, Siegel JE, Russell LB, Weinstein MC. Appendix A: summary recommendations. In: Gold MR, Siegel JE, Russell LB, Weinstein MC, eds. *Cost-effectiveness in Health and Medicine*. New York, NY: Oxford University Press; 1996:425.

26. Garber AM, Phelps CE. Economic foundations of cost-effectiveness analysis. *J Health Economics*. 1997;16:1–31.

27. Montgomery WH. *Program Management Guidelines*. Dallas, Tex: American Heart Association; 1984.

28. Safar P, Bircher NG, World Federation of Societies of Anaesthesiologists, Committee on Cardiopulmonary Resuscitation and Critical Care, European Academy of Anaesthesiology, Committee on Cardiopulmonary Resuscitation. *Cardiopulmonary Cerebral Resuscitation: Basic and Advanced Cardiac and Trauma Life Support: An Introduction to Resuscitation Medicine*. 3rd ed. Philadelphia, Pa: WB Saunders; 1988.

29. Rosomoff HL, Kochanek PM, Clark R, DeKosky ST, Ebmeyer U, Grenvik AN, Marion DW, Obrist W, Palmer AM, Safer P, White RJ. Resuscitation from severe brain trauma. *Crit Care Med*. 1996;24:S48–S56.

30. Eisenberg MS, Bergner L, Hallstrom A. Cardiac resuscitation in the community: importance of rapid provision and implications for program planning. *JAMA*. 1979;241:1905–1907.

31. Weaver WD, Copass MK, Bufi D, Ray R, Hallstrom AP, Cobb LA. Improved neuralgic recovery and survival after early defibrillation. *Circulation*. 1984;69:1905–1907.

32. Weaver WD, Cobb LA, Hallstrom AP, Fahrenbruch C, Copass MK, Ray R. Factors influencing survival after out-of-hospital cardiac arrest. *J Am Coll Cardiol*. 1986;7:752–757.

33. White RD, Vukov LF, Bugliosi TF. Early defibrillation by police: initial experience with measurement of critical time intervals and patient outcome. *Ann Emerg Med*. 1994;23:1009–1013.

34. White RD, Asplin BR, Bugliosi TF, Hankins DG. High discharge survival rate after out-of-hospital ventricular fibrillation with rapid defibrillation by police and paramedics. *Ann Emerg Med*. 1996;28:480–485.

35. White RD, Hankins DG, Bugliosi TF. Seven years' experience with early defibrillation by police and paramedics in an emergency medical services system. *Resuscitation*. 1998;39:145–151.

36. Davis EA, Mosesso VN Jr. Performance of police first responders in utilizing automated external defibrillation on victims of sudden cardiac arrest. *Prehosp Emerg Care*. 1998;2:101–107.

37. Mosesso VN Jr, Davis EA, Auble TE, Paris PM, Yealy DM. Use of automated external defibrillators by police officers for treatment of out-of-hospital cardiac arrest. *Ann Emerg Med*. 1998;32:200–207.

38. Davis EA, McCrorry J, Mosesso VN Jr. Institution of a police automated external defibrillation program: concepts and practice. *Prehosp Emerg Care*. 1999;3:60–65.

39. O'Rourke MF, Donaldson E, Geddes JS. An airline cardiac arrest program [see comments]. *Circulation*. 1997;96:2849–2853.

40. Wolbrink A, Borrillo D. Airline use of automatic external defibrillators: shocking developments [see comments]. *Aviat Space Environ Med*. 1999;70:87–88.

41. Emergency Cardiac Care Committee. *Basic Life Support Heartsaver Guide*. Dallas, Tex: American Heart Association; 1997.

42. Emergency Cardiac Care Committee. *Pediatric Basic Life Support*. Dallas, Tex: American Heart Association; 1997.

43. Chandra NC, Hazinski MF. *Basic Life Support for Healthcare Providers*. Dallas, Tex: American Heart Association; 1997.

44. Chandra J, Hazinski MF, Stapleton ER. *Instructor's Manual for Basic Life Support for Healthcare Providers*. Dallas, Tex: American Heart Association; 1997.

45. Kaye W, Rallis SF, Mancini ME, Linhares KC, Angell ML, Donovan DS, Zajano NC, Finger JA. The problem of poor retention of cardiopulmonary resuscitation skills may lie with the instructor, not the learner or the curriculum. *Resuscitation*. 1991;21:67–87.

46. Brennan RT, Braslow A. Skill mastery in cardiopulmonary resuscitation training classes. *Am J Emerg Med*. 1995;13:505–508.

47. Liberman M, Lavoie A, Mulder D, Sampalis J. Cardiopulmonary resuscitation: errors made by pre-hospital emergency medical personnel. *Resuscitation*. 1999;42:47–55.

48. Kaye W, Mancini ME. Retention of cardiopulmonary skills by physicians, registered nurses, and the general public. *Crit Care Med*. 1986;14:620–622.

49. Wilson E, Brooks B, Tweed WA. CPR skills retention of lay basic rescuers. *Ann Emerg Med*. 1983;12:482–484.

50. Mancini ME, Kaye W. The effect of time since training on house officers' retention of cardiopulmonary resuscitation skills. *Am J Emerg Med*. 1985;3:31–32.

51. Mandel LP, Cobb LA. Initial and long term competency of citizens trained in CPR. *Emerg Health Serv Q*. 1982;1:49–63.

52. Mancini ME, Kaye W. Measuring cardiopulmonary performance: a comparison of the Heartsaver checklist to manikin strip. *Resuscitation*. 1990;19:135–141.

53. Brennan RT, Braslow A, Batcheller AM, Kaye W. A reliable and valid method for evaluating cardiopulmonary resuscitation training outcomes. *Resuscitation*. 1996;32:85–93.

54. Sigsbee M, Geden EA. Effects of anxiety on family members of patients with cardiac disease learning cardiopulmonary resuscitation. *Heart Lung*. 1990;19:662–665.

55. Tweed WA, Wilson E, Isfeld B. Retention of cardiopulmonary resuscitation skills after initial overtraining. *Crit Care Med*. 1980;8:651–653.

56. Mandel LP, Cobb LA. Reinforcing CPR skills without mannequin practice. *Ann Emerg Med.* 1987;16:1117–1120.

57. Eisenberg M, Damon S, Mandel L, Tewodros A, Meischke H, Beaupied E, Bennett J, Guildner C, Ewell C, Gordon M. CPR instruction by videotape: results of a community project. *Ann Emerg Med.* 1995;25:198–202.

58. Schluger J, Hayes JG, Turino GM, Fishman S, Fox AC. The effectiveness of film and videotape in teaching cardiopulmonary resuscitation to the lay public. *N Y State J Med.* 1987;87:382–385.

59. Braslow A, Brennan RT, Newman MM, Bircher NG, Batcheller AM, Kaye W. CPR training without an instructor: development and evaluation of a video self-instructional system for effective performance of cardiopulmonary resuscitation. *Resuscitation.* 1997;34:207–220.

60. Todd KH, Braslow A, Brennan RT, Lowery DW, Cox RJ, Lipscomb LE, Kellermann AL. Randomized, controlled trial of video self-instruction versus traditional CPR training. *Ann Emerg Med.* 1998;31:364–369.

61. Todd KH, Heron SL, Thompson M, Dennis R, O'Connor J, Kellermann AL. Simple CPR: a randomized, controlled trial of video self-instructional cardiopulmonary resuscitation training in an African American church congregation [see comments]. *Ann Emerg Med.* 1999;34:730–737.

62. Starr LM. An effective CPR home learning system: a program evaluation. *Am Assoc Occupat Health Nurses J.* 1998;46:289–295.

63. Doherty A, Damon S, Hein K, Cummins RO. Evaluation of CPR Prompt & Home Learning System for teaching CPR to lay rescuers. *Circulation.* 1998;98(suppl I):I-410. Abstract.

64. Starr LM. Electronic voice boosts CPR responses. *Occup Health Saf.* 1997;66:30–37.

65. Kaye W, Dubin HG, Rallis SF. A core advanced cardiac life support (ACLS) course for junior house officers. *Clin Res.* 1988;36:371A.

66. Wik L, Brennan RT, Braslow A. A peer-training model for instruction of basic cardiac life support. *Resuscitation.* 1995;29:119–128.

67. Guidelines for cardiopulmonary resuscitation (CPR) and emergency cardiac care (ECC). *JAMA.* 1992;286:2135–2302.

68. Dracup K, Moser DK, Guzy PM, Taylor SE, Marsden C. Is cardiopulmonary resuscitation training deleterious for family members of cardiac patients? *Am J Public Health.* 1994;84:116–118.

69. Dracup K, Moser DK, Taylor SE, Guzy PM. The psychological consequences of cardiopulmonary resuscitation training for family members of patients at risk for sudden death. *Am J Public Health.* 1997;87:1434–1439.

70. Dracup K, Heaney DM, Taylor SE, Guzy PM, Breu C. Can family members of high-risk cardiac patients learn cardiopulmonary resuscitation? *Arch Intern Med.* 1989;149:61–64.

71. Schlessel JS, Rappa HA, Lesser M, Pogge D, Ennis R, Mandel L. CPR knowledge, self-efficacy, and anticipated anxiety as functions of infant/child CPR training. *Ann Emerg Med.* 1995;25:618–623.

72. Dracup K, Doering LV, Moser DK, Evangelista L. Retention and use of cardiopulmonary resuscitation skills in parents of infants at risk for cardiopulmonary arrest. *Pediatr Nurs.* 1998;24:219–225.

73. Moser DK, Dracup K, Guzy PM, Taylor SE, Breu C. Cardiopulmonary resuscitation skills retention in family members of cardiac patients. *Am J Emerg Med.* 1990;8:498–503.

74. Becker L, Vath J, Eisenberg M, Meischke H. The impact of television public service announcements on the rate of bystander CPR. *Prehosp Emerg Care.* 1999;3:353–356.

75. *10 Leading Causes of Death in the United States.* Washington, DC: National Center for Injury Prevention; 1995.

76. Lester C, Donnelly P, Weston C. Is peer tutoring beneficial in the context of school resuscitation training? *Health Educ Res.* 1997;12:347–354.

77. Van Kerschaver E, Delooz HH, Moens GF. The effectiveness of repeated cardiopulmonary resuscitation training in a school population. *Resuscitation.* 1989;17:211–222.

78. Vanderschmidt H, Burnap TK, Thwaites JK. Evaluation of a cardiopulmonary resuscitation course for secondary schools retention study. *Med Care.* 1976;14:181–184.

79. Vanderschmidt H, Burnap TK, Thwaites JK. Evaluation of a cardiopulmonary resuscitation course for secondary schools. *Med Care.* 1975;13:763–774.

80. Moore PJ, Plotnikoff RC, Preston GD. A study of school students' long term retention of expired air resuscitation knowledge and skills. *Resuscitation.* 1992;24:17–25.

81. Lewis RM, Fulstow R, Smith GB. The teaching of cardiopulmonary resuscitation in schools in Hampshire. *Resuscitation.* 1997;35:27–31.

Part 2: Ethical Aspects of CPR and ECC

Introduction

CPR and ECC have the same goals as other medical interventions: to preserve life, restore health, relieve suffering, and limit disability. One goal unique to CPR is the reversal of clinical death, an outcome achieved in only a minority of patients. The performance of CPR, however, may conflict with the patient's own desires and requests or may not be in his or her best interest.[1,2] Decisions concerning CPR are complicated and often must be made within seconds by rescuers who may not know the patient or know of the existence of an advance directive. Resuscitative efforts may be inappropriate if goals of patient care cannot be achieved. In some instances resuscitation may not be the best use of limited medical resources. Concern about costs associated with prolonged intensive care, however, should not preclude emergency resuscitative attempts in individual patients.

The purpose of this section is to guide ECC healthcare professionals in making difficult decisions to start or stop CPR and ECC. These are general guidelines. Each decision must be made for the individual, with compassion, based on ethical principles and available scientific information.

Ethical Principles

When beginning and ending resuscitation attempts, differences in ethical and cultural norms must be considered. Although the broad principles of *beneficence, nonmaleficence, autonomy,* and *justice* appear to be accepted across cultures, the priority of these principles may vary among different cultures. In the United States the greatest emphasis is placed on individual patient autonomy. In Europe a greater emphasis on the autonomy of healthcare providers and their duty to make informed decisions about their patients is emerging. In some societies the benefits to society at large outweigh the autonomy of the individual. Physicians must play a role in decision making regarding resuscitation. Scientifically proven data and societal values should guide resuscitative efforts, while at the same time we strive to maintain cultural autonomy.

The Principle of Patient Autonomy

Patient autonomy is generally respected ethically and in most countries legally. This, however, requires a patient who can communicate and can consent to or refuse an intervention, including CPR. In many countries, including the United States, adult patients are presumed to have decision-making capacity unless a court of law has declared them incompetent to make such decisions. In other countries court decisions are not necessary to establish incompetence based on psychiatric illness.

Truly informed decisions require that patients receive and understand accurate information about their condition and prognosis, the nature of the proposed intervention, the alternatives, and the risks and benefits. The patient must be able to deliberate and choose among alternatives and be able to relate the decision to a stable framework of values. When in doubt, the patient should be regarded as competent. When decision-making capacity is temporarily impaired by such factors as concurrent illness, medications, or depression, treatment of these conditions may restore that capacity. In an emergency, patient preferences may be uncertain, with little time to determine them. In this instance it is prudent to give standard medical care.

People rarely plan for future illness. Many do not wish to prepare advance directives or to discuss CPR. Physicians seldom discuss advance directives, even with their seriously ill patients. Many patients have only a vague understanding of CPR and its consequences. The public generally overestimates the probability of survival from cardiac arrest. Some patients will decline CPR because of the possibility of severe residual neurological deficit with survival. In fact, in many studies the quality of life for survivors of cardiac arrest has been described as acceptable.[3]

The physician and patient, however, may differ in their perceptions of quality of life. Physicians have an obligation to determine a patient's understanding of CPR and resuscitation outcomes. Appropriate decision making rests on a good understanding and, if necessary, a discussion of perceptions and outcomes. This goal also can be complicated by physicians' misconceptions. Many physicians, for example, cannot accurately predict chance of survival from cardiac arrest. Enabling patients to give truly informed consent for resuscitation continues to be a challenge for healthcare providers.

There is some evidence that surrogates, acting on behalf of patients who have lost their decision-making capacity, do not always accurately reflect the patients' preferences. Approximately one third of patients with chronic renal disease would accept the decisions of a surrogate, even if those decisions conflicted with their own expressed wishes.[4] It is most helpful to establish patient preferences in advance by discussing the subject with the patient at admission to the hospital, but patients must not be coerced into providing advance directives.

Advance Directives and Living Wills

Advance directive is the term applied to any expression of a person's thoughts, wishes, or preferences for his or her

Circulation. 2000;102(suppl I):I-12–I-21.
© 2000 American Heart Association, Inc.

Circulation is available at http://www.circulationaha.org

end-of-life care. Most often advance directives provide instructions on limitation of care, including resuscitation from cardiac arrest. Advance directives can be based on conversations, written directives, living wills, or durable powers of attorney for health care. While still competent, the patient's conversations with relatives, friends, or physicians are the most common form of advance directives. In the United States and some other countries the courts consider written advance directives more trustworthy than recollections of conversations. Following the advance directives of patients who have lost their decision-making capacity respects their autonomy and is widely recommended.

Legal precedents in the United States have held that an advance directive cannot be used to withhold life-sustaining treatment unless these conditions are met:

- A surrogate has given authorization.
- The patient has a terminal condition certified by 2 physicians **or**
- The patient is in a persistent vegetative state certified by 2 physicians, including 1 with special expertise in evaluating cognitive function.

In a *living will* the patient gives directions to physicians about provision of medical care should the patient become terminally ill and unable to make decisions. A living will constitutes clear evidence of the patient's wishes and can be legally enforced in most areas of the United States. Most other countries do not recognize a legal requirement that caregivers follow the directions in the living will.

Living wills and advance directives, once stated, should be reconsidered periodically. As they decline or recover from a chronic illness, people inevitably change their perceptions about their quality of life and about the importance of living days and weeks longer. Patient preferences may not be consistent over even a 2-month period. In the SUPPORT study,[4] patients who initially chose a "Do Not Attempt Resuscitation" (DNAR) order changed their mind more often than those who initially chose to have CPR. Sick patients hold a deep desire not to die. Healthcare providers have an orientation to underestimate this desire. Every individual should be able to provide an advance directive, which then can be reassessed at regular intervals.

Patient Self-Determination Act
The Patient Self-Determination Act of 1991 requires healthcare institutions and managed-care organizations to inquire whether patients have advance directives. Healthcare institutions are required to facilitate the completion of advance directives if patients desire them. Although this Act was designed to encourage the use of advance directives, there is little evidence that this has occurred. Despite laws and education, advance directives have had minimal impact on resuscitation decisions in the United States. Such laws do not exist in most other countries.

In the SUPPORT study,[5] advance directives had little impact on patient care despite an intensive education program for healthcare providers and patients. Fewer than 40% of 9000 seriously ill patients discussed their CPR preferences with their physician, and only 20% had prepared advance

directives. Advance directives did not affect resuscitation decisions.[4] Advance directives still provide useful information for clinicians by helping them understand patient preferences and guide clinical decisions.

Surrogate Decision Makers
In the United States, when patients have lost normal mental capacities, a close relative or friend can become a *surrogate decision maker* for that patient. Legal proceedings, however, can follow and may result in long delays or superficial review of a case, even when procedures are expedited.

Competent patients in anticipation of later incompetence can designate a surrogate decision maker or grant durable power of attorney for health care. Durable power of attorney, typically given to a relative or close friend, allows that person to make medical decisions for the patient if he or she loses the capacity to make reasonable decisions. Surrogates should base their decisions on the patient's previously expressed preferences if known; otherwise, surrogates decide on the basis of the patient's best interest. In some countries, relatives have no legal rights to be surrogates. Surrogate decision makers are rare in Europe and many other countries. Unlike a living will, which applies only to terminal illnesses, surrogate status and durable powers of attorney apply to any situation in which the patient is incapable of making medical decisions.

At some time, all adults should provide a written advance directive that names surrogate decision makers and people to receive durable power of attorney for health issues and states preferences about life-sustaining treatment.

Children should be involved in decision making as their level of maturity allows and should be asked to consent to healthcare decisions when able. Some cases are difficult or controversial. In such cases the attending physician should consult a knowledgeable colleague who is not directly involved in the patient's care. Consultation helps ensure that hidden assumptions and value judgments are made explicit and that caregivers' personal values and attitudes are not imposed on the patient. Consultants ensure that all viewpoints and alternatives are carefully considered. The opinion of the family's primary care physician may be of particular value.

Hospital Ethics Committees
In the United States and some other countries, hospitals are required to have advisers for clinicians. These advisers are usually members of the ethics committee or bioethicists qualified to assist in the resolution of medical/ethical questions and to serve in a consultative and advisory capacity. Ethics committees have been effective in organizing educational programs and developing hospital policies and guidelines. There is considerable variation among hospitals with respect to committee responsibilities, authority, membership, access, and procedural protocols. Hospitals should develop explicit statements on these issues.

The Principle of Futility
Medical treatment is futile if its purpose cannot be achieved. The 2 major determinants of medical futility are *length of life* and *quality of life*. An intervention that cannot establish any increase in length or quality of life is futile. In resuscitation a

qualitative definition of futility must include low chance of survival and low quality of life afterward. Key factors are the underlying disease before cardiac arrest and expected state of health after resuscitation. The term *qualitative futility* implies the possibility of hidden value judgments. The correlation between quality-of-life evaluations by physicians and survivors can be poor.

A careful balance of the patient's prognosis for both length of life and quality of life will determine whether CPR is appropriate. CPR is inappropriate when survival is not expected or if the patient is expected to survive without the ability to communicate. The issue becomes more difficult with changes in legal, cultural, or personal perspectives. The value of life in a patient who is completely unable to communicate is viewed differently by different cultures.

The major dilemma in making decisions about the futility of treatment centers on the patient's chance of survival and those making the decision. When is a rate of survival to hospital discharge so low that resuscitation should not be offered to a patient who requests it—5%, 1%, 0.5%? Although prolonging life and restoring consciousness are appropriate medical goals, who determines the goal for an individual patient? Is the chance of 1 or 2 more months of life for a patient who is terminally ill an acceptable goal for resuscitation?[6] Who decides what is appropriate as a goal or what constitutes futility—the healthcare provider at the patient's bedside? The patient or family? A consensus of experts in the field? The values of patients, healthcare providers, and local society are all factors in the answer to this key question.

Ideally the initial decision about these very difficult questions should not be made during cardiac arrest. As noted above, physicians may be inaccurate in predicting the outcome of resuscitation from cardiac arrest, and individual bias may be of concern. The framework for decisions about futility can be best achieved by a social consensus.[7] Discussion and debate among healthcare professionals and the public are encouraged so as to reach a consensus based on the values of society.

Patients or families may ask physicians to provide care that is inappropriate. Physicians are not obliged to provide such care when there is scientific and social consensus that such treatment is ineffective. Some examples are CPR for patients with signs of irreversible death, such as rigor mortis, decapitation, dependent lividity, or decomposition. In addition, healthcare providers are not obliged to provide CPR if no benefit from CPR and advanced cardiovascular life support (ACLS) can be expected. For example, CPR would not restore effective circulation in a patient whose cardiac arrest is terminal and occurs despite optimal treatment for progressive septic or cardiogenic shock.

Beyond these clinical circumstances, resuscitation should be offered to all patients who want it unless there is clear evidence of quantitative futility. Quantitative futility implies that survival is not expected after CPR under given circumstances. Several factors that predict a patient's prognosis after resuscitation have been investigated in well-designed studies from multiple institutions. Patient variables include comorbid diseases and medications. Cardiac arrest variables include witnessed arrest, initial rhythm, and system factors, including time to CPR, defibrillation, and ACLS. No single factor or combination of factors, such as morbidity scores or unwitnessed asystolic arrest, meets the criteria for quantitative futility. A patient with metastatic cancer could be in relatively good health and have an incidental cardiac arrest. Recent studies have demonstrated a 10% rate of survival to hospital discharge for patients with metastatic cancer. Of these patients, 4% survived for 1 year.[8-10] A scoring system using patient or resuscitation variables with acceptable sensitivity for accurately predicting a universally poor outcome is not available.

For the newly born, antenatal information about gestational age or congenital anomalies may be uncertain and prediction of outcome may not be accurate. In these cases a trial of therapy and additional assessment of the infant may yield more accurate diagnostic and prognostic data to present to the family, allowing better-informed discussions about continuation or withdrawal of support. New developments in neonatal intensive care and changing neonatal outcomes require continued reevaluation of gestational age and birthweight criteria for noninitiation of resuscitation. Current data, however, supports the belief that resuscitation of extremely immature or extremely low birthweight infants and infants with certain chromosomal or anatomic defects is unlikely to result in survival or survival without extreme disability. This constitutes both quantitative and qualitative futility. For these infants, noninitiation of resuscitation in the delivery room, ideally after discussion with the family, is appropriate.

Criteria for Not Starting CPR

Scientific evaluation has shown that there are no clear criteria to predict the futility of CPR accurately. Therefore, it is recommended that all patients in cardiac arrest receive resuscitation unless

- The patient has a valid DNAR order.
- The patient has signs of irreversible death: rigor mortis, decapitation, or dependent lividity.
- No physiological benefit can be expected because the vital functions have deteriorated despite maximal therapy for such conditions as progressive septic or cardiogenic shock.
- Withholding attempts to resuscitate in the delivery room is appropriate for newly born infants with
  —Confirmed gestation <23 weeks or birthweight <400 g
  —Anencephaly
  —Confirmed trisomy 13 or 18

Criteria for Terminating Resuscitative Efforts

In the hospital the decision to terminate resuscitative efforts rests with the treating physician. Healthcare professionals must understand the patient, the arrest features, and the system factors that have prognostic importance for resuscitation. These include time to CPR, time to defibrillation, comorbid disease, prearrest state, and initial arrest rhythm. None of these factors alone or in combination is clearly predictive of outcome.[11] The most important factor associated with poor outcome is time of resuscitative efforts.[12-16] The chance of discharge from the hospital alive and neurologically intact diminishes as resuscitation time increases.[17–20] Clinicians must constantly reassess patient status. The responsible clinician should stop the resuscitative effort when he or she determines with a high degree of certainty that the arrest victim will not respond to further ACLS efforts. (See below for further discussion.) No reliable criteria are available to determine neurological outcome during cardiac arrest.

Available scientific studies have shown that, in the absence of mitigating factors, prolonged resuscitative efforts for adults and children are unlikely to be successful and can be discontinued if there is no return of spontaneous circulation at any time during 30 minutes of cumulative ACLS. If return of spontaneous circulation of any duration occurs at any time, however, it may be appropriate to consider extending the resuscitative effort. Other issues, such as drug overdose and severe prearrest hypothermia (eg, near-drowning in icy water), should be considered when determining whether to extend resuscitative efforts.

For the newly born infant, discontinuation of resuscitative efforts may be appropriate if spontaneous circulation has not returned after 15 minutes. Lack of response to intensive resuscitation for >10 minutes carries an extremely poor prognosis for survival or survival without disability.[21–24]

DNAR Orders

Unlike other medical interventions, CPR is initiated without a physician's order under the theory of implied consent for emergency treatment. In the United States a physician's order is necessary to withhold CPR, but this may not apply in other countries in specific circumstances. For example, since physician-staffed ambulances are much more common in Europe, those physicians are able to make such decisions themselves, without having to place a telephone call to a separate medical control person. Many patients will discuss resuscitative options, but physicians often hesitate to initiate discussion because of inappropriate concern about provoking severe anxiety or undermining a patient's hope. There is good evidence that this is not the case.

The commonly used term *do not resuscitate* (DNR) may be misleading. It suggests that resuscitation would be successful if undertaken. The term *do not attempt resuscitation* (DNAR) may more clearly indicate that success at resuscitation often is not achieved. The terms *DNR, DNAR,* and *no CPR* are currently in use, and local custom determines the preferred term. The term *DNAR* is used throughout the remainder of this chapter.

In the United States, legal precedent has defined very specific requirements before an advance directive can be used to withhold CPR. DNAR orders written in the hospital are not advance directives, and these legal requirements do not apply. The scope of a DNAR order may be ambiguous. A DNAR order does not preclude interventions such as administration of parenteral fluids, nutrition, oxygen, analgesia, sedation, antiarrhythmic agents, or vasopressors. Some patients may choose to accept defibrillation and chest compressions but not intubation and artificial ventilation. The DNAR order can be written for an individual in specific clinical circumstances and should be reviewed at regular intervals.

Some physicians discuss CPR when patients are thought to be at risk of cardiopulmonary arrest. Typically the possibility of cardiopulmonary arrest becomes clear as a patient's condition worsens. Then the patient may no longer be capable of decision making. Targeting sicker patients also reinforces the belief that discussion of DNAR orders signifies a bleak prognosis. Selective discussions may also be inequitable. Physicians discuss DNAR orders more frequently with patients who have AIDS or cancer than with patients who have coronary artery disease, cirrhosis, or other diseases with a similarly poor prognosis.[8] Physicians must, within reason, consider initiating CPR discussions with all adults admitted for medical and surgical care or with their surrogates.

Terminally ill patients may fear abandonment and pain more than death. In discussions with such patients, physicians need to emphasize their plans to control pain and provide comfort and general overall care even if resuscitation is withheld.

All decision making begins with the physician making a recommendation based on sound medical judgment to the patient. Patients and their surrogates have a right to choose from medically appropriate options on the basis of their assessment of the relative benefits, risks, and burdens of the proposed intervention. This does not imply the right to demand care beyond options based on appropriate medical judgment and accepted standards of care. Physicians also are not required to provide care that violates their own ethical principles. In such cases they may choose to transfer care to other healthcare providers.

Conflicts of interest may lead parents to make decisions that are not in the best interest of their child. Outside consultation should be obtained if patients, surrogates, or parents cannot agree with physicians on a course of action. In such an instance the physician may seek the assistance of another consultant, the family physician, the hospital ethics committee, or—as a last resort in pediatric cases—a governmental child protection agency. A growing number of children with chronic and potentially life-threatening conditions are living in foster care under state jurisdiction. Ambiguities about the scope of decision-making authority vested in custodial guardians, especially decisions about CPR and prolonged life support, must be resolved.

Decisions to limit resuscitative efforts should be communicated to all professionals involved in the care of the patient. Such interactions provide a wider information base, ensure that staff is fully informed, and offer an opportunity for discussion and resolution of conflicts. DNAR orders carry no inherent implications for limiting other forms of treatment. Other aspects of the treatment plan should be documented separately and communicated. Admitting a patient with a DNAR order to an intensive care unit is consistent with the attitude that all patients deserve the best available care, regardless of the existence of a DNAR order.

DNAR orders should be reviewed before surgery by the anesthesiologist, attending surgeon, and patient or surrogate to determine their applicability in the operating room and postoperative recovery room.

Ethical Issues Around
Out-of-Hospital Resuscitation

Withholding CPR at the Start Versus
Withdrawing CPR at the End?

Basic life support training urges the average citizen responding first to a cardiac arrest to perform CPR. Healthcare professionals are expected to provide BLS and ACLS as part of their professional duty to respond. There are, however, several exceptions:

- When a person lies dead, with obvious clinical signs of irreversible death
- When attempts to perform CPR would place the rescuer at risk of physical injury
- When the patient or surrogate has indicated that resuscitation is not desired

Neither citizens nor professionals should make a judgment about the present or future quality of life of a cardiac arrest victim on the basis of current or anticipated neurological status. Such "snap" judgments are often inaccurate. Quality of life should never be used as a criterion to withhold CPR. Conditions such as irreversible brain damage or brain death cannot be reliably assessed or predicted.

In Europe and other non-US countries, the widespread use of doctor-staffed ambulances precludes many problems with advance directives, DNAR statements, and death pronouncement. In the United States, however, EMS protocols must recognize and plan for adults and children who have advance directives limiting resuscitation. Such out-of-hospital DNAR protocols must be clear to physicians, patients, family members and loved ones, and prehospital healthcare professionals. Decision making by family and patient can be distorted regarding end-of-life events, expectations, and the value of CPR. Advance directives can take many forms, such as written bedside orders from physicians, wallet identification cards, identification bracelets, and other mechanisms approved by the local EMS authority.

Honoring Advance Directives Outside the Hospital

The Washington State EMS system in the United States has adopted a "No CPR" bracelet system that allows EMS personnel to provide care and comfort at the end of a person's life without the obligation to attempt an inappropriate resuscitation. A study in King County, Washington, showed that the No CPR bracelet stopped the EMS system from providing a full resuscitation response when a person wearing the bracelet had a cardiac arrest. On the negative side, the study revealed that few patients or their families and friends knew of the system. Furthermore, few family physicians, oncologists, internists, or other healthcare professionals knew of the system or implemented it in their own practice.

In certain cases it may be difficult to determine whether resuscitation should be initiated. For example, family members, a surrogate, or the family physician may request CPR for a patient despite the presence of a DNAR order. EMS professionals should initiate CPR and ACLS if there is good reason to believe that a DNAR order is invalid, that the patient may have changed his or her mind, or that the best interests of the patient are in question. They should initiate CPR and ACLS in cases in which there is reasonable doubt. CPR or other life support measures may be discontinued later when further information becomes available. Sometimes, within a few minutes of resuscitation being initiated, relatives or other medical personnel arrive and confirm that the patient had clearly expressed a wish that resuscitation not be attempted.

Out-of-hospital DNAR orders should not be confused with advance directives or living wills. Advance directives are statements by individuals about the level of medical care they want if they lose decision-making capacity. Advance directives and living wills require interpretation by a physician and need to be formulated into the treatment plan with specific orders for resuscitation that are consistent with the patient's wishes. The existence of a living will does not necessarily indicate that a patient wishes to forgo aggressive medical care or CPR. A living will may, for example, specify that the patient would choose aggressive medical treatment, including CPR. In contrast, the will may specify no resuscitative attempts in a terminal illness.

The EMS professional should not be required to determine immediately whether the provisions of a living will are in effect. In the United States, resuscitation must be instituted at once if the patient does not have a clear DNAR order approved by the EMS authority. Unclear issues are clarified later in hospital. In other countries, EMS professionals can review and make these decisions without involvement of a physician.

Family members may be concerned that EMS personnel will not follow advance directives written in the hospital if an out-of-hospital arrest occurs. Families and physicians often fail to provide an advance directive or DNAR order for the out-of-hospital setting when a patient returns home. Thus, an out-of-hospital DNAR order is not available. In countries where this is applicable, EMS personnel must convey sensitively and emphatically their responsibility to initiate treatment. Families should be counseled that more definitive direction will be obtained when the patient reaches the hospital. The key to preventing these dilemmas rests with the patient's regular physician who has been providing prearrest care.

An inappropriate out-of-hospital tracheal intubation, for example, can be corrected by responsible physicians in the Emergency Department (ED) or the hospital. It is ethical for ED personnel to discontinue treatment initiated by EMS personnel in the prehospital setting, provided that there is valid, after-the-fact evidence that these interventions are now inappropriate. This includes withdrawing the tracheal tube, removing intravenous access, and stopping infusion solutions and intravenous medications. Remember—and international ethicists are in complete agreement on this point—decisions either to not start CPR or to stop CPR once started are ethically and legally similar, without distinction. Stated more prosaically, "*withholding resuscitative efforts at the initial collapse*" is ethically and morally equivalent to "*withdrawing resuscitative efforts at the terminal event.*"

Terminating Attempted Resuscitation in Prehospital Systems That Lack ACLS Providers

BLS rescuers who start BLS should continue until one of the following occurs:

- Restoration of effective, spontaneous circulation and ventilation
- Care is transferred to a more senior level of emergency medical professional who may determine unresponsiveness to resuscitation
- Recognition of reliable criteria indicating irreversible death
- The rescuer is unable to continue resuscitation because exhaustion, the presence of dangerous environmental hazards, or continuation of resuscitation places other lives in jeopardy
- Presentation of a valid DNAR order to the rescuers

Chances of successful resuscitation decline as resuscitation time increases. Rescuers in remote environments and BLS ambulance services in some locales may have prolonged transport times before ACLS can be instituted. The risk of vehicular crashes during high-speed emergency transport must be weighed against the likelihood of a successful resuscitation after prolonged BLS fails to rescue the victim at the scene. State or local EMS authorities need to develop protocols for initiation and withdrawal of BLS in areas in which ACLS is not rapidly available or may be significantly delayed. Local circumstances, resources, and risk to rescuers should be considered. Defibrillators are now recommended as standard equipment on all ambulances. The absence of a "shockable" rhythm on the defibrillator after an adequate trial of CPR can be the key criterion for withdrawing BLS in the absence of timely ACLS arrival.

Time for Termination: Transporting Cardiac Arrest Patients Who Fail BLS and ACLS Efforts in the Out-Of-Hospital Setting

In a number of countries around the world, but especially in the United States, advanced-level personnel operate under protocols that prohibit death certification in the field. For a doctor-staffed ambulance, as in much of Europe, this does not pose a problem—the ambulance doctor pronounces death on the scene, where the arrest took place. The problem becomes more difficult in those areas in which only nonphysician personnel respond. If the EMS system does not allow nonphysicians to pronounce death and stop all resuscitative efforts, the personnel are forced to perform an unethical act—transporting from home to hospital a dead cardiac arrest victim proven refractory to proper BLS and ACLS care.

This situation creates the following contradiction: carefully executed BLS and ACLS care protocols fail in the out-of-hospital setting. How could the same protocols possibly succeed in the ED? Only in research settings such as academic centers will the ED offer interventions not already available outside the hospital. A number of studies over the past decade observe consistently that <1% of patients transported with continuing CPR survive to hospital discharge.

The new ACLS asystole algorithm has been modified to bring the issues of termination of resuscitation to the forefront for scrutiny and discussion. This new algorithm recognizes that some people in asystole can be resuscitated, and therefore it presents recommendations to follow for resuscitation. The asystole algorithm, however, also recognizes that when people have died, the heart monitor displays a flat line, or "asystole." Therefore, the International Guidelines 2000 asystole algorithm contains notes about what to do if asystole persists, that is, when the patient is dead. The asystole algorithm focuses on the following questions:

Asystole Persists

- Time to terminate resuscitative efforts?
- Are all BLS/ACLS interventions completed? (CPR, ventilation and oxygenation, defibrillation, intravenous access obtained, and indicated medications given?)
- Has asystole persisted for several minutes? (documented electrical silence; no specific time criteria imposed, but default approach should be shorter time requirements, not longer)
- Consider opposing family attitudes toward stopping efforts.

Clinical Features That Change Predictive Accuracy

- Young age
- Toxins or electrolyte abnormalities
- Profound hypothermia
- Drug overdose

The criteria for terminating ACLS resuscitative efforts are defined above. Some EMS systems are authorized to terminate resuscitation out of hospital. Protocols for pronouncement of death and appropriate transport of the body by non-EMS vehicles should be established or available. EMS personnel must be trained to deal sensitively with family members and others at the scene. Notification and involvement of a member of the clergy or social worker should be considered when appropriate.

Ambulance and rescue personnel commonly encounter terminally ill patients in private homes, hospice programs, or nursing homes. These patients may require treatment for acute medical illness or traumatic injuries, measures to relieve suffering, or transport by ambulance to a medical facility. Local EMS authorities should adopt policies allowing patients to decline resuscitative attempts while maintaining access to other emergency medical treatment and ambulance transport.

Personal physicians should help patients who are entering the terminal stages of an illness to plan for death. Physicians must be familiar with local laws related to certification and pronouncement of death, the role of the coroner and police, and disposal of the body. Physicians may not realize that in-hospital DNAR orders are usually not transferable outside the hospital. An additional out-of-hospital DNAR form must be completed. Failure to address these issues may result in unnecessary confusion and inappropriate care.

Many patients prefer to die at home surrounded by their loved ones. The hospice movement and many societies for specific diseases (eg, multiple sclerosis, AIDS, and muscular dystrophy) provide excellent guidelines for planning an expected death at home and answering questions from physicians and families. Physicians, patients, and family members should discuss measures of comfort, pain control, terminal support, and hygiene; when (and when not) to call the EMS system; use of a local hospice; and when and how to contact the personal physician. Funeral plans, disposition of the body, psychological concerns surrounding death and dying, and availability of bereavement counseling and ministerial support should be discussed. Such knowledge and discussions will reduce and even eliminate many ethical and medicolegal issues related to CPR.

Nursing home facilities should develop and implement guidelines for providing CPR to their residents. A nursing home is considered an out-of-hospital setting, and residents are provided with emergency medical services if medically indicated. Advance directives and out-of-hospital DNAR orders should be considered when developing treatment plans for residents who lack decision-making capacity if this is in accord with their request.

Resuscitation in the Hospital

Hospitalized patients should be periodically evaluated to determine the appropriate level of care. Levels of care are usually defined as (1) aggressive emergency resuscitation; (2) intensive care monitoring and prolonged life support; (3) general medical care, including medication, surgery, artificial nutrition, and hydration; (4) general nursing care; and (5) terminal care. Selection of the appropriate level of care is a medical decision made in accordance with information from the patient or surrogate.

Withdrawal of Life Support

Withdrawal of life support is an emotionally complex decision for family and staff. Withholding and withdrawing life support are ethically similar. A decision to withdraw life support is justifiable if the physician and patient or surrogate agree that treatment goals cannot be met or the burden to the patient of continued treatment would exceed any benefits.

There are no reliable criteria for clinicians to use during resuscitation to predict neurological outcome for a patient in cardiac arrest. Determination of brain death must be governed by nationally accepted guidelines. Once a patient is determined to be brain dead, life-sustaining treatment is withdrawn unless consent for vascular organ donation has been given. If such consent has been given, previous DNAR orders are replaced with standard cadaver-care transplant protocols until the organ(s) has been procured. It is recommended that hospitals develop policies and guidelines for determination of death that reflect current consensus and address areas of controversy.

Some patients do not regain consciousness after cardiac arrest and restoration of spontaneous circulation by CPR and ACLS. The prognosis for adults who remain deeply comatose (Glasgow Coma Scale <5) after cardiac arrest can be predicted with accuracy after 2 to 3 days in most cases.[25] Specific investigations may be helpful to assist with this process. A recent meta-analysis of 33 studies of outcome of anoxic-ischemic coma documented the following 3 factors to be associated with poor outcome: absence of pupillary response to light on the third day, absence of motor response to pain by the third day, and bilateral absence of cortical response to median somatosensory evoked potentials with the first week.[26] Withdrawal of life support is ethically permissible under these circumstances.

Patients in the end stage of an incurable disease, whether responsive or unresponsive, should have care that ensures their comfort and dignity. Care is provided to minimize suffering associated with pain, dyspnea, delirium, convulsions, and other terminal complications. For such patients it is ethically acceptable to gradually increase the dosage of narcotics and sedatives to relieve pain and other symptoms, even to levels that might concomitantly shorten the patient's life.

Hospital DNAR Policies

In the United States, hospitals must have written policies for limitation-of-treatment orders such as DNAR. The Joint Commission on the Accreditation of Healthcare Organizations requires such policies. These policies should be reviewed periodically to reflect developments in care and technology, changes in ECC and ACLS guidelines, and changes in the law. In other countries the situation is not drawn up in formal or legalistic terms.

The attending physician should write the DNAR order in the patient's chart with a note explaining the rationale for the DNAR order and any other specific limitations of care. Some countries require the signatures of 2 attending physicians on the DNAR order. The limitation-of-treatment order is best if it contains guidelines for specific emergency interventions that may arise during hospitalization, such as the use of pressor agents, blood products, or antibiotics. Oral DNAR orders are not acceptable. If the attending physician is not physically present, nursing staff may accept a DNAR order by telephone with the understanding that the physician will sign the order promptly. DNAR orders should be reviewed periodically, particularly if the patient's condition changes.

Delayed or token efforts (knowingly providing ineffective resuscitation) that appear to provide CPR and ACLS are inappropriate. This practice compromises the ethical integrity of healthcare professionals and undermines the physician-patient and nurse-patient relationship.

Orders to limit some but not all resuscitative efforts, such as withholding defibrillation or tracheal intubation, are rarely appropriate. An informed patient or surrogate may choose only limited resuscitative efforts, with the understanding that the chances of successful resuscitation are decreased.

A DNAR order is restricted to initiation of CPR, including the ACLS cascade that may follow. A DNAR order does not limit other appropriate nonresuscitative care. Orders to not attempt resuscitation should not lead to abandonment of patients or denial of appropriate and indicated medical and nursing care. DNAR orders should not convey a sense of "giving up" to the patient, family, and healthcare providers. Limitation of specific additional care, however, may be appropriate. The attending physician should clarify both the DNAR order and plans for further care with nurses, consultants, house staff, and the patient or surrogate. Interventions for diagnosis or treatment always remain appropriate after a DNAR order is written. In the intensive care unit or critical care unit, attending physicians should clarify orders for antiarrhythmia therapy and pressor therapy for hypotension. Basic nursing and comfort care, such as oral hygiene, skin care, patient positioning, and measures to relieve pain and other symptoms, is always continued.

Working With the Family

Notifying Survivors of a Loved One's Death

Despite our best efforts, most resuscitations fail. Survival to discharge after an in-hospital cardiac arrest has seldom been reported at rates >15%. People would not be in the hospital unless they were already ill. In some out-of-hospital reports the survival rate from out-of-hospital arrest has been as high as 20% to 25% for specific subsets of patients (usually witnessed ventricular fibrillation/ventricular tachycardia arrest with immediate bystander CPR).

Notifying family and friends of the death of their loved one from cardiac arrest is an important aspect of the resuscitation continuum.[27,28] Notification of death and the discussions that follow are difficult, even for experienced healthcare providers. Survivors should be informed with compassion by a knowledgeable healthcare professional.

Healthcare professionals can be sensitive to survivors' needs by using appropriate words and body language. Many hospitals in ethnically diverse areas now use standard protocols customized for different cultures, locales, or institutions. These protocols provide recommendations for choice of vocabulary and approaches that are appropriate for specific cultures. A packet of materials containing information on transportation of the body from a home or hospital, death certification, and autopsy and medical examiner requirements is useful. Information on body, organ, and tissue donation should be included.[28]

Family Presence During Resuscitation Attempts

A growing number of hospitals and institutions, most often following a local "grassroots effort" by emergency and critical care nurses, have started programs to ask family members whether they wish to be in the same room with the patient during the resuscitation attempts. Accompanied by a calm, experienced social worker or nurse, families can view the professional efforts made by medical personnel attempting to save their loved one. Afterward they rarely ask the recurring question that so often accompanies an unsuccessful resuscitation attempt: Was everything done?[27]

Retrospective reports on these efforts note positive reactions from family members,[29-31] many of whom said that they felt a sense of having helped their loved one and of easing their own grieving process.[29] When surveyed before they had observed resuscitative efforts and a loved one's death, the majority of family members stated a preference for being present during attempted resuscitation. This has been confirmed by several surveys in the United States and the United Kingdom.[29-35]

Parents and caretakers of chronically ill children are often knowledgeable about and comfortable with medical equipment and emergency procedures. Family members with no medical background have reported that being at a loved one's side and saying goodbye during their final moments of life

was comforting.[30,36,37] Family members who were present during resuscitative efforts reported that it helped them adjust to the death of their loved one,[30,31] and most indicated they would do so again.[30] Standard psychological questionnaires suggest that family members who were present during resuscitative efforts demonstrated less anxiety and depression and more constructive grief behavior than family members who were not present during the resuscitation attempt.[33]

Parents or family members seldom ask if they can be present unless they have been encouraged to do so. Healthcare providers should offer the opportunity to family members whenever possible.[32,36,38,39] Medical and nursing staff should discuss the presence of family members during resuscitation attempts before bringing a spouse or other family member into such an emotional situation. Advance roleplaying by resuscitation team members, with a focus on team response to a number of scenarios, is recommended by the nursing and medical staffs of hospitals that pioneered this concept. Resuscitation team members should be sensitive to the presence of family members during resuscitative efforts. One team member should be assigned to the family to answer questions, clarify information, and offer comfort.[40]

The Ethics of How We Allocate Resources

Lack of consistent access to ECC and the quality of ACLS should be a major concern for healthcare providers. Efforts should continue to reduce response times and improve the quality of resuscitation attempts through all links in the Chain of Survival. Justice dictates a minimum level of emergency care for all persons who require it. Resources should be fairly allocated to ensure that ECC is available to all persons. Physicians must serve as leaders in achieving the maximum benefit from available medical resources. They should also serve as advocates for all patients, acting in the best interest of each one. Recent ethical deliberations have expressed concern about overly aggressive treatment of patients with a poor prognosis. When resources are inadequate to meet immediate patient care needs, rationing (ie, triage) of medical services occurs. Rationing, or the distribution of a scarce resource, should be based on ethically oriented criteria.

Organ and Tissue Donation

The ECC community supports efforts to respond to the increased need for organ and tissue donations. EMS agencies should consider contacting the organ procurement organization in their region to discuss the need for tissue from donors pronounced dead in the field. In the United States, permission for organ and tissue donations must be obtained from the patient's relatives. Guidelines for organ and tissue procurement in hospitals and throughout the EMS system should be clearly defined and available to all healthcare professionals. There may be differences between applicable laws and societal values in procedures for organ procurement.

Research and Training on Newly Dead Patients: Informed Consent?

The use of newly dead patients for research and training raises important ethical and, in the United States, legal issues. Whether family consent is necessary or practical is central to the controversy. The consent of family members is ideal and respectful of the newly dead. However, this is not always possible or practical in the immediate cardiac arrest period. Advocates of research on the newly dead claim that a greater good is served, which benefits the living. Some have claimed that consent is unnecessary because the body is "non persona" and without autonomy. This position is questionable because it is the family who suffers after death, not the deceased.

Presumed consent implies that consent is assumed if a reasonable person (in the United Kingdom a reasonable physician) would consent under the same circumstances. In many countries, including Austria, Belgium, France, and Norway, presumed consent is the basis for harvesting of organs. An extrapolation from these laws to cover training and research is probably excessive. In a Norwegian study, 60% of parents who recently had lost a newly born infant opposed presumed consent.[41] Presumed consent for research and training using the newly dead should require a well-informed community, public discussion, and debate. Individuals should have the right to decline consent.

Seeking consent can be a considerable strain on both the family and physician. Of parents of newly born infants who had recently died, 8% said they would have been angry if they had been approached for permission to practice tracheal intubation on the infant. Alternatively, a consent rate of 59% was obtained for retrograde tracheal intubation and a rate of 39% for cricothyrotomy. Mandated choice on a variety of healthcare issues that might later apply is considered unethical.[42] Neither the Helsinki declaration or statutes in most countries nor common law precedents in the United States or the United Kingdom cover research on the newly dead.

Ownership of the newly dead has not been established. In the United States, a quasi property right, which pertains only to the eventual disposal of the body, has been claimed. In the United Kingdom, unauthorized research or training on a cadaver is not a crime unless the body is dissected or dismembered. In the United States, someone not authorized by law who treats a cadaver in a manner he or she knows would outrage the family has committed a misdemeanor. There are significant cultural differences in the acceptance or nonacceptance of the use of cadavers.

In the United States, unlike most other countries, the issue of informed consent for resuscitation research has become one of the most crucial barriers to future progress in ECC. When first learning that resuscitation researchers almost never obtained prearrest signed informed consent from arrest subjects, regulatory agencies in the federal government simply stopped all resuscitation research. The decision to stop the research was made before there was a solution to the obvious fact that a person in cardiac arrest cannot give informed consent for interventions that need to be used within minutes of the victim's becoming a candidate for enrollment. Having next of kin give early consent has proved to be impractical, if not impossible. It is usually not feasible or practical to obtain consent from the next of kin.

Research on such patients has attracted much public attention in the United States, and the potential for unethical studies casts a pall of public suspicion on all medical research in this country. Nonetheless, this type of research usually is well conducted and has led to significant benefits for society in general and individual patients in particular. After much public discussion and in recognition of the value of this type of human research, the US government, through the Food and Drug Administration and the National Institutes of Health, recently adopted new regulations that allow a waiver of the need to obtain informed consent in certain limited circumstances. Stringent preresearch directives require the researchers to consult with experts plus representative laypersons who might be study patients. The researchers also must make full public disclosure of the details of the study methodology and disclose this information in a public manner. Newspaper articles and radio and TV announcements have been used in several projects. The study investigators must arrange for candid public discussion of the need for resuscitation research, acknowledge the lack of an evidence-based foundation for many current practices, and detail the many potential benefits of the research.

During the Guidelines 2000 Conference, experts and attendees from Europe, Australia, Canada, and other countries discussed their different approaches to these problems. These discussions revealed a deep influence of culture and history, rather than science and clinical outcomes, on these issues.

Conclusions

Clear institutional guidelines and mechanisms are needed to address and guide the management of these sensitive issues. The work of hospital ethics committees, made up of representatives of several disciplines, has been particularly beneficial. All advance directives should be entered into the patient's record and should be subject to routine review. The newly dead should be treated with respect and their known wishes followed. It is important to consider cultural and religious factors. Healthcare providers who require training and experience should practice lifesaving procedures on newly dead patients only in defined educational programs under the supervision of a specialist. If informed consent is not requested, the relevant ethics committee should approve this practice.

References

1. United States President's Commission for the Study of Ethical Problems in Medicine and Biomedical and Behavioral Research. *Deciding to Forego Life-Sustaining Treatment: a Report on the Ethical, Medical, and Legal Issues in Treatment Decisions/President's Commission for the Study of Ethical Problems in Medicine and Biomedical and Behavioral Research.* Washington, DC: The Commission: For sale by the Superintendent of Documents, US Government Publishing Office; 1983.

2. Bossaert LERC. *European Resuscitation Council Guidelines for Resuscitation.* Edited by Leo Bossaert for the European Resuscitation Council. The Ethics of Resuscitation in Clinical Practice. Amsterdam, New York: Elsevier; 1998:206–217.

3. Nichol G, Stiell IG, Hebert P, Wells GA, Vandemheen K, Laupacis A. What is the quality of life for survivors of cardiac arrest? A prospective study [see comments]. *Acad Emerg Med.* 1999;6:95–102.

4. Hines SC, Glover JJ, Holley JC, Babrow AS, Badzek LA, Moss AH. Dialysis patients' preferences for family-based advance care planning *Ann Intern Med.* 2000;133:825–8.

5. The SUPPORT Principal Investigators. A controlled trial to improve care for seriously ill hospital patients: the study to understand prognoses and

preferences for outcomes and risks of treatments (SUPPORT). *JAMA.* 1995;274:1591–8.

6. Iserson KV. Law versus life: the ethical imperative to practice and teach using the newly dead emergency department patient [see comments]. *Ann Emerg Med.* 1995;25:91–4.

7. Callahan D. Medical futility, medical necessity: the-problem-without-a-name [see comments]. *Hastings Cent Rep.* 1991;21:30–5.

8. Hofman JC, Wenger NS, Davis EB, et al. Patient preferences for communication with physicians about end-of-life decisions. *Ann Intern Med.* 1997;127:1–12.

9. Kennedy BJ. Communicating with patients about advanced cancer. *JAMA.* 1998;280:1403–4.

10. De Vos R, Haes HC, Koster RW, de Haan RJ. Quality of survival after cardiopulmonary resuscitation. *Arch Intern Med.* 1999;159:249–54.

11. Sirbaugh PE, Pepe PE, Shook JE, Kimball KT, Goldman MJ, Ward MA, Mann DM. A prospective, population-based study of the demographics, epidemiology, management, and outcome of out-of-hospital pediatric cardiopulmonary arrest [see comments] [published erratum appears in *Ann Emerg Med.* 1999;33:358]. *Ann Emerg Med.* 1999;33:174–84.

12. Barzilay Z, Somekh M, Sagy M, Boichis H. Pediatric cardiopulmonary resuscitation outcome. *J Med.* 1998;19:229–241.

13. Kuisma M, Suominen P, Korpela R. Paediatric out-of-hospital cardiac arrests: epidemiology and outcome. *Resuscitation.* 1995;30:141–50.

14. Innes PA, Summers CA, Boyd IM, Molyneux EM. Audit of paediatric cardiopulmonary resuscitation. *Arch Dis Child.* 1993;68:487–91.

15. Quan L, Wentz KR, Gore EJ, Copass MK. Outcome and predictors of outcome in pediatric submersion victims receiving prehospital care in King County, Washington [see comments]. *Pediatrics.* 1990;86:586–93.

16. Zaritsky A, Nadkarni V, Getson P, Kuehl K. CPR in children. *Ann Emerg Med.* 1987;16:1107–11.

17. Ronco R, King W, Donley DK, Tilden SJ. Outcome and cost at a children's hospital following resuscitation for out-of-hospital cardiopulmonary arrest. *Arch Pediatr Adolesc Med.* 1995;149:210–4.

18. Schindler MB, Bohn D, Cox PN, McCrindle BW, Jarvis A, Edmonds J, Barker G. Outcome of out-of-hospital cardiac or respiratory arrest in children [see comments]. *N Engl J Med.* 1996;335:1473–9.

19. Torphy DE, Minter MG, Thompson BM. Cardiorespiratory arrest and resuscitation of children. *Am J Dis Child.* 1984;138:1099–102.

20. O'Rourke PP. Outcome of children who are apneic and pulseless in the emergency room. *Crit Care Med.* 1986;14:466–8.

21. Davis DJ. How aggressive should delivery room cardiopulmonary resuscitation be for extremely low birth weight neonates? [see comments]. *Pediatrics.* 1993;92:447–50.

22. Jain L, Ferre C, Vidyasagar D, Nath S, Sheftel D. Cardiopulmonary resuscitation of apparently stillborn infants: survival and long-term outcome [see comments]. *J Pediatr.* 1991;118:778–82.

23. Yeo CL, Tudehope DI. Outcome of resuscitated apparently stillborn infants: a ten year review. *J Paediatr Child Health.* 1994;30:129–33.

24. Casalaz DM, Marlow N, Speidel BD. Outcome of resuscitation following unexpected apparent stillbirth. *Arch Dis Child Fetal Neonatal Ed.* 1998;78:F112–F115.

25. Attia J, Cook DJ. Prognosis in anoxic and traumatic coma. *Crit Care Clin.* 1998;14:497–511.

26. Zandenberg EGJ, de Haan RJ, Soutenberg CP, Koelman JHTM, Hijdra A. Systematic review of early prediction of poor outcome of anoxic-ischemic coma. *Lancet.* 1998;352:1808–12.

27. Iserson KV. *Grave Words: Notifying Survivors About Sudden, Unexpected Deaths.* Tucson, Ariz: Galen Press Ltd; 1999.

28. *Bereavement.* Resuscitation Council UK Advanced Life Support Course Manual. 1998.

29. Hanson C, Strawser D. Family presence during cardiopulmonary resuscitation: Foote Hospital emergency department's nine-year perspective. *J Emerg Nurs.* 1992;18:104–6.

30. Doyle CJ, Post H, Burney RE, Maino J, Keefe M, Rhee KJ. Family participation during resuscitation: an option. *Ann Emerg Med.* 1987;16:673–5.

31. Barratt F, Wallis DN. Relatives in the resuscitation room: their point of view [see comments]. *J Accid Emerg Med.* 1998;15:109–11.

32. Meyers TA, Eichhorn DJ, Guzzetta CE. Do families want to be present during CPR? A retrospective survey. *J Emerg Nurs.* 1998;24:400–5.

33. Robinson SM, Mackenzie-Ross S, Campbell Hewson GL, Egleston CV, Prevost AT. Psychological effect of witnessed resuscitation on bereaved relatives [see comments]. *Lancet.* 1998;352:614–7.

34. Boie ET, Moore GP, Brummett C, Nelson DR. Do parents want to be present during invasive procedures performed on their children in the emergency department? A survey of 400 parents. *Ann Emerg Med.* 1999;34:70–4.

35. Adams S, Whitlock M, Higgs R, Bloomfield P, Baskett PJ. Should relatives be allowed to watch resuscitation? [see comments]. *BMJ.* 1994;308:1687–92.

36. Boyd R. Witnessed resuscitation by relatives. *Resuscitation.* 2000;43:171–6.

37. Hampe SO. Needs of the grieving spouse in a hospital setting. *Nurs Res.* 1975;24:113–20.

38. Offord RJ. Should relatives of patients with cardiac arrest be invited to be present during cardiopulmonary resuscitation? *Intens Crit Care Nurs.* 1998;14:288–93.

39. Shaner K, Eckle N. Implementing a program to support the option of family presence during resuscitation. *Assoc Care Child Health (ACCH) Advocate.* 1997;3:3–7.

40. Eichhorn DJ, Meyers TA, Mitchell TG, Guzzetta CE. Opening the doors: family presence during resuscitation. *J Cardiovasc Nurs.* 1996;10:59–70.

41. Games MK, Vassbo K, Forde R. Intubation training on the deceased newborn: parents' opinion? [Norwegian]. *Tidsskr nor legeforn.* 1999;265:2360–3.

42. Skegg PD. Medical uses of corpses and the "no property" rule. *Med Sci Law.* 1992;32:311–8.

Part 3: Adult Basic Life Support

Major Guidelines Changes

Following are the major guidelines changes related to adult basic life support, with the rationale for the change.

BLS Role in Stroke and ACS Management

1. Rescuers should "phone first" for unresponsive adults. Exceptions: "phone fast" (provide CPR first) for adult victims of submersion, trauma, and drug intoxication (Class Indeterminate).
2. Prehospital BLS providers should identify possible stroke victims (through use of stroke scales or screens) and provide rapid transport and prearrival notification to the receiving hospital to increase the likelihood of their eligibility for intravenous fibrinolytic therapy (Class I).
3. Patients with suspected stroke merit the same priorities for dispatch as patients with acute myocardial infarction (AMI) or major trauma (Class IIb).
4. Victims of suspected ischemic stroke (with prearrival notification) should be transported to a facility capable of initiating fibrinolytic therapy within 1 hour of arrival unless that facility is >30 minutes away by ground ambulance (Class IIb).

BLS Sequence

Rescue Breathing and Bag-Mask Ventilation

5. Change ventilation volumes and inspiratory times for mouth-to-mask or bag-mask ventilation as follows:
   a. Without oxygen supplement: tidal volume approximately 10 mL/kg (700 to 1000 mL) over 2 seconds (Class IIa).
   b. With oxygen supplement (≥40%): a smaller tidal volume of 6 to 7 mL/kg (approximately 400 to 600 mL) may be delivered over 1 to 2 seconds (Class IIb).
6. Alternative airway devices (ie, laryngeal mask airway and the esophageal-tracheal Combitube) may be acceptable when rescuers are trained in their use (Class IIb).

Pulse Check

7. Lay rescuers will no longer be taught or expected to perform a pulse check. The signal for lay rescuers to begin chest compressions (and attach an AED) is the absence of signs of circulation (normal breathing, coughing, or movement). *Healthcare providers* should continue to perform a pulse check with assessment of signs of circulation (breathing, coughing, or movement).

Chest Compressions

8. The compression rate for adult CPR is approximately 100 per minute (Class IIb).
9. The compression-ventilation ratio for 1- and 2-rescuer CPR is 15 compressions to 2 ventilations when the victim's airway is unprotected (not intubated) (Class IIb).
10. Chest compression–only CPR is recommended for use in dispatch-assisted CPR or when the rescuer is unwilling or unable to perform mouth-to-mouth rescue breathing (Class IIa).
11. Audio prompts that guide action sequences and the timing of chest compressions and ventilations increase learning and retention of CPR skills and improve CPR performance (Class IIb).

Relief of Foreign-Body Airway Obstruction

12. *Lay rescuers* will no longer be taught the sequence for management of foreign-body airway obstruction (FBAO) for unresponsive adults (Class IIb). If FBAO is suspected in the victim who has become unresponsive or who is found unresponsive, lay rescuers should perform the sequence of CPR. When rescue breathing is performed, the lay rescuer should look for a foreign body in the mouth and if one is seen, remove it. Healthcare providers should still perform the sequence for relief of FBAO in the unresponsive victim.

Introduction

The actions taken during the first few minutes of an emergency are critical to victim survival. BLS defines this sequence of actions and saves lives. BLS includes

- Prompt recognition and action for myocardial infarction and stroke to prevent respiratory and cardiac arrest
- Rescue breathing for victims of respiratory arrest
- Chest compressions and rescue breathing for victims of cardiopulmonary arrest
- Attempted defibrillation of patients with ventricular fibrillation (VF) or ventricular tachycardia (VT) with an automated external defibrillator (AED)
- Recognition and relief of FBAO

With the inclusion of AED use in BLS skills, BLS is now defined by the first 3 links in the Chain of Survival: early access, early CPR, and early defibrillation (Figure 1).[1] Each link must be strong throughout the community; this approach is consistent with the concept that the community is the "ultimate coronary care unit."[2]

Early access requires prompt recognition of emergencies that require time-critical BLS interventions, such as heart attack, stroke, FBAO, and respiratory and cardiac arrest. Early access of the EMS system quickly alerts EMS providers, who can respond with a defibrillator.[3–5] Emergency Medical Dispatchers (EMDs) can lead callers through the steps of CPR until EMS personnel arrive.[6–11]

Circulation. 2000;102(suppl I):I-22–I-59.
© 2000 American Heart Association, Inc.

Circulation is available at http://www.circulationaha.org

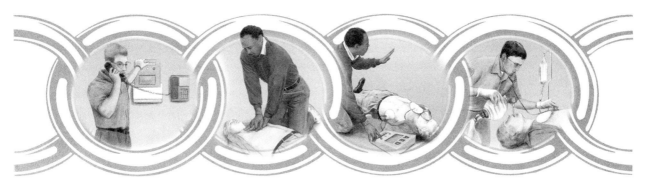

Figure 1. The Chain of Survival. The Chain of Survival consists of 4 links or actions: early access, early CPR, early defibrillation, and early advanced care.

Early CPR is the best treatment for cardiac arrest until the arrival of an AED and advanced cardiovascular life support (ACLS) care.[12,13] Early CPR prevents VF from deteriorating to asystole, may increase the chance of defibrillation, contributes to preservation of heart and brain function, and significantly improves survival.[13–15] Early defibrillation is the single greatest determinant of survival for adult victims of cardiac arrest.[1,12,16–23] Public access defibrillation (PAD) is a healthcare initiative to make AEDs available throughout the community for use by trained laypersons. PAD holds promise to be the single greatest advance in the treatment of VF arrest since the development of CPR.[1,12,16–23] PAD programs, including trained flight attendants and police officers, have achieved resuscitation success rates as high as 49%.[21,24–28] This nearly doubles the resuscitation rates previously achieved by the most successful EMS programs.[29,30]

Three BLS actions—early access, early CPR, and early defibrillation—serve as the foundation for emergency cardiovascular care throughout the community.[2] Each community should identify weaknesses in its Chain of Survival and strengthen the Chain through CPR training programs, effective PAD initiatives, and an optimized EMS.[31–37]

BLS Response to Cardiopulmonary Emergencies

Epidemiology of Adult Cardiopulmonary Arrest: "Phone First" (Adult)/"Phone Fast" (Infants and Children)

When the initial ECG is obtained, most adults with sudden (witnessed), nontraumatic cardiac arrest are found to be in VF.[38] For these victims, *the time from collapse to defibrillation is the single greatest determinant of survival.*[1,3,27,38–46] The window of opportunity is small. Survival from cardiac arrest caused by VF declines by approximately 7% to 10% for each minute without defibrillation.[47] More than 12 minutes after collapse, the cardiac arrest survival rate is only 2% to 5%.[1,3,27,28,38–47] Structured EMS systems that can be quickly accessed by telephoning an emergency telephone number (such as 911 in the United States, 112 in Europe, or 119 in Japan) have been shown to improve survival from sudden cardiac death by providing early defibrillation (see "Part 12: From Science to Survival: Strengthening the Chain of Survival in Every Community," for international emergency EMS contact numbers).[1,3,28,39,43,47] Because of this compel-

ling data in adult victims, both trained and untrained bystanders should be instructed to activate the EMS system as soon as they have determined that an adult victim requires emergency care.

In sharp contrast to cardiac arrest in adults, most causes of cardiopulmonary arrest in infants (aged <1 year) or children (aged 1 to 8 years) are related to airway or ventilation problems rather than sudden cardiac arrest.[48] In these victims, rescue support (especially rescue breathing) is essential and should be attempted first—before activation of the EMS system—if the rescuer is trained.[49] This respiratory etiology of cardiopulmonary arrest in children provides the rationale for the "phone fast" approach to resuscitation in children: the rescuer provides approximately 1 minute of CPR and then activates the EMS system.

There are exceptions to the "phone first/phone fast" recommendation for unresponsive adults and children. Some studies suggest that VT/VF may be more common in pediatric and adolescent victims of cardiac arrest (up to 15% of cases) than previously believed, and in some pediatric studies, VF represents the most treatable terminal arrhythmia.[50–52] Conversely, noncardiac causes of cardiac arrest can occur in adults and can have favorable outcomes.[53] Ideally the lay rescuer should learn a rescue sequence that is tailored to the cause of the victim's arrest. However, a rescuer may become confused attempting to learn and remember a variety of rescue sequences, and this confusion could create barriers to action during a real emergency. Consequently, these guidelines continue to recommend a "phone first" approach for adult victims and children ≥8 years old and a "phone fast" approach for unresponsive victims <8 years old. However, training materials for BLS laypersons will identify exceptions to the "phone first/phone fast" recommendation (Class Indeterminate). Healthcare providers should be familiar with these exceptions. Exceptions to the "phone first/phone fast" rule include

1. Submersion/near-drowning ("phone fast," all ages)
2. Arrest associated with trauma ("phone fast," all ages)
3. Drug overdoses ("phone fast," all ages)
4. Cardiac arrest in children known to be at high risk for arrhythmias ("phone first," all ages)

If an FBAO is present in a *responsive* adult victim, the trained rescuer should attempt to clear the airway (the Heimlich maneuver is recommended by most resuscitation councils) before activating the EMS system.[49] The *untrained* rescuer should activate the EMS system immediately in an emergency; trained dispatchers can then instruct the rescuer to perform CPR or provide other assistance until EMS personnel arrive.

If a second rescuer is available when a victim of cardiac or respiratory arrest *of any age* is discovered, the first rescuer should begin CPR (open airway, rescue breathing, chest compressions as needed) while the second rescuer activates the EMS system and retrieves the AED if appropriate.

Throughout "Part 3: Adult Basic Life Support," an "adult" is defined as anyone ≥8 years of age.

Out-of-Hospital EMS Care, Including Emergency Medical Dispatch

Emergency medical dispatch has evolved over the past 25 years to become a sophisticated and integral component of a comprehensive EMS response.[6–9,54,55] EMDs provide the first link between the victim and bystanders and EMS personnel.[6–9,54,55] Trained medical dispatchers may provide prearrival instructions to bystanders using standard, medically approved telephone instructions.[56] Dispatchers should receive formal training in emergency medical dispatch,[10,57] and they should use medical dispatch protocols, including prearrival telephone instructions for airway control, CPR, relief of FBAO, and use of an AED.[6–9,11,54,55,58]

Dispatchers play an important role in early triage and dispatch for patients with AMI.[59] Dispatchers are able to accurately identify victims of cardiac arrest.[55] However, they may need specialized training to improve their ability to correctly identify and prioritize victims of stroke.[54,60] In one recent study, only 41% of ambulances responding to calls for victims of stroke were dispatched with a high priority.[60] If emergency facilities are available for administration of fibrinolytic therapy, EMS policies should set the same high dispatch, treatment, and transport priorities for patients with signs and symptoms of an acute ischemic stroke as those for patients with signs and symptoms of an AMI or major trauma. Patients with suspected stroke with airway compromise or altered level of consciousness should be given the same high priority for dispatch, treatment, and transport as similar patients without stroke symptoms (Class IIb).

Using a script based on written protocols for cardiac arrest, dispatchers can question callers, rapidly assess the condition of the victim, and activate the necessary emergency service.[8–11,55] To dispatch appropriate rescue personnel to the scene of a cardiac arrest, the dispatcher needs to know whether the victim is unresponsive, whether CPR is in progress, or whether an AED is in use. If a bystander does not know how to perform CPR or does not remember what steps to take, an EMD can instruct the rescuer in appropriate emergency interventions.[8–11,55]

Dispatch protocols are evolving as new resuscitation science emerges.[61] For example, when providing dispatcher-assisted CPR, some centers have simplified the technique for untrained bystanders to reduce time to bystander intervention.[62,63] Dispatchers instruct rescuers to locate the lower half of the victim's sternum by placing their hands in the center of the chest at the nipple line.[62,63] In a single study of dispatcher-

assisted CPR, chest compression–only bystander CPR was associated with survival equivalent to chest compressions plus ventilations for victims of witnessed arrest.[63] Several studies have demonstrated that chest compression–only CPR is better than *no* CPR for adult cardiac arrest.[64–68] For these reasons of simplicity and elimination of barriers to action, we recommend chest compression–only CPR for use in dispatcher-assisted CPR instructions to untrained bystanders (Class IIa). Continued evaluation of simplified protocols and methods to encourage bystander CPR is needed.

Dispatcher-assisted CPR is practical and effective and can increase the percentage of cardiac arrests in which bystander CPR is performed.[10,11,55,58] Because dispatch instructions can be lifesaving, EMD assistance has rapidly become the standard of care in EMS systems.[6–11,54,55,57–60,62,69]

Some evidence suggests that priority dispatch triage systems that tier the EMS response to send BLS ambulance responders to less urgent calls and reserve paramedics (ACLS responders) for more critical incidents may significantly improve use of paramedic skills.[11,70] Although studies of patient outcome are only inferential, traditional systems with high survival rates have used such an approach.[6,11,70,71] Research into this concept should continue.

No scientific studies have documented improved survival with use of computerized systems that automatically provide the EMD with the caller's location and telephone number (called "enhanced 911" in the United States). Such systems, however, expedite the EMD process, and their use should be strongly encouraged.[6]

Recognition and Actions for Acute Coronary Syndromes

Each year millions of patients around the world are evaluated for chest pain in Emergency Departments (EDs).[72] Of these, approximately half will be diagnosed as having an acute coronary syndrome (ACS), including unstable angina, non–Q-wave myocardial infarction (MI), and ST-elevation MI.[72,73] Of all patients with ACS, approximately half will die before reaching the hospital. Of patients who reach the hospital, an additional 25% will die within the first year.[74] In 17% of patients, ischemic pain is the first, last, and only symptom.[75]

Current management of ACS contrasts dramatically with the approach used 2 decades ago. Fibrinolytic agents and percutaneous coronary interventions (including angioplasty/stent) may reopen the blocked coronary vessels that cause myocardial ischemia. These treatments save lives and improve quality of life.[76–83] Early diagnosis and treatment of AMI significantly reduces mortality,[76] decreases infarct size,[77] improves regional[78] and global[79–81] left ventricular function, and decreases the incidence of resultant heart failure.[82,83] To be most effective, these interventions must be administered within the first few hours of symptom onset.[76–83]

The time-limited treatments now available for ACS have highlighted the important role of lay rescuers, first responders, and EMS personnel. Early recognition, early intervention, and early transport of victims with suspected ACS from the scene to the hospital can substantially reduce morbidity and mortality.

Presentation of ACS
Early access to the EMS system is often delayed because both victim and bystanders fail to recognize the signs and symptoms of ACS.[84–88] Public education is needed to increase recognition of the signs and symptoms of ACS and encourage the public to access the EMS system quickly.

The classic symptom associated with ACS is a dull, substernal discomfort variably described as a pressure or tightness, often radiating to the left arm, neck, or jaw. It may be associated with shortness of breath, palpitations, nausea, vomiting, or sweating. Symptoms of angina pectoris typically last <15 minutes. In contrast, the symptoms of AMI are characteristically more intense and last >15 minutes.

Some victims of ACS have atypical or vague chest discomfort. The victim may feel light-headed, short of breath, nauseous, or faint, or have a cold sweat. The discomfort may be more diffuse than classic chest pain and may radiate to the back or may be concentrated between the shoulder blades. The elderly,[89] women,[90–92] and persons with diabetes and ACS are more likely to present with vague complaints rather than classic descriptions of chest pain.

The patient with new onset of chest discomfort should rest quietly. Both angina pectoris and AMI are caused by a lack of adequate blood supply to the heart, so activity should be kept to a minimum. If chest discomfort lasts more than a few minutes, initiate emergency action. The action steps for lay rescuers include (1) recognize the signs and symptoms of ACS, (2) have the victim sit or lie down, and (3) if discomfort persists for ≥5 minutes, activate the EMS system.

After activating the EMS system, give the victim supportive care, including rest, reassurance, and use of a recovery position. If the victim becomes unresponsive, be prepared to provide rescue breathing, chest compressions, and (when possible and appropriate) attempted defibrillation with an AED.

Denial is a common reaction to emergencies such as AMI. The victim's first tendency may be to deny the possibility of a heart attack. This response is not limited to the victim; the lay rescuer may also deny such a possibility. In an emergency, those involved, whether victims or bystanders, are inclined to deny or downplay the seriousness of the problem. This response, while natural, must be overcome to give victims the greatest chance of survival. Denial of the serious nature of symptoms delays treatment and increases risk of death.[93,94]

The elderly, women, and persons with diabetes, hypertension, or known coronary artery disease are most likely to delay calling the EMS system.[82] Because the victim may deny the possibility of a heart attack, lay rescuers must be prepared to activate the EMS system themselves and provide additional BLS as needed. Public education campaigns have been effective in increasing public awareness of this important issue.[95,96]

Out-of-Hospital Care for ACS
There are many benefits to early access of the EMS system as soon as you recognize the signs and symptoms of ACS. EMDs can send the appropriate emergency team and provide instructions for patient care before EMS personnel arrive.[8]

BLS ambulance providers can provide CPR; use an AED; support airway, oxygenation, and ventilation; and administer nitroglycerin and aspirin out of the hospital.[97,98] The EMS provider should also obtain a significant medical history and inquire about risk factors for ACS.

Nitroglycerin is effective for relief of symptoms, and it dilates coronary arteries and reduces ventricular preload and oxygen requirements.[99] If the patient with chest pain has nitroglycerin and his systolic blood pressure is >90 mm Hg, the BLS ambulance provider can help the patient take the nitroglycerin. The patient can take up to 3 nitroglycerin tablets at intervals of 3 to 5 minutes. After administration of each nitroglycerin tablet, monitor blood pressure closely for signs of hypotension.

If local protocol permits, the BLS ambulance provider should administer aspirin (160 to 325 mg) en route. Aspirin inhibits coronary reocclusion and recurrent events after fibrinolytic therapy and reduces mortality in ACS.[100] Routine out-of-hospital administration of nitroglycerin and aspirin by BLS ambulance providers is expected to reduce morbidity and mortality from AMI.[101]

Some ACLS ambulance providers are authorized to administer morphine to reduce pain and decrease myocardial oxygen requirements and left ventricular preload and afterload. ACLS providers also monitor the heart rhythm and can immediately detect potentially lethal cardiac arrhythmias. ACLS ambulance providers may administer medications to manage arrhythmias, shock, and pulmonary congestion; they may initiate transcutaneous pacing as well. The mnemonic "MONA" (morphine, oxygen, nitroglycerin, and aspirin) is a reminder of the core out-of-hospital therapies for ACS.

In many systems, ACLS ambulance providers can attach a 12-lead ECG to the victim and transmit the findings to the receiving facility. This allows diagnosis of a heart attack in progress and significantly reduces time to treatment, which may include fibrinolytic therapy, in the hospital.[102–110] This prearrival ECG and notification has been shown to improve outcome.[111] In the event of a complication (either at the scene or en route to the hospital), ACLS ambulance providers can administer lifesaving therapies, including CPR, rapid defibrillation, airway management, and intravenous medications.

The BLS algorithm for EMS out-of-hospital management of patients with ACS is shown in Figure 2. (For further information about the management of ACS, see "Part 7, Section 1: Acute Coronary Syndromes.")

Recognition of Stroke and Actions for Patients With Suspected Stroke
Stroke is a leading cause of death and brain injury in adults. Each year millions of adults suffer a new or recurrent stroke, and nearly a quarter of them die.[112] Until recently, care of the stroke patient was largely supportive, with therapy focused on treatment of complications.[113] Because no treatment was directed toward altering the course of the stroke itself, little emphasis was placed on rapid identification, transport, or intervention.[113]

Now fibrinolytic therapy offers the opportunity to limit neurological insult and improve outcome in ischemic stroke patients.[114–121] Fibrinolytic therapy reduces disability and

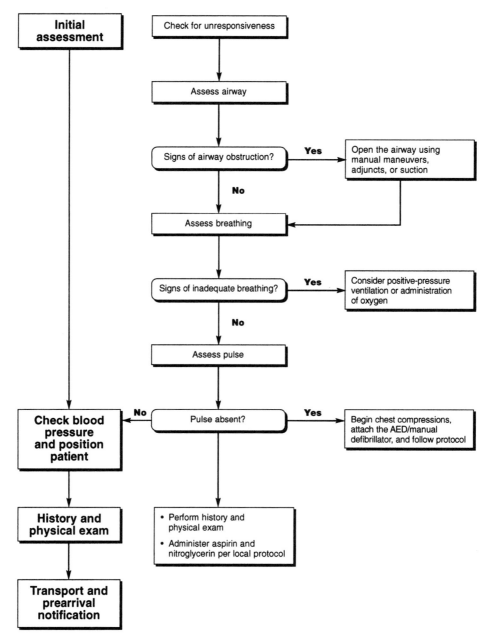

Figure 2. The algorithm reviews the out-of-hospital management of patients with acute coronary syndromes for BLS ambulance providers.

death from stroke in eligible patients.[114–121] Furthermore, patients treated with fibrinolytics are more likely to be discharged home and less likely to be discharged to a rehabilitative or chronic care facility. Fibrinolytic therapy is cost-effective and results in sustained improvement in quality of life.[118,122] For these reasons, intravenous fibrinolytic therapy should be considered for all patients presenting to the hospital within 3 hours of the onset of signs and symptoms consistent with acute ischemic stroke (Class I).[114,117,118,121] Use of intra-arterial fibrinolytic agents within 3 to 6 hours of symptom onset may also be beneficial for patients with stroke caused by middle cerebral artery occlusion (Class IIb).[115,119,120]

The window of opportunity to provide this beneficial therapy is small. For most stroke victims, definitive hospital-

based intervention must occur *within 3 hours of symptom onset.* The time-limited treatments now available for stroke have emphasized the important role of lay rescuers, first responders, and emergency rescue service personnel. Early recognition, early intervention, and early transport of victims with suspected stroke from the scene to the hospital can substantially reduce morbidity and mortality from stroke.

Presentation of Stroke

A transient ischemic attack (TIA) is a reversible episode of focal neurological dysfunction that typically lasts a few minutes to a few hours. It is impossible to distinguish between a TIA and a stroke at the time of onset. If the neurological symptoms completely resolve within 24 hours, the event is classified as a TIA. Most TIAs, however, last

<15 minutes.[123,124] TIAs are a significant indicator of stroke risk. Approximately one fourth of patients presenting with stroke have had a previous TIA.[125] In addition, approximately 5% of patients with a TIA will develop a stroke within 1 month if untreated.[113,126]

A stroke is a neurological impairment caused by disruption of blood supply to the brain. Approximately 75% of strokes are ischemic, the result of complete occlusion of a cerebral artery caused by cerebral thrombosis or embolism. Hemorrhagic strokes are caused by cerebral artery rupture with bleeding into the surface of the brain (subarachnoid hemorrhage) or bleeding into the tissue of the brain (intracerebral hemorrhage). The most common cause of a subarachnoid hemorrhage is an aneurysm.[127,128] Hypertension is the most common cause of intracerebral hemorrhage.[129,130]

Although both ischemic and hemorrhagic stroke can be life-threatening, ischemic stroke rarely leads to death within the first hour. In comparison, hemorrhagic stroke can be fatal at onset. Patients with ischemic strokes can often be treated with fibrinolytic therapy if they are able to receive the drug within 3 hours of symptom onset. Fibrinolytic therapy cannot be given to patients with hemorrhagic stroke because it would worsen intracerebral bleeding. Some patients with hemorrhagic stroke can benefit from surgical intervention.[131,132]

In both stroke and heart attack, blood supply is inadequate, often the result of an obstructing blood clot. Rapid intervention with fibrinolytic therapy can improve outcome after an ischemic stroke just as it can after an AMI.[114]

Recognition of the signs and symptoms of stroke is critical to early intervention and treatment. The presentation of stroke may be subtle. Signs and symptoms of stroke may include only mild facial paralysis or difficulty speaking that may go unnoticed or be denied by the patient or family members.[133] Other signs and symptoms of stroke include alteration in consciousness (confusion, stupor, or coma); sudden weakness or numbness of the face, arm, or leg on one side of the body; slurred or incoherent speech; unexplained dizziness; unsteadiness; sudden falls; and dimness or loss of vision, particularly in one eye. The lay rescuer should immediately activate the EMS system as soon as signs or symptoms of stroke are suspected.

Stroke victims may either be unable to understand that they are having a stroke or, like AMI victims, deny their symptoms by rationalization.[134] Most stroke victims delay access to care for hours after symptom onset.[123,133–142] Tragically, this delay often eliminates the possibility of fibrinolytic therapy. Because the victim may deny having symptoms of a stroke or be unable to understand, lay rescuers must take the initiative and rapidly activate the EMS system, providing additional BLS as necessary.

The 7 "D's" of Stroke Management
Management of the stroke patient can be remembered by use of the mnemonic of the 7 "D's": Detection, Dispatch, Delivery, Door, Data, Decision, and Drug.[143] Delay may occur at any of these points of management, so response to and management of the stroke victim must be skilled and efficient at each point. The first 3 D's (detection, dispatch, and delivery) are the responsibility of BLS providers in the community, including the lay public and EMS responders. A patient, family member, or bystander recognizes (detects) the signs and symptoms of a stroke or TIA and activates the EMS system. EMDs then prioritize the call for a patient with suspected stroke just as they would for a victim of AMI or serious trauma, and they dispatch the appropriate EMS team with high transport priority. EMS providers must respond rapidly, confirm signs and symptoms of a suspected stroke, and provide transport (delivery) of the patient to a stroke center (a hospital that can provide fibrinolytic therapy within 1 hour after arrival at the ED door). The remaining 4 D's are initiated in the hospital, including rapid triage at the door (in the ED), neurological examination, and performance and interpretation of a CT scan to diagnose type of stroke (data), identifying candidates eligible for fibrinolytic therapy (decision), and treating with fibrinolytic therapy (drug).

Layperson BLS Care for Stroke
Rapid access of the EMS system is essential as soon as signs and symptoms of a stroke appear. When the EMS is used for transport, stroke patients arrive at the hospital faster than those who do not use the EMS (a major advantage for time-critical treatment).[133,135,144–149] Furthermore, EMDs can send the appropriate emergency team with a priority dispatch response and provide instructions for patient care before EMS personnel arrive.[150–152] The EMS system can then rapidly transport the victim to a stroke center and notify the facility before arrival to ensure rapid hospital-based evaluation and treatment. Delays in transport and initial hospital evaluation occur if the victim or family contacts the family physician or transports the stroke victim by private car to the hospital. Such delays may make the victim ineligible for fibrinolytic treatment.[133,146,148]

Currently, in the United States only half of stroke victims use the EMS system for transport to the hospital.[133,136] If a stroke occurs while the victim is alone or sleeping, this further delays prompt recognition of symptoms and initiation of therapy.[153] Eighty-five percent of strokes occur at home.[136] As a result, public education programs have focused on persons at risk for stroke and their friends and family members.[136] Public education has been successful in reducing time to arrival at the ED.[136,137]

After accessing the EMS system, provide supportive care, including reassurance. Place the victim in a recovery position. If the victim becomes unresponsive, provide rescue breathing and other steps of CPR if needed.

Out-of-Hospital Care for Stroke
BLS ambulance providers now play a critical role in recognition, stabilization, and rapid transport of the stroke victim as well as selection of a receiving hospital capable of administering fibrinolytic therapy. In the past, these providers received minimal training in stroke assessment and care.[7,150–152,154] Programs are now needed to train EMS personnel to accurately recognize and prioritize stroke victims.[54,60,155–164]

If emergency facilities are available for administration of fibrinolytic therapy, emergency ambulance service policies should require the same high dispatch, treatment, and transport priorities for patients with signs and symptoms of an

TABLE 1.   Cincinnati Prehospital Stroke Scale

Facial droop (have patient show teeth or smile)

   Normal—both sides of face move equally

   Abnormal—one side of face does not move as well as the other side

Arm drift (patient closes eyes and holds both arms straight out for 10 seconds)

   Normal—both arms move the same or both arms do not move at all (other findings, such as pronator grip, may be helpful)

   Abnormal—one arm does not move or one arm drifts down compared with the other

Abnormal speech (have the patient say "you can't teach an old dog new tricks")

   Normal—patient uses correct words with no slurring

   Abnormal—patient slurs words, uses the wrong words, or is unable to speak

Interpretation: If any of these 3 signs is abnormal, the probability of a stroke is 72%.

From Reference 158.

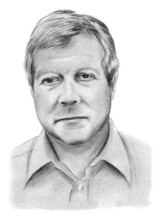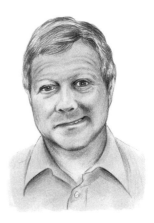

Figure 3. Right-sided facial droop. Left, patient in repose. Right, patient after the command "Look up and smile and show your teeth."

acute ischemic stroke as those for patients with signs and symptoms of an AMI or major trauma. Patients with suspected stroke with airway compromise or altered level of consciousness should be given the same high dispatch, treatment, and transport priorities as other nonstroke patients with similar problems (Class IIb). Airway compromise after stroke is relatively common. Cardiac arrest is relatively uncommon, although many stroke victims demonstrate arrhythmias, including ventricular tachyarrhythmias and atrial fibrillation, in the first hours and days after a stroke.[165–167]

   The goals of out-of-hospital management by BLS ambulance providers of patients with suspected stroke include (1) priority dispatch and response; (2) initial assessment and management, including support of airway, oxygenation, ven-

tilation, and circulation; (3) rapid identification of stroke (by use of a standardized stroke scale); (4) rapid transport of the victim to a stroke center capable of delivering fibrinolytics within 1 hour of arrival; and (5) prearrival notification of the hospital.

   The clinical presentations of ischemic and hemorrhagic stroke often overlap, making a diagnosis on the basis of symptoms alone impossible. In general, headaches (often described by the victim as the sudden onset of "the worst headache of my life"), disturbances in consciousness, nausea, and vomiting are more severe in association with intracranial hemorrhages. Loss of consciousness may be transient, with resolution by the time the patient receives medical attention. Patients with subarachnoid hemorrhage may have an intense headache without focal neurological signs.

   The patient with an *ischemic* stroke may be eligible for in-hospital treatment with fibrinolytic therapy. The diagnosis

TABLE 2.   Los Angeles Prehospital Stroke Screen (LAPSS)

For evaluation of acute, noncomatose, nontraumatic neurological complaint: If items 1 through 6 are **ALL checked "yes"** (or "unknown"), notify the receiving hospital before arrival of the potential stroke patient. If any are checked "no," follow appropriate treatment protocol.

Interpretation: Ninety-three percent of patients with stroke will have positive findings (all items checked "yes" or "unknown") on the LAPSS (sensitivity=93%), and 97% of those with positive findings will have a stroke (specificity=97%). The patient may still be having a stroke if LAPSS criteria are not met.

Criteria	Yes	Unknown	No
1. Age >45 years	[ ]	[ ]	[ ]
2. History of seizures or epilepsy **absent**	[ ]	[ ]	[ ]
3. Symptom duration <24 hours	[ ]	[ ]	[ ]
4. At baseline, patient is **not** wheelchair bound or bedridden	[ ]	[ ]	[ ]
5. Blood glucose between 60 and 400	[ ]	[ ]	[ ]
6. ***Obvious asymmetry*** (right vs left) in **any** of the following 3 categories (***must be unilateral***)	[ ]	[ ]	[ ]

	Equal	R Weak	L Weak
Facial smile/grimace	[ ]	[ ] Droop	[ ] Droop
Grip	[ ]	[ ] Weak grip	[ ] Weak grip
	[ ]	[ ] No grip	[ ] No grip
Arm strength	[ ]	[ ] Drifts down	[ ] Drifts down
	[ ]	[ ] Falls rapidly	[ ] Falls rapidly

From References 149 and 159.

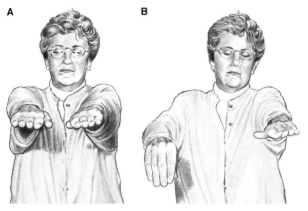

Figure 4. Arm drift. The patient is instructed to extend arms with eyes closed. Note the right-sided drift related to motor weakness.

of ischemic stroke and determination of eligibility, however, require several time-consuming steps once the victim arrives at the hospital: a treatment team is mobilized, the patient is assessed and eligibility determined, a CT scan is obtained and interpreted to rule out intracranial hemorrhage, and therapy is administered. All of these steps must be completed to allow drug delivery *within 3 hours after onset of patient symptoms.* BLS ambulance providers can maximize the likelihood of patient eligibility for fibrinolytic therapy by rapidly identifying a possible stroke victim, rapidly transporting the victim to a stroke center, and providing prearrival notification to the receiving hospital. Emphasis on the time-critical nature of this management should be included in out-of-hospital assessment and management protocols.

BLS ambulance providers should establish the time of onset of signs and symptoms of stroke: this timing has important implications for potential therapy. The onset of symptoms is viewed as the beginning (onset) of the stroke, and eligibility for fibrinolytic therapy ends 3 hours from that time. If the victim is unable to estimate the time of onset of signs and symptoms, question family members or friends at the scene. It may be possible to determine when the victim was last observed, what the victim was doing when symptoms developed (eg, preparing lunch), and any other information that will give the receiving hospital an estimate of the time of symptom onset.

Brief Neurological Evaluation: Stroke Scale and
Stroke Screen
It is impractical to perform an extensive neurological examination out of hospital because it delays the patient's transport to the ED. The abbreviated out-of-hospital neurological examination should include a validated tool such as the Cincinnati Prehospital Stroke Scale[158] (Table 1) or the Los Angeles Prehospital Stroke Screen (LAPSS) (Table 2).[149,159] Providers using the Cincinnati Prehospital Stroke Scale attempt to elicit any of 3 major physical findings suggestive of stroke: facial droop (Figure 3), arm drift (Figure 4), and abnormal speech.[158] The LAPSS includes several items designed to rule out other causes of altered level of consciousness (history of seizures, severe hyperglycemia or hypogly-

cemia). The provider using the LAPSS attempts to identify asymmetry in facial weakness/grimace, hand grip, or arm strength; asymmetry (right versus left) in any category indicates that the victim has had a possible stroke (Table 2).[149,159] These scales are both sensitive and specific in identifying stroke patients[149,158,159] and can be quickly applied.

Assess the patient's level of consciousness. The Glasgow Coma Scale (GCS) can be used to score the patient's responsiveness when the level of consciousness is depressed. This scale evaluates eye opening, best motor response, and best verbal response to simple stimuli, such as voice and pain. The highest possible score is 15; a score of 13 to 14 indicates mild neurological impairment; 11 to 13, moderate impairment; and <11, severe impairment. The GCS is well known, reproducible, and reliable when applied to patients with stroke.[160]

EMS personnel can identify stroke patients with reasonable sensitivity and specificity.[150,156,158,159,161–164] *Once the diagnosis of stroke is suspected, time in the field should be minimized and the patient prepared for immediate transport to a stroke center.* (For further information, please see "Part 7, Section 2: Acute Stroke."

EMS physicians should work with neurologists and local hospitals to establish clear destination protocols for patients suspected of having an acute stroke.[144–146,154–156] EMS ambulance services should transport a patient with stroke symptoms to an emergency receiving facility with proven capability to initiate fibrinolytic therapy for eligible stroke patients within 1 hour of arrival unless the emergency facility is >30 minutes away by ground ambulance (Class IIb). A Canadian study revealed that the vast majority of residents live within a 30-minute drive of a hospital with 24-hour CT scanning capability.[164]

Prearrival notification to the receiving facility shortens the time to definitive hospital-based evaluation and intervention for patients with stroke.* In addition to standard information, *EMS systems should communicate the results of the stroke scale or stroke screen, the GCS, and the estimated time of symptom onset to the receiving hospital before arrival.* The receiving facility should have a written plan to initiate therapy as quickly as possible (see Figure 5). Figure 5 summarizes BLS ambulance provider out-of-hospital assessment and management of patients with possible stroke.

Indications for BLS

Respiratory Arrest
Respiratory arrest can result from a number of causes, including submersion/near-drowning, stroke, FBAO, smoke inhalation, epiglottitis, drug overdose, electrocution, suffocation, injuries, myocardial infarction, lightning strike, and coma from any cause. When primary respiratory arrest occurs, the heart and lungs can continue to oxygenate the blood for several minutes, and oxygen will continue to circulate to the brain and other vital organs.[168] Such patients initially demonstrate signs of circulation. When respiratory

---

*References 7, 114, 134, 136–142, 144–146, 149–155, 164.

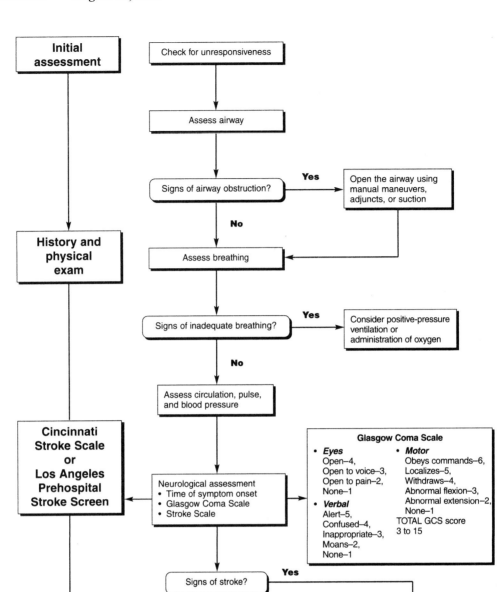

Figure 5. The algorithm reviews the out-of-hospital management of patients with stroke for BLS ambulance providers.

arrest occurs or spontaneous respirations are inadequate, establishment of a patent airway and rescue breathing can be lifesaving because it can maintain oxygenation and may prevent cardiac arrest.

Cardiac Arrest

In cardiac arrest, circulation ceases and vital organs are deprived of oxygen. Ineffective "gasping" breathing efforts ("agonal" respirations) may occur early in cardiac arrest and should not be confused with effective respirations.[66,169,170] Because lay rescuers rely on evaluation of breathing to determine cardiac arrest, they should be carefully trained to differentiate between adequate versus inadequate ventilation.

Cardiac arrest can be accompanied by the following cardiac rhythms: VF, VT, asystole, or pulseless electrical activity.

AED Use

The cardiac arrest rhythms of VT and VF are treated most effectively with early defibrillation. AED use is now considered an important and lifesaving addition to BLS and provides the trained lay rescuer or healthcare provider with the opportunity to implement the first 3 links in the Chain of Survival (early access, early CPR, and early defibrillation).[33,34] The sequence of action for a rescuer with training and access to an AED is identical to that of CPR except for the added step of attaching and using the AED. AEDs are

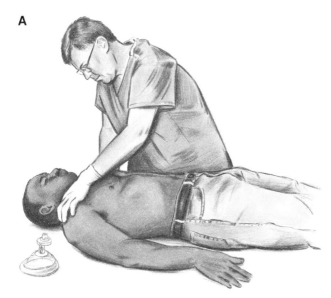

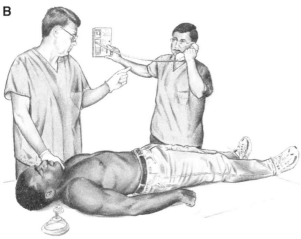

Figure 6. Check for unresponsiveness and EMS activation. The rescuer should tap the victim's shoulder and shout "Are you all right?" If the victim does not respond, the rescuer directs someone to activate the emergency medical response system (telephone 911 or appropriate emergency telephone number).

effective and easy to use.[171] (See "Part 4: The Automated External Defibrillator" later in the guidelines.)

The Sequence of BLS: Assessment, EMS Activation, the ABCs of CPR, and the "D" of Defibrillation

The BLS sequence described in this section applies to victims ≥8 years old. This sequence will be applied to older children, adolescents, and adults. For simplicity, the victim is consistently referred to as an "adult" to differentiate the victim from a "pediatric" victim who is <8 years old.

Resuscitation Sequence

BLS consists of a series of skills performed sequentially. These skills include assessment skills and support/intervention skills. The assessment phases of BLS are crucial. No victim should undergo the more intrusive procedures of CPR (positioning, opening the airway, rescue breathing, or chest compressions) until need has been established by the appropriate assessment. Assessment also in-

volves a more subtle, constant process of observing the victim and the victim's response to rescue support. The importance of the assessment phases should be stressed in teaching CPR.

Each of the ABCs of CPR—airway, breathing, and circulation—begins with an assessment phase: assess responsiveness, breathing, and signs of circulation. In the United States, the EMS system should be activated if any adult is found to be suddenly unresponsive. Outside the United States, EMS activation may be recommended if the victim is found to be unresponsive and not breathing, or activation may be delayed until after delivery of rescue breaths and determination that the victim has no signs of circulation. In all countries the EMS system should be activated as soon as it has been established that emergency care is needed. Whenever ≥2 rescuers are present, 1 rescuer remains with the victim to provide CPR while the second rescuer activates the EMS.

Hospitals and medical facilities and some businesses or building complexes will have an established emergency medical response system that provides a first response or early response on site. Such a response system notifies rescuers of the location of an emergency and the type of response needed. If the cardiopulmonary emergency occurs in a facility with an established medical response system, that system should be notified of the emergency, because it will provide more rapid response than EMS personnel arriving from outside the facility. For rescuers in these facilities, the emergency medical response system should replace the EMS system in the sequences below.

Assess Responsiveness
After determining that the scene is safe, the rescuer arriving at the side of the collapsed victim must quickly assess any injury and determine whether the person is responsive. Tap or gently shake the victim and shout, "Are you all right?" (Figure 6). If the victim has sustained trauma to the head and neck or if neck trauma is suspected, move the victim only if absolutely necessary. Improper movement may cause paralysis in the victim with injury to the spine or spinal cord.

Activate the EMS System
Activate the EMS system by calling the appropriate local emergency response system telephone number. This number should be widely publicized in each community. The person who calls the EMS system should be prepared to give the following information as calmly as possible[172]:

1. Location of the emergency (with names of office or room number or cross streets or roads, if possible)
2. Telephone number from which the call is being made
3. What happened: heart attack, auto crash, etc
4. Number of persons who need help
5. Condition of the victim(s)
6. What aid is being given to the victim(s) (eg, "CPR is being performed" or "we're using an AED")
7. Any other information requested. To ensure that EMS personnel have no more questions, the caller should hang up only when instructed to do so by the EMD.

The stage in the rescue process at which EMS activation is appropriate is determined by each country's resuscitation council and is based on the facilities available, the remoteness

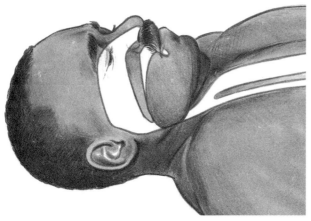

Figure 7. Obstruction by the tongue and epiglottis. When a victim is unconscious, the tongue and epiglottis can block the upper airway. The head tilt–chin lift opens the airway by lifting the tongue and epiglottis.

from those facilities of the scene of collapse, and national and local practice. In the United States, for example, the EMS should be activated as soon as the adult victim is found to be unresponsive. In many countries in Europe, the EMS system is activated after the airway is opened, breathing is assessed, and the unresponsive victim is found to be not breathing. In Australia, the EMS system is activated after the rescuer delivers rescue breaths.

Airway
If the victim is unresponsive, the rescuer will need to determine whether the victim is breathing adequately. To assess breathing, the victim should be supine (lying on his or her back) with an open airway.

Position the Victim
For resuscitative efforts and evaluation to be effective, the victim must be supine and on a firm, flat surface. If the victim is lying face down, roll the victim as a unit so that the head, shoulders, and torso move simultaneously without twisting. The head and neck should remain in the same plane as the torso, and the body should be moved as a unit. The non-breathing victim should be supine with the arms alongside the body. The victim is now appropriately positioned for CPR.

Rescuer Position
The trained rescuer should be at the victim's side, positioned to perform both rescue breathing and chest compression. The rescuer should anticipate the arrival of an AED, if appropriate, and should be prepared to operate it when it arrives.

Open the Airway
When the victim is unresponsive/unconscious, muscle tone is decreased and the tongue and epiglottis may obstruct the pharynx (Figure 7).[172–175] The tongue is the most common cause of airway obstruction in the unresponsive victim. Because the tongue is attached to the lower jaw, when you move the lower jaw forward you will lift the tongue away from the back of the throat and open the airway. The tongue or the epiglottis,[175] or both, may also create an obstruction when negative pressure is created in the airway by spontane-

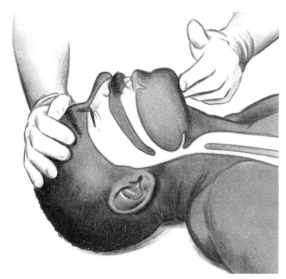

Figure 8. Head tilt–chin lift. This maneuver lifts the tongue to relieve airway obstruction.

ous inspiratory effort; this creates a valve-type mechanism that can occlude the entrance to the trachea.

If there is no evidence of head or neck trauma, use the head tilt–chin lift maneuver described below (Figure 8) to open the airway. Remove any visible foreign material or vomitus from the mouth. Wipe liquids or semiliquids out of the mouth with fingers covered with a glove or piece of cloth. Extract solid material with a hooked index finger while keeping the tongue and jaw supported with the other hand.

Head Tilt–Chin Lift Maneuver
To accomplish the head tilt maneuver, place one hand on the victim's forehead and apply firm, backward pressure with your palm, tilting the head back. To complete the head tilt–chin lift maneuver, place the fingers of your other hand under the bony part of the lower jaw near the chin. Lift the jaw upward to bring the chin forward and the teeth almost to occlusion (Figure 8). This maneuver supports the jaw and helps tilt the head back. Do not press deeply into the soft tissue under the chin, because this might obstruct the airway. Do not use your thumb to lift the chin. Open the victim's mouth to facilitate spontaneous breathing and to prepare for mouth-to-mouth breathing.

If the victim's dentures are loose, head tilt–chin lift facilitates creation of a solid mouth-to-mouth seal.[176] Remove the dentures if they cannot be kept in place.

Jaw-Thrust Maneuver
The jaw-thrust without head tilt maneuver for airway opening should be taught to both lay rescuers and healthcare providers. Place one hand on each side of the victim's head, resting your elbows on the surface on which the victim is lying. Grasp the angles of the victim's lower jaw and lift with both hands (Figure 9). If the lips close, you can retract the lower lip with your thumb. If mouth-to-mouth breathing is necessary while you maintain the jaw thrust, close the victim's nostrils by placing your cheek tightly against them. This technique is very effective for opening the airway[177] but fatiguing and technically difficult for the rescuer.[176]

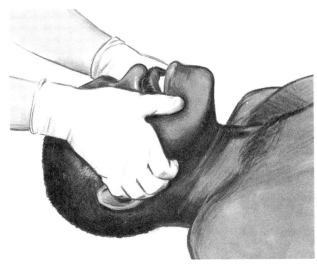

Figure 9. Jaw thrust without head tilt. The jaw is lifted without tilting the head. This is the airway maneuver of choice for a victim suspected of having sustained a cervical spine injury.

The jaw-thrust technique *without* head tilt is the safest initial approach to opening the airway of the victim with suspected neck injury because it usually can be done without extending the neck. Carefully support the head without tilting it backward or turning it from side to side.

Recommendations for Opening the Airway
The recommended technique for opening the airway must be simple, safe, easily learned, and effective. Because head tilt–chin lift meets these criteria, it should be the method of choice for lay rescuers performing BLS, and lay rescuers should use this technique unless trauma is suspected. Although all rescuers are taught both head tilt–chin lift and jaw thrust methods of opening the airway, the professional rescuers (BLS ambulance providers and other healthcare providers) should be proficient in both head tilt–chin lift and jaw thrust.

Breathing

Assessment: Check for Breathing
To assess breathing, place your ear near the victim's mouth and nose while maintaining an open airway. Then, while observing the victim's chest, (1) *look* for the chest to rise and fall, (2) *listen* for air escaping during exhalation, and (3) *feel* for the flow of air. If the chest does not rise and fall and no air is exhaled, the victim is not breathing. This evaluation procedure should take no more than 10 seconds.

Most victims with respiratory or cardiac arrest have no signs of breathing. Occasionally, however, the victim will demonstrate abnormal and inadequate breathing. Some victims demonstrate apparent respiratory efforts with signs of upper airway obstruction. These victims may resume effective breathing when you open the airway. Some victims may have a patent airway but may make only weak, inadequate attempts to breathe. Reflex gasping respiratory efforts (agonal respirations) are another form of inadequate breathing that may be observed early in the course of primary cardiac arrest. Absent or inadequate respirations require rapid intervention with rescue breathing. If you are not *confident* that respira-

tions are adequate, proceed immediately with rescue breathing. Lay rescuers are taught to provide rescue breathing if "normal" breathing is absent.

If a victim resumes breathing and regains signs of circulation (pulse, normal breathing, coughing, or movement) during or after resuscitation, continue to help the victim maintain an open airway. Place the victim in a recovery position if the victim maintains breathing and signs of circulation.

Recovery Position
The recovery position is used in the management of victims who are unresponsive but are breathing and have signs of circulation (Class Indeterminate). When an unresponsive victim is lying supine and breathing spontaneously, the airway may become obstructed by the tongue or mucus and vomit. These problems may be prevented when the victim is placed on his or her side, because fluid can drain easily from the mouth.

Some compromise is needed between ideal position for maximum airway patency and optimal position to allow monitoring and support with good body alignment. A modified lateral position is used because a true lateral posture tends to be unstable, involves excessive lateral flexion of the cervical spine, and results in less free drainage from the mouth. A near-prone position, on the other hand, can hinder adequate ventilation because it splints the diaphragm and reduces pulmonary and thoracic compliance.[178] Several versions of the recovery position exist, each with its own advantages. No single position is perfect for all victims. When deciding which position to use, consider 6 principles[179]:

1. The victim should be in as near a true lateral position as possible, with the head dependent to allow free drainage of fluid.
2. The position should be stable.
3. Avoid any pressure on the chest that impairs breathing.
4. It should be possible to turn the victim on his or her side and to return to the back easily and safely, with concern for a possible cervical spine injury.
5. Good observation of and access to the airway should be possible.
6. The position itself should not cause an injury to the victim.

It is particularly important to avoid injury to the victim when turning the victim.[180,181] If trauma is present or suspected, the victim should be moved only if an open airway cannot otherwise be maintained. This might be the case if, for example, a lone rescuer needs to leave the victim to get help. Monitor the victim, particularly for impairment of blood flow in the lowermost arm.[182,183] If the victim remains in the recovery position for >30 minutes, turn the victim to the opposite side. Although no single specific recovery position can be recommended, the one illustrated (Figure 10) is suitable for training purposes.

Provide Rescue Breathing
When providing rescue breathing, you must inflate the victim's lungs adequately with each breath.

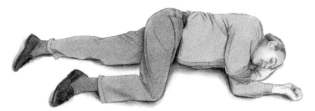

Figure 10. The recovery position.

Mouth-to-Mouth Breathing

Mouth-to-mouth rescue breathing is a quick, effective way to provide oxygen and ventilation to the victim.[184] Your exhaled breath contains enough oxygen to supply the victim's needs.[184] To provide rescue breaths, hold the victim's airway open, pinch the nose, and make a seal with your mouth over the victim's mouth. Rest the palm of one hand on the victim's forehead and pinch the victim's nose closed with your thumb and index finger. Pinching the nose will prevent air from escaping through the victim's nose. Take a deep breath and seal your lips around the victim's mouth, creating an airtight seal. Give slow breaths, delivering each breath over 2 seconds, making sure the victim's chest rises with each breath. Be prepared to deliver approximately 10 to 12 breaths per minute (1 breath every 4 to 5 seconds) if rescue breathing alone is required (see Figure 11).

The number of breaths delivered to initiate rescue breathing/ventilation varies throughout the world, and there is no data to suggest superiority of one number over the other. In the United States, 2 breaths are provided. In Europe, Australia, and New Zealand, 5 breaths are provided to initiate resuscitation. Each approach has its advantages. Delivery of fewer breaths will shorten the time to assessment of circulation/pulse and attachment of an AED (and possible defibrillation), but delivery of a greater number of breaths may help to correct hypoxia and hypercarbia. In the absence of data to support one number of breaths over another, it is appropriate to deliver 2 to 5 initial breaths, according to local custom.

Gastric inflation frequently develops during mouth-to-mouth ventilation.[185,186] Gastric inflation can produce serious

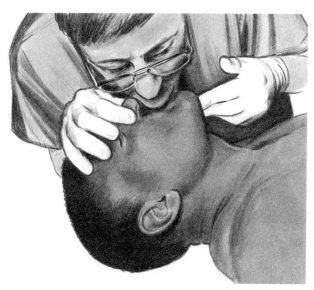

Figure 11. Mouth-to-mouth rescue breathing.

complications, such as regurgitation,[187–189] aspiration,[190] or pneumonia.[191] It also increases intragastric pressure,[185,186,190–195] elevates the diaphragm, restricts lung movements, and decreases respiratory system compliance.[185,196,197] Gastric inflation occurs when the pressure in the esophagus exceeds the lower esophageal sphincter opening pressure, causing the sphincter to open so that air delivered during rescue breaths enters the stomach instead of the lungs.[185,196–201] During cardiac arrest, the likelihood of gastric inflation increases because the lower esophageal sphincter relaxes.[198] Factors that contribute to creation of a high esophageal pressure and gastric inflation during rescue breathing include a short inspiratory time, a large tidal volume, and a high peak airway pressure.

Previous guidelines recommended that rescue breaths provide a tidal volume of 800 to 1200 mL delivered over 1 to 2 seconds.[49] With respect to gastric inflation, a substantially smaller tidal volume would be safer but is ineffective in maintaining adequate arterial oxygen saturation unless supplemental oxygen can be delivered via a face mask or bag-valve mask.[202,203]

To reduce the risk of gastric inflation during mouth-to-mouth ventilation, deliver slow breaths at the lowest tidal volume that will still make the chest visibly rise with each ventilation. For mouth-to-mouth ventilation in most adults, this volume will be approximately 10 mL/kg (approximately 700 to 1000 mL) and should be delivered over 2 seconds (Class IIa). This recommendation represents a slightly decreased range of tidal volume compared with previous guidelines, and it uses the upper limit of inspiratory time recommended in the previous guidelines. This new recommendation is intended to reduce the risk of gastric inflation (and its serious consequences) while maintaining adequate arterial oxygen saturation during respiratory and cardiac arrest.

If you take a deep breath before each ventilation, you will optimize your exhaled gas composition, ensuring that you will provide as much oxygen as possible to the victim.[204] You are providing adequate ventilation if you see the chest rise and fall with each breath and you hear and feel the air escape during exhalation. When possible (eg, during 2-rescuer CPR), maintain airway patency to allow unimpeded exhalation between rescue breaths.

If initial (or subsequent) attempts to ventilate the victim are unsuccessful, reposition the victim's head and reattempt rescue breathing. Improper chin and head positioning is the most common cause of difficulty with ventilation. If the victim cannot be ventilated after repositioning of the head, the healthcare provider (but *not* the lay rescuer) should proceed with maneuvers to relieve FBAO (see "Foreign-Body Airway Obstruction Management" below).

Mouth-to-Nose Breathing

The mouth-to-nose method of ventilation is recommended when it is impossible to ventilate through the victim's mouth, the mouth cannot be opened (trismus), the mouth is seriously injured, or a tight mouth-to-mouth seal is difficult to achieve.[205] Mouth-to-nose breathing may be the best method of providing ventilation while rescuing a submersion victim

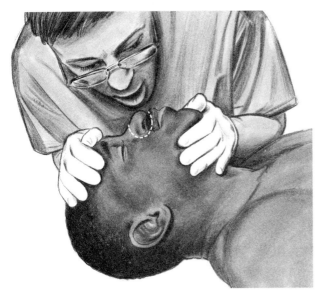

Figure 12. Mouth-to-nose rescue breathing.

from the water. The rescuer's hands often will be used to support the victim's head and shoulders during rescue. The mouth-to-nose technique may enable the rescuer to begin rescue breathing as soon as the victim's head is out of the water.

To provide mouth-to-nose breathing, tilt the victim's head back with one hand on the forehead and use the other hand to lift the victim's mandible (as in head tilt–chin lift) and close the victim's mouth.[175] Take a deep breath, seal your lips around the victim's nose, and exhale into the victim's nose. Then remove your lips from the victim's nose, allowing passive exhalation (Figure 12). It may be necessary to open the victim's mouth intermittently and separate the lips with the thumb to allow free exhalation; this is particularly important if partial nasal obstruction is present.[206]

Mouth-to-Stoma Breathing
A tracheal stoma is a permanent opening at the front of the neck that extends from the surface of the skin into the trachea (Figure 13A).[207] When a person with a tracheostomy requires rescue breathing, direct mouth-to-stoma ventilation should be performed. Place your mouth over the stoma, making an airtight seal around the stoma. Blow into the stoma until the chest rises (Figure 13B). Then remove your mouth from the patient, allowing passive exhalation.

A tracheostomy tube may be present in the tracheal stoma. This tube must be patent for either spontaneous ventilation or rescue breathing to occur. If the tube is not patent and you are unable to clear an obstruction or any secretions, remove and replace the tube. If a second tube is unavailable and the original tube is obstructed, remove the tube and provide rescue breathing through the stoma. If a significant volume of air escapes through the victim's nose and mouth during ventilation through the tracheostomy, seal the victim's mouth and nose with your hand or a tightly fitting face mask. Air escape is alleviated if you can provide ventilation through a tracheostomy tube with an inflated cuff.

A

B

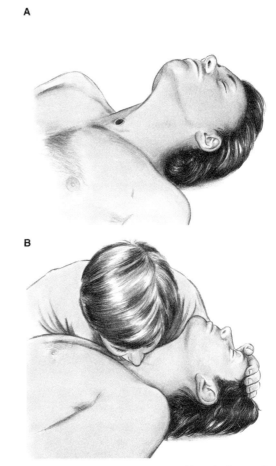

Figure 13. Mouth-to-stoma rescue breathing. A, Stoma; B, mouth-to-stoma.

Mouth-to–Barrier Device Breathing
Some rescuers prefer to use a barrier device during mouth-to-mouth ventilation. The use of barrier devices should be encouraged for rescuers who may perform CPR in areas outside the home, such as the workplace. Two broad categories of barrier devices are available: mouth-to-mask devices and face shields. Mouth-to-mask devices typically have a 1-way valve so that the victim's exhaled air does not enter the rescuer's mouth. Face shields usually have no exhalation valve, and the victim's expired air escapes between the shield and the victim's face. Barrier devices should have a low resistance to gas flow so that they do not impede ventilation.

Mouth-to–Face Shield Rescue Breathing
Unlike mouth-to-mask devices, face shields have only a clear plastic or silicone sheet that separates the rescuer from the victim. The opening of the face shield is placed over the victim's mouth. In some models a short (1- to 2-inch) tube is part of the shield. If a tube is present, insert the tube in the victim's mouth, over the tongue. Pinch the victim's nose closed and seal your mouth around the center opening of the face shield while maintaining head tilt–chin lift or jaw thrust. Provide slow breaths (2 seconds each) through the 1-way valve or filter in the center of the face shield, allowing the victim's exhaled air to escape between the shield and the victim's face when you lift your mouth off the shield between breaths (Figure 14).

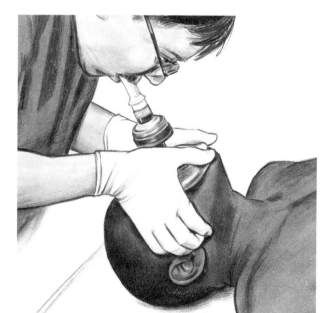

Figure 14. Face shield. The shield is placed over the mouth and nose with the opening at the center of the shield placed over the victim's mouth. The technique of rescue breathing is the same as for mouth-to-mouth.

The face shield should remain on the victim's face during chest compressions and ventilations. If the victim begins to vomit during rescue efforts, immediately turn the victim onto his side, remove the face shield, and clear the airway. Proximity to the victim's face and the possibility of contamination if the victim vomits are major disadvantages of face shields.[208,209] In addition, the efficacy of face shields has not been documented conclusively. For these reasons, healthcare professionals and rescuers with a duty to respond should use face shields only as a substitute for mouth-to-mouth breathing

and should use mouth-to-mask or bag-mask devices at the first opportunity.[210,211]

Tidal volumes and inspiratory times for rescuer breathing through barrier devices should be the same as those for mouth-to-mouth breathing (in an adult, a tidal volume of approximately 10 mL/kg or 700 to 1000 mL delivered over 2 seconds and sufficient to make the chest rise clearly).

Mouth-to-Mask Rescue Breathing
A transparent mask with or without a 1-way valve is used in mouth-to-mask breathing. The 1-way valve directs the rescuer's breath into the victim while diverting the victim's exhaled air away from the rescuer. Some devices include an oxygen inlet that permits administration of supplemental oxygen.

Mouth-to-mask ventilation is particularly effective because it allows the rescuer to use 2 hands to create a mask seal. There are 2 possible techniques for using the mouth-to-mask device. The first technique positions the rescuer above the victim's head (cephalic technique). This technique can be used by a single rescuer when the patient is in respiratory arrest (but not cardiac arrest) or during performance of 2-rescuer CPR. A jaw thrust is used in the cephalic technique, which has the advantage of positioning the rescuer so that the rescuer is facing the victim's chest while performing rescue breathing (see Figure 15A and 15B).

In the second technique (lateral technique), the rescuer is positioned at the victim's side and uses head tilt–chin lift. The lateral technique is ideal for performing 1-rescuer CPR, because the rescuer can maintain the same position for both rescue breathing and chest compressions (see Figure 16).

Cephalic technique. Position yourself directly above the victim's head and perform the following steps:

A

B

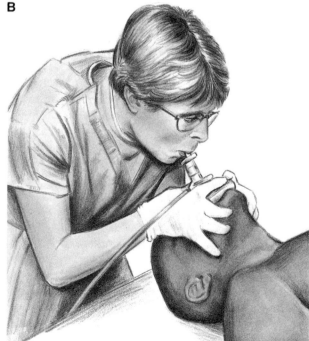

Figure 15. Mouth-to-mask, cephalic technique. A, Using thumb and thenar eminence on the top of the mask. B, Circling the thumb and first finger around the top of the mask.

- Apply the mask to the victim's face, using the bridge of the nose as a guide for correct position.
- Place your thumbs and thenar eminence (portion of the palm at the base of the thumb) along the lateral edges of the mask.
- Place the index fingers of both hands under the victim's mandible and lift the jaw into the mask as you tilt the head back. Place your remaining fingers under the angle of the jaw (Figure 15A).
- While lifting the jaw, squeeze the mask with your thumbs and thenar eminence to achieve an airtight seal (see jaw thrust).
- Provide slow rescue breaths (2 seconds) while observing for chest rise.

An alternative method for the cephalic technique is to use the thumb and first finger of each hand to make a complete seal around the edges of the mask. Use the remaining fingers to lift the angle of the jaw and extend the neck (Figure 15B). With either variation of the cephalic technique, the rescuer uses both hands to hold the mask and open the airway. In victims with suspected head or neck (potential cervical spine) injury, lift the mandible at the angles of the jaw but do not tilt the head.

Lateral technique. Position yourself beside the victim's head to provide rescue breathing and chest compressions:

- Apply the mask to the victim's face, using the bridge of the nose as a guide for correct position.
- Seal the mask by placing your index finger and thumb of the hand closer to the top of the victim's head along the border of the mask and placing the thumb of your other hand along the lower margin of the mask.
- Place your remaining fingers on the hand closer to the victim's feet along the bony margin of the jaw and lift the jaw while performing a head tilt–chin lift (Figure 16).
- Compress firmly and completely around the outside margin of the mask to provide a tight seal.
- Provide slow rescue breaths while observing for chest rise.

Effective use of the mask requires instruction and supervised practice. During 2-rescuer CPR, the mask can be used in a variety of ways. The most appropriate method will depend on the experience of personnel and equipment available. Oral airways and cricoid pressure may be used with mouth-to-mask and any other form of rescue breathing.

If oxygen is not available, tidal volumes and inspiratory times for mouth-to-mask ventilation should be the same as for mouth-to-mouth breathing (in an adult, a tidal volume of approximately 10 mL/kg or 700 to 1000 mL delivered over 2 seconds and sufficient to make the chest rise clearly). If supplemental oxygen is used with the face mask, a minimum flow rate of 10 L/min provides an inspired concentration of oxygen ≥40%.[212] When oxygen is provided, lower tidal volumes are recommended (tidal volume of approximately 6 to 7 mL/kg or 400 to 600 mL given over 1 to 2 seconds until the chest rises) (Class IIb).[3] The smaller tidal volumes are effective for maintaining adequate arterial oxygen saturation, provided that supplemental oxygen is delivered to the device, but these smaller volumes will not maintain normocarbia.[202] These volumes will reduce the risk of gastric inflation[185,186] and its serious consequences.[185,187–191,196,197]

Bag-Mask Device
Bag-mask devices used in the prehospital setting consist of a self-inflating bag and a nonrebreathing valve attached to a face mask. These devices provide the most common method of delivering positive-pressure ventilation in both the EMS and hospital settings. Most commercially available adult bag-mask units have a volume of approximately 1600 mL, which is usually adequate to produce lung inflation. In several studies, however, many rescuers were unable to deliver adequate tidal volumes to unintubated manikins.[213–217] Adult bag-mask units may provide a smaller tidal volume than mouth-to-mouth or mouth-to-mask ventilation because the lone rescuer may have difficulty obtaining a leak-proof seal to the face while squeezing the bag and maintaining an open airway. For this reason, self-inflating bag-mask units are most effective when 2 trained and experienced rescuers work together, one sealing the mask to the face and the other squeezing the bag slowly over 2 seconds (Figure 17). In fact,

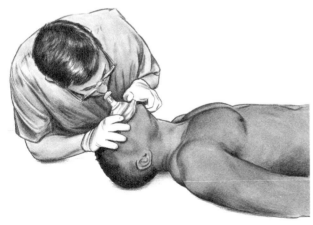

Figure 16. Mouth-to-mask, lateral technique. The lateral technique allows the rescuer to perform 1-rescuer CPR from a fixed position at the side of the victim.

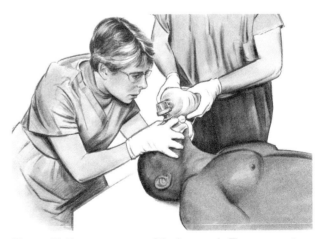

Figure 17. Two-rescuer use of the bag mask. The rescuer at the head uses the thumb and first finger of each hand to provide a complete seal around the edges of the mask. Use the remaining fingers to lift the mandible and extend the neck while observing chest rise. The other rescuer slowly squeezes the bag (over 2 seconds) until he observes chest rise.

in some countries (eg, Australia), bag-mask ventilation during BLS CPR is performed by 2 rescuers.

There are significant advantages to the use of small tidal volumes during resuscitation. Small tidal volume will reduce the risk of gastric inflation and its consequences, but it does risk the development of hypoxia and hypercarbia and their complications.[217a] The use of small tidal volumes with oxygen supplementation during resuscitation has been evaluated in laboratory[186,193–195,218,219] and clinical[194,218–220] settings. With smaller tidal volumes, airway pressure does not exceed the victim's lower esophageal sphincter pressure,[185,196–198] so lower tidal volumes will reduce gastric inflation and its potential consequences of regurgitation,[187–189] aspiration,[190] and pneumonia.[191] Supplementary oxygen will ensure maintenance of oxygen saturation at these smaller tidal volumes.[202]

If supplementary oxygen (minimum flow rate of 8 to 12 L/min with oxygen concentration ≥40%) is available, the rescuer skilled in bag-mask ventilation should attempt to deliver a smaller tidal volume (6 to 7 mL/kg or approximately 400 to 600 mL) over 1 to 2 seconds (Class IIb). Of course, in the clinical setting, the actual tidal volume delivered is impossible to determine. Tidal volume can be titrated to provide sufficient ventilation to maintain oxygen saturation and produce visible chest expansion. The tidal volume should be sufficient to make the chest rise. It is important to note that this smaller tidal volume may be associated with the development of hypercarbia.[217a]

If oxygen is not available, the rescuer should attempt to deliver the same tidal volume recommended for mouth-to-mouth ventilation (10 mL/kg, 700 to 1000 mL) over 2 seconds. This tidal volume should result in very obvious chest rise.

An adult bag-mask device should have the following features:

- A nonjam inlet valve system allowing a maximum oxygen inlet flow of 30 L/min
- Either no pressure relief valve or, if a pressure relief valve is present, the pressure relief valve must be capable of being closed
- Standard 15-mm/22-mm fittings
- An oxygen reservoir to allow delivery of high concentrations of oxygen[221]
- A nonrebreathing outlet valve that cannot be obstructed by foreign material
- Ability to function satisfactorily under common environmental conditions and extremes of temperature

Technique. Bag-mask ventilation technique requires instruction and practice. The rescuer should be able to use the equipment effectively in a variety of situations.

If you are the only rescuer providing respiratory support, position yourself at the top of the victim's head. If there is no concern about neck injury, tilt the victim's head back and place it on a towel or pillow to achieve the sniffing position. Apply the mask to the victim's face with one hand, using the bridge of the nose as a guide for correct position. Place the third, fourth, and fifth fingers of that hand along the bony portion of the mandible, and place the thumb and index

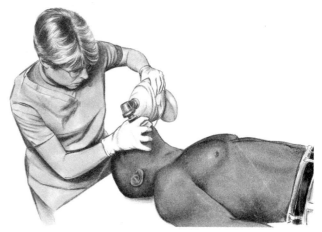

Figure 18. One-rescuer use of the bag mask. The rescuer circles the top edges of the mask with her index and first finger and lifts the jaw with the remaining fingers. The bag is squeezed while the rescuer observes chest rise. Mask seal is key to the successful use of the bag mask.

fingers of the same hand on the mask. Maintain head tilt and jaw thrust to keep the airway patent and snug against the mask (Figure 18).

Compress the bag with your other hand and watch the chest to be sure it rises, indicating that ventilation is adequate. Deliver each breath over 2 seconds (using 1 to 2 seconds when you deliver smaller tidal volumes with oxygen supplementation). You may want to compress the bag against your body to achieve the selected tidal volume. It is critical to maintain an airtight seal during delivery of each breath.

Effective ventilation is more likely to be provided when 2 rescuers use the bag-mask system: 1 rescuer holds the mask and 1 rescuer squeezes the bag (Figure 17). The techniques for holding the mask are the same as for mouth-to-mask devices described above. If a third rescuer is available, cricoid pressure may be applied.

Bag-mask ventilation is a complex technique that requires considerable skill and practice. Such skill is difficult to maintain when used infrequently. Accordingly, alternative airway devices such as the laryngeal mask airway and the esophageal-tracheal Combitube are being introduced within the scope of BLS practice for healthcare providers. These devices are generally easier to insert than tracheal tubes, but they allow similar support of ventilation. These devices may provide acceptable alternatives to bag-mask ventilation for healthcare providers who are well trained and have sufficient opportunities to use these devices (Class IIb). A detailed explanation of these devices is found in Part 6 of this document (see "Adjuncts for Oxygenation, Ventilation, and Airway Control").

Cricoid Pressure
The cricoid pressure technique applies pressure to the victim's cricoid cartilage. This pushes the trachea posteriorly, compressing the esophagus against the cervical vertebrae during rescue breathing. Cricoid pressure is effective in preventing gastric inflation, reducing the risk of regurgitation and aspiration.[222–225] It should be used only if the victim is unconscious. Proper use of the cricoid pressure technique

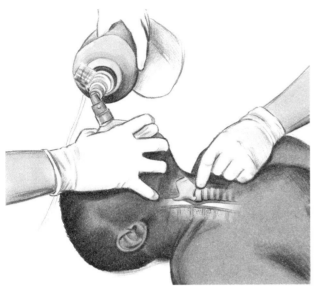

Figure 19. Cricoid pressure (Sellick maneuver).

requires an additional rescuer to provide cricoid pressure alone, without diversion to other resuscitation activities. As a result, this technique should be used only by healthcare professionals when an extra rescuer is present. This means that during "2"-rescuer CPR, 3 rescuers would actually be required: 1 rescuer to perform rescue breathing, 1 to perform chest compressions, and 1 to apply cricoid pressure.

The technique for applying cricoid pressure is as follows:

1. Locate the thyroid cartilage (Adam's apple) with your index finger.

2. Slide your index finger to the base of the thyroid cartilage and palpate the prominent horizontal ring below (cricoid cartilage).

3. Using the tips of your thumb and index finger, apply firm backward pressure to the cricoid cartilage (Figure 19).

Apply moderate rather than excessive pressure on the cricoid. Use of moderate pressure is particularly important if the victim is small.

Rescue Breathing Without Chest Compressions

Deliver 2 initial breaths slowly over 2 seconds each, allowing complete exhalation between breaths to diminish the likelihood of exceeding the esophageal opening pressure. This technique should result in less gastric inflation, regurgitation, and aspiration. For respiratory arrest, when chest compressions are not being performed, provide approximately 10 to 12 breaths per minute (1 breath every 4 to 5 seconds). Check every few minutes to ensure that the victim continues to show signs of circulation (see next section).

Circulation

Assessment: No Pulse Check for Lay Rescuers

Since the first resuscitation guidelines were published in 1968, the pulse check has been the "gold standard" method of determining whether the heart was beating. In the sequence of CPR, the absence of a pulse indicates cardiac arrest and the need to provide chest compressions. In the current era of early defibrillation, absence of a pulse is an indication for the attachment of the AED. Since 1992 several published studies have called into question the validity of the pulse check as a

TABLE 3. Sensitivity, Specificity, and Reliability of Pulse Check: Performance of Pulse Check as a Diagnostic Test

	Pulse Is Present	Pulse Is Absent	Totals
Rescuer thinks pulse is present	81 (Sensitivity: correct positive result of pulse check÷all times a pulse was actually present) **a**	6 **b**	87 (No. of times rescuer thought pulse present=a+b)
Rescuer thinks pulse is absent	66 **c**	53 (Specificity: correct negative result of pulse check÷all times there actually was no pulse) **d**	119 (No. of times rescuer thought pulse absent=c+d)
Totals	147 (Total number of study opportunities where a pulse was actually present=a+c)	59 (Total number of study opportunities where a pulse was actually absent=b+d)	206 (Total study opportunities=a+b+c+d)

Calculations derived from above:

   a. Positive predictive value: Of the total times the rescuer thinks a pulse is present (total=87 times), a pulse *is* present=81/87 times=93%.

   b. Negative predictive value: Of the total times the rescuer thinks a pulse is absent (total=119 times), a pulse *is* absent=53/119=45%.

   c. Sensitivity: Rescuer's ability to detect a pulse when one actually is present=81/147=55%.

   d. Specificity: Rescuer's ability to recognize that a pulse is absent when a pulse actually is absent=53/59=90%.

   e. Accuracy="rescuer correct"/total=(81 pulse correctly found+53 pulse correctly thought absent)/206=65%.

Modified from Cummins RO, Hazinski MF. Cardiopulmonary resuscitation techniques and instruction: when does evidence justify revision? *Ann Emerg Med.* 1999;34:780–784. Based on data from Eberle B, Dick WF, Schneider T, Wisser G, Doetsch S, Tzanova I. Checking the carotid pulse: diagnostic accuracy of first responders in patients with and without a pulse. *Resuscitation.* 1996;33:107–116.

test for cardiac arrest, particularly when used by laypersons.[226–235] This research has used manikin simulation,[231] unconscious patients undergoing cardiopulmonary bypass,[235] unconscious mechanically ventilated patients,[232] and conscious "test persons."[227,232] These studies conclude that as a diagnostic test for cardiac arrest, the pulse check has serious limitations in accuracy, sensitivity, and specificity.

When lay persons use the pulse check, they require a long time to decide whether a pulse is present. They then fail in 1 of 10 times to recognize the absence of a pulse or cardiac arrest (poor sensitivity). When lay rescuers assess unresponsive victims who do have a pulse, the rescuers miss the pulse in 4 of 10 times (poor specificity). Details of the published studies include the following conclusions:

1. Rescuers require far too much time to perform the pulse check: The majority of all rescue groups, including laypersons, medical students, paramedics, and physicians, take much longer than the recommended 5 to 10 seconds to check for the carotid pulse. In one study, half of the rescuers required more than 24 seconds to decide whether a pulse was present. With survival from VF falling by 7% to 10% for every minute defibrillation is delayed, time allotted to assessment of circulation must be brief. Only 15% of the participants correctly confirmed the presence of a pulse within 10 seconds, the maximum time currently allotted for a pulse check.[235]
2. When considered as a diagnostic test, the pulse check is extremely inaccurate. This accuracy can be expressed in a classic 2×2 matrix, based on results from a representative study[235] (Table 3) and summarized as follows:
   a. Specificity (ability to correctly identify victims who have NO pulse and ARE in cardiac arrest) is only 90%: When *subjects were pulseless*, rescuers thought a pulse was present approximately 10% of the time. By mistakenly thinking a pulse IS present when it is not, rescuers will fail to provide chest compressions and will not attach an AED for 10 of every 100 people in cardiac arrest. The consequences of such errors would be death without possibility of resuscitation for 10 of every 100 victims of cardiac arrest.
   b. Sensitivity (ability to correctly recognize victims who HAVE a pulse and ARE NOT in cardiac arrest) was only 55%. When the pulse was *present*, the rescuers assessed the pulse as being *absent* approximately 45% of the time. By erroneously thinking a pulse was absent, rescuers would provide chest compressions for approximately 4 of 10 potential victims who do not need them and would attach an AED, if available.
3. The overall accuracy was only 65%, leaving an error rate of 35%.

On review of this and other data, the experts and delegates at the 1999 Evidence Evaluation Conference and the International Guidelines 2000 Conference concluded that the pulse check could not be recommended as a tool for lay rescuers to identify victims of cardiac arrest in the CPR sequence. If rescuers use the pulse check to identify victims of cardiac arrest, they will "miss" true cardiac arrest at least 10 times out of 100. In addition, rescuers will provide unnecessary chest compressions (and may attach an AED) for many victims who are not in cardiac arrest and do not require such intervention. This error is less serious but still undesirable. The more serious error in this situation is clearly the potential failure to intervene for victims of cardiac arrest who require immediate intervention to survive.

Therefore, *the lay rescuer should not rely on the pulse check to determine the need for chest compressions* or use of an AED. Lay rescuers should not perform the pulse check and will not be taught the pulse check in CPR courses (Class IIa). Instead, lay rescuers will be taught to assess for "signs of circulation," including normal breathing, coughing, or movement, in response to the rescue breaths. This guideline recommendation applies to *victims of any age. Healthcare providers should continue to use the pulse check as one of several signs of circulation.* Other signs of circulation include breathing, coughing, or movement.

It is expected that this guideline change will result in more rapid and more accurate identification of cardiac arrest. It should eliminate delays in provision of chest compressions and use of the AED. Most important, it should reduce the missed opportunities to provide CPR and early defibrillation for victims in cardiac arrest.

Assessment: Check for Signs of Circulation

These guidelines often refer to assessment of "signs of circulation." For the *lay rescuer,* this means the following: deliver initial rescue breaths and evaluate the victim for normal breathing, coughing, or movement in response to the rescue breaths. The lay rescuer will look, listen, and feel for breathing while scanning the victim for signs of other movement. Lay rescuers should look for "normal breathing" to minimize confusion with agonal respirations.

When healthcare professionals assess signs of circulation, they add a pulse check while simultaneously evaluating the victim for breathing, coughing, or movement. Professional rescuers are instructed to look for "breathing" because they are trained to distinguish between agonal breathing and other forms of ventilation not associated with cardiac arrest.

In practice, the assessment for signs of circulation for the lay rescuer is performed as follows:

1. Provide initial rescue breaths to the unresponsive, nonbreathing victim.
2. Look for signs of circulation.
   a. With your ear near the victim's mouth, look, listen, and feel for normal breathing or coughing.
   b. Quickly scan the victim for any signs of movement.
3. If the victim is not breathing normally, coughing, or moving, immediately begin chest compressions.

This assessment should take no more than 10 seconds. Healthcare providers should perform a pulse check in conjunction with assessment for signs of circulation. If you are not *confident* that circulation is present, begin chest compressions immediately.

When a pulse check is performed for the victim >1 year of age, the carotid artery is the preferred artery to palpate, although the femoral artery may be used as an alternative. Pulses will persist in these arteries even when hypotension and poor perfusion cause peripheral pulses to disappear. To

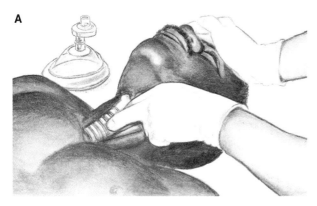

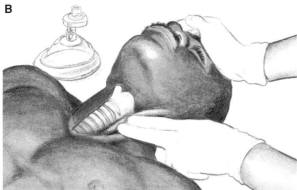

Figure 20. Checking the carotid pulse. A, Locate the trachea. B, Gently feel for the carotid pulse.

locate the carotid artery, maintain a head tilt with one hand on the victim's forehead and locate the trachea with 2 or 3 fingers of the other hand (Figure 20A). Slide these 2 or 3 fingers into the groove between the trachea and the muscles at the side of the neck, where the carotid pulse can be felt (Figure 20B). Use only gentle pressure so that you do not compress the artery. The artery on the side of the neck toward you is typically most readily palpated.

Provide Chest Compressions

Chest compressions for CPR are serial, rhythmic applications of pressure over the lower half of the sternum.[236] These compressions create blood flow by increasing intrathoracic pressure or directly compressing the heart.[237,238] Blood circulated to the lungs by chest compressions, accompanied by properly performed rescue breathing, will most likely deliver adequate oxygen to the brain and other vital organs until defibrillation can be performed.

Theoretical,[239,240] animal,[237,241–244] and human[245,246] data supports a rate of chest compression >80 per minute to achieve optimal forward blood flow during CPR. For this reason, a compression rate of 100 per minute is recommended (Class IIb). The compression rate refers to the *speed* of compressions, *not to the actual number* of compressions delivered in 1 minute. A compression rate of approximately 100 per minute will result in delivery of *fewer than* 100 compressions per minute by the single rescuer who must interrupt chest compressions to deliver rescue breaths. The actual number of chest compressions delivered per minute depends on the accuracy and consistency of the rate of chest

compressions and the time the rescuer requires to open the airway and deliver rescue breaths.

Previous versions of the adult BLS guidelines recommended a ratio of 15 compressions to 2 ventilations for 1-rescuer CPR and a ratio of 5 compressions to 1 ventilation for 2-rescuer CPR.[49,179] A ratio of 15:2 provides more chest compressions per minute (approximately 64 versus 50) than a ratio of 5:1.[247] There is evidence to suggest that adult cardiac arrest victims are more likely to be saved if a higher number of chest compressions are delivered during CPR, even if the victims receive fewer ventilations.[68,248] The quality of rescue breathing and chest compressions is not affected by compression-ventilation ratio.[247]

During cardiac arrest, the coronary perfusion pressure gradually rises with the performance of sequential compressions.[248] This pressure is higher after 15 uninterrupted chest compressions than it is after 5 chest compressions.[248] Therefore, after each pause for ventilation, several compressions must be performed before previous levels of brain and coronary perfusion are reestablished.[248] For these reasons, a ratio of 15 compressions to 2 ventilations is recommended for 1 *or* 2 rescuers (Class IIb) until the airway is secured. This applies to adult BLS provided by both laypersons and healthcare providers. Research is ongoing to determine the benefits of further increasing the number of compressions between ventilations during CPR. Once the airway is secured (protected) with a cuffed tracheal tube (as discussed in the ACLS guidelines), compressions may be continuous and ventilations may be asynchronous, with a ratio of 5 compressions to 1 ventilation.

During actual CPR, rescuers often compress at a slower rate than 100 per minute.[248,249] For teaching and during performance of CPR, therefore, some form of audio timing prompt may help to achieve the recommended compression rate of approximately 100 per minute (Class IIb).[250,251]

The victim must be in the horizontal, supine position on a firm surface during chest compressions to optimize the effect of the compressions and blood flow to the brain. When the head is elevated above the heart, blood flow to the brain is reduced or eliminated. If the victim cannot be removed from a bed, place a rigid board, preferably the full width of the bed, under the victim's back to avoid diminished effectiveness of chest compression.

Chest Compression Technique

Proper hand placement is established by identifying the lower half of the sternum. The guidelines below may be used, or you may choose alternative techniques to identify the lower sternum.

1. Place your fingers on the lower margin of the victim's rib cage on the side nearer you (Figure 21A).
2. Slide your fingers up the rib cage to the notch where the ribs meet the lower sternum in the center of the lower part of the chest.
3. Place the heel of one hand on the lower half of the sternum (Figure 21B) and the other hand on top of the first, so that the hands are parallel (Figure 21C). Be sure the long axis of the heel of your hand is placed on the long axis of the sternum. This will keep the main force

A

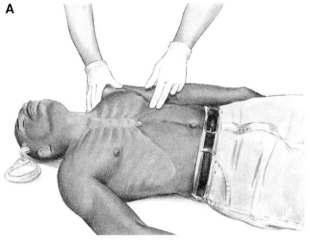

B

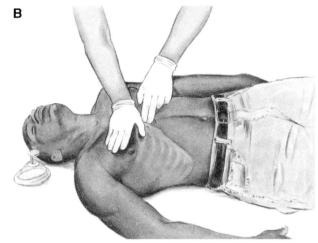

C

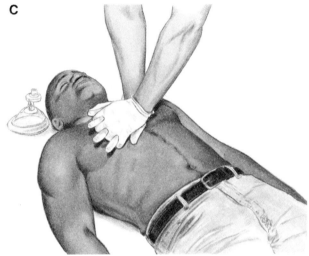

Figure 21. Positioning the rescuer's hands on the lower half of the sternum. The rescuer should (A) locate the margin of the rib using first and second finger of the hand closer to the victim's feet, (B) follow the rib margin to the base of the sternum (xiphoid process) and place his or her hand above the fingers (on the lower half of the sternum), and (C) place the other hand directly over the hand on the sternum.

of compression on the sternum and decrease the chance of rib fracture. Do not compress over the lowest portion of the base of the sternum (the xiphoid process).

4. Your fingers may be either extended or interlaced but should be kept off the chest.

If you have difficulty creating sufficient force during compressions, an acceptable alternative hand position is to grasp the wrist of the hand on the chest with your other hand and push downward with both. This technique is helpful for rescuers with arthritic hands and wrists.

A simplified method of achieving correct hand position has also been used in various settings for teaching laypersons the chest compression technique.* To find a position on the lower half of the sternum, the rescuer is instructed to place the heel of one hand in the center of the chest between the nipples. This method has been used with success for >10 years in dispatcher-assisted CPR and other settings.*

Effective compression is accomplished by attention to the following guidelines:

_____

*References 35–37, 55, 56, 62, 63, 69, 252–254.

1. Lock the elbows in position, with the arms straightened. Position your shoulders directly over your hands so that the thrust for each chest compression is straight down on the sternum (Figure 22). If the thrust is not in a straight downward direction, the victim's torso has a tendency to roll; if this occurs, a part of the force of compressions will be lost, and the chest compressions may be less effective.

2. Depress the sternum approximately 1½ to 2 inches (4 to 5 cm) for the normal-sized adult. Rarely, in very small victims, lesser degrees of compression may be sufficient to generate a palpable carotid or femoral pulse. Alternatively, in large victims, sternal compression depth of 1½ to 2 inches (4 to 5 cm) may be inadequate, and a slightly greater depth of chest compression may be needed to generate a carotid or femoral pulse. Optimal sternal compression is generally gauged by identifying the compression force that generates a palpable carotid or femoral pulse.[168] However, this validation of pulses requires at least 2 healthcare providers (one provides compressions while the other attempts to palpate the pulse), and it may yield misleading results. Detection of a pulse during CPR does not necessarily mean that there is optimal or even adequate

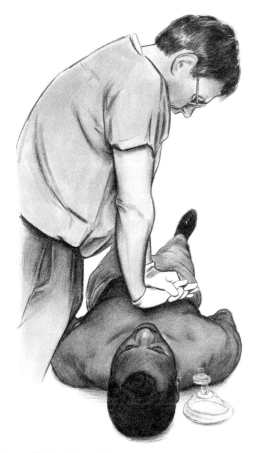

Figure 22. Position of the rescuer during compressions.

blood flow, because a compression wave may be palpated in the absence of effective blood flow. The best method of providing adequate compression force is to depress the sternum 1½ to 2 inches (4 to 5 cm) with each compression.

3. Release the pressure on the chest to allow blood to flow into the chest and heart. You must release the pressure completely and allow the chest to return to its normal position after each compression. Keep your hands in contact with the victim's sternum to maintain proper hand position. Chest compressions should be performed at a rate of approximately 100 per minute.

4. Effective cerebral and coronary perfusion has been shown to occur when 50% of the duty cycle is devoted to the chest compression phase and 50% to the chest relaxation phase.[239,249,255,256] Rescuers find this ratio reasonably easy to achieve with practice.[249]

5. To maintain correct hand position throughout the 15-compression cycle, do not lift your hands from the chest or change their position in any way. However, do allow the chest to recoil to its normal position after each compression.

Rescue breathing and chest compression must be combined for effective resuscitation of the victim of cardiopulmonary arrest. Research over the past 40 years has helped identify the mechanisms for blood flow during chest compression. In both animal models and humans, it appears that blood flow during CPR probably results from manipulation of intrathoracic pressure (thoracic pump mechanism) or direct cardiac com-

pression.[236–238] The duration of CPR affects the mechanism of CPR.[257–261] In CPR of short duration, blood flow is generated more by the cardiac pump mechanism. When the duration of cardiac arrest or resuscitation with chest compressions is prolonged, the heart becomes less compliant. Only in this setting does the thoracic pump mechanism dominate. When the thoracic pump mechanism dominates, however, the cardiac output generated by chest compression decreases significantly.[256–261]

Over the past 20 years, there has been important research regarding techniques and devices to improve blood flow during CPR, including pneumatic vest CPR,[262] interposed abdominal compression CPR (IAC-CPR),[263–265] and active compression-decompression CPR (ACD-CPR).[266–272] Recent evaluation of these devices in humans[254,262–272] has resulted in more specific recommendations for their use. The interested reader will find a more expanded discussion of this topic in Part 6 of this publication.

During cardiac arrest, properly performed chest compressions can produce systolic arterial blood pressure peaks of 60 to 80 mm Hg, but diastolic blood pressure is low.[261] Mean blood pressure in the carotid artery seldom exceeds 40 mm Hg.[261] Cardiac output resulting from chest compressions is probably only one fourth to one third of normal and decreases during the course of prolonged conventional CPR.[261] You can optimize blood flow during chest compression if you use the recommended chest compression force and chest compression duration and maintain a chest compression rate of approximately 100 per minute.[255]

Airway-breathing-circulation ("ABC") is the specific sequence used to initiate CPR in the United States and in the ILCOR Guidelines. In The Netherlands, however, "CAB" (compression-airway-breathing) is the common sequence of CPR, with resuscitation outcomes similar to those reported for the ABC protocol in the United States.[273] No human studies have directly compared the ABC technique of resuscitation with CAB. Hence, a statement of relative efficacy cannot be made and a change in present teaching is not warranted. Both techniques are effective.

Compression-Only CPR

Mouth-to-mouth rescue breathing is a safe and effective technique that has saved many lives. Despite decades of experience indicating its safety for victims and rescuers alike, some published surveys have documented reluctance on the part of professional and lay rescuers to perform mouth-to-mouth ventilation for unknown victims of cardiac arrest. This reluctance is related to fear of infectious disease transmission.[274–278] If a person is unwilling or unable to perform mouth-to-mouth ventilation for an adult victim, chest compression–only CPR should be provided rather than no attempt at CPR being made (Class IIa).

Current evidence indicates that the outcome of chest compression without mouth-to-mouth ventilation is significantly better than *no* CPR at all in the setting of adult cardiac arrest.[64–68] Some evidence in animal models and limited adult clinical trials suggests that positive-pressure ventilation is not essential during the initial 6 to 12 minutes of adult CPR.[64–67] The Cerebral Resuscitation Group of Belgium also showed no difference in outcome of CPR between victims who received mouth-to-mouth ventilation with chest compression and those who received compressions only.[68]

Several mechanisms may account for the effectiveness of chest compression alone. Studies have demonstrated that spontaneous gasping can maintain near-normal minute ventilation, $PaCO_2$, and PaO_2 during CPR without positive-pressure ventilation.[66,279] Because the cardiac output generated during chest compression is only 25% of normal, there is also a reduced requirement for ventilation to maintain optimal ventilation/perfusion relationships.[280,281]

Chest compression–only CPR is recommended *only* in the following circumstances:

1. When a rescuer is unwilling or unable to perform mouth-to-mouth rescue breathing (Class IIa), or
2. For use in dispatcher-assisted CPR instructions where the simplicity of this modified technique allows untrained bystanders to rapidly intervene (Class IIa).

Cough CPR

Self-initiated CPR is possible. Its use, however, is limited to clinical situations in which the patient has a monitored cardiac arrest, the arrest was recognized before loss of consciousness, and the patient can cough forcefully.[257–260] These conditions are typically present during only the first 10 to 15 seconds of the cardiac arrest. The increase in intrathoracic pressure that occurs with coughing will generate blood flow to the brain and maintain consciousness.

Defibrillation

Most adults with sudden, witnessed, nontraumatic cardiac arrest are found to be in VF.[38] For these victims the time from collapse to defibrillation is the single greatest determinant of survival.[1,3,27,38,46] Survival from VF cardiac arrest declines by approximately 7% to 10% for each minute without defibrillation.[47] Healthcare providers should be trained and equipped to provide defibrillation at the earliest possible moment for victims of sudden cardiac arrest.

Early defibrillation in the community is defined as a shock delivered within 5 minutes of EMS call receipt. This 5-minute call-to-defibrillation interval in the community is a Class I recommendation.

Early defibrillation also must be provided in hospitals and medical facilities. First responders in medical facilities should be able to provide early defibrillation to collapsed patients in VF in all areas of the hospital and ambulatory care facilities (Class I recommendation). In these areas healthcare providers should be able to deliver a shock within 3 ± 1 minutes of arrest for a high percentage of patients. To achieve these goals, BLS providers must be trained and equipped to use defibrillators and must rehearse use of the defibrillator present in their clinical area.

For further information, refer to "Part 4: The Automated External Defibrillator" and "Part 6, Section 2: Defibrillation."

CPR Performed by 1 and 2 Rescuers

CPR Performed by 1 Rescuer

Laypersons with no specific duty or expectation to respond to emergencies in the workplace should be taught 1-rescuer CPR only, because the 2-rescuer technique is infrequently used by laypersons in rescue situations. If 2 rescuers are present, they can alternate performing 1-rescuer CPR. Whether 1- or 2-rescuer CPR is performed, rescuers should ensure scene safety. One-rescuer CPR should be performed as follows:

1. **Assessment:** Determine unresponsiveness (tap or gently shake the victim and shout). If unresponsive,
2. **Activate the EMS system:** This should be performed according to local practice. In many countries and regions, activation of the EMS system is delayed until it has been determined that the victim is not breathing.
3. **Airway:** Position the victim and open the airway by the head tilt–chin lift or jaw-thrust maneuver.
4. **Breathing:** Assess breathing to identify absent or inadequate breathing.
   - If the victim is unresponsive *with normal breathing*, and spinal injury is not suspected, place the victim in a recovery position, maintaining an open airway.
   - If the adult victim is unresponsive and *not breathing*, begin rescue breathing. In the United States and many other countries, 2 initial breaths are provided, but up to 5 breaths are recommended in areas such as Europe, Australia, and New Zealand. If you are unable to give the initial breaths, reposition the head and reattempt ventilation. If you are still unsuccessful in making the chest rise with each ventilation after an attempt and reattempt:
     —Lay rescuers should provide chest compressions and begin the cycle of 15 compressions and 2 ventilations. Each time you open the airway to attempt ventilation, look for an object in the throat. If you see an object (such as a foreign body), remove it.
     —Healthcare providers follow the unresponsive FBAO sequence.
   - Be sure the victim's chest rises with each rescue breath you provide.
   - Once you deliver the effective breaths, assess for signs of circulation.
5. **Circulation.** Check for signs of circulation: after the initial breaths, look for normal breathing, coughing, or movement by the victim in response to the initial breaths. Healthcare providers should also feel for a carotid pulse—take no more than 10 seconds to do this. If there are no signs of circulation, begin chest compressions:
   - Locate proper hand position.
   - Perform 15 chest compressions at a rate of approximately 100 per minute. Depress the chest $1\frac{1}{2}$ to 2 inches (4 to 5 cm) with each compression. Make sure you allow the chest to rebound to its normal position after each compression by removing all pressure from the chest (while still maintaining contact with the sternum and proper hand position). Count "1 and, 2 and, 3 and, 4 and, 5 and, 6 and, 7 and, 8 and, 9 and, 10 and, 11, 12, 13, 14, 15." (Any mnemonic that accomplishes the same compression rate is acceptable. For ease of recollection, use the "and" only up to the number 10.)
   - Open the airway and deliver 2 slow rescue breaths (2 seconds each).

- Find the proper hand position and begin 15 more compressions at a rate of 100 per minute.
- Perform 4 complete cycles of 15 compressions and 2 ventilations.

6. **Reassessment:** Reevaluate the victim according to local protocol. In the United States, this will be after 4 cycles of compressions and ventilations (15:2 ratio); elsewhere, reevaluation may be recommended only if the victim shows some sign of recovery. Check for signs of circulation (10 seconds). If there are no signs of circulation, resume CPR, beginning with chest compressions. If signs of circulation are present, check for breathing.

  - If breathing is present, place the victim in a recovery position and monitor breathing and circulation.
  - If breathing is absent but signs of circulation are present, provide rescue breathing at 10 to 12 times per minute (1 breath every 4 to 5 seconds) and monitor for signs of circulation every few minutes.
  - If there are no signs of circulation, continue compressions and ventilations in a 15:2 ratio.
  - Stop and check for signs of circulation and spontaneous breathing every few minutes (according to local protocol).
  - Do not interrupt CPR except in special circumstances.
  - If adequate spontaneous breathing is restored and signs of circulation are present, maintain an open airway and place the patient in a recovery position.

Entrance of a Second Rescuer to Replace the First Rescuer

When another rescuer is available at the scene, that rescuer should activate the EMS system (if not done previously) and perform 1-rescuer CPR when the first rescuer becomes fatigued. This should be done with as little interruption of CPR as possible. When the second rescuer arrives, you should assess the victim's responsiveness, breathing, and signs of circulation before CPR is resumed.

CPR Performed by 2 Rescuers

All professional rescuers (BLS ambulance providers, healthcare professionals, and appropriate laypersons who have a duty or obligation to respond, such as lifeguards or police) should learn both the 1-rescuer and the 2-rescuer techniques. When possible, airway adjunct methods such as mouth-to-mask devices should be used.

In 2-rescuer CPR, one person is positioned at the victim's side and performs chest compressions. The other professional rescuer remains at the victim's head, maintains an open airway, monitors the carotid pulse to assess effectiveness of chest compressions, and provides rescue breathing. The compression rate for 2-rescuer CPR is 100 per minute. The compression-ventilation ratio is 15:2, with a pause for ventilation of 2 seconds each until the airway is secured by a cuffed tracheal tube. Exhalation occurs between the 2 breaths and during the first chest compression of the next cycle. When the person performing chest compressions becomes fatigued, the rescuers should change positions with minimal interruption of chest compressions.

Reassessment During 2-Rescuer CPR

The rescuers must monitor the victim's condition to assess the effectiveness of the rescue effort. The person ventilating the victim assumes the responsibility for monitoring signs of circulation and breathing.

To assess the effectiveness of the partner's chest compressions, the professional rescuer should check the pulse during compressions. To determine whether the victim has resumed spontaneous breathing and circulation, chest compressions must be stopped for 10 seconds at approximately the end of the first minute of CPR (or per local protocol) and every few minutes thereafter. (See No. 6, Reassessment, above.)

Epidemiology, Recognition, and Management of FBAO

Complete airway obstruction is an emergency that will result in death within minutes if not treated. The most common cause of upper-airway obstruction is obstruction by the tongue during loss of consciousness and cardiopulmonary arrest. An unresponsive victim can develop airway obstruction from intrinsic (tongue and epiglottis) and extrinsic (foreign body) causes. The tongue may fall backward into the pharynx, obstructing the upper airway. The epiglottis can block the entrance of the airway in unconscious victims. Blood from head and facial injuries or regurgitated stomach contents may also obstruct the upper airway, particularly if the victim is unconscious. Extrinsic causes may also produce airway obstruction, although the frequency is difficult to determine.

FBAO is a relatively uncommon but preventable cause of cardiac arrest. This form of death is much less common than death caused by other emergencies (1.2 deaths from choking per 100 000 population versus 1.7 per 100 000 for drowning, 16.5 per 100 000 for motor vehicle crashes, and 198 per 100 000 for coronary heart disease).[282–285]

FBAO is *not* a common problem among submersion/near-drowning victims. Water does not act as a (solid) foreign body and does not obstruct the airway.[286] Many submersion victims do not aspirate water at all, and any aspirated water will be absorbed in the upper airway and trachea. Near-drowning victims require immediate provision of CPR, particularly rescue breathing, to correct hypoxia. Therefore, efforts to relieve FBAO are not recommended for treatment of the victim of near-drowning. Such efforts may produce complications and will delay CPR, the most important treatment for the submersion victim.[286] (For further information, see "Part 8, Section 3: Special Challenges in ECC: Submersion or Near-Drowning.")

Causes and Precautions

FBAO should be considered as a cause of deterioration in any victim, especially a younger victim, who suddenly stops breathing, becomes cyanotic, and falls unconscious for no apparent reason.

FBAO in adults usually occurs during eating,[287,288] and meat is the most common cause of obstruction. A variety of other foods and foreign bodies, however, have caused choking in children and some adults.[289–294] Common factors associated with choking on food include attempts to swallow large, poorly chewed pieces of food, elevated blood alcohol levels, and dentures.[289–295] Elderly patients with dysphagia are also at risk for FBAO and should take care while drinking and eating. In restaurants, choking emergencies have been

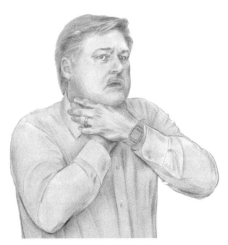

Figure 23. Universal choking sign.

mistaken for a heart attack, giving rise to the term "café coronary."[287,288]

The following precautions may help modify the risks and prevent FBAO:

1. Cut food into small pieces and chew slowly and thoroughly, especially if wearing dentures.
2. Avoid laughing and talking during chewing and swallowing.
3. Avoid excessive intake of alcohol.
4. Prevent children from walking, running, or playing when they have food in their mouths.
5. Keep foreign objects (eg, marbles, beads, thumbtacks) away from infants and children.
6. Do not give foods that must be thoroughly chewed (eg, peanuts, peanut butter, popcorn, hot dogs, etc) to young children.

Recognition of FBAO

Because recognition of airway obstruction is the key to successful outcome, it is important to distinguish this emergency from fainting, stroke, heart attack, seizure, drug overdose, or other conditions that may cause sudden respiratory failure but require different treatment.

Foreign bodies may cause either *partial* or *complete* airway obstruction. With partial airway obstruction, the victim may be capable of either "good air exchange" or "poor air exchange." With good air exchange, the victim is responsive and can cough forcefully, although frequently there is wheezing between coughs. As long as good air exchange continues, encourage the victim to continue spontaneous coughing and breathing efforts. At this point the rescuer should not interfere with the victim's own attempts to expel the foreign body but should stay with the victim and monitor these attempts. If partial airway obstruction persists, activate the EMS system.

The victim with FBAO may immediately demonstrate poor air exchange or may demonstrate initially good air exchange that progresses to poor air exchange. Signs of *poor* air exchange include a weak, ineffective cough, high-pitched noise while inhaling, increased respiratory difficulty, and possibly cyanosis. *Treat a victim with partial obstruction and poor air exchange as if he had a complete airway obstruction—you must act immediately.*

With *complete* airway obstruction the victim is unable to speak, breathe, or cough and may clutch the neck with the thumb and fingers. Movement of air is absent. The public should be encouraged to use the universal distress signal for choking emergencies (Figure 23). Ask the victim whether he or she is choking. If the victim nods, ask the victim if he or she can speak—if the victim is unable to speak, this indicates that a complete airway obstruction is present and you must act immediately.

If complete airway obstruction is not relieved, the victim's blood oxygen saturation will fall rapidly because the obstructed airway prevents entry of air into the lungs. If you do not succeed in removing the obstruction, the victim will become unresponsive, and death will follow rapidly.

Relief of FBAO

Several techniques are used throughout the world to relieve FBAO, and it is difficult to compare the effectiveness of any one method with another.[296] Most resuscitation councils recommend one or more of the following: the Heimlich abdominal thrusts, back blows, or chest thrusts. The level of evidence regarding any of these methods is weak, largely contained in case reports,[288,297] cadaver studies,[298] small studies involving animals,[288,299] or mechanical models.[300] Unfortunately, implementation of a randomized, prospective study to compare techniques for relief of FBAO in humans would be extremely difficult. Mechanical models of choking have been unsatisfactory.[300] Cadaver studies can provide excellent models of unresponsive/unconscious victims,[298] but they cannot replicate awake, responsive choking victims. Therefore, current recommendations are based on a low level of evidence (LOE 5 to 8), with an emphasis on the need to simplify information taught to the lay rescuer.

The Heimlich maneuver (also known as subdiaphragmatic abdominal thrusts or abdominal thrusts) is recommended for lay rescuer relief of FBAO in responsive adult (≥8 years of age) and child (1 to 8 years of age) victims in the United States, Canada, and many other countries.[288–295] It is not recommended for relief of FBAO in infants. The Heimlich maneuver is also recommended by the AHA and several other resuscitation councils for use *by healthcare providers* for *unresponsive* adult and child (but not infant) victims.

Some resuscitation councils (eg, the European Resuscitation Council) recommend that the rescuer provide up to 5 back blows/slaps as the initial maneuver, with the back slaps delivered between the shoulder blades with the heel of the rescuer's hand. If back slaps fail, up to 5 abdominal thrusts are then attempted, and groups of back slaps and abdominal thrusts are repeated. In countries such as Australia, back slaps and lateral chest thrusts are recommended for relief of FBAO in adults.

The Heimlich abdominal thrusts elevate the diaphragm and increase airway pressure, forcing air from the lungs. This may be sufficient to create an artificial cough and expel a foreign body from the airway.[288,297] Successful relief of FBAO in responsive victims has been reported in the lay press and in medical case studies. Abdominal thrusts, however, may cause complications. For this reason, the Heimlich maneuver should never be performed unless it is necessary. Reported

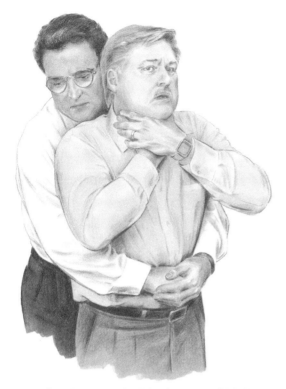

Figure 24. Subdiaphragmatic abdominal thrust (Heimlich maneuver), victim standing.

complications of the Heimlich maneuver include damage to internal organs, such as rupture or laceration of abdominal or thoracic viscera.[301–305] In fact, victims who receive the Heimlich maneuver should be medically evaluated to rule out any life-threatening complications.[303] To minimize the possibility of complications, do not place your hands on the xiphoid process of the sternum or on the lower margins of the rib cage. Your hands should be below this area but above the navel and in the midline. Some complications may develop even if the Heimlich maneuver is performed correctly. Regurgitation may occur as a result of abdominal thrusts and may be associated with aspiration.[306]

Heimlich Maneuver With Responsive Victim Standing or Sitting

Stand behind the victim, wrap your arms around the victim's waist, and proceed as follows (Figure 24). Make a fist with one hand. Place the thumb side of your fist against the victim's abdomen, in the midline slightly above the navel and well below the tip of the xiphoid process. Grasp the fist with your other hand and press the fist into the victim's abdomen with a quick inward and upward thrust. Repeat the thrusts until the object is expelled from the airway or the victim becomes unresponsive. Each new thrust should be a separate and distinct movement administered with the intent of relieving the obstruction.[288]

The Heimlich maneuver is repeated until the object is expelled or the victim becomes unresponsive (loses consciousness). When the victim becomes unresponsive, the EMS system should be activated, and the lay rescuer will attempt CPR. The healthcare provider will proceed with the

sequence of actions to relieve FBAO in the unconscious victim (see below).

The Self-Administered Heimlich Maneuver

To treat his or her own complete FBAO, the victim makes a fist with one hand, places the thumb side on the abdomen above the navel and below the xiphoid process, grasps the fist with the other hand, and then presses inward and upward toward the diaphragm with a quick motion. If this is unsuccessful, the victim should press the upper abdomen quickly over any firm surface, such as the back of a chair, side of a table, or porch railing. Several thrusts may be needed to clear the airway.

Chest Thrusts for Responsive Pregnant or Obese Victim

Chest thrusts may be used as an alternative to the Heimlich maneuver when the victim is in the late stages of pregnancy or is markedly obese. Stand behind the victim, with your arms directly under the victim's armpits, and encircle the victim's chest. Place the thumb side of one fist on the middle of the victim's breastbone, taking care to avoid the xiphoid process and the margins of the rib cage. Grab the fist with your other hand and perform backward thrusts until the foreign body is expelled or the victim becomes unresponsive.

If you cannot reach around the pregnant or extremely obese person, you can perform chest thrusts with the victim supine. Place the victim on his or her back and kneel close to the victim's side. The hand position and technique for the application of chest thrusts are the same as for chest compressions during CPR. In the adult, for example, the heel of the hand is on the lower half of the sternum. Deliver each thrust with the intent of relieving the obstruction.

Lay Rescuer Actions for Relief of FBAO in the Unresponsive Victim

Previous Guidelines recommendations for treatment of FBAO in the unresponsive victim were long, they took considerable time to teach, and they were often confusing for the student.[49] When training programs attempt to teach large amounts of material, they fail to achieve core educational objectives (eg, the psychomotor skills of CPR), and the result is poor skills retention and performance.[307–312] Focused training on small amounts of information results in superior levels of student performance compared with traditional CPR courses.[313–316] This compelling data indicates a need to simplify CPR training for laypersons.

Epidemiological data[282–285] does not distinguish between FBAO fatalities in which the victim is *responsive* when first encountered and those in which the victim is *unresponsive* when first encountered by rescuers. The total number of all deaths caused by choking is small, however, so the likelihood that a rescuer will encounter an unconscious victim of FBAO is small. Cardiac arrest caused by VF is far more common than cardiac arrest caused by complete FBAO.

Expert panelists at the 1999 Evidence Evaluation Conference and at the International Guidelines 2000 Conference agreed that lay rescuer BLS courses should focus on teaching a small number of essential skills. These essential skills were identified as relief of FBAO in the responsive/conscious victim and the skills of CPR. Teaching the complex skills of

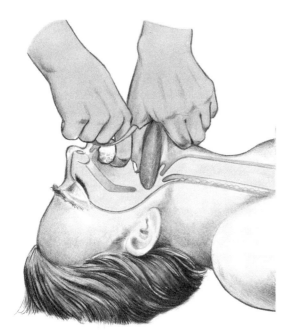

Figure 25. Finger sweep.

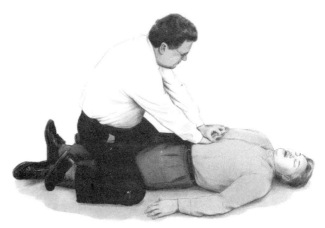

Figure 26. Healthcare provider provision of subdiaphragmatic abdominal thrust (Heimlich maneuver) in unresponsive/unconscious victim.

relief of FBAO in the *unresponsive/unconscious* victim *to lay rescuers* is no longer recommended (Class IIb). If the adult choking victim becomes unresponsive/unconscious during attempts to relieve FBAO, the lone lay rescuer should activate the EMS system (or send someone to do it) and begin CPR. In fact, chest compressions may be effective for relief of FBAO in the unresponsive victim.[298,317] A recent study using cadaver subjects (an acceptable model of the unresponsive/unconscious victim of FBAO) has shown that chest compressions may create a peak airway pressure that is equal to or superior to that created by abdominal thrusts.[298] If the lay rescuer appears to encounter an unsuspected airway obstruction in the unresponsive victim during the sequence of CPR after attempting and reattempting ventilation, the rescuer should continue the sequence of CPR, with chest compressions and cycles of compressions and ventilations.

The lay rescuer should attempt CPR with a single addition—each time the airway is opened, look for the obstructing object in the back of the throat. *If you see an object*, remove it. This recommendation is designed to simplify layperson CPR training and ensure the acquisition of the core skills of rescue breathing and compression while still providing treatment for the victim with FBAO.

Finger Sweep and Tongue-Jaw Lift
The finger sweep should be used by healthcare providers only in the *unresponsive/unconscious* victim with complete FBAO. This sweep should not be performed if the victim is responsive or is having seizures.

With the victim face up, open the victim's mouth by grasping both the tongue and lower jaw between the thumb and fingers and lifting the mandible (tongue-jaw lift). This action draws the tongue away from the back of the throat and from a foreign body that may be lodged there. This maneuver alone may be sufficient to relieve an obstruction. Insert the index finger of your other hand down along the

inside of the cheek and deeply into the victim's throat, to the base of the tongue. Then use a hooking action to dislodge the foreign body and maneuver it into the mouth so that it can be removed (Figure 26). It is sometimes necessary to use the index finger to push the foreign body against the opposite side of the throat to dislodge and remove it. Be careful to avoid forcing the object deeper into the airway.

Healthcare Provider Sequence for Relief of FBAO in the Unresponsive Victim
Victims of FBAO may initially be responsive when encountered by the rescuer and then become unresponsive. In this circumstance the rescuer will know that FBAO is the cause of the victim's symptoms. Victims of FBAO may be unresponsive when initially encountered by the rescuer. In this circumstance the rescuer will probably not know that the victim has FBAO until repeated attempts at rescue breathing are unsuccessful.

Healthcare Provider Relief of FBAO in a Responsive Victim Who Becomes Unresponsive
If you observe the victim's collapse and you *know* it is caused by FBAO, the following sequence of actions is recommended:

1. Activate the emergency response system at the proper time in the CPR sequence. If a second rescuer is available, send the second rescuer to activate the EMS system while you remain with the victim. Be sure the victim is supine.
2. Perform a tongue-jaw lift, followed by a finger sweep to remove the object.
3. Open the airway and try to ventilate; if you are unable to make the victim's chest rise, reposition the head and try to ventilate again.
4. If you cannot deliver effective breaths (the chest does not rise) even after attempts to reposition the airway consider FBAO. Straddle the victim's thighs (see Figure 26) and perform the Heimlich maneuver (up to 5 times).
5. Repeat the sequence of tongue-jaw lift, finger sweep, attempt (and reattempt) to ventilate, and Heimlich maneuver (steps 2 through 4) until the obstruction is cleared and the chest rises with ventilation or advanced

procedures are available (ie, Kelly clamp, Magill forceps, cricothyrotomy) to establish a patent airway.

6. If the FBAO is removed and the airway is cleared, check breathing. If the victim is not breathing, provide slow rescue breaths. Then check for signs of circulation (pulse check and evidence of breathing, coughing, or movement). If there are no signs of circulation, begin chest compressions.

To deliver abdominal thrusts to the unresponsive/unconscious victim, kneel astride the victim's thighs and place the heel of one hand against the victim's abdomen, in the midline slightly above the navel and well below the tip of the xiphoid. Place your second hand directly on top of the first. Press both hands into the abdomen with quick upward thrusts (Figure 27). If you are in the correct position, you will be positioned over the midabdomen, unlikely to direct the thrust to the right or left. You can use your body weight to perform the maneuver.

Two types of conventional forceps are acceptable for removal of a foreign body, the Kelly clamp and the Magill forceps. Forceps should be used only if the foreign body is seen. Either a laryngoscope or tongue blade and flashlight can be used to permit direct visualization. The use of such devices by untrained or inexperienced persons is unacceptable. Cricothyrotomy should be performed only by healthcare providers trained and authorized to perform this surgical procedure.

Healthcare Provider Relief of FBAO in Victims Found Unresponsive
If the victim is found to be unresponsive and the cause is unknown, the following sequence of actions is recommended:

1. Activate the emergency response system at the appropriate time in the CPR sequence. If a second rescuer is available, send that rescuer to activate the EMS system while you remain with the victim.
2. Open the airway and attempt to provide rescue breaths. If you are unable to make the chest rise, reposition the victim's head (reopen the airway) and try to ventilate again.
3. If the victim cannot be ventilated even after attempts to reposition the airway, straddle the victim's knees (see Figure 27) and perform the Heimlich maneuver (up to 5 times).
4. After 5 abdominal thrusts, open the victim's airway using a tongue-jaw lift and perform a finger sweep to remove the object.
5. Repeat the sequence of attempts (and reattempts) to ventilate, Heimlich maneuver, and tongue-jaw lift and finger sweep (steps 2 through 4) until the obstruction is cleared or advanced procedures are available to establish a patent airway (eg, Kelly clamps, Magill forceps, or cricothyrotomy).
6. If the FBAO is removed and the airway is cleared, check breathing. If the victim is not breathing, provide 2 rescue breaths. Then check for signs of circulation (pulse check and evidence of breathing, coughing, or movement). If there are no signs of circulation, begin chest compressions.

Unique CPR Situations

Changing Locations During CPR Performance
If the location is unsafe, such as a burning building, move the victim to a safe area and then immediately start CPR. Do not move a victim for convenience from a cramped or busy location until effective CPR is provided and the victim shows a return of signs of circulation or until help arrives. Whenever possible, perform CPR without interruption.

Stairways
In some instances a victim must be transported up or down a flight of stairs. It is best to perform CPR at the head or foot of the stairs and, at a predetermined signal, to interrupt CPR and move as quickly as possible to the next level, where CPR can be resumed. Interruptions should be brief and must be avoided if possible.

Litters
Do not interrupt CPR while transferring a victim to an ambulance or other mobile emergency care unit. If the victim is placed on a low-wheeled litter, the rescuer can stand alongside, providing chest compressions with the locked-arm position. If the victim is placed on a high litter or bed, it may be necessary for the rescuer to kneel beside the victim on the bed or litter to gain the needed height over the victim's sternum.

Generally, CPR should be interrupted only when tracheal intubation is being performed by trained personnel, an AED or manual defibrillator is being applied or used, or there are problems with transportation. If the rescuer is alone, a momentary delay of CPR is necessary to activate the EMS system.[11]

Pitfalls and Complications of BLS
CPR can support life when it is performed properly. Even properly performed CPR, however, can result in complications.[318] Fear of complications should not prevent potential rescuers from providing CPR to the best of their ability.

Potential Complications of Rescue Breathing
The most common complication of rescue breathing is gastric inflation resulting from excess ventilation volume and rapid flow rates.[185,186] Rescue breathing frequently causes gastric inflation, especially in children.[186,193,194–196] This inflation can be minimized by maintaining an open airway and limiting ventilation volumes to just the point at which the chest rises adequately.[208] This is best achieved by providing slow rescue breaths (allow 2 seconds per breath in adults). Gastric inflation can be further minimized by ensuring that the airway remains open during inspiration and expiration. Unfortunately, in 1-rescuer CPR this is difficult, but it can be performed during 2-rescuer CPR. When possible, an additional rescuer should apply cricoid pressure to minimize gastric inflation.

Marked inflation of the stomach may promote regurgitation[187–189] and reduce lung volume by elevating the diaphragm.[187,196,197] If the stomach becomes distended during rescue breathing, recheck and reopen the airway and look for the rise and fall of the chest. Avoid factors (rapid breaths, short inspiratory times, forceful breaths) that may contribute to the development of high airway pressure. Continue slow rescue breathing and do not attempt to expel the stomach contents. Experience has shown that attempts to relieve stomach inflation with application of manual pressure over the victim's upper abdomen is almost certain to cause regurgitation if the stomach is full. If regurgitation does occur, turn the victim's entire body to the side, wipe out the mouth, return the body to the supine position, and continue CPR.

Potential Complications of Chest Compression

Proper CPR techniques lessen the possibility of complications. Assess for signs of circulation before performing compressions, but allow only 10 seconds to do this. If in any doubt, assume that there is no circulation and begin chest compressions.

Even properly performed chest compressions can cause rib fractures in adult patients.[319] However, rib fractures and other injuries rarely complicate CPR in infants and children.[320,321] Other complications may occur despite proper CPR technique, including fracture of the sternum, separation of the ribs from the sternum, pneumothorax, hemothorax, lung contusions, lacerations of the liver and spleen, and fat emboli.[318] These complications may be minimized by use of proper hand position during chest compressions, but they cannot be prevented entirely. Concern for injuries that may complicate CPR should not impede prompt and energetic application of CPR. The only alternative to timely initiation of effective CPR for the victim of cardiac arrest is death.

Rescuer Safety During CPR Training and CPR Performance

Safety during CPR training and in actual rescue situations has gained increased attention. The following recommendations should minimize possible risk of infectious complications to instructors and students during CPR training and actual CPR performance. The recommendations for manikin decontamination and rescuer safety originally established in 1978 by the Centers for Disease Control[322] have been updated twice by the AHA, the American Red Cross, and the Centers for Disease Control and Prevention.[49,323] Additional recommendations for manikin decontamination have been developed by such organizations as the Australian National Health and Medical Research Council.

Disease Transmission During CPR Training

The risk of disease transmission during CPR training is extremely low. Use of CPR manikins has never been shown to be responsible for an outbreak of infection, and a literature search through March 2000 revealed no reports of infection associated with CPR training.[323,324] To date, an estimated 70 million people in the United States have had direct contact with manikins during CPR training courses without reported infectious complications.[324]

Under certain circumstances, manikin surfaces can present a very small risk of disease transmission. Therefore, manikin surfaces should be cleaned and disinfected in a consistent way after each rescuer use and after each class.[325]

Two important practices are needed to minimize risk of transmission of infectious agents during CPR training. First, rescuers should avoid any contact with any saliva or body fluids present on the manikins.

Second, internal manikin parts, such as the valve mechanisms and artificial lungs in manikin airways, invariably become contaminated during use and must be thoroughly cleaned between uses. A wide variety of manikins are commercially available, and it is impossible here to detail the cleaning required for each model and type. Instructors and training agencies should carefully follow the manufacturers' recommendations for manikin use and maintenance.[325–328]

There is no evidence to date that HIV can be transmitted by casual personal contact, indirect contact with inanimate surfaces, or an airborne route.[324] The primary retroviral agent that causes acquired immunodeficiency syndrome (AIDS), HIV, is comparatively delicate and is inactivated in <10 minutes at room temperature by a number of disinfectants, including those agents recommended for manikin cleaning.[329–333] If current recommendations published by the AHA[49,322,323] and manikin manufacturers for manikin cleaning and decontamination are carefully followed, risk of transmission of HIV and hepatitis B virus (HBV), as well as bacterial and fungal infections, should be minimized.

Disease Transmission During Actual Performance of CPR

The vast majority of CPR performed internationally is provided by healthcare and public safety personnel, many of whom assist in ventilation of respiratory and cardiac arrest victims who are unknown to the rescuer. A layperson is far less likely to perform CPR than healthcare providers, and the layperson is most likely to perform CPR in the home, where 70% to 80% of respiratory and cardiac arrests occur.[49]

The actual risk of disease transmission during mouth-to-mouth ventilation is quite small; only 15 reports of CPR-related infection were published between 1960 and 1998,[324] and no reports have been published in scientific journals from 1998 through March 2000.[324,334] Researchers have found that there is little reluctance by lay rescuers to perform CPR on family members, even in the presence of vomitus or alcohol on the breath.[335] At last report (1998),[324] the cases of disease transmission during CPR include *Helicobacter pylori*,[210] *Mycobacterium tuberculosis*,[211] meningococcus,[336] herpes simplex,[337–339] *Shigella*,[340] *Streptococcus*,[341] *Salmonella*,[342] and *Neisseria gonorrhoeae*.[324] No reports on transmission of HIV, HBV, hepatitis C virus, or cytomegalovirus were found.[324] Nevertheless, despite the remote chances of its occurring, fears regarding disease transmission are common in the current era of universal precautions. Indeed, not only laypersons but also physicians, nurses, and even BLS instructors are extremely reluctant to perform mouth-to-mouth ventilation.[274,277,278,343–346] The most commonly stated reason for not performing mouth-to-mouth ventilation is fear of contracting AIDS. In one survey, only 5% of 975 respondents reported a willingness to perform chest compression with mouth-to-mouth ventilation on a stranger, whereas 68% would "definitely" perform chest compression alone if it was offered as an effective alternative CPR technique.[338] The attitude of rescuers who have actually performed mouth-to-mouth ventilation is much different regarding fear of infectious disease. Of bystanders who performed CPR in one study, 92% stated that they had no fear of infectious disease.[347] Of 425 interviewed rescuers from the same group, 99.5% indicated that if called on they would perform CPR again.[347]

The rescuer who responds to an emergency for an unknown victim should be guided by individual moral and ethical values and knowledge of risks that may exist in various rescue situations. The rescuer should assume that any emergency situation involving exposure to certain body fluids has the potential for disease transmission for both the rescuer and victim. If a rescuer is unwilling or unable to perform mouth-to-mouth breathing, chest compressions alone should be attempted, because it may increase the chances for survival (Class IIa). This is particularly true if the victim is exhibiting gasping breaths or if the time to defibrillation is likely to be short.[64–67,348]

The greatest concern over the risk of disease transmission should be directed to persons who perform CPR frequently, particularly healthcare providers, both in hospital and out of hospital. If appropriate precautions are taken to prevent exposure to blood or other body fluids, the risk of disease transmission from infected persons to providers of out-of-hospital emergency health care should be no higher than that for those providing emergency care in the hospital.

The probability that a rescuer (lay or professional) will become infected with HBV or HIV as a result of performing CPR is minimal.[349] Although transmission of HBV and HIV between healthcare workers and patients has been documented as a result of blood exchange or penetration of the skin by blood-contaminated instruments,[350] transmission of HBV and HIV infection during mouth-to-mouth resuscitation has not been documented.[324,351] There is evidence that some face masks are experimentally impermeable to the HIV-1 virus.[352]

Direct mouth-to-mouth breathing will probably result in exchange of saliva between the victim and rescuer. HBV-positive saliva, however, has not been shown to be infectious even to oral mucous membranes, through contamination of shared musical instruments, or through HBV carriers.[349] In addition, saliva has not been implicated in the transmission of HIV after bites, percutaneous inoculation, or contamination of cuts and open wounds with saliva from HIV-infected patients.[353,354] The theoretical risk of infection is greater for salivary or aerosol transmission of herpes simplex, *Neisseria meningitidis*, and airborne diseases such as tuberculosis and other respiratory infections. Rare instances of herpes transmission during CPR have been reported.[339]

The emergence of multidrug-resistant tuberculosis[355,356] and the risk of tuberculosis to emergency workers[357] is a cause for concern. Rescuers with impaired immune systems may be particularly at risk. In most instances, transmission of tuberculosis requires prolonged close exposure as is likely to occur in households, but transmission to emergency workers can occur during resuscitative efforts by either the airborne route[357] or direct contact. The magnitude of the risk is unknown but probably low. After performing mouth-to-mouth resuscitation on a person suspected of having tuberculosis, the caregiver should be evaluated for tuberculosis by standard approaches based on the caregiver's baseline skin tests.[358] Caregivers with negative baseline skin tests should be retested 12 weeks later. Preventive therapy should be considered for all persons with positive tests and should be started on all converters.[358,359] In areas where multidrug-re-

sistant tuberculosis is common or after exposure to known multidrug-resistant tuberculosis, the optimal preventive therapeutic agent has not been established. Some authorities suggest use of 2 or more agents.[360]

Performance of mouth-to-mouth resuscitation or invasive procedures can result in the exchange of blood between the victim and rescuer. This is especially true in cases of trauma or if either victim or rescuer has breaks in the skin on or around the lips or soft tissues of the oral cavity mucosa. Thus, a theoretical risk of HBV and HIV transmission during mouth-to-mouth resuscitation exists.[361]

Because of the concern about disease transmission between victim and rescuer, rescuers with a duty to provide CPR should follow precautions and guidelines such as those established by the Centers for Disease Control and Prevention[349] and the Occupational Safety and Health Administration.[362] These guidelines include the use of barriers, such as latex gloves, and manual ventilation equipment, such as a bag mask and other resuscitation masks with valves capable of diverting the victim's expired air away from the rescuer. Rescuers who have an infection that may be transmitted by blood or saliva should not perform mouth-to-mouth resuscitation if circumstances allow other immediate or effective methods of ventilation.

Several studies confirm that there is a risk of transmission of pathogens (diseases) during exposure to blood, saliva, and other body fluids.* OSHA supports this observation. Several devices have been developed to minimize risk of pathogen exposure to the rescuer. Participants in BLS courses should be taught to use a barrier device (face shield or face masks) when a mouth-to-mask device is not available and mouth-to-mouth ventilation would place the rescuer at risk. Face masks may be more effective barriers to oral bacteria than face shields. In fact, all face masks with 1-way valves prevent the transmission of bacteria to the rescuer side of the mask. Face shields, on the other hand, contaminated the rescuer side of the shield in 6 of 8 tests.[356]

Because the efficacy of face shields has not been proven, those with a duty to respond should learn during CPR training how to use masks with 1-way valves and other manual ventilation devices.[210,211] Masks without 1-way valves and inline filters (including those with S-shaped devices) offer little, if any, protection and should not be considered for routine use.[210,211] Intubation with tracheal tubes and other airway adjuncts obviates the need for mouth-to-mouth resuscitation and enables ventilation that is equal to or more effective than the use of masks alone.[366–371] Early intubation is encouraged when equipment and trained professionals are available. Resuscitation equipment known or suspected to be contaminated with blood or other body fluids should be discarded or thoroughly cleaned and disinfected after each use.[372]

CPR: The Human Dimension

Since 1973, millions of people throughout the world have learned CPR. Although CPR is considered by some to be the most successful public health initiative in recent times, the cardiac arrest survival rate to hospital discharge averages

---

*References 209, 336, 337, 339, 340, 362–364.

15%, with some studies reporting a favorable neurological status among such survivors.[273]

Serious long-lasting physical and emotional symptoms may occur in rescuers who participate in unsuccessful resuscitation attempts. Rescuers may experience grief reactions, stress, and anxiety. The stress of the experience often leaves the rescuer feeling fatigued and uncertain, which may result in chronic anxiety and depression.

A "critical incident debriefing" may allow rescuers to work through their feelings and their grief. Debriefings are most useful after an unsuccessful CPR attempt, and efforts should be made to include all members of the resuscitation team. In these sessions, rescuers discuss their thoughts, feelings, and performance. Participants should analyze what was done and why, with a discussion of things that went right and things that went wrong. The critical incident debriefing is also a time for learning something that may be useful next time. The human dimension of CPR is often not discussed. Because of its importance, it should be incorporated into CPR training and practice.

For additional information, see "Part 6, Section 7A: The Resuscitation Attempt as a 'Critical Incident': Code Critique and Debriefing."

BLS Research Initiatives

Continued improvement of BLS programs requires ongoing scientific research. This resuscitation research must ultimately translate into effective programs to teach CPR to anyone who may witness a cardiac arrest, so that if cardiac arrest occurs, the EMS system is activated immediately, CPR is skillfully performed, and survival is maximized. In many critical areas, insufficient data is available to guide resuscitation experts and clinicians. Because scientific data is lacking in some areas, portions of the current guidelines are based on information derived from limited published data, some clinical experience, and consensus of experts.

BLS is a fundamental therapy, yet many questions remain to be answered about circumstances of arrest that are fundamental to development of CPR skill sequences. To develop optimal sequences for CPR action, it is important to know how often rescuers are alone and how often second rescuers are present. Research is needed about a variety of aspects of programs of public access to defibrillation: what is the optimum retraining interval for anticipated rescuers? What factors should guide placement of AEDs in communities? Should rescuers perform 1 minute of CPR before defibrillation? Further research is needed to identify optimal chest compression–ventilation rates and ratios and methods to differentiate victims who require chest compression from those who do not. In addition, research is needed to increase the number of people who learn CPR and to identify optimal ways to teach CPR to lay rescuers and healthcare providers. CPR programs must be simplified to remove distracting information and emphasize core elements, and then simplified programs must be evaluated to ensure that participants can learn, remember, and demonstrate the steps of CPR. Future changes and advances in CPR based on sound scientific investigation will undoubtedly improve the quality, delivery, and outcome of BLS.

References

1. Cummins RO, Ornato JP, Thies WH, Pepe PE. Improving survival from sudden cardiac arrest: the "chain of survival" concept: a statement for health professionals from the Advanced Cardiac Life Support Subcommittee and the Emergency Cardiac Care Committee, American Heart Association. *Circulation.* 1991;83:1832–1847.
2. McIntyre KM. Cardiopulmonary resuscitation and the ultimate coronary care unit. *JAMA.* 1980;244:510–511.
3. Calle PA, Verbeke A, Vanhaute O, Van Acker P, Martens P, Buylaert W. The effect of semi-automatic external defibrillation by emergency medical technicians on survival after out-of-hospital cardiac arrest: an observational study in urban and rural areas in Belgium. *Acta Clin Belg.* 1997;52:72–83.
4. Martens P, Calle P, Mullie A. Do we know enough to introduce semi-automated defibrillation by ambulancemen in Belgium? *Eur J Med.* 1993;2:430–434.
5. Richless LK, Schrading WA, Polana J, Hess DR, Ogden CS. Early defibrillation program: problems encountered in a rural/suburban EMS system. *J Emerg Med.* 1993;11:127–134.
6. Becker LB, Pepe PE. Ensuring the effectiveness of community-wide emergency cardiac care. *Ann Emerg Med.* 1993;22(2 pt 2):354–365.
7. Zachariah BS, Pepe PE. The development of emergency medical dispatch in the USA: a historical perspective. *Eur J Emerg Med.* 1995;2:109–112.
8. Rossi R. The role of the dispatch centre in preclinical emergency medicine. *Eur J Emerg Med.* 1994;1:27–30.
9. Nemitz B. Advantages and limitations of medical dispatching: the French view. *Eur J Emerg Med.* 1995;2:153–159.
10. Calle PA, Lagaert L, Vanhaute O, Buylaert WA. Do victims of an out-of-hospital cardiac arrest benefit from a training program for emergency medical dispatchers? *Resuscitation.* 1997;35:213–218.
11. Curka PA, Pepe PE, Ginger VF, Sherrard RC, Ivy MV, Zachariah BS. Emergency medical services priority dispatch. *Ann Emerg Med.* 1993; 22:1688–1695.
12. Larsen MP, Eisenberg MS, Cummins RO, Hallstrom AP. Predicting survival from out-of-hospital cardiac arrest: a graphic model. *Ann Emerg Med.* 1993;22:1652–1658.
13. Swor RA, Jackson RE, Cynar M, Sadler E, Basse E, Boji B, Rivera-Rivera EJ, Maher A, Grubb W, Jacobson R, et al. Bystander CPR, ventricular fibrillation, and survival in witnessed, unmonitored out-of-hospital cardiac arrest. *Ann Emerg Med.* 1995;25:780–784.
14. Eisenberg MS, Hallstrom AP, Copass MK, et al. Treatment of ventricular fibrillation: emergency medical technician defibrillation and paramedic services. *JAMA.* 1984;251:1723–1726.
15. Weaver WD, Copass MK, Bufi D, et al. Improved neurologic recovery and survival after early defibrillation. *Circulation.* 1984;69:943–948.
16. White RD, Vukov LF, Bugliosi TF. Early defibrillation by police: initial experience with measurement of critical time intervals and patient outcome. *Ann Emerg Med.* 1994;23:1009–1013.
17. Auble TE, Menegazzi JJ, Paris PM. Effect of out-of-hospital defibrillation by basic life support providers on cardiac arrest mortality: a meta-analysis. *Ann Emerg Med.* 1995;25:642–648.
18. Chadda KD, Kammerer R. Early experiences with the portable automatic external defibrillator in the home and public places. *Am J Cardiol.* 1987;60:732–733.
19. Holmberg M, Holmberg S, Herlitz J, Gardelov B. Survival after cardiac arrest outside hospital in Sweden. *Resuscitation.* 1998;36:29–36.
20. Nichol G, Hallstrom AP, Ornato JP, Riegel B, Stiell IG, Valenzuela T, Wells GA, White RD, Weisfeldt ML. Potential cost-effectiveness of public access defibrillation in the United States. *Circulation.* 1998;97: 1315–1320.
21. O'Rourke MF, Donaldson E, Geddes JS. An airline cardiac arrest program. *Circulation.* 1997;96:2849–2853.
22. Page RL, Hamdan MH, McKenas DK. Defibrillation aboard a commercial aircraft. *Circulation.* 1998;97:1429–1430.
23. Valenzuela TD, Roe DJ, Cretin S, Spaite DW, Larsen MP. Estimating effectiveness of cardiac arrest interventions: a logistic regression survival model. *Circulation.* 1997;96:3308–3313.
24. White RD, Asplin BR, Bugliosi TF, Hankins DG. High discharge survival rate after out-of-hospital ventricular fibrillation with rapid defibrillation by police and paramedics. *Ann Emerg Med.* 1996;28: 480–485.
25. Davis EA, Mosesso VN Jr. Performance of police first responders in utilizing automated external defibrillation on victims of sudden cardiac arrest. *Prehosp Emerg Care.* 1998;2:101–107.

26. Davis EA, McCrorry J, Mosesso VN Jr. Institution of a police automated external defibrillation program: concepts and practice. *Prehosp Emerg Care.* 1999;3:60–65.

27. Mosesso VN, Davis EA, Auble TE, Paris PM, Yealy DM. Use of automated external defibrillators by police officers for treatment of out-of-hospital cardiac arrest. *Ann Emerg Med.* 1998;32:200–207.

28. White RD, Hankins DG, Bugliosi TF. Seven years' experience with early defibrillation by police and paramedics in an emergency medical services system. *Resuscitation.* 1998;39:145–151.

29. Eisenberg MS, Cummins RO. Defibrillation performed by the emergency medical technician. *Circulation.* 1986;74(suppl IV):IV-9–IV-12.

30. Eisenberg MS, Bergner L, Hallstrom A. Cardiac resuscitation in the community: importance of rapid provision and implications for program planning. *JAMA.* 1979;241:1905–1907.

31. Stiell IG, Wells GA, DeMaio VJ, Spaite DW, Field BJ III, Munkley DP, Lyver MB, Luinstra LG, Ward R. Modifiable factors associated with improved cardiac arrest survival in a multicenter basic life support/defibrillation system: OPALS Study phase I results. Ontario Prehospital Advanced Life Support. *Ann Emerg Med.* 1999;33:44–50.

32. Stiell IG, Wells GA, Field BJ, et al. Improved out-of-hospital cardiac arrest survival through the inexpensive optimization of an existing defibrillation program: OPALS study phase II. Ontario Prehospital Advanced Life Support. *JAMA.* 1999;281:1175–1181.

33. Weisfeldt ML, Kerber RE, McGoldrick RP, et al. American Heart Association report on the Public Access Defibrillation Conference, December 8–10, 1994. Automatic External Defibrillation Task Force. *Circulation.* 1995;92:2740–2747.

34. Weisfeldt ML, Kerber RE, McGoldrick RP, et al. Public access defibrillation: a statement for healthcare professionals from the American Heart Association Task Force on Automatic External Defibrillation. *Circulation.* 1995;92:2763.

35. Aufderheide TP, Stapleton ER, Hazinski MF, Cummins RO. *Heartsaver AED for the Lay Rescuer and First Responder.* Dallas, Tex: American Heart Association; 1998.

36. Emergency Cardiac Care Committee, American Heart Association. *Heartsaver ABC.* Dallas, Tex: American Heart Association; 1999.

37. Emergency Cardiac Care Committee, American Heart Association. *Heartsaver CPR in Schools.* Dallas, Tex: American Heart Association; 1999.

38. Bayes de Luna A, Coumel P, Leclercq JF. Ambulatory sudden cardiac death: mechanisms of production of fatal arrhythmia on the basis of data from 157 cases. *Am Heart J.* 1989;117:151–159.

39. Weaver WD, Hill D, Fahrenbruch CE, et al. Use of the automatic external defibrillator in the management of out-of-hospital cardiac arrest. *N Engl J Med.* 1988;319:661–666.

40. Cummins RO, Graves JR. Critical results of standard CPR: Prehospital and inhospital. In: Kaye W, Bircher N, eds. *Cardiopulmonary Resuscitation.* Clinics in Critical Care Medicine. New York, NY: Churchill-Livingstone; 1989.

41. Cummins RO, Eisenberg MS. Prehospital cardiopulmonary resuscitation: is it effective? *JAMA.* 1985;253:2408.

42. Cummins RO, Eisenberg MS, Hallstrom AP, Litwin PE. Survival of out-of-hospital cardiac arrest with early initiation of cardiopulmonary resuscitation. *Am J Emerg Med.* 1985;3:114–119.

43. Ladwig KH, Schoefinius A, Danner R, Gurtler R, Herman R, Koeppel A, Hauber P. Effects of early defibrillation by ambulance personnel on short and long-term outcome of cardiac arrest survival: the Munich experiment. *Chest.* 1997;112:1584–1591.

44. Sweeney TA, Runge JW, Gibbs MA, Raymond JM, Schafermeyer RW, Norton HJ, Boyle-Whitesel MJ. EMT defibrillation does not increase survival from sudden cardiac death in a two-tiered urban-suburban EMS system. *Ann Emerg Med.* 1998;31:234–240.

45. Kellermann AL, Hackman BB, Somes G, Kreth TK, Nail L, Dobyns P. Impact of first-responder defibrillation in an urban emergency medical services system. *JAMA.* 1993;270:1708–1713.

46. Shuster M, Keller JL. Effect of fire department first responder automated defibrillation. *Ann Emerg Med.* 1993;4:721–727.

47. Cummins RO. From concept to standard-of-care? Review of the clinical experience with automated external defibrillators. *Ann Emerg Med.* 1989;18:1269–1275.

48. Zaritsky A, Nadkarni V, Getson P, Kuehl K. CPR in children. *Ann Emerg Med.* 1987;16:1107–1111.

49. Emergency Cardiac Care Committee and Subcommittees, American Heart Association. Guidelines for cardiopulmonary resuscitation and emergency cardiac care. *JAMA.* 1992;268:2171–2295.

50. Safranek DJ, Eisenberg MS, Larsen MP. The epidemiology of cardiac arrest in young adults. *Ann Emerg Med.* 1992;21:1102.

51. Appleton GO, Cummins RO, Larson MP, Graves JR. CPR and the single rescuer: at what age should you "call first" rather than "call fast?" *Ann Emerg Med.* 1995;25(4):492–494.

52. Mogayzel C, Quan L, Graves JR, Tiedeman D, Fahrenbruch C, Herndon P. Out-of-hospital ventricular fibrillation in children and adolescents: causes and outcomes. *Ann Emerg Med.* 1995;25:484–491.

53. Kuisma M, Alaspaa A. Out-of-hospital cardiac arrests of non-cardiac origin: epidemiology and outcome [see comments]. *Eur Heart J.* 1997;18:1122–1128.

54. Pepe PE, Zachariah BS, Sayre MR, Floccare D, Chain of Recovery Writing Group. Ensuring the chain of recovery for stroke in your community. *Prehosp Emerg Care.* 1998;2:89–95.

55. Bang A, Biber B, Isaksson L, Lindqvist J, Herlitz J. Evaluation of dispatcher-assisted cardiopulmonary resuscitation. *Eur J Emerg Med.* 1999;6:175–183.

56. National Association of EMS Physicians. Emergency medical dispatching. *Prehospital Disaster Med.* 1989;4:163–166.

57. Nordberg M. NAEMD (National Academy of Emergency Medical Dispatch) strives for universal certification. *Emerg Med Serv.* 1999;28:45–46.

58. Clawson JJ, Sinclair B. "Medical Miranda": –improved emergency medical dispatch information from police officers. *Prehospital Disaster Med.* 1999;14:93–96.

59. National Heart Attack Alert Program Coordinating Committee Access to Care Subcommittee. Emergency medical dispatching: rapid identification and treatment of acute myocardial infarction. *Am J Emerg Med.* 1995;13:67–73.

60. Porteous GH, Corry MD, Smith WS. Emergency medical services dispatcher identification of stroke and transient ischemic attack. *Prehosp Emerg Care.* 1999;3:211–216.

61. Nordberg M. Emergency medical dispatch: a changing profession. *Emerg Med Serv.* 1998;27:25–6, 28–34.

62. *Standard Practice for Emergency Medical Dispatch.* Philadelphia, Pa: American Society for Testing and Materials; 1990. Publication F1258–F1290.

63. Hallstrom A, Cobb L, Johnson E, Copass M. Cardiopulmonary resuscitation by chest compression alone or with mouth-to-mouth ventilation. *N Engl J Med.* 2000;342:1546–1553.

64. Berg RA, Kern KB, Sanders AB, Otto CW, Hilwig RW, Ewy GA. Bystander cardiopulmonary resuscitation: is ventilation necessary? *Circulation.* 1993;88(4 pt 1):1907–1915.

65. Chandra NC, Gruben KG, Tsitlik JE, Brower R, Guerci AD, Halperin HH, Weisfeldt ML, Permutt S. Observations of ventilation during resuscitation in a canine model. *Circulation.* 1994;90:3070–3075.

66. Tang W, Weil MH, Sun SJ, Kette D, Kette F, Gazmuri RJ, O'Connell F. Cardiopulmonary resuscitation by precordial compression but without mechanical ventilation. *Am J Respir Crit Care Med.* 1994;150:1709–1713.

67. Noc M, Weil MH, Tang W, Turner T, Fukui M. Mechanical ventilation may not be essential for initial cardiopulmonary resuscitation. *Chest.* 1995;108:821–827.

68. Van Hoeyweghen RJ, Bossaert LL, Mullie A, Calle P, Martens P, Buylaert WA, Delooz H. Quality and efficiency of bystander CPR: Belgian Cerebral Resuscitation. *Resuscitation.* 1993;26:47–52.

69. Clawson JJ, Hauert SA. Dispatch life support: establishing standards that work. *J Emerg Med Serv.* 1990;15:82–84, 86–88.

70. Stout J, Pepe PE, Mosesso VN. All-advanced life support vs tiered-response ambulance systems. *Prehosp Emerg Care.* 2000;4:1–6.

71. Nichol G, Detsky AS, Stiell IG, O'Rourke K, Wells G, Laupacis A. Effectiveness of emergency medical services for victims of out-of-hospital cardiac arrest: a meta-analysis. *Ann Emerg Med.* 1996;27:700–710.

72. Graves EJ. National hospital discharge survey, 1991. *Vital Health Statistics, vol 13.* Hyattsville, Md: US Department of Health and Human Services; 1993.

73. *Heart and Stroke Facts. 1996 Statistical Supplement.* Dallas, Tex: American Heart Association; 1995.

74. Gillum RF. Trends in acute myocardial infarction and coronary heart disease death in the United States. *J Am Coll Cardiol.* 1994;23:1273–1277.

75. Kannel WB, Schatzkin A. Sudden death: lessons from subsets in population studies. *J Am Coll Cardiol.* 1985;5(suppl):141B–149B.

76. Brouwer MA, Martin JS, Maynard C, et al. Influence of early prehospital thrombolysis on mortality and event-free survival (the Myocardial Infarction Triage and Intervention [MITI] Randomized Trial): MITI Project Investigators. *Am J Cardiol.* 1996;78:497–502.

77. Raitt MH, Maynard C, Wagner GS, et al. Relation between symptom duration before thrombolytic therapy and final myocardial infarct size. *Circulation.* 1996;93:48–53.

78. Wackers FJ, Terrin ML, Kayden DS, et al. Quantitative radionuclide assessment of regional ventricular function after thrombolytic therapy for acute myocardial infarction: results of phase I Thrombolysis in Myocardial Infarction (TIMI) trial. *J Am Coll Cardiol.* 1989;13: 998–1005.

79. Res JC, Simoons ML, van der Wall EE, et al. Long term improvement in global left ventricular function after early thrombolytic treatment in acute myocardial infarction: report of a randomised multicentre trial of intracoronary streptokinase in acute myocardial infarction. *Br Heart J.* 1986;56:414–421.

80. Mathey DG, Sheehan FH, Schofer J, Dodge HT. Time from onset of symptoms to thrombolytic therapy: a major determinant of myocardial salvage in patients with acute transmural infarction. *J Am Coll Cardiol.* 1985;6:518–525.

81. Serruys PW, Simoons ML, Suryapranata H, et al. Preservation of global and regional left ventricular function after early thrombolysis in acute myocardial infarction. *J Am Coll Cardiol.* 1986;7:729–742.

82. Newby LK, Rutsch WR, Califf RM, et al. Time from symptom onset to treatment and outcomes after thrombolytic therapy: GUSTO-1 Investigators. *J Am Coll Cardiol.* 1996;27:1646–1655.

83. Anderson JL, Karagounis LA, Califf RM. Metaanalysis of five reported studies on the relation of early coronary patency grades with mortality and outcomes after acute myocardial infarction. *Am J Cardiol.* 1996; 78:1–8.

84. Zapka J, Estabrook B, Gilliland J, Leviton L, Meischke H, Melville S, Taylor J, Daya M, Laing B, Meshack A, Reyna R, Robbins M, Hand M, Finnegan J. Health care providers' perspectives on patient delay for seeking care for symptoms of acute myocardial infarction. *Health Educ Behav.* 1999;26:714–733.

85. Goldberg RJ, Gurwitz JH, Gore JM. Duration of, and temporal trends (1994–1997) in prehospital delay in patients with acute myocardial infarction: the second National Registry of Myocardial Infarction. *Arch Intern Med.* 1999;159:2141–2147.

86. Raczynski JM, Finnegan JR Jr, Zapka JG, Meischke H, Meshack A, Stone EJ, Bracht N, Sellers DE, Daya M, Robbins M, McAlister A, Simons-Morton D. REACT theory-based intervention to reduce treatment-seeking delay for acute myocardial infarction. Rapid Early Action for Coronary Treatment. *Am J Prev Med.* 1999;16:325–334.

87. Ashton KC. How men and women with heart disease seek care: the delay experience. *Prog Cardiovasc Nurs.* 1999;14:53–60, 74.

88. Zerwic JJ. Patient delay in seeking treatment for acute myocardial infarction symptoms. *J Cardiovasc Nurs.* 1999;13:21–32.

89. Solomon CG, Lee TH, Cook EF, et al. Comparison of clinical presentation of acute myocardial infarction in patients over 65 years of age to younger patients: the Multicenter Chest Pain Study experience. *Am J Cardiol.* 1989;63:772–776.

90. Peberdy MA, Ornato JP. Coronary artery disease in women. *Heart Dis Stroke.* 1992;1:315–319.

91. Douglas PS, Ginsburg GS. The evaluation of chest pain in women. *N Engl J Med.* 1996;334:1311–1315.

92. Sullivan AK, Holdright DR, Wright CA, et al. Chest pain in women: clinical, investigative, and prognostic features. *BMJ.* 1994;308: 883–886.

93. Kereiakes DJ, Weaver WD, Anderson JL, et al. Time delays in the diagnosis and treatment of acute myocardial infarction: a tale of eight cities. Report from the Pre-hospital Study Group and the Cincinnati Heart Project. *Am Heart J.* 1990;120:773–780.

94. Weaver WD. Time to thrombolytic treatment: factors affecting delay and their influence on outcome. *J Am Coll Cardiol.* 1995;25(suppl): 3S–9S.

95. Blohm M, Herlitz J, Schroder U, et al. Reaction to a media campaign focusing on delay in acute myocardial infarction. *Heart Lung.* 1991;20: 661–666.

96. Blohm MB, Hartford M, Karlson BW, Luepker RV, Herlitz J. An evaluation of the media and educational campaigns designed to shorten the time taken by patients with acute myocardial infarction to decide to go to hospital. *Heart.* 1996;76:430–434.

97. Haynes BE, Pritting J. A rural emergency medical technician with selected advanced skills. *Prehosp Emerg Care.* 1999;3:343–346.

98. Funk D, Groat C, Verdile VP. Education of paramedics regarding aspirin use. *Prehosp Emerg Care.* 2000;4:62–64.

99. Held P. Effects of nitrates on mortality in acute myocardial infarction and in heart failure. *Br J Clin Pharmacol.* 1992;34(suppl 1):25S–28S.

100. Verheugt FW, van der Laarse A, Funke-Kepper AJ, Sterkman LG, Galema TW, Roos JP. Effects of early intervention with low-dose aspirin (100 mg) on infarct size, reinfarction and mortality in anterior wall acute myocardial infarction. *Am J Cardiol.* 1990;66:267–277.

101. Tan WA, Moliterno DJ. Aspirin, ticlopidine, and clopidogrel in acute coronary syndromes: underused treatments could save thousands of lives. *Cleve Clin J Med.* 1999;66:615–618, 621–624, 627–628.

102. Kereiakes DJ, Gibler WB, Martin LH, et al. Relative importance of emergency medical system transport and the prehospital electrocardiogram on reducing hospital time delay to therapy for acute myocardial infarction: a preliminary report from the Cincinnati Heart Project. *Am Heart J.* 1992;23:835–840.

103. Karagounis L, Ipsen SK, Jessop MR, et al. Impact of field-transmitted electrocardiography on time to in-hospital thrombolytic therapy in acute myocardial infarction. *Am J Cardiol.* 1990;66:786–791.

104. Aufderheide TP, Hendley GE, Woo J, et al. A prospective evaluation of prehospital 12-lead ECG application in chest pain patients. *J Electrocardiol.* 1992;24S:8–13.

105. Aufderheide TP, Keelan MH, Hendley GE, et al. Milwaukee Prehospital Chest Pain Project: phase 1: feasibility and accuracy of prehospital thrombolytic candidate selection. *Am J Cardiol.* 1992;69:991–996.

106. Hayes OW. Emergency management of acute myocardial infarction: focus on pharmacologic therapy. *Emerg Med Clin North Am.* 1998;16: 541–563, vii-viii.

107. Selker HP, Zalenski RJ, Antman EM, Aufderheide TP, et al. An evaluation of technologies for identifying acute cardiac ischemia in the emergency department: a report from a National Heart Attack Alert Program Working Group. *Ann Emerg Med.* 1997;29:13–87.

108. Weaver WD, Eisenberg MS, Martin JS, et al. Myocardial Infarction Triage and Intervention Project: phase 1: patient characteristics and feasibility of prehospital initiation of thrombolytic therapy. *J Am Coll Cardiol.* 1990;15:925–931.

109. Aufderheide TP, Kereiakes DJ, Weaver WD, et al. Planning, implementation, and process monitoring for prehospital 12-lead ECG diagnostic programs. *Prehosp Disaster Med.* 1996;11:162–171.

110. National Heart Attack Alert Program Coordinating Committee, 60 Minutes to Treatment Working Group. Emergency department: rapid identification and treatment of patients with acute myocardial infarction. *Ann Emerg Med.* 1994;23:311–329.

111. Canto JG, Rogers WJ, Bowlby LJ, et al. The prehospital electrocardiogram in acute myocardial infarction: is its full potential being realized? *J Am Coll Cardiol.* 1997;29:498–505.

112. *1997 Heart and Stroke Statistical Update.* Dallas, Tex: American Heart Association; 1996.

113. Easton JD, Hart RG, Sherman DG, Kaste M. Diagnosis and management of ischemic stroke, I: threatened stroke and its management. *Curr Probl Cardiol.* 1983;8:1–76.

114. The National Institute of Neurological Disorders, and Stroke rt-PA Stroke Study Group. Tissue plasminogen activator for acute ischemic stroke. *N Engl J Med.* 1995;333:1581–1587.

115. Del Zoppo GJ, Higashida RT, Furlan AJ, Pessin MS, Rowley HA, Gent M, and the ProAct Investigators. ProAct: a phase II randomization trial of recombinant pro-urokinase by direct arterial delivery in acute middle cerebral artery stroke. *Stroke.* 1998;29:4–11.

116. Bendzus M, Urbach H, Ries F, Solymosi L. Outcome after local intra-arterial fibrinolysis compared with the natural course of patients with a dense middle cerebral artery on early CT. *Neuroradiology.* 1998;40: 54–58.

117. Wardlaw JM, del Zoppo G, Yamaguchi T. Thrombolysis for acute ischaemic stroke. Cochrane Database of Systematic Reviews: 4th issue; 1999.

118. Kwiatkowski TG, Libman RB, Frankel M, Tilley BC, Morgenstern LB, Lu M, Broderick JP, Lewandowski CA, Marler JR, Levine SR, Brott T, for the NINDS r-tPA Stroke Study Group. Effects of tissue plasminogen activator for acute ischemic stroke at one year. *N Engl J Med.* 1999; 340:1781–1787.

119. Furlan A, Higashida R, Wechsler L, Gent M, Rowley H, Kase C, Pessin M, Ahuja A, Callahan F, Clark WM, Silver F, Rivera F, for the PROACT investigators. Intra-arterial prourokinase for acute ischemic stroke: the PROACT II Study: a randomized controlled trial. *JAMA.* 1999;282:2003–2011.

120. Lewandowski CA, Frankel M, Tomsick TA, Broderick J, Frey J, Clark W, Starkman S, Grotta J, Spilker J, Khoury J, Brott T, and the EMS Bridging Trial Investigators. Combined intravenous and intra-arterial r-TPA versus intra-arterial therapy of acute ischemic stroke: Emergency Management of Stroke (EMS) Bridging Trial. *Stroke.* 1999;30:2598–2605.

121. Albers GW, Bates VE, Clark WM, Bell R, Verro P, Hamilton SA. Intravenous tissue-type plasminogen activator for treatment of acute stroke: the Standard Treatment with Alteplase to Reverse Stroke (STARS) Study. *JAMA.* 2000;283:1145–1150.

122. Fagan SC, Morgenstern LB, Petitta A, Ward RE, Tilley BC, Marler JR, Levine SR, Broderick JP, Kwiatkowski TG, Frankel M, Brott TG, Walker MD, and the NINDS rt-PA Study Group. Cost-effectiveness of tissue plasminogen activator for acute ischemic stroke. *Neurology.* 1998;50:883–890.

123. Pepe PE. The initial links in the chain of recovery for brain attack: access, prehospital care, notification, and transport. In: *Proceedings of the National Symposium on Rapid Identification and Treatment of Acute Stroke.* Bethesda, Md: National Institute of Neurological Disorders and Stroke; 1997:17–28.

124. Barnett HJ. The pathophysiology of transient cerebral ischemic attacks. *Med Clin North Am.* 1979;63:649–679.

125. Antiplatelet Trialists' Collaboration. Collaborative overview of randomized trials of antiplatelet therapy, I: prevention of death, myocardial infarction, and stroke by prolonged antiplatelet therapy in various categories of patients. *BMJ.* 1994;308:81–106.

126. Viitanen M, Eriksson S, Asplund K. Risk of recurrent stroke, myocardial infarction and epilepsy during long-term follow-up after stroke. *Eur Neurol.* 1988;28:227–231.

127. Weir B, ed. *Aneurysms Affecting the Nervous System.* Baltimore, Md: Williams & Wilkins; 1987.

128. Broderick JP, Brott T, Tomsick T, Huster G, Miller R. The risk of subarachnoid and intracerebral hemorrhages in blacks as compared with whites. *N Engl J Med.* 1992;326:733–736.

129. Brott T, Thalinger K, Hertzberg V. Hypertension as a risk factor for spontaneous intracerebral hemorrhage. *Stroke.* 1986;17:1078–1083.

130. Furlan AJ, Whisnant JP, Elveback LR. The decreasing incidence of primary intracerebral hemorrhage: a population study. *Ann Neurol.* 1979;5:365–373.

131. Kassell NF, Torner JC, Haley EC Jr, Jane JA, Adams HP, Kongable GL. The International Cooperative Study on the Timing of Aneurysm Surgery, I: overall management results. *J Neurosurg.* 1990;73:18–36.

132. Kassell NF, Torner JC, Jane JA, Haley EC Jr, Adams HP. The International Cooperative Study on the Timing of Aneurysm Surgery, II: surgical results. *J Neurosurg.* 1990;73:37–47.

133. Barsan WG, Brott TG, Broderick JP, et al. Time of hospital presentation in patients with acute stroke. *Arch Intern Med.* 1993;2558–2561.

134. Feldmann E, Gorson N, Books JM, et al. Factors associated with early presentation of acute stroke. *Stroke.* 1993;24:1805–1809.

135. Alberts MJ, Perry A, Dawson DV, Bertels C. Effects of professional and public education on reducing the delay in presentation and referral of stroke patients. *Stroke.* 1992;23:352–356.

136. Lyden PD, Rapp K, Babcock T, Rothrock J. Ultra-rapid identification, triage, and enrollment of stroke patients into clinical trials. *J Stroke Cerebrovasc Dis.* 1994;4:106–107.

137. Spilker JA. The importance of patient and public education in acute ischemic stroke. In: *Proceedings of the National Symposium on Rapid Identification and Treatment of Acute Stroke.* Bethesda, Md: The National Institute of Neurological Disorders and Stroke; 1996:73–87.

138. Grotta JC. The importance of time. In: *Proceedings of the National Symposium on Rapid Identification and Treatment of Acute Stroke.* Bethesda, Md: National Institute of Neurological Disorders and Stroke; 1997:5–9.

139. Kwiatkowski T, Silverman R, Paiano R, et al. Delayed hospital arrival in patients with acute stroke. *Acad Emerg Med.* 1996;3:538.

140. Morris DL, Fordon RA, Hinn AR, et al. Delay in seeking care for stroke: demographic determinants. —The Delay in Accessing Stroke Healthcare Study. *Acad Emerg Med.* 1996;3:539.

141. Kay R, Woo J, Poon WS. Hospital arrival time after onset of stroke. *J Neurol Neurosurg Psychiatry.* 1992;55:973–974.

142. Biller J, Shephard A. Delay between onset of ischemic stroke and hospital arrival. *Neurology.* 1992;42(suppl I):390P.

143. Hazinski MF. Demystifying recognition and management of stroke. *Curr Emerg Cardiac Care.* 1996;7:8.

144. The National Institute of Neurological Disorders and Stroke (NINDS) rt-PA Stroke Study Group. A systems approach to immediate evaluation and management of hyperacute stroke: experience at eight centers and implications for community practice and patient care. *Stroke.* 1997;28:1530–1540.

145. Crocco TJ, Kothari RU, Sayre MR, Liu T. A nationwide prehospital stroke survey. *Prehosp Emerg Care.* 1999;3:201–206.

146. Ferro JM, Melo TP, Oliveira V, Crespo M, Canhao P, Pinto AN. An analysis of the admission delay of acute strokes. *Cerebrovasc Dis.* 1994;4:72–75.

147. Kothari R, Jauch E, Broderick J, Brott T, Sauerbeck L, Khoury J, Liu T. Acute stroke: delays to presentation and emergency department evaluation. *Ann Emerg Med.* 1999;33:3–8.

148. Morris DL, Rosamond WD, Hinn AR, Gorton RA. Time delays in accessing stroke care in the emergency department. *Acad Emerg Med.* 1999;6:218–223.

149. Kidwell CS, Saver JL, Schubert GB, Eckstein M, Starkman S. Design and retrospective analysis of the Los Angeles Prehospital Stroke Screen (LAPSS). *Prehosp Emerg Care.* 1998;2:267–273.

150. Kothari R, Barsan W, Brott T, Broderick J, Ashbrock S. Frequency and accuracy of prehospital diagnosis of acute stroke. *Stroke.* 1993;26:937–941.

151. Zachariah B, Dunford J, Van Cott CC. Dispatch life support and the acute stroke patient: making the right call. In: *Proceedings of the National Symposium on Rapid Identification and Treatment of Acute Stroke.* Bethesda, Md: The National Institute of Neurological Disorders and Stroke; 1991:88–96.

152. Dávalos A, Castillo J, Martinez-Villa E. Delay in neurological attention and stroke outcome: Cerebrovascular Disease Study Group of the Spanish Society of Neurology. *Stroke.* 1995;26:2233–2237.

153. Bornstein NM, Gur AY, Fainshtein P, Korczyn AD. Stroke during sleep: epidemiological and clinical features. *Cerebrovasc Dis.* 1999;9:320–2.

154. Sayre MR, Swor RA, Honeykutt LK. Prehospital identification and treatment. In: *Proceedings of the National Symposium on Rapid Identification and Treatment of Acute Stroke.* Bethesda, Md: National Institute of Neurological Disorders and Stroke; 1997:35–43.

155. Zweifler RM, Drinkard R, Cunningham S, Brody ML, Rothrock JF. Implementation of a stroke code system in Mobile, Alabama: diagnostic and therapeutic yield. *Stroke.* 1997;28:981–983.

156. Smith WS, Isaacs M, Corry MD. Accuracy of paramedic identification of stroke and transient ischemic attack in the field. *Prehosp Emerg Care.* 1998;2:170–175.

157. Williams LS, Bruno A, Rouch D, Marriott DJ. Stroke patients' knowledge of stroke: influence on time to presentation. *Stroke.* 1997;28:912–915.

158. Kothari R, Pancioli A, Liu T, et al. Cincinnati Prehospital Stroke Scale: reproducibility and validity. *Ann Emerg Med.* 1999;33:373–378.

159. Kidwell CS, Starkman S, Eckstein M, Weems K, Saver JL. Identifying stroke in the field: prospective validation of the Los Angeles Prehospital Stroke Screen (LAPSS). *Stroke.* 2000;31:71–76.

160. Prasad K, Menon GR. Comparison of the three strategies of verbal scoring of the Glasgow Coma Scale in patients with stroke. *Cerebrovasc Dis.* 1998;8:79–85.

161. Kothari R, Hall K, Brott T, Broderick J. Early stroke recognition: developing an out-of-hospital NIH Stroke Scale. *Acad Emerg Med.* 1997;4:986–990.

162. Kothari R, Pio BJ, Sayre MR, Liu T. A prospective evaluation of the accuracy of prehospital diagnosis of acute stroke. *Prehosp Emerg Care.* 1999;3:82. Abstract.

163. Kothari R, Sauerbeck L, Jauch E, Broderick J, Brott T, Khoury J, Liu T. Patients' awareness of stroke signs, symptoms, and risk factors. *Stroke.* 1997;28:1871–1875.

164. Scott PA, Temovsky CJ, Lawrence K, Gudaitis E, Lowell MJ. Analysis of Canadian population with potential geographic access to intravenous thrombolysis for acute ischemic stroke. *Stroke.* 1998;29:2304–2310.

165. Oppenheimer SM, Hachinski VC. The cardiac consequences of stroke. *Neurol Clin.* 1992;10:167–176.

166. Goldstein DS. The electrocardiogram in stroke: relationship to pathophysiological type and comparison with prior tracings. *Stroke.* 1979;10:253–259.

167. European Ad Hoc Consensus Group, Hacke W, Chair. Optimizing intensive care in stroke: a European perspective. *Cerebrovasc Dis.* 1997;7:113–128.

168. Mackenzie GJ, Taylor SH, McDonald AH, Donald KW. Haemodynamic effects of external cardiac compression. *Lancet.* 1964;1:1342–1345.

169. Noc M, Weil MH, Sun SJ, Tang W, Bisera J. Spontaneous gasping during cardiopulmonary resuscitation without mechanical ventilation. *Am J Respir Crit Care Med.* 1994;150:861–864.

170. Clark JJ, Larsen MP, Cully LL, Graves JR, Eisenberg MS. Incidence of agonal respirations in sudden cardiac arrest. *Ann Emerg Med.* 1991;21: 1464–1467.

171. Gundry JW, Comess KA, DeRook FA, Jorgenson D, Bardy GH. Comparison of naive sixth-grade children with trained professionals in the use of an automated external defibrillator. *Circulation.* 1999;100: 1703–1707.

172. Chandra NC, Hazinski MF, Stapleton E. *Instructor's Manual for Basic Life Support.* Dallas, Tex: American Heart Association; 1997.

173. Safar P. Ventilatory efficacy of mouth-to-mouth artificial respiration: airway obstruction during manual and mouth-to-mouth artificial respiration. *JAMA.* 1958;167:335–341.

174. Safar P, Escarraga LA, Chang F. Upper airway obstruction in the unconscious patient. *J Appl Physiol.* 1959;14:760–764.

175. Ruben HM, Elam JO, Ruben AM, Greene DG. Investigation of upper airway problems in resuscitation: studies of pharyngeal x-rays and performance by laymen. *Anesthesiology.* 1961;22:271–279.

176. Guildner CW. Resuscitation: —opening the airway: a comparative study of techniques for opening an airway obstructed by the tongue. *JACEP.* 1976;5:588–590.

177. Elam JO, Greene DG, Schneider MA, et al. Head-tilt method of oral resuscitation. *JAMA.* 1960;172:812–815.

178. Safar P, Escarrage LA. Compliance in apneic anesthetized adults. *Anesthesiology.* 1959;20:283–289.

179. Handley AJ, Becker LB, Allen M, van Drenth A, Kramer EB, Montgomery WH. Single rescuer adult basic life support: an advisory statement from the Basic Life Support Working Group of the International Liaison Committee on Resuscitation (ILCOR). *Resuscitation.* 1997;34:101–108.

180. Turner S, Turner I, Chapman D, Howard P, Champion P, Hatfield J, James A, Marshal S, Barber S. A comparative study of the 1992 and 1997 recovery positions for use in the UK. *Resuscitation.* 1998;39: 153–160.

181. Doxey J. Comparing 1997 Resuscitation Council (UK) recovery position with recovery position of 1992 European Resuscitation Council guidelines: a user's perspective. *Resuscitation.* 1998;39:161–169.

182. Fulstow R, Smith GB. The new recovery position: a cautionary tale. *Resuscitation.* 1993;26:89–91.

183. Rathgeber J, Panzer W, Gunther U, Scholz M, Hoeft A, Bahr J, Kettler D. Influence of different types of recovery positions on perfusion indices of the forearm. *Resuscitation.* 1996;32:13–17.

184. Wenzel V, Idris AH, Banner MJ, Fuerst RS, Tucker KJ. The composition of gas given by mouth-to-mouth ventilation during CPR. *Chest.* 1994;106:1806–1810.

185. Wenzel V, Idris AH, Banner MJ, Kubilis PS, Band R, Williams JL, Lindner KH. Respiratory system compliance decreases after cardiopulmonary resuscitation and stomach inflation: impact of large and small tidal volumes on calculated peak airway pressure. *Resuscitation.* 1998; 38:113–118.

186. Idris AH, Wenzel V, Banner MJ, Melker RJ. Smaller tidal volumes minimize gastric inflation during CPR with an unprotected airway. *Circulation.* 1995;92(suppl I):I-759. Abstract.

187. Morton HJV, Wylie WD. Anaesthetic deaths due to regurgitation or vomiting. *Anaesthesia.* 1951;6:192–205.

188. Ruben A, Ruben H. Artificial respiration: flow of water from the lung and the stomach. *Lancet.* 1962;780:81.

189. Stone BJ, Chantler PJ, Baskett PJ. The incidence of regurgitation during cardiopulmonary resuscitation: a comparison between the bag valve mask and laryngeal mask airway. *Resuscitation.* 1998;38:3–6.

190. Lawes EG, Baskett PJF. Pulmonary aspiration during unsuccessful cardiopulmonary resuscitation. *Intens Care Med.* 1987;13:379–382.

191. Bjork RJ, Snyder BD, Campion BC, Loewenson RB. Medical complications of cardiopulmonary arrest. *Arch Intern Med.* 1982;142:500–503.

192. Spence AA, Moir DD, Finlay WIE. Observations on intragastric pressure. *Anaesthesia.* 1967;22:249–256.

193. Wenzel V, Idris AH, Banner MJ, Kubilis PS, Williams JL. The influence of tidal volume on the distribution of gas between the lungs and stomach

194. Wenzel V, Keller C, Idris AH, Dörges V, Lindner KH, Brimacombe JR. Effects of smaller tidal volumes during basic life support ventilation in patients with respiratory arrest: good ventilation, less risk? *Resuscitation.* 1999;43:25–29.

195. Weiler N, Heinrichs W, Dick W. Assessment of pulmonary mechanics and gastric inflation pressure during mask ventilation. *Prehospital Disaster Med.* 1995;10:101–105.

196. Cheifetz IM, Craig DM, Quick G, McGovern JJ, Cannon ML, Ungerleider RM, Smith PK, Meliones JN. Increasing tidal volumes and pulmonary overdistension adversely affect pulmonary vascular mechanics and cardiac output in a pediatric swine model. *Crit Care Med.* 1998;26:710–716.

197. Berg MD, Idris AH, Berg RA. Severe ventilatory compromise due to gastric distension during cardiopulmonary resuscitation. *Resuscitation.* 1998;36:71–73.

198. Bowman FP, Menegazzi JJ, Check BD, Duckett TM. Lower esophageal sphincter pressure during prolonged cardiac arrest and resuscitation. *Ann Emerg Med.* 1995;26:216–219.

199. Melker RJ. Recommendations for ventilation during cardiopulmonary resuscitation: time for change? *Crit Care Med.* 1985;13(pt 2):882–883.

200. Baskett P, Nolan J, Parr M, Tidal volumes which are perceived to be adequate for resuscitation. *Resuscitation.* 1996;31:231–234.

201. Baskett P, Bossaert LL, Carli P, Chamberlain D, Dick W, Nolan JP, Parr MJA, Schneidegger D, Zideman D. Guidelines for the basic management of the airway and ventilation during resuscitation: a statement by the Airway and Ventilation Management Working Group of the European Resuscitation Council. *Resuscitation.* 1996;31:187–200.

202. Idris AH, Gabrielli A, Caruso L. Smaller tidal volume is safe and effective for bag-valve-ventilation, but not for mouth-to-mouth ventilation: an animal model for basic life support. *Circulation.* 1999; 100(suppl I):I-644. Abstract.

203. Dörges V, Ocker H, Hagelberg S, Wenzel V, Idris AH. Smaller tidal volumes with room air are not sufficient to ensure adequate oxygenation during basic life support. *Resuscitation.* 2000;44:37–41.

204. Htin KJ, Birenbaum DS, Idris AH, Banner MJ, Gravenstein N. Rescuer breathing pattern significantly affects O_2 and CO_2 received by the patient during mouth-to-mouth ventilation. *Crit Care Med.* 1998;26(suppl 1):A56–A60.

205. Ruben H. The immediate treatment of respiratory failure. *Br J Anaesth.* 1964;36:542–549.

206. Safar P, Redding J. The "tight jaw" in resuscitation. *Anesthesiology.* 1959;20:701–702.

207. International Association of Laryngectomees. *First Aid for (Neck Breathers) Laryngectomees.* New York, NY: American Cancer Society; 1971.

208. Figura N. Mouth-to-mouth resuscitation and *Helicobacter pylori* infection. *Lancet.* 1996;347:1342. Letter.

209. Heilman KM, Muscheheim C. Primary cutaneous tuberculosis resulting from mouth-to-mouth respiration. *N Engl J Med.* 1965;273:1035–1036.

210. Simmons M, Deao D, Moon L, et al. Bench evaluation: three face-shield CPR barrier devices. *Respir Care.* 1995;40:618–623.

211. Exhaled-air pulmonary resuscitators (EAPRs), and disposable manual pulmonary resuscitators (DMPRs). *Health Devices.* 1989;18:333–352.

212. Johannigman JA, Branson RD. Oxygen enrichment of expired gas for mouth-to-mask resuscitation. *Respir Care.* 1991;36:99–103.

213. Elling R, Politis J. An evaluation of emergency medical technicians' ability to use manual ventilation devices. *Ann Emerg Med.* 1983;12: 765–768.

214. Hess D, Baran C. Ventilatory volumes using mouth-to-mouth, mouth-to-mask, and bag-valve-mask techniques. *Am J Emerg Med.* 1985;3:292–296.

215. Cummins RO, Austin D, Graves JR, Litwin PE, Pierce J. Ventilation skills of emergency medical technicians: a teaching challenge for emergency medicine. *Ann Emerg Med.* 1986;15:1187–1192.

216. Johannigman JA, Branson RD, Davis K Jr, Hurst JM. Techniques of emergency ventilation: a model to evaluate tidal volume, airway pressure, and gastric insufflation. *J Trauma.* 1991;31:93–98.

217. Fuerst RS, Banner MJ, Melker RJ. Gastric inflation in the unintubated patient: a comparison of common ventilating devices. *Ann Emerg Med.* 1992;21:636. Abstract.

217a. Langhelle A, Sunde K, Wik L, Steen PA. Arterial blood gases with 500- versus 1000-mL tidal volume during out-of-hospital CPR. *Resuscitation.* 2000;45:27–33.

218. Dörges V, Sauer C, Ocker H, Wenzel V, Schmucker P. Airway management during cardiopulmonary resuscitation: a comparative study of

bag-valve-mask, laryngeal mask airway and Combitube in a bench model. *Resuscitation.* 1999;41:63–69.

219. Dörges V, Sauer C, Ocker H, Wenzel V, Schmucker P. Smaller tidal volumes during cardiopulmonary resuscitation: comparison of adult and pediatric size self-inflatable bags with three different ventilatory devices. *Resuscitation.* 1999;43:31–37.

220. Winkler M, Mauritz W, Hackl W, Gilly H, Weindlmayr-Goettel M, Steinbereithner K, Schindler I. Effects of half the tidal volume during cardiopulmonary resuscitation on acid-base balance and haemodynamics in pigs. *Eur J Emerg Med.* 1998;5:201–206.

221. Elam JO. Bag-valve-mask O$_2$ ventilation. In: Safer P, Elam JO, eds. *Advances in Cardiopulmonary Resuscitation: The Wolf Creek Conference on Cardiopulmonary Resuscitation.* New York, NY: Springer-Verlag Inc; 1977:73–79.

222. Sellick BA. Cricoid pressure to control regurgitation of stomach contents during induction of anesthesia. *Lancet.* 1961;2:404–406.

223. Dailey RH, Simon B, Young GP, Steward RD. *The Airway: Emergency Management.* St Louis, Mo: Mosby Year Book; 1992.

224. Salem MR, Joseph NJ, Heyman HJ, Belani B, Paulissian R, Ferrara TP. Cricoid pressure is effective in obliterating the esophageal lumen in the presence of a nasogastric tube. *Anesthesiology.* 1985;4:443–446.

225. Petito SP, Russell WJ. The prevention of gastric inflation: –a neglected benefit of cricoid pressure. *Anaesth Intensive Care.* 1998;16:139–143.

226. Mather C, O'Kelly S. The palpation of pulses. *Anaesthesia.* 1996;51:189–191.

227. Bahr J, Klingler H, Panzer W, Rode H, Kettler D. Skills of lay people in checking the carotid pulse. *Resuscitation.* 1997;35:23–26.

228. Ochoa FJ, Ramalle-Gomara E, Carpintero JM, Garcia A, Saralegui I. Competence of health professionals to check the carotid pulse. *Resuscitation.* 1998;37:173–175.

229. Flesche CW, Zucker TP, Lorenz C, Nerudo B, Tarnow J. The carotid pulse check as a diagnostic tool to assess pulselessness during adult basic life support. *Euroanaesthesia '95.* 1995; Abstract. Presented at the European Resuscitation Council.

230. Cummins RO, Hazinski MF. Cardiopulmonary resuscitation techniques and instruction: when does evidence justify revision? *Ann Emerg Med.* 1999;34:780–784.

231. Flesche C, Neruda B, Breuer S, et al. Basic cardiopulmonary resuscitation skills: a comparison of ambulance staff and medical students in Germany. *Resuscitation.* 1994;28:S25. Abstract.

232. Flesche C, Neruda B, Noetages T, et al. Do cardiopulmonary skills among medical students meet current standards and patients' needs? *Resuscitation.* 1994;28:S25. Abstract.

233. Monsieurs KG, De Cauwer HG, Bossaert LL. Feeling for the carotid pulse: is five seconds enough? *Resuscitation.* 1996;31:S3.

234. Flesche CW, Breuer S, Mandel LP, Brevik H, Tarnow J. The ability of health professionals to check the carotid pulse. *Circulation.* 1994;90(suppl I):I-288. Abstract.

235. Eberle B, Dick WF, Schneider T, Wisser G, Doetsch S, Tzanova I. Checking the carotid pulse: diagnostic accuracy of first responders in patients with and without a pulse. *Resuscitation.* 1996;33:107–116.

236. Kouwenhoven WB, Jude JR, Knickerbocker GG. Closed-chest cardiac massage. *JAMA.* 1960;173:1064–1067.

237. Maier GW, Tyson GS Jr, Olsen CO, et al. The physiology of external cardiac massage: high-impulse cardiopulmonary resuscitation. *Circulation.* 1984;70:86–101.

238. Rudikoff MT, Maughan WL, Effron M, Freund P, Weisfeldt ML. Mechanisms of blood flow during cardiopulmonary resuscitation. *Circulation.* 1980;61:345–352.

239. Fitzgerald KR, Babbs CF, Frissora HA, Davis RW, Silver DI. Cardiac output during cardiopulmonary resuscitation at various compression rates and durations. *Am J Physiol.* 1981;241:H442–H448.

240. Babbs CF, Thelander K. Theoretically optimal duty cycles for chest and abdominal compression during external cardiopulmonary resuscitation. *Acad Emerg Med.* 1995;2:698–707.

241. Maier GW, Newton JR, Wolfe JA, Tson GS, Olsen CO, Glower DD, Spratt JA, Davis JW, Feneley MPRJS. The influence of manual chest compression rate on hemodynamic support during cardiac arrest; high-impulse cardiopulmonary resuscitation. *Circulation.* 1986;74(suppl IV):IV-51–IV-59.

242. Feneley MP, Maier GW, Kern KB, Gaynor JW, Gall SA, Sanders AB, Raessler K, Muhlbaier LH, Scott Rankin J, Ewy GA. Influence of compression rate on initial success of resuscitation and 24 hour survival after prolonged manual cardiopulmonary resuscitation in dogs. *Circulation.* 1988;77:240–250.

243. Wolfe JA, Maier GW, Newton JR, Glower DD, Tyson GS, Spratt JA, Rankin JS, Olsen CO. Physiologic determinants of coronary blood flow during external cardiac massage. *J Thorac Cardiovasc Surg.* 1988;95:523–532.

244. Sanders AB, Kern KB, Fonken S, Otto CW, Ewy GA. The role of bicarbonate and fluid loading in improving resuscitation from prolonged cardiac arrest with rapid manual chest compression CPR. *Ann Emerg Med.* 1990;19:1–7.

245. Swenson RD, Weaver D, Niskanen RA, Martin J, Dahlberg S. Hemodynamics in humans during conventional and experimental methods of cardiopulmonary resuscitation. *Circulation.* 1988;78:630–639.

246. Kern KB, Sanders AB, Raife J, Milander MM, Otto CW, Ewy GA. A study of chest compression rates during cardiopulmonary resuscitation in humans. *Arch Intern Med.* 1992;152:145–149.

247. Wik L, Steen PA. The ventilation-compression ratio influences the effectiveness of two rescuer advanced cardiac life support on a manikin. *Resuscitation.* 1996;31:113–119.

248. Kern KB, Hilwig RW, Berg RA, Ewy GA. Efficacy of chest compression-only BLS CPR in the presence of an occluded airway. *Resuscitation.* 1998;39:179–188.

249. Handley AJ, Handley JA. The relationship between rate of chest compression and compression:relaxation ratio. *Resuscitation.* 1995;30:237–241.

250. Berg RA, Sanders AB, Milander M, Tellez D, Liu P, Beyda D. Efficacy of audio-prompted rate guidance in improving resuscitator performance of cardiopulmonary resuscitation on children. *Acad Emerg Med.* 1994;1:35–40.

251. Milander MM, Hiscok PS, Sanders AB, Kern KB, Berg RA, Ewy GA. Chest compression and ventilation rates during cardiopulmonary resuscitation: the effects of audible tone guidance. *Acad Emerg Med.* 1995;2:708–713.

252. Clawson JJ. Dispatch priority training: strengthening the weak link. *J Emerg Med Serv.* 1981;6:32–36.

253. Clawson JJ. Telephone treatment protocols: reach out and help someone. *J Emerg Med Serv.* 1986;11:43–46.

254. Culley LL, Clark JJ, Eisenberg MS, Larsen MP. Dispatcher-assisted telephone CPR: common delays and time standards for delivery. *Ann Emerg Med.* 1991;20:362–366.

255. Halperin HR, Tsitlik JE, Guerci AD, Mellits ED, Levin HR, Shi A-Y, Chandra N, Weisfeldt ML. Determinants of blood flow to vital organs during cardiopulmonary resuscitation in dogs. *Circulation.* 1986;73:539–550.

256. Swart GL, Mateer JR, DeBehnke DJ, Jameson SJ, Osborn JL. The effect of compression duration on hemodynamics during mechanical high-impulse CPR. *Acad Emerg Med.* 1994;1:430–437.

257. Criley JM, Blaufuss AH, Kissel GL. Cough-induced cardiac compression: self-administered form of cardiopulmonary resuscitation. *JAMA.* 1976;236:1246–1250.

258. Petelenz T, Iwinski J, Chlebowczyk J, Czyz Z, Flak Z, Fiutowski L, Zaorski K, Petelenz T, Zeman S. Self-administered cough cardiopulmonary resuscitation (c-CPR) in patients threatened by MAS events of cardiovascular origin. *Wiad Lek.* 1998;51:326–336.

259. Saba SE, David SW. Sustained consciousness during ventricular fibrillation: case report of cough cardiopulmonary resuscitation. *Cathet Cardiovasc Diagn.* 1996;37:47–48.

260. Miller B, Cohen A, Serio A, Bettock D. Hemodynamics of cough cardiopulmonary resuscitation in a patient with sustained torsades de pointes/ventricular flutter. *J Emerg Med.* 1994;12:627–632.

261. Paradis NA, Martin GB, Goetting MG, et al. Simultaneous aortic, jugular bulb, and right atrial pressures during cardiopulmonary resuscitation in humans: insights into mechanisms. *Circulation.* 1989;80:361–368.

262. Guerci AD, Chandra NC, Gelfand MI, et al. Vest CPR increases aortic pressure in humans. *Circulation.* 1989;80(suppl II):II-496. Abstract.

263. Sack JB, Kesselbrenner MB, Bregman D. Survival from in-hospital cardiac arrest with interposed abdominal counterpulsation during cardiopulmonary resuscitation. *JAMA.* 1992;267:379–385.

264. Sack JB, Kesselbrenner MB, Jarrad A. Interposed abdominal compression-cardiopulmonary resuscitation and resuscitation outcome during asystole and electromechanical dissociation. *Circulation.* 1992;86:1692–1700.

265. Barranco F, Lesmes A, Irles JA, et al. Cardiopulmonary resuscitation with simultaneous chest and abdominal compression: comparative study in humans. *Resuscitation.* 1990;20:67–77.

266. Cohen TJ, Tucker KJ, Lurie KG, et al. Active compression-decompression: a new method of cardiopulmonary resuscitation. *JAMA.* 1992;267:2916–2923.

267. Plaisance P, Lurie K, Vicaut E, et al. Comparison of standard cardiopulmonary resuscitation and active compression decompression for out-of-hospital cardiac arrest. *N Engl J Med.* 1999;341:569–575.

268. Plaisance P, Adnet F, Vicaut E, et al. Benefit of active compression-decompression cardiopulmonary resuscitation as a prehospital advanced cardiac life support: a randomized multicenter study. *Circulation.* 1997;95:955–961.

269. Mauer D, Schneider T, Dick W, et al. Active compression-decompression resuscitation: a prospective, randomized study in a two-tiered EMS system with physicians in the field. *Resuscitation.* 1996;33:125–134.

270. Plaisance P, Lurie KG, Payden D. Inspiratory impedance during active compression-decompression cardiopulmonary resuscitation: a randomized evaluation in patients in cardiac arrest. *Circulation.* 2000;101:989–994.

271. Lurie KG, Coffeen PR, Shultz JJ, McKnite SH, Deltoid BS. Improving active compression-decompression cardiopulmonary resuscitation with an inspiratory impedance valve. *Circulation.* 1995;91:1629–1632.

272. Lurie KG, Mulligan K, McKnite S, Deltoid B, Lindner K. Optimizing standard cardiopulmonary resuscitation with an inspiratory threshold valve. *Chest.* 1998;113:1084–1090.

273. Simoons ML, Kimman GP, Ivens EMA, Hartman JAM, Hart HN. Follow up after out of hospital resuscitation. Paper presented at: XIIth Annual Congress of the European Society of Cardiology; September 16–20, 1990; Stockholm, Sweden.

274. Ornato JP, Hallagan LF, McMahan SB, Peeples EH, Rostafinski AG. Attitudes of BCLS instructors about mouth-to-mouth resuscitation during the AIDS epidemic. *Ann Emerg Med.* 1990;19:151–156.

275. Brenner BE, Van DC, Cheng D, Lazar EJ. Determinants of reluctance to perform CPR among residents and applicants: the impact of experience on helping behavior. *Resuscitation.* 1997;35:203–211.

276. Hew P, Brenner B, Kaufman J. Reluctance of paramedics and emergency medical technicians to perform mouth-to-mouth resuscitation. *J Emerg Med.* 1997;15:279–284.

277. Brenner BE, Kauffman J. Reluctance of internists and medical nurses to perform mouth-to-mouth resuscitation. *Arch Intern Med.* 1993;153:1763–1769.

278. Locke CJ, Berg RA, Sanders AB, Davis MF, Milander MM, Kern KB, Ewy GA. Bystander cardiopulmonary resuscitation: concerns about mouth-to-mouth. *Arch Intern Med.* 1995;155:938–943.

279. Berg RA, Kern KB, Hilwig RW, Berg MD, Sanders AB, Otto CW, Ewy GA. Assisted ventilation does not improve outcome in a porcine model of single-rescuer bystander cardiopulmonary resuscitation. *Circulation.* 1997;95:1635–1641.

280. Weil MH, Rackow EC, Trevino R, Grundler W, Falk JL, Griffel MI. Difference in acid-base state between venous and arterial blood during cardiopulmonary resuscitation. *N Engl J Med.* 1986;315:153–156.

281. Sanders AB, Otto CW, Kern KB, Rogers JN, Perrault P, Ewy GA. Acid-base balance in a canine model of cardiac arrest. *Ann Emerg Med.* 1988;17:667–671.

282. Fingerhut LA, Cox CS, Warner M. International Comparative Analysis of Injury Mortality. Findings from the International Collaborative Effort (ICE) on Injury Statistics. *Advance Data from Vital and Health Statistics of the Centers for Disease Control and Prevention.* Number 303; October 7, 1998.

283. National Center for Health Statistics and National Safety Council. *Data on odds of death due to choking.* May 7, 1998.

284. National Safety Council. *Accident Facts 1997.* Chicago, Ill: National Safety Council; 1997.

285. Canadian Hospitals Injury Reporting and Prevention Program. *Summary Statistics CHIRPP Database for the Year 1997.*

286. Rosen P, Stoto M, Harley J. The use of the Heimlich maneuver in near drowning: Institute of Medicine report. *J Emerg Med.* 1995;13:397–405.

287. Haugen RK. The café coronary: sudden death in restaurants. *JAMA.* 1963;186:142–143.

288. Heimlich HJ. A life-saving maneuver to prevent food-choking. *JAMA.* 1975;234:398–401.

289. Ekberg O, Feinberg M. Clinical and demographic data in 75 patients with near-fatal choking episodes. *Dysphagia.* 1992;7:205–208.

290. Fioritti A, Giaccotto L, Melega V. Choking incidents among psychiatric patients: retrospective analysis of thirty-one cases from the Bologna psychiatric wards. *Can J Psychiatry.* 1997;42:515–520.

291. Lan RS. Non-asphyxiating tracheobronchial foreign bodies in adults. *Eur Respir J.* 1994;7:510–514.

292. Fitzpatrick PC, Guarisco JL. Pediatric foreign bodies. *J La State Med Soc.* 1998;150:138–141.

293. Jacob B, Wiebrauck C, Lamprecht J, Bonte W. Laryngologic aspects of bolus asphyxiation-bolus death. *Dysphagia.* 1992;7:313–5.

294. Chen CH, Lai CL, Tsai TT, Lee YC, Perng RP. Foreign body aspirations into the lower airway in Chinese adults. *Chest.* 1997;112:129–133.

295. Jones TM, Luke LC. Life threatening airway obstruction: a hazard of concealed eating disorders. *J Accid Emerg Med.* 1998;15:332–333.

296. Committee on Emergency Medical Services, Assembly of Life Sciences, National Research Council. *Report on Emergency Airway Management.* Washington, DC: National Academy of Sciences; 1976:296.

297. Redding JS. The choking controversy: critique of evidence on the Heimlich maneuver. *Crit Care Med.* 1979;7:475–479.

298. Langhelle A, Sunde K, Wik L, Steen PA. Airway pressure during chest compression vs Heimlich manoeuvre in newly dead adults with complete airway obstruction. *Resuscitation.* 2000;44:105–108.

299. Gordon AS, Belton MK, Ridolpho PF. Emergency management of foreign body airway obstruction. In: Safer P, Elam JO, eds. *Advances in Cardiopulmonary Resuscitation.* New York, NY: Springer-Verlag; 1977.

300. Day RL, Crelin ES, DuBois AB. Choking: the Heimlich abdominal thrust vs back blows: an approach to measurement of inertial and aerodynamic forces. *Pediatrics.* 1982;70:113–119.

301. Nowitz A, Lewer BM, Galletly DC. An interesting complication of the Heimlich manoeuvre. *Resuscitation.* 1998;39:129–131.

302. Majumdar A, Sedman PC. Gastric rupture secondary to successful Heimlich manoeuvre. *Postgrad Med J.* 1998;74:609–610.

303. Bintz M, Cogbill TH. Gastric rupture after the Heimlich maneuver. *J Trauma.* 1996;40:159–160.

304. Dupre MW, Silva E, Brotman S. Traumatic rupture of the stomach secondary to Heimlich maneuver. *Am J Emerg Med.* 1993;11:611–612.

305. Anderson S, Buggy D. Prolonged pharyngeal obstruction after the Heimlich manoeuvre. *Anaesthesia.* 1999;54:308–309. Letter.

306. Orlowski JP. Vomiting as a complication of the Heimlich maneuver. *JAMA.* 1987;258:512–513.

307. Kaye W, Rallis SF, Mancini ME, Linhares KC, Angell ML, Donovan DS, Zajano NC, Finger JA. The problem of poor retention of cardiopulmonary resuscitation skills may lie with the instructor, not the learner or the curriculum. *Resuscitation.* 1991;21:67–86.

308. Brennan RT, Braslow A. Skill mastery in cardiopulmonary resuscitation training classes. *Am J Emerg Med.* 1995;13:505–508.

309. Liberman M, Lavoie A, Mulder D, Sampalis J. Cardiopulmonary resuscitation: errors made by pre-hospital emergency medical personnel. *Resuscitation.* 1999;42:47–55.

310. Kaye W, Mancini ME. Retention of cardiopulmonary skills by physicians, registered nurses and the general public. *Crit Care Med.* 1986;14:620–622.

311. Mancini ME, Kaye W. The effect of time since training on house officers' retention of cardiopulmonary resuscitation skills. *Am J Emerg Med.* 1985;3:31–32.

312. Mandel LP, Cobb LA. Initial and long term competency of citizens trained in CPR. *Emerg Health Serv Q.* 1982;1:49–63.

313. Braslow A, Brennan RT, Newman MM, Bircher NG, Batcheller AM, Kaye W. CPR training without an instructor: development and evaluation of a video self-instructional system for effective performance of cardiopulmonary resuscitation. *Resuscitation.* 1997;34:207–220.

314. Todd KH, Braslow A, Brennan RT, Lowery DW, Cox RJ, Lipscomb LE, Kellermann AL. Randomized, controlled trial of video self-instruction versus traditional CPR training. *Ann Emerg Med.* 1998;31:364–369.

315. Todd KH, Heron SL, Thompson M, Dennis R, O'Connor J, Kellermann AL. Simple CPR: a randomized, controlled trial of video self-instructional cardiopulmonary resuscitation training in an African American church congregation. *Ann Emerg Med.* 1999;34:730–737.

316. Handley JA, Handley AJ. Four-step CPR: improving skill retention. *Resuscitation.* 1998;36:3–8.

317. Skulberg A. Chest compressions: an alternative to the Heimlich manoeuver? *Resuscitation.* 1992;24:91.

318. Krischer JP, Fine EG, Davis JH, Nagel EL. Complications of cardiac resuscitation. *Chest.* 1987;92:287–291.

319. Scholz KH, Tebbe U, Herrmann C, Wojcik J, Lingen R, Chemnitius JM, Brune S, Kreuzer H. Frequency of complications of cardiopulmonary resuscitation after thrombolysis during acute myocardial infarction [see comments]. *Am J Cardiol.* 1992;69:724–728.

320. Bush CM, Jones JS, Cohle SD, Johnson H. Pediatric injuries from cardiopulmonary resuscitation. *Ann Emerg Med.* 1996;28:40–44.

321. Spevak MR, Kleinman PK, Belanger PL, Primack C, Richmond JM. Cardiopulmonary resuscitation and rib fractures in infants: a post-mortem. *JAMA.* 1994;272:617–618.

322. Centers for Disease Control. *Recommendations for Decontaminating Manikins Used in Cardiopulmonary Resuscitation.* Hepatitis Surveillance, Report 42. Atlanta, Ga: Centers for Disease Control; 1978;34–36.

323. The Emergency Cardiac Care Committee of the American Heart Association. Risk of infection during CPR training and rescue: supplemental guidelines. *JAMA.* 1989;262:2714–2715.

324. Mejicano GC, Maki DG. Infections acquired during cardiopulmonary resuscitation: estimating the risk and defining strategies for prevention. *Ann Intern Med.* 1998;129:813–828.

325. Stern A, Dickenson E. Don't be a dummy: staying safe with mannequin training. *J Emerg Med Serv JEMS.* 1994;19:85–86.

326. Corless IB, Lisker A, Buckheit RW. Decontamination of an HIV-contaminated CPR manikin. *Am J Public Health.* 1992;82:1542–1543.

327. Q & A: disinfecting Resusci Annes. *Healthcare Hazardous Materials Management.* 1992;5:11.

328. Bond WW, Favero MS, Petersen NJ, Ebert JW. Inactivation of hepatitis B virus by intermediate-to-high-level disinfectant chemicals. *J Clin Microbiol.* 1983;18:535–538.

329. Favero MS, Bond WW. Sterilization, disinfection and antisepsis in the hospital. In: Balows A, Hausler WJ Jr, Hermann KL, Eisenberg HD, Shadomy HJ, eds. *Manual of Clinical Microbiology.* 5th ed. Washington, DC: American Society for Microbiology; 1991:183–200.

330. Resnick L, Veren K, Salahuddin SZ, Tondreau S, Markham PD. Stability and inactivation of HTLV-III/LAV under clinical and laboratory environments. *JAMA.* 1986;255:1887–1891.

331. Martin LS, McDougal JS, Loskoski SL. Disinfection and inactivation of the human T lymphotropic virus type III/lymphadenopathy-associated virus. *J Infect Dis.* 1985;152:400–403.

332. McDougal JS, Cort SP, Kennedy MS, et al. Immunoassay for the detection and quantitation of infectious human retrovirus, lymphadenopathy-associated virus (LAV). *J Immunol Methods.* 1985;76:171–183.

333. Spire B, Dormont D, Barre-Sinoussi F, Montagnier L, Chermann JC. Inactivation of lymphadenopathy-associated virus by heat, gamma rays, and ultraviolet light. *Lancet.* 1985;1:188–189.

334. Sun D, Bennett RB, Archibald DW. Risk of acquiring AIDS from salivary exchange through cardiopulmonary resuscitation courses and mouth-to-mouth resuscitation. *Semin Dermatol.* 1995;14:205–211.

335. McCormack AP, Damon SK, Eisenberg MS. Disagreeable physical characteristics affecting bystander CPR. *Ann Emerg Med.* 1989;18:283–285.

336. Feldman HA. Some recollections of the meningococcal disease: the first Harry F. Dowling lecture. *JAMA.* 1972;220:1107–1112.

337. Finkelhor RS, Lampman JH. Herpes simplex infection following mouth-to-mouth resuscitation. *JAMA.* 1980;243:650. Letter.

338. Mannis MJ, Wendel RT. Transmission of herpes simplex during cardiopulmonary resuscitation training. *Compr Ther.* 1984;10:15–17.

339. Hendricks AA, Shapiro EP. Primary herpes simplex infection following mouth-to-mouth resuscitation. *JAMA.* 1980;243:257–258.

340. Todd MA, Bell JS. Shigellosis from cardiopulmonary resuscitation. *JAMA.* 1980;243:331. Letter.

341. Valenzuela TD, Hooten TM, Kaplan EL, Schlievert P. Transmission of "toxic strep" syndrome from an infected child to a firefighter during CPR. *Ann Emerg Med.* 1991;20:90–92.

342. Ahmad F, Senadhira DC, Charters J, Acquilla S. Transmission of salmonella via mouth-to-mouth resuscitation. *Lancet.* 1990;335:787–788. Letter.

343. Brenner B, Stark B, Kauffman J. The reluctance of house staff to perform mouth-to-mouth resuscitation in the inpatient setting: what are the considerations? *Resuscitation.* 1994;28:185–193.

344. Brenner B, Kauffman J, Sachter JJ. Comparison of the reluctance of house staff of metropolitan and suburban hospitals to perform mouth-to-mouth resuscitation. *Resuscitation.* 1996;32:5–12.

345. Michael AD, Forrester JS. Mouth-to-mouth ventilation: the dying art. *Am J Emerg Med.* 1992;10:156–161.

346. Bierens JJLM, Berden HJJM. Basic-CPR and AIDS. Are volunteer life-savers prepared for a storm? *Resuscitation.* 1996;32:185–191.

347. Axelsson A, Herlitz J, Ekstrom L, Holmberg S. Bystander-initiated cardiopulmonary resuscitation out-of-hospital: a first description of the bystanders and their experiences. *Resuscitation.* 1996;33:3–11.

348. Becker LB, Berg RA, Pepe PE, Idris AH, Aufderheide TP, Barnes TA, Stratton SJ, Chandra NC. A reappraisal of mouth-to-mouth ventilation during bystander-initiated cardiopulmonary resuscitation: a statement for healthcare professionals from the Ventilation Working Group of the Basic Life Support and Pediatric Life Support Subcommittees, American Heart Association. *Resuscitation.* 1997;35:189–201.

349. Centers for Disease Control. Guidelines for prevention of transmission of human immunodeficiency virus and hepatitis B virus to health-care and public-safety workers. *MMWR.* 1989;38(suppl 6):1–37.

350. Marcus R. Surveillance of health care workers exposed to blood from patients infected with the human immunodeficiency virus. *N Engl J Med.* 1988;319:1118–1123.

351. Sande MA. Transmission of AIDS: the case against casual contagion. *N Engl J Med.* 1986;314:380–382.

352. Lightsey DM, Shah PK, Forrester JS, Micheal TA. A human immunodeficiency virus-resistant airway for cardiopulmonary resuscitation. *Am J Emerg Med.* 1992;10:73–77.

353. Friedland GH, Saltzman BR, Rogers MF, et al. Lack of transmission of HTLV-III/LAV infection to household contacts of patients with AIDS or AIDS-related complex with oral candidiasis. *N Engl J Med.* 1986;314:344–349.

354. Fox PC, Wolff A, Yeh CK, Atkinson JC, Baum BJ. Saliva inhibits HIV-1 infectivity. *J Am Dent Assoc.* 1988;116:635–637.

355. Centers for Disease Control. Outbreak of multidrug-resistant tuberculosis—Texas, California, and Pennsylvania. *MMWR.* 1990;39:369–372.

356. Centers for Disease Control. Nosocomial transmission of multidrug-resistant tuberculosis among HIV-infected persons—Florida and New York, 1988–1991. *MMWR.* 1991;40:585–591.

357. Haley CE, McDonald RC, Rossi L, Jones WD Jr, Haley RW, Luby JP. Tuberculosis epidemic among hospital personnel. *Infect Control Hosp Epidemiol.* 1989;10:204–210.

358. Dooley SW Jr, Castro KG, Hutton MD, Mullan RJ, Polder JA, Snider DE Jr. Guidelines for preventing the transmission of tuberculosis in healthcare settings, with special focus on HIV-related issues. *MMWR.* 1990;39:1–29.

359. Centers for Disease Control. The use of preventive therapy for tuberculosis infection in the United States: recommendations of the Advisory Committee for Elimination of Tuberculosis. *MMWR.* 1990;39:9–12.

360. Steinberg JL, Nardell EA, Kass EH. Antibiotic prophylaxis after exposure to antibiotic-resistant *Mycobacterium* tuberculosis. *Rev Infect Dis.* 1988;10:1208–1219.

361. Piazza M, Chirianni A, Picciotto L, Guadagnino V, Orlando R, Cataldo PT. Passionate kissing and microlesions of the oral mucosa: possible role in AIDS transmission. *JAMA.* 1989;261:244–245. Letter.

362. Occupational Safety and Health Administration of Labor. Occupational exposure to bloodborne pathogens-final rule. 29 CFR Part 1910.1030, Part II (excerpts). *Fed Register.* 1991;56:64175–64182.

363. Harris MJ, Wendl RT. Transmission of herpes simplex during cardiopulmonary resuscitation. *Compr Ther.* 1984;10:15–17.

364. Ahmad F, et al. Transmission of salmonella via mouth-to-mouth resuscitation. *Lancet.* 1990;335:787.

365. Cydulka RK, Connor PJ, Myers TF, Pavza G, Parker M. Prevention of oral bacterial flora transmission by using mouth-to-mask. *J Emerg Med.* 1991;9:317–321.

366. Rumball CJ, MacDonald D. The PTL, Combitube, laryngeal mask, and oral airway: a randomized prehospital comparative study of ventilatory device effectiveness and cost effectiveness in 470 cases of cardiopulmonary arrest. *Prehosp Emerg Care.* 1997;1:1–10.

367. Staudinger T, Brugger S, Watschinger B, Roggla M, Dielacher C, Lobl T, et al. Emergency intubation with the Combitube: comparison with the endotracheal airway. *Ann Emerg Med.* 1993;22:1573–1575.

368. Staudinger T, Brugger S, Roggla M, Rintelen C, Atherton GL, Johnson JC, et al. Comparison of the Combitube with the endotracheal tube in cardiopulmonary resuscitation in the prehospital phase [in German]. *Wien Klin Wochenschr.* 1994;106:412–415.

369. Atherton GL, Johnson JC. Ability of paramedics to use the Combitube in prehospital cardiac arrest. *Ann Emerg Med.* 1993;22:1263–1268.

370. Bartlett RL, Martin SD, McMahon JM Jr, Schafermeyer RW, Vukich DJ, Hornung CA. A field comparison of the pharyngeotracheal lumen airway and the endotracheal tube. *J Trauma.* 1992;32:280–284.

371. Frass M, Frenzer R, Rauscha F, Schuster E, Glogar D. Ventilation with the esophageal tracheal Combitube in cardiopulmonary resuscitation: promptness and effectiveness. *Chest.* 1988;93:781–784.

372. Recommendation for prevention of HIV transmission in healthcare settings. *MMWR.* 1987;36:1S–18S.

Part 4: The Automated External Defibrillator
Key Link in the Chain of Survival

Major Guidelines Changes

Following are the major guidelines changes related to use of automated external defibrillators (AEDs) in basic life support:

1. Early defibrillation (shock delivery within 5 minutes of EMS call receipt) is a high-priority goal.
2. Healthcare providers with a duty to perform CPR should be trained, equipped, and authorized to perform defibrillation (Class IIa).
3. For in-hospital defibrillation:
   a. Early defibrillation capability, which is defined as having appropriate equipment and trained first responders, should be available throughout hospitals and affiliated outpatient facilities (Class IIa).
   b. The goal of early defibrillation by first responders is a collapse-to-shock interval, when appropriate, of <3 minutes in all areas of the hospital and ambulatory care facilities (Class I).
   c. Response time intervals for in-hospital resuscitation events are often inaccurate and must be corrected before documented times to defibrillation can be considered reliable (Class IIa).
4. Evidence supports establishment of public access defibrillation (PAD) programs in the following cases:
   a. The frequency of cardiac arrest events is such that there is a reasonable probability of one AED use in 5 years (estimated event rate of 1 sudden cardiac arrest per 1000 person-years).
   b. An EMS call–to-shock time interval of <5 minutes cannot be reliably achieved with conventional EMS services. In many communities, this EMS call–to-shock time interval can be achieved by training and equipping laypersons to
      • Function as first responders in the community
      • Recognize cardiac arrest
      • Activate the EMS system (phoning 911 or another appropriate emergency response number) at appropriate times
      • Provide CPR
      • Attach/operate an AED safely.
   c. For BLS responders such as police, firefighters, security personnel, sports marshals, ski patrol members, ferryboat crews, and airline flight attendants (referred to as level 1 responders in this document), education in CPR and the use of an AED is a Class IIa recommendation. For level 2 targeted responders such as citizens at worksites or in public places, this is a Class Indeterminate recommendation at this time. Likewise, for level 3 responders (family and friends of persons at high risk) this is a Class Indeterminate recommendation.
5. Use of AEDs in children >8 years of age (approximately >25 kg body weight) is a Class IIb recommendation.
6. Use of AEDs in infants and children <8 years of age is not recommended (Class Indeterminate).
7. Biphasic waveform defibrillation with shocks ≤200 J is safe and has equivalent or higher efficacy for termination of ventricular fibrillation (VF) compared with higher-energy escalating monophasic-waveform shocks (Class IIa).

Introduction

Public access defibrillation, which places AEDs in the hands of trained laypersons, has the potential to be the single greatest advance in the treatment of VF cardiac arrest since the development of CPR.[1–11] Time to defibrillation is the most important determinant of survival from cardiac arrest.[1–16] PAD provides the opportunity to defibrillate victims of cardiac arrest within a few minutes, even at sites remote from traditional EMS responders. Extraordinary survival rates—as high as 49%—have been reported in PAD programs.[17–24] These rates are twice those previously reported for the most effective EMS systems.[25]

AEDs are sophisticated, computerized devices that are reliable and simple to operate, enabling lay rescuers with minimal training to administer this lifesaving intervention.[1–24,26] Flight attendants, security personnel, sports marshals, police officers, firefighters, lifeguards, family members, and many other trained laypersons have used AEDs successfully.[15–24] AEDs are located in airports, airplanes, casinos, high-rise office buildings, housing complexes, recreational facilities, shopping malls, golf courses, and numerous other public locations.[15,16,23,24,27–29] AEDs are also used by healthcare professionals in ambulances, hospitals, dental clinics, and physicians' offices.[29–34]

With the inclusion of AED use as a BLS skill, BLS now encompasses the first 3 links in the Chain of Survival (early access, early CPR, and early defibrillation).[35] AEDs widely used by the public and distributed throughout the community significantly advance the concept proposed more than 2 decades ago: the community should become the "ultimate coronary care unit."[36]

Principle of Early Defibrillation

Early defibrillation is critical to survival from cardiac arrest for several reasons: (1) the most frequent initial rhythm in witnessed sudden cardiac arrest is VF; (2) the most effective treatment for VF is electrical defibrillation; (3) the probability of successful defibrillation diminishes rapidly over time; and

Circulation. 2000;102(suppl I):I-60–I-76.
© 2000 American Heart Association, Inc.

Circulation is available at http://www.circulationaha.org

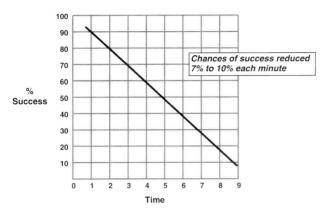

Figure 1. Composite data illustrating relationship between probability of survival to hospital discharge (indicated as "success" in figure) after VF cardiac arrest and interval between collapse and defibrillation. Based on data from Reference 41.

(4) VF tends to convert to asystole within a few minutes.[25,37–46] Many adults in VF can survive neurologically intact even if defibrillation is performed as late as 6 to 10 minutes after sudden cardiac arrest, particularly if CPR is provided.[25,37–46] The performance of CPR while awaiting the arrival of the AED appears to prolong VF, contributing to preservation of heart and brain function.[39,40] Basic CPR, however, is unlikely to convert VF to a normal rhythm.

The speed with which defibrillation is performed is the major determinant of the success of resuscitative attempts for treatment of VF cardiac arrest.[38–56] Survival rates after VF cardiac arrest decrease approximately 7% to 10% with every minute that defibrillation is delayed.[25,37–52] (See Figure 1.[41]) A survival rate as high as 90% has been reported when defibrillation is achieved within the first minute of collapse.[43–46] When defibrillation is delayed, survival rates decrease to approximately 50% at 5 minutes, approximately 30% at 7 minutes, approximately 10% at 9 to 11 minutes, and approximately 2% to 5% beyond 12 minutes.[25,37–52] One historical observational study suggests that survival may be improved if CPR is performed by first responders for 1 minute before defibrillation when defibrillation is delayed ≥4 minutes[57] and no bystander CPR is performed.

Survival rates from cardiac arrest can be remarkably high if the event is witnessed. For example, when people in supervised cardiac rehabilitation programs experience a witnessed cardiac arrest, defibrillation is usually performed within minutes; in 4 studies of cardiac arrest in this setting, 90 of 101 victims (89%) were resuscitated.[43–46] This is the highest survival rate reported for a defined out-of-hospital population.

Communities with no out-of-hospital ACLS services but with early defibrillation programs have reported improved survival rates among patients with cardiac arrest when survival rates for EMT care with and without AEDs were compared.[47–51] The most impressive results were reported by King County, Washington, where the survival rate of patients with VF improved from 7% to 26%,[47] and rural Iowa, where the survival rate rose from 3% to 19%.[48] More modest results have been observed in rural communities in southeastern Minnesota,[49] northeastern Minnesota,[50] and Wisconsin.[51] Af-

ter implementation of early defibrillation programs by EMS personnel in 5 European regions, survival to discharge from VF cardiac arrest was as high as 27% to 55%.[58]

Clearly the earlier defibrillation occurs, the better the prognosis.[38–56] Emergency personnel have only a few minutes after a victim's collapse to reestablish a perfusing rhythm. CPR can sustain a patient for a short time but cannot directly restore an organized rhythm. Restoration of an adequate perfusing rhythm requires defibrillation and advanced cardiovascular care, which must be administered within a few minutes of the initial arrest.[37] The use of AEDs increases the range of personnel who can use a defibrillator, shortening the time between collapse and defibrillation.[47–51,53–56] This exciting prospect accounts for the addition of this intervention as an integral component of BLS.

Early defibrillation (shock within 5 minutes of EMS call receipt) is a high-priority goal of EMS care. Every community should assess its capability to provide this intervention and institute whatever measures are necessary to make this recommendation a reality.

History of AEDs

In a prophetic report of what was to follow in the next 2 decades, Diack and colleagues[59] described experimental and clinical experience with the first AED. Subsequently, other studies provided supportive evidence for the potential role of such a device for widespread provision of rapid defibrillation.[60–62]

In the ensuing years, clinical studies have documented various aspects of AED performance, confirming the high sensitivity and specificity of the AED algorithms as well as the safety and efficacy of the devices.[62–76]

Another major advance in the use of AEDs was the development of a small (6.25-lb) AED specifically designed for home use. This AED delivered up to 3 nonescalating 180-J monophasic damped sinusoidal shocks and instructed the operator with easy-to-follow audible prompts. New AED models and manufacturers soon entered the field. Clinical evaluation confirmed the safety and efficacy of this AED in termination of out-of-hospital VF arrest.[72,76,77] Home trials were conducted and reported, but the concept of home defibrillation for patients at high risk was not yet ready for acceptance.[15,16,78–81]

In the last few years there has been a significant increase in the use of AEDs in early defibrillation programs in a variety of settings, including EMS systems, police departments, casinos, airport terminals, and commercial aircraft, among others.[12,13,17,18,20–24,82–84] In most of these settings, use of AEDs by BLS ambulance providers or first responders (PAD level 1 responders) in early defibrillation programs has been associated with a significant increase in survival rates. In some cases no benefit from such early defibrillation has been observed, usually in rural areas or systems in which EMS response is rapid enough to preclude benefit.[14,85,86] Also, improved survival will not be likely when infrequent bystander CPR and delays in dispatch impose weaknesses in other aspects of the Chain of Survival.[87] Long arrest-to-shock times (mean 23.8 minutes) and a low occurrence of bystander CPR (9%) were accompanied by a low survival rate (6%)

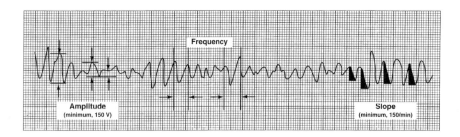

Figure 2. Features of an ECG analyzed by an AED.

from VF after introduction of AEDs in a large Asian city.[88] These and similar studies suggest that the introduction of AEDs into ambulance services may not significantly improve outcome unless other links in the Chain of Survival are optimized.[87] Guidelines for implementation of early defibrillation programs have been published that emphasize the components that are likely to result in improved patient outcomes, especially the critical links in the Chain of Survival.[89–91]

Advances in defibrillation waveform technology have been incorporated into AEDs, following the transition from monophasic to biphasic waveforms with implantable cardioverter-defibrillators (ICDs).[91a] Experimental and clinical evidence supporting the transition to biphasic waveforms in ICDs was abundant and consistent.[92–101] The use of biphasic defibrillation waveforms permits a reduction in the size and weight of AEDs, a major consideration in many settings, such as aircraft. Recommendations for specifying algorithm performance and demonstrating the equivalence of alternative waveforms were published by the American Heart Association Subcommittee on AED Safety and Efficacy in 1997.[102]

Contemporary AEDs

The term "AED" refers to an automated external defibrillator that incorporates a rhythm analysis system and a shock-advisory system.[103,104] The AED "advises" a shock and the operator must take the final action (press the SHOCK button) to deliver the shock. Fully automated external defibrillators do not require pressing the SHOCK button, and they are available only for special situations.

Automated Analysis of Cardiac Rhythms

Current AEDs are highly sophisticated, microprocessor-based devices that analyze multiple features of the surface ECG signal, including frequency, amplitude, and some integration of frequency and amplitude, such as slope or wave morphology (Figure 2). Various filters check for QRS-like signals, radio transmission, or 50- or 60-cycle interference as well as loose electrodes and poor electrode contact. Some intermittent radio transmissions can produce an ECG artifact if a transmitter or receiver is used within 6 feet of a patient during rhythm analysis. Some devices are programmed to detect spontaneous movement by the patient or movement of the patient by others.[103,104]

AEDs have been extensively tested, both in vitro against libraries of recorded cardiac rhythms[105] and clinically in numerous field trials.[59,60,62–64,67,68,72] Their accuracy in rhythm analysis is high.[62–64] The rare errors noted in field trials have been almost solely errors of omission (sensitivity) in which the device failed to recognize certain varieties of VF or tachycardia or when operators failed to follow recommended operating procedures, such as avoidance of patient movement.[66]

Inappropriate Shocks or Failure to Shock

Extensive clinical experience has revealed that AEDs are infrequently affected by movement of the patient (eg, seizures and agonal respirations), repositioning of the patient, or artifactual signals, although some rare difficulties have been reported.[59,60,62–64,66–68,72] Failure to follow the manufacturer's instructions for use of a fully automated external defibrillator has in rare instances (<0.1%) resulted in delivery of inappropriate electrical countershocks.[12] AEDs should be placed in the analysis mode only when full cardiac arrest has been confirmed and *only* when all movement, particularly patient transport, has ceased. Agonal respiration poses a problem because some devices may not be able to complete analysis cycles if the patient continues to have gasping respirations. Use of radio receivers and transmitters should be avoided during rhythm analysis. The major errors reported in clinical trials have been occasional failures to deliver shocks to rhythms that may benefit from electrical therapy, such as extremely fine or coarse VF.[62,64,66] Occasionally the analysis and treatment cycles of implanted and automated defibrillators can conflict.[64,66,106]

Ventricular Tachycardia

Although AEDs are not designed to deliver synchronized shocks, all AEDs will shock monomorphic and polymorphic ventricular tachycardia (VT) if the rate exceeds preset values. AEDs should be operated *only* on patients who are unresponsive, not breathing, and have no signs of circulation.

With this approach, the operator serves as a second verification system to confirm that the patient has suffered a cardiac arrest. In an apneic patient without signs of life, electrical shocks are indicated whether the rhythm is supraventricular tachycardia (SVT), VT, or VF. There have been rare reports of shocks delivered to responsive patients with perfusing ventricular or supraventricular arrhythmias.[12,62] These are operator errors, not device errors, and are preventable when rescuers are well trained and possess good patient assessment skills.[67]

Throughout this chapter, for laypersons the term "signs of circulation" means quickly evaluating the victim for normal breathing, coughing, or movement. For healthcare professionals the term "signs of circulation" means quickly performing a pulse check while simultaneously evaluating the victim for breathing, coughing, or movement.

Waveforms and Energy Levels

The energy settings for defibrillators are designed to provide the lowest effective energy needed to terminate VF. If energy and current are too low, the shock will not terminate the arrhythmia; if energy and current are too high, myocardial damage may result.[107–111] There is no clear relation between body size and energy requirements for defibrillation in adults. Modern AEDs fall into 2 broad categories of waveforms: monophasic and biphasic. Energy levels vary by type of device. Monophasic waveforms deliver current that is primarily of 1 polarity (ie, direction of current flow). They are further subdivided by the rate at which the current pulse decreases to zero; namely, either gradually (damped sinusoidal or instantaneously (truncated exponential). The waveforms of biphasic defibrillators indicate a sequence of 2 current pulses; the polarity of the second is opposite that of the first.

In a prospective out-of-hospital study of monophasic manual defibrillators, defibrillation rates and the proportion of patients resuscitated and later discharged from the hospital were virtually identical in patients who received initial monophasic damped sine (MDS) waveform shocks of 175 J and 320 J.[112] The recommended first-shock energy for monophasic waveform defibrillation is 200 J.[112] For monophasic devices the recommended second shock is 200 to 300 J; the recommended third shock is 360 J.[112] The intent of this escalating energy dosage protocol is to maximize shock success (termination of VF) while minimizing shock toxicity.[107–111]

The first biphasic waveform for use in an AED was approved in the United States in 1996. This impedance-compensating biphasic truncated exponential (BTE) waveform was incorporated into an AED that discharged nonescalating 150-J shocks. Impedance compensation was achieved by adjusting first-phase tilt, relative duration of the 2 phases, and total duration to a maximum of 20 ms. Experimental work in animals suggested the superiority of this waveform over monophasic truncated exponential (MTE) waveforms.[113] In-hospital studies during ICD testing compared 115-J and 130-J shocks using the BTE waveform with MDS waveform shocks of 200 J and 360 J.[114,115] This in-hospital data indicated that for short-duration VF, BTE shocks at low energy (115 J and 130 J) were as effective as the 200-J MDS shocks traditionally used for the first shock.[114,115] Fewer ST-segment changes were observed after transthoracic defibrillation of short-duration VF with the 115- and 130-J BTE shocks compared with those after 200-J MDS shocks.[116]

Another in-hospital study comparing an MDS waveform with a damped sinusoidal version of a biphasic waveform ("Gurvich") concluded that this biphasic waveform was likewise superior to the MDS waveform in terminating short-duration VT and VF.[117]

Early clinical experience with the 150-J, impedance-compensated BTE waveform for treatment of out-of-hospital long-duration VF was also positive.[118,119] This experience, along with in-hospital clinical data, formed the basis for the AHA evidence-based review of this low-energy biphasic waveform defibrillation, which led to an initial Class IIb recommendation.[120] Since then, cumulative experience with this waveform in 100 patients with VF was reported, con-

firming its efficacy in terminating VF arrest outside the hospital.[121] The aggregate data with this waveform in VF arrest from one EMS system (Rochester, Minn) also affirmed the efficacy of this waveform for terminating VF.[82] This experience was compared retrospectively with that of the MDS waveform in the same EMS system.[82] The growing body of evidence is now considered sufficient to support a Class IIa recommendation for this low-energy, BTE waveform.

Other versions of biphasic waveforms have been introduced and have undergone initial evaluation during electrophysiology study and ICD implantation and testing. Experience with short-duration VF, in which a low-energy (120- to 170-J), constant-current, rectilinear biphasic waveform was used has recently been reported.[122] This waveform has also been very effective in terminating atrial fibrillation during elective cardioversion with energies as low as 70 J.[123] At this time no studies have reported experience with other biphasic waveforms in long-duration VF in out-of-hospital arrest. When such data becomes available, it will need to be assessed by the same evidence-evaluation process as used for the biphasic AED and this guidelines process.

The data indicates that biphasic waveform shocks of relatively low energy (≤ 200 J) are safe and have equivalent or higher efficacy for termination of VF compared with higher-energy escalating monophasic waveform shocks (Class IIa). The safety and efficacy data related to specific biphasic waveforms must be evaluated on an individual basis in both in-hospital (electrophysiology studies, ICD testing) and out-of-hospital settings.

Evaluation of Defibrillation Waveform Performance

The evaluation of defibrillation shock waveform efficacy requires the adoption of standard descriptors of defibrillation and postshock rhythms.[124] Clinical investigators should uniformly apply such descriptors in the assessment of defibrillation waveforms. The term "defibrillation" means reversal of the action of fibrillation. Defibrillation is not a synonym for "shock." Thus, defibrillation should be understood to mean termination of fibrillation and should not be confused with other resuscitation outcomes, such as restoration of a perfusing rhythm, admission to hospital, or discharge survival.[125] These additional end points may occur during resuscitation as a consequence of many variables, including time from collapse to shock and other interventions, such as CPR and drug therapy.

In several recent studies,[82,119,126] a successful defibrillatory shock was defined as the absence of VF 5 seconds after shock delivery. This definition of shock outcome was one of several considered by the 1999 Evidence Evaluation experts as acceptable to define "success" in evaluation of defibrillator waveforms. Thus, asystole or non-VF electrical activity at the postshock end point constitutes "success" because VF has been terminated. This is consistent with data from electrophysiological mapping studies confirming the time course of termination of VF after shock delivery, and clinically it is an easily measurable point in time after a shock.[127,128] At this point the direct effect of the shock on VF is not influenced by many other interventions that may ensue after shock delivery, such as chest compressions, ventilation, and administration of drugs, which themselves have an impact on cardiac rhythm after shocks. Examining the rhythm 5 seconds after each of the first series of shocks, before any drugs or other advanced life support interventions are initiated, will yield the most useful specific information about shock efficacy. In addition, tracking the postshock rhythm during the first minute after shock delivery will provide additional data, such as whether an organized rhythm is supraventricular or idioventricular and whether or not a perfusing rhythm accompanies restoration of organized electrical activity.

As new defibrillation waveforms evolve and are evaluated in out-of-hospital arrest, it is essential that standardized definitions of shock efficacy be accepted and uniformly applied by clinical investigators engaged in waveform research. The definitions proposed here help meet that need.

Operation of the AED

Before attaching the AED, the operator should first determine whether special situations exist that contraindicate the use of the AED or require additional actions before its use.

Special Situations That May Require Additional Actions

While preparing to use the AED, the operator must identify 4 possible circumstances (special situations) that may require rescuers to modify their actions before or during AED use. These situations include victims in water, those <8 years of age or <25 kg, those with transdermal medication patches, and those with implanted pacemakers or ICDs. Metal surfaces are *not* included as a special circumstance because they pose no shock hazard to either victim or rescuer.

Water

Water is a good conductor of electricity and may provide a pathway for energy from the AED to rescuers and bystanders treating the victim. There is a small possibility that rescuers or bystanders may receive shocks or minor burns if they are within such a pathway. Water on the skin of the chest can also provide a direct path of energy from one electrode pad to the other (arcing) and can decrease the effectiveness of the shock delivered to the heart. It is critical to quickly remove the victim from freestanding water and dry the victim's chest before using the AED. If the victim has a diving injury or other possible spinal injury, care should be taken to maintain cervical spine immobilization while moving the victim and performing resuscitation.

Children

Cardiac arrest is less common in children than adults, and its causes are more diverse.[129–132] Approximately 50% of pediatric cardiac arrests occur in children <1 year old.[129] Most of these are caused by sudden infant death syndrome and respiratory disease.[129–132] Beyond the first 6 months of life, injuries and drowning are the major causes of cardiac arrest.[129–132] The most common terminal rhythm observed in patients ≤17 years of age is asystole or pulseless electrical activity.[129,131–137] When pediatric cardiac arrest rhythms are reported, estimates of VF range from 7% to 15%.[129,131,133–135,138] In some studies, pediatric patients with VF who receive defibrillation at the scene have a

higher initial resuscitation rate and are more likely to be discharged from the hospital with good neurological outcomes than pediatric patients who present with non-VF rhythms.[131,133]

Experience with AEDs in children is very limited. The sensitivity and specificity for children of the AED algorithm need further study. The data suggests that AEDs can accurately detect VF in children of all ages (sensitivity),[139–141] but there is inadequate data on the ability of AEDs to correctly identify nonshockable tachycardic rhythms in infants (specificity).[141] Although the available data is encouraging, more data in larger pediatric populations is needed to define AED algorithm sensitivity and specificity.

More studies are also needed to determine AED energy doses that are safe and effective for children. In adults, clinical reports of biphasic waveform AED use have described energy doses as low as 120 J, with success rates equal to 200-J monophasic shocks for termination of VF; less postresuscitation myocardial dysfunction was observed after lower-energy shocks.[122,142,143] Currently available AEDs deliver energy doses that exceed the recommended monophasic dose of 2 to 4 J/kg in most children <8 years of age. The median weight of children more than 8 years of age is typically >25 kg; therefore, the delivered *initial* dose from a monophasic or biphasic AED (150 to 200 J) will be <10 J/kg for this age group. Data from animals suggests that this may be a safe dose, although human pediatric data is extremely limited.[144] At this time attempted defibrillation of VF/pulseless VT detected by an AED may be considered in older children (≥8 years old, approximately >25 kg body weight), particularly in the out-of-hospital setting. A weight of 25 kg corresponds to a body length of approximately 50 in (128 cm) using a Broselow color-coded tape.[144a]

In summary, although VF is not a common arrhythmia in children, it is observed in as many as 15% of pediatric and adolescent arrests.[129,131,133–135,137] In these patients rapid defibrillation may improve outcomes.[131,133,138] Multicenter or controlled studies of AED algorithm sensitivity and specificity are needed, as well as a clearer definition of appropriate energy doses for children of all ages and sizes.

For these reasons, use of AEDs in children ≥8 years old (approximately >25 kg body weight) is a Class IIb recommendation. Use of AEDs in infants and children <8 years old is not recommended, primarily because of the lack of data concerning sensitivity, specificity, safety, and efficacy (Class Indeterminate). Healthcare providers who routinely care for children at risk for arrhythmias and cardiac arrest (eg, in-hospital settings) should continue to use defibrillators capable of appropriate energy adjustment. For infants and children <8 years old who are in cardiac arrest, the initial priorities continue to be support of the airway, oxygenation, and ventilation.

Transdermal Medications

AED electrodes should not be placed directly on top of a transdermal medication patch (eg, nitroglycerin, nicotine, analgesics, hormone replacements, antihypertensives), because the patch may block delivery of energy from the electrode pad to the heart and may cause small burns to the skin.[145] The only problems reported with shocks over a transdermal patch have involved patches with a metal backing. Metal backing for patches is no longer being used, so this potential problem has been eliminated. Medication patches should be removed and the area wiped clean before the AED electrode pad is attached.

Implanted Pacemakers/ICDs

Defibrillators that deliver a limited number of low-energy shocks directly to the myocardium have been implanted in selected patients with a history of malignant arrhythmias. These devices create a hard lump beneath the skin of the upper chest or abdomen (usually on the victim's left side). The lump is about half the size of a pack of cards and usually has a small overlying scar. Placement of an AED electrode pad directly over an implanted medical device may reduce the effectiveness of defibrillation attempts.[146] Instead, place the pad at least 1 inch (2.5 cm) away from the implanted device. Then follow the usual steps for operating an AED.[146] However, if the ICD is delivering shocks to the patient (ie, the patient's muscles contract in a manner like that observed during external defibrillation), allow 30 to 60 seconds for the ICD to complete the treatment cycle. Occasionally the analysis and shock cycles of automatic ICDs and AEDs will conflict.[106] (See "Part 6, Section 2: Defibrillation" for guidelines for management of patients with ICDs.)

The "Universal AED": Common Steps to Operate All AEDs

It is recommended that AEDs used in PAD programs (eg, large buildings, shopping malls, or homes) be stored next to a telephone. This allows the rescuer to activate the EMS system (by phoning 911 or another appropriate emergency telephone number) and retrieve the AED quickly. In some settings (eg, airports), security personnel or the local EMS system are automatically notified when the AED is retrieved from its storage case.

Position the AED close to the supine victim's ear. Performing defibrillation protocols from the victim's *left* side allows better access to the AED controls and easier placement of electrode pads. The left-side position also provides space for a second rescuer to perform CPR from the victim's right side. This position, however, may not be accessible in all clinical settings. Alternative positions and operator roles may be used with equal success.

AEDs are available in several models. There are small differences from model to model, but all AEDs operate in basically the same way.[103,104] The 4 universal steps of AED operation are as follows:

Step 1: POWER ON the AED

The first step in operating an AED is to turn the power on. This initiates voice prompts, which guide the operator through subsequent steps. To turn the AED on, press a power switch or lift the monitor cover or screen to the "up" position.

Step 2: Attach electrode pads

Quickly open and attach the self-adhesive monitor-defibrillator electrode pads directly to the skin of the victim's chest. In some models the pads and cables are preconnected

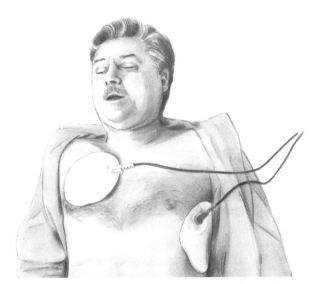

Figure 3. AED electrode pad placement on the victim.

to the AED. Other devices may require a connection between the cable and AED or between the cable and electrode pads.

Place the electrode pads on the upper-right sternal border (directly below the clavicle) and lateral to the left nipple, with the top margin of the pad a few inches (approximately 7 cm) below the axilla (Figure 3). The correct position of the electrode pads is often illustrated on the pads themselves or another part of the AED. Stop CPR just before attaching the pads.

If the victim is noticeably diaphoretic, dry the chest with a cloth or towel before attaching the electrode pads.

If the victim has a hairy chest, the adhesive electrode pads may stick to the hair on the chest, preventing effective contact with the skin of the chest and causing transthoracic impedance to be high,[147] leading to a *"check electrodes"* or *"check electrode pads"* message from the AED. This problem may be resolved by pressing firmly on each pad. If the error message continues, briskly remove the original pads (this will remove the hair under the pad) and apply a second set of electrodes. If the problem continues, shave the chest in the area of the pads before attaching a third set of electrodes. Alternatively, clip hair close to the chest or shave the chest hair before applying the second set of electrodes.

Step 3: Analyze the rhythm

Clear rescuers and bystanders from the victim and ensure that no one is touching the victim. To prevent artifactual errors, avoid all movement affecting the patient during rhythm analysis.[12,52] In some devices the operator presses an ANALYZE button to initiate rhythm analysis. Other devices automatically begin analysis when the electrode pads are attached to the chest. Rhythm analysis requires from 5 to 15 seconds, depending on the brand of AED. If VF is present, the device will announce it through a displayed message, visual or auditory alarm, or voice-synthesized statement that a shock is indicated.

Step 4: Clear the victim and press the SHOCK button

Before pressing the SHOCK button, ensure that no one is touching the victim. Always loudly state a "Clear the patient" message, such as "I'm clear, you're clear, everybody clear" or simply "Clear." At the same time perform a visual check to ensure that no one is in contact with the patient. In most devices, the capacitors charge automatically if a treatable rhythm is detected. A tone, voice-synthesized message, or light indicates that charging has started. Delivery of a shock should occur only after the victim is "cleared."[148] The shock will produce a sudden contraction of the patient's musculature (like that seen with a conventional defibrillator).

After the first shock, do not restart CPR. Some AED models require that the rescuer immediately press the ANA-LYZE button. In other models the AED will automatically begin rhythm analysis after shock delivery. If VF persists, the AED will indicate it, and the *"shock indicated"* and *"charging"* sequence will repeat for a second and, if needed, third shock. The AED is programmed to reanalyze the victim's rhythm and provide a shock as quickly as possible after each shock, to a total of 3 shocks. The purpose of this cluster or series of 3 shocks is to identify and treat a shockable rhythm as quickly as possible. Therefore, during the series of 3 shocks the rescuer should not interrupt or interfere with the rapid analysis and shock pattern. AEDs are programmed to pause after each group of 3 shocks to allow 1 minute for CPR. Therefore, after 3 shocks, check signs of circulation and prepare to provide chest compressions and continue compressions and ventilations for 1 minute (see below).

Outcomes and Actions After Attempted Defibrillation

"Shock Indicated" Message: Recurrent VF

If signs of circulation do not return after 3 shocks, rescuers without immediate ACLS backup should resume CPR for 60 seconds. After 60 seconds most devices will prompt a check for signs of circulation. If VF continues, deliver additional rounds of 3 "stacked" shocks after appropriate analysis. Provide sets of 3 stacked shocks followed by 1 minute of CPR until the AED gives a *"no shock indicated"* message or ACLS is available.

Do not check for signs of circulation between stacked shocks, ie, after shocks 1 and 2, 4 and 5, 7 and 8, etc. Checking for signs of circulation between shocks will delay rapid identification and shocking of persistent VF. The rapid sequence of shocks has the additional advantage of modestly reducing transthoracic impedance; this reduction will increase the effective energy delivered.

"No Shock Indicated" Message

Signs of Circulation Absent

When the AED gives a *"no shock indicated"* message, check for signs of circulation, and if there are no signs of circulation, resume CPR. Three *"no shock indicated"* messages suggest that there is a low probability that the rhythm can be successfully defibrillated. Therefore, rhythm analysis should be repeated only after 1- to 2-minute intervals of CPR. CPR should then be discontinued during rhythm analysis. No one should touch the victim during analysis.

Signs of Circulation Present

If signs of circulation are present, check breathing. If the victim is not breathing, provide rescue breathing at a rate of 10 to 12 breaths per minute. If the victim is breathing adequately, place him or her in a recovery position. The AED should always be left attached. If VF recurs, most AEDs will prompt the rescuer to check for signs of circulation (or *"check patient"*). The device will then charge automatically and advise the rescuer to deliver an additional shock.

AEDs in a Moving Ambulance

AEDs can be left in place during transport of the patient in a moving vehicle. But never push the ANALYZE button while the patient is in transport, because the movement of the ambulance can interfere with rhythm assessment and artifact can simulate VF.[12,52] Some devices continuously analyze the patient. If rhythm analysis is necessary during transport or if the AED prompts the rescuer to check the patient or recommends a shock, stop the vehicle, then reanalyze.

One Rescuer With an AED

In some situations, 1 rescuer with immediate access to an AED may respond to a cardiac arrest. The rescuer should quickly activate the EMS system or the emergency medical response system on the premises (eg, airport security personnel or the hospital resuscitation team) to summon ACLS providers. The recommended BLS rescue sequence for adults is as follows:

1. Verify unresponsiveness.
2. Activate EMS (or the emergency medical response system) at the appropriate time.
3. Open the airway, check breathing.
4. If the victim is not breathing, provide initial ventilations (2 in the United States; up to 5 in other countries).
5. Check for signs of circulation. If there are no signs of circulation, attach the AED and follow the AED treatment algorithm.

Reasonable variations in this sequence are acceptable.

Integration of CPR and AED Use

When arriving at the scene of a suspected cardiac arrest, rescuers must rapidly integrate CPR with use of the AED. In most out-of-hospital and in-hospital situations, rescuers will have the benefit of having 1 or more additional rescuers to assist with the multiple actions needed to resuscitate a victim of sudden cardiac death. In general, 3 actions must occur simultaneously at the scene of a cardiac arrest: (1) activation of the EMS system (or emergency medical response system, such as the hospital resuscitation team), (2) CPR, and (3) operation of the AED. When 2 or more rescuers are present, these functions can be initiated simultaneously. AED operators should be trained in scene leadership and team management to ensure timely and effective actions by multiple rescuers.[149]

Care After Successful Defibrillation

When signs of circulation and breathing return, place the patient in a recovery position and leave the AED attached. Continue to monitor the victim. Many AEDs monitor rhythm continuously and advise the operator if fibrillation recurs. It is

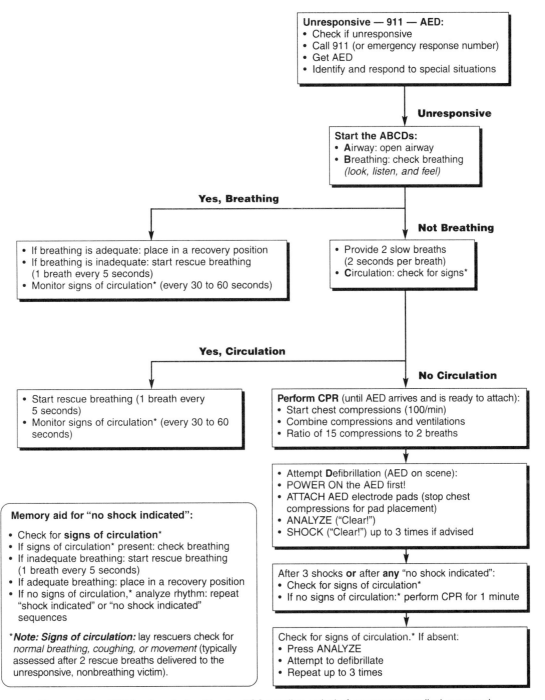

Figure 4. The AED treatment algorithm for ECC pending arrival of emergency medical personnel.

important to check breathing and signs of circulation frequently.

AED programs should coordinate with the local EMS system to ensure seamless transfer of care after the arrival of BLS or ACLS healthcare providers.

The AED treatment algorithm (Figure 4) summarizes the approach to the cardiac arrest victim while using an AED.

Device Maintenance and Quality Assurance

Appropriate maintenance of the AED is vital for proper operation.[150,151] AED manufacturers provide specific recommendations for maintenance and readiness, which should be followed carefully. Checklists have been developed to help identify and prevent maintenance deficiencies and suggest methods of uniform device testing. Use of these checklists will increase user familiarity with the equipment.[152] Newer AED models require almost no maintenance. These devices conduct a self-check of operation and indicate "readiness to use." Nonetheless, operators trained to use an AED must still ensure that the AED is ready to use at any time.

Medical Direction

Legislation and regulations regarding EMS authority and the use of AEDs vary from country to country and even from one

EMS system to another. In general, ambulance providers can perform some medical procedures in emergencies, but only with a physician's medical authorization.[153] The authorizing physician assumes medical direction and takes legal responsibility for the activity of BLS ambulance providers, including the use of AEDs. The authorizing physician for a PAD program oversees implementation of the program, issues standing orders for BLS personnel who operate AEDs, and monitors the system to ensure continuous quality improvement. In areas such as the United States, where AEDs are considered medical equipment, the rescuer must operate the AED under the authority of either the medical director or administrative codes of the state or commonwealth.[153]

Case-by-Case Review
Ideally the medical director or designated representative should review every event in which an AED is used (or could have been used). This means every incident in which CPR was performed or an AED used should undergo a medical review to establish whether the patient was treated according to professional standards and local standing orders. Medical reviews should also determine whether VF and other rhythms were treated appropriately with defibrillation and BLS. Other dimensions of performance that can be evaluated include command of the scene, safety, efficiency, speed, professionalism, ability to troubleshoot, completeness of patient care, and interactions with other professionals and bystanders.[65]

Quality Assurance
Organized collection and review of patient data can identify systemwide problems and allow assessment of each link in the Chain of Survival for the adult victim of sudden cardiac death. The Utstein Guidelines for reporting out-of-hospital cardiac arrest data present the recommended data to enable quality assurance monitoring for EMS and resuscitation programs (see also "Part 12: From Science to Survival").[154] This data collection constitutes quality assurance activities and as such should not expose clinical providers or organizations to increased risk of liability. Adult victims of witnessed cardiac arrest of presumed cardiac etiology caused by VF appear to be the best group on which to focus. A lower-than-expected hospital discharge rate in this group may be explained by long ambulance response times, delayed activation of EMS, infrequent witnessed arrests, rare bystander CPR, or slow on-scene times to defibrillation. Each of these problems can be addressed with a specific programwide effort. Continued systematic and uniform data collection will determine whether the new efforts succeed.

Emergency Cardiovascular Care Systems and the AED

The ECC Systems Concept
The term "Chain of Survival"[35] provides a useful metaphor for the elements of the ECC systems concept, summarizing the best approach to treatment of persons in sudden cardiac arrest.[155] The 4 links in the chain are early access to the EMS system, early CPR, early defibrillation, and early advanced cardiovascular life support. Epidemiological and clinical research have established that effective emergency cardiovascular care, whether in or out of hospital, requires that each of these links be strong, yet all are interconnected.[35,41,156,157] The effectiveness of early defibrillation and PAD programs also depends on a strong Chain of Survival in the community.

Early Defibrillation
Early defibrillation with an AED has established benefit. The principle of early defibrillation[53–56] suggests that the first person to arrive at the scene of a cardiac arrest should have a defibrillator.[52] This principle is now internationally accepted.[89] Healthcare providers with a duty to perform CPR should be trained, equipped, and authorized to attempt defibrillation[155] (Class IIa). Healthcare providers who may be first responders include BLS ambulance providers,[58,158–160] hospital-based healthcare providers,[30–34] and trained laypersons in PAD programs.[161,162]

Out-of-Hospital BLS Providers and AEDs
BLS emergency medical responders have different names in different countries, but BLS providers are the most common type of emergency responder in the world. These rescuers provide BLS but do not provide invasive interventions such as tracheal intubation, IV access, or IV medications. In Europe, BLS providers are often called "ambulancemen," "ambulance drivers," or "ambulance personnel." In the United States they are usually called "emergency medical technicians" (EMTs). In these Guidelines they are referred to as "BLS personnel," "BLS rescuers," "BLS providers," or "BLS ambulance personnel." Because BLS providers are typically the first emergency personnel to reach the scene of an out-of-hospital cardiac arrest, they can provide rapid defibrillation with an AED.

Early studies demonstrated a trend to superior survival rates with the use of AEDs in out-of-hospital cardiac arrest by BLS ambulance providers.[42,72] These studies also established many practical advantages of AED use by BLS ambulance providers, including easy, brief, and inexpensive initial training and continuing education, as well as evidence that AEDs can be operated more quickly than conventional defibrillators.[64,66,72] Subsequent studies have confirmed these findings, including AED accuracy,[163] shorter times to defibrillation,[69,70,164] faster application of subsequent ACLS interventions,[69] and comparable[165–167] or improved[12,71,168–171] survival. Taken together, these studies stand as powerful confirmation of the value of early defibrillation by out-of-hospital emergency personnel.[172]

The clinical benefits and practical superiority of the AED are well established. Early defibrillation is recommended as a standard of care for EMS[28,90,172] except in sparsely populated and remote settings, where the frequency of cardiac arrest is low and rescuer response times are excessively long.[173–175]

In-Hospital Use of AEDs
An approach pioneered by William Kaye and others[30–34] is now being used by many hospitals: general care nurses are being trained to use AEDs in resuscitation attempts. Hospital records were examined in several hospitals before AED placement to determine the average in-hospital time to first shock. This examination documented an unexpected and disturbing performance problem in many medical facilities:

long delays (5 to 10 minutes) before conventional in-hospital response teams first attempt defibrillation.[176,177] Delayed defibrillation occurs infrequently in monitored beds and critical care units, but it occurs more often in unmonitored hospital beds and outpatient and diagnostic facilities, which hundreds of patients enter and leave each day. In such areas several minutes may elapse before centralized response teams arrive with a defibrillator, attach it, and deliver shocks.[176] Resuscitation committees may inappropriately place more emphasis on arrival of the resuscitation team than on delivery of the first defibrillatory shock.[30] As with out-of-hospital care, in-hospital practice must shift from a focus on CPR as the core of BLS care.[30,178]

In recognition of the new AED technology, BLS has expanded to include CPR *and* defibrillation. An unacceptably high percentage of hospitals lack methods to assess resuscitation performance, underuse personnel in resuscitative efforts, and have not made significant attempts to improve the availability of early defibrillation by placing AEDs in non–critical care areas.[179,180]

Several obstacles must be overcome before a quality early defibrillation program in which AEDs are used can be successfully implemented in the hospital. Nurses can be trained to use an AED and retain the skills needed for its safe and effective operation.[30,181]

Strategic deployment of AEDs throughout hospital areas and authorization and training of first-responding personnel in their use is necessary to bring in-hospital use of AEDs up to the level of the out-of-hospital setting.[32,33]

Documentation of in-hospital resuscitation events is often inaccurate and therefore unreliable in making quantitative assessments of such critical components as time to defibrillation and other interventions during resuscitation. This must be corrected before any data can be considered reliable enough to provide accurate assessment of resuscitation practices.

The absence of in-hospital early defibrillation programs is evident in the scarcity of data related to deployment of AEDs in hospital and its impact on patient outcome.[32] Some studies have documented the components of a successful program such as acquisition and retention of skills in AED use by nurses, including a recommendation that AED use be incorporated into BLS training of all hospital personnel expected to respond to a cardiac arrest.[30] Early defibrillation capability should be available in ambulatory care facilities as well as throughout hospital inpatient areas.

The International Liaison Committee on Resuscitation and the European Resuscitation Council have included in their guidelines formal recommendations for establishing in-hospital early defibrillation programs.[89,90,182]

One regulatory organization is attempting to improve systemwide response to resuscitation. In the United States, the Joint Commission for the Accreditation of Healthcare Organizations (JCAHO) altered its standards for individual in-hospital resuscitation capabilities by evaluating the following characteristics[183]:

1. Appropriate policies, procedures, processes, or protocols for provision of resuscitation services

2. Appropriate equipment placed strategically throughout the hospital close to areas where patients are likely to need resuscitation services
3. Ongoing review of outcomes related to resuscitation in the aggregate to identify opportunities for improvement of resuscitative efforts
4. Appropriate staff trained and competent to recognize the need for and use of designated equipment in resuscitative efforts
5. Appropriate data collection related to the process and outcomes of resuscitation, particularly the ability to track trends and changes over several years

The AHA has established the National Registry of Cardiopulmonary Resuscitation to assist participating hospitals with systematic data collection of resuscitative efforts. The objectives of the registry are to develop a well-defined database documenting resuscitation performance of hospitals over time. This information can establish a hospital's baseline performance, target problem areas, and identify opportunities for improvement in data collection and the resuscitation program in general. The registry is also the largest repository of information on in-hospital cardiopulmonary arrest. Patterned after the highly respected British Resuscitation Study (Bresus), the registry is based on the Utstein Guidelines for collecting and reporting information from in-hospital resuscitation events.[184] Further guidelines for in-hospital resuscitation will emerge from future analyses of the large database provided by the registry. Participation in the registry will also allow hospitals to fully comply with the new JCAHO standards.

The capability to provide early defibrillation within patient-care areas is an obligation of the modern hospital. Early defibrillation is achieved by having defibrillators (including AEDs), ventilation equipment, and trained responders available throughout hospitals and affiliated outpatient facilities (Class IIa). The goal for all hospitals should be to have first responders provide *early* defibrillation to collapsed patients in VF in all areas of the hospital and ambulatory care facilities (Class I). The principle of early defibrillation should be "the earlier the better," and evaluation and intervention should occur when prolonged collapse-to-shock intervals are documented. Experts at the international Guidelines 2000 Conference endorsed a goal of 3 ± 1 minutes for the collapse-to-shock interval for a high percentage of in-hospital arrests.

When medical quality assurance monitoring is instituted, it is important to note that recorded response-time intervals for in-hospital resuscitation events are notoriously inaccurate. The most common methods used to time events are unsynchronized wristwatches and wall and bedside clocks. This asynchrony must be corrected before documentation of times to defibrillation will be consistently reliable. In many countries AEDs could easily be equipped with a timing mechanism that is synchronized with governmental atomic clock satellites. The AED clock could then become the gold standard for timing resuscitation events. Accurate time-interval data must be obtained because it is the key to future high-quality research (Class IIa).

Public Access Defibrillation

The concept of early defibrillation with AEDs was originally developed and explored by Douglas Chamberlain in Brighton, England, where AEDs were placed in train stations and commercial aircraft, and by Mickey Eisenberg in King County, Washington, who placed AEDs with families of high-risk patients. To develop strategies to implement programs of *early* defibrillation in the community, the AHA Task Force on Early Defibrillation hosted 2 conferences (in 1994 and 1997) on the subject of PAD.[27,28]

The recommendations that emerged from those conferences included the recognition that AEDs are the most promising method for achieving rapid defibrillation and that AEDs and training in their use should be accessible to the community.[27,28,185] Advisory statements from ILCOR (1997)[185] and the European Resuscitation Council (1998)[182] affirmed the importance of early defibrillation programs.

Placement of AEDs in selected locations for immediate use by trained laypersons may be the key intervention to significantly increase survival from out-of-hospital cardiac arrest. The demonstrated safety and effectiveness of the AED make it an ideal source of early defibrillation by trained laypersons.[52,62] Conceptually the AED and rescuer function as a sharp diagnostic and therapeutic probe searching for just 1 phenomenon—VF/pulseless (no circulation) VT—and providing a potentially lifesaving therapy over just a few seconds. AEDs are of no value for non-VF/pulseless VT arrest and provide no benefit after VF/pulseless VT has been terminated. Therefore, the rescuer must also be trained to open the airway and support ventilation and circulation with chest compressions as needed. For this reason, all persons who operate an AED still must be trained to recognize emergencies, including cardiac arrest, and to provide effective CPR.

PAD Rescuers

PAD implies expanded use of AEDs in the community to the broadest possible number of rescuers while maintaining safety and effectiveness.[27,28,186] Within the next few years an increasing range of laypersons and healthcare professionals will learn the combined skills of CPR and AED use. These diverse groups can be roughly categorized into 3 levels of PAD responders, although the number and type of such responders change daily.

Level 1: Nontraditional Responders

Nontraditional responders are persons other than healthcare personnel, such as police, firefighters, security personnel, sports marshals, ski patrol members, ferryboat crews, and flight attendants, whose job duties require them to respond to an emergency. Traditionally, however, they have not been asked or expected to take any action other than to perform basic CPR.

Level 2: Targeted Responders

Targeted, or worksite, responders, who may also be called "citizen responders," frequently participate in PAD programs. These responders are employees of companies, corporations, or public facilities with established PAD programs. Their location at the worksite (eg, central reception area staff) makes them a natural choice to be the primary responder with the AED. PAD programs can shorten the time to defibrillation

and improve the chance of survival from sudden cardiac death in the workplace or community.

Level 3: Responders to Persons at High Risk

Family members and friends living with or visiting persons at high risk for cardiac emergencies are another potential category of responders. They often participate in early defibrillation programs and are taught CPR and use of an AED when a friend or loved one is at high risk for sudden cardiac death.

Deployment Strategies for PAD Programs

Before deploying AEDs, PAD program directors should determine whether the population in the geographic area covered by the program will be likely to benefit from it. Some PAD planners target locations with a large concentration of persons >50 years old, such as senior citizen centers.[187] Implementation of AED programs in places where >10 000 people gather has been recommended for consideration.[188] Ideally program planners should review communitywide cardiac arrest data, identify sites with the highest incidence of cardiac arrest, and target those locations for AED placement.

Location

Some data is available on the location and frequency of cardiac arrest events in metropolitan areas. In Seattle and King County, Washington, for example, the incidence of cardiac arrest is greatest at the international airport, then (in decreasing order of frequency) county correctional facilities, shopping malls, public sports venues, industrial sites, golf courses, shelters, ferries/train terminals, health clubs/gyms, and community/senior centers.[189] The site-specific incidence and need for specific distribution of AEDs within those sites is likely to vary with each community. To optimize the benefit of limited healthcare resources in each community, program planners must provide AEDs and make trained rescuers available in locations with the highest incidence of cardiac arrest.

Accordingly, the evidence supports establishment of PAD programs at sites in which

1. The frequency of cardiac arrest events is such that there is a reasonable probability of AED use (an estimated event rate of 1 sudden cardiac arrest per 1000 person-years).
2. An EMS call–to-shock time interval of <5 minutes cannot be reliably achieved with conventional EMS services.
3. An EMS call–to-shock time interval of <5 minutes can be reliably achieved (in >90% of cases) by training and equipping laypersons to function as first responders in the community EMS system, recognizing cardiac arrest, phoning 911 (or another appropriate emergency telephone number), initiating CPR, and attaching/operating an AED.

For level 1 responders, such as police, firefighters, security personnel, ski patrol members, ferryboat crews, and flight attendants, this is a Class IIa recommendation. For level 2 targeted responders, such as citizens at worksites or in public places, this is a Class Indeterminate recommendation at this time. It is hoped that data from a prospective, randomized multicenter trial regarding PAD will justify a change in this class of recommendation. For level 3 responders (family and friends of persons at high risk), the above recommendation is a Class Indeterminate recommendation.

Coordination With EMS Systems

PAD program planners should attempt to coordinate PAD programs with the local EMS system. This may include but is not limited to medical direction, assistance in planning AED deployment and AED protocols, training, continuous quality improvement, monitoring, and review of AED events. Integration with the local EMS dispatch system is important because many dispatch systems use phone-directed protocols to assist rescuers in the use of the AED if needed and will notify EMS en route that an AED is being used at the scene.[190,191] The American College of Emergency Physicians has issued a policy statement endorsing coordination with EMS systems to ensure medical direction of AED programs, including those in which bystanders use AEDs.[192] Many other international organizations have issued similar recommendations.[89,90,182]

Elements of Successful PAD Programs

Objective data on details of successful PAD programs is lacking. Nonetheless, rational conjecture plus data extrapolated from other sources have identified many elements as keys to successful PAD programs. There must be a strong Chain of Survival within the community. Innovative methods of providing effective, quality training to laypersons in the use of AEDs is important.[149] Incorporating EMS dispatch into PAD programs allows dispatchers to direct a caller to the nearest AED location and provide instruction by telephone if needed. It also allows the EMS personnel to learn to operate specific types of AEDs in advance, enabling seamless patient care.[190,191]

Careful planning, training, communication with the EMS system, and continuous quality improvement are vital to a successful PAD program. The program director should carefully select AED users who are motivated, available during the expected response period, and capable of performing their duties. A specific response plan should be implemented within each site, targeting a collapse-to-defibrillation time ≤4 to 5 minutes (eg, AEDs located throughout the facility so that the walk to retrieve an AED is no more than 1.5 minutes). Frequent unannounced practice drills and evaluations of performance and response time are recommended.

The most frequent cause of AED malfunction is lack of maintenance.[150,151] Maintaining the device according to the manufacturer's specifications is essential.[152] Regular system evaluations should be conducted.

PAD program directors must also attend to the emotional needs of lay rescuers, who are not accustomed to providing lifesaving care in an emergency.[193] Case-by-case review with laypersons and critical incident stress debriefing provide important support for PAD program participants.[193] Medical direction includes responsibility for quality of training and medical care provided by PAD lay responders. PAD programs must comply with local or regional regulation and legislation.

Effectiveness of PAD Programs

Several studies have demonstrated the cost-effectiveness of AED use by BLS ambulance providers and PAD programs compared with other medical interventions.[53,187,194,195] This data establishes the substantial survival benefits and attractive cost-effectiveness of a well-designed and well-implemented PAD program.

The National Heart, Lung, and Blood Institute (NHLBI), in partnership with the AHA and industry, has embarked on a multisite, controlled, prospective clinical trial to determine the efficacy and cost-effectiveness of placing AEDs in a variety of public settings. Such definitive scientific evidence is essential for decision making related to the potentially huge PAD initiative. Final results from the PAD trial are not expected for at least 3 years. The results of a large, controlled, randomized, multicenter, prospective clinical trial will eventually be needed for PAD to be considered a Class I recommendation.

Education and Training

Skills Maintenance

Survey results and experience in rural communities have demonstrated that emergency responders may go several years without treating a patient in cardiac arrest.[173–175] Therefore, every program director must determine how to ensure correct performance of BLS and automated external defibrillation. Principles of adult education suggest that frequent practice of psychomotor skills such as use of an AED in a simulated cardiac arrest offers the best opportunity for skills maintenance.

Frequency of Practice

The frequency and content of these practice sessions have been established by several successful programs.[6,51,173] At present many programs provide practice drills every 3 to 6 months and have found this interval satisfactory. Many EMS personnel and systems drill as often as once a month. The most successful long-term skills maintenance occurs when individual rescuers perform a quick check of the equipment frequently and regularly. This check includes a visual inspection of the defibrillator components and controls and a mental review of the steps to take and controls to operate during a cardiac arrest.

The AHA ECC Committee and international expert panels encourage routine skills review and practice sessions at least every 6 months.

Future of PAD

The future of PAD is likely to include further improvements in device design, making AEDs easier to use, lighter, and less expensive. Public access to AEDs is increasing, and implementation of AEDs in a diversity of settings is growing as well. Automated external defibrillation will continue to increase survival from VF if AED programs are well implemented and AEDs are used within the first few minutes after cardiac arrest.

References

1. Atkins JM. Emergency medical service systems in acute cardiac care: state of the art. *Circulation.* 1986;74(suppl IV):IV-4–IV-8.

2. Cummins RO, Eisenberg MS, Stults KR. Automatic external defibrillators: clinical issues for cardiology. *Circulation.* 1986;73:381–385.

3. White RD. EMT-defibrillation: time for controlled implementation of effective treatment. *AHA Emergency Cardiac Care Newsletter.* 1986; 8:1–3.

4. Atkins JM, Murphy D, Allison EJ, Graves JR. Toward earlier defibrillation: first responders are next. *J Emerg Med Serv.* 1986;11:50–57.

5. Eisenberg MS, Cummins RO. Defibrillation performed by the emergency medical technician. *Circulation.* 1986;74(suppl IV):IV-9–IV-12.

6. Cummins RO. EMT-defibrillation: national guidelines for implementation. *Am J Emerg Med.* 1987;5:254–257.

7. Ruskin JN. Automatic external defibrillators and sudden cardiac death[editorial]. *N Engl J Med.* 1988;319:713–715.

8. Cummins RO, Eisenberg MS. EMT-defibrillation: a proven concept. *American Heart Association Emergency Cardiac Care National Faculty Newsletter.* 1984;1:1–3.

9. Cummins RO, Eisenberg MS, Moore JE, Hearne TR, Andresen E, Wendt R, Litwin PE, Graves JR, Hallstrom AP, Pierce J. Automatic external defibrillators: clinical, training, psychological, and public health issues. *Ann Emerg Med.* 1985;14:755–760.

10. Newman MM. National EMT-D study. *J Emerg Med Serv.* 1986;11: 70–72.

11. Newman MM. The survival advantage: early defibrillation programs in the fire service. *J Emerg Med Serv.* 1987;12:40–46.

12. Sedgwick ML, Watson J, Dalziel K, Carrington DJ, Cobbe SM. Efficacy of out of hospital defibrillation by ambulance technicians using automated external defibrillators: the Heartstart Scotland Project. *Resuscitation.* 1992;24:73–87.

13. Mols P, Beaucarne E, Bruyninx J, Labruyere JP, De Myttenaere L, Naeije N, Watteeuw G, Verset D, Flamand JP. Early defibrillation by EMTs: the Brussels experience. *Resuscitation.* 1994;27:129–136.

14. Stapczynski JS, Svenson JE, Stone CK. Population density, automated external defibrillator use, and survival in rural cardiac arrest. *Acad Emerg Med.* 1997;4:552–558.

15. Cummins RO, Eisenberg MS, Bergner L, Hallstrom A, Hearne T, Murray JA. Automatic external defibrillation: evaluations of its role in the home and in emergency medical services. *Ann Emerg Med.* 1984; 13:798–801.

16. Jacobs L. Medical, legal, and social implications of automatic external defibrillators[editorial]. *Ann Emerg Med.* 1986;15:863–864.

17. White RD, Vukov LF, Bugliosi TF. Early defibrillation by police: initial experience with measurement of critical time intervals and patient outcome. *Ann Emerg Med.* 1994;23:1009–1013.

18. White RD, Asplin BR, Bugliosi TF, Hankins DG. High discharge survival rate after out-of-hospital ventricular fibrillation with rapid defibrillation by police and paramedics. *Ann Emerg Med.* 1996;28: 480–485.

19. White RD, Hankins DG, Bugliosi TF. Seven years' experience with early defibrillation by police and paramedics in an emergency medical services system. *Resuscitation.* 1998;39:145–151.

20. Davis EA, Mosesso VN Jr. Performance of police first responders in utilizing automated external defibrillation on victims of sudden cardiac arrest. *Prehosp Emerg Care.* 1998;2:101–107.

21. Mosesso VN Jr, Davis EA, Auble TE, Paris PM, Yealy DM. Use of automated external defibrillators by police officers for treatment of out-of-hospital cardiac arrest. *Ann Emerg Med.* 1998;32:200–207.

22. Davis EA, McCrorry J, Mosesso VN Jr. Institution of a police automated external defibrillation program: concepts and practice. *Prehosp Emerg Care.* 1999;3:60–65.

23. O'Rourke MF, Donaldson E, Geddes JS. An airline cardiac arrest program [see comments]. *Circulation.* 1997;96:2849–2853.

24. Wolbrink A, Borrillo D. Airline use of automatic external defibrillators: shocking developments [see comments]. *Aviat Space Environ Med.* 1999;70:87–88.

25. Eisenberg MS, Horwood BT, Cummins RO, Reynolds-Haertle R, Hearne TR. Cardiac arrest and resuscitation: a tale of 29 cities. *Ann Emerg Med.* 1990;19:179–186.

26. Gundry JW, Comess KA, DeRook FA, Jorgenson D, Bardy GH. Comparison of naive sixth-grade children with trained professionals in the use of an automated external defibrillator. *Circulation.* 1999;100: 1703–1707.

27. Nichol G, Hallstrom AP, Kerber R, Moss AJ, Ornato JP, Palmer D, Riegel B, Smith S Jr, Weisfeldt ML. American Heart Association report

28. on the Second Public Access Defibrillation Conference, April 17–19, 1997. *Circulation.* 1998;97:1309–1314.

28. Weisfeldt ML, Kerber RE, McGoldrick RP, Moss AJ, Nichol G, Ornato JP, Palmer DG, Riegel B, Smith SC Jr. Public access defibrillation: a statement for healthcare professionals from the American Heart Association Task Force on Automatic External Defibrillation. *Circulation.* 1995;92:2763.

29. Wassertheil J, Keane G, Fisher N, Leditschke GF. Cardiac arrest outcomes at the Melbourne Cricket Ground and Shrine of Remembrance, using a tiered response strategy: a forerunner to public access defibrillation. *Resuscitation.* 2000;44:97–104.

30. Kaye W, Mancini ME, Giuliano KK, Richards N, Nagid DM, Marler CA, Sawyer-Silva S. Strengthening the in-hospital chain of survival with rapid defibrillation by first responders using automated external defibrillators: training and retention issues. *Ann Emerg Med.* 1995;25: 163–168.

31. Kaye W, Mancini ME, Richards N. Organizing and implementing a hospital-wide first-responder automated external defibrillation program: strengthening the in-hospital chain of survival. *Resuscitation.* 1995;30: 151–156.

32. Destro A, Marzaloni M, Sermasi S, Rossi F. Automatic external defibrillators in the hospital as well? *Resuscitation.* 1996;31:39–43; discussion 43–44.

33. Kaye W, Mancini ME. Improving outcome from cardiac arrest in the hospital with a reorganized and strengthened chain of survival: an American view [editorial]. *Resuscitation.* 1996;31:181–186.

34. Mancini ME, Kaye W. In-hospital first-responder automated external defibrillation: what critical care practitioners need to know. *Am J Crit Care.* 1998;7:314–319.

35. Cummins RO, Ornato JP, Thies WH, Pepe PE. Improving survival from sudden cardiac arrest: the "chain of survival" concept. A statement for health professionals from the Advanced Cardiac Life Support Subcommittee and the Emergency Cardiac Care Committee, American Heart Association. *Circulation.* 1991;83:1832–1847.

36. McIntyre KM. Cardiopulmonary resuscitation and the ultimate coronary care unit[editorial] *JAMA.* 1980;244:510–511.

37. Eisenberg MS, Cummins RO, Damon S, Larsen MP, Hearne TR. Survival rates from out-of-hospital cardiac arrest: recommendations for uniform definitions and data to report. *Ann Emerg Med.* 1990;19: 1249–1259.

38. Eisenberg MS, Copass MK, Hallstrom A, Cobb LA, Bergner L. Management of out-of-hospital cardiac arrest: failure of basic emergency medical technician services. *JAMA.* 1980;243:1049–1051.

39. Eisenberg MS, Hallstrom AP, Copass MK, Bergner L, Short F, Pierce J. Treatment of ventricular fibrillation: emergency medical technician defibrillation and paramedic services. *JAMA.* 1984;251:1723–1726.

40. Weaver WD, Copass MK, Bufi D, Ray R, Hallstrom AP, Cobb LA. Improved neurologic recovery and survival after early defibrillation. *Circulation.* 1984;69:943–948.

41. Larsen MP, Eisenberg MS, Cummins RO, Hallstrom AP. Predicting survival from out-of-hospital cardiac arrest: a graphic model. *Ann Emerg Med.* 1993;22:1652–1658.

42. Eisenberg MS, Bergner L. Paramedic programs and cardiac mortality: description of a controlled experiment. *Public Health Rep.* 1979;94: 80–84.

43. Fletcher GF, Cantwell JD. Ventricular fibrillation in a medically supervised cardiac exercise program: clinical, angiographic, and surgical correlations. *JAMA.* 1977;238:2627–2629.

44. Haskell WL. Cardiovascular complications during exercise training of cardiac patients. *Circulation.* 1978;57:920–924.

45. Hossack KF, Hartwig R. Cardiac arrest associated with supervised cardiac rehabilitation. *J Cardiac Rehab.* 1982;2:402–408.

46. Van Camp SP, Peterson RA. Cardiovascular complications of outpatient cardiac rehabilitation programs. *JAMA.* 1986;256:1160–1163.

47. Eisenberg MS, Copass MK, Hallstrom AP, Blake B, Bergner L, Short FA, Cobb LA. Treatment of out-of-hospital cardiac arrests with rapid defibrillation by emergency medical technicians. *N Engl J Med.* 1980; 302:1379–1383.

48. Stults KR, Brown DD, Schug VL, Bean JA. Prehospital defibrillation performed by emergency medical technicians in rural communities. *N Engl J Med.* 1984;310:219–223.

49. Vukov LF, White RD, Bachman JW, O'Brien PC. New perspectives on rural EMT defibrillation. *Ann Emerg Med.* 1988;17:318–321.

50. Bachman JW, McDonald GS, O'Brien PC. A study of out-of-hospital cardiac arrests in northeastern Minnesota. *JAMA.* 1986;256:477–483.

51. Olson DW, LaRochelle J, Fark D, Aprahamian C, Aufderheide TP, Mateer JR, Hargarten KM, Stueven HA. EMT-defibrillation: the Wisconsin experience [see comments]. *Ann Emerg Med.* 1989;18:806–811.

52. Cummins RO. From concept to standard-of-care? Review of the clinical experience with automated external defibrillators. *Ann Emerg Med.* 1989;18:1269–1275.

53. Valenzuela TD, Roe DJ, Cretin S, Spaite DW, Larsen MP. Estimating effectiveness of cardiac arrest interventions: a logistic regression survival model. *Circulation.* 1997;96:3308–3313.

54. Holmberg M, Holmberg S, Herlitz J, Gardelov B. Survival after cardiac arrest outside hospital in Sweden: Swedish Cardiac Arrest Registry. *Resuscitation.* 1998;36:29–36.

55. Valenzuela TD, Spaite DW, Meislin HW, Clark LL, Wright AL, Ewy GA. Case and survival definitions in out-of-hospital cardiac arrest: effect on survival rate calculation [see comments]. *JAMA.* 1992;267:272–274.

56. Valenzuela TD, Spaite DW, Meislin HW, Clark LL, Wright AL, Ewy GA. Emergency vehicle intervals versus collapse-to-CPR and collapse-to-defibrillation intervals: monitoring emergency medical services system performance in sudden cardiac arrest. *Ann Emerg Med.* 1993;22:1678–1683.

57. Cobb LA, Fahrenbruch CE, Walsh TR, Copass MK, Olsufka M, Breskin M, Hallstrom AP. Influence of cardiopulmonary resuscitation prior to defibrillation in patients with out-of-hospital ventricular fibrillation [see comments]. *JAMA.* 1999;281:1182–1188.

58. Herlitz J, Bahr J, Fischer M, Kuisma M, Lexow K, Thorgeirsson G. Resuscitation in Europe. a tale of five European regions. *Resuscitation.* 1999;41:121–131.

59. Diack AW, Welborn WS, Rullman RG, Walter CW, Wayne MA. An automatic cardiac resuscitator for emergency treatment of cardiac arrest. *Med Instrum.* 1979;13:78–83.

60. Jaggarao NS, Heber M, Grainger R, Vincent R, Chamberlain DA, Aronson AL. Use of an automated external defibrillator-pacemaker by ambulance staff. *Lancet.* 1982;2:73–75.

61. Rozkovec A, Crossley J, Walesby R, Fox KM, Maseri A. Safety and effectiveness of a portable external automatic defibrillator-pacemaker. *Clin Cardiol.* 1983;6:527–533.

62. Cummins RO, Eisenberg M, Bergner L, Murray JA. Sensitivity, accuracy, and safety of an automatic external defibrillator. *Lancet.* 1984;2:318–320.

63. Cummins RO, Eisenberg MS, Litwin PE, Graves JR, Hearne TR, Hallstrom AP. Automatic external defibrillators used by emergency medical technicians: a controlled clinical trial. *JAMA.* 1987;257:1605–1610.

64. Stults KR, Brown DD, Kerber RE. Efficacy of an automated external defibrillator in the management of out-of-hospital cardiac arrest: validation of the diagnostic algorithm and initial clinical experience in a rural environment. *Circulation.* 1986;73:701–709.

65. Cummins RO, Austin D Jr, Graves JR, Hambly C. An innovative approach to medical control: semiautomatic defibrillators with solid-state memory modules for recording cardiac arrest events. *Ann Emerg Med.* 1988;17:818–824.

66. Dickey W, Dalzell GW, Anderson JM, Adgey AA. The accuracy of decision-making of a semi-automatic defibrillator during cardiac arrest. *Eur Heart J.* 1992;13:608–615.

67. Jakobsson J, Nyquist O, Rehnqvist N. Effects of early defibrillation of out-of-hospital cardiac arrest patients by ambulance personnel. *Eur Heart J.* 1987;8:1189–1194.

68. Gray AJ, Redmond AD, Martin MA. Use of the automatic external defibrillator-pacemaker by ambulance personnel: the Stockport experience. *Br Med J.* 1987;294:1133–1135.

69. Hoekstra JW, Banks JR, Martin DR, Cummins RO, Pepe PE, Stueven HA, Jastremski M, Gonzalez E, Brown CG, the Multicenter High Dose Epinephrine Study Group. Effect of first-responder automated defibrillation on time to therapeutic interventions during out-of-hospital cardiac arrest. [see comments]. *Ann Emerg Med.* 1993;22:1247–1253.

70. Shuster M, Keller JL. Effect of fire department first-responder automated defibrillation. *Ann Emerg Med.* 1993;22:721–727.

71. Auble TE, Menegazzi JJ, Paris PM. Effect of out-of-hospital defibrillation by basic life support providers on cardiac arrest mortality: a metaanalysis [see comments]. *Ann Emerg Med.* 1995;25:642–648.

72. Weaver WD, Hill D, Fahrenbruch CE, Copass MK, Martin JS, Cobb LA, Hallstrom AP. Use of the automatic external defibrillator in the management of out-of-hospital cardiac arrest. *N Engl J Med.* 1988;319:661–666.

73. Kroll MW, Brewer JE. Automated external defibrillators: design considerations. *New Horiz.* 1997;5:128–136.

74. Niskanen RA. Automated external defibrillators: experiences with their use and options for their further development. *New Horiz.* 1997;5:137–144.

75. Sunde K, Eftestol T, Askenberg C, Steen PA. Quality assessment of defibrillation and advanced life support using data from the medical control module of the defibrillator. *Resuscitation.* 1999;41:237–247.

76. Weaver WD, Copass MK, Hill DL, Fahrenbruch C, Hallstrom AP, Cobb LA. Cardiac arrest treated with a new automatic external defibrillator by out-of-hospital first responders. *Am J Cardiol.* 1986;57:1017–1021.

77. Weaver WD, Hill DL, Fahrenbruch C, Cobb LA, Copass MK, Hallstrom AP, Martin J. Automatic external defibrillators: importance of field testing to evaluate performance. *J Am Coll Cardiol.* 1987;10:1259–1264.

78. Moore JE, Eisenberg MS, Andresen E, Cummins RO, Hallstrom A, Litwin P. Home placement of automatic external defibrillators among survivors of ventricular fibrillation. *Ann Emerg Med.* 1986;15:811–812.

79. Moore JE, Eisenberg MS, Cummins RO, Hallstrom A, Litwin P, Carter W. Lay person use of automatic external defibrillation. *Ann Emerg Med.* 1987;16:669–672.

80. Eisenberg MS, Moore J, Cummins RO, Andresen E, Litwin PE, Hallstrom AP, Hearne T. Use of the automatic external defibrillator in homes of survivors of out-of-hospital ventricular fibrillation. *Am J Cardiol.* 1989;63:443–446.

81. Cummins RO, Schubach JA, Litwin PE, Hearne TR. Training lay persons to use automatic external defibrillators: success of initial training and one-year retention of skills. *Am J Emerg Med.* 1989;7:143–149.

82. Gliner BE, White RD. Electrocardiographic evaluation of defibrillation shocks delivered to out-of-hospital sudden cardiac arrest patients. *Resuscitation.* 1999;41:133–144.

83. Karch SB, Graff J, Young S, Ho CH. Response times and outcomes for cardiac arrests in Las Vegas casinos. *Am J Emerg Med.* 1998;16:249–253.

84. Page RL, Hamdan MH, McKenas DK. Defibrillation aboard a commercial aircraft. *Circulation.* 1998;97:1429–1430.

85. Kellermann AL, Hackman BB, Somes G, Kreth TK, Nail L, Dobyns P. Impact of first-responder defibrillation in an urban emergency medical services system [see comments]. *JAMA.* 1993;270:1708–1713.

86. Joyce SM, Davidson LW, Manning KW, Wolsey B, Topham R. Outcomes of sudden cardiac arrest treated with defibrillation by emergency medical technicians (EMT-Ds) or paramedics in a two-tiered urban EMS system. *Prehosp Emerg Care.* 1998;2:13–17.

87. Sweeney TA, Runge JW, Gibbs MA, Raymond JM, Schafermeyer RW, Norton HJ, Boyle-Whitesel MJ. EMT defibrillation does not increase survival from sudden cardiac death in a two-tiered urban-suburban EMS system. *Ann Emerg Med.* 1998;31:234–240.

88. Liu JCZ. Evaluation of the use of automatic external defibrillation in out-of-hospital cardiac arrest in Hong Kong. *Resuscitation.* 1999;41:113–119.

89. Bossaert L, Handley A, Marsden A, Arntz R, Chamberlain D, Ekstrom L, Evans T, Monsieurs K, Robertson C, Steen P. European Resuscitation Council guidelines for the use of automated external defibrillators by EMS providers and first responders: a statement from the Early Defibrillation Task Force, with contributions from the Working Groups on Basic and Advanced Life Support, and approved by the Executive Committee. *Resuscitation.* 1998;37:91–94.

90. Kloeck W, Cummins RO, Chamberlain D, Bossaert L, Callanan V, Carli P, Christenson J, Connolly B, Ornato JP, Sanders A, Steen P. Early defibrillation: an advisory statement from the Advanced Life Support Working Group of the International Liaison Committee on Resuscitation. *Circulation.* 1997;95:2183–2184.

91. McDowell R, Krohmer J, Spaite DW, Benson N, Pons P, American College of Emergency Physicians. Guidelines for implementation of early defibrillation/automated external defibrillator programs. *Ann Emerg Med.* 1993;22:740–741.

91a. Gurvich NL, Makarychev VA. Defibrillation of the heart with biphasic electrical impulses. *Kardiologiya.* 1967;7:109–112.

92. Jones JL, Jones RE, Balasky G. Microlesion formation in myocardial cells by high-intensity electric field stimulation. *Am J Physiol.* 1987;253:H480–H486.

93. Walcott GP, Walcott KT, Knisley SB, Zhou X, Ideker RE. Mechanisms of defibrillation for monophasic and biphasic waveforms. *Pacing Clin Electrophysiol.* 1994;17:478–498.

94. Bardy GH, Ivey TD, Allen MD, Johnson G, Mehra R, Greene HL. A prospective randomized evaluation of biphasic versus monophasic waveform pulses on defibrillation efficacy in humans. *J Am Coll Cardiol.* 1989;14:728–733.

95. Kwaku KF, Dillon SM. Shock-induced depolarization of refractory myocardium prevents wave-front propagation in defibrillation. *Circ Res.* 1996;79:957–973.

96. Jones JL, Tovar OH. The mechanism of defibrillation and cardioversion. *Proc IEEE.* 1996;84:392–403.

97. Jones JL, Tovar OH. Threshold reduction with biphasic defibrillator waveforms: role of charge balance. *J Electrocardiol.* 1995;28(suppl):25–30.

98. Tovar OH, Jones JL. Biphasic defibrillation waveforms reduce shock-induced response duration dispersion between low and high shock intensities. *Circ Res.* 1995;77:430–438.

99. Jones JL, Swartz JF, Jones RE, Fletcher R. Increasing fibrillation duration enhances relative asymmetrical biphasic versus monophasic defibrillator waveform efficacy. *Circ Res.* 1990;67:376–384.

100. Winkle A, Mead R, Ruder M, Gaudiani V, Buch W, Pless B, Sweeney M, Schmidt P. Improved low energy defibrillation efficacy in man with the use of a biphasic truncated exponential waveform. *Am Heart J.* 1989;117:122–127.

101. Sweeney RJ, Gill RM, Steinberg MI, Reid PR. Ventricular refractory period extension caused by defibrillation shocks [see comments]. *Circulation.* 1990;82:965–972.

102. Kerber R, Becker L, Bourland J, Cummins R, Hallstrom A, Michos M, Nichol G, Ornato J, Thies W, White R, Zuckerman B. Automatic external defibrillators for public access defibrillation: recommendations for specifying and reporting arrhythmia analysis, algorithm performance, incorporating new waveforms, and enhancing safety. *Circulation.* 1997;95:1677–1682.

103. Stults KR, Cummins RO. Fully automatic versus shock advisory defibrillators: what are the issues? *J Emerg Med Services.* 1987;12:71–73.

104. Stults KR, Brown DD, Cooley F, Kerber RE. Self-adhesive monitor/defibrillation pads improve prehospital defibrillation success. *Ann Emerg Med.* 1987;16:872–877.

105. Cummins RO, Stults KR, Haggar B, Kerber RE, Schaeffer S, Brown DD. A new rhythm library for testing automatic external defibrillators: performance of three devices. *J Am Coll Cardiol.* 1988;11:597–602.

106. Monsieurs KG, Conraads VM, Goethals MP, Snoeck JP, Bossaert LL. Semiautomatic external defibrillation and implanted cardiac pacemakers: understanding the interactions during resuscitation. *Resuscitation.* 1995;30:127–131.

107. Kerber RE, Martins JB, Kienzle MG, Constantin L, Olshansky B, Hopson R, Charbonnier F. Energy, current, and success in defibrillation and cardioversion: clinical studies using an automated impedance-based method of energy adjustment. *Circulation.* 1988;77:1038–1046.

108. Geddes LA, Tacker WA, Rosborough JP, Moore AG, Cabler PS. Electrical dose for ventricular defibrillation of large and small animals using precordial electrodes. *J Clin Invest.* 1974;53:310–319.

109. Gutgesell HP, Tacker WA, Geddes LA, Davis S, Lie JT, McNamara DG. Energy dose for ventricular defibrillation of children. *Pediatrics.* 1976;58:898–901.

110. Dahl C, Ewy G, Warner E, et al. Myocardial necrosis from direct current countershock. *Circulation.* 1974;50:956.

111. Pantridge JF, Adgey AA, Webb SW, Anderson J. Electrical requirements for ventricular defibrillation. *BMJ.* 1975;2:313–315.

112. Weaver WD, Cobb LA, Copass MK, Hallstrom AP. Ventricular defibrillation: a comparative trial using 175-J and 320-J shocks. *N Engl J Med.* 1982;307:1101–1106.

113. Gliner B, Lyster T, Dillion S, Bardy G. Transthoracic defibrillation of swine with monophasic and biphasic waveforms. *Circulation.* 1995;92:1634–1643.

114. Bardy GH, Gliner BE, Kudenchuk PJ, Poole JE, Dolack GL, Jones GK, Anderson J, Troutman C, Johnson G. Truncated biphasic pulses for transthoracic defibrillation. *Circulation.* 1995;91:1768–1774.

115. Bardy GH, Marchlinski FE, Sharma AD, Worley SJ, Luceri RM, Yee R, Halperin BD, Fellows CL, Ahern TS, Chilson DA, Packer DL, Wilber DJ, Mattioni TA, Reddy R, Kronmal RA, Lazzara R, Transthoracic Investigators. Multicenter comparison of truncated biphasic shocks and standard damped sine wave monophasic shocks for transthoracic ventricular defibrillation. *Circulation.* 1996;94:2507–2514.

116. Reddy RK, Gleva MJ, Gliner BE, Dolack GL, Kudenchuk PJ, Poole JE, Bardy GH. Biphasic transthoracic defibrillation causes fewer ECG ST-segment changes after shock. *Ann Emerg Med.* 1997;30:127–134.

117. Greene HL, DiMarco JP, Kudenchuk PJ, Scheinman MM, Tang AS, Reiter MJ, Echt DS, Chapman PD, Jazayeri MR, Chapman FW, et al, for the Biphasic Waveform Defibrillation Investigators. Comparison of monophasic and biphasic defibrillating pulse waveforms for transthoracic cardioversion. *Am J Cardiol.* 1995;75:1135–1139.

118. White RD. Early out-of-hospital experience with an impedance-compensating low-energy biphasic waveform automatic external defibrillator. *J Intervent Card Electrophysiol.* 1997;1:203–208; discussion 209–210.

119. Poole JE, White RD, Kanz KG, Hengstenberg F, Jarrard GT, Robinson JC, Santana V, McKenas DK, Rich N, Rosas S, Merritt S, Magnotto L, Gallagher JV III, Gliner BE, Jorgenson DB, Morgan CB, Dillon SM, Kronmal RA, Bardy GH, LIFE Investigators. Low-energy impedance-compensating biphasic waveforms terminate ventricular fibrillation at high rates in victims of out-of-hospital cardiac arrest. *J Cardiovasc Electrophysiol.* 1997;8:1373–1385.

120. Cummins RO, Hazinski MF, Kerber RE, Kudenchuk P, Becker L, Nichol G, Malanga B, Aufderheide TP, Stapleton EM, Kern K, Ornato JP, Sanders A, Valenzuela T, Eisenberg M. Low-energy biphasic waveform defibrillation: evidence-based review applied to emergency cardiovascular care guidelines: a statement for healthcare professionals from the American Heart Association Committee on Emergency Cardiovascular Care and the Subcommittees on Basic Life Support, Advanced Cardiac Life Support, and Pediatric Resuscitation. *Circulation.* 1998;97:1654–1667.

121. Gliner BE, Jorgenson DB, Poole JE, White RD, Kanz KG, Lyster TD, Leyde KW, Powers DJ, Morgan CB, Kronmal RA, Bardy GH, LIFE Investigators. Treatment of out-of-hospital cardiac arrest with a low-energy impedance-compensating biphasic waveform automatic external defibrillator. *Biomed Instrum Technol.* 1998;32:631–644.

122. Mittal S, Ayati S, Stein KM, Knight BP, Morady F, Schwartzman D, Cavlovich D, Platia EV, Calkins H, Tchou PJ, Miller JM, Wharton JM, Sung RJ, Slotwiner DJ, Markowitz SM, Lerman BB, ZOLL Investigators. Comparison of a novel rectilinear biphasic waveform with a damped sine wave monophasic waveform for transthoracic ventricular defibrillation. *J Am Coll Cardiol.* 1999;34:1595–1601.

123. Mittal S, Ayati S, Stein KM, Schwartzman D, Cavlovich D, Tchou PJ, Markowitz SM, Slotwiner DJ, Scheiner MA, Lerman BB. Transthoracic cardioversion of atrial fibrillation: comparison of rectilinear biphasic versus damped sine wave monophasic shocks. *Circulation.* 2000;101:1282–1287.

124. White RD. External defibrillation: the need for uniformity in analyzing and reporting results [editorial; comment]. *Ann Emerg Med.* 1998;32:234–236.

125. Cummins RO, Eisenberg MS, Hallstrom AP, Hearne TR, Graves JR, Litwin PE. What is a "save"? Outcome measures in clinical evaluations of automatic external defibrillators. *Am Heart J.* 1985;110:1133–1138.

126. White RD, Blanton DM. Biphasic truncated exponential waveform defibrillation. *Prehosp Emerg Care.* 1999;3:283–289.

127. Chen PS, Shibata N, Dixon EG, Wolf PD, Danieley ND, Sweeney MB, Smith WM, Ideker RE. Activation during ventricular defibrillation in open-chest dogs: evidence of complete cessation and regeneration of ventricular fibrillation after unsuccessful shocks. *J Clin Invest.* 1986;77:810–823.

128. Usui M, Callihan RL, Walker RG, Walcott GP, Rollins DL, Wolf PD, Smith WM, Ideker RE. Epicardial sock mapping following monophasic and biphasic shocks of equal voltage with an endocardial lead system. *J Cardiovasc Electrophysiol.* 1996;7:322–334.

129. Eisenberg M, Bergner L, Hallstrom A. Epidemiology of cardiac arrest and resuscitation in children. *Ann Emerg Med.* 1983;12:672–674.

130. Kuisma M, Suominen P, Korpela R. Paediatric out-of-hospital cardiac arrests: epidemiology and outcome. *Resuscitation.* 1995;30:141–150.

131. Hickey RW, Cohen DM, Strausbaugh S, Dietrich AM. Pediatric patients requiring CPR in the prehospital setting [see comments]. *Ann Emerg Med.* 1995;25:495–501.

132. Sirbaugh PE, Pepe PE, Shook JE, Kimball KT, Goldman MJ, Ward MA, Mann DM. A prospective, population-based study of the demographics, epidemiology, management, and outcome of out-of-hospital pediatric cardiopulmonary arrest [see comments] [published erratum appears in *Ann Emerg Med.* 1999;33:358]. *Ann Emerg Med.* 1999;33:174–184.

133. Mogayzel C, Quan L, Graves JR, Tiedeman D, Fahrenbruch C, Herndon P. Out-of-hospital ventricular fibrillation in children and adolescents: causes and outcomes [see comments]. *Ann Emerg Med.* 1995;25:484–491.

134. Appleton GO, Cummins RO, Larson MP, Graves JR. CPR and the single rescuer: at what age should you "call first" rather than "call fast"? [see comments]. *Ann Emerg Med*. 1995;25:492–494.

135. Ronco R, King W, Donley DK, Tilden SJ. Outcome and cost at a children's hospital following resuscitation for out-of-hospital cardiopulmonary arrest. *Arch Pediatr Adolesc Med*. 1995;149:210–214.

136. Walsh CK, Krongrad E. Terminal cardiac electrical activity in pediatric patients. *Am J Cardiol*. 1983;51:557–561.

137. Safranek DJ, Eisenberg MS, Larsen MP. The epidemiology of cardiac arrest in young adults. *Ann Emerg Med*. 1992;21:1102–1106.

138. Losek JD, Hennes H, Glaeser P, Hendley G, Nelson DB. Prehospital care of the pulseless, nonbreathing pediatric patient. *Am J Emerg Med*. 1987;5:370–374.

139. Atkins DL, Hartley LL, York DK. Accurate recognition and effective treatment of ventricular fibrillation by automated external defibrillators in adolescents. *Pediatrics*. 1998;101:393–397.

140. Cecchin F, Perry JC, Berul CI, Jorgenson DB, Brian DW, Lyster T, Snider DE, Zimmerman AA, Lupinetti FM, Rosenthal GL, Rule D, Atkins DL. Accuracy of automatic external defibrillator analysis algorithm in young children. *Circulation*. 1999;100(suppl I):I-663. Abstract.

141. Hazinski MF, Walker C, Smith J, Deshpande J. Specificity of automatic external defibrillator (AED) rhythm analysis in pediatric tachyarrhythmias. *Circulation*. 1997;96(suppl I):I-561. Abstract.

142. Clark CB, Davies LR, Kerber RE. Pediatric defibrillation: biphasic vs. monophasic waveforms in an experimental model. *Circulation*. 1999; 200(suppl I):I-90. Abstract.

143. Tang W, Weil MH, Sun S, Yamaguchi H, Povoas HP, Pernat AM, Bisera J. The effects of biphasic and conventional monophasic defibrillation on postresuscitation myocardial function. *J Am Coll Cardiol*. 1999;34:815–822.

144. Babbs CF, Tacker WA, VanVleet JF, Bourland JD, Geddes LA. Therapeutic indices for transchest defibrillator shocks: effective, damaging, and lethal electrical doses. *Am Heart J*. 1980;99:734–738.

144a. Lubitz DS, Seidel JS, Chameides L, Luten RC, et al. A rapid method for estimating weight and resuscitation drug dosages from length in the pediatric age group. *Ann Emerg Med*. 1988;17:576–581.

145. Panacek EA, Munger MA, Rutherford WF, Gardner SF. Report of nitropatch explosions complicating defibrillation. *Am J Emerg Med*. 1992;10:128–129.

146. Calle PA, Buylaert W. When an AED meets an ICD... automated external defibrillator: implantable cardioverter defibrillator. *Resuscitation*. 1998;38:177–183.

147. Bissing JW, Kerber RE. Effect of shaving the chest of hirsute subjects on transthoracic impedance to self-adhesive defibrillation electrode pads. *Am J Cardiol*. In press.

148. Gibbs W, Eisenberg M, Damon SK. Dangers of defibrillation: injuries to emergency personnel during patient resuscitation. *Am J Emerg Med*. 1990;8:8:101–104.

149. Aufderheide T, Stapleton ER, Hazinski MF, Cummins RO. *Heartsaver AED for the Lay Rescuer and First Responder*. Dallas, Tex: American Heart Association; 1999.

150. Emergency Care Research Institute. Hazard: user error and defibrillator discharge failures. *Health Devices*. 1986;15.

151. Cummins RO, Chesemore K, White RD, Defibrillator Working Group. Defibrillator failures: causes of problems and recommendations for improvement. [see comments]. *JAMA*. 1990;264:1019–1025.

152. White RD. Maintenance of defibrillators in a state of readiness. *Ann Emerg Med*. 1993;22:302–306.

153. White RD. AED (automated external defibrillators): a physician's responsibility. *J Emerg Med Serv*. 1992;17:8–9.

154. Cummins RO. The Utstein style for uniform reporting of data from out-of-hospital cardiac arrest. *Ann Emerg Med*. 1993;22:37–40.

155. Emergency Cardiac Care Committees and Subcommittees AHA. Guidelines for cardiopulmonary resuscitation and emergency cardiac care. *JAMA*. 1992;268:2171–2302.

156. Murphy DM. Rapid defibrillation: fire service to lead the way. *J Emerg Med Serv*. 1987;12:67–71.

157. Newman M. Chain of Survival concept takes hold. *J Emerg Med Serv*. 1989;14:11–13.

158. Walters G, Glucksman E, Evans TR. Training St John Ambulance volunteers to use an automated external defibrillator. *Resuscitation*. 1994;27:39–45.

159. Weaver WD, Sutherland K, Wirkus MJ, Bachman R. Emergency medical care requirements for large public assemblies and a new

160. Watts DD. Defibrillation by basic emergency medical technicians: effect on survival [see comments]. *Ann Emerg Med*. 1995;26:635–639.

161. Fenner P, Leahy S. Successful defibrillation on a beach by volunteer surf lifesavers. *Med J Aust*. 1998;168:169.

162. Riegel B. Training nontraditional responders to use automated external defibrillators. *Am J Crit Care*. 1998;7:402–410.

163. Herlitz J, Bang A, Axelsson A, Graves JR, Lindqvist J. Experience with the use of automated external defibrillators in out of hospital cardiac arrest. *Resuscitation*. 1998;37:3–7.

164. Calle P, Van Acker P, Buylaert W, Quets A, Corne L, Delooz H, Bossaert L, Martens P, Mullie A, the Belgian Cerebral Resuscitation Study Group. Should semi-automatic defibrillators be used by emergency medical technicians in Belgium? *Acta Clin Belg*. 1992; 47:6–14.

165. Calle PA, Verbeke A, Vanhaute O, Van Acker P, Martens P, Buylaert W. The effect of semi-automatic external defibrillation by emergency medical technicians on survival after out-of-hospital cardiac arrest: an observational study in urban and rural areas in Belgium. *Acta Clin Belg*. 1997;52:72–83.

166. Martens P, Calle P, Mullie A. Do we know enough to introduce semi-automatic defibrillation by ambulancemen in Belgium? *Eur J Med*. 1993;2:430–434.

167. Richless LK, Schrading WA, Polana J, Hess DR, Ogden CS. Early defibrillation program: problems encountered in a rural/suburban EMS system. *J Emerg Med*. 1993;11:127–134.

168. Ho J, Held T, Heegaard W, Crimmins T. Automatic external defibrillation and its effects on neurologic outcome in cardiac arrest patients in an urban, two-tiered EMS system. *Prehospital Disaster Med*. 1997;12: 284–287.

169. Herlitz J, Bang A, Holmberg M, Axelsson A, Lindkvist J, Holmberg S. Rhythm changes during resuscitation from ventricular fibrillation in relation to delay until defibrillation, number of shocks delivered and survival. *Resuscitation*. 1997;34:17–22.

170. Hamer DW, Gordon MW, Cusack S, Robertson CE. Survival from cardiac arrest in an accident and emergency department: the impact of out of hospital advisory defibrillation. *Resuscitation*. 1993;26:31–37.

171. Arntz HR, Oeff M, Willich SN, Storch WH, Schroder R. Establishment and results of an EMT-D program in a two-tiered physician-escorted rescue system: the experience in Berlin, Germany. *Resuscitation*. 1993; 26:39–46.

172. National Heart Attack Alert Program Coordinating Committee Access to Care Subcommittee. Staffing and equipping emergency medical services system: rapid identification and treatment of acute myocardial infarction. *Am J Emerg Med*. 1995;13:58–66.

173. Stults KR, Brown DD. Special considerations for defibrillation performed by emergency medical technicians in small communities. *Circulation*. 1986;74(suppl IV):IV-13–IV-17.

174. Ornato JP, McNeill SE, Craren EJ, Nelson NM. Limitation on effectiveness of rapid defibrillation by emergency medical technicians in a rural setting. *Ann Emerg Med*. 1984;13:1096–1099.

175. Cummins RO, Eisenberg MS, Graves JR, Damon SK. EMT-defibrillation: is it right for you? *J Emerg Med Serv*. 1985;10:60–64.

176. Lazzam C, McCans J. Predictors of survival of in-hospital cardiac arrest. *Can J Cardiol*. 1991;7:113–116.

177. Dickey W, Adgey A. Mortality within hospital after resuscitation from ventricular fibrillation outside the hospital. *Br Heart J*. 1992;67: 334–338.

178. Cummins RO, Sanders A, Mancini E, Hazinski MF. In-hospital resuscitation: a statement for healthcare professionals from the American Heart Association Emergency Cardiac Care Committee and the Advanced Cardiac Life Support, Basic Life Support, Pediatric Resuscitation, and Program Administration Subcommittees. *Circulation*. 1997; 95:2211–2212.

179. Nelson ME, Zenas CS. Losing the race to resuscitate. *Nurs Management*. 1998;29:36D–36E, 36G.

180. Mancini ME, Kaye W. AEDs: changing the way you respond to cardiac arrest : automatic external defibrillators. *Am J Nurs*. 1999;99:26–30; quiz 31.

181. Warwick JP, Mackie K, Spencer I. Towards early defibrillation: a nurse training programme in the use of automated external defibrillators [see comments]. *Resuscitation*. 1995;30:231–235.

182. Bossaert EL. *European Resuscitation Council Guidelines for Resuscitation*. Amsterdam, Netherlands: Elsevier Science; 1998.

strategy for managing cardiac arrest in this setting. *Ann Emerg Med*. 1989;18:155–160.

183. Anonymous Joint Commission on Accreditation of Healthcare Organizations. In-hospital resuscitation requirements reinstated for hospitals. *Joint Commission Perspectives*. 1998;18:5.

184. Cummins RO, Chamberlain D, Hazinski MF, Nadkarni V, Kloeck W, Kramer E, Becker L, Robertson C, Koster R, Zaritsky A, Bossaert L, Ornato JP, Callanan V, Allen M, Steen P, Connolly B, Sanders A, Idris A, Cobbe S. Recommended guidelines for reviewing, reporting, and conducting research on in-hospital resuscitation: the in-hospital "Utstein style": a statement for healthcare professionals from the American Heart Association, the European Resuscitation Council, the Heart and Stroke Foundation of Canada, the Australian Resuscitation Council, and the Resuscitation Councils of Southern Africa. *Resuscitation*. 1997;34:151–183.

185. Kloeck W, Cummins RO, Chamberlain D, Bossaert L, et al. Early defibrillation: an advisory statement from the advanced life support working group of the International Liaison Committee on Resuscitation. *Circulation*. 1997;95:2183–2184.

186. Stoddard FG. Public access defibrillation comes of age. *Currents*. 1997; 7:1–3.

187. Nichol G, Hallstrom AP, Ornato JP, Riegel B, Stiell IG, Valenzuela T, Wells GA, White RD, Weisfeldt ML. Potential cost-effectiveness of public access defibrillation in the United States. *Circulation*. 1998;97:1315–1320.

188. Cobb LA, Eliastam M, Kerber RE, Melker R, Moss AJ, Newell L, Paraskos JA, Weaver WD, Weil M, Weisfeldt ML. Report of the American Heart Association Task Force on the Future of Cardiopulmonary Resuscitation. *Circulation*. 1992;85:2346–2355.

189. Becker L, Eisenberg M, Fahrenbruch C, Cobb L. Public locations of cardiac arrest: implications for public access defibrillation. *Circulation*. 1998;97:2106–2109.

190. Zachariah BS, Pepe PE. The development of emergency medical dispatch in the U S A: a historical perspective. *Eur J Emerg Med*. 1995;2:109–112.

191. Rossi R. The role of the dispatch centre in preclinical emergency medicine. *Eur J Emerg Med*. 1994;1:27–30.

192. American College of Emergency Physicians. Early defibrillation programs. *Ann Emerg Med*. 1999;33:371.

193. Axelsson A, Herlitz J, Karlsson T, Lindqvist J, Reid Graves J, Ekstrom L, Holmberg S. Factors surrounding cardiopulmonary resuscitation influencing bystanders' psychological reactions. *Resuscitation*. 1998;37:13–20.

194. Ornato JP, Craren EJ, Gonzalez ER, Garnett AR, McClung BK, Newman MM. Cost-effectiveness of defibrillation by emergency medical technicians. *Am J Emerg Med*. 1988;6:108–112.

195. Stiell IG, Wells GA, Field BJ, Spaite DW, De Maio VJ, Ward R, Munkley DP, Lyver MB, Luinstra LG, Campeau T, Maloney J, Dagnone E. Improved out-of-hospital cardiac arrest survival through the inexpensive optimization of an existing defibrillation program: OPALS study phase II. Ontario Prehospital Advanced Life Support. [see comments]. *JAMA*. 1999;281:1175–1181.

Part 5: New Guidelines for First Aid

Background

Since their initial publication in 1974,[1] the Guidelines on Cardiopulmonary Resuscitation (CPR) and Emergency Cardiac Care (ECC) have earned the reputation of an authoritative document. The reputation of the guidelines has been enhanced by the gradual move toward evidence-based recommendations, which provide information about the strength of the scientific evidence behind each recommendation. If the scientific basis for a recommendation is weak and based mainly on accepted practice, it is hoped that the clear indication of a paucity of scientific evidence will stimulate research.

The initial impetus for the ECC Guidelines was resuscitation of the victim of a cardiac event. It immediately became evident that in emergency situations it was not always clear which events were cardiac in origin. Furthermore, many emergency events, if left unattended, would eventually become cardiac events. Recommendations for the immediate care of the choking victim, the so-called "café coronary," were added, as were sections on special situations, such as lightning strike and near-drowning, in which CPR recommendations were applicable. Tentatively in 1980[2] and more definitively in 1986,[3] guidelines were developed for resuscitation of infants, children, and neonates in the delivery room. The development of pediatric guidelines necessitated expanding the scope of the guidelines into such areas as injury prevention, asphyxia, shock, and respiratory failure.

As early as the 1960s[4] and as recently as 1999,[5] Peter Safar called for extending ECC educational programs into what he calls "life-supporting first aid," the few simple measures that are crucial for making a difference in the patient's immediate survival while awaiting professional help.

In 1999 the American Heart Association introduced the Heartsaver FACTS Course, which combined a first aid course developed by the National Safety Council with the AHA course on automated external defibrillators (AEDs) and CPR.[6] Organizations in other countries, such as St John Ambulance and the British Red Cross, have developed courses with similar goals.

A task force on first aid* was appointed in October 1999 to develop evidence-based guidelines for first aid. Its purpose is to ensure consistency with the AHA practice of offering courses developed from guidelines that are based on evidence. Since 1992 it has been the goal of various worldwide resuscitation organizations to make the guidelines international in scope. Task forces have worked to reconcile differences[7] and have collaborated in the preparation of the International Guidelines 2000, including these first aid recommendations. The goals of the first aid task force were to reduce morbidity and mortality due to emergency events and to analyze the scientific evidence that answers the following questions:

- What are the most common emergency conditions that lead to significant morbidity and mortality?
- In which of these emergency conditions will morbidity or mortality be reduced by the intervention of a trained lay rescuer?
- How strong is the scientific evidence showing that interventions performed by a lay rescuer are both safe and effective?

The task force defined first aid as assessments and interventions that can be performed by a bystander with minimal equipment until appropriate medical personnel arrive. Administration of first aid must never delay activation of the EMS system or other medical or professional assistance. The task force strongly believes that education in first aid should be universal: everyone can learn first aid and everyone should.

The task force initially addressed emergencies in adults, including those at the worksite, where the availability of personnel trained in first aid is mandated. The Occupational Safety and Health Administration[8,9] requires that "at least one person, and preferably two or more, trained in first aid, must be available at the worksite. In areas where accidents resulting in suffocation, severe bleeding, or other life-threatening injury or illness can be expected, a 3- to 4-minute response time, from time of injury to time of administering first aid, is required. In other circumstances, ie, where a life-threatening injury is an unlikely outcome of an accident, a 15-minute response time is acceptable. If an employer can take employees to an infirmary, clinic, or hospital, or if outside emergency assistance can arrive within the allotted times, the employer is not required to train employees in first aid." Most countries have standards of first aid for the workplace (employment legislation) and organizations that train personnel in first aid.

A number of organizations, including the American Red Cross,[10] the National Safety Council,[11] the National Highway Traffic Safety Administration of the US Department of Transportation,[12] and St John Ambulance,[13] have developed first aid curricula and courses. In Europe and Australia, similar organizations provide first aid training based on

*Leon Chameides, MD, Chair; Paul Berlin, MS, NREMT-P; Richard O. Cummins, MD, MPH, MSc; Louis Gonzales, BS, NREMT-P; Judy Goodman; Mary Fran Hazinski, RN, MSN; Mark C. Henry, MD; Lenworth M. Jacobs, MD, MPH; Robb S. Rehberg, MS, ATC, NREMT; Donna Seger, MD; Adam Singer, MD; Edward Stapleton, EMT-P; Lark Stewart, MS, NREMT; David A. Zideman, MD.

Circulation. 2000;102(suppl I):I-77–I-85.
© 2000 American Heart Association, Inc.

Circulation is available at http://www.circulationaha.org

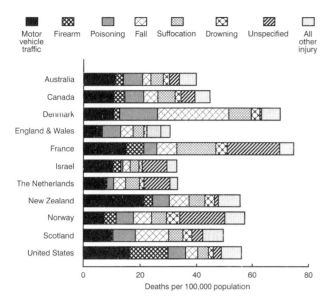

Figure 1. Average annual injury-related death rates by mechanism for 11 countries.[21]

locally developed national protocols. The previous first aid guidelines,[14] however, were developed as a consensus document. It is hoped that this document will become the foundation on which future evidence-based guidelines for first aid are built.

The Evidence: What Really Works in First Aid?

The task force consulted first aid texts and performed a thorough review of published studies to identify, evaluate, and classify the scientific basis for first aid recommendations. Previous studies[15–17] have noted the paucity of scientific evidence to support many interventions in prehospital emergency care. Many first aid practices rest on an equally precarious scientific foundation. The resuscitation councils that developed the International Guidelines 2000 used a

"class of recommendations" scheme to indicate the evidence supporting each recommendation (see "Part 1: Introduction"). Most of the evidence supporting the value of first aid assessment and management was found to be in Levels 6, 7, and 8, namely, astute clinical observations, extrapolations from other data sources, and common sense.

Scope of the Problem

Unintentional injury continues to be a major cause of morbidity and mortality. It is the fifth leading cause of death (92 000 in 1998) in the United States, exceeded only by heart disease, cancer, stroke, and chronic obstructive lung disease. Injuries in the United States are responsible for approximately 2.6 million people being hospitalized, 34.9 million people being treated in hospital emergency departments, and 87.6 million visits to medical offices each year.[18]

In 1998 there were 5100 work-related deaths and 3 800 000 work-related disabling injuries in the United States.[19] In 1997 there were 429 800 occupational illnesses, including those due to repeated trauma (276 600), skin diseases (58 000), and respiratory conditions due to toxic agents (20 000).[20] Figure 1 shows comparative data from 11 countries[21] for all age groups. There is considerable variation between countries, with more than 100% variation between the country with the lowest injury death rate (England and Wales) and the country with the highest rate (France).

Many adult workers have sudden medical emergencies that are not associated with their occupation, such as heart attacks, strokes, and asthma attacks. First aid training and skills for such conditions can be lifesaving. Specific statistics are lacking, however, to estimate the frequency with which first aid maneuvers are necessary or how often their timely application is effective.

Faced with this dilemma, the task force examined the leading causes of death in the United States in persons 25 to 64 years old.[22] Chronic conditions, such as malignancies, liver disease, and human immunodeficiency virus infection,

TABLE 1.   Leading Causes of Death in Persons 25 to 64 Years Old: First Aid Assessments and Interventions Related to Specific Causes of Death

Rank	Cause of Death	First Aid Assessments and Interventions
1	Malignancy	Mechanism of death (cardiac arrest, shock, CNS event); may require first aid interventions
2	Heart disease	Heart attack, sudden death; CPR, AED
3	Unintentional injury	Hemorrhage, spine immobilization, ALOC, fractures, soft-tissue injury; CPR
4	Suicide	Hemorrhage, spine immobilization, ALOC, fractures, poisoning, soft-tissue injury; CPR
5	Cerebrovascular accident	Stroke, seizures, ALOC, airway protection; CPR
6	Diabetes	Hypoglycemia, seizures
7	Liver disease	Mechanism of death (cardiac arrest, shock, CNS event) may require first aid interventions
8	Human immunodeficiency virus	Mechanism of death (cardiac arrest, shock, CNS event) may require first aid interventions
9	Bronchitis, emphysema, asthma	Breathing difficulties; CPR
10	Homicide	Hemorrhage, spine immobilization, ALOC, fractures, soft-tissue injury; CPR

CNS indicates central nervous system; AED, automated external defibrillator; and ALOC, altered level of consciousness.

TABLE 2.   Leading Causes of Work-Related Fatalities (1992–1997)[23]: Assessments and Interventions Related to Specific Causes of Death

Rank	Cause	First AidAssessments and Interventions
1	Transportation incidents (41%)	Hemorrhage, spine immobilization, ALOC, fractures, soft-tissue injury; CPR
2	Assaults and violence (20%)	Hemorrhage, spine immobilization, ALOC, fractures, soft-tissue injury; CPR
3	Contact with objects and equipment (16%)	Hemorrhage, spine immobilization, ALOC, fractures, soft-tissue injury, eye injury, poisoning; CPR
4	Environmental exposure (12%)	Hypothermia, hyperthermia, electrocution, caustic and allergenic substances
5	Falls (10%)	Hemorrhage, spine immobilization, ALOC, fractures, soft-tissue injury; CPR
6	Fires and explosions (3%)	Burns; CPR

ALOC indicates altered level of consciousness.

were excluded, for they are unlikely to require first aid maneuvers. These causes of death and the first aid assessments and interventions related to each cause are listed in Table 1.[23]

The task force then examined the leading causes of work-related deaths in a similar manner (Table 2).

The international resuscitation councils do not intend for these first aid guidelines to be comprehensive or to cover all the first aid assessments and interventions listed in Tables 1 and 2. These guidelines are a beginning, an initial attempt to develop evidence-based guidelines that will be expanded in the future. Our goal is for these guidelines to encourage research related to first aid so that we can remedy the current paucity of scientific evidence.

Some essential first aid topics, such as basic life support, including CPR, recognition of heart attack, and use of automated external defibrillators, are covered elsewhere in these guidelines (see Parts 3 and 4).

Specific Evidence-Based Guidelines: Some Examples

Burns
In the United States, fires and burns are the fifth leading cause of unintentional death related to injury (3700 deaths per year).[24] A large number of burns that cause injuries ranging from discomfort to severe disability occur at work, at home, and in recreational areas. Injuries from burns may be due to chemicals, electrocution, or contact with hot objects (thermal burns).

Thermal Burns
To treat a thermal burn, remove the victim from the source of injury as soon as possible, being careful not to place yourself in danger. The degree of care needed is related to the circumstances of the burn. If the victim's clothing is on fire, have the victim "stop, drop, and roll" and soak the flames with water or smother them with a blanket. Immediately cool the burn with cold—but not ice-cold—water (Class IIa). Immediate cooling of burns with cold water is supported by a large number of observational clinical studies[25–28] and controlled animal experiments.[28–45] Although no results from randomly controlled trials are available, findings from a small controlled trial in volunteers support this recommendation.[46] Cooling of burns has many beneficial effects, including pain

relief,[25–27,46,47] reduced formation of edema,* reduced infection rates,[27,30] reduced depth of injury,[29,30,33] more rapid healing,[25,34] reduced need for grafting,[27] and reduced mortality.[26,32,34,36,37] Although cooling should begin as soon as possible, delayed cooling may still be beneficial.[29,31] The temperature and duration of recommended cooling for burns vary considerably among reported studies. The most comprehensive data available is from Ófeigsson's[28–30] studies on rats. Optimal healing and the lowest mortality rates were noted with water temperatures of 20°C to 25°C (68°F to 77°F). Other studies in which the water temperature ranged from 10°C to 15°C (50°F to 59°F) have also noted beneficial results in both healing and mortality rates,[31,32,34,36,37] even in dogs with extensive burns covering 50% of total body surface area.[32] This temperature range of 10°C to 15°C (50°F to 59°F) is typical of cold water available in household taps in North America.

Excessive cooling with ice water at 0°C (32°F) resulted in hypothermia and increased mortality rates in rats with burns to 20% of total body surface area compared with noncooled controls.[29] Although brief exposure to ice or ice water may be beneficial,[35] prolonged cooling may cause additional local injury as a result of ischemia.[47] The duration of cooling is also controversial, but cooling should continue at least until pain is relieved and probably for a total duration of 15 to 30 minutes. Cooling should not delay transfer to a medical facility.

Remove all nonadhering clothing and jewelry that can be removed without force from the burn area. Leave blisters intact (Class IIb). Cover the burn area with a clean dressing if one is available. Do not apply lotions, creams, ointments, or home remedies to the burn area (Class IIb).

Although the results of several in vitro studies have shown that the fluid in blisters contains agents that are detrimental to wound healing,[48,49] others have demonstrated that the fluid in blisters contains agents beneficial to wound healing.[50–52] Furthermore, a controlled volunteer experiment[53] and controlled animal experiments[54–56] have shown a benefit of leaving blisters intact. Unroofing of blisters under less than sterile conditions clearly exposes the patient to significant risk of contamination.

Carefully brush powdered chemicals off the skin with a gloved hand or piece of cloth. Remove all contaminated clothing from the victim, while avoiding contaminating

---

*References 25, 27, 30, 31, 34, 36, 38, 40–46.

yourself. Flush chemical burns with large amounts of cool running water (Class IIa)[57–60] and continue flushing until EMS personnel arrive.

Electrocution and Electrical Burns

Electric shock caused 482 deaths in the United States in 1997.[61] The Centers for Disease Control and Prevention estimates that 52 000 trauma admissions per year are due to electrical injuries.

The severity of electrical injuries can vary widely, from an unpleasant tingling sensation caused by low-intensity current to thermal burns, cardiopulmonary arrest, and death. Thermal burns may result from burning clothing in contact with the skin or from electric current traversing a portion of the body, in which case thermal burns may be present at the points where the current entered and exited the body and internally along its pathway. Burns can result from both low-voltage (<1000 V) and high-voltage (>1000 V) injuries.[62]

Cardiopulmonary arrest is the primary cause of immediate death in persons who have sustained an electrical injury.[63] Cardiac arrhythmias, including ventricular fibrillation, ventricular asystole, and ventricular tachycardia, that progress to ventricular fibrillation may occur as a result of exposure to low- or high-voltage current.[64] Respiratory arrest may result from electrical injury to the respiratory center in the brain or from tetanic contractions or paralysis of the respiratory muscles.

Factors that determine the nature and severity of injury include the magnitude of energy delivered, voltage, resistance to current flow, type of current, duration of contact, and current pathway. High-tension current causes the most serious injuries, but fatal electrocutions may also occur with low-voltage household current.[65] Skin resistance, the most important factor impeding current flow, can be reduced substantially by moisture, converting a low-voltage injury into a life-threatening one.

Do not place yourself in danger by touching the victim while the electricity is on. Turn off the power at its source; at home the switch is usually near the fuse box.

In case of high-voltage electrocution, such as that caused by fallen power lines, immediately notify the appropriate authorities (the electric company and fire department). Everything will conduct electricity if the voltage is high enough, so do not enter the area around the victim or attempt to remove wires or other materials with any object, including wooden ones, until the power has been turned off by knowledgeable personnel.

Once the power is off, assess the victim, who may need CPR, defibrillation, and treatment for shock and thermal burns. Appropriate precautions must be taken because musculoskeletal and spinal cord injuries (see below) may be present. All victims of electric shock require medical assessment.

Poisoning

Poisoning can be caused by solids, liquids, gases, and vapors. Gases and vapors are inhaled; solids and liquids are ingested or absorbed through the skin. Ingestion may be unintentional or self-inflicted. In 1997, in the United States, 9000 deaths

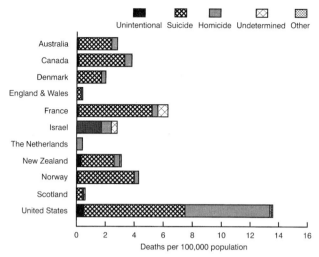

Figure 2. Average annual poisoning death rates by intent from 11 countries.[21]

were caused by poisons,[66] as were almost 4% of work-related deaths. Figure 2 shows data from 11 countries[21]; again the data shows considerable variation. The poisoning rate in the United States is more than twice that of any other country. This is due to a rate of homicidal posioning that alone is as high as the *total* poisoning rate in any other country.

The number of poisonous substances available at work and home is very large. It is important to understand the toxic nature of chemicals in the environment, proper use of protective equipment, and emergency procedures for toxic exposure. In the United States, access to poison control centers is available to the public, but in other countries, access may be available only through the EMS system or hospital. The telephone number of the local poison control center should be prominently displayed at home and at worksites where poisonous substances are present. If poisoning occurs, contact the poison control center for advice and recommendations. In the United States, material safety data sheets should not be used to determine first aid treatment, nor should the use of these sheets take the place of a call to the poison control center. The sheets may be of value, however, in determining actual exposure, and the agents listed on them should be relayed to the specialist in poison information.

Rescuers must protect themselves before administering first aid, especially if the poison can be inhaled or absorbed through the skin. Do not enter any area where victims are unconscious without knowledge of the agents to which the victims have been exposed and without the required protective equipment.

If the poison is a gas or vapor, remove the victim from the contaminated area as soon as possible. If the victim's skin has been exposed, thoroughly flush it with running water until EMS personnel arrive.

Evaluate victims of poisoning for adequacy of airway, breathing, and circulation and provide basic life support (see "Part 3: Adult Basic Life Support," in these guidelines) as required. Place symptomatic victims who are breathing spontaneously in a recovery position. EMS personnel will transport most poisoning victims or will recommend that you transport them to the nearest Emergency Department. Regardless of symptoms, transport all victims who ingest a poison in a suicide attempt to the nearest Emergency Department.

Do not administer anything by mouth unless advised by a poison control center (Class IIb). The results of some animal studies[67–69] suggest that dilution or neutralization of a caustic agent by water or milk after ingestion reduces tissue injury, but no human studies have demonstrated a clinical benefit of this practice. Administration of milk or water may be considered if a large amount of an industrial-strength caustic or a solid caustic has been ingested, but call the poison control center first.

Some controversy continues about the role of gastrointestinal decontamination by inducing vomiting with syrup of ipecac or by adsorption of the toxin by activated charcoal, gastrointestinal decontamination has not been shown to change outcome (defined as morbidity, mortality, cost, or length of hospital stay).[70]

At this time there is insufficient data to support or exclude administration of ipecac to induce vomiting in poisoning victims (Class Indeterminate). The potential danger of aspiration and the lack of clear-cut evidence of a benefit support our recommendation: do not administer ipecac unless specifically directed by a poison control center or other authority (eg, local emergency department physician). If ipecac is administered, it should be given only within 30 minutes of ingestion and only to victims who are alert and responsive (Class IIb). The decontamination effects of ipecac have been extrapolated from studies performed in dogs,[71–73] but the findings are probably not applicable to humans. Results of studies performed in human volunteers[74–77] are not applicable to poisonings because the volunteers were given nontoxic drugs.

Administration of activated charcoal by first aid rescuers is not recommended (Class Indeterminate). Animal studies[78] suggest that administration of activated charcoal immediately after drug ingestion decreases the amount of drug absorbed, but the amount varies and decreases with time.[79,80] Activated charcoal is unpalatable and difficult to administer, and death due to its aspiration has been reported.[81]

Hemorrhage

Because hemorrhage is a potential component of both intentional and unintentional injuries, it is a major health problem in terms of both morbidity and mortality. First aid responders have a responsibility to protect themselves and must understand and practice protection against blood-borne diseases. Consider all body fluids from victims to be infectious. Wear gloves and, if possible, protective shields and gowns when providing assistance in which exposure to droplets of blood, saliva, or other body fluids[82] is likely. After the hemorrhage is controlled, wash your hands thoroughly and change blood-soaked clothing. Avoid touching your mouth, nose, or eyes or eating before you have washed your hands.

Minor bleeding such as bruises or abrasions can be treated as soft-tissue injuries (see below). To treat a nose bleed, have the victim bend forward at the waist and pinch the nasal alae

with the thumb and index finger[83–86] (Class IIb). Continued bleeding may require medical intervention.

To control any active bleeding, apply direct pressure with the flat portion of your fingers or the palm of your hand over a sterile dressing or clean pad (Class IIb). If the bleeding does not stop, apply more pressure. If the dressing becomes saturated, apply a second dressing over the first. If a barrier is unavailable and the victim is conscious, have the victim apply pressure directly to the bleeding source.

If bleeding is from an extremity, elevate the extremity above the level of the heart (Class IIb). If severe bleeding continues despite application of firm pressure, add arterial pressure by applying pressure to the brachial artery if bleeding is from the upper extremity and over the femoral artery if bleeding is from the lower extremity (Class Indeterminate).

The use of tourniquets is controversial. Tourniquets are widely used in operating rooms under controlled conditions and have been studied for safety, effectiveness, and related complications under those conditions.[87–94] Arterial tourniquets, however, cause injury as a result of ischemia after 90 minutes of compression. Complications include bleeding, injury to soft tissues, nerve and vascular injury, and paralysis.[95–97] Tourniquets applied by first aid providers usually cause venous rather than arterial occlusion and often increase rather than decrease hemorrhage.[98–100] Because of these potentially serious complications, tourniquets should be used only as a last resort for massive hemorrhage that is not controlled by other methods and only by persons skilled in their use.

Every precaution must be taken to maintain normal body temperature in the bleeding victim. Remove wet clothing and use blankets or other material to protect the victim from hypothermia.

Altered Mental States

An altered mental state may be due to trauma or a medical condition such as diabetes or stroke. Signs and symptoms of an altered mental state include loss of consciousness, confusion, combativeness, disorientation, headache, inability to move a body part, dizziness, problems with balance, and double vision. Any sudden change in level of consciousness requires medical evaluation. First aid measures include removing the victim from a potentially dangerous environment; evaluating airway, breathing, and circulation; maintaining body temperature; and placing the victim in a recovery position. If the victim is known to have diabetes and is able to swallow, give him or her a drink containing glucose. Note that drinks with artificial sweeteners (diet drinks) do not contain glucose.

Fainting is a momentary loss of consciousness. Minor pain, sudden fright, or standing in one position for prolonged periods, especially in a hot environment, are precipitating factors in susceptible persons. First aid measures include protecting the victim from injury, placing the victim in a supine position, and checking airway, breathing, and circulation. If airway and breathing are adequate and the victim is not injured, you may place the victim in a recovery position. The victim usually regains consciousness within a few seconds and has no alteration in mental status once consciousness is regained.

Head Trauma

In the United States the head, neck, and spine are the parts of the body most commonly involved in unintentional injuries. Injuries to the head, neck, and spine are most frequently associated with falls (21%), violence (13%), and sports (13%). Many of these injuries are preventable, and many states have regulations that require workers to use head and neck protection at specific worksites.

Head injury should be suspected when any of the following has occurred:

- The victim fell from a height greater than his or her own.
- When found, the victim was unconscious.
- The victim sustained a blunt force injury (eg, from impact with or ejection from a car).
- The victim's injury was caused by diving, lightning strike, or electrocution, or the victim's head protection or helmet was broken or insufficient.
- The victim sustained a high-impact sports injury.

First aid responders should gather information on the mechanism of injury, whether an alteration in mental status has occurred, and the presence and duration of unconsciousness. This information is important for early treatment of the victim and is used in several protocols to classify the severity of the injury and the risk of progressive brain injury and to guide treatment during the first 24 hours. A concussion is an alteration in mental status, especially confusion and amnesia, and may or may not include a loss of consciousness. Because the signs and symptoms may be transient, the first aid responder's observations at the scene provide EMS personnel with important information for subsequent treatment. Information about whether to obtain a head CT or cervical spine radiographs is beyond the scope of first aid actions. The interested reader should consult 2 important new studies.[100a,100b]

If head injury is suspected

- Determine whether the victim's location poses a danger to the victim or you, and remove the victim from the site if it does.
- Assess and provide CPR to an unconscious, nonbreathing, pulseless victim.
- Assess the victim's risk of vomiting and ability to protect the airway.
- Assess and control bleeding.
- Maintain the victim's body temperature.
- Stabilize the cervical spine in high-risk situations (see next section).

Spinal Cord Injuries and Cervical Spine Immobilization

In the United States approximately 11 000 people sustain spinal cord injuries each year.[101] Motor vehicle crashes are the cause of 40% of such injuries; violence, 25%; falls, 21%; diving accidents, 10%; and work- or sports-related accidents, 4%.

An overwhelming majority of spinal cord injuries occur during the primary traumatic event. Some evidence indicates that spinal cord injuries may occur after the primary trauma. Some injuries are presumably due to extension of the original damage from edema, swelling, and hemorrhage. Some are caused by additional injury to the spinal cord from movement of the spinal column after the original trauma. Movement of the spinal column relative to the spinal cord may occur during initial stabilization, movement, or transport of the victim.

Even minimal degrees of force can injure the spinal cord. At the time of injury it is difficult to identify victims with an unstable spine, who are at risk for spinal cord injury. In the past, emergency personnel considered the mechanism of injury, independent of subjective complaints and physical findings, to be the best predictor of spine and spinal cord injury. They have since abandoned their reliance on mechanism of injury alone.[102] Current practice incorporates evaluation of specific pain, distribution of tenderness, neurological deficits, and mechanisms of injury to assess the risk of spine and spinal cord injuries.[103] Most first aid providers lack the training and experience to conduct these more sophisticated evaluations. Furthermore, extensive physical examination may be inappropriate or inaccurate when carried out in the prehospital environment.

First aid responders should suspect an unstable spine or spinal cord injury with any of the following (all Class Indeterminate):

- Injury was caused by force sufficient to result in loss of consciousness.
- Injury occurred on the upper part of the body, especially the head and neck.[104]
- Injury resulted in altered mental status.
- There is evidence of drug or alcohol intoxication.[103]

If spinal cord injury is suspected, do not allow the victim to move in any direction. Immobilize the victim's head, neck, and trunk. If CPR is required, open the airway with jaw thrust (see "Part 3: Adult BLS") rather than head extension. If the victim is stable and does not require CPR or lifesaving first aid, such as hemorrhage control, do not move him or her until EMS personnel arrive. If movement is necessary (to provide CPR or lifesaving first aid or because of potential danger), support the victim's head, neck, and trunk securely so that the head and neck do not move in any direction. (See previous section and References 100a and 100b regarding diagnostic studies.)

Seizures

Approximately 10% of all people will have a seizure during their lifetime, and 1% to 2% will have recurrent seizures.[105] Although seizures are rarely fatal,[106,107] injuries related to seizures are relatively common.[108–110] Severe injuries include fractures, dislocations, burns, brain concussion, subdural hematoma, and intracerebral hemorrhage. Dental injuries are also fairly common.[111]

The general principles of first aid management of seizures are (1) prevention of injury, (2) assurance of an open airway, and (3) reassurance of an open airway after the seizure has ended.

The person having a seizure must be protected from injuring himself or herself. Try to keep the victim from falling. Protect the head with a pillow or other soft material. Do not restrain the victim during a seizure or place an object in the victim's mouth. Restraining the victim may cause musculoskeletal or soft-tissue injury. Placing an object in the victim's mouth is futile because most tongue biting occurs at the onset of seizure activity; doing so is also dangerous because it may result in dental damage or aspiration.

To prevent aspiration of secretions, place the seizure victim in a recovery position as soon as possible after the seizure has stopped.[112]

After a seizure it is not unusual for the victim to be unresponsive or confused for a short time. Activate the EMS system if (1) a seizure lasts more than 5 minutes or is recurrent, (2) the victim exhibits any respiratory problems, (3) the victim has sustained an injury, or (4) unresponsiveness or confusion lasts more than 5 minutes after the seizure has stopped.

When able to do so, the victim should be allowed to decide whether to seek additional medical assistance.

Musculoskeletal Trauma: Soft-Tissue Sprains and Contusions, Ligament and Tendon Strains, and Fractures

Closed soft-tissue injuries include joint sprains and muscle contusions. The basic principle in first aid for soft-tissue injuries is to decrease hemorrhage, edema, and pain. Numerous human studies have shown that the application of ice is effective for reducing pain and duration of disability (Class IIa).[113–118] The best way to apply ice is to use a plastic bag. Refreezable packs of gelled solutions are inefficient.[119,120] To prevent cold injury to the skin, it is best to limit application of ice to 20 minutes at a time. In contrast to cold therapy, application of heat leads to an increase in blood flow, hemorrhage, and inflammatory response.[115]

Compression of closed soft-tissue injury with a circumferential elastic bandage appears to decrease the amount of edema formation (Class Indeterminate).

Assume that any injury to an extremity includes a bone fracture. Cover open wounds with a sterile dressing if one is available. Stabilize the extremity, but do not straighten it if it is deformed. If a deformed (injured) extremity appears blue and there is no distal pulse, this is a critical emergency. Report such findings to medical control or responders with a higher skill level and follow their instructions. The victim should not bear any weight on the extremity and preferably should rest in a supine or recovery position. Maintain body temperature to prevent shock.

References

1. Standards for cardiopulmonary resuscitation (CPR) and emergency cardiac care (ECC). *JAMA.* 1974;227(suppl):883–868.
2. Standards and guidelines for cardiopulmonary resuscitation (CPR) and emergency cardiac care (ECC). *JAMA.* 1980;244:472–476, 495–500.
3. Standards and guidelines for cardiopulmonary resuscitation (CPR) and emergency cardiac care (ECC). *JAMA.* 1986;255:2954–2973.
4. Safar P, Bircher NG. *Cardiopulmonary Cerebral Resuscitation: An introduction to Resuscitation Medicine: Guidelines by the World Federation of Societies of Anaesthesiologists (WFSA).* Stavanger, Norway: Laerdal; 1968.
5. Eisenburger P, Safar P. Life supporting first aid training of the public: review and recommendations. *Resuscitation.* 1999;41:3–18.
6. National Safety Council/American Heart Association. *Heartsaver FACTS.* Sudbury, Mass: Jones and Bartlett Publishers; 1999.
7. Cummins RO, Chamberlain DA. Advisory statements of the international liaison committee on resuscitation. *Circulation.* 1997;95:2172–2273.
8. *Medical Services and First Aid.* OSHA Standard 1910.151.
9. OSHA Standards Interpretation, and Compliance Letters: First Aid Training (01/27/1976).
10. American Red Cross. *First Aid Manual.* 1998.
11. Aufderheide T, Stapleton E, Hazinski MF, Cummins R (Heartsaver AED), Thygerson AL, Lochhaas T (First Aid). *Heartsaver FACTS.* American Heart Association and National Safety Council: 1999.
12. National Highway and Traffic Safety Administration. *National Standard First Responder Curriculum.* 1998.
13. St John Ambulance. *First Aid Manual.* 1998.
14. *National Guidelines for First Aid Training in Occupational Settings, First Aid Provider Core Elements, Course Guide.* November 1998. [Online] Available at www.pitt.edu/~cemwp/education/ngfatos/ngfatos.htm.
15. Callaham M. Quantifying the scanty science of prehospital emergency care. *Ann Emerg Med.* 1997;30:785–790.
16. Neely K, Drake M, Moorhead JC, et al. Multiple options and unique pathways: a new direction for EMS? *Ann Emerg Med* 1997;30:797–799.
17. Spaite D, Criss E, Valenzuela J, et al. Developing a foundation for the evaluation of expanded scope EMS: a window of opportunity that cannot be ignored. *Ann Emerg Med.* 1997;30:791–796.
18. National Safety Council. *1999 Injury Facts, 1999 Edition.* Itasca, Ill: National Safety Council; 1999:iv.
19. National Safety Council. *1999 Injury Facts, 1999 Edition.* Itasca, Ill: National Safety Council; 1999:48.
20. National Safety Council. *1999 Injury Facts, 1999 Edition.* Itasca, Ill: National Safety Council; 1999:72.
21. Fingerhut LA, Cox CS, Warner M, et al. *International Comparative Analysis of Injury Mortality: Findings From the ICE on Injury Statistics. Advance Data From Vital and Health Statistics; No. 303.* Hyattsville, Md: National Center for Health Statistics; 1998.
22. National Safety Council. *1999 Injury Facts, 1999 Edition.* Itasca, Ill: National Safety Council; 1999:13.
23. National Safety Council. *1999 Injury Facts, 1999 Edition.* Itasca, Ill: National Safety Council; 1999:59.
24. National Safety Council. *1999 Injury Facts, 1999 Edition.* Itasca, Ill: National Safety Council; 1999:9–15.
25. Shulman AG. Ice water as primary treatment of burns: Simple method of emergency treatment of burns to alleviate pain, reduce sequelae, and hasten healing. *JAMA.* 1960;173:1916–1919.
26. Rose HW. Initial cold water treatment for burns. *Northwest Med.* 1936;35:267–270.
27. Iung OS, Wade FV. The treatment of burns with ice water, Phisohex, and partial hypothermia. *Industrial Med Surg.* 1963;365–370.
28. Ófeigsson J. Observations and experiments on the immediate cold water treatment for burns and scalds. *Br J Plast Surg.* 1959;12:104–119.
29. Ófeigsson J. Water cooling: first aid treatment for scalds and burns. *Surgery.* 1965;57:391–400.
30. Ófeigsson J, Mitchell R, Patrick RS. Observations on the cold water treatment of cutaneous burns. *J Pathol.* 1972;108:145–150.
31. King TC, Zimmerman JM. First aid cooling of the fresh burn. *Surg Gynecol Obstet.* 1965;120:1271–1273.
32. King TC, Zimmerman JM, Price PB. Effect of immediate short-term cooling on extensive burns. *Surg Forum.* 1962;13:487–488.
33. Moserova J, Behounkova E. Subcutaneous temperature measurements in a thermal injury. *Burns.* 1975;1:267–268.
34. Shulman AG, Wagner K. Effect of cold water immersion on burn edema in rabbits. *Surg Gynecol Obstet.* 1962;115:557–560.
35. Sawada Y, Urushidate S, Yotsuyanagi T, Ishita K. Is prolonged and excessive cooling of a scalded wound effective? *Burns.* 1997;23:55–58.
36. Reynolds LE, Brown CR, Price PB. Effects of local chilling in the treatment of burns. *Surg Forum.* 1956;6:85–87.
37. King TC, Price PB. Surface cooling following extensive burns. *JAMA.* 1963;183:677–678.
38. Jandera V, Hudson DA, de Wet PM, Innes DM, Rode H. Cooling the burn wound: evaluation of different modalities. *Burns.* 2000;26:265–270.
39. Wiedeman MP, Brigham MP. The effects of cooling on the microvasculature after thermal injury. *Microvasc Res.* 1991;3:154–161.
40. King TC, Reynolds LE, Price PB. Local edema and capillary permeability associated with burn wounds. *Surg Forum.* 1956;6:80–84.

41. Courtice FC. The effect of local temperature on fluid loss in thermal burns. *J Physiol.* 1946;104:321–345.

42. Moore DH, Worf DL. Effect of temperature on the transfer of serum proteins into tissues injured by tourniquet and by scald. *Am J Physiol.* 1952;170:616–623.

43. Demling RH, Mazess RB, Wolberg W. The effect of immediate and delayed cold immersion on burn edema formation and resorption. *J Trauma.* 1979; 19:56–60.

44. Raine TJ, Heggers JP, Robson MC, et al. Cooling the burn wound to maintain microcirculation. *J Trauma.* 1981;21:394–397.

45. Boykin JV, Eriksson E, Sholley MM, et al. Cold water treatment of scald injury and inhibition of histamine-mediated burn edema. *J Surg Res.* 1981; 31:111–123.

46. Raghupati AG. First-aid treatment of burns: efficacy of water cooling. *Br J Plast Surg.* 1968;21:68–72.

47. Purdue GF, Layton TR, Copeland CE. Cold injury complicating burn therapy. *J Trauma.* 1985;25:167–168.

48. Deitch EA. Opsonic activity of blister fluid from burn patients. *Infect Immun.* 1983;41:1184–1189.

49. Rockwell WB, Ehrlich HP. Fibrinolysis inhibition in human burn blister fluid. *J Burn Care Rehabil.* 1990;11:1–6.

50. Wilson Y, Goberdhan N, Dawson RA, et al. Investigation of the presence and role of calmodulin and other mitogens in human burn blister fluid. *J Burn Care Rehabil.* 1994;15:303–314.

51. Garner WL, Zuccaro C, Marcelo C, et al. The effects of burn blister fluid on keratinocyte replication and differentiation. *J Burn Care Rehabil.* 1993;14: 127–131.

52. Deitch EA, Smith BJ. The effect of blister fluid from thermally injured patients on normal lymphocyte transformation. *J Trauma.* 1983;23: 106–110.

53. Gimbel NS, Kapetansky DI, Weissman F, et al. A study of epithelization in blistered burns. *Arch Surg.* 1957;74:800–803.

54. Wheeler ES, Miller TA. The blister and the second degree burn in guinea pigs: the effect of exposure. *Plast Reconstr Surg.* 1976;57:74–83.

55. Singer AJ, Thode JC Jr, McCain SA. The effects of epidermal debridement of partial-thickness burns on infection and reepithelialization in swine. *Acad Emerg Med.* 2000;7:114–119.

56. Singer AJ, Mohammad M, Tortora G, et al. Octylcyanoacrylate for the treatment of contaminated partial-thickness burns in swine: a randomized controlled experiment. *Acad Emerg Med.* 2000;7:222–227.

57. Bromberg BE, Song IC, Walden RH. Hydrotherapy of chemical burns. *Plast Reconstr Surg.* 1965;35:85–95.

58. van Rensburg LCJ. An experimental study of chemical burns. *S Africa Med J.* 1962;36:754–759.

59. Gruber RP, Laub DR, Vistnes LM. The effect of hydrotherapy on the clinical course and pH of experimental cutaneous chemical burns. *Plast Reconstr Surg.* 1975;55:200–204.

60. Yano K, Hosokawa K, Kakibuchi M, et al. Effects of washing acid injuries to the skin with water: an experimental study using rats. *Burns.* 1995;21: 500–502.

61. National Safety Council. *1999 Injury Facts, 1999 Edition.* Itasca, Ill: National Safety Council; 1999:17.

62. Garcia-Sanchez V, Gomez Morell P. Electric burns: high and low tension injuries. *Burns.* 1999;25:357–360.

63. Homma S, Gillam LD, Weyman AE. Echocardiographic observations in survivors of acute electric injury. *Chest.* 1990;97:103–105.

64. Jensen PJ, Thomsen PE, Bagger JP, et al. Electrical injury causing ventricular arrhythmias. *Br Heart J.* 1987;57:279–283.

65. Budnick LD. Bathtub-related electrocutions in the United States, 1979–1982. *JAMA.* 1984;252:918–920.

66. National Safety Council. *1999 Injury Facts, 1999 Edition.* Itasca, Ill: National Safety Council; 1999:8.

67. Homan CS, Maitra SR, Lane BP, et al. Esophageal acid injury. *Acad Emerg Med.* 1995;2:587–591.

68. Homan CS, Maitra SR, Lane BP, et al. Effective treatment for acute alkali injury to the esophagus using weak-acid neutralization therapy: an ex-vivo study. *Acad Emerg Med.* 1995;2:952–958.

69. Homan CS, Singer AJ, Thomajan C, et al. Thermal characteristics of neutralization therapy and water dilution for strong acid ingestion: an in-vivo canine model. *Acad Emerg Med.* 1998;5:286–292.

70. Pond SM, Lewis-Driver DJ, Williams GM, et al. Gastric emptying in acute overdose: a prospective randomized controlled trial. *Med J Aust.* 1995;163: 345–349.

71. Arnold FJ, Hodges JB Jr, Barta RA Jr. Evaluation of the efficacy of lavage and induced emesis in treatment of salicylate poisoning. *Pediatrics.* 1959; 23:286–301.

72. Abdallah AH, Tye A. A comparison of the efficacy of emetic drugs and stomach lavage. *Am J Dis Child.* 1967;113:571–575.

73. Corby DG, Lisciandro RC, Lehman RH, Decker WJ. The efficiency of methods used to evacuate the stomach after acute ingestions. *Pediatrics.* 1967;40:871–874.

74. Tandberg D, Diven BG, McLeod JW. Ipecac-induced emesis versus gastric lavage. *Am J Emerg Med.* 1986;4:205–209.

75. Tenenbein M, Cohen S, Sitar DS. Efficacy of ipecac induced emesis, orogastric lavage, and activated charcoal for acute drug overdose. *Ann Emerg Med.* 1987;16:838–841.

76. Vasquez TE, Evans DG, Ashburn WL. Efficacy of syrup of ipecac-induced emesis for emptying gastric contents. *Clin Nucl Med.* 1988;13:638–639.

77. Danel V, Henry JA, Glucksman E. Activated charcoal, emesis, and gastric lavage in aspirin overdose. *BMJ.* 1988;296:1507.

78. Cooney DO. *Activated Charcoal in Medicinal Applications.* New York, NY: Marcel Dekker; 1995.

79. Galinsky RE, Levy G. Evaluation of activated charcoal-sodium sulfate combination of inhibition of acetaminophen absorption and repletion of inorganic sulfate. *J Toxicol Clin Toxicol.* 1984;22:21–30.

80. Levy G, Houston JB. Effect of activated charcoal on acetaminophen absorption. *Pediatrics.* 1976;58:432–435.

81. Toore D, Sampietro C, Quadrelli C. Effects of orally administered activated charcoal on ciprofloxacin pharmacokinetics in healthy volunteers. *Chemioterapia.* 1988;7:382–386.

82. Centers for Disease Control. Guidelines for prevention of transmission of human immunodeficiency virus and hepatitis B virus to health care and public safety workers. *MMWR.* 1989;38(suppl 6):1–37.

83. McGarry GW, Moulton C. The first aid management of epistaxis by accident and emergency department staff. *Arch Emerg Med.* 1993;10: 298–300.

84. Lavy JA, Koay CB. First aid treatment of epistaxis: are the patients well informed? *J Accid Emerg Med.* 1996;13:193–195.

85. Strachan D, England J. First-aid treatment of epistaxis: confirmation of widespread ignorance. *Postgrad Med J.* 1998;863:113–114.

86. Tan LKS, Calhoun KH. Epistaxis. *Otolaryngol Internist.* 1999;83:43–57.

87. Romanoff H, Goldberger S. Prognostic factors in peripheral vascular injuries. *J Cardiovasc Surg (Torino).* 1977;18:485–491.

88. Moore MR, Garfin SR, Hargens AR. Wide tourniquets eliminate blood flow at low inflation pressures. *J Hand Surg.* 1987;12A:1006–1011.

89. Jeyaseelan S, Stevenson TM, Pfitzner J. Tourniquet failure and arterial calcification: case report and theoretical dangers. *Anaesthesia.* 1981;36: 48–50.

90. Savvidis E, Parsch K. Prolonged transitory paralysis after pneumatic tourniquet use on the upper arm. *Unfallchirurg.* 1999;102:141–144.

91. Mohler LR, Pedowitz RA, Lopez MA, Gershuni DH. Effects of tourniquet compression on neuromuscular function. *Clin Orthop.* 1999;(359):213–220.

92. Ogino Y, Tatsuoka Y, Matsuoka R, Nakamura K, Nakamura H, Tanaka C, Kamiya N, Matsuoka Y. Cerebral infarction after deflation of a pneumatic tourniquet during total knee replacement. *Anesthesiology.* 1999;90: 297–298.

93. Jorn LP, Lindstrand A, Toksvig-Larsen S. Tourniquet release for hemostasis increases bleeding. *Acta Orthop Scand.* 1999;70:265–267.

94. Landi A, Saracino A, Pinelli M, Caserta G, Facchini MC. Tourniquet paralysis in microsurgery. *Ann Acad Med Singapore.* 1995;24(4 suppl): 89–93.

95. Forbes TL, Carson M, Harris KA, et al. Skeletal muscle injury induced by ischemia-reperfusion. *Can J Surg.* 1995;38:56–63.

96. Petrasek PF, Shervanti HV, Walker PM. Determinants of ischemic injury to skeletal muscle. *J Vasc Surg.* 1994;19:623–630.

97. Odeh M. The role of reperfusion-induced injury in the pathogenesis of the crush syndrome. *N Engl J Med.* 1991;324:1417–1422.

98. Fasol R, Sheena I, Zilla Å. Vascular injuries caused by anti-personnel mines. *J Cardiovasc Surg.* 1989;30:467–472.

99. Mellesmo S, Pillgram-Larsen J. Primary care of amputation injuries. *JEUR.* 1995;8:131–135.

100. Husum H. Effects of early prehospital life support to war injured: the battle of Jalalabad, Afghanistan. *Prehospital Disaster Med.* 1999;14:75–80.

100a.Hoffman JR, Mower WR, Wolfson AB, Todd KH, Zucker MI, for the National Emergency X-Radiography Utilization Study Group. Validity of a set of clinical criteria to rule out injury to the cervical spine in patients with blunt trauma. *N Engl J Med.* 2000;343:94–99.

100b. Haydel MJ, Prestor CA, Mills TJ, Luber S, Blaudeau E, DeBlieux PMC. Indications for computed tomography in patients with minor head injury. *N Engl J Med.* 2000;343:100–105.

101. The Christopher Reeve Paralysis Foundation. http://www.apacure.com.

102. Domeier RM, Evans RW, Swor RA. The reliability of prehospital clinical evaluation for potential spinal injury is not affected by the mechanism of injury. *Prehosp Emerg Care.* 1999;3:332–337.

103. Domeier RM. Position paper National Association of EMS Physicians: indications for prehospital spinal immobilization. *Prehosp Emerg Care.* 1999;3:251–253.

104. Worsing RA Jr. Principles of prehospital care of musculoskeletal injuries. *Emerg Med Clin North Am.* 1984;2:205–217.

105. Pelligrino TR. Seizures and status epilepticus in adults. In: Titinalli JE, Ruiz E, Krome RL, eds. *Emergency Medicine: A Comprehensive Study Guide.* American College of Emergency Physicians. New York, NY: McGraw-Hill; 1996:1026–1033.

106. Kirby S, Sadler RM. Injury and death as a result of seizures. *Epilepsia.* 1995;36:25–28.

107. Jallon P. Sudden death of epileptic patients [in French]. *Presse Med.* 1999; 28:605–611.

108. Gur S, Yilmaz H, Tuzuner S, Aydin AT, et al. Fractures due to hypocalcemic convulsion. *Int Orthop.* 1999;23:308–309.

109. Vestergaard P, Tigaran S, Rejnmark L, et al. Fracture risk is increased in epilepsy. *Acta Neurol Scand.* 1999;99:269–275.

110. Neufeld MY, Vishne T, Chistik V, et al. Life-long history of injuries related to seizures. *Epilepsy Res.* 1999;34:123–127.

111. Buck D, Baker GA, Jacoby A, et al. Patients' experiences of injury as a result of epilepsy. *Epilepsia.* 1997;38:439–444.

112. Lip GY, Brodie MJ. Sudden death in epilepsy: an avoidable outcome? *J R Soc Med.* 1992;85:609–611.

113. Hocutt JE, Jaffe R, Rylander CR, et al. Cryotherapy in ankle sprains. *Am J Sports Med.* 1982;10:316–319.

114. Barnes L. Cryotherapy: putting injury on ice. *Phys Sports Med.* 1979;3: 130–136.

115. Kalenak A, Medlar CE, Fleagle SB, et al. Athletic injuries: heat vs cold. *Am Fam Physician.* 1975;12:131–134.

116. Starkey JA. The treatment of ankle sprains by the simultaneous use of intermittent compression and ice packs. *Am J Sports Med.* 1976;4:142–144.

117. Kalenak A, Medlar CE, Fleagle SB, et al. Treating thigh contusions with ice. *Phys Sports Med.* 1975;3:65–67.

118. Meeusen R, Lievens P. The use of cryotherapy in sports injuries. *Sports Med.* 1986;3:398–414.

119. McMaster WC, Liddle S, Waugh TR. Laboratory evaluation of various cold therapy modalities. *Am J Sports Med.* 1978;6:291–294.

120. Hocutt JE. Cryotherapy. *Am Fam Physician.* 1981;23:141–144.

Part 6: Advanced Cardiovascular Life Support
Section 1: Introduction to ACLS 2000: Overview of Recommended Changes in ACLS From the Guidelines 2000 Conference

Evidence-Based International Resuscitation Guidelines

At the Second American Heart Association International Evidence Evaluation Conference and the international Guidelines 2000 Conference on CPR and ECC, the high level of participation of international experts changed profoundly the way all future resuscitation guidelines will be developed. Future resuscitation guidelines cannot achieve validity and consensus without international input. Enrichment comes when experts from different countries—with different systems, different personnel, and different resources—share their ideas, perspectives, and experiences. Our guidelines are no longer just *descriptive*—"This is how we do it here"—but now can also be *prescriptive*—"This is how we should be doing it in the future."

The experts at the conferences reached a strong consensus to change a number of the CPR and ECC guidelines. Large portions of the earlier guidelines remain unaltered or have been refined on the basis of new data. Many topics, however, have been updated to reflect consensus opinions developed according to the principles of evidence-based medicine. While the evidence-based approach constrains the number of new guidelines endorsed, it clarifies perspectives on the evidence reviewed—and on the amount of research still needed.

New Topics, New Problems, New Guidelines

Because of rapid development of new therapies and strategies, the sections on acute myocardial infarction (MI) (now *acute coronary syndromes*) and stroke have undergone major change. We have expanded the section on special resuscitation situations for experienced providers. This includes new topics that are known to be important causes of cardiac arrest but that we have not addressed before, for example, cardiac arrest and altered vital signs caused by drug overdoses and toxins, life-threatening electrolyte abnormalities, near-fatal asthma, and anaphylaxis. These problems challenge ACLS providers all over the world.

This introductory ACLS section discusses these changes in recommendations, based on evidence review and consensus opinion. The reasons for the class recommendations and the evidence-based approach are reviewed briefly with comments from the Evidence Evaluation Conference and the Guidelines 2000 Conference. The full details of this intense process will be published in the *Proceedings of the Guidelines 2000 Conference* and in the journal *Annals of Emergency Medicine*.

The new recommendations include the following:

Pharmacology of Resuscitation

- **Amiodarone** (Class IIb) and **procainamide** (Class IIb) are recommended ahead of lidocaine and adenosine for the initial treatment of hemodynamically stable wide-complex tachycardia, especially in patients with compromised cardiac function.

- **Amiodarone** and **sotalol** (a drug that awaits Food and Drug Administration approval for US use) are new agents recommended as Class IIa agents for the treatment of *stable* monomorphic and polymorphic ventricular tachycardia (VT).

- References to **bretylium** have been dropped from the ventricular fibrillation (VF)/pulseless VT algorithm. In 1998 through 2000, severe problems with obtaining the raw materials to produce bretylium stopped the supply for a number of months. These guidelines must avoid generating a demand that cannot be met by an undependable source. The world's natural sources of bretylium appear to be nearly exhausted. Bretylium remains acceptable to use, but it is no longer recommended. Bretylium has a high incidence of side effects, particularly hypotension, in the postresuscitation setting. Bretylium stays as a Class IIb recommendation because no new, supportive information is available and some studies question its efficacy.

- **Lidocaine** is an established agent that suffered during our new emphasis on evidence. Although lidocaine remains acceptable as an antiarrhythmic to use for the treatment of shock-refractory VF and pulseless VT, the evidence supporting its efficacy is poor and methodologically weak (levels 6, 7, and 8 only). The evidence supporting amiodarone is much stronger (one level 1 study) and justifies use of amiodarone before lidocaine in the opinion of many. The conference experts concluded that lidocaine could continue to be used for VF/VT but that given the antiquated evidence, it merits only an Indeterminate class of recommendation (Class Indeterminate).

Lidocaine has not been recommended for routine prophylaxis of ventricular arrhythmias in the setting of acute MI for >8 years. Conference experts reexamined this topic and concluded that the data do not justify changing the

Circulation. 2000;102(suppl I):I-86–I-89.
© 2000 American Heart Association, Inc.

Circulation is available at http://www.circulationaha.org

classification of lidocaine to a Class III (*evidence-of-harm*) agent.

- **Amiodarone,** a respected and effective agent in the hospital, catheterization suite, and critical care unit, is included only in the notes for the VF/pulseless VT algorithm. The algorithm states "consider antiarrhythmics," referring the reader to several notes. Methodological problems in studying out-of-hospital VF/VT arrest limit the conclusions that can be drawn about any antiarrhythmic. The evidence supporting antiarrhythmics in general is only fair, and this accounts for the fact that all antiarrhythmics are lumped into one Class IIb "consider" category. However, on the strength of design and execution in the ARREST study (Kudenchuk PJ, Cobb LA, Copass MK, Cummins RO, Doherty AM, et al. *N Engl J Med.* 1999;341:871–878), amiodarone does have better evidence-based support than any other antiarrhythmic. The expert panel members would have no problem with clinicians routinely using amiodarone as the first-choice antiarrhythmic for shock-refractory VF/VT. This practice decision, however, must be made with a clear awareness that the evidence—powerful in the design—was weak in the conclusions.

- **Magnesium** has shown effectiveness only in the treatment of known hypomagnesemic states and torsades de pointes, for which it still has a Class IIb recommendation.

- **Vasopressin (arginine vasopressin)** may be a more effective pressor agent than epinephrine for promoting the return of spontaneous circulation in cardiac arrest. The evidence from prospective clinical trials in humans is limited but consistently positive (Class IIb). Vasopressin (40 U IV, not repeated) may be substituted for epinephrine as an alternative Class IIb agent. The lower adverse effects profile may be the major indication for vasopressin.

- Research on **high-dose epinephrine** has not yet shown that routine use of initial and repeated or escalating doses of epinephrine can improve survival in cardiac arrest (Class Indeterminate). Nor has high-dose epinephrine (0.1 mg/kg) in adults been shown to improve survival or neurological outcomes. Some troublesome evidence indicates that cardiac arrest survivors who received high-dose epinephrine have more postresuscitation complications than survivors who received the standard dose. Because of the potential for harm, high-dose epinephrine (0.1 mg/kg) is not recommended (Class Indeterminate).

Ventilation

- The experts on the Ventilation Panels recommend a reduction in the ventilation tidal volume for patients *not* in cardiovascular collapse to approximately one half of that recommended previously. Volume should approximate 6 to 7 mL/kg over 1.5 to 2 seconds (Class IIa). Higher volumes increase risk of gastric inflation without improving blood oxygenation. For clinical guidance, resuscitation professionals can use the "chest rise" sign as a rough indication of ventilation tidal volumes that are in the range of 6 to 7 mL/kg. Smaller tidal volumes, however, raise the risk of inducing both hypoxia and hypercarbia. Consequently, a widespread recommendation to provide supplemental oxygen, adjusted on the basis of oxygen saturation readings, appears laudable, although specific, high-level evidence to support this recommendation has not yet become available.

- **Tracheal intubation** in unconscious patients should be attempted only by healthcare providers experienced in performing this skill. Such persons should increase their experience in tracheal intubations steadily by performing intubations frequently or by retraining regularly. Only personnel with advanced life support training and documented skills should attempt tracheal intubation. Furthermore, ALS providers unable to obtain regular field experience (non–evidence-based guideline: 6 to 12 times per year) should use alternative, noninvasive techniques for airway management.

- In the absence of a bag-mask device or authorization to perform tracheal intubation, healthcare providers may use alternative airways (laryngeal mask airway, esophageal-tracheal Combitube, pharyngotracheal lumen airway) (Class IIb).

- In the opinion of many experts the single most important new recommendation from the Guidelines 2000 is long overdue: emergency responders must **confirm tracheal tube position** by using nonphysical examination techniques. These include **esophageal detector devices, qualitative end-tidal CO_2 indicators, and capnographic and capnometric devices.** In patients not in full cardiac arrest these devices are Class IIa. In cardiac arrest and conditions of low pulmonary flow, these devices are lowered to Class IIb because the devices may falsely indicate esophageal placement, leading to unnecessary removal of a properly placed tube.

- Growing evidence suggests that **tracheal tube dislodgments** after a successful tracheal tube insertion may be occurring at much higher rates than previously suspected. Emphasis should be placed on securing the tube carefully with a tie or tape. With little evidence to directly support any specific commercial device, tracheal tube holders are a Class IIb recommendation. During long transport efforts in the out-of-hospital setting, restless intubated patients can be fitted with a cervical collar and immobilized with sandbags (or some other validated technique) to prevent accidental tube dislodgment. With little evidence to directly support any specific commercial device, tracheal tube holders are a Class IIb recommendation. During long transport efforts in the out-of-hospital setting, intubated patients are at high risk for tracheal tube dislodgment. Monitors for oxygen saturation and end-tidal CO_2 levels can detect tube dislodgments. The best technique, however, to prevent, detect, and correct tube dislodgment is the constant vigilance of care providers.

Defibrillation

- Healthcare providers with a duty to perform CPR need to be trained, equipped, and authorized to use an automated external defibrillator (AED) (Class IIa).

- Hospitals need to establish a comprehensive program for in-hospital early CPR and early defibrillation. Hospital staff members trained in CPR need to be capable of providing early defibrillation.

- Hospitals need to establish programs to achieve early defibrillation throughout the facilities and in related patient care areas (Class I).

Public Access Defibrillation Programs

- Public access defibrillation (PAD) programs have the potential to reduce one of the major health problems—VF-induced cardiac arrest.
- AEDs are recommended for public sites with a high probability of at least one use every 5 years (1 arrest per 5 years). Select sites for AED deployment that are within a 5-minute radius of the majority of expected arrests but outside a 5-minute radius of the closest EMS units (Class IIb).

Acute Coronary Syndromes

- **The prehospital 12-lead ECG** improves prehospital diagnosis, reduces hospital-based time to treatment, identifies patients requiring reperfusion, contributes to mortality reduction, and facilitates triage to cardiac centers with interventional facilities. The prehospital ECG is useful and effective in prehospital urban/suburban EMS systems and should become standard equipment on all ACLS units that handle acute coronary syndrome patients (Class IIa).
- **Prehospital fibrinolytic therapy** is beneficial when the transport of patients with acute infarction from home to the hospital is prolonged and should be considered by busy EMS systems (Class IIa). At present, prehospital screening of chest pain patients allows ambulance personnel to notify hospital personnel that a person with a probable acute MI is en route for further evaluation and care.
  - If the total time of the following 2 intervals exceeds 60 minutes, consider prehospital fibrinolytics: (1) onset of chest pain to contact of ACLS personnel with the patient, and (2) arrival of ACLS personnel at the patient's side to arrival at the hospital.
  - In Europe a prehospital fibrinolytic program is considered whenever the above intervals exceed 30 minutes. Moreover, if the Emergency Department has a door-to-fibrinolytic interval consistently >60 minutes, prehospital fibrinolytic treatment should offer superior outcomes.
- **Angioplasty is an alternative to fibrinolytic therapy** (Class I) in centers with high volume and experienced operators. Patients in cardiogenic shock who are <75 years of age need transportation to cardiac interventional centers for initiation of primary angioplasty and intra-aortic balloon placement. Benefit occurs, however, only when door-to-balloon times average ≤90 minutes (Class I). Patients who are not eligible for fibrinolytic therapy because of increased risk of intracranial bleeding need to be transported or transferred to these centers (Class IIa). Patients with large anterior infarctions, low blood pressure (systolic blood pressure ≤100 mm Hg), increased heart rate (≥100 beats per minute), or rales more than one third of the way

up are also candidates (Class IIa). Prehospital EMS systems should develop triage policies where applicable.
  - Antiplatelet therapy with glycoprotein IIb/IIIa inhibitors for patients with non–Q-wave MI and high-risk unstable angina provides clinically significant benefit (Class IIa). Antithrombin therapy with low-molecular-weight heparins is now an alternative to unfractionated heparin in high-risk unstable angina/non–Q-wave MI patients. Data for this class of agents, however, is heterogeneous, in part because of variable anti–factor Xa inhibition (Class Indeterminate). The dose of unfractionated heparin, when used as adjunctive therapy with fibrin-specific lytics (alteplase, reteplase) is now reduced to a bolus of 60 U/kg (maximum 4000 U) and an infusion of 12 IU/kg per hour. This dose reduction will help to minimize the incidence of intracerebral hemorrhage.
  - Metabolic manipulation of the infarct with glucose-potassium-insulin is under continuing investigation. This therapy is acceptable and of some benefit for diabetic patients and patients undergoing reperfusion (Class IIb).
  - All patients with acute MI, including non–Q-wave MI, need aspirin and β-blockers in the absence of contraindications (Class I). Patients with a large anterior infarction, left ventricular dysfunction, and ejection fraction <40% need early angiotensin-converting enzyme inhibition in the absence of hypotension.

Stroke

- **Intravenous recombinant tissue plasminogen activator (rtPA)** improves neurological outcome when administered within 3 hours of stroke onset in patients who meet fibrinolytic criteria (Class I). Patients with stroke presenting within 3 hours require emergent triage. The urgency should equal that of an acute MI, with ST-segment elevation.
- The use of **rtPA** in patients with symptom onset between 3 and 6 hours of presentation at an Emergency Department is under investigation. While subgroups of such patients may benefit from fibrinolytic treatment, routine use is not currently recommended (Class Indeterminate).
- **Prourokinase** has been found to improve neurological outcome in patients treated within 3 to 6 hours in one completed but unpublished study. Review of the published data and additional studies are needed before this fibrinolytic agent can be recommended (Class Indeterminate).
- EMS systems should implement a **prehospital stroke protocol** to rapidly identify patients who may benefit from **fibrinolytic therapy.** This approach is similar to the protocol for chest pain patients (Class IIb). Transport patients who may be candidates for fibrinolytic therapy to hospitals identified as acute stroke treatment facilities with 24-hour availability of computerized tomography and interpretation (Class IIb).

Postresuscitation Care

- Following cardiac arrest, do not actively rewarm patients who are mildly hypothermic (Class IIb). Active initiation of hypothermia after cardiac arrest is under clinical investigation (Class Indeterminate). Treat febrile patients to achieve normothermia, a goal of early therapy (Class IIa).

- Following cardiac arrest, ventilatory values in patients who require mechanical ventilation should be maintained within the normal range (Class IIa). Hyperventilation may be harmful and should be avoided (Class III). An exception is the use of hyperventilation in patients who have signs of cerebral herniation after resuscitation.

Toxicology

- Cocaine use is associated with serious ventricular arrhythmias and acute coronary syndromes. The use of β-blockers in patients with cocaine-associated acute coronary syndromes has caused coronary vasoconstriction and should be avoided (Class III). Nitrates should be first-line therapy (Class I) together with benzodiazepines (Class IIa). α-Adrenergic blocking agents may induce tachycardia and hypotension and should be reserved for patients who do not respond to nitrates and benzodiazepines (Class IIb).
- Hypotension or ventricular arrhythmias occur with tricyclic overdose. The induction of systemic alkalosis (pH of 7.50 to 7.55) is the treatment of choice (Class IIa). Antiarrhythmic agents such as lidocaine or procainamide have not been studied in this setting (Class Indeterminate).
- Acute respiratory failure (respiratory acidosis and hypoxemia) may occur with opiate overdose. Reverse these abnormalities by mechanical ventilation before the administration of naloxone. This will reduce the incidence of pulmonary edema and serious arrhythmias associated with abrupt catecholamine elevation (Class IIa).

Overview of ACLS

ACLS includes the knowledge and skills necessary to provide the appropriate early treatment for cardiopulmonary arrest. Additional important areas include the proper management of situations likely to lead to cardiac arrest and stabilization of the patient in the early period following successful resuscitation. ACLS includes (1) basic life support; (2) use of advanced equipment and special techniques for establishing and maintaining effective ventilation and circulation; (3) ECG monitoring, 12-lead ECG interpretation, and arrhythmia recognition; (4) establishment and maintenance of intravenous access; (5) therapies for the treatment of patients with cardiac or respiratory arrest (including stabilization in the postarrest phase); (6) treatment of patients with suspected acute coronary syndromes, including acute MI; and (7) strategies for rapid assessment and treatment with tPA of eligible stroke patients. ACLS includes the knowledge, training, and judgment required to use these skills and the ability to perform them.

Communities should provide rapid and effective ACLS. Every community should strive continually to implement the Chain of Survival and provide as many high-quality ACLS components as possible, in particular very early defibrillation using AEDs (see "Part 4: The Automated External Defibrillator: Key Link in the Chain of Survival") and noninvasive airway support.

BLS and ACLS should be integrated into a community as part of an EMS system. This system should have sufficient laypersons trained in BLS to ensure immediate ventilatory and circulatory assistance to any cardiac arrest victim within 5 minutes and immediate entry of that victim into the EMS system. We strongly encourage implementation of public access defibrillation in high-risk settings. In turn the emergency care system, under medical supervision, should provide rescue personnel adequately trained in BLS and ACLS to respond promptly when summoned. ACLS must be continued either until the patient has been admitted to a medical facility capable of continuing care or until life support efforts have been terminated by order of the responsible physician or by a properly executed advance directive.

The same level of training, commitment, and medical supervision should be applied to in-hospital ACLS. In particular, prompt BLS and rapid defibrillation should be available in all areas of a healthcare facility (Class IIa).

BLS and Early Defibrillation

For people in cardiac arrest, *rapid defibrillation in <5 minutes* is a high-priority goal. Community and in-hospital ACLS must be supported by a well-established BLS program that can provide immediate emergency CPR. The Evidence Evaluation Conference and Guidelines 2000 Conference again affirmed and endorsed the principle of early defibrillation from 1991—the recommendation that healthcare providers with a duty to respond to cardiac arrest should be educated, equipped, and authorized to perform automated external defibrillation (Class IIa). The ideal response time is achieved when people collapse in front of a person who has an AED. Such cases occur in many locations, and in general the survival rate can be 70% to 80%.

For respiratory arrest, airway adjuncts and ventilation devices should be readily available. In cardiac arrest, the need for early defibrillation is clear and should have the highest priority. Today, with the availability of AEDs, defibrillation is considered part of BLS. Adjunctive equipment should not divert attention or effort from basic resuscitative measures. Rescue personnel should know the indications for and techniques of using adjunctive equipment. Such equipment should be tested periodically according to prescribed regulations and each periodic test documented.

Section 2: Defibrillation

For a person in VF the probability of successful defibrillation and subsequent survival to hospital discharge is directly and negatively related to the time interval between onset of VF and delivery of the first shock.[1-3] Early defibrillation by first rescuers and trained lay responders is a rational implementation of the concept that the earlier defibrillation is performed, the better the rate of survival to hospital discharge. Early defibrillation has reversed VF cardiac arrest in a number of small case series (American Airlines, QANTAS Airlines,[4] Chicago's O'Hare Airport,[4a] and Las Vegas casinos[5]). These dramatic examples of the effectiveness of early defibrillation by nontraditional responders have provided a driving force for PAD in the United States.[6-10]

For more than a decade the AHA has recommended that every ambulance vehicle be equipped with a defibrillator and personnel trained in defibrillation.[11] All healthcare providers with a duty to perform CPR should be trained, equipped, and encouraged to perform defibrillation (Class IIa). The Guidelines 2000 Conference recommends that early defibrillation be available throughout all hospital and outpatient medical facilities (Class IIa). The use of defibrillation now transcends both ACLS and BLS care. This section addresses use of standard defibrillators, including cardioversion, for the experienced healthcare provider in the ACLS environment. Early defibrillation, automated external defibrillation, and PAD are also discussed in "Part 4: The Automated External Defibrillator: Key Link in the Chain of Survival."

Energy Requirements for Defibrillation

Defibrillation depends on the successful selection of energy to generate sufficient current flow through the heart (transmyocardial current) to achieve defibrillation while at the same time causing minimal electrical injury to the heart. A shock will not terminate the arrhythmia if the energy and current are too low. Functional and morphological damage may result if energy and current are too high.[12,13] Selection of appropriate current also reduces the number of repetitive shocks and limits myocardial damage.[14] There is no definite relationship between body size and energy requirements for defibrillation in adults. Transthoracic impedance does play an important role (see below).

Biphasic Waveform Defibrillators

Modern defibrillators, including AEDs, deliver energy or current in "waveforms." Energy levels vary with the type of device and type of waveform. Several types of monophasic waveforms have been used in modern defibrillators. Biphasic waveforms have recently been developed and approved for marketing and clinical use. The body of evidence about the efficacy and safety of devices using biphasic waveforms has increased dramatically in the 4 years since the first such device was marketed. The first biphasic AED approved for use in the United States used a waveform set at a lower energy (150 to 175 J) than that recommended by the AHA (200 J) for the first shock. This first device also was fixed-nonescalating, meaning the energy level of shocks could not be increased. In a recent review of evidence through 1997 for nonescalating low-energy biphasic waveforms in out-of-hospital arrest,[15] the reviewers concluded that lower-energy biphasic shocks, delivered without an increase in energy, achieved clinical outcomes equivalent to those of monophasic shocks with increasing energy levels.

Monophasic waveforms deliver current in one direction. Monophasic defibrillators vary the speed and amount of waveform fall and the speed of the return to zero voltage point. If the monophasic waveform falls to zero gradually, the term *damped sinusoidal* is used. If the waveform falls instantaneously, the term *truncated exponential* is used. Biphasic waveforms, in contrast, deliver current that flows in a positive direction for a specified duration. The current then reverses and flows in a negative direction for the remaining milliseconds of the electrical discharge. Biphasic waveforms have proved superior to monophasic waveforms for defibrillation by implantable defibrillators.[15,17] (See the Figure.)

In 1996 the Food and Drug Administration approved the first AED that used a biphasic waveform.. This was a biphasic truncated exponential (BTE) waveform with impedance compensation. This AED delivered only nonescalating 150-J shocks. Studies compared this waveform with conventional monophasic damped sinusoidal (MDS) waveform shocks at 200 and 360 J. These studies were conducted in electrophysiology stimulation suites during implantation of automatic implantable cardioverter-defibrillators (ICDs). In projects funded by defibrillator manufacturers, researchers observed that 150-J BTE shocks achieved first-shock defibrillation at the same rate as 200-J MDS shocks. BTE 150-J shocks also produced less ST-segment change than 200-J MDS shocks.[18] Researchers have collected data both in-hospital (electrophysiological studies and ICD testing) and out of hospital.[19] This research indicates that repetitive lower-energy biphasic waveform shocks (repeated shocks at ≤200 J) have equivalent or higher success for eventual termination of VF than defibrillators that increase the current (200, 300, 360 J) with successive shocks (escalating).

Biphasic Waveform Defibrillation

The optimal energies for biphasic defibrillation have not been determined. Importantly, the biphasic first-shock energy level

Circulation. 2000;102(suppl I):I-90–I-94.
© 2000 American Heart Association, Inc.

Circulation is available at http://www.circulationaha.org

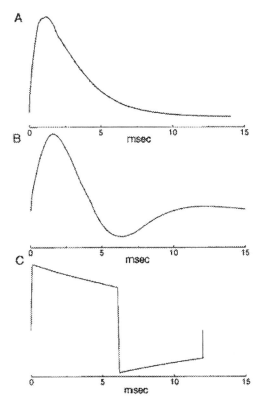

Relative efficacy of monophasic and biphasic waveforms for transthoracic defibrillation after short and long durations of ventricular fibrillation. Reprinted with permission from Walcott GP, Melnick SB, Chapman FW, Jones JL, Smith WM, Ideker RE. Relative efficacy of monophasic and biphasic waveforms for transthoracic defibrillation after short and long durations of ventricular fibrillation. *Circulation.* 1998;98:2210–2215.

yielding the highest termination rate for VF is unknown. The percentage of patients who fail to respond to a first or successive biphasic shock at a constant energy of ≤200 J remains unknown. Do patients in VF that is unresponsive to multiple "lower-energy" shocks then require higher-energy (escalating) biphasic shocks? Or will these patients require only repetition of low-energy biphasic shocks?

Research has not yet determined the *optimal* biphasic waveform. The potential advantages of new biphasic waveform variants, such as a *rectilinear first pulse waveform,* are also unknown. Researchers need to study the efficacy of "impedance compensation." Compensation for patient-to-patient differences in impedance may be achieved by changes in duration and voltage of shocks or by releasing the residual membrane charge (called *burping*). Whether there is an optimal ratio of first-phase to second-phase duration and leading-edge amplitude is unclear. The threshold for the start and extent of cardiac damage from biphasic waveforms compared with monophasic waveforms remains a mystery. Finally, it will be important to determine whether a waveform more effective for *immediate outcomes* (defibrillation) and *short-term outcomes* (spontaneous circulation, admission to the hospital) results in better *long-term outcomes* (survival to hospital discharge, survival for 1 year). These are critical questions in communities in which the interval from collapse to first shock remains long.

Shock Energies

The traditional recommended energy for the first monophasic shock is 200 J.[20] The energy level for second and third shocks can be either the same (200 J) or as high as 360 J. Even a failed shock at one energy may be successful if simply repeated. Clinically the energy does not need to increase simply because the first shock failed to defibrillate. Any given energy has a constant probability to achieve defibrillation. Repeated shocks, even at the same energy level, *add* to the probability of successful defibrillation. This is not immediately obvious but can be clarified with a brief example. A waveform with a defibrillation rate of 80% will leave 20% of the victims in VF with each successive shock: of 100 people, first shock=20 in VF; second shock=4 in VF (20% of 20); third shock=1 in VF (20% of 4). Thus, this waveform, with a 1-shock success rate of 80%, will achieve a 99% success rate if the 3 successive, nonescalating shocks are considered a single intervention.

Higher current flow will occur with subsequent shocks even at the same energy, because transthoracic impedance declines with repeated shocks.[21,22] These arguments favor repeating the second shock at the same energy level as the first if VF persists, but reductions in human transthoracic impedance are only modest.[21] A more predictable increase in current occurs when shock energy is increased. This supports second shocks of higher energy. A compromise between these positions is the use of a range of energies (200 to 300 J) for the second monophasic shock.

Increase the current/voltage and deliver a third shock of 360 J immediately if 2 *monophasic* shocks fail to defibrillate the heart. If VF is initially terminated by a shock but then recurs later in the arrest, deliver subsequent shocks at the previously successful energy level.

We cannot make a definitive recommendation for the energy for first and subsequent nonescalating biphasic defibrillation attempts. Current research confirms that biphasic shock energies ≤200 J are safe and effective. Even though both escalating- and nonescalating-energy defibrillators are available, there is insufficient data to recommend one approach over another. Any claim of superiority at this time is unsupported. Nonescalating biphasic energies appear to have success rates for VF termination equivalent to or better than monophasic shocks (Class IIa) that increase in energy with each shock.

The most important determinant of survival in adult VF is rapid defibrillation. Give shocks as soon as a defibrillator is available.[1,2] If the first 3 shocks fail to achieve defibrillation immediately, continue CPR and follow the ACLS guidelines for sudden VF/VT: IV access, tracheal intubation, epinephrine; shock if still in VF; consider amiodarone or lidocaine.

Cardioversion

Atrial Fibrillation

The recommended initial energy for cardioversion of atrial fibrillation is 100 to 200 J MDS. Atrial flutter and paroxysmal supraventricular tachycardia (PSVT) generally require less energy. An initial energy of 50 to 100 J MDS is often sufficient, with stepwise increases in energy if initial shocks fail.[23-25] Transthoracic cardioversion of atrial fibrillation with a low-energy (120-J), rectilinear, first-pulse biphasic waveform was superior to 200 J MDS in a recent controlled trial.[26] Cardioversion with biphasic waveform is now available, but more data is needed before specific comparative recommendations can be made.

Ventricular Tachycardia

The amount of energy required for cardioversion of VT depends on the morphological characteristics and rate of the arrhythmia.[27] Monomorphic VT (regular form and rate) with or without a pulse responds well to cardioversion shocks at initial energies of 100 J MDS. Polymorphic VT (irregular morphology and rate) responds similarly to VF. The initial shock energy should be 200 J MDS. Give stepwise increases if the first shock fails to cardiovert.[27]

Transthoracic Impedance

Defibrillation is accomplished by passage of sufficient electric current (amperes) through the heart. The energy chosen (joules) and the transthoracic impedance (ohms), or resistance to current flow, determine the current flow. Factors that determine transthoracic impedance include energy selected, electrode size, paddle-skin coupling material, number and time interval of previous shocks, phase of ventilation, distance between electrodes (size of the chest), and paddle electrode pressure.[21,22,28] The average adult human impedance is approximately 70 to 80 Ω.[13,21,22,29-31] When transthoracic impedance is too high, a low-energy shock will not generate enough current to achieve defibrillation.[13,24,30] To reduce transthoracic impedance, the defibrillator operator should always press firmly on handheld electrode paddles and use a gel or cream or saline-soaked gauze pads between handheld electrode paddles and the chest. Self-adhesive monitor/defibrillator electrode pads do not require additional pressure. Use of "bare" handheld paddles without a coupling material between electrodes and the chest wall creates high transthoracic impedance.[22] Male patients with a hirsute chest have poor electrode-to-chest contact plus air trapping. This results in high impedance, with occasional "arcing." (Although extremely rare, in oxygen-rich environments such as critical care units this arcing has been known to produce fires if an accelerant is present.) Rapid shaving of the area of intended pad placement may be necessary. The AHA textbook *Heartsaver AED for the Lay Rescuer and First Responder* contains an excellent description of successful approaches to removal of chest hair.

Current-Based Defibrillation

VF and other cardiac arrhythmias can be terminated by electric shock when sufficient current passes through the myocardium. A promising alternative approach to defibrillation is the use of electric current (amperes) instead of energy (joules). This approach would prevent attempts to deliver inappropriately low energy levels to a patient with high impedance. Current-based therapy would also prevent high-energy shocks to patients with low impedance, which result in excessive current flow, myocardial damage, and failure to defibrillate.[13,24]

Clinical studies using MDS waveform shocks have attempted to identify the range of current necessary to achieve defibrillation and cardioversion. The optimal current for ventricular defibrillation appears to be 30 to 40 A MDS.[29-31] Comparable information on current dosage for biphasic waveform shocks is under investigation.

Electrode Position

Place electrodes in positions to maximize current flow through the myocardium. The standard placement is one electrode just to the right of the upper sternal border below the clavicle. Place the second electrode to the left of the nipple with the center of the electrode in the midaxillary line. An acceptable alternative is to place the "apex" paddle anterior, over the left precordium, and the other paddle (labeled "sternum") posterior to the heart in the *right* infrascapular location.[32,33] Take care that the electrodes are well separated and that paste or gel is not smeared on the chest between the paddles, because the current may follow a superficial pathway along the chest wall, "missing" the heart. Self-adhesive monitor/defibrillator electrode pads are also effective and can be used in any of these locations.[31]

When performing cardioversion or defibrillation in patients with permanent pacemakers or ICDs, do not place the electrodes near the device generator, because defibrillation can cause malfunction. A pacemaker or ICD also may block some current to the myocardium during defibrillation, delivering suboptimal energy to the heart. Finally, because some of the defibrillation current flows down the pacemaker leads, always reevaluate the pacing threshold after shock(s) to patients with permanent pacemakers.[34] ICD function also should be evaluated.

Electrode Size

The Association for the Advancement of Medical Instrumentation recommends a minimum electrode size of 50 cm^2 for individual electrodes.[35] The sum of the electrode areas should be a minimum of 150 cm^2. Larger electrodes have lower impedance, but excessively large electrodes may result in less transmyocardial current flow.[36]

For adult defibrillation, both handheld paddle electrodes and self-adhesive pad electrodes 8 to 12 cm in diameter are used and perform well.[21,31,37] Even smaller pads have been found effective[38] in VF of brief duration.

Synchronized Cardioversion

Delivered energy should be *synchronized* with the QRS complex to reduce the possibility of inducing VF, which can occur when a shock "hits" the relative refractory portion of the cardiac cycle.[32] *Synchronization* to prevent this complication is recommended for hemodynamically stable wide-complex tachycardia requiring cardioversion, supraventricular tachycardia, atrial fibrillation, and atrial flutter. VF requires *unsynchronized* defibrillation mode. It is important to note that synchronization in VT may be difficult and misleading because of the wide-complex and variable forms of ventricular arrhythmia. The VT patient who is pulseless, unconscious, hypotensive, or in severe pulmonary edema should receive unsynchronized shocks to avoid the delay associated with attempts to synchronize. The healthcare provider should be prepared to deliver another unsynchronized shock within seconds if VF or pulseless VT remains or recurs.

Blind Defibrillation

Administration of shocks without a monitor or an ECG rhythm diagnosis is referred to as "blind" defibrillation. Blind defibrillation is rarely necessary. Handheld paddles with "quick-look" monitoring capabilities on modern manually operated defibrillators are universally available. AEDs use reliable and proven decision algorithms to identify VF.

"Occult" Versus "False" Asystole

There is no evidence that attempting to "defibrillate" asystole is beneficial. In rare patients, however, coarse VF can be present in some leads, with very small undulations seen in the orthogonal leads, which is called *occult VF*. A flat line that may resemble asystole is displayed. Examine the rhythm in 2 leads to help differentiate this technical artifact.[39] Of more importance, one study noted that "false" asystole, a flat line produced by technical errors (eg, no power, leads unconnected, gain set to low, or incorrect lead selection), was far more frequent than occult VF.[40]

Maintaining Defibrillators in a State of Readiness

User checklists have been developed to reduce equipment malfunction and operator errors. Failure to properly maintain the defibrillator or power supply is responsible for the majority of reported malfunctions. Checklists are useful when designed to identify and prevent such deficiencies. Checklists help most when (1) users are trained in their proper use, (2) healthcare providers who actually use the defibrillators perform the check, and (3) checklists are completed with every change in personnel.

References

1. Eisenberg MS, Copass MK, Hallstrom AP, Blake B, Bergner L, Short F, Cobb L. Treatment of out-of-hospital cardiac arrest with rapid defibrillation by emergency medical technicians. *N Engl J Med*. 1980;302: 1379–1383.
2. Stults KR, Brown DD, Schug VL, Bean JA. Prehospital defibrillation performed by emergency medical technicians in rural communities. *N Engl J Med*. 1984;310:219–223.
3. Larsen MP, Eisenberg MS, Cummins RO, Hallstrom AP. Predicting survival from out-of-hospital cardiac arrest: a graphic model. *Ann Emerg Med*. 1993;22:1652–1658.
4. O'Rourke MF, Donaldson E, Geddes JS. An airline cardiac arrest program [see comments]. *Circulation*. 1997;96:2849–2853.
4a. Help is only one minute away. *Currents in Emergency Cardiovascular Care*. Fall 1999;10:1, 4.
5. Valenzuela TD, Bjerke HS, Clark LL, et al. Rapid defibrillation by nontraditional responders: the Casino Project. *Acad Emerg Med*. 1998;5: 414–415.
6. Cummins RO, Graves JR, Horan S, Larsen MP, Crump K. The relative contributions of early defibrillation and ACLS interventions to resuscitation and survival from prehospital cardiac arrest. *Ann Emerg Med*. 1989;18:468–469. Abstract.
7. Bossaert L, Callanan V, Cummins RO. Early defibrillation: an advisory statement by the Advanced Life Support Working Group of the International Liaison Committee on Resuscitation. *Resuscitation*. 1997;34: 113–114.
8. Wilcox-Gok VL. Survival from out-of-hospital cardiac arrest: a multivariate analysis. *Med Care*. 1991;29:104–114.
9. White R, Asplin B, Bugliosi T, Hankins D. High discharge survival rate after out-of-hospital ventricular fibrillation with rapid defibrillation by police and paramedics. *Ann Emerg Med*. 1996;28:480–485.
10. Weisfeldt ML, Kerber RE, McGoldrick RP, Moss AJ, Nichol G, Ornato JP, Palmer DG, Riegel B, Smith SC Jr, Automatic External Defibrillation Task Force. American Heart Association report on the Public Access Defibrillation Conference December 8–10, 1994 [see comments]. *Circulation*. 1995;92:2740–2747.
11. Kerber R, members of Emergency Cardiac Care Committee. Statement on early defibrillation from the American Heart Association. *Circulation*. 1991;83:2233.
12. Dahl CF, Ewy GA, Warner ED, Thomas ED. Myocardial necrosis from direct current countershock: effect of paddle electrode size and time interval between discharges. *Circulation*. 1974;50:956–961.
13. Kerber RE, Kouba C, Martins J, Kelly K, Low R, Hoyt R, Ferguson D, Bailey L, Bennett P, Charbonnier F. Advance prediction of transthoracic impedance in human defibrillation and cardioversion: importance of impedance in determining the success of low-energy shocks. *Circulation*. 1984;70:303–308.
14. Joglar JA, Kessler DJ, Welch PJ, Keffer JH, Jessen ME, Hamdan MH, Page RL. Effects of repeated electrical defibrillations on cardiac troponin I levels. *Am J Cardiol*. 1999;83:270–272, A6.
15. Cummins RO, Hazinski MF, Kerber RE, Kudenchuk P, Becker L, Nichol G, Malanga B, Aufderheide TP, Stapleton EM, Kern K, Ornato JP, Sanders A, Valenzuela T, Eisenberg M. Low-energy biphasic waveform defibrillation: evidence-based review applied to emergency cardiovascular care guidelines: a statement for healthcare professionals from the American Heart Association Committee on Emergency Cardiovascular Care and the Subcommittees on Basic Life Support, Advanced Cardiac Life Support, and Pediatric Resuscitation. *Circulation*. 1998;97:1654–1667.
16. Deleted in proof.
17. Fain E, Sweeney M, Franz M. Improved internal defibrillation efficacy with a biphasic waveform. *Am Heart J*. 1989;117:358–364.
18. Bardy GH, Marchlinski FE, Sharma AD, Worley SJ, Luceri RM, Yee R, Halperin BD, Fellows CL, Ahern TS, Chilson DA, Packer DL, Wilber DJ, Mattioni TA, Reddy R, Kronmal RA, Lazzara R, Transthoracic Investigators. Multicenter comparison of truncated biphasic shocks and standard damped sine wave monophasic shocks for transthoracic ventricular defibrillation. *Circulation*. 1996;94:2507–2514.
19. Poole JE, White RD, Kanz KG, Hengstenberg F, Jarrard GT, Robinson JC, Santana V, McKenas DK, Rich N, Rosas S, Merritt S, Magnotto L, Gallagher JV III, Gliner BE, Jorgenson DB, Morgan CB, Dillon SM, Kronmal RA, Bardy GH. Low-energy impedance-compensating biphasic waveforms terminate ventricular fibrillation at high rates in victims of out-of-hospital cardiac arrest. *J Cardiovasc Electrophysiol*. 1997;8:1373–1385.
20. Weaver WD, Cobb LA, Copass MK, Hallstrom AP. Ventricular defibrillation: a comparative trial using 175-J and 320-J shocks. *N Engl J Med*. 1982;307:1101–1106.
21. Kerber RE, Grayzel J, Hoyt R, Marcus M, Kennedy J. Transthoracic resistance in human defibrillation: influence of body weight, chest size, serial shocks, paddle size and paddle contact pressure. *Circulation*. 1981;63: 676–682.
22. Sirna SJ, Ferguson DW, Charbonnier F, Kerber RE. Factors affecting transthoracic impedance during electrical cardioversion. *Am J Cardiol*. 1988;62:1048–1052.
23. Deleted in proof.
24. Kerber R, Martins J, Kienzle M, Constantin L, Olshansky B, Hopson R, Charbonnier F. Energy, current, and success in defibrillation and cardioversion: clinical studies using an automated impedance-based method of energy adjustment. *Circulation*. 1988;77:1038–1046.
25. Pinski SL, Sgarbossa EB, Ching E, Trohman RG. A comparison of 50-J versus 100-J shocks for direct-current cardioversion of atrial flutter. *Am Heart J*. 1999;137:439–442.
26. Mittal S, Ayati S, Stein KM, Schwartzman D, Cavlovich D, Tchou PJ, Markowitz SM, Slotwiner DJ, Scheiner MA, Lerman BB. Transthoracic cardioversion of atrial fibrillation: comparison of rectilinear biphasic versus damped sine wave monophasic shocks. *Circulation*. 2000;101: 1282–1287.
27. Kerber RE, Kienzle MG, Olshansky B, Waldo AL, Wilber D, Carlson MD, Aschoff AM, Birger S, Fugatt L, Walsh S, et al. Ventricular tachycardia rate and morphology determine energy and current requirements for transthoracic cardioversion. *Circulation*. 1992;85:158–163.
28. Ewy GA, Hellman DA, McClung S, Taren D. Influence of ventilation phase on transthoracic impedance and defibrillation effectiveness. *Crit Care Med*. 1980;8:164–166.

29. Lerman BB, DiMarco JP, Haines DE. Current-based versus energy-based ventricular defibrillation: a prospective study. *J Am Coll Cardiol*. 1988; 12:1259–1264.

30. Dalzell GW, Cunningham SR, Anderson J, Adgey AA. Electrode pad size, transthoracic impedance and success of external ventricular defibrillation. *Am J Cardiol*. 1989;64:741–744.

31. Kerber RE, Martins JB, Kelly KJ, Ferguson DW, Kouba C, Jensen SR, Newman B, Parke JD, Kieso R, Melton J. Self-adhesive preapplied electrode pads for defibrillation and cardioversion. *J Am Coll Cardiol*. 1984;3:815–820.

32. Lown B. Electrical reversion of cardiac arrhythmias. *Br Heart J*. 1967; 29:469–489.

33. Kerber RE, Jensen SR, Grayzel J, Kennedy J, Hoyt R. Elective cardioversion: influence of paddle-electrode location and size on success rates and energy requirements. *N Engl J Med*. 1981;305:658–662.

34. Levine PA, Barold SS, Fletcher RD, Talbot P. Adverse acute and chronic effects of electrical defibrillation and cardioversion on implanted unipolar cardiac pacing systems. *J Am Coll Cardiol*. 1983;1:1413–1422.

35. Association for the Advancement of Medical Instrumentation. *American National Standard: Automatic External Defibrillators and Remote Controlled Defibrillators (DF39)*. Arlington, Va: Association for the Advancement of Medical Instrumentation; 1993.

36. Hoyt R, Grayzel J, Kerber RE. Determinants of intracardiac current in defibrillation: experimental studies in dogs. *Circulation*. 1981;64: 818–823.

37. Stults KR, Brown DD, Cooley F, Kerber RE. Self-adhesive monitor/defibrillation pads improve prehospital defibrillation success. *Ann Emerg Med*. 1987;16:872–877.

38. Wilson RF, Sirna S, White CW, Kerber RE. Defibrillation of high-risk patients during coronary angiography using self-adhesive, preapplied electrode pads. *Am J Cardiol*. 1987;60:380–382.

39. Ewy GA, Dahl CF, Zimmermann M, Otto C. Ventricular fibrillation masquerading as ventricular standstill. *Crit Care Med*. 1981;9:841–844.

40. Cummins RO, Austin D Jr. The frequency of "occult" ventricular fibrillation masquerading as a flat line in prehospital cardiac arrest. *Ann Emerg Med*. 1988;17:813–817.

Section 3: Adjuncts for Oxygenation, Ventilation, and Airway Control

Oxygenation Devices

During cardiopulmonary emergencies use supplemental oxygen as soon as it is available. Rescue breathing (ventilation using exhaled air) will deliver approximately 16% to 17% inspired oxygen concentration to the patient, ideally producing an alveolar oxygen tension of 80 mm Hg. During cardiac arrest and CPR, tissue hypoxia occurs because of low cardiac output with reduced peripheral oxygen delivery and a resulting wide arteriovenous oxygen difference. Additional factors that cause hypoxia are intrapulmonary shunting with attendant ventilation-perfusion abnormalities and underlying respiratory disease. Tissue hypoxia leads to anaerobic metabolism and metabolic acidosis. Acid-base imbalance frequently blunts the beneficial effects of chemical and electrical therapy. For these reasons 100% inspired oxygen ($Fio_2 = 1.0$) is recommended during BLS and ACLS when available. High inspired oxygen tensions will tend to maximize arterial blood oxygen saturation and, in turn, systemic oxygen delivery (cardiac output × blood oxygen content). Short-term therapy with 100% oxygen is beneficial and not toxic. Oxygen toxicity occurs during prolonged therapy with a high Fio_2.

In patients with acute MI, supplemental oxygen reduces both the magnitude and the extent of ST-segment changes on the ECG. We recommend oxygen administered at 4 L/min by nasal cannula for the first 2 to 3 hours for all patients with suspected acute coronary syndromes (Class IIa). The use of oxygen beyond 3 to 6 hours is indicated for patients with continuing or recurrent ischemia, complicated infarcts with congestive heart failure, or arrhythmia until hypoxemia has resolved and the patient is clinically stable.

Ventilatory Devices

Masks

A well-fitting mask can be an effective, simple adjunct for use in artificial ventilation by appropriately trained rescuers. Masks should be made of transparent material to allow detection of regurgitation. They should be capable of a tight seal on the face, covering both mouth and nose. Masks should be fitted with an oxygen (insufflation) inlet and have a standard 15-/22-mm connector[1] and should be available in one average size for adults with additional sizes for infants and children. For mouth-to-mask ventilation we recommend masks equipped with a 1-way valve that diverts the victim's exhaled gas. Mouth-to-mask ventilation has been shown to be superior to that with bag-mask devices in delivering adequate tidal volumes on manikins. These devices are not to be confused with face-shield devices, which do not have an exhalation port. The efficacy of face shields has not been compared with that of other devices, and at this time face shields are recommended for BLS lay rescuers only (Class IIb).[2]

An adequate seal is best achieved with a mouth-to-mask device when the rescuer is positioned at the top of the patient's head (Figure 1). The rescuer ventilates the victim by sealing his or her lips around the coupling adapter of the mask. Use both hands to hold the mask securely in position and maintain airway patency with head tilt. Manikin practice with masks should be required of all personnel who are likely to use a mask for mouth-to-mask ventilation.

Bag-Valve Devices

Bag-valve devices consist of a bag (self-inflating) and a valve (nonrebreathing). They may be used with a mask, a tracheal tube, or other alternative airway adjuncts. Most commercially available adult bag-mask units have a volume of approximately 1600 mL. This volume is much greater than currently recommended tidal volumes for CPR (10 mL/kg, 700 to 1000 mL). When the airway is unsecured (as with a mask versus a tracheal tube), the possibility of overventilation with gastric inflation, subsequent regurgitation, and aspiration becomes a significant concern. In several studies many rescuers were able to deliver adequate tidal volumes (6 to 7 mL/kg, approximately 500 mL) with a bag-valve and mask to unintubated manikins (Class IIa).[2]

To optimize bag-valve and mask performance, one rescuer must be positioned at the top of the victim's head. Generally an oral airway should be inserted (see below) and, if possible, the head elevated if no concern for neck injury exists. While the head is maintained in position, deliver the selected tidal volume (preferably 6 to 7 mL/kg) over 2 seconds.[3] Slow, gentle ventilation minimizes risk of gastric inflation. A bag-valve device may be used with any airway adjunct, such as tracheal tube, laryngeal mask airway, or esophageal-tracheal Combitube. Proper use of these combinations requires training, practice, and demonstrated proficiency.

A satisfactory bag-valve unit should have (1) a self-refilling bag, (2) a nonjam valve system allowing for a maximum oxygen inlet flow of 30 L/min, (3) a no–pop-off valve, (4) standard 15-/22-mm fittings, (5) a system for delivering high concentrations of oxygen through an ancillary oxygen reservoir, (6) a true nonrebreathing valve, and (7) the capability to perform satisfactorily under all common environmental conditions and extremes of temperature (Figure 2).

Automatic Transport Ventilators

Automatic patient transport ventilators (ATVs) specifically designed for prehospital care and portability have been used in Europe since the early 1980s.[4] Their acceptance in the

Circulation. 2000;102(suppl I):I-95–I-104.
© 2000 American Heart Association, Inc.

Circulation is available at http://www.circulationaha.org

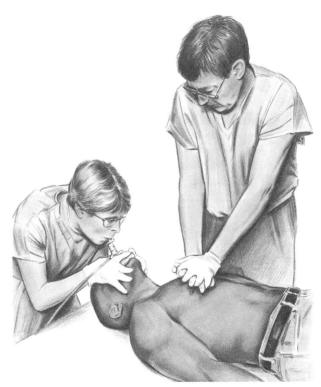

Figure 1. Rescuer using mouth-to-mask ventilation. Rescuer providing rescue breathing using face mask with supplementary oxygen during CPR. Rescuer is using cephalic technique (rescuer positioned at top of patient's head). Both of the rescuer's hands are used to hold the mask securely in position while keeping the victim's airway open. The rescuer's thumbs and forefingers hold the mask in place while the third, fourth, and fifth fingers of each hand lift the jaw (jaw thrust) and maintain an open airway with the head tilted (as shown). Alternatively, the thumbs and a portion of the rescuer's palms can anchor the mask and the index and remaining fingers can lift the jaw, holding it against the mask.

United States has been slow, partly because of concerns that ventilation cannot be synchronized with external chest compression during cardiac arrest. These concerns are unwarranted. First, in unintubated patients it is easy to interpose compressions between mechanically delivered ventilator breaths. If necessary, the rescuer controlling the airway can indicate to the other rescuer when the device is triggered "ON." Second, in intubated patients it is unnecessary to synchronize ventilation with compression.

A number of ATVs are commercially available.[5-9] Studies comparing ATVs with self-inflating bag-ventilation devices during intrahospital transport show that both devices can maintain a satisfactory minute ventilation and appropriate arterial blood gas exchange.[10-13] Bag-ventilation devices are accurate only when tidal volume and minute ventilation are constantly monitored, an impractical approach in prehospital care.[14] Although not as accurate, ATVs remain effective without measures of tidal volume and minute ventilation.

Studies have also revealed that ATVs are as effective as other devices used in prehospital care in intubated patients.[5,15] In addition, studies on mechanical models and in animals demonstrate the superiority of ATVs for ventilating unintubated patients in respiratory arrest.[16] Further studies evaluating the use of these devices are warranted. At the present

time, ATVs are considered to provide advantages over alternative methods of ventilation:

- In intubated patients they free the rescuer for other tasks.
- In unintubated patients the rescuer has both hands free for mask application and airway maintenance.
- Cricoid pressure can be applied with one hand while the other seals the mask on the face.
- Once set, they provide a specific tidal volume, respiratory rate, and minute ventilation.

Studies have observed improved lung inflation or absent gastric inflation when ATVs were compared with other devices, including mouth-to-mask, bag-mask, and manually triggered devices.[12,13] This is due to the lower inspiratory flow and longer inspiratory times (2 seconds) provided by ATVs.

Disadvantages of ATVs include the need for an oxygen source and electric power. In addition, some ATVs may be inappropriate for children under 5 years of age. Because most ATVs require either an oxygen source or an electric power source, a self-inflating bag-valve device or a simple mask should always be available in case the oxygen source is depleted, or no oxygen or electric power source is available, or the ventilator malfunctions.

ATVs used for prehospital care should be simple and time- or volume-cycled. Avoid pressure-cycled devices.[12] Delivered tidal volumes should be relatively unaffected by changes in lung-thorax impedance (<10% change).[7] Operational gas consumption should be <5 L/min. ATVs should have the following minimum features:

- A lightweight connector with a standard 15-/22-mm coupling for a face mask, tracheal tube, or other airway adjunct
- A lightweight (≤4 kg), compact, rugged design, with a carrying or mounting bracket
- Capability of operating under likely extremes of temperature
- A default peak inspiratory pressure limit of 60 cm H_2O, adjustable from 20 to 80 cm H_2O, that is easily accessible to the user
- An audible alarm that sounds when the peak inspiratory limiting pressure is generated. This alerts the rescuer that low compliance or high airway resistance is resulting in a diminished tidal volume delivery
- Minimal gas compression volume in the breathing circuit
- Ability to deliver an F_{IO_2} of 0.5 to 1.0
- A default inspiratory time of 2 seconds in adults and 1 second in children and default inspiratory flow of approximately 30 L/min in adults and 15 L/min in children, with the ability to adjust inspiratory time and flow once the patient is intubated with a tracheal tube or alternative airway[4,6,7]
- A default rate of 10 breaths per minute for adults and 20 breaths per minute for children, with the ability to adjust the rate once the patient is intubated with a tracheal tube or alternative airway

A demand-flow valve may be incorporated into the ATV to reduce the work of breathing should spontaneous breathing

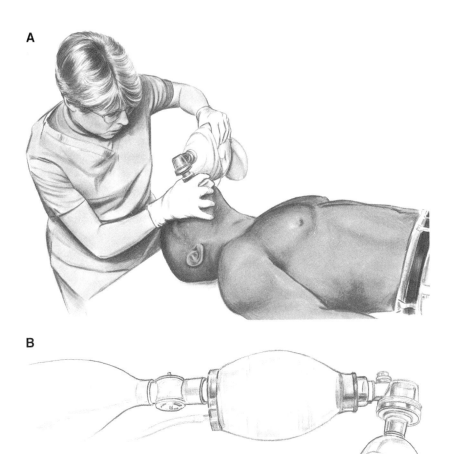

A

B

Figure 2. Detailed view of bag-mask. A, Rescuer provides ventilation with bag and mask attached to oxygen supply. The rescuer is using the E-C technique to hold the mask to the face (creating a "C" with the thumb and forefinger) while lifting the jaw along the bony portion of the mandible with the last 3 fingers of the same hand (these fingers make the "E"). The second hand squeezes the bag while the rescuer watches the victim's chest to ensure that the chest rises with each ventilation. The rescuer is keeping the victim's airway open with both a head tilt and a jaw thrust. B, Details of a bag-mask system with supplementary oxygen. The system consists of a self-refilling bag with an oxygen inlet, either no pop-off valve or (as shown) a pop-off valve that can be disabled during resuscitation to ensure delivery of adequate tidal volumes despite high pressures, and standard fittings (in this case, the bag is joined with a standard fitting to a mask). This system is capable of delivering high concentrations of oxygen because it contains an oxygen reservoir. If additional gas is required during ventilation, the gas is drawn from the oxygen reservoir rather than from room air, so a high concentration of oxygen can be delivered during ventilation.

return. The valve should be able to deliver a peak inspiratory flow rate of at least 120 L/min (2 L/s) on demand. The pressure to trigger spontaneous flow should not exceed −1 to −2 cm H_2O.

Some ATVs allow higher preselected ventilator breathing rates. During CPR use caution in selecting ventilation rates more frequent than 10 per minute in adults or 20 per minute in children, because adequate time for exhalation is necessary to prevent air trapping and a positive end-expiratory pressure (auto-PEEP) effect. Auto-PEEP may reduce forward blood flow (ie, effective cardiac output) because pulmonary perfusion pressures are very low during CPR. Pulmonary capillary flow is easily impeded by high alveolar pressure. An appropriate exhalation time to maintain a 1:2 inhalation-to-exhalation time (I:E) ratio is necessary to minimize air trapping.[17]

Additional desirable features include a pressure manometer, provision for PEEP in more sophisticated ventilators, at least two controls (one for rate and one for tidal volume), and alarms to indicate depletion of oxygen cylinders, ventilator disconnect, or low battery.

Directors of prehospital or transport programs need to ensure that ATVs are used only by personnel who have received adequate ATV training. Monitoring of use and complication rates is essential to ensure safe and effective use of ATVs.

Correct Placement of Tube Confirmed: Next Actions

Ventilate with tidal volume of 10 to 15 mL/kg.

Ventilate with rate of 12 to 15 breaths per minute.

Ventilate with duration of 2 seconds.

Ventilate with 100% oxygen.

Insert oropharyngeal airway.

Insert bite protector.

Secure the tube in place (use tape or purpose-made devices); note depth marking on tube at front teeth.

Consider C-spine collar, backboard, and C-spine collar–to-backboard if transfer is required.

Oxygen-Powered, Manually Triggered Devices

Oxygen-powered, manually triggered devices have been used in prehospital care for >25 years despite a paucity of high-level scientific evidence supporting their use. When used with a face mask, high inspiratory flow and pressure may cause massive gastric inflation. When used with other airway adjuncts, high flow and pressure may cause barotrauma. In an effort to limit the damage caused by these devices, in 1986 a recommendation was made to limit flow to 40 L/min. Oxygen-powered manually triggered devices are not recommended at this time (Class Indeterminate). Further in vivo studies are needed to compare their efficacy with that of bag-valve devices and ATVs.

Airway Adjuncts

Oropharyngeal Airways

Oropharyngeal airways should be reserved for obtunded unconscious patients who are not intubated (Class IIa). Care is required in placement of the oral airway because incorrect insertion can displace the tongue into the hypopharynx and result in airway obstruction. In conscious patients oropharyngeal airways can promote retching, vomiting, or laryngospasm caused by activation of the gag reflex. Oral airways should be inserted only by persons trained adequately in their use. Oropharyngeal airways should be available in various infant, child, and adult sizes.

Nasopharyngeal Airways

Nasopharyngeal airways are especially useful in patients with trismus, biting, clenched jaws, or maxillofacial injuries, which prevent placement of an oral airway (Class IIa). They should be used with caution in patients with suspected fracture at the base of the skull. In patients who are not deeply unconscious, nasopharyngeal airways are better tolerated than oropharyngeal ones. Insertion can cause damage to the nasal mucosa, resulting in bleeding. If the tube is too long, it may stimulate the laryngeal or glossopharyngeal reflexes to produce laryngospasm, retching, or vomiting. As with all adjunctive equipment, safe use of nasopharyngeal airways requires adequate training, practice, and retraining.

Alternative Airways

In some communities tracheal intubation is not permitted, or patients are so few that practitioners obtain little experience. Alternative airways that require blind passage of the device into the airway may be simpler to master than passage of a tracheal tube under direct vision. Alternative airways include the laryngeal mask airway (LMA), the esophageal-tracheal Combitube (ETC), and the pharyngotracheal lumen airway (PTL). When used by adequately trained healthcare providers, the LMA and the ETC provide superior ventilation compared with face masks in patients in cardiac arrest (Class IIa). To achieve good outcomes with these devices, healthcare providers must maintain a high level of knowledge and skills through frequent practice and field use.

Esophageal-Tracheal Combitube

The ETC is an invasive double-lumen airway with 2 inflatable balloon cuffs that is inserted without visualization of the vocal cords. Assessment of the location of the distal orifice[18] is then made, and the patient is ventilated through the appropriate opening. One lumen contains ventilating side holes at the hypopharyngeal level and is closed at the distal end; the other lumen has a distal open end with a cuff similar to a tracheal tube. When inflated the large pharyngeal balloon fills the space between the base of the tongue and the soft palate, anchoring the ETC into position, and isolates the oropharynx from the hypopharynx. The tube most commonly finds its way into the esophagus because of the stiffness and curve of the tube and the shape and structure of the pharynx. The tube is advanced until the patient's teeth lie between 2 marks printed on the tube. The pharyngeal and distal balloons are then inflated, thus isolating the oropharynx above the upper balloon and the esophagus (or trachea) below the lower balloon.

The advantages of the ETC over the face mask are similar to those of the tracheal tube over the face mask: isolation of the airway, reduction in the risk of aspiration, and more reliable ventilation. The advantages of the ETC over the tracheal tube relate chiefly to ease of training and maintenance of placement skills, because laryngoscopy and visualization of the vocal cords are not necessary for insertion of the ETC. Ventilation and oxygenation with the ETC compare favorably with those achieved with the tracheal tube. Successful insertion rates with the ETC range from 69% to 100%.[19–25] Because successful insertion is not ensured, providers should have a strategy for airway management when they are unable to ventilate with their first-choice adjunct. Fatal complications with the ETC may occur if the position of the distal lumen of the ETC in the esophagus or the trachea is identified incorrectly. In one EMS system a retrospective review reported that the incorrect port was used for ventilation in 3.5% of cases.[20] For this reason use the ETC in conjunction with an end-tidal CO_2 or esophageal detector device.[26,27]

Another possible complication from the ETC is esophageal trauma.[28] Eight cases of subcutaneous emphysema were retrieved from a retrospective review of 1139 patients resuscitated with the ETC by emergency medical technicians. Four patients underwent autopsy, and 2 were found to have esophageal lacerations.[29] To optimize insertion rates and to minimize complications, providers should receive adequate initial training in use of the ETC and should practice with the device regularly. To ensure optimal outcomes, we also highly recommend that EMS and other healthcare providers monitor their success rates and the occurrence of complications.

Laryngeal Mask Airway

The LMA is an adjunctive airway device composed of a tube with a cuffed mask-like projection at the distal end (see Figure 3A).[30] The LMA is introduced into the pharynx (Figure 3B) and advanced until resistance is felt as the distal portion of the tube locates in the hypopharynx. The cuff is then inflated, which seals the larynx, leaving the distal opening of the tube just above the glottis, providing a clear, secure airway (Figure 3C and 3D).

The LMA provides a more secure and reliable means of ventilation than the face mask.[31,32] Although the LMA does not ensure absolute protection against aspiration, studies have shown that regurgitation is less likely with the LMA than with the bag-mask device and that aspiration is uncommon.[33,34] In comparison with the tracheal tube, the LMA provides equivalent ventilation. Training in the placement and use of an LMA is simpler than tracheal intubation because laryngoscopy and visualization of the vocal cords are unnecessary for insertion of the LMA.[35–37] The LMA may have advantages over the tracheal tube when access to the patient is limited,[38] there is a possibility of unstable neck injury,[39] or appropriate positioning of the patient for tracheal intubation is impossible.

Studies have examined the use of the LMA by nurses, respiratory therapists, and EMS personnel, many of whom

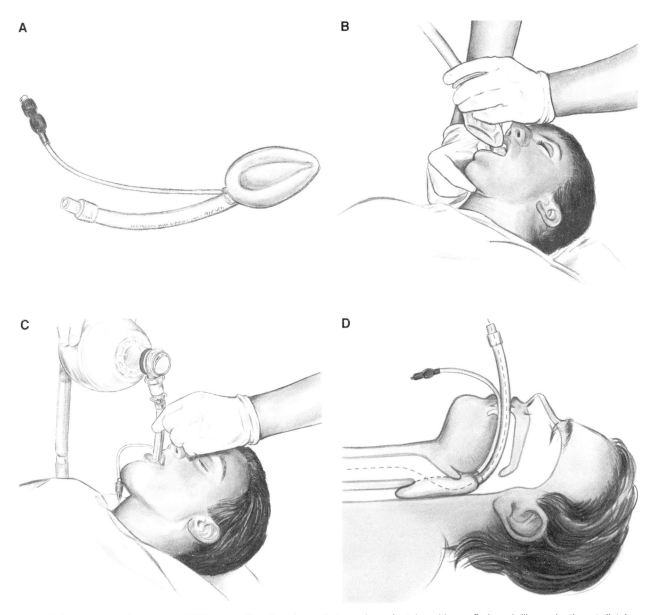

Figure 3. Laryngeal mask airway. A, LMA is an adjunctive airway that consists of a tube with a cuffed mask-like projection at distal end. B, LMA is introduced through mouth into pharynx. C, Once LMA is in position, a clear, secure airway is present. D (Anatomic detail), During insertion, LMA is advanced until resistance is felt as distal portion of tube locates in hypopharynx. Cuff is then inflated. This seals larynx and leaves distal opening of tube just above glottis, providing a clear, secure airway (see arrow).

had not previously used either an LMA or a tracheal tube. Successful insertion rates with the LMA range from 64% to 100%.[25,34,40–44]

Even when the LMA can be inserted, studies report that a small proportion of patients cannot be ventilated with the LMA. Because insertion and ventilation are not ensured, it is important for providers to have an alternative strategy for management of the airway. Providers should receive adequate initial training in the use of the LMA and should practice with the device regularly to optimize insertion rates and to minimize complications. To ensure optimal outcomes we also highly recommend that EMS and other healthcare providers monitor their success rates and the occurrence of complications.

Transtracheal (Translaryngeal) Catheter Ventilation

In those rare cases when airway obstruction is not relieved by any of the methods described above, additional procedures are necessary. These include transtracheal catheter or translaryngeal ventilation. Only specially trained and experienced personnel should attempt such procedures.

Pharyngotracheal Lumen Airway

The PTL is a double-lumen tube similar in structure and function to the ETC.[45] The tube is inserted blindly into the pharynx, ending in either the esophagus or the trachea. Assessment of its location is then made, and the patient is ventilated through the proper lumen. In the only published study since 1992 in which use of the PTL was examined, the tube performed well but was preferred less than the ETC.[21] The PTL is not currently in wide use (Class Indeterminate).

Cuffed Oropharyngeal Airway

The cuffed oropharyngeal airway (COPA) was first described in 1992.[46] Although designed originally for spontaneous ventilation in anesthetized subjects, it may represent a useful adjunct during resuscitation. The device is a modified oropharyngeal airway with a distal inflatable cuff and proximal standard 15-mm connector to which a self-inflating bag can be attached. Recent data suggests that the COPA is relatively easy to use and may offer an effective method of providing an adequate airway during resuscitation by personnel not trained in more advanced techniques.[47]

Tracheal Intubation

In the absence of a protected airway, providing adequate lung inflations may require pharyngeal pressures sufficient to cause gastric inflation, subsequent regurgitation, and the potential for aspiration of gastric contents into the lungs.[48–51] In extreme cases, gastric inflation may elevate the diaphragm sufficiently to interfere with lung inflation.[52,53] Therefore, as soon as practical during the resuscitative process, trained personnel should intubate the trachea or insert an alternative airway (LMA or ETC).

Tracheal intubation should be preceded by preoxygenation of the patient. If the patient is ventilating spontaneously, preoxygenation is achieved by providing 3 minutes of high-flow oxygen. If spontaneous ventilation is insufficient, assist ventilation with a bag-mask device.[54]

Currently the tracheal tube is considered the ventilation adjunct of choice because it keeps the airway patent, permits suctioning of airway secretions, ensures delivery of a high concentration of oxygen, provides a route for the administration of certain drugs, facilitates delivery of a selected tidal volume, and protects the airway from aspiration of gastric contents or blood and mucus from the oropharynx.[55] Repeated safe and effective placement of the tracheal tube, over the wide range of patient and environmental conditions encountered in resuscitation, requires considerable skill and experience. Unless initial training is sufficient and ongoing practice and experience are adequate, fatal complications may result.

Multiple or unsuccessful intubation attempts may affect outcome from cardiac arrest adversely. Rates for failure to intubate are as high as 50% in EMS systems with a low patient volume and providers who do not perform intubation frequently.[56,57] When tracheal intubation is attempted by providers with insufficient skill, the following complications may be seen: trauma to the oropharynx, ventilation withheld for unacceptably long periods, delayed or withheld chest compressions, esophageal or bronchial intubation, failure to secure the tube, and failure to recognize misplacement of the tube. Therefore, inexperienced providers should use only those airway management devices for which they have been adequately trained. Those who

perform tracheal intubation require either frequent experience or frequent retraining. EMS systems should keep a record for each provider, documenting the number of intubations performed and success rates and complications (Class IIa).

Indications for tracheal intubation include (1) inability of the rescuer to ventilate the unconscious patient with less invasive methods and (2) absence of protective reflexes (coma or cardiac arrest).

During the process of tracheal intubation, the maximum interruption to ventilation should be 30 seconds. If more than 1 attempt at intubation is required, adequate ventilation and oxygenation must be provided between attempts. If the patient has a perfusing rhythm, use pulse oximetry and ECG monitoring continuously during intubation attempts.

Whenever possible a second rescuer should apply cricoid pressure during tracheal intubation in adults to protect against regurgitation of gastric contents and to help ensure tube placement in the tracheal orifice. Apply pressure with the thumb and index fingers to the right and left anterolateral aspects of the cricoid cartilage just lateral to the midline. Avoid overzealous pressure; it will occlude the airway and impair tracheal intubation.[58,59] Maintain cricoid pressure until the cuff of the tracheal tube is inflated.[60,61] The BURP (*B*ackward, *U*pward, *R*ightward *P*ressure) technique may be useful in bringing the vocal cords into the field of vision of the intubator.

Tracheal tubes should be available in a variety of sizes. They should have standard 15-/22-mm connectors and should have high-volume, low-pressure cuffs suitable for adults and older children. The size of tracheal tube required typically is 8 mm for average adult women and 8 mm for average adult men. Because of the variation in size of adults, a range of tubes should be available.

A stylet should be available and may be used to assist with tracheal tube insertion by providing some stiffness to the tube and by allowing the direction of the tube to be controlled better during manipulation. When used, the stylet should not extend beyond the distal end of the tube.

Another excellent device to assist with placement of the tracheal tube is the gum elastic bougie. Because of its size and flexibility, the bougie is easier to place in the trachea than a tracheal tube. Once the bougie is placed in the trachea, the tracheal tube is passed over the bougie and into position in the trachea.[62–66]

Difficulties in achieving tracheal intubation usually occur because of inability to bring the vocal cords into view through the laryngoscope. Visualization is best accomplished by flexing the neck and extending the head at the atlanto-occipital joint (the "sniffing position"). Once the vocal cords are seen, the tube should be placed so that the cuff is just beyond the cords. In the average adult this position usually results in the tube lying at a depth marked on the side of the tube between the 19- and 23-cm marks at the front teeth. The cuff is then inflated with just enough air to occlude the airway (usually 10 mL). An adequate seal is confirmed by listening over the larynx while ventilation is continued and air is added to the cuff. While a normal tidal volume is delivered, air is added to the cuff just until the audible air leak around the tube disappears.

Immediately after insertion of the tracheal tube, confirm placement by auscultating over the epigastrium, the midaxillary, and the anterior chest line on the right and left sides of the chest. Even when the tracheal tube is seen to pass through the vocal cords and is verified in the trachea by auscultation, make secondary confirmation of placement with an end-tidal CO_2 or esophageal detection device (Class IIa).[67] Extensive data shows that clinical signs of proper tube placement (such as condensation in the tube, auscultation over the lungs and abdomen, and chest rise) are not always reliable indicators of correct tube placement.[68–72]

To protect against unrecognized esophageal intubation, confirmation of tube placement by an expired CO_2 or esophageal detection device is necessary. In the out-of-hospital setting, unrecognized misplacement of the tracheal tube has been reported in as many as 17% of patients.[73] Once the tube is placed, especially out of hospital, the location of the tracheal tube must be monitored closely.

The esophageal detector device depends on the ability to aspirate air from the lower airways through a tracheal tube placed in the cartilage-supported rigid trachea. When the tube is in the esophagus, air cannot be aspirated because the esophagus collapses when aspiration is attempted. The esophageal detector device is generally reliable in patients with both a perfusing and a nonperfusing rhythm (Class IIa),[74–80] but it may yield misleading results in patients with morbid obesity, late pregnancy, or status asthmaticus or when there are copious tracheal secretions.[78,81,82] With some of these conditions, the trachea tends to collapse. In the case of status asthmaticus, the airway secretions or the small-airway obstruction that characterizes severe asthma blocks air aspiration from the lower airways.

How to Confirm Accurate Placement of Tracheal Tube: Primary Confirmation
Confirm tube placement immediately, assessing the first breath delivered by the bag-valve unit.

- As the bag is squeezed, listen over the epigastrium and observe the chest wall for movement. If you hear stomach gurgling and see no chest wall expansion, you have intubated the esophagus. Deliver no further ventilations. Remove the tracheal tube at once.
- Reattempt intubation after reoxygenating the victim (15 to 30 seconds of bag ventilations using 100% oxygen).
- If the chest wall rises appropriately and stomach gurgling is not heard, listen to the lung fields: left and right anterior, left and right midaxillary, and once again over the stomach. Document in the medical records where you heard breath sounds. If you have any doubt, stop ventilations through the tube.
- If there is continued doubt about correct tube placement, use the laryngoscope and look directly to see whether the tube is passing through the vocal cords.
- If the tube seems to be in place, reconfirm the tube mark at the front teeth (this was noted after the tube was inserted 1 to 2 cm past the vocal cords.

- Secure the tube with a purpose-built commercial device, although most traditional taping patterns are acceptable.
- Once the tube is secured, insert an oropharyngeal airway or add a bite block, or both, to prevent the patient from biting down and occluding the airway.

How to Confirm Accurate Placement of Tracheal Tube: Secondary Confirmation
A variety of electronic and mechanical devices, ranging from simple and inexpensive to complex and costly, are available for both in-hospital and out-of-hospital use. These include several models of end-tidal CO_2 detectors (qualitative, quantitative, and continuous) and a variety of esophageal detector devices.

End-Tidal CO_2 Detectors
Several commercial devices measure the concentration of exhaled CO_2 from the lungs. The presence of exhaled CO_2 indicates proper tracheal tube placement. A lack of CO_2 on the detector generally means that the tube is in the esophagus, particularly in patients with spontaneous circulation.

False-positive readings* (tube is really in the trachea; device indicates in the esophagus; leads to unnecessary tube removal) may occur because CO_2 delivery is low in cardiac arrest patients with low blood flow to the lungs or in patients with a large amount of dead space (eg, significant pulmonary embolus). False-negative readings (tube is really in the esophagus; device indicates in the trachea) have been reported from patients who had ingested carbonated liquids before the arrest.

Continuous (usually quantitative as well) end-tidal CO_2 monitors can confirm successful tracheal tube placement within seconds of an intubation attempt. These monitors can also detect subsequent tracheal tube dislodgment, an event that is more likely to occur during out-of-hospital transportation of a patient.

Esophageal Detector Devices
These devices create a suction force at the tracheal end of the tracheal tube, either from pulling back the plunger on a large syringe or compressing a flexible bulb. If the tube is in the esophagus, the suction will pull the esophageal mucosa against the distal end of the detector and prevent movement of the device plunger or reexpansion of the suction bulb.

Expired CO_2 detectors are very reliable in patients with perfusing rhythms and are recommended to confirm tube position in these patients (Class IIa).[83,84] During cardiac arrest, pulmonary blood flow may be so low that there is insufficient expired CO_2, so a correctly placed tracheal tube is not identified by the expired CO_2 detector. When expired CO_2 is detected in cardiac arrest, it is a reliable indicator of tube position, but when it is absent, we recommend adding a second method of confirming tracheal tube placement, such as the esophageal detector device (Class IIb).[85–89]

---

*The use of the terms "false-positive" and "false-negative" when applied to a diagnostic technique can be confusing. The meanings can flip-flop depending on whether the esophageal detector device is "positive" when it detects proper tracheal tube placement, or "positive" when it detects esophageal placement. There is no widely accepted convention in discussing such tools. See the editorial on the carotid pulse check as a diagnostic test.—Editors

A variety of electronic as well as simple, inexpensive, colorimetric detectors that detect exhaled CO_2 are available for both in-hospital and out-of-hospital use.

After you confirm the position of the tube in the trachea, careful auscultation is needed to avoid inadvertent right main bronchial intubation. Once you achieve the correct positioning of the tube, record the depth of the tube as marked at the front teeth and secure the tube. Once the tube is secured, place an oropharyngeal airway or bite block. The respiratory rate during cardiac or respiratory arrest when the patient has been intubated should be 12 to 15 breaths per minute (1 breath every 4 to 5 seconds). Once a tracheal tube is in place, ventilation need not be synchronized with chest compressions. Once spontaneous circulation is restored after cardiac arrest, continue to provide 12 to 15 breaths per minute.

After tube confirmation and fixation, obtain a chest x-ray to confirm proper position of the end of the tracheal tube above the carina.

In patients with severe obstructive pulmonary disease with increased resistance to exhalation, care should be taken not to induce air trapping, which may result in auto-PEEP. In patients with hypovolemia this may cause a profound reduction in blood pressure. Lower respiratory rates (6 to 8 per minute) should be used, allowing more time for complete exhalation of gas.

Suction Devices

Both portable and installed suction equipment should be available for resuscitative emergencies. The portable unit should provide vacuum and flow adequate for pharyngeal suction. It should be fitted with large-bore, nonkinking suction tubing and semirigid pharyngeal tips. Several sterile suction catheters of various sizes should be available for suctioning through tracheostomy tubes, along with a nonbreakable collection bottle and a supply of sterile water for cleaning tubes and catheters.

The installed suction unit should be powerful enough to provide an airflow of >40 L/min at the end of the delivery tube and a vacuum of >300 mm Hg when the tube is clamped. The amount of suction should be adjustable for use in children and intubated patients. Hand-powered suction units lack the problems associated with electric pumps and have had considerable anecdotal clinical success, although no formal evaluations have been published.

An additional set of rigid pharyngeal suction tips (tonsil suction tips) and sterile, curved tracheal suction catheters of various sizes should be available. For tracheal suction, a Y-piece or T-piece or a lateral opening should lie between the suction tube and the source of the on-off suction control. The suction yoke, collection bottle, water for rinsing, and suction tube should be readily accessible to the attendant in charge of the airway. Suction apparatus must be designed for easy cleaning and subsequent decontamination.

Airway Summary

Airway control using an invasive airway device is fundamental to ACLS. Determining rapidly whether the tracheal tube is in the esophagus or trachea should be one of the primary end points of training and clinical use of invasive airway techniques. This key skill is required for the safe and effective use of these devices. Training, frequency of use, and monitoring of success and complications influence the long-term impact of any device more than the choice of the specific device.

References

1. Johannigman JA, Branson RD. Oxygen enrichment of expired gas for mouth-to-mask resuscitation. *Respir Care.* 1991;36:99–103.
2. Melker RJ, Banner MJ. Ventilation during CPR: two-rescuer standards reappraised. *Ann Emerg Med.* 1985;14:397–402.
3. Dorges V, Ocker H, Hagelberg S, Wenzel V, Idris AH, Schmucker P. Smaller tidal volumes with room-air are not sufficient to ensure adequate oxygenation during bag-valve-mask ventilation. *Resuscitation.* 2000;44:37–41.
4. Harber T, Lucas BG. An evaluation of some mechanical resuscitators for use in the ambulance service. *Ann R Coll Surg Engl.* 1980;62:291–203.
5. Branson RD, McGough EK. Transport ventilators. *Probl Crit Care.* 1990;4:254–274.
6. Nolan JP, Baskett PJF. Gas-powered and portable ventilators: an evaluation of six models. *Prehospital Disaster Med.* 1992;7:25–34.
7. McGough EK, Banner MJ, Melker RJ. Variations in tidal volume with portable transport ventilators. *Respir Care.* 1992;37:233–239.
8. Johannigman JA, Branson RD, Davis K, Hurst JM. Techniques of emergency ventilation: a model to evaluate tidal volume, airway pressure, and gastric insufflation. *Trauma.* 1991;31:93–98.
9. Davis K, Johannigman JA, Johnson RC, Branson RD. Lung compliance following cardiac arrest. *Acad Emerg Med.* 1995;2:874–878.
10. Braman SS, Dunn SM, Amico CA, Millman RP. Complications of intrahospital transport in critically ill patients. *Ann Intern Med.* 1987;107:469–473.
11. Gervais HW, Eberle B, Konietzke D, Hennes HJ, Dick W. Comparison of blood gases of ventilated patients during transport. *Crit Care Med.* 1987;15:761–763.
12. Johannigman JA, Branson RD, Johnson DJ, Davis K Jr, Hurst JM. Out-of-hospital ventilation: bag-valve device vs transport ventilator. *Acad Emerg Med.* 1995;2:719–724.
13. Updike G, Mosesso VN Jr, Auble TE, Delgado E. Comparison of bag-valve-mask, manually triggered ventilator, and automated ventilator devices used while ventilating a nonintubated manikin model. *Prehosp Emerg Care.* 1998;2:52–55.
14. Weg JG, Haas CF. Safe intrahospital transport of critically ill ventilator-dependent patients. *Chest.* 1989;96:631–635.
15. Hurst JM, Davis K Jr, Branson RD, Johannigman JA. Comparison of blood gases during transport using two methods of ventilatory support. *J Trauma.* 1989;29:1637–1640.
16. Fuerst RS, Banner MJ, Melker RJ. Gastric inflation in the unintubated patient: a comparison of ventilating devices. *Ann Emerg Med.* 1992;21:636.
17. Pepe PE, Marini JJ. Occult positive end-expiratory pressure in mechanically ventilated patients with airflow obstruction: the auto-PEEP effect. *Am Rev Respir Dis.* 1982;126:166–170.
18. Frass M, Frenzer R, Rauscha F, Weber H, Packer R, Leithner C. Evaluation of esophageal tracheal Combitube in cardiopulmonary resuscitation. *Crit Care Med.* 1986;15:609–611.
19. Atherton GL, Johnson JC. Ability of paramedics to use the Combitube in prehospital cardiac arrest. *Ann Emerg Med.* 1993;22:1263–1268.
20. Lefrancois D. Use of the esophageal-tracheal Combitube (ETC) in prehospital cardiorespiratory arrest (CRA) in an EMT-D level EMS system. *Resuscitation.* 1998;37:544. Abstract.
21. Rumball CJ, Macdonald D. The PTL, Combitube, laryngeal mask, and oral airway: a randomized prehospital comparative study of ventilatory device effectiveness and cost-effectiveness in 470 cases of cardiorespiratory arrest. *Prehosp Emerg Care.* 1997;1:1–10.
22. Staudinger T, Brugger S, Watschinger B. Emergency intubation with the Combitube: comparison with the endotracheal tube. *Ann Emerg Med.* 1993;22:1573–1575.

23. Staudinger T, Brugger S, Roggla M. Comparison of the Combitube with the endotracheal tube in cardiopulmonary resuscitation in the prehospital phase. *Wien Klin Wochenschr.* 1994;106:412–415.

24. Frass M, Frenzer R, Rauscha F. Ventilation with esophageal tracheal Combitube in cardiopulmonary resuscitation: promptness and effectiveness. *Chest.* 1988;93:781–784.

25. Tanigawa K, Shigematsu A. A choice of airway device for 12,020 cases of non-traumatic cardiac arrest in Japan. *Prehosp Emerg Care.* 1998;2:96–100.

26. Butler BD, Little T, Drtil S. Combined use of the esophageal-tracheal Combitube with a colorimetric carbon dioxide detector for emergency intubation/ventilation. *Clin Monit.* 1995;11:311–316.

27. Wafai Y, Salem MR, Baraka A. Effectiveness of the self-inflating bulb for verification of proper placement of the esophageal tracheal Combitube. *Anesth Analg.* 1995;80:122–126.

28. Klein H, Williamson M, Sue-Ling HM. Esophageal rupture associated with the use of the Combitube. *Anesth Analg.* 1997;85:937–939.

29. Vezina D, Lessard MR, Bussieres J. Complications associated with the use of the esophageal tracheal Combitube. *Can J Anaesth.* 1998;45:76–80.

30. Brain AI. The laryngeal mask: a new concept in airway management. *Br J Anaesth.* 1983;55:801–805.

31. Martin PD, Cyna AM, Hunter WAH. Training nursing staff in airway management for resuscitation: a clinical comparison of the facemask and laryngeal mask. *Anaesthesia.* 1993;48:33–37.

32. Alexander R, Hodgson P, Lomax D. A comparison of laryngeal mask airway and Guedel airway, bag and facemask for manual ventilation. *Anaesthesia.* 1993;48:231–234.

33. Stone BJ, Chantler PJ, Basket PJ. The incidence of regurgitation during cardiopulmonary resuscitation: a comparison between the bag valve mask and laryngeal mask airway. *Resuscitation.* 1998;38:3–6.

34. Baskett PJF. The use of the laryngeal mask airway by nurses during cardiopulmonary resuscitation: results of a multicentre trial. *Anaesthesia.* 1994;49:3–7.

35. Pennant JH, Walker MB. Comparison of the endotracheal tube and laryngeal mask in airway management by paramedical personnel. *Anesth Analg.* 1992;74:531–534.

36. Reinhart DJ. Laryngeal mask airway (LMA) vs endotracheal tube by paramedics and respiratory therapists. *Ann Emerg Med.* 1994;24:260–263.

37. Davies PRF, Tighe SQ, Greenslade GL. Laryngeal mask and tracheal tube insertion by unskilled personnel. *Lancet.* 1990;336:977–979.

38. Greene MK, Radon R, Hinchley G. The laryngeal mask airway: two cases of prehospital care. *Anaesthesia.* 1992;47:686–689.

39. Pennant H, Pace NA, Gajraj NM. Role of the laryngeal mask airway in the immobile cervical spine. *J Clin Anesth.* 1993;5:226–230.

40. Kokkinis K. The use of the laryngeal mask in CPR. *Resuscitation.* 1994;27:9–12.

41. Kokkinis K, Leach A, Alexander CA, Stone B. The laryngeal mask in cardiopulmonary resuscitation in a district general hospital: a preliminary communication. Multicentre Trial (Co-ordinator Baskett PJF). *Resuscitation.* 1993;25:245–248.

42. Samarkandi AH, Seraj MA, el Dawlatly A. The role of the laryngeal mask airway in cardiopulmonary resuscitation. *Resuscitation.* 1994;28:103–106.

43. Verghese C, Prior Willeard PFS, Baskett PJF. Immediate management of the airway during cardiopulmonary resuscitation in a hospital without a resident anaesthesiologist. *Eur J Emerg Med.* 1994;1:123–125.

44. Grantham H, Phillips G, Gilligan JE. The laryngeal mask in prehospital emergency care. *Emerg Med.* 1994;6:193–197.

45. Niemann JT, Rosborough JP, Myers R, Scarberry EN. The pharyngeotracheal lumen airway: preliminary investigation of a new adjunct. *Ann Emerg Med.* 1984;13:591–596.

46. Asai T, Koga K, Stacey MR. Use of the cuffed oropharyngeal airway after difficult ventilation through a facemask. *Anaesthesia.* 1997;52:1236–1237.

47. Rees SG, Gabbott DA. Use of the cuffed oropharyngeal airway for manual ventilation by nonanaesthetists. *Anaesthesia.* 1999;54:1089–1093.

48. Bowman FP, Menegazzi JJ, Check BD, Duckett TM. Lower esophageal sphincter pressure during prolonged cardiac arrest and resuscitation. *Ann Emerg Med.* 1995;26:216–219.

49. Ruben H, Knudsen EJ, Carugati G. Gastric inflation in relation to airway pressure. *Acta Anaesthesiol Scand.* 1961;5:107–114.

50. Weiler N, Heinrichs W, Dick W. Assessment of pulmonary mechanics and gastric inflation pressure during mask ventilation. *Prehospital Disaster Med.* 1995;10:101–105.

51. Ruben H, Johansen SH. Gastric inflation due to artificial respiration. *Acta Anaesthesiol Scand.* 1970;14:281–285.

52. Wenzel V, Idris AH, Banner MJ. Respiratory system compliance decreases after cardiopulmonary resuscitation and stomach inflation: impact of large and small tidal volumes on calculated peak airway pressure. *Resuscitation.* 1998;38:113–118.

53. Berg MD, Idris AH, Berg RA. Severe ventilatory compromise due to gastric distension during cardiopulmonary resuscitation. *Resuscitation.* 1998;36:71–73.

54. McGowan P, Skinner A. Preoxygenation: the importance of a good facemask seal. *Br J Anaesth.* 1995;75:777–778.

55. Pepe PE, Copass MK, Joyce TH. Prehospital endotracheal intubation: rationale for training emergency medical personnel. *Ann Emerg Med.* 1985;14:1085–1092.

56. Bradley JS, Billows GL, Olinger ML, Boha SP, Cordell WH, Nelson DR. Prehospital oral endotracheal intubation by rural basic emergency medical technicians. *Ann Emerg Med.* 1998;32:26–32.

57. Sayre MR, Sakles JC, Mistler AF, Evans JL, Kramer AT, Panicioli AM. Field trial of endotracheal intubation by basic EMTs. *Ann Emerg Med.* 1998;31:228–233.

58. Hartsilver EL, Vanner RG. Airway obstruction with cricoid pressure. *Anaesthesia.* 2000;55:208–211.

59. MacG Palmer JH, Ball DR. The effect of cricoid pressure on the cricoid cartilage and vocal cords: an endoscopic study in anaesthetised patients. *Anaesthesia.* 2000;55:263–268.

60. Sellick BA. Cricoid pressure to control regurgitation of stomach contents during induction of anaesthesia. *Lancet.* 1961;2:2404–2406.

61. Wraight WJ, Chamney AR, Howells TH. The determination of an effective cricoid pressure. *Anaesthesia.* 1983;38:461–466.

62. Nolan JP, Wilson ME. Orotracheal intubation in patients with potential cervical spine injuries: an indication for the gum elastic bougie. *Anaesthesia.* 1993;48:630–633.

63. Viswanathan S, Campbell C, Wood DG. The Eschmann tracheal tube introducer (gum elastic bougie). *Anesthesiol Rev.* 1992;19:29–34.

64. Kidd JF, Dyson A, Latto IP. Successful difficult intubation use of the gum elastic bougie. *Anaesthesia.* 1988;43:437–438.

65. Nolan JP, Wilson ME. An evaluation of the gum elastic bougie: intubation times and incidence of sore throat. *Anaesthesia.* 1992;47:878–881.

66. Dogra S, Falconer R, Latto IP. Successful difficult intubation: tracheal tube placement over a gum elastic bougie. *Anaesthesia.* 1990;45:774–776.

67. White SJ, Slovis CM. Inadvertent esophageal intubation in the field: reliance on a fool's "gold standard." *Acad Emerg Med.* 1997;4:89–91.

68. Charters P. Normal chest expansion with esophageal placement of a tracheal tube. *Anaesthesia.* 1989;44:365.

69. Andersen KH, Hald A. Assessing the position of the tracheal tube: the reliability of different methods. *Anaesthesia.* 1989;44:984–985.

70. Vaghadia II, Jenkins LC, Ford RW. Comparison of end-tidal carbon dioxide, oxygen saturation and clinical signs for the detection of esophageal intubation. *Can J Anaesth.* 1989;36:560–564.

71. Kelly JJ. Use of tube condensation as an indicator of endotracheal tube placement. *Ann Emerg Med.* 1998;31:575–578.

72. Anderson KH, Schultz-Lebahn T. Esophageal intubation can be undetected by auscultation of the chest. *Acta Anaesthesiol Scand.* 1994;38:580–582.

73. Katz SH, Falk JL. Misplaced endotracheal tubes by paramedics in an urban emergency medical services system. *Acad Emerg Med.* 1998;5:429.

74. Zaleski L, Abello D, Gold MI. The esophageal detector device: does it work? *Anesthesiology.* 1993;79:244–247.

75. Williams KN, Nunn JF. The oesophageal detector device: a prospective trial on 100 patients. *Anaesthesia.* 1989;44:412–414.

76. Wee MY, Walker AK. The oesophageal detector device: an assessment with uncuffed tubes in children. *Anaesthesia.* 1991;46:869–871.

77. Marley CD Jr, Eitel DR, Anderson TE. Evaluation of a prototype esophageal detection device. *Acad Emerg Med.* 1995;2:503–507.

78. Baraka A, Khoury PJ, Siddik SS. Efficacy of the self-inflating bulb in differentiating esophageal from tracheal intubation in the parturient undergoing cesarean section. *Anesth Analg.* 1997;84:533–537.

79. Salem MR, Wafai Y, Joseph NJ. Efficacy of the self-inflating bulb in detecting esophageal intubation: does the presence of a nasogastric tube or cuff deflation make a difference? *Anesthesiology.* 1994;80:42–48.

80. Kasper CL, Deem S. The self-inflating bulb to detect esophageal intubation during emergency airway management. *Anesthesiology.* 1998;88:898–902.

81. Lang DJ, Wafai Y, Salem MR. Efficacy of the self-inflating bulb in confirming tracheal intubation in the morbidly obese. *Anesthesiology.* 1996;85:246–253.

82. Davis DP, Stephen KA, Vilke GM. Inaccuracy in endotracheal tube verification using a Toomey syringe. *Emerg Med.* 1999;17:35–38.

83. MacLeod BA, Heller MB, Gerard J, Yealy DM, Menegazzi JJ. Verification of endotracheal tube placement with colorimetric end-tidal CO_2 detection. *Ann Emerg Med.* 1991;20:267–270.

84. Chow LH, Lui PW, Cheung EL, Jong HR, Yang TC, Chen YC. Verification of endotracheal tube misplacement with the colorimetric carbon dioxide detector during anesthesia. *Chung Hua I Hsueh Tsa Chih.* 1993;51:415–418.

85. Hayden SR, Sciammarella J, Viccellio P. Colorimetric end-tidal CO_2 detector for verification of endotracheal tube placement in out-of-hospital cardiac arrest. *Acad Emerg Med.* 1995;2:499–502.

86. Anton WR, Gordon RW, Jordan TM. A disposable end-tidal CO_2 detector to verify endotracheal intubation. *Ann Emerg Med.* 1991;20:271–275.

87. Bozeman WP, Hexter D, Liang HK, Kelen GD. Esophageal detector device versus detection of end-tidal carbon dioxide level in emergency intubation. *Ann Emerg Med.* 1996;27:595–599.

88. Schaller RJ, Huff JS, Zahn A. Comparison of a colorimetric end-tidal CO_2 detector and an esophageal aspiration device for verifying endotracheal tube placement in the prehospital setting: a six-month experience. *Prehospital Disaster Med.* 1997;12:57–63.

89. Jenkins WA, Verdile VP, Paris PM. The syringe aspiration device technique to verify endotracheal tube position. *Am J Emerg Med.* 1994;12:413–416.

Section 4: Devices to Assist Circulation

Alternative CPR Techniques

Alternative techniques to standard manual CPR have been developed to improve perfusion during CPR. These include interposed abdominal compression (IAC) CPR, high-frequency CPR, active compression-decompression (ACD) CPR, vest CPR, mechanical (piston) CPR, simultaneous ventilation-compression (SVC) CPR, phased thoracic-abdominal compression-decompression (PTACD) CPR, and invasive CPR. Each of these approaches has been evaluated initially in animal models and then in patients. For some the data is sufficient to recommend them as alternatives to standard CPR in specific clinical settings as described below.

Compared with standard CPR, CPR adjuncts generally require additional personnel, training, or equipment. The added effort may increase forward blood flow during CPR from 20% to 100%—levels that are still significantly less than normal cardiac output. Maximum benefits are reported when adjuncts are begun early in the treatment of cardiac arrest,[1] so their use is often limited to in-hospital settings. Adjunctive techniques produce little benefit when started late in a prolonged resuscitative effort or when performed as a last-ditch measure after failed ACLS.[2-4] To date no adjunct has been shown to be universally superior to standard manual CPR for prehospital BLS.

IAC-CPR

IAC-CPR includes manual compression of the abdomen by an extra rescuer during the relaxation phase of chest compression.[5-10] The abdominal compression point is located in the midline, halfway between the xiphoid process and the umbilicus (Figure). The recommended force of abdominal compression should be sufficient to generate approximately 100 mm Hg external pressure on the abdominal aorta and vena cava and is equivalent to that required to optimally palpate the aortic pulse when the heart is beating normally.[11-13]

Two randomized clinical trials of IAC-CPR for in-hospital cardiac arrest have shown statistically significant improvement in outcome measures.[14] Results of the first trial found improved return of spontaneous circulation (ROSC), 24-hour survival, and hospital discharge in 48 of 103 patients randomly assigned to IAC-CPR. Results of the second trial also found improved ROSC and 24-hour survival with IAC-CPR, although none of the patients with an initial rhythm of asystole or pulseless electrical activity survived to hospital discharge. Pooled data from these 2 randomized in-hospital studies shows a difference in 24-hour survival of 33% versus 13%. One smaller trial randomly assigned patients on arrival at the emergency department. If spontaneous circulation

could not be successfully restored within 20 minutes, patients were assigned to the other therapy, with each patient acting as his or her own control. Mean end-tidal P_{CO_2} was 17.1 mm Hg during IAC-CPR versus 9.6 mm Hg during standard CPR. Six of 16 patients were resuscitated before crossover with IAC-CPR versus 3 of 17 with standard CPR ($P=0.19$).[10] One randomized trial of prehospital IAC-CPR showed no difference in outcome or complications.[7] In this study, however, most patients randomly assigned to IAC-CPR received both standard CPR and IAC-CPR during at least some of the resuscitative attempt.

Analysis of all available data for both prehospital and in-hospital resuscitations shows improvement in ROSC with IAC-CPR compared with standard CPR. When only in-hospital studies are examined, the effect of IAC becomes much greater. Data from 2 studies that examined long-term, neurologically intact survival following in-hospital resuscitations shows a positive benefit of IAC-CPR compared with standard CPR. This clinical data is consistent with a series of theoretical and animal studies documenting the "abdominal pump" mechanism for hemodynamic augmentation.[15,16]

The safety of IAC has been reviewed.[17] Increased emesis and aspiration from IAC have not been reported. In fact, there is evidence that positive abdominal pressure applied during ventilations from the beginning of an arrest reduces the rate of gastric inflation before tracheal intubation.[18]

In summary, randomized clinical studies have demonstrated improved outcome when IAC-CPR was compared with standard CPR for *in-hospital* resuscitation, but no survival benefit for *out-of-hospital* arrest has been shown.[19] CPR-induced injuries do not appear to be more common with IAC-CPR than with standard CPR. Because of the positive hemodynamic advantages, safety record, and encouraging in-hospital results, the use of IAC-CPR for in-hospital resuscitations is recommended as an alternative intervention to standard CPR whenever sufficient personnel trained in the technique are available (Class IIb). The safety and efficacy of IAC-CPR has not been studied in patients with aortic aneurysms, pregnancy, or recent abdominal surgery.

High-Frequency ("Rapid Compression Rate") CPR

High-frequency (>100 compressions per minute) manual CPR has been advocated as a technique for improving resuscitation from cardiac arrest.[20-23] Studies in some, but not all, laboratories have shown that rapid compression rates improve cardiac output, aortic and myocardial perfusion pressures, coronary blood flow, and 24-hour survival compared with standard CPR.[20,21] Clinical studies on the use of high-frequency CPR are limited. There is evidence for

Circulation. 2000;102(suppl I):I-105–I-111.
© 2000 American Heart Association, Inc.

Circulation is available at http://www.circulationaha.org

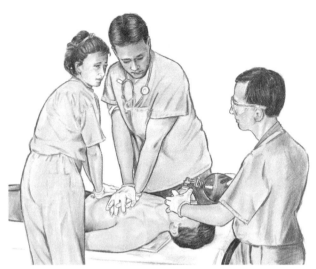

Figure 1. IAC-CPR. In practice it is more convenient when chest and abdominal compressions are performed from opposite sides of the victim.

improved hemodynamics with manual but not mechanical rapid chest compression rates in patients.[22-24] Thus, high-frequency CPR shows some promise for improving CPR. Outcome studies in humans are needed to determine the efficacy of this technique in the management of patients in cardiac arrest (Class Indeterminate).

ACD-CPR

ACD-CPR is another technique developed to improve the efficiency of CPR.[16,25-35] Decreasing intrathoracic pressure during the decompression phase of CPR is thought to enhance venous return and thereby "prime the pump" for the next compression. ACD-CPR is performed with a hand-held device equipped with a suction cup to actively lift the anterior chest during decompression. Early laboratory and clinical data showed that acute hemodynamic parameters such as arterial blood pressure and vital organ perfusion are superior with use of ACD-CPR compared with standard CPR.[36-40] Clinical outcome data is less consistent and suggests that technique and training are critical. The most promising results are from Paris, France, where 1-year survival rates increased from 2% (7 of 377 patients) to 5% (17 of 373 patients) with the use of ACD-CPR.[41] A number of clinical studies, however, have found no significant benefit from the use of ACD-CPR.[42-45] Factors associated with clinical improvement with ACD-CPR include rigorous and repetitive training, concurrent use of low- rather than high-dose epinephrine,[35] use of the force gauge, and performance of CPR for a duration sufficient to prime the pump.

There is some concern that the extra force and energy applied to the chest wall during ACD-CPR tends to induce a higher incidence of rib fractures than that which occurs during standard CPR.[46,47] One case report describes massive cardiac injury in an area of myocardial infarction with pericardial tamponade.[48] In women with large breasts, the presence of a deeper sternum may cause greater force to be transmitted to the lateral rims of the ACD device, enhancing the likelihood of rib fracture.[49] Design improvements, such as

the inclusion of cushions, may well eliminate this problem, which should not be considered fundamental. Other published concerns include difficulties with application of the technique and increased energy expenditure by rescuers.

In summary, laboratory and clinical studies to date have demonstrated that there is often measurable improvement in resuscitation hemodynamics with ACD-CPR compared with standard CPR. Clinical long-term results with ACD-CPR have been favorable (4 studies)[26,28,30,50] or at least neutral (4 studies)[32,51-53] compared with standard CPR. Complications of ACD are noteworthy but not of major concern. ACD-CPR is considered an acceptable alternative to standard CPR when rescue personnel adequately trained in use of the device are available (Class IIb).

(Note: In hearings conducted several years ago the FDA concluded that the evidence did not support the labeling information included with the device. On that basis the FDA did not approve the device for sale and distribution. This conclusion does not conflict with the International Guidelines 2000 recommendations noted above: not proved effective in the out-of-hospital setting; acceptable but weak data supports in-hospital use—Class IIb.)

Vest CPR

The CPR vest was an earlier attempt to take advantage of the thoracic pump mechanism of blood flow.[24,54-59] Vest CPR uses a circumferential thoracic vest, analogous to a large blood pressure cuff, that is cyclically inflated and deflated, vest CPR produces increases in intrathoracic pressure. Vest CPR has shown improved myocardial and cerebral blood flow in animals and improved peak aortic and coronary perfusion pressures during CPR in animals and humans.[60,61] A preliminary report of vest CPR did find improved 6-hour survival but not 24-hour survival.[62] Large randomized trials have not been completed. One such trial was unfortunately interrupted secondary to a lack of continued funding.[63]

There is no evidence of increased resuscitation trauma with vest CPR. The present size and energy requirements for operation of the device continue to be substantial barriers for its widespread use. The size and weight of the device require that it be used for patients who can readily undergo vest CPR without substantial delay in either the hospital or emergency vehicle settings. Long-term survival studies of this approach are needed.

Vest CPR may be considered an alternative to standard CPR in-hospital or during ambulance transport, because vest CPR (1) shows hemodynamic improvement in animal and clinical studies, (2) does not substantially delay starting CPR, (3) presents no significant known disadvantages, (4) has been assessed for hemodynamic effect in patients in cardiac arrest, and (5) does not interfere with defibrillation efforts. Vest CPR should be used only when there are an adequate number of well-trained, in-hospital personnel to properly perform CPR (Class IIb). The manufacturer of the vest-CPR device has not yet sought and obtained FDA permission for its distribution and sale.

Mechanical (Piston) CPR

Mechanical devices that depress the sternum are not a substitute for manual external chest compression but rather an adjunct to be used by trained personnel to optimize compression and reduce rescuer fatigue in prolonged resuscitative efforts.[64] The efficacy and safety of these devices have not been demonstrated in infants and children; their use should be limited to adults. A disadvantage of any mechanical chest compression device is the potential for interrupting chest compressions for extended periods while setting up and initiating compressions. Mechanical chest compressors can be manual or automatic.

Simple, manually operated mechanical chest compressors can provide effective external chest compressions. Automatic mechanical chest compressors such as the Mechanical Thumper consist of a compressed gas-powered plunger mounted on a backboard. The devices can be programmed to deliver standard CPR in a compression-ventilation ratio of 5:1, with a compression duration that is 50% of the cycle length, or other ratios. Most animal and clinical studies have shown variable hemodynamic results compared with other CPR techniques (standard, ACD, and SVC CPR).[57,65] Results of the 2 most recent clinical trials both showed improved expired end-tidal CO_2 compared with standard manual CPR.[66] The limited clinical data has thus far shown no improvement in survival outcome when mechanical CPR was compared with standard CPR in patients with cardiac arrest.

An advantage of the mechanical devices is delivery of a consistent rate and depth of compression by eliminating such variables as operator technique and fatigue. Problems related to the use of automatic mechanical chest compressors, however, include sternal fracture, expense, size, weight, restrictions on mobility, and dislocation of the plunger in relation to the sternum. Ventilation or chest compression, or both, may be inadequate when these devices are improperly positioned or operated. In addition, the weight of the compressor on the chest may limit chest wall recoil and venous return during decompression, especially after one or more rib fractures have occurred. There is no consistent measurable improvement in hemodynamics and no observed survival outcome data showing that mechanical resuscitators similar to mechanical chest compressors are superior to standard CPR. The mechanical resuscitator is an acceptable alternative to standard manual CPR in circumstances that make manual chest compressions difficult, ie, certain transport situations or lack of adequate personnel (Class IIb).

Simultaneous Ventilation-Compression CPR
The technique of SVC-CPR was conceived to take advantage of the entire thorax as a pump in producing blood flow during cardiac arrest.[24,55,57,67–72] Pressure gradients are developed between intrathoracic and extrathoracic vascular beds. Studies in experimental models showed that SVC-CPR resulted in improved peak compression ("systolic") pressures and carotid artery blood flows.[67–69] On the basis of these studies, a mechanical CPR device that provides simultaneous ventilation and chest compression was developed and tested clinically. Laboratory studies showed improvement in short-term survival when SVC-CPR was compared with standard CPR in some laboratories[55,73] but not others.[57,71] Clinical studies have failed to identify any benefits of SVC-CPR. Instead the studies show standard CPR to be superior to SVC-CPR in

hemodynamics[24,72] and survival. SVC-CPR is not currently available for clinical use.

Phased Thoracic-Abdominal Compression-Decompression CPR
PTACD-CPR uses a hand-held device that alternates chest compression and abdominal decompression with chest decompression and abdominal compression. This innovative technique basically combines the concepts of IAC-CPR and ACD-CPR. Theoretically the combined 4-phase approach, including both compression and decompression of the chest and abdomen, could increase blood flow during cardiac arrest and CPR.[16]

The use of PTACD-CPR has led to hemodynamic improvement in animal and clinical studies.[74,75] PTACD-CPR does not substantially delay starting CPR and presents no significant known disadvantages or harm when used correctly. No clinical outcome data is available, and the device is not yet approved by the FDA (Class Indeterminate).

Other Adjunctive CPR Devices
Several mechanical devices have been developed as adjuncts to CPR. These devices do not replace basic CPR but rather are additions to the ongoing resuscitative effort. They can be combined with a variety of CPR techniques, eg, standard CPR, IAC-CPR, ACD-CPR, vest CPR, and mechanical CPR. Such adjunctive CPR devices can be recommended only after they have been shown to improve the efficacy of CPR in patients in cardiac arrest (hemodynamic changes are equal or better) and to have no significant increase in complications compared with standard manual CPR.

Impedance Threshold Valve
The impedance threshold valve (ITV, or ResQ-Valve) is associated with lower intrathoracic pressure.[76,77] When used with a compression/decompression device, the valve is inserted into a standard tracheal tube ventilation circuit and does not disrupt CPR performance. The airway must be secured with a cuffed tracheal tube. By preventing inspiration during chest decompression, the impedance threshold valve produces more negative intrathoracic pressure, enhancing blood return to the thorax.

The impedance threshold valve (ResQ-Valve) is not intended for use with standard CPR. Future clinical studies may indicate efficacy of the impedance valve during standard CPR, but no recommendation can now be made for this device as an adjunct for standard CPR (Class Indeterminate). Observations from 2 animal studies and 1 small (n=11) human trial[77a] showed significant improvements in hemodynamic **parameters** when this device was used as an adjunct to ACD-CPR. Despite better hemodynamics, no improvement in short- or long-term outcome occurred, and no complications were noted in the 11 study patients. The impedance threshold valve is acceptable as an adjunct to be used with a cardiac compression/decompression device to augment hemodynamic parameters (Class IIb).

Invasive CPR
Direct cardiac compression is a special technique that may provide near-normal perfusion of the brain and heart.[3,4,78–80]

Experimental studies have shown that direct cardiac massage used early in cardiac arrest after a short period of ineffective closed-chest CPR can improve survival from cardiac arrest.[81] Limited clinical series have shown similar beneficial hemodynamic effects with open-chest massage. Experimental and clinical studies have shown that direct cardiac massage does not improve outcome when applied late (after >25 minutes of total arrest time) in the treatment of patients in cardiac arrest.[3,4] One prospective, nonrandomized, historically controlled series, however, did show improved ROSC with the use of open-chest direct cardiac massage.[82]

In the emergency thoracotomy, open-chest cardiac massage is, by necessity, associated with some morbidity. An experienced team is needed to successfully perform this technique and optimally care for the patient afterward. We do not recommend its routine use for cardiac arrest victims. *In particular, it should not be used as a last effort at the end of a lengthy resuscitation treatment sequence.* Outcome studies assessing the use of open-chest direct cardiac massage early in the cardiac arrest treatment sequence are needed.

Specific indications for the use of open-chest direct cardiac compression in the clinical setting are changing. Previous recommendations included cardiac arrest from nonpenetrating, blunt trauma. Blunt abdominal trauma associated with cardiac arrest does not respond to invasive resuscitative efforts and should not be considered an indication. A thoracotomy is indicated for patients with penetrating chest trauma who develop cardiac arrest. Other clinical circumstances in which a thoracotomy could be considered include (1) cardiac arrest caused by hypothermia, pulmonary embolism, or pericardial tamponade; (2) chest deformity where closed-chest CPR is ineffective; and (3) penetrating abdominal trauma with deterioration and cardiac arrest. The use of open-chest direct cardiac massage can be considered under special circumstances but should not be done simply as a late last-ditch effort (Class IIb).

Emergency cardiopulmonary bypass has been advocated as a circulatory adjunct for treatment of patients in cardiac arrest.[83-85] The bypass pump can be applied by using the femoral artery and vein without requiring a thoracotomy. Experimental studies have shown improved hemodynamics and survival when cardiopulmonary bypass is used after prolonged cardiac arrest.[83,84] Clinical studies have shown the feasibility of cardiopulmonary bypass in the treatment of patients in cardiac arrest from specific, potentially reversible causes (such as drug overdoses and poisonings).[84] No outcome studies of significance have been done to date. Further clinical studies are needed to define the role of cardiopulmonary bypass in the treatment of patients in cardiac arrest (Class Indeterminate). Its success in the special situations of drug overdoses and hypothermic arrest may be sufficient justification alone for its use in specific hospital settings.

Assessment of CPR

At present there are no good prognostic criteria that clinicians can use to assess the efficacy of CPR. Clinical outcome—either resuscitation or death—is often the only way to judge the adequacy of CPR efforts. Assessment of ongoing CPR efforts would allow clinicians to modify resuscitative efforts and individualize treatment protocols for patients in cardiac arrest. Ideally clinicians could judge the value of specific adjuncts in individual patients. If a less-than-optimal response were documented, a new strategy could be attempted and individualized, depending on such real-time feedback during the resuscitative effort. Several adjuncts may be useful in the assessment of ongoing CPR efforts.

Assessment of Hemodynamics

Perfusion pressures. Studies in experimental models have repeatedly shown the importance of the aortic diastolic and myocardial perfusion (aortic-to–right atrial diastolic gradient) pressures during CPR for successful resuscitation from cardiac arrest.[86-92] The aortic diastolic and myocardial perfusion pressures have been correlated with coronary blood flow during CPR.[93] Much CPR research has focused on drugs or adjuncts that improve these pressures. Although the placement of arterial and central venous lines during resuscitative efforts has been accomplished by a resuscitation research team in some settings, placement of these lines is impractical in most clinical settings.[86,94] When arterial lines are available, the clinician should attempt to optimize the aortic diastolic and myocardial perfusion pressures during the resuscitative effort.

Pulses. Clinicians frequently use the presence or absence of pulses resulting from chest compressions during the resuscitative effort to assess the adequacy of artificial perfusion during CPR. The presence of pulses does not indicate any meaningful arterial blood flow during CPR. No studies have shown the clinical utility of checking pulses during ongoing CPR. A palpable pulse represents the difference between the peak pressure and nadir pressure within a vascular bed. The important factor for perfusion of the myocardium is coronary perfusion pressure (aortic minus right atrial pressure during the relaxation phase of chest compressions). The difference in peak and nadir pressures does not correlate with perfusion. It is important to remember that because there are no valves in the inferior vena cava, retrograde blood flow may occur in the femoral vein. Palpation of a pulse in the femoral area may be misleading and may indicate venous rather than arterial blood flow. In summary, the presence of carotid pulses during CPR may indicate the presence of a pulse wave and perhaps some forward blood flow, but it cannot be used to gauge the efficacy of myocardial or cerebral perfusion from ongoing CPR efforts.

Assessment of Respiratory Gases

Some clinicians use *arterial blood gases* to gauge the efficacy of ongoing CPR efforts. Adequate oxygen concentration in arterial blood during low-flow states may not imply adequate oxygen delivery to the peripheral tissue beds. Physiologically, arterial blood gases do not reflect tissue pH and Pco_2. Mixed venous gases often show severe hypercarbia despite normal arterial gases.[95] No correlation between arterial blood gases and resuscitation success has been demonstrated in experimental models of cardiac arrest.[96] Thus, arterial blood gases can be useful for evaluating oxygenation but should not be used to assess adequacy of CPR efforts.

Studies on the use of *oximetry* for assessing tissue perfusion during CPR have shown that transconjunctival oxygen tension falls rapidly when a patient goes into cardiac arrest and returns to baseline when spontaneous circulation is restored.[97] Oximetry, however, has not been shown to be a useful prognostic guide for predicting resuscitation from cardiac arrest. Pulse oximetry is commonly used in emergency departments and critical care units. However, measurements depend on the presence of a peripheral pulse, and the technique is unreliable when used on patients in cardiac arrest.

Capnometry shows the most promise as a measurement of CPR effectiveness. Measuring expired end-tidal CO_2 is a noninvasive technique for monitoring cardiac output generated during ongoing CPR.[98] During cardiac arrest CO_2 continues to be generated throughout the body. Once delivered to the lungs, it is excreted. The major determinant of CO_2 excretion is its rate of delivery from the peripheral production sites to the lungs. If ventilation is reasonably constant, then end-tidal CO_2 concentration reflects cardiac output. Capnometry measures CO_2 excretion through the tracheal tube. In experimental models, end-tidal CO_2 concentration during ongoing CPR correlated with cardiac output, coronary perfusion pressure, and successful resuscitation from cardiac arrest.[98–101] Clinical studies have shown that patients who were successfully resuscitated from cardiac arrest had significantly higher end-tidal CO_2 levels than patients who could not be resuscitated.[102–106] Capnometry can also be used as an early indicator of ROSC.[102–104]

Despite these promising studies, other variables can cause changes in CO_2 excretion. Large changes in the minute ventilations will affect the end-tidal CO_2 reading. Ventilations must be held relatively constant during the resuscitative effort. Administration of bicarbonate will increase CO_2 excretion for several minutes before it returns to stable conditions for measurement.[104,105] High doses of pressor agents such as epinephrine will increase myocardial perfusion pressure but decrease cardiac output. CO_2 excretion will decrease with decreased blood flow to the lungs.[107,108] In summary, end-tidal CO_2 monitoring during cardiac arrest can be useful as a noninvasive indicator of cardiac output generated during CPR (Class IIa). Research is needed to define the ability of end-tidal CO_2 monitoring to predict cardiac arrest victims who could be resuscitated with more aggressive interventions or prolonged resuscitations.

Assessment of Chest Compression

The quality of chest compressions and resuscitative effort is an important aspect of CPR. Even physicians recently trained in ACLS have difficulty meeting the recommended compression and ventilatory rates. Simple metronome guidance can correct this.[109] Guaranteeing the depth of chest compressions has been even more difficult to ensure.

A device called CPR-Plus has been developed to improve the rescuer's performance of chest compression. When this device is placed on the victim's chest and used as a baseplate for chest compressions, the rescuer obtains feedback that includes a metronome-guided rate and force of compression performed. To date, only manikin studies using the CPR-Plus device have been reported.[110,111] These studies showed that performance of chest compressions was significantly improved when rescuers used the CPR-Plus device rather than standard CPR alone. Animal and clinical studies, however, are needed to assess whether CPR-Plus improves or detracts from resuscitation hemodynamics in animal models and patients with cardiac arrest. Until such studies are available, informed commentary on this promising device is not possible. We do not recommend the use of CPR-Plus during CPR (Class Indeterminate).

References

1. Walker LI, MacMath T, Chipman H, Bayne E. MAST application in the treatment of paroxysmal supraventricular tachycardia in a child. *Ann Emerg Med.* 1988;17:529–531.
2. Adams CP, Martin GB, Rivers EP, Ward KR, Smithline HA, Rady MY. Hemodynamics of interposed abdominal compression during human cardiopulmonary resuscitation. *Acad Emerg Med.* 1994;1:498–502.
3. Geehr EC, Lewis FR, Auerbach PS. Failure of open-heart massage to improve survival after prehospital nontraumatic cardiac arrest. *N Engl J Med.* 1986;314:1189–1190. Letter.
4. Bodai BI, Smith JP, Ward RE, O'Neill MB, Auborg R. Emergency thoracotomy in the management of trauma. *JAMA.* 1983;249:1891–1896.
5. Ralston SH, Babbs CF, Niebauer MJ. Cardiopulmonary resuscitation with interposed abdominal compression in dogs. *Anesth Analg.* 1982;61:645–651.
6. Sack JB, Kesselbrenner MB, Jarrad A. Interposed abdominal compression–cardiopulmonary resuscitation and resuscitation outcome during asystole and electromechanical dissociation [see comments]. *Circulation.* 1992;86:1692–1700.
7. Mateer JR, Stueven HA, Thompson BM, Aprahamian C, Darin JC. Interposed abdominal compression CPR versus standard CPR in prehospital cardiopulmonary arrest: preliminary results. *Ann Emerg Med.* 1984;13:764–766.
8. Barranco F, Lesmes A, Irles JA, Blasco J, Leal J, Rodriguez J, Leon C. Cardiopulmonary resuscitation with simultaneous chest and abdominal compression: comparative study in humans. *Resuscitation.* 1990;20:67–77.
9. Berryman CR, Phillips GM. Interposed abdominal compression-CPR in human subjects. *Ann Emerg Med.* 1984;13:226–229.
10. Ward KR, Sullivan RJ, Zelenak RR, Summer WR. A comparison of interposed abdominal compression CPR and standard CPR by monitoring end-tidal P_{CO_2} [see comments]. *Ann Emerg Med.* 1989;18:831–837.
11. Babbs CF, Ralston SH, Geddes LA. Theoretical advantages of abdominal counterpulsation in CPR as demonstrated in a simple electrical model of the circulation. *Ann Emerg Med.* 1984;13:660–671.
12. Beyar R, Kishon Y, Kimmel E, Neufeld H, Dinnar U. Intrathoracic and abdominal pressure variations as an efficient method for cardiopulmonary resuscitation: studies in dogs compared with computer model results. *Cardiovasc Res.* 1985;19:335–342.
13. Voorhees WD, Niebauer MJ, Babbs CF. Improved oxygen delivery during cardiopulmonary resuscitation with interposed abdominal compressions. *Ann Emerg Med.* 1983;12:128–135.
14. Sack JB, Kesselbrenner MB, Bregman D. Survival from in-hospital cardiac arrest with interposed abdominal counterpulsation during cardiopulmonary resuscitation [see comments]. *JAMA.* 1992;267:379–385.
15. Babbs CF, Sack JB, Kern KB. Interposed abdominal compression as an adjunct to cardiopulmonary resuscitation. *Am Heart J.* 1994;127:412–421.
16. Babbs CF. CPR techniques that combine chest and abdominal compression and decompression: hemodynamic insights from a spreadsheet model. *Circulation.* 1999;100:2146–2152.
17. Sack JB, Kesselbrenner MB. Hemodynamics, survival benefits, and complications of interposed abdominal compression during cardiopulmonary resuscitation. *Acad Emerg Med.* 1994;1:490–497.
18. Babbs CF, Schoenlein WE, Lowe MW. Gastric insufflation during IAC-CPR and standard CPR in a canine model. *Am J Emerg Med.* 1985;3:99–103.
19. Mateer JR, Stueven HA, Thompson BM, Aprahamian C, Darin JC. Prehospital IAC-CPR versus standard CPR: paramedic resuscitation of cardiac arrests. *Am J Emerg Med.* 1985;3:143–146.
20. Feneley MP, Maier GW, Kern KB, Gaynor JW, Gall SA Jr, Sanders AB, Raessler K, Muhlbaier LH, Rankin JS, Ewy GA. Influence of compression rate on initial success of resuscitation and 24 hour survival after prolonged

manual cardiopulmonary resuscitation in dogs. *Circulation*. 1988;77: 240–250.

21. Halperin HR, Tsitlik JE, Guerci AD, Mellits ED, Levin HR, Shi AY, Chandra N, Weisfeldt ML. Determinants of blood flow to vital organs during cardiopulmonary resuscitation in dogs. *Circulation*. 1986;73: 539–550.

22. Kern KB, Sanders AB, Raife J, Milander MM, Otto CW, Ewy GA. A study of chest compression rates during cardiopulmonary resuscitation in humans: the importance of rate-directed chest compressions. *Arch Intern Med*. 1992; 152:145–149.

23. Ornato JP, Gonzalez ER, Garnett AR, Levine RL, McClung BK. Effect of cardiopulmonary resuscitation compression rate on end-tidal carbon dioxide concentration and arterial pressure in man. *Crit Care Med*. 1988;16: 241–245.

24. Swenson RD, Weaver WD, Niskanen RA, Martin J, Dahlberg S. Hemodynamics in humans during conventional and experimental methods of cardiopulmonary resuscitation. *Circulation*. 1988;78:630–639.

25. Tucker KJ, Redberg RF, Schiller NB, Cohen TJ, Cardiopulmonary Resuscitation Working Group. Active compression-decompression resuscitation: analysis of transmitral flow and left ventricular volume by transesophageal echocardiography in humans. *J Am Coll Cardiol*. 1993;22:1485–1493.

26. Cohen T, Goldner B, Maccaro P, et al. A comparison of active compression-decompression cardiopulmonary resuscitation with standard cardiopulmonary resuscitation for cardiac arrests occurring in the hospital. *N Engl J Med*. 1993;329:1918–1921.

27. Shultz JJ, Coffeen P, Sweeney M, Detloff B, Kehler C, Pineda E, Yakshe P, Adler SW, Chang M, Lurie KG. Evaluation of standard and active compression-decompression CPR in an acute human model of ventricular fibrillation. *Circulation*. 1994;89:684–693.

28. Tucker KJ, Galli F, Savitt MA, Kahsai D, Bresnahan L, Redberg RF. Active compression-decompression resuscitation: effect on resuscitation success after in-hospital cardiac arrest. *J Am Coll Cardiol*. 1994;24:201–209.

29. Orliaguet GA, Carli PA, Rozenberg A, Janniere D, Sauval P, Delpech P. End-tidal carbon dioxide during out-of-hospital cardiac arrest resuscitation: comparison of active compression-decompression and standard CPR. *Ann Emerg Med*. 1995;25:48–51.

30. Plaisance P, Adnet F, Vicaut E, Hennequin B, Magne P, Prudhomme C, Lambert Y, Cantineau JP, Leopold C, Ferracci C, Gizzi M, Payen D. Benefit of active compression-decompression cardiopulmonary resuscitation as a prehospital advanced cardiac life support: a randomized multicenter study. *Circulation*. 1997;95:955–961.

31. Malzer R, Zeiner A, Binder M, Domanovits H, Knappitsch G, Sterz F, Laggner AN. Hemodynamic effects of active compression-decompression after prolonged CPR. *Resuscitation*. 1996;31:243–253.

32. Stiell IG, Hebert PC, Wells GA, Laupacis A, Vandemheen K, Dreyer JF, Eisenhauer MA, Gibson J, Higginson LA, Kirby AS, Mahon JL, Maloney JP, Weitzman BN. The Ontario trial of active compression-decompression cardiopulmonary resuscitation for in-hospital and prehospital cardiac arrest [see comments]. *JAMA*. 1996;275:1417–1423.

33. Urban P, Cereda J. Glasgow coma score one hour after cardiac arrest. *Lancet*. 1985;2:1012–1014.

34. Lindner KH, Pfenninger EG, Lurie KG, Schurmann W, Lindner IM, Ahnefeld FW. Effects of active compression-decompression resuscitation on myocardial and cerebral blood flow in pigs. *Circulation*. 1993;88: 1254–1263.

35. Gueugniaud PY, Vaudelin T, Gaussorgues P, Petit P. Out-of-hospital cardiac arrest: the teaching of experience at the SAMU of Lyon. *Resuscitation*. 1989;17(suppl):S79–S98; discussion S199–S206.

36. Tzivoni D, Banai S, Schuger C, et al. Treatment of torsades de pointes with magnesium sulfate. *Circulation*. 1988;77:392–399.

37. Tucker KJ, Idris A. Clinical and laboratory investigations of active compression-decompression cardiopulmonary resuscitation [editorial]. *Resuscitation*. 1994;28:1–7.

38. Tresch D, Wetherbee J, Siegel R, Troup P, Keelan MJ, Olinger G, Brooks H. Long-term follow-up of survivors of prehospital sudden cardiac death treated with coronary bypass surgery. *Am Heart J*. 1985;110:1139–1145.

39. Clinton J, McGill J, Irwin G, Peterson G, Lilja G, Ruiz E. Cardiac arrest under age 40: etiology and prognosis. *Ann Emerg Med*. 1984;13: 1011–1015.

40. Tuggle D. Meeting the emotional needs of survivors of sudden cardiac arrest. *Cardiovasc Nurs*. 1982;18:25–30.

41. Plaisance P, Lurie KG, Vicaut E, Adnet F, Petit JL, Epain D, Ecollan P, Gruat R, Cavagna P, Biens J, Payen D, French Active Compression-Decompression Cardiopulmonary Resuscitation Study Group. A comparison of standard cardiopulmonary resuscitation and active compression-

decompression resuscitation for out-of-hospital cardiac arrest. *N Engl J Med*. 1999;341:569–575.

42. Timerman A, Piegas L, Sousa J. Results of cardiopulmonary resuscitation in a cardiology hospital. *Resuscitation*. 1989;18:75–84.

43. Tonkin A. Prevention of sudden cardiac death: the ICD, or an electrical end-point with preceding opportunities for intervention? *Aust N Z J Med*. 1992;22:631–635.

44. Tomlinson T, Brody H. Futility and the ethics of resuscitation. *JAMA*. 1990;264:1276–1280.

45. Thies W. Risk of infection during CPR training and rescue: supplemental guidelines. *JAMA*. 1989;262:2714–2715.

46. Siscovick DS, Raghunathan TE, Psaty BM, Koepsell TD, Wicklund KG, Lin X, Cobb L, Rautaharju PM, Copass MK, Wagner EH. Diuretic therapy for hypertension and the risk of primary cardiac arrest [see comments]. *N Engl J Med*. 1994;330:1852–1857.

47. Rabl W, Baubin M, Broinger G, Scheithauer R. Serious complications from active compression-decompression cardiopulmonary resuscitation. *Int J Legal Med*. 1996;109:84–89.

48. Klintschar M, Darok M, Radner H. Massive injury to the heart after attempted active compression-decompression cardiopulmonary resuscitation. *Int J Legal Med*. 1998;111:93–96.

49. Haid C, Rabl W, Baubin M. Active compression-decompression resuscitation: the influence of different chest geometries on the force transmission. *Resuscitation*. 1997;35:83–85.

50. Lurie KG, Shultz JJ, Callaham ML, Schwab TM, Gisch T, Rector T, Frascone RJ, Long L. Evaluation of active compression-decompression CPR in victims of out-of-hospital cardiac arrest [see comments]. *JAMA*. 1994;271:1405–1411.

51. Schwab T, Callaham M, Madsen C, Utecht T. A randomized clinical trial of active compression-decompression CPR vs standard CPR in out-of-hospital cardiac arrest in two cities. *JAMA*. 1995;273:1261–1268.

52. Mauer D, Schneider T, Dick W, Withelm A, Elich D, Mauer M. Active compression-decompression resuscitation: a prospective, randomized study in a two-tiered EMS system with physicians in the field. *Resuscitation*. 1996;33:125–134.

53. Luiz T, Ellinger K, Denz C. Active compression-decompression cardiopulmonary resuscitation does not improve survival in patients with prehospital cardiac arrest in a physician-manned emergency medical system [see comments]. *J Cardiothorac Vasc Anesth*. 1996;10:178–186.

54. Babbs CF. New versus old theories of blood flow during CPR. *Crit Care Med*. 1980;8:191–195.

55. Niemann JT, Rosborough JP, Niskanen RA, Alferness C, Criley JM. Mechanical "cough" cardiopulmonary resuscitation during cardiac arrest in dogs. *Am J Cardiol*. 1985;55:199–204.

56. Krischer JP, Fine EG, Weisfeldt ML, Guerci AD, Nagel E, Chandra N. Comparison of prehospital conventional and simultaneous compression-ventilation cardiopulmonary resuscitation. *Crit Care Med*. 1989;17: 1263–1269.

57. Kern KB, Carter AB, Showen RL, Voorhees WD III, Babbs CF, Tacker WA, Ewy GA. Comparison of mechanical techniques of cardiopulmonary resuscitation: survival and neurologic outcome in dogs [published erratum appears in *Am J Emerg Med*. 1987;5:304]. *Am J Emerg Med*. 1987;5: 190–195.

58. Niemann JT, Rosborough JP, Niskanen RA, Criley JM. Circulatory support during cardiac arrest using a pneumatic vest and abdominal binder with simultaneous high-pressure airway inflation. *Ann Emerg Med*. 1984;13: 767–770.

59. Halperin HR, Guerci AD, Chandra N, Herskowitz A, Tsitlik JE, Niskanen RA, Wurmb E, Weisfeldt ML. Vest inflation without simultaneous ventilation during cardiac arrest in dogs: improved survival from prolonged cardiopulmonary resuscitation. *Circulation*. 1986;74:1407–1415.

60. Weinstein M, Stason W. Foundations of cost-effectiveness analysis for health and medical practice. *N Engl Med*. 1977;296:716–721.

61. Marley CD Jr, Eitel DR, Anderson TE, Mum AJ, Patterson GA. Evaluation of a prototype esophageal detection device. *Acad Emerg Med*. 1995;2: 503–507.

62. Cummins RO, Chamberlain DA. Advisory statements of the International Liaison Committee on Resuscitation. *Circulation*. 1997;95:2172–3217.

63. Chamberlain D, Bossaert L. Personal communication.

64. Taylor GJ, Rubin R, Tucker M, Greene HL, Rudikoff MT, Weisfeldt ML. External cardiac compression: a randomized comparison of mechanical and manual techniques. *JAMA*. 1978;240:644–646.

65. McDonald JL. Systolic and mean arterial pressures during manual and mechanical CPR in humans. *Crit Care Med*. 1981;9:382–383.

66. Ward KR, Menegazzi JJ, Zelenak RR, Sullivan RJ, McSwain NE Jr. A comparison of chest compressions between mechanical and manual CPR by monitoring end-tidal P_{CO_2} during human cardiac arrest. *Ann Emerg Med.* 1993;22:669–674.

67. Rudikoff MT, Maughan WL, Effron M, Freund P, Weisfeldt ML. Mechanisms of blood flow during cardiopulmonary resuscitation. *Circulation.* 1980;61:345–352.

68. Chandra N, Snyder LD, Weisfeldt ML. Abdominal binding during cardiopulmonary resuscitation in man. *JAMA.* 1981;246:351–353.

69. Chandra N, Rudikoff M, Weisfeldt ML. Simultaneous chest compression and ventilation at high airway pressure during cardiopulmonary resuscitation. *Lancet.* 1980;1:175–178.

70. Niemann JT, Rosborough JP, Hausknecht M, Garner D, Criley JM. Pressure-synchronized cineangiography during experimental cardiopulmonary resuscitation. *Circulation.* 1981;64:985–991.

71. Sanders AB, Ewy GA, Alferness CA, Taft T, Zimmerman M. Failure of one method of simultaneous chest compression, ventilation, and abdominal binding during CPR. *Crit Care Med.* 1982;10:509–513.

72. Martin GB, Carden DL, Nowak RM, Lewinter JR, Johnston W, Tomlanovich MC. Aortic and right atrial pressures during standard and simultaneous compression and ventilation CPR in human beings. *Ann Emerg Med.* 1986;15:125–130.

73. Kern KB, Carter AB, Showen RL, Voorhees WD III, Babbs CF, Tacker WA, Ewy GA. Twenty-four hour survival in a canine model of cardiac arrest comparing three methods of manual cardiopulmonary resuscitation. *J Am Coll Cardiol.* 1986;7:859–867.

74. Tang W, Weil MH, Schock RB, Sato Y, Lucas J, Sun S, Bisera J. Phased chest and abdominal compression-decompression: a new option for cardiopulmonary resuscitation. *Circulation.* 1997;95:1335–1340.

75. Sterz F, Behringer W, Berzlanovich A, Wernigg H, Domanovits H, Muellner M, Schreiber W, Ohley WJ, Schoerkhuber W, Laggner AN. Active compression-decompression of thorax and abdomen (Lifestick™-CPR) in patients with cardiac arrest. *Circulation.* 1996;94(suppl I):I-9. Abstract.

76. Lurie KG, Mulligan KA, McKnite S, Detloff B, Lindstrom P, Lindner KH. Optimizing standard cardiopulmonary resuscitation with an inspiratory impedance threshold valve. *Chest.* 1998;113:1084–1090.

77. Tresch D, Grove J, Siegal R, Keelan M, Brooks H. Survivors of prehospitalization sudden death: characteristic clinical and angiographic features. *Arch Intern Med.* 1981;141:1154–1157.

77a. Plaisance P, Lurie KG, Payen D. Inspiratory impedance during active compression-decompression cardiopulmonary resuscitation: a randomized evaluation of patients in cardiac arrest. *Circulation.* 2000;101:989–994.

78. Robertson C. The value of open chest CPR for non-traumatic cardiac arrest. *Resuscitation.* 1991;22:203–208.

79. Babbs CF. Hemodynamic mechanisms in CPR: a theoretical rationale for resuscitative thoracotomy in non-traumatic cardiac arrest. *Resuscitation.* 1987;15:37–50.

80. Shocket E, Rosenblum R. Successful open cardiac massage after 75 minutes of closed massage. *JAMA.* 1967;200:333–335.

81. Kern KB, Sanders AB, Badylak SF, Janas W, Carter AB, Tacker WA, Ewy GA. Long-term survival with open-chest cardiac massage after ineffective closed-chest compression in a canine preparation. *Circulation.* 1987;75:498–503.

82. Takino M, Okada Y. The optimum timing of resuscitative thoracotomy for non-traumatic out-of-hospital cardiac arrest. *Resuscitation.* 1993;26:69–74.

83. Cogbill TH, Moore EE, Millikan JS, Cleveland HC. Rationale for selective application of emergency department thoracotomy in trauma. *J Trauma.* 1983;23:453–460.

84. Danne PD, Finelli F, Champion HR. Emergency bay thoracotomy. *J Trauma.* 1984;24:796–802.

85. Roberge RJ, Ivatury RR, Stahl W, Rohman M. Emergency department thoracotomy for penetrating injuries: predictive value of patient classification. *Am J Emerg Med.* 1986;4:129–135.

86. Paradis NA, Martin GB, Rivers EP, Goetting MG, Appleton TJ, Feingold M, Nowak RM. Coronary perfusion pressure and the return of spontaneous circulation in human cardiopulmonary resuscitation [see comments]. *JAMA.* 1990;263:1106–1113.

87. Redding JS. Abdominal compression in cardiopulmonary resuscitation. *Anesth Analg.* 1971;50:668–675.

88. Redding JS, Pearson JW. Resuscitation from ventricular fibrillation: drug therapy. *JAMA.* 1968;203:255–260.

89. Sanders AB, Ewy GA, Taft TV. Prognostic and therapeutic importance of the aortic diastolic pressure in resuscitation from cardiac arrest. *Crit Care Med.* 1984;12:871–873.

90. Ditchey RV, Winkler JV, Rhodes CA. Relative lack of coronary blood flow during closed-chest resuscitation in dogs. *Circulation.* 1982;66:297–302.

91. Michael JR, Guerci AD, Koehler RC, Shi AY, Tsitlik J, Chandra N, Niedermeyer E, Rogers MC, Traystman RJ, Weisfeldt ML. Mechanisms by which epinephrine augments cerebral and myocardial perfusion during cardiopulmonary resuscitation in dogs. *Circulation.* 1984;69:822–835.

92. Ralston SH, Voorhees WD, Babbs CF. Intrapulmonary epinephrine during prolonged cardiopulmonary resuscitation: improved regional blood flow and resuscitation in dogs. *Ann Emerg Med.* 1984;13:79–86.

93. Sanders A, Ewy G, Taft T. Prognostic and therapeutic importance of the aortic diastolic pressure in resuscitation from cardiac arrest. *Crit Care Med.* 1984;12:871–873.

94. Sanders AB, Ogle M, Ewy GA. Coronary perfusion pressure during cardiopulmonary resuscitation. *Am J Emerg Med.* 1985;3:11–14.

95. Weil MH, Rackow EC, Trevino R, Grundler W, Falk JL, Griffel MI. Difference in acid-base state between venous and arterial blood during cardiopulmonary resuscitation. *N Engl J Med.* 1986;315:153–156.

96. Sanders AB, Ewy GA, Taft TV. Resuscitation and arterial blood gas abnormalities during prolonged cardiopulmonary resuscitation. *Ann Emerg Med.* 1984;13:676–679.

97. Abraham E, Fink S. Conjunctival oxygen tension monitoring in emergency department patients. *Am J Emerg Med.* 1988;6:549–554.

98. Weil MH, Bisera J, Trevino RP, Rackow EC. Cardiac output and end-tidal carbon dioxide. *Crit Care Med.* 1985;13:907–909.

99. Sanders AB, Atlas AB, Ewy GA, Kern KB, Bragg S. Expired P_{CO_2} as an index of coronary perfusion pressure. *Am J Emerg Med.* 1985;3:147–149.

100. Sanders AB, Ewy GA, Bragg S, Atlas AB, Kern KB. Expired P_{CO_2} as a prognostic indicator of successful resuscitation from cardiac arrest. *Ann Emerg Med.* 1985;14:948–952.

101. Gudipati CV, Weil MH, Bisera J, Deshmukh HG, Rackow EC. Expired carbon dioxide: a noninvasive monitor of cardiopulmonary resuscitation. *Circulation.* 1988;77:234–239.

102. Kalenda Z. The capnogram as a guide to the efficacy of cardiac massage. *Resuscitation.* 1978;6:259–263.

103. Garnett AR, Ornato JP, Gonzalez ER, Johnson EB. End-tidal carbon dioxide monitoring during cardiopulmonary resuscitation. *JAMA.* 1987;257:512–515.

104. Falk JL, Rackow EC, Weil MH. End-tidal carbon dioxide concentration during cardiopulmonary resuscitation. *N Engl J Med.* 1988;318:607–611.

105. Sanders AB, Kern KB, Otto CW, Milander MM, Ewy GA. End-tidal carbon dioxide monitoring during cardiopulmonary resuscitation: a prognostic indicator for survival [see comments]. *JAMA.* 1989;262:1347–1351.

106. Callaham M, Barton C. Prediction of outcome of cardiopulmonary resuscitation from end-tidal carbon dioxide concentration [see comments]. *Crit Care Med.* 1990;18:358–362.

107. Callaham M, Barton C, Matthay M. Effect of epinephrine on the ability of end-tidal carbon dioxide readings to predict initial resuscitation from cardiac arrest. *Crit Care Med.* 1992;20:337–343.

108. Martin GB, Gentile NT, Paradis NA, Moeggenberg J, Appleton TJ, Nowak RM. Effect of epinephrine on end-tidal carbon dioxide monitoring during CPR. *Ann Emerg Med.* 1990;19:396–398.

109. Milander M, Hiscok P, Sanders A, Kern K, Berg R, Ewy G. Chest compression and ventilation rates during cardiopulmonary resuscitation: the effects of audible tone guidance. *Acad Emerg Med.* 1995;1:708–713.

110. Jones BR, Dorsey MJ. Sensitivity of a disposable end-tidal carbon dioxide detector. *J Clin Monit.* 1991;7:268–270.

111. Thomas BW, Falcone RE. Confirmation of nasogastric tube placement by colorimetric indicator detection of carbon dioxide: a preliminary report. *J Am Coll Nutr.* 1998;17:195–197.

Section 5: Pharmacology I: Agents for Arrhythmias

Cardiac Monitoring

Arrhythmias, serious electrical abnormalities of the heart, cause most sudden coronary deaths. Establish ECG monitoring as soon as possible for all patients who collapse suddenly or who have symptoms of coronary ischemia or infarction. To avoid delay, use the "quick-look paddles" feature available on most conventional defibrillators. For patients with acute myocardial infarction (AMI) or severe ischemia, the greatest risk for serious arrhythmias occurs during the first hour after the start of symptoms. Healthcare professionals must start cardiac monitoring as soon as possible during this critical period.

Arrhythmia Recognition

Interpret all ECG and rhythm information within the context of total patient assessment. Inaccurate diagnoses and inappropriate therapy occur when ACLS providers base their decisions solely on cardiac rhythm and neglect to evaluate the patient's clinical signs, such as ventilation, oxygenation, heart rate, blood pressure, level of consciousness, and other signs of inadequate organ perfusion. In addition, full diagnosis requires assessment of the patient's metabolic and acid-base status. In specific clinical settings consider the possibility of proarrhythmic drug effects, adverse drug effects from intentional or unintentional overdose, or drug toxicity occurring with normal dosing patterns.

Providers of ACLS should participate in training and evaluation sessions that will establish their ability to detect and treat serious arrhythmias. After initial training, ACLS providers require regular updates in their rhythm expertise combined with evaluation sessions. Providers of ACLS must know how to use ECG monitoring equipment and be able to troubleshoot the most common technical problems.

Rhythms to Recognize

Professionals at the ACLS level should be able to recognize the following arrhythmias.

Normal sinus rhythm

- Sinus bradycardia
- Atrioventricular (AV) blocks of all degrees
- Premature atrial complexes (PACs)
- Supraventricular tachycardia (SVT)
- Preexcited arrhythmias (associated with an accessory pathway)
- Premature ventricular complexes (PVCs)
- Ventricular tachycardia (VT)
- Ventricular fibrillation (VF)
- Ventricular asystole

Classification of tachycardias

The tachycardias listed above can be classified in a number of ways. One useful system is described below.

- Narrow QRS complex (supraventricular) tachycardias
  —Sinus tachycardia
  —Atrial fibrillation (AF)
  —Atrial flutter
  —Atrial tachycardia (ectopic and reentrant)
  —Multifocal atrial tachycardia (MAT)
  —AV nodal reentry tachycardia (AVNRT)
  —Junctional tachycardia
  —Accessory pathway–mediated tachycardia (see below)
- Wide-QRS–complex tachycardias
  —Ventricular tachycardia
  —Ventricular fibrillation
  —Any supraventricular tachycardias (SVT) with aberrancy (bundle-branch block or intraventricular conduction delay)
- Preexcited tachycardias (supraventricular arrhythmias associated with or mediated by the presence of an accessory pathway)
  —Atrial tachycardia with accessory pathway conduction
  —Atrial flutter or AF with accessory pathway conduction
  —AV reentry tachycardia (AVRT)

ACLS providers must be able to distinguish between supraventricular and ventricular rhythms and be aware that most wide-complex (broad-complex) tachycardias are ventricular in origin. If a patient is pulseless, in shock, or in congestive heart failure, such rhythms should always be presumed to be VT. Initial management should proceed under the presumption of VT. Obtain a 12-lead ECG as soon as practicable. An esophageal lead may be helpful if the origin of the arrhythmia remains in doubt. ACLS providers must also be able to identify various artifacts that may mimic arrhythmias and know the clinical significance and appropriate treatment of all common rhythm disorders.

Administration of Medications During Cardiac Arrest: Correct Priorities

The 1992 Guidelines coincided with a reductionist period in cardiac resuscitation in regard to the value of medications. In 1992 evidence review led to recommendations to reduce the indications for calcium chloride, sodium bicarbonate, epinephrine, and isoproterenol. The International Guidelines 2000 continue this pattern. On close evidence review we recognize that few drugs are supported by strong evidence. This includes drugs used for cardiac arrest as well as drugs for prearrest arrhythmias. Therefore, during cardiac arrest, drug

Circulation. **2000;102(suppl I):I-112–I-128.**
© 2000 American Heart Association, Inc.

Circulation is available at http://www.circulationaha.org

administration is secondary to other interventions. Rescuers must place primary priorities on basic CPR, defibrillation when indicated, and proper airway management. Once these interventions are initiated, emergency personnel can start an IV infusion and consider which drugs might be useful.

Central Versus Peripheral Infusions

If no vein has been cannulated before the arrest, a peripheral vein (antecubital or external jugular) should be the first choice. Central line access (internal jugular or subclavian) requires interruption of chest compressions. Peak drug concentrations, however, are lower and circulation times are longer when drugs are administered via peripheral sites compared with central sites.[1–3] When given via a peripheral vein, drugs require 1 to 2 minutes to reach the central circulation, but the delay is appreciably shorter with a central venous route. Peripheral venous cannulation, however, is easier to learn, results in fewer complications, and does not require interruption of CPR. If peripheral venous access is used during resuscitative efforts, administer IV drugs rapidly by bolus injection; follow with a 20-mL bolus of IV fluid and elevate the extremity for 10 to 20 seconds.[4]

If spontaneous circulation does not return after defibrillation and administration of drugs via peripheral vein and experienced providers are available, consider placement of a central line unless there are contraindications. Placement of a central line, however, can produce complications, so consider the risk-benefit ratio.

Central lines may be associated with an increase in the rate of complications for patients who receive fibrinolytic therapy. A punctured central vascular structure or noncompressible vessel—regardless of whether a catheter was inserted—is a relative contraindication for fibrinolytic therapy, although in experienced hands and with no obvious bleeding or hematoma, it is not an absolute contraindication. Avoid attempts at central line placement in patients who are candidates for pharmacological reperfusion.

Tracheal Drug Administration

If a tracheal tube has been placed before venous access is achieved, epinephrine,[6,7] lidocaine, and atropine[8] can be administered via the tracheal tube. Administer all tracheal medications at 2 to 2.5 times the recommended IV dose, diluted in 10 mL of normal saline or distilled water. Tracheal absorption is greater with distilled water as the diluent than with normal saline, but distilled water has a greater adverse effect on PaO_2. Pass a catheter beyond the tip of the tracheal tube, stop chest compressions, spray the drug solution quickly down the tracheal tube, follow immediately with several quick insufflations to create a rapidly absorbed aerosol, then resume chest compressions.[6]

Arrhythmias and the Drugs Used to Treat Them

Researchers have gathered important new information since previous resuscitation guidelines. This information has prompted a critical reevaluation of the treatment recommendations for arrhythmias, especially the tachyarrhythmias. The International Guidelines 2000 experts who performed this reevaluation searched for evidence of clinical efficacy. This

TABLE 1.   Classification of Most Common Forms of Wide-Complex Tachycardia

Ventricular tachycardia

Supraventricular tachycardia with aberrancy due to intraventricular conduction delay. These include

   Sinus tachycardia

   Atrial tachycardia (ectopic or reentrant)

   Atrial flutter, with fixed AV block

   AV nodal reentry tachycardia

   Junctional tachycardia

Preexcited tachycardias (associated with or mediated by an accessory pathway) including

   Atrial tachycardia

   Atrial flutter

   AV reentry tachycardia

has resulted in several new international recommendations for the treatment of common tachyarrhythmias. As of 2000, arrhythmia specialists and clinical cardiologists advocate a new emphasis on existing hemodynamic instability and on the degree of impaired ventricular function. The experts restricted the evidence evaluation to parenteral medications used during arrest or during the periarrest period. Because the guidelines are evidence-based, the experts expanded their search to include all drugs supported by clinical research, not just agents approved and available in each country. In addition, the AHA has dropped references to bretylium because of its limited utility and availability.

Hemodynamically Stable Wide-/Broad-Complex Tachycardias

Wide-/broad-complex tachycardias (see the Tachycardias Overview Algorithm in Part 6, Section 7D) present a diagnostic challenge. When defining tachycardias with a prolonged QRS or QRST interval, "wide" is the common term in the United States, whereas in the United Kingdom "broad" is preferred. A clinician needs to make a specific diagnosis because he or she will treat the different types of wide-complex tachycardias with different interventions. Establish whether a wide complex tachycardia is stable or unstable. The criteria for hemodynamically *stable* wide-complex tachycardia are

- *Regular* tachycardia at a rate greater than the upper limit of sinus tachycardia at rest (>120 bpm)
- *Uniform* (monomorphic) QRS configuration of ≥120 ms in duration
- No signs or symptoms of impaired consciousness or tissue hypoperfusion

The patient must be stable enough to allow time for rhythm diagnosis or transport to a facility more capable of diagnosing the rhythm. The drugs used for most tachycardias lower the blood pressure. Therefore, patients should have blood pressures high enough to permit use of these drugs. Otherwise the drug-induced drop in blood pressure will require immediate electrical cardioversion to end the abnormal rhythm. Table 1 lists the most common forms of wide-complex tachycardia.

Treatment of Wide-Complex Tachycardias

Previous treatment recommendations for wide-complex tachycardias in adults listed lidocaine as the treatment of choice. Lidocaine was recommended as well for all wide-complex tachyarrhythmias not known with certainty to be supraventricular in origin. The international Guidelines 2000 Conference, however, focused on the need to establish a rhythm diagnosis before initiating treatment in stable patients. This change in treatment approach is based on new evidence that debunks 2 axioms about wide-complex tachycardias: (1) if the true rhythm is ventricular tachycardia, then only lidocaine will convert the rhythm to a sinus complex; (2) if the true rhythm is supraventricular tachycardia with aberrancy, then only adenosine will convert the rhythm to a sinus complex. By 2000 most cardiologists who specialize in arrhythmias think that adenosine has been overused for wide-complex tachycardias, certainly in the case of VT unresponsive to lidocaine. This overuse has often delayed more appropriate treatment.

When circumstances and expertise allow, ACLS providers should make a reasonable attempt to distinguish hemodynamically stable VT from SVT with aberrancy. A history of coronary artery disease or other structural heart disease suggests ventricular origin. A history of previous aberrant rhythms, accessory pathways, preexisting bundle-branch block, or rate-dependent bundle-branch blocks suggests supraventricular aberrancy if the QRS matches that observed with the tachycardia.

The 12-lead ECG

Always obtain a 12-lead ECG before and during pharmacological interventions and after conversion to a regular rhythm. If the 12-lead ECG is not diagnostic, an esophageal lead may be helpful if the equipment and experts who can interpret esophageal lead tracings are available.[9–12] A carefully evaluated 12-lead ECG, monitor tracing, or esophageal lead permits identification of AV dissociation. The loss of a 1-to-1 relationship between atrial electrical activity (P waves) and ventricular response (QRS complexes) is a highly specific criterion for VT.

When initial care providers state whether a wide-complex tachycardia is ventricular or supraventricular in origin, they are wrong in more than 50% of the cases. Their most frequent error is to evaluate true VT and then misdiagnose it as *SVT with aberrancy (a false-negative or type II error: see the editorial "Guidelines Based on the Principle 'First, Do No Harm'")*. The clinician then proceeds to treat true VT with agents meant for SVT with aberrancy.[13,14] The QRS configuration of the 12-lead ECG can help in the differentiation of SVT from VT, but accuracy requires experience.[13,15–19] Complex rules exist for making the correct rhythm diagnosis by QRS morphology *alone*. These rules, however, are difficult to teach, learn, remember, and apply repeatedly, and they may complicate the diagnosis of acute MI.[14,20–24] The 12-lead ECG is, therefore, most useful for looking for AV dissociation. As a practical matter, 12-lead ECGs are often unavailable in many out-of-hospital EMS systems, where out of necessity paramedics will be treating numerous people with

rapid VT. The bottom line is to keep it simple and not puzzle over complex rhythm interpretive algorithms.

Lidocaine

Lidocaine is used frequently as a first-line agent to treat wide-complex tachycardias. There is a widely held, albeit incorrect, idea that lidocaine, like adenosine (see below), has diagnostic utility. In fact, lidocaine is not an effective or appropriate treatment for SVT. Evidence does not support the use of lidocaine to discriminate between perfusing VT and wide-complex tachycardia of uncertain origin.

Lidocaine will effectively suppress ventricular arrhythmias associated with acute myocardial ischemia and infarction once they occur.[25] But the prophylactic use of lidocaine to prevent the arrhythmias in the first place causes higher mortality and has been abandoned.[26–29] Two studies suggest that lidocaine is ineffective for termination of hemodynamically stable sustained VT,[30,31] and 2 have found lidocaine to be less effective against VT than IV procainamide[32] or IV sotalol.[33]

In summary, lidocaine appears in the algorithm for stable VT, monomorphic or polymorphic (in Part 6, Section 7D). Lidocaine is acceptable for all 4 possible VT scenarios: stable, monomorphic VT with (1) normal cardiac function and (2) with impaired cardiac function; polymorphic VT with either (3) normal baseline QT interval or (4) prolonged QT interval. Note carefully, however, that for all 4 of these indications lidocaine is a second-tier choice. Other drugs are preferred over lidocaine in each VT scenario.

Adenosine

The principal therapeutic effect of adenosine is to slow AV nodal conduction. Adenosine is not an effective agent for common forms of ventricular arrhythmias or for preexcited atrial arrhythmias such as atrial fibrillation or atrial flutter.[34–38] Although adenosine has vasodilatory effects that are short-lived, instances of worsened hypotension have been reported in patients with barely compensated blood pressure after inappropriate treatment with adenosine for VT.[36] Adenosine also carries the theoretical risk of causing angina, bronchospasm, proarrhythmia, and acceleration of accessory pathway conduction.[36] Adenosine is used for narrow-complex tachycardias (see The Tachycardia Overview Algorithm, column 2); for narrow-complex supraventricular tachycardia, *stable* (see the Narrow-Complex Algorithm); and for wide-complex tachycardias that are confirmed as supraventricular in origin (The Tachycardia Overview Algorithm, column 3). These algorithms are in Part 6, Section 7D.

Procainamide

Antiarrhythmic agents such as procainamide have shown efficacy in treating a broad variety of arrhythmias, including supraventricular arrhythmias, with and without aberrancy, and VT.[32,39,40] Procainamide is effective at terminating SVT because of its ability to alter conduction across an accessory pathway (Class IIa).[41–52]

Amiodarone

Amiodarone also is effective for supraventricular tachycardias because it alters conduction through the accessory pathway (Class IIa if LV function is normal and IIb if ventricular function is impaired).[53–81] (See the Narrow-Complex Tachycardia Algorithm, Part 6, Section 7D.) Note that amiodarone becomes the antiarrhythmic of choice (after failure of adenosine) if the patient's cardiac function is impaired and the ejection fraction is <40% or there are signs of congestive heart failure.

Amiodarone has not been studied specifically for the pharmacological termination of hemodynamically stable VT, but it is effective in treating hemodynamically unstable VT and VF.[78,81–91] Both procainamide and amiodarone have vasodilatory effects and negative inotropic properties, which can destabilize hemodynamic status.[87,92,93] These effects seem to depend on the dose given and the rate of administration. IV amiodarone may be better tolerated hemodynamically than procainamide.

Intravenous sotalol, IV propafenone, and IV flecainide are each effective against SVT, including atrial arrhythmias with and without preexcitation. These agents, however, are not available in all countries, nor have they been studied against wide-complex tachycardias. I_C agents (Vaughn-Williams classification) such as flecainide and propafenone are associated with a higher mortality in patients with ischemic heart disease. Avoid using flecainide or propafenone in such patients.

New Concerns From the International Guidelines 2000 Conference: Impaired Hearts and "Proarrhythmic Antiarrhythmics"

The evidence presented at the Guidelines 2000 Conference has dramatically changed the recommended approach to the treatment of tachycardias. The tachycardia algorithm from 1992, complex by necessity, has undergone extensive revisions to accommodate the 2 concerns of proarrhythmias and the effects of antiarrhythmics on impaired hearts.

Proarrhythmias are serious tachyarrhythmias or bradyarrhythmias seemingly generated by antiarrhythmic agents. All antiarrhythmic agents have some degree of proarrhythmic effects. Tachyarrhythmias account for most proarrhythmia events. The rhythm called torsades de pointes accounts for the majority of tachycardic proarrhythmic episodes. The interactions between agents are complex. Sequential use of 2 or more antiarrhythmic drugs compounds the adverse effects, particularly for bradycardia, hypotension, and torsades de pointes. Never use more than 1 agent unless absolutely necessary. In most patients, when an appropriate dose of a single antiarrhythmic medication fails to terminate an arrhythmia, turn to electrical cardioversion rather than a second antiarrhythmic medication. The Stable Ventricular Tachycardia Algorithm implements this conservative approach to VT.

Patients with clinical congestive heart failure or depressed LV function should be treated cautiously with antiarrhythmic therapy. In these patients, many antiarrhythmic agents depress LV function further, often precipitating or worsening congestive heart failure. Amiodarone and lidocaine cause the least additional impairment of LV function. Because of its broad antiarrhythmic spectrum and lesser negative inotropic effect, amiodarone now dominates the management of tachycardias. If amiodarone fails to produce the desired

response, the preferred next intervention is to attempt early electrical cardioversion.

Summary: Treatment of Hemodynamically Stable, Wide-Complex Tachycardias

In summary, faced with ECG-confirmed or strongly suspected *SVT with aberrancy,* treat according to the tachycardia overview and narrow-complex tachycardia algorithms. If a specific rhythm (eg, atrial flutter) is diagnosed, then treat using the tachycardia overview algorithm and rate and rhythm control recommendations for tachycardias (table accompanying the overview algorithm).

Treat confirmed or strongly suspected VT (*hemodynamically stable* VT) according to the tachycardia overview algorithm and the stable ventricular tachycardia algorithm. DC cardioversion is the definitive therapy, but in some circumstances electrical cardioversion is not possible, desirable, or successful.

In these patients, empirical pharmacological therapy may be necessary for a hemodynamically stable wide-complex tachycardia of unknown origin. (See Tachycardia Overview Algorithm, column 3.) Empirical treatment of wide-complex tachycardia of unknown origin involves broad-spectrum antiarrhythmic agents. Agents such as procainamide, amiodarone, and sotalol possess efficacy against VT, SVT with accessory pathway conduction, and SVT. However, agents that block the AV node (such as adenosine, β-adrenergic receptor blockers, and calcium channel blockers) are hazardous in patients with VT or preexcited atrial arrhythmias. These agents should not be used for the empirical treatment of wide–QRS-complex tachyarrhythmias. Consequently, column 3 of the Tachycardia Overview Algorithm limits the therapeutic options to DC cardioversion, or procainamide or amiodarone.

Hemodynamically Stable (Monomorphic) VT (See Algorithm)

Consider VT "hemodynamically stable" if there are no symptoms or clinical evidence of tissue hypoperfusion or shock. Hemodynamically unstable VT requires immediate termination with synchronized cardioversion. With clinical stability and adequate blood pressure there is sufficient time to allow pharmacological intervention.

Previous guidelines recommended use of lidocaine followed by procainamide, bretylium, and electrical cardioversion. In cases in which electrical cardioversion is not possible, desirable, or successful, the International Guidelines 2000 now recommend treatment of hemodynamically stable VT with IV procainamide, IV sotalol, IV amiodarone, or IV β-blockers. Each of these is considered preferable to IV lidocaine. The Stable Ventricular Tachycardia Algorithm shows how the specific choice of agent is based on considerations of normal versus impaired cardiac function and long versus short QT intervals. Although lidocaine can be administered rapidly with minimal effect on blood pressure, studies suggest that it is relatively ineffective for termination of VT[30,31] and less effective against VT than IV procainamide[32] or IV sotalol.[33]

Twelve studies have evaluated amiodarone for the treatment of hemodynamically *unstable* VT and VF.[78,81–91] Although amiodarone has not been specifically evaluated for the pharmacological termination of hemodynamically stable VT, by extrapolation from other studies amiodarone remains acceptable (see the Stable Ventricular Tachycardia Algorithm), and for monomorphic VT with impaired cardiac function, amiodarone is the agent of first choice.

Electrical cardioversion is a highly effective and recommended therapy for hemodynamically stable VT. In adults, when electrical cardioversion is not inappropriate, any one of the following drugs is preferred over IV lidocaine: IV procainamide (Class IIa), IV sotalol (Class IIa), IV amiodarone (Class IIb), or disopyramide (Class IIb). (Disopyramide is not approved in the United States.)

Polymorphic VT

VT with varying QRS morphology is called polymorphic VT. Polymorphic VT is usually irregular in rate, hemodynamically unstable, and likely to quickly degenerate to VF. It is often associated with ischemic heart events or electrolyte or toxic conditions. A unique form of polymorphic VT is called torsades de pointes, which usually occurs in a setting of bradycardia and prolongation of the QT interval. A continuously changing VT morphology is often described as appearing to rotate or turn around the ECG baseline. Polymorphic VT, including torsades, frequently terminates, *but the arrhythmia will recur and seldom remains stable.*

There is limited data regarding treatment of polymorphic VT with or without suspected torsades de pointes. The algorithm for stable ventricular tachycardia, monomorphic or polymorphic, displays a reasonably evidence-based approach, supported largely by extrapolation from less-specific studies. Hemodynamically unstable polymorphic VT should be treated using the VF/Pulseless VT Algorithm.[94] These patients and those with hemodynamically *stable* polymorphic VT are treated according to the presence or absence of torsades de pointes.

Polymorphic VT of the torsades de pointes type should be treated immediately (Stable Ventricular Tachycardia Algorithm) because of the frequent transition to unstable VT. The first step is to stop medications known to prolong the QT interval. Correct electrolyte imbalance and any other acute precipitants.

Other interventions that may be helpful but have not been adequately evaluated in controlled trials include administration of IV magnesium (Class Indeterminate) and temporary atrial or ventricular pacing ("overdrive pacing") (Class Indeterminate).[95] If patients are free of coronary artery disease, ischemic syndromes, or other contraindications, then isoproterenol (Class Indeterminate) may be administered as an interim measure to accelerate heart rate while temporary pacing is initiated (Class Indeterminate).[96] After pacing has been initiated, β-blockers may be used as adjunctive therapy. Limited studies of lidocaine have shown uncertain efficacy (Class Indeterminate).[96,97] These recommendations are incorporated into the Stable Ventricular Tachycardia Algorithm.

Polymorphic VTs other than torsades de pointes do not respond to magnesium. For patients in whom polymorphic

VT may be precipitated by acute coronary syndromes, use β-blockers (in the absence of bradycardia) and anti-ischemic agents. (See the Stable Ventricular Tachycardia Algorithm.) Lidocaine may be more effective in patients with myocardial ischemia[25,98–100] than in patients without ischemia. In other circumstances, effective antiarrhythmic drugs include IV amiodarone (Class IIb), lidocaine (Class IIb), procainamide (Class IIb), IV sotalol (Class IIb), β-blockers (Class Indeterminate), or phenytoin (Class Indeterminate). These agents are recommended only as Class IIb or indeterminate agents because supportive evidence comes only from extrapolation of results from the treatment of hemodynamically stable and unstable monomorphic VT.

VF/Pulseless VT

Efficacy studies of antiarrhythmic drugs in VF/VT arrest have addressed only short-term outcomes. The recommendations for antiarrhythmic agents are based on surrogate, or immediate, or intermediate outcome measures that may not correlate with the preferred outcome of neurologically intact survival for 1 or more years after the cardiac arrest.

The optimal number of defibrillation shocks that should be administered for refractory VF/VT before pharmacological therapy is initiated is also unknown. However, given the established efficacy of early defibrillation (a Class I intervention), it is reasonable to add pharmacological therapy after at least 3 precordial shocks, delivered in rapid sequence, fail to restore a stable perfusing rhythm. In particular, patients in whom a perfusing rhythm can be transiently restored but not successfully maintained between repeated shocks (recurrent VT/VF) are highly appropriate candidates for early treatment with antiarrhythmic medications. In such patients the antiarrhythmics will facilitate and stabilize the return of circulation. Patients with shock-refractory arrhythmias should be considered for pharmacological therapies sooner rather than later, for the likelihood of benefit declines rapidly with the duration of cardiac arrest.

The VF/Pulseless VT Algorithm (Part 6, Section 7C) emphasizes this greater value of defibrillation over pharmacology. The algorithm shows that after 3 unsuccessful defibrillation attempts the rescuers must move quickly to accomplish tracheal intubation and to gain access to the circulation with an intravenous line. Once the IV is established, vasopressors (epinephrine or vasopressin) are administered, followed by another attempt to defibrillate. This fourth shock usually follows a period of many minutes during which the tracheal tube was placed, confirmed, and secured and the intravenous line established. Delivery of the fourth shock is based more on the passage of time than on any requirement that epinephrine or vasopressin *must* be administered before the fourth shock can be given. In scenarios where an intravenous line is not in place before arrest, long delays to the fourth shock would ensue if rescuers think a specific sequence of medications *must* be given before further defibrillation attempts. *Shocks must not be delayed until an IV line is established and medications have been delivered.*

The details of the ARREST study confirm that a mandate that amiodarone (or any antiarrhythmic) must be given before the fourth shock would undoubtedly produce profound delays in the fourth shock. The ARREST study observed that the time from medic arrival on the scene to IV access obtained was 4.7 minutes and from arrival to tracheal intubation was 5.2 minutes; however, from arrival of medics to administration of amiodarone took a full 13 minutes. With amiodarone administration requiring so much extra time, it would be unacceptable to require amiodarone before a fourth shock. In addition, an average of 5 shocks were given before amiodarone was administered, and an average of 4 more were given after the amiodarone was given.

The use of lidocaine for ventricular arrhythmias was supported by initial studies in animals[99–104] and extrapolation from the historical use of the drug to suppress PVCs and prevent VF after acute MI.[25] Lidocaine improved resuscitation rate and admission alive to the hospital rate in 1 retrospective prehospital study,[105] but other trials comparing lidocaine and bretylium found no statistically significant differences in outcome.[106–108] A randomized comparison between amiodarone and lidocaine found a greater likelihood of successful resuscitation with amiodarone.[109] A randomized comparison between lidocaine and epinephrine showed a higher incidence of asystole with lidocaine use and no difference in return of spontaneous circulation.[110] Numerous animal studies, as well as a retrospective, uncontrolled trial, suggested that lidocaine reduced short-term resuscitation success.[111] Some studies have observed an elevated defibrillation threshold after treatment.[112–119] No benefit and increased morbidity (serious arrhythmias) have been associated with prophylactic administration of lidocaine to patients with acute MI.[26–29]

Use of procainamide in cardiac arrest is supported by only a retrospective comparison study involving only 20 patients.[120] Procainamide administration in cardiac arrest is limited by the need for slow infusion and uncertain efficacy in emergent circumstances.

Use of magnesium in torsades de pointes may be beneficial.[121,122] They are comparably effective in patients with cardiac arrest due to monomorphic, polymorphic, or torsades VT.[94] Routine administration of magnesium in resuscitation does not affect outcome and may be associated with a higher incidence of hypotension despite a potential for improved neurological outcome in survivors.[123,124]

In summary, evidence supports the use of IV amiodarone, following epinephrine, to treat shock-refractory cardiac arrest due to VF or pulseless VT (Class IIb).[125] Amiodarone restored spontaneous circulation and improved early survival to the hospital in adults. However, no pharmacological interventions for cardiac arrest have yet been found to improve survival to hospital discharge. Disadvantages of amiodarone include its side effects (hypotension and bradycardia), its relatively high cost, and difficulties in administration. As currently available, the drug must be drawn up from a 6-mL glass ampule into a syringe and then diluted with 5% dextrose in water to 20 mL before injection. Preloaded syringes are not available because amiodarone adheres to the plastic surface of preloaded syringes.

Lidocaine, an alternative antiarrhythmic of long standing and widespread familiarity, has fewer immediate side effects and lower cost and is available in prefilled syringes. Lidocaine, however, has no proven short- or long-term efficacy in cardiac arrest. Lidocaine and magnesium (for suspected torsades de pointes or hypomagnesemic states) should be considered alternative treatments (Class Indeterminate) on the basis of less supportive evidence for their efficacy.

Paroxysmal Supraventricular Tachycardia (See the Narrow-Complex Tachycardia Algorithm)

Paroxysmal SVT (PSVT) is a *regular* tachycardia exceeding the expected limits of sinus tachycardia at rest (>120 bpm) with or without discernible P waves that is usually of abrupt onset and abrupt termination. The arrhythmia is of *known* supraventricular origin (QRS complex <100 ms, or if wide [broad], bundle-branch aberrancy is *known* to be present). PSVT may include AVNRT or AVRT mediated by a concealed or manifest accessory pathway. PSVT can be distinguished from junctional tachycardia (which can also appear "P-less") or ectopic atrial tachycardia by the relative rarity of such tachycardia in adults and by the often gradual onset ("warm-up") and termination of automatic tachyarrhythmias (versus the abrupt onset and termination of reentrant PSVT).

Previous guidelines recommended vagal maneuvers to initially attempt termination of PSVT. If the patient was unresponsive, adenosine was given if the patient remained clinically stable. Further treatment was based on the duration of the QRS complex (wide- versus narrow-complex tachycardia) and hemodynamic stability.

New parenteral drugs have completed clinical study and are now available for the treatment of PSVT. New recommendations also include treatment strategies that are modified by the presence of clinical congestive heart failure and the status of LV function, when known.

Initial use of vagal maneuvers and IV adenosine in all patients (without contraindications) with PSVT continues to be recommended. Adenosine can provoke bronchospasm and should be used cautiously in patients with reactive airway disease. Cardiac denervation after cardiac transplantation may render patients hypersensitive to the bradycardic effects of adenosine. Patients treated with methylxanthines (theophylline) may be less sensitive to the effects of adenosine. Use of dipyridamole (Persantine) may enhance sensitivity to adenosine. In patients with preserved LV function, calcium channel blockers (verapamil, diltiazem) and β-blockers (esmolol, metoprolol) remain supported by previous evidence. Digitalis (digoxin) is a time-honored drug for treatment of PSVT, but indirect evidence from treatment of AF and atrial flutter suggests that digitalis has a slower onset of action and lower potency relative to other treatment agents.

In addition to procainamide, newly available parenteral antiarrhythmic agents for treatment of PSVT refractory to vagal maneuvers, adenosine, and AV nodal blocking agents include amiodarone, propafenone, flecainide, and sotalol. Use of IV procainamide for PSVT (in the presence or absence of an accessory pathway) is effective.[69] IV amiodarone is effective in AVNRT or accessory pathway–mediated AVRT[53,57,60,63,79] and is comparable to procainamide[69] and magnesium[126] but has less efficacy than propafenone.[58] IV flecainide[127] and IV sotalol[128,129] have also been useful in terminating PSVT due to AVNRT.

Primary antiarrhythmic agents (such as amiodarone, procainamide, sotalol, flecainide, propafenone, and disopyramide) require slow administration and can destabilize marginally compensated patients by hypotensive effects. They also have the potential for proarrhythmic effects, including the provocation of life-threatening ventricular arrhythmias. Antiarrhythmic agents should be considered only when AV nodal blocking agents or electrical cardioversion is not feasible, desirable, or successful. *Serial* use of calcium channel blockers, β-blockers, and primary antiarrhythmic agents should be discouraged because of the potential additive hypotensive, bradycardic, and proarrhythmic effects of these drugs in combination.

In the setting of significantly impaired LV function (clinical evidence of congestive heart failure or moderately to severely reduced LV ejection fraction), caution should be exercised in administering drugs with negative inotropic effects to patients with PSVT. These include verapamil, β-blockers, procainamide, propafenone, flecainide, and sotalol but not digitalis, amiodarone,[86,90] or perhaps diltiazem. Life-threatening ventricular proarrhythmias may be higher with primary antiarrhythmic medications in patients with congestive heart failure. In addition, some antiarrhythmic agents have been shown to increase mortality in patients with ischemic heart disease.[130] Thus, flecainide, and perhaps propafenone, should be avoided in patients with documented coronary heart disease.

In summary, in the absence of contraindications, vagal maneuvers or adenosine should be used in an effort to initially terminate PSVT. With preserved LV function, additional treatment options include calcium channel blockers (verapamil or diltiazem; Class I), β-blockers (Class I), or digitalis (Class IIb). Strong consideration should be given to electrical cardioversion when AV nodal agents are unsuccessful in terminating PSVT. When electrical cardioversion is not feasible, desirable, or successful, patients who "fail" AV nodal blocking agents with either persistent or recurrent PSVT may be treated with antiarrhythmic agents, including procainamide (Class IIa), amiodarone (Class IIa), flecainide (Class IIa), propafenone (Class IIa), and sotalol (Class IIa). The proarrhythmic potential of this group of medications makes them less desirable options, however, than AV nodal blocking drugs.

The serial or combined use of parenteral calcium channel blockers, β-adrenergic blockers, and primary antiarrhythmic agents is discouraged. In patients with significantly impaired LV function, verapamil, β-blockers, procainamide, flecainide, propafenone, and sotalol should be avoided in favor of digitalis (Class IIb), amiodarone (Class IIb), or perhaps diltiazem (Class IIb). By itself digitalis is a relatively slow-acting and less effective AV nodal blocking agent. When given in combination with other agents, however, initial use of digitalis may allow for lower doses of subsequently administered agents for rhythm termination or potential blunting of their negative inotropic properties by the positive inotropic effects of digitalis.

Atrial Tachycardia (Ectopic Atrial Tachycardia, MAT)

See the Narrow-Complex Tachycardia Algorithm. Atrial arrhythmias, including ectopic atrial tachycardia and MAT, are the result of increased automaticity of a single or multiple (MAT) atrial focus. Ectopic atrial tachycardia can be distinguished from sinus tachycardia on the 12-lead ECG by the presence of an abnormal P-wave configuration and P-wave axis. It is important to distinguish MAT from AF, because both can result in an irregularly irregular rhythm. MAT is distinguished from AF by the presence of P waves having 3 or more different morphologies preceding QRS complexes. By contrast, atrial activity in AF continuously undulates or is incessant between QRS complexes, without individually identifiable P waves. Automatic arrhythmias such as ectopic atrial tachycardia can be distinguished from reentry-caused PSVT (such as AVNRT or AVRT mediated by an accessory pathway) by their often gradual onset (warm-up) and termination (versus the abrupt onset and termination of reentrant PSVT) and by their continuation even when their conduction is blocked through the AV node.

The 1992 guidelines did not specify treatment for atrial tachycardias, apart from AF and atrial flutter. By 2000 evidence suggests that automatic atrial tachycardias are due to increased automaticity and require a different treatment from the reentrant supraventricular arrhythmias (PSVT, AF, and atrial flutter).

Diagnosis of an atrial tachycardia is made by identifying P-wave morphology on the 12-lead ECG. Vagal maneuvers or adenosine may be used to demonstrate AV block with persistence of the atrial arrhythmia. Automatic rhythms (ectopic atrial tachycardia, MAT, sinus tachycardia), unlike reentry arrhythmias, are not responsive to electrical cardioversion. Many of these arrhythmias are secondary phenomena, requiring supportive measures and treatment of precipitating causes. MAT, for example, typically is seen in patients with decompensated chronic obstructive pulmonary disease. With preserved LV function, β-blockers or calcium channel blockers (verapamil or diltiazem) may provide improved rate control by enhancing AV block or conversion of the arrhythmia to normal sinus rhythm. Digitalis may be effective in slowing heart rate but not in terminating ectopic atrial arrhythmias.[59] Digitalis also has been associated with provoking ectopic atrial tachycardia. Other useful drugs for ectopic atrial tachycardia or MAT include amiodarone,[59,60,80] flecainide,[131,132] and propafenone.[133,134] Quinidine, procainamide, and phenytoin are not effective.[59] In summary, synchronized electrical cardioversion is ineffective for the treatment of automatic atrial arrhythmias (Class III). In patients with preserved LV function, acceptable treatments include calcium channel blockers (Class IIb), β-blockers (Class IIb), digitalis (Class Indeterminate), amiodarone (Class IIb), intravenous flecainide (Class IIb), and IV propafenone (Class IIb). In patients with impaired LV function, drugs with significant negative inotropic properties (verapamil, β-blockers, flecainide, and propafenone) are contraindicated. In the presence of LV impairment, preferred agents include diltiazem (Class IIb), amiodarone (Class IIb), and digitalis (Class Indeterminate).

Atrial Fibrillation/Flutter

New evidence allows more specific recommendations for acute management of AF and atrial flutter (see The Tachy-

TABLE 2. Management Principles for Atrial Fibrillation/Flutter

Hemodynamically unstable, rapid-response atrial fibrillation or flutter should be electrically cardioverted immediately, regardless of the duration of the arrhythmia (Class I).

Pharmacological rate control is the recommended initial treatment for stable, rapid atrial fibrillation/flutter (≥120 bpm) regardless of its duration. Specific drug treatment depends on the presence or absence of impaired LV function (ejection fraction <40%)

Adenosine is an inappropriate drug to use for atrial fibrillation/flutter because of its ultrashort duration of action (Class III).

In patients with preserved LV function, β-blockers (Class I), calcium blockers (Class I), and digitalis (Class IIb) are reasonable agents for rate control.

In patients with congestive heart failure, digitalis (Class IIb), diltiazem (Class IIb), and amiodarone (Class IIb) are recommended.

In patients with preexcited atrial fibrillation/flutter, β-blockers, calcium channel blockers, and digitalis are contraindicated (Class III). If electrical cardioversion is not feasible, desirable, or successful, such patients with preserved LV function may be treated with procainamide (Class IIb) or amiodarone (Class IIb), IV flecainide (Class IIb), propafenone (Class IIb), or sotalol (Class IIb) (not all available in all countries).

In patients with congestive heart failure and preexcited atrial fibrillation/flutter, IV amiodarone (Class IIb) is recommended over other drugs.

Efforts should be made to minimize the risk of *thromboembolic complications* that are strongly related to the duration of the arrhythmia before cardioversion (>48 hours).

Electrical cardioversion is the preferred treatment for restoration of sinus rhythm.

Pharmacological cardioversion is recommended if electrical cardioversion is not feasible or desirable or is unsuccessful in maintaining sinus rhythm.

cardia Overview Algorithm, Table). Additional considerations include pharmacological control of the rate, pharmacological control of the rhythm, guidelines on the use of anticoagulation, and different treatment approaches for patients with significantly impaired LV function. Impaired ventricular function is defined as clinical congestive heart failure or a depressed LV ejection fraction (moderate impairment 0.30 to 0.40; severe impairment <0.30). Table 2 discusses the management principles for atrial fibrillation/flutter.

Major goals in the management of AF are ventricular rate control, assessment of anticoagulation needs, and restoration of sinus rhythm. Reversible and underlying causes of AF should be investigated and corrected, if possible. These include hypoxemia, anemia, hypertension, congestive heart failure, mitral regurgitation, thyrotoxicosis, hypokalemia, hypomagnesemia, and other toxic and metabolic causes. Ischemia is an uncommon cause but may result from AF.

IV verapamil,[135–143] β-blockers,[144–150] and diltiazem[151–157] are recommended for rate control in patients with AF or atrial flutter, preserved LV function, and a heart rate ≥120 bpm.[136] Available evidence suggests that digitalis,[158] though effective, is the least potent and has the slowest onset of action of the available pharmacological options for ventricular rate control. In patients with clinical evidence of congestive heart failure, greater caution should be exercised in use of calcium channel and β-blocking agents because of their recognized negative inotropic properties and because in trials of efficacy,

patients with congestive heart failure were usually excluded. This risk may be less with diltiazem than with verapamil or β-blockers.[154,159] Digoxin remains the only parenteral AV nodal blocking drug with positive inotropic properties, but its usefulness is limited by its relative impotence and slow onset of action, particularly in high adrenergic states such as congestive heart failure.

New evidence also suggests that IV amiodarone is also effective for rate control[160] in patients resistant to conventional heart rate control measures[62] or in combination with digitalis.[55] Conversion to normal sinus rhythm may occur with amiodarone. Therefore, in patients at risk for systemic emboli, amiodarone is recommended only when other medications for rate control have proved ineffective or are contraindicated and the risk of possible pharmacological cardioversion is felt to be justified. Some studies have found that whereas amiodarone was effective for rate control, conversion to sinus rhythm was no greater with conventional doses of IV amiodarone than placebo or digitalis,[55–67,160] particularly in refractory AF and clinical shock. Because of this concern amiodarone should be reserved for use within the first 48 hours of arrhythmia onset[62,78] or in patients in whom other rate-control measures are ineffective or contraindicated.

In some patients a conduction pathway bypasses the AV node. Such a conduction pathway is called an accessory bypass tract. In a few patients who have downward conduction through this pathway, there is the potential for extremely rapid ventricular responses during AF with degeneration to VF. Digitalis, verapamil, diltiazem, adenosine, and possibly intravenous β-blockers can cause a paradoxical increase in ventricular response rates in these patients with Wolff-Parkinson-White syndrome. If patients are clinically unstable, synchronized electrical cardioversion is indicated. Otherwise, when Wolff-Parkinson-White syndrome is known or suspected, cardiology consultation is indicated for the selection of the most appropriate management strategy. Antiarrhythmic agents that have direct effects on accessory pathway conduction and refractoriness (such as procainamide, propafenone,[127] flecainide,[127,161] or amiodarone) are more likely to slow ventricular response during preexcited AF or atrial flutter as well as convert the arrhythmia to sinus rhythm.

If AF has been present for >48 hours, a risk of systemic embolization exists with conversion to sinus rhythm unless patients are adequately anticoagulated for at least 3 weeks. Electrical cardioversion and the use of antiarrhythmic agents should be avoided unless the patient is unstable or hemodynamically compromised. In marginal patients, heparinization and cardiology consultation with the use of transesophageal echocardiography to exclude atrial thrombi is indicated to assess the risk and benefits of therapeutic strategies.

Electrical cardioversion is the technique of choice for cardioversion of patients with AF or atrial flutter to sinus rhythm. The recommended initial energy using a damped sinusoidal waveform defibrillator is 100 to 200 J. Atrial flutter and PSVT may require less energy, 50 to 100 J. The optimal AF energy protocol and the efficacy of other shock waveforms for cardioversion of AF and atrial flutter will require additional clinical trials, now ongoing.

Efforts to slow the ventricular rate response or to convert AF to sinus rhythm can lead to profound bradycardia and even asystole, especially in patients with significant underlying conduction system disease or sick sinus syndrome. Consequently, it is advisable to have temporary pacing capability (transcutaneous or transvenous) or pharmacological support (atropine, dopamine, or isoproterenol) available.

After satisfactory rate control and anticoagulation measures (if AF is >48 hours in duration), electrical cardioversion of AF or atrial flutter remains the technique of choice for conversion of patients with either preserved or significantly impaired LV function, particularly in patients with preexcitation. If not feasible, desirable, or successful, a number of pharmacological alternatives are available for cardioversion of patients with preserved LV function, including ibutilide (Class IIa), IV flecainide (Class IIa), IV propafenone (Class IIa), IV procainamide (Class IIa), IV amiodarone (Class IIa), IV sotalol (Class IIb), and IV disopyramide (Class IIb). In patients with impaired LV function, the negative inotropic effects of flecainide, propafenone, sotalol, and procainamide as well as the potential proarrhythmic potential of ibutilide make these agents less desirable. IV amiodarone is a preferable agent in such circumstances (Class IIb). For preexcited AF or atrial flutter, IV procainamide (Class IIb), IV amiodarone (Class IIb), IV flecainide (Class IIb), IV propafenone (Class IIb), and IV sotalol (Class IIb) are acceptable treatments. Preexcited arrhythmias in patients with significantly impaired LV function should be treated preferably with IV amiodarone (Class IIb).

Junctional Tachycardia

In adults true junctional tachycardia is rare. Apparent junctional tachycardia is most commonly due to misdiagnosed PSVT and should be treated according to the Narrow-Complex Tachycardia algorithm. True junctional tachycardia in adults is usually a manifestation of digitalis toxicity (best treated by withdrawal of digitalis) or of exogenous catecholamines or theophylline (best treated with reduction or withdrawal of such infusions). If no apparent cause is found, symptomatic junctional tachycardia may respond to IV amiodarone or to β-blockers or calcium channel blockers. This recommendation, however, has no specific human evidence to provide support. Instead, the recommendation is based on rational extrapolations from the known antisympathetic and nodal effects of β-blockers and calcium channel blockers (Class Indeterminate) or IV amiodarone (Class IIb).

Antiarrhythmic Drugs and the Arrhythmias They Treat

Adenosine

Adenosine is an endogenous purine nucleoside that depresses AV node and sinus node activity. Most common forms of PSVT involve a reentry pathway including the AV node. Adenosine is effective in terminating these arrhythmias. If the arrhythmias are not due to reentry involving the AV node or sinus node (eg, atrial flutter, AF, atrial or ventricular tachycardias), adenosine will not terminate the arrhythmia but may produce transient AV or retrograde (ventriculoatrial)

block that may clarify the diagnosis. Adenosine produces a short-lived pharmacological response because it is rapidly metabolized by enzymatic degradation in blood and peripheral tissue. The half-life of adenosine is <5 seconds. The recommended initial dose is a 6-mg rapid bolus over 1 to 3 seconds. The dose should be followed by a 20-mL saline flush.

If no response is observed within 1 to 2 minutes, a 12-mg repeated dose should be administered in the same manner. Experience with larger doses is limited, but patients taking theophylline are less sensitive to adenosine and may require larger doses. Side effects with adenosine are common but transient; flushing, dyspnea, and chest pain are the most frequently observed.[162] Because of the short half-life of adenosine, PSVT may recur. Repeated episodes may be treated with additional doses of adenosine or with a calcium channel blocker. Adenosine is more likely to precipitate persistent hypotension if the arrhythmia does not terminate.

Adenosine has several important drug interactions. Therapeutic concentrations of theophylline or related methylxanthines (caffeine and theobromine) block the receptor responsible for the electrophysiological and hemodynamic effects of adenosine. Dipyridamole blocks adenosine uptake and potentiates its effects. The effects of adenosine are also prolonged in patients on carbamazepine and in denervated transplanted hearts. Dose adjustment or alternative therapy should be selected in such patients.

Use of adenosine to discriminate VT from SVT with aberrancy in hemodynamically stable wide-complex tachycardia of uncertain origin is controversial, and such a practice should be discouraged. Adenosine should be used only when a supraventricular origin is strongly suspected.

Amiodarone (IV)

Intravenous amiodarone is a complex drug with effects on sodium, potassium, and calcium channels as well as α- and β-adrenergic blocking properties. The drug is useful for treatment of atrial and ventricular arrhythmias.

- Amiodarone is also helpful for ventricular rate control of rapid atrial arrhythmias in patients with severely impaired LV function when digitalis has proved ineffective (Class IIb).
- Amiodarone is recommended after defibrillation and epinephrine in cardiac arrest with persistent VT or VF (Class IIb).
- Amiodarone is effective for control of hemodynamically stable VT (Class IIb), polymorphic VT (Class IIb), and wide-complex tachycardia of uncertain origin (Class IIb).
- Amiodarone is an adjunct to electrical cardioversion of refractory PSVTs (Class IIa), atrial tachycardia (Class IIb), and pharmacological cardioversion of AF (Class IIa).
- Amiodarone can control rapid ventricular rate due to accessory pathway conduction in preexcited atrial arrhythmias (Class IIb).

In patients with severely impaired heart function, IV amiodarone is preferable to other antiarrhythmic agents for atrial and ventricular arrhythmias. Amiodarone has both greater efficacy and a lower incidence of proarrhythmic effects than other antiarrhythmic drugs under similar circumstances. IV amiodarone is administered as 150 mg over 10 minutes, followed by 1 mg/min infusion for 6 hours, and then 0.5 mg/min. Supplementary infusions of 150 mg can be repeated as necessary for recurrent or resistant arrhythmias to a maximum manufacturer-recommended total daily dose of 2 g. One study found amiodarone to be effective in patients with AF when administered at relatively high doses of 125 mg/h for 24 hours (total dose 3 g).[160] In cardiac arrest due to pulseless VT or VF, IV amiodarone is initially administered as a 300-mg rapid infusion diluted in a volume of 20 to 30 mL of saline or dextrose in water. Based on extrapolation from studies in patients with hemodynamically unstable VT, supplementary doses of 150 mg by rapid infusion may be administered for recurrent or refractory VT/VF, followed by an infusion of 1 mg/min for 6 hours and then 0.5 mg/min, to a maximum daily dose of 2 g.

The major adverse effects from amiodarone are hypotension and bradycardia, which can be prevented by slowing the rate of drug infusion or can be treated with fluids, pressors, chronotropic agents, or temporary pacing.

Atropine

Atropine sulfate reverses cholinergic-mediated decreases in heart rate, systemic vascular resistance, and blood pressure. Atropine is useful in treating symptomatic sinus bradycardia (Class I). Atropine may be beneficial in the presence of AV block at the nodal level (Class IIa) or ventricular asystole but should not be used when infranodal (Mobitz type II) block is suspected.

The recommended dose of atropine sulfate for asystole and slow pulseless electrical activity is 1.0 mg IV and repeated in 3 to 5 minutes if asystole persists. For bradycardia the dose is 0.5 to 1.0 g IV every 3 to 5 minutes to a total dose of 0.04 mg/kg. A total dose of 3 mg (0.04 mg/kg) results in full vagal blockade in humans. Because atropine increases myocardial oxygen demand and can initiate tachyarrhythmias, the administration of a total vagolytic dose of atropine should be reserved for asystolic cardiac arrest. Doses of atropine sulfate of <0.5 mg may be parasympathomimetic and further slow the cardiac rate. Atropine also is well absorbed through the tracheal route of administration.

Atropine should be used cautiously in the presence of AMI or infarction because excessive increases in rate may worsen ischemia or increase the zone of infarction. Rarely, VF and VT have followed IV administration of atropine. Atropine is not indicated in bradycardia from AV block at the His-Purkinje level (type II AV block and third-degree block with new wide-QRS complexes). In such instances atropine can rarely accelerate sinus rate and AV node conduction.

β-Adrenergic Blockers

β-Adrenergic blockers have potential benefits in patients with acute coronary syndromes, including patients with non–Q-wave MI and unstable angina (Class I). In the absence of contraindications, β-blockers should be given to all patients with suspected AMI and high-risk unstable angina. β-Blockers are also effective antiarrhythmia agents and have been shown to reduce the incidence of VF in studies preceding the reperfusion era. As an adjunctive agent with fibrinolytic therapy, β-blockade may reduce the rate of nonfatal reinfarction and recurrent ischemia. β-Blockers also reduce mortality if administered early to fibrinolytic-ineligible patients.

Atenolol, metoprolol, and propranolol have been shown to reduce the incidence of VF significantly in post-MI patients who did not receive fibrinolytic agents. The recommended dose is 5 mg *slow* IV (over 5 minutes); wait 10 minutes, then if the first dose was well tolerated, give a second dose of 5 mg slow IV (over 5 minutes). An oral regimen is then initiated at 50 mg every 12 hours. Metoprolol is given in doses of 5 mg by slow IV push at 5-minute intervals to a total of 15 mg. An oral regimen is then initiated 15 minutes after the last IV dose at 50 mg twice daily for 24 hours and increased to 100 mg twice a day, as tolerated. An alternative agent is propranolol (now used uncommonly), to a total dose of 0.1 mg/kg by slow IV push divided into 3 equal doses at 2- to 3-minute intervals. The rate of administration should not exceed 1 mg/min. The oral maintenance regimen is 180 to 320 mg/d, given in divided doses.

IV esmolol is a short-acting (half-life of 2 to 9 minutes) β_1-selective β-blocker that is recommended for the acute treatment of supraventricular tachyarrhythmias, including PSVT (Class I), rate control in nonpreexcited AF or atrial flutter (Class I), ectopic atrial tachycardia (Class IIb), inappropriate sinus tachycardia (Class IIb), and polymorphic VT due to torsades de pointes (as adjunctive therapy to cardiac pacing) or myocardial ischemia (Class IIb). It is metabolized by erythrocyte esterases and requires no dose adjustment in patients with renal or hepatic impairment. Esmolol has a complicated dosing regimen and requires an IV infusion pump. Esmolol is administered as an IV loading dose of 0.5 mg/kg over 1 minute, followed by a maintenance infusion of 50 μg/kg per minute for 4 minutes. If the response is inadequate a second bolus of 0.5 mg/kg is infused over 1 minute, with an increase of the maintenance infusion to 100 μg/kg. The bolus dose (0.5 mg/kg) and titration of the infusion dose (addition of 50 μg/kg per minute) can be repeated every 4 minutes to a maximum infusion of 300 μg/kg per minute. Infusions can be maintained for up to 48 hours if necessary. Esmolol 50 to 200 μg/kg per minute IV has an effect equivalent to that of 3 to 6 mg IV propranolol.

Side effects related to β-blockade include bradycardias, AV conduction delays, and hypotension. Cardiovascular decompensation and cardiogenic shock after β-adrenergic blocker therapy are infrequent provided that administration to patients with severe congestive heart failure is avoided and patients with mild and moderate congestive heart failure are monitored closely with appropriate diuresis. β-Blocker therapy should be withheld from patients with absolute contraindications to these agents. Contraindications to the use of β-adrenergic blocking agents include second- or third-degree heart block, hypotension, severe congestive heart failure, and lung disease associated with bronchospasm. β-Adrenergic blocking agents should be used cautiously in patients with preexisting sinus bradycardia and sick sinus syndrome.

Bretylium

Bretylium tosylate is a quaternary ammonium compound used in the treatment of resistant VT and VF unresponsive to attempts at defibrillation and epinephrine. The cardiovascular actions of bretylium are complex and include a release of catecholamines initially on injection. Postganglionic adrenergic blocking follows and frequently induces hypotension. In 1999 bretylium was unavailable from the manufacturer. This stimulated a review of the evidence supporting continued use of bretylium for VF/VT arrest and the other indications for bretylium, such as its value as an anti-VF agent in hypothermic cardiac arrest. Subsequently bretylium has been removed from ACLS treatment algorithms and guidelines because of a high occurrence of side effects, the availability of safer agents at least as efficacious, and the limited supply and availability of the drug.

Calcium Channel Blockers: Verapamil and Diltiazem

Verapamil and diltiazem are calcium channel blocking agents that slow conduction and increase refractoriness in the AV node. These actions may terminate reentrant arrhythmias that require AV nodal conduction for their continuation. Verapamil and diltiazem may also control ventricular response rate in patients with AF, atrial flutter, or MAT. Verapamil and diltiazem may decrease myocardial contractility and may exacerbate congestive heart failure in patients with severe LV dysfunction.

Intravenous verapamil is effective for terminating narrow-complex PSVT and may also be used for rate control in AF. Adenosine, however, is the drug of choice for terminating narrow-complex PSVT. Adenosine has an ultrashort half-life and is not effective for ventricular rate control of AF or atrial flutter. The initial dose of verapamil is 2.5 to 5 mg IV given over 2 minutes. In the absence of a therapeutic response or drug-induced adverse event, repeated doses of 5 to 10 mg may be administered every 15 to 30 minutes to a maximum of 20 mg. Verapamil should be given *only* to patients with narrow-complex PSVT or arrhythmias known with certainty to be of supraventricular origin. Verapamil should not be given to patients with impaired ventricular function or heart failure.

Diltiazem at a dose of 0.25 mg/kg, followed by a second dose of 0.35 mg/kg, seems to be equivalent in efficacy to verapamil. Diltiazem offers the advantage of producing less myocardial depression than verapamil. Diltiazem may also be used as a maintenance infusion of 5 to 15 mg/h to control the ventricular rate in AF and atrial flutter.

Disopyramide

Disopyramide is a Vaughn Williams classification I_A antiarrhythmic agent that acts both to slow conduction velocity and to prolong the effective refractory period, similar to procainamide. It has potent anticholinergic, negative inotropic, and hypotensive effects that limit its use. IV disopyramide is given as 2 mg/kg over 10 minutes, followed by a continuous infusion of 0.4 mg/kg per hour. IV disopyramide is limited by its need to be infused relatively slowly, which may be impractical and of uncertain efficacy in emergent circumstances, particularly under compromised circulatory conditions.

Dopamine

Dopamine hydrochloride is an endogenous catecholamine agent with dose-related dopaminergic and β- and α-adrenergic agonist activity. At doses between 3 and 7.5 μg/kg per minute, dopamine acts as a β-agonist, increasing cardiac output and heart rate. The β-agonist effects of dopamine are less pronounced than those of isoproterenol, and titration is easier. The inotropic effects of dopamine are modest compared with those of dobutamine. Dopamine is now regarded as a safer agent and has displaced isoproterenol as the preferred catecholamine for bradycardias in which atropine is either ineffective or contraindicated. Dopamine-induced constriction of pulmonary veins is evidenced by a dose-dependent increase in pulmonary capillary wedge pressure. LV filling pressures are spuriously elevated. As catecholamine stores are depleted, tachyphylaxis to the drug occurs.

Dopamine has been used in low doses (2 μg/kg per minute) as a renal vasodilator. Dopamine, however, has shown no benefit when used in acute oliguric renal failure.[163–165] Low-dose dopamine is no longer recommended for the management of acute oliguric renal failure.[165,166]

Flecainide

Flecainide hydrochloride is approved in oral form in the United States (and in intravenous form outside the United States) for ventricular arrhythmias and for supraventricular arrhythmias in patients without structural heart disease. Flecainide is a potent sodium channel blocker with significant conduction-slowing effects (antiarrhythmic Vaughn Williams classification I_C agent). IV flecainide (not approved for use in the United States) has been effective for termination of atrial flutter and AF, ectopic atrial tachycardia, AV nodal reentrant tachycardia, and SVTs associated with an accessory pathway (Wolff-Parkinson-White syndrome), including preexcited AF. Because of significant negative inotropic effects, flecainide should be avoided in patients in impaired LV function. It has also been observed to increase mortality in patients who have had MI, and its use should be avoided when coronary artery disease is suspected.

Flecainide is usually administered as 2 mg/kg body weight at 10 mg/min. Reported adverse side effects include bradycardia, hypotension, and neurological symptoms, such as oral paresthesias and visual blurring. Flecainide is limited by its need to be infused relatively slowly, which may be impractical and of uncertain efficacy in emergent circumstances, particularly under compromised circulatory conditions.

Ibutilide

Ibutilide is a short-acting antiarrhythmic, available only in parenteral form. Ibutilide acts by prolonging the action potential duration and increasing the refractory period of cardiac tissue (antiarrhythmic Vaughn Williams classification III effect). Ibutilide is recommended for *acute* pharmacological conversion of atrial flutter or AF or as an adjunct to electrical cardioversion in patients in whom electrical cardioversion alone has been ineffective. Ibutilide has a relatively short duration of action, making it less effective than other antiarrhythmic agents for maintaining sinus rhythm once restored. Ibutilide seems most effective for the pharmacological conversion of AF or atrial flutter of relatively brief duration.

For adults weighing ≥60 kg, ibutilide is administered intravenously, diluted or undiluted, as 1 mg (10 mL) over 10 minutes. If that is unsuccessful in terminating the arrhythmia, a second 1-mg dose can be administered at the same rate 10 minutes after the first. In patients weighing <60 kg, an initial dose of 0.01 mg/kg is recommended. Ibutilide has minimal effects on blood pressure and heart rate. Its major limitation is a relatively high incidence of ventricular proarrhythmia (polymorphic VT) including torsades de pointes. Patients receiving ibutilide should be *continuously monitored* for arrhythmias at the time of its administration and for *at least 4 to 6 hours* after drug administration (longer in patients with hepatic dysfunction in whom the clearance of ibutilide may be prolonged). Patients with significantly impaired LV function may be at higher risk of ibutilide-induced proarrhythmia.

Isoproterenol

Isoproterenol hydrochloride is a pure β-adrenergic agonist with potent inotropic and chronotropic effects. It increases myocardial oxygen consumption, cardiac output, and myocardial work and can exacerbate ischemia and arrhythmias in patients with ischemic heart disease, congestive heart failure, or impaired ventricular function. On the basis of limited evidence, isoproterenol is recommended as a temporizing measure before pacing for torsades de pointes (Class Indeterminate) and immediate temporary control of hemodynamically significant bradycardia when atropine and dobutamine have failed and transcutaneous and transvenous pacing are not available (Class IIb). Isoproterenol is not the treatment of choice for either of these conditions. At low doses the chronotropic effect (increase in heart rate) of isoproterenol raises blood pressure and compensates for its vasodilatory effects. The recommended infusion rate is 2 to 10 μg/min titrated according to the heart rate and rhythm response. An isoproterenol infusion is prepared by adding 1 mg of isoproterenol hydrochloride to 500 mL of D₅W; this produces a concentration of 2 μg/mL. For symptomatic bradycardia isoproterenol should be used, *if at all*, with extreme caution. Isoproterenol should be administered only in low doses (Class IIb). Higher doses are associated with increased myocardial oxygen consumption, increased infarct size, and malignant ventricular arrhythmias (Class III). Isoproterenol is not indicated in patients with cardiac arrest or hypotension.

Lidocaine

Lidocaine is one of a number of antiarrhythmic drugs available for treatment of ventricular ectopy, VT, and VF. Lidocaine seems to be more effective during AMI. In the presence of AMI, prophylactic administration of lidocaine reduces the incidence of primary VF but does not lower mortality. The toxic-to-therapeutic balance is delicate. The routine prophylactic use of lidocaine in patients suspected of having AMI is not recommended. Lidocaine may be used in uncomplicated AMI or ischemia when facilities for defibrillation are not readily available or when circulation is compromised by a high frequency of ventricular premature beats.

Such use should be balanced against the potential toxicity of the drug as well as the lack of evidence that prophylactic administration of lidocaine to suppress ventricular premature ectopy reduces mortality. On the basis of established use, historical precedent, and no evidence of significant harm, lidocaine is acceptable for

- VF/pulseless VT that persists after defibrillation and administration of epinephrine (Class Indeterminate)
- Control of hemodynamically compromising PVCs (Class Indeterminate)
- Hemodynamically stable VT (Class IIb)

However, lidocaine remains a second choice behind other alternative agents (amiodarone, procainamide, or sotalol) in many of these circumstances.

In cardiac arrest, an initial bolus of 1.0 to 1.5 mg/kg IV is necessary to rapidly achieve and maintain therapeutic lidocaine levels. For refractory VT/VF an additional bolus of 0.5 to 0.75 mg/kg can be given over 3 to 5 minutes if necessary. Total dose should not exceed 3 mg/kg (or >200 to 300 mg during a 1-hour period). The more aggressive dosing approach (1.5 mg/kg) is recommended in cardiac arrest due to VF or pulseless VT after failure of defibrillation and epinephrine. Only bolus therapy should be used in cardiac arrest. Administering a continuous infusion of (prophylactic) antiarrhythmic agents to maintain circulation *after* it has been successfully restored is controversial. However, until data is available supporting the prophylactic administration of antiarrhythmic agents after return of circulation, it is reasonable to continue an infusion of the drug associated with the restoration of a stable rhythm (Class Indeterminate). A continuous infusion of lidocaine should be initiated at 1 to 4 mg/min. Reappearance of arrhythmias during a constant infusion of lidocaine should be treated with a small bolus dose (0.5 mg/kg) and an increase in the infusion rate in incremental doses (maximal infusion rate of 4 mg/min).

The half-life of lidocaine increases after 24 to 48 hours as the drug, in effect, inhibits its own hepatic metabolism. With prolonged infusions, the dosage should be reduced after 24 hours or blood levels should be monitored. The dose should be reduced in the presence of decreased cardiac output (eg, in AMI with hypotension or shock, congestive cardiac failure, or poor peripheral perfusion states), in patients older than 70 years, and in those with hepatic dysfunction. These patients should receive the usual bolus dose first, followed by half the normal maintenance infusion. Lidocaine reaches the central circulation after bolus peripheral administration in approximately 2 minutes. Patients should be observed closely for signs of drug efficacy and toxicity. Toxic reactions and side effects include slurred speech, altered consciousness, muscle twitching, seizures, and bradycardia. Lidocaine blood levels may assist in guiding therapy.

Magnesium

Severe magnesium deficiency is associated with cardiac arrhythmias, symptoms of cardiac insufficiency, and sudden cardiac death. Hypomagnesemia can precipitate refractory VF and can hinder the replenishment of intracellular potassium. Magnesium deficiency should be corrected if present. In emergent circumstances, magnesium sulfate 1 to 2 g is diluted in 100 mL D₅W and administered over 1 to 2 minutes. Rapid administration of magnesium may cause clinically significant hypotension or asystole and should be avoided.

Anecdotal experience suggests that magnesium may be an effective treatment for antiarrhythmic drug-induced torsades de pointes even in the absence of magnesium deficiency. A variety of dosing regimens for magnesium sulfate have been described. Magnesium may be administered as a loading dose of 1 to 2 g (8 to 16 mEq), mixed in 50 to 100 mL D₅W, given over 5 to 60 minutes, followed by an infusion of 0.5 to 1.0 g (4 to 8 mEq) per hour. The rate and duration of the infusion should be determined by the clinical situation. The routine prophylactic administration of magnesium in patients with AMI is no longer recommended. Magnesium is not recommended in cardiac arrest except when arrhythmias are suspected to be caused by magnesium deficiency or when the monitor displays torsades de pointes.

Procainamide

Procainamide hydrochloride suppresses both atrial and ventricular arrhythmias. Procainamide is acceptable for the pharmacological conversion of supraventricular arrhythmias (particularly AF and atrial flutter) to sinus rhythm (Class IIa), for control of rapid ventricular rate due to accessory pathway conduction in preexcited atrial arrhythmias (Class IIb), and for wide-complex tachycardias that cannot be distinguished as being of supraventricular or ventricular origin (Class IIb).

Procainamide hydrochloride may be given in an infusion of 20 mg/min until the arrhythmia is suppressed, hypotension ensues, the QRS complex is prolonged by 50% from its original duration, or a total of 17 mg/kg (1.2 g for a 70-kg patient) of the drug has been given. Bolus administration of the drug can result in toxic concentrations and significant hypotension. Delay resulting from recommendations to infuse procainamide slowly presents the major barrier to its use in life-threatening situations. In urgent situations, up to 50 mg/min may be administered to a total dose of 17 mg/kg. Use of procainamide in pulseless VT/VF is supported by a retrospective comparison study involving only 20 patients[120] and is limited by the need to infuse the agent relatively slowly. The potential hazard of more rapid (bolus) administration during overt cardiac arrest must be balanced against the attendant risks and requires further study. The maintenance infusion rate of procainamide hydrochloride is 1 to 4 mg/min. The maintenance dosage should be reduced in the presence of renal failure. Blood levels should be monitored in patients with renal failure and in patients receiving a constant infusion of more than 3 mg/min for more than 24 hours.

Procainamide should be avoided in patients with preexisting QT prolongation and torsades de pointes. The ECG and blood pressure must be monitored continuously during procainamide administration. Precipitous hypotension may occur if the drug is injected too rapidly.

Propafenone

Propafenone hydrochloride, like flecainide, is a Vaughn Williams classification I$_C$ antiarrhythmic agent with signifi-

cant conduction-slowing and negative inotropic effects. In addition, propafenone has nonselective β-blocking properties. Oral propafenone is approved for use in the United States against ventricular arrhythmias and supraventricular arrhythmias in patients without structural heart disease. Intravenous propafenone (not approved for use in the United States) is used abroad for the same indications as flecainide. Because of significant negative inotropic effects, propafenone, like flecainide, should be avoided in patients with impaired LV function. Propafenone also falls into the same Vaughn Williams classification as flecainide (which has been observed to increase mortality in patients who have had MI), and by extrapolation of this data, its use should also probably be avoided when coronary artery disease is suspected.

Intravenous propafenone is customarily administered as 1 to 2 mg/kg body weight at 10 mg/min. Reported side effects include bradycardia, hypotension, and gastrointestinal upset. Propafenone is limited by its need to be infused relatively slowly, which may be impractical and of uncertain efficacy in emergent circumstances, particularly under compromised circulatory conditions.

Sotalol

Sotalol hydrochloride is a Vaughn Williams classification III antiarrhythmic agent that, like amiodarone, prolongs action potential duration and increases cardiac tissue refractoriness. In addition, it has nonselective β-blocking properties. Sotalol is approved in oral form in the United States for ventricular arrhythmias. Sotalol is used orally and intravenously for both ventricular and supraventricular arrhythmias.

Intravenous sotalol is usually administered as 1 to 1.5 mg/kg body weight at a rate of 10 mg/min. Side effects include bradycardia, hypotension, and proarrhythmia (torsades de pointes). IV sotalol is limited by its need to be infused relatively slowly. This may be impractical and has uncertain efficacy in emergent circumstances, particularly under compromised circulatory conditions.

References

1. Kuhn GJ, White BC, Swetnam RE, Mumey JF, Rydesky MF, Tintinalli JE, Krome RL, Hoehner PJ. Peripheral vs central circulation times during CPR: a pilot study. *Ann Emerg Med.* 1981;10:417–419.
2. Hedges JR, Barsan WB, Doan LA, Joyce SM, Lukes SJ, Dalsey WC, Nishiyama H. Central versus peripheral intravenous routes in cardiopulmonary resuscitation. *Am J Emerg Med.* 1984;2:385–390.
3. Barsan WG, Levy RC, Weir H. Lidocaine levels during CPR: differences after peripheral venous, central venous, and intracardiac injections. *Ann Emerg Med.* 1981;10:73–78.
4. Emerman CL, Pinchak AC, Hancock D, Hagen JF. Effect of injection site on circulation times during cardiac arrest [see comments]. *Crit Care Med.* 1988;16:1138–1141.
5. Emerman CL, Bellon EM, Lukens TW. A prospective study of femoral versus subclavian vein catheterization during cardiac arrest. *Ann Emerg Med.* 1990;19:26–30.
6. Jasani MS, Nadkarni VM, Finkelstein MS, Mandell GA, Salzman SK, Norman ME. Effects of different techniques of endotracheal epinephrine administration in pediatric porcine hypoxic-hypercarbic cardiopulmonary arrest [see comments]. *Crit Care Med.* 1994;22:1174–1180.
7. Mazkereth R, Paret G, Ezra D, Aviner S, Peleg E, Rosenthal T, Barzilay Z. Epinephrine blood concentrations after peripheral bronchial versus endotracheal administration of epinephrine in dogs. *Crit Care Med.* 1992;20:1582–1587.
8. Johnston C. Endotracheal drug delivery. *Pediatr Emerg Care.* 1992;8: 94–97.

9. Schnittger I, Rodriguez IM, Winkle RA. Esophageal electrocardiography: a new technology revives an old technique. *Am J Cardiol.* 1986; 57:604–607.

10. Shaw M, Niemann JT, Haskell RJ, Rothstein RJ, Laks MM. Esophageal electrocardiography in acute cardiac care: efficacy and diagnostic value of a new technique. *Am J Med.* 1987;82:689–696.

11. Katz A, Guetta V, Ovsyshcher IA. Transesophageal electrocardiography using a temporary pacing balloon-tipped electrode in acute cardiac care. *Ann Emerg Med.* 1991;20:961–963.

12. Lopez JA, Lufschanowski R, Massumi A. Transesophageal electrocardiography and adenosine in the diagnosis of wide complex tachycardia. *Tex Heart Inst J.* 1994;21:130–133.

13. Stewart RB, Bardy GH, Greene HL. Wide complex tachycardia: misdiagnosis and outcome after emergent therapy. *Ann Intern Med.* 1986; 104:766–771.

14. Akhtar M, Shenasa M, Jazayeri M, Caceres J, Tchou PJ. Wide QRS complex tachycardia: reappraisal of a common clinical problem. *Ann Intern Med.* 1988;109:905–912.

15. Brugada P, Brugada J, Mont L, Smeets J, Andries EW. A new approach to the differential diagnosis of a regular tachycardia with a wide QRS complex [see comments]. *Circulation.* 1991;83:1649–1659.

16. Antunes E, Brugada J, Steurer G, Andries E, Brugada P. The differential diagnosis of a regular tachycardia with a wide QRS complex on the 12-lead ECG: ventricular tachycardia, supraventricular tachycardia with aberrant intraventricular conduction, and supraventricular tachycardia with anterograde conduction over an accessory pathway [see comments]. *Pacing Clin Electrophysiol.* 1994;17:1515–1524.

17. Steurer G, Gursoy S, Frey B, Simonis F, Andries E, Kuck K, Brugada P. The differential diagnosis on the electrocardiogram between ventricular tachycardia and preexcited tachycardia. *Clin Cardiol.* 1994;17:306–308.

18. Wellens HJ, Bar FW, Lie KI. The value of the electrocardiogram in the differential diagnosis of a tachycardia with a widened QRS complex. *Am J Med.* 1978;64:27–33.

19. Kindwall KE, Brown J, Josephson ME. Electrocardiographic criteria for ventricular tachycardia in wide complex left bundle branch block morphology tachycardias. *Am J Cardiol.* 1988;61:1279–1283.

20. Halperin BD, Kron J, Cutler JE, Kudenchuk PJ, McAnulty JH. Misdiagnosing ventricular tachycardia in patients with underlying conduction disease and similar sinus and tachycardia morphologies. *West J Med.* 1990;152:677–682.

21. Littmann L, McCall MM. Ventricular tachycardia may masquerade as supraventricular tachycardia in patients with preexisting bundle-branch block. *Ann Emerg Med.* 1995;26:98–101.

22. Alberca T, Almendral J, Sanz P, Almazan A, Cantalapiedra JL, Delcan JL. Evaluation of the specificity of morphological electrocardiographic criteria for the differential diagnosis of wide QRS complex tachycardia in patients with intraventricular conduction defects. *Circulation.* 1997; 96:3527–3533.

23. Herbert ME, Votey SR, Morgan MT, Cameron P, Dziukas L. Failure to agree on the electrocardiographic diagnosis of ventricular tachycardia [see comments]. *Ann Emerg Med.* 1996;27:35–38.

24. Andrade FR, Eslami M, Elias J, Kinoshita O, Nakazato Y, Marcus FI, Frank R, Tonet J, Fontaine G. Diagnostic clues from the surface ECG to identify idiopathic (fascicular) ventricular tachycardia: correlation with electrophysiologic findings. *J Cardiovasc Electrophysiol.* 1996;7:2–8.

25. Lie KI, Wellens HJ, van Capelle FJ, Durrer D. Lidocaine in the prevention of primary ventricular fibrillation: a double-blind, randomized study of 212 consecutive patients. *N Engl J Med.* 1974;291:1324–1326.

26. MacMahon S, Collins R, Peto R, Koster RW, Yusuf S. Effects of prophylactic lidocaine in suspected acute myocardial infarction: an overview of results from the randomized, controlled trials. *JAMA.* 1988; 260:1910–1916.

27. Hine LK, Laird N, Hewitt P, Chalmers TC. Meta-analytic evidence against prophylactic use of lidocaine in acute myocardial infarction. *Arch Intern Med.* 1989;149:2694–2698.

28. Sadowski ZP, Alexander JH, Skrabucha B, Dyduszynski A, Kuch J, Nartowicz E, Swiatecka G, Kong DF, Granger CB. Multicenter randomized trial and a systematic overview of lidocaine in acute myocardial infarction [see comments]. *Am Heart J.* 1999;137:792–798.

29. Alexander JH, Granger CB, Sadowski Z, Aylward PE, White HD, Thompson TD, Califf RM, Topol EJ, the GUSTO-I and GUSTO-IIb Investigators. Prophylactic lidocaine use in acute myocardial infarction: incidence and outcomes from two international trials [see comments]. *Am Heart J.* 1999;137:799–805.

30. Armengol RE, Graff J, Baerman JM, Swiryn S. Lack of effectiveness of lidocaine for sustained, wide QRS complex tachycardia. *Ann Emerg Med.* 1989;18:254–257.

31. Nasir N Jr, Taylor A, Doyle TK, Pacifico A. Evaluation of intravenous lidocaine for the termination of sustained monomorphic ventricular tachycardia in patients with coronary artery disease with or without healed myocardial infarction. *Am J Cardiol.* 1994;74:1183–1186.

32. Gorgels AP, van den Dool A, Hofs A, Mulleneers R, Smeets JL, Vos MA, Wellens HJ. Comparison of procainamide and lidocaine in terminating sustained monomorphic ventricular tachycardia [see comments]. *Am J Cardiol.* 1996;78:43–46.

33. Ho DS, Zecchin RP, Richards DA, Uther JB, Ross DL. Double-blind trial of lignocaine versus sotalol for acute termination of spontaneous sustained ventricular tachycardia [see comments]. *Lancet.* 1994;344:18–23.

34. Griffith MJ, Linker NJ, Ward DE, Camm AJ. Adenosine in the diagnosis of broad complex tachycardia. *Lancet.* 1988;1:672–675.

35. Griffith MJ, Linker NJ, Garratt CJ, Ward DE, Camm AJ. Relative efficacy and safety of intravenous drugs for termination of sustained ventricular tachycardia. *Lancet.* 1990;336:670–673.

36. Sharma AD, Klein GJ, Yee R. Intravenous adenosine triphosphate during wide QRS complex tachycardia: safety, therapeutic efficacy, and diagnostic utility. *Am J Med.* 1990;88:337–343.

37. Garratt CJ, Griffith MJ, O'Nunain S, Ward DE, Camm AJ. Effects of intravenous adenosine on antegrade refractoriness of accessory atrioventricular connections. *Circulation.* 1991;84:1962–1968.

38. Brodsky MA, Hwang C, Hunter D, Chen PS, Smith D, Ariani M, Johnston WD, Allen BJ, Chun JG, Gold CR. Life-threatening alterations in heart rate after the use of adenosine in atrial flutter. *Am Heart J.* 1995;130:564–571.

39. Callans DJ, Marchlinski FE. Dissociation of termination and prevention of inducibility of sustained ventricular tachycardia with infusion of procainamide: evidence for distinct mechanisms. *J Am Coll Cardiol.* 1992;19:111–117.

40. Giardina EG, Heissenbuttel RH, Bigger JT Jr. Intermittent intravenous procaine amide to treat ventricular arrhythmias: correlation of plasma concentration with effect on arrhythmia, electrocardiogram, and blood pressure. *Ann Intern Med.* 1973;78:183–193.

41. Mattioli AV, Lucchi GR, Vivoli D, Mattioli G. Propafenone versus procainamide for conversion of atrial fibrillation to sinus rhythm. *Clin Cardiol.* 1998;21:763–766.

42. Kochiadakis GE, Igoumenidis NE, Solomou MC, Parthenakis FI, Christakis-Hampsas MG, Chlouverakis GI, Tsatsakis AM, Vardas PE. Conversion of atrial fibrillation to sinus rhythm using acute intravenous procainamide infusion. *Cardiovasc Drugs Ther.* 1998;12:75–81.

43. Heisel A, Jung J, Stopp M, Schieffer H. Facilitating influence of procainamide on conversion of atrial flutter by rapid atrial pacing. *Eur Heart J.* 1997;18:866–869.

44. Stambler BS, Wood MA, Ellenbogen KA. Comparative efficacy of intravenous ibutilide versus procainamide for enhancing termination of atrial flutter by atrial overdrive pacing. *Am J Cardiol.* 1996;77:960–966.

45. Hjelms E. Procainamide conversion of acute atrial fibrillation after open-heart surgery compared with digoxin treatment. *Scand J Thorac Cardiovasc Surg.* 1992;26:193–196.

46. Fulham MJ, Cookson WO, Sher M. Procainamide infusion and acute atrial fibrillation. *Anaesth Intensive Care.* 1984;12:121–124.

47. Fenster PE, Comess KA, Marsh R, Katzenberg C, Hager WD. Conversion of atrial fibrillation to sinus rhythm by acute intravenous procainamide infusion. *Am Heart J.* 1983;106:501–504.

48. Mandel WJ, Laks MM, Obayashi K, Hayakawa H, Daley W. The Wolff-Parkinson-White syndrome: pharmacologic effects of procaine amide. *Am Heart J.* 1975;90:744–754.

49. Leitch JW, Klein GJ, Yee R, Feldman RD, Brown J. Differential effect of intravenous procainamide on anterograde and retrograde accessory pathway refractoriness. *J Am Coll Cardiol.* 1992;19:118–124.

50. Boahene KA, Klein GJ, Yee R, Sharma AD, Fujimura O. Termination of acute atrial fibrillation in the Wolff-Parkinson-White syndrome by procainamide and propafenone: importance of atrial fibrillatory cycle length [see comments]. *J Am Coll Cardiol.* 1990;16:1408–1414.

51. Wellens HJ, Braat S, Brugada P, Gorgels AP, Bar FW. Use of procainamide in patients with the Wolff-Parkinson-White syndrome to disclose a short refractory period of the accessory pathway. *Am J Cardiol.* 1982;50:1087–1089.

52. Sellers TD Jr, Campbell RW, Bashore TM, Gallagher JJ. Effects of procainamide and quinidine sulfate in the Wolff-Parkinson-White syndrome. *Circulation.* 1977;55:15–22.

53. Gomes JA, Kang PS, Hariman RJ, El-Sherif N, Lyons J. Electrophysiologic effects and mechanisms of termination of supraventricular tachycardia by intravenous amiodarone. *Am Heart J*. 1984;107:214–221.

54. Noc M, Stajer D, Horvat M. Intravenous amiodarone versus verapamil for acute conversion of paroxysmal atrial fibrillation to sinus rhythm [see comments]. *Am J Cardiol*. 1990;65:679–680.

55. Galve E, Rius T, Ballester R, Artaza MA, Arnau JM, Garcia-Dorado D, Soler-Soler J. Intravenous amiodarone in treatment of recent-onset atrial fibrillation: results of a randomized, controlled study [see comments]. *J Am Coll Cardiol*. 1996;27:1079–1082.

56. Cochrane AD, Siddins M, Rosenfeldt FL, Salamonsen R, McConaghy L, Marasco S, Davis BB. A comparison of amiodarone and digoxin for treatment of supraventricular arrhythmias after cardiac surgery. *Eur J Cardiothorac Surg*. 1994;8:194–198.

57. Vietti-Ramus G, Veglio F, Marchisio U, Burzio P, Latini R. Efficacy and safety of short intravenous amiodarone in supraventricular tachyarrhythmias. *Int J Cardiol*. 1992;35:77–85.

58. Bertini G, Conti A, Fradella G, Francardelli L, Giglioli C, Mangialavori G, Margheri M, Moschi G. Propafenone versus amiodarone in field treatment of primary atrial tachydysrhythmias. *J Emerg Med*. 1990;8:15–20.

59. Mehta AV, Sanchez GR, Sacks EJ, Casta A, Dunn JM, Donner RM. Ectopic automatic atrial tachycardia in children: clinical characteristics, management and follow-up. *J Am Coll Cardiol*. 1988;11:379–385.

60. Holt P, Crick JC, Davies DW, Curry P. Intravenous amiodarone in the acute termination of supraventricular arrhythmias. *Int J Cardiol*. 1985;8:67–79.

61. Kochiadakis GE, Igoumenidis NE, Simantirakis EN, Marketou ME, Parthenakis FI, Mezilis NE, Vardas PE. Intravenous propafenone versus intravenous amiodarone in the management of atrial fibrillation of recent onset: a placebo-controlled study. *Pacing Clin Electrophysiol*. 1998;21:2475–2479.

62. Clemo HF, Wood MA, Gilligan DM, Ellenbogen KA. Intravenous amiodarone for acute heart rate control in the critically ill patient with atrial tachyarrhythmias. *Am J Cardiol*. 1998;81:594–598.

63. Cybulski J, Kulakowski P, Makowska E, Czepiel A, Sikora-Frac M, Ceremuzynski L. Intravenous amiodarone is safe and seems to be effective in termination of paroxysmal supraventricular tachyarrhythmias. *Clin Cardiol*. 1996;19:563–566.

64. Larbuisson R, Venneman I, Stiels B. The efficacy and safety of intravenous propafenone versus intravenous amiodarone in the conversion of atrial fibrillation or flutter after cardiac surgery. *J Cardiothorac Vasc Anesth*. 1996;10:229–234.

65. Kerin NZ, Faitel K, Naini M. The efficacy of intravenous amiodarone for the conversion of chronic atrial fibrillation: amiodarone vs quinidine for conversion of atrial fibrillation [see comments]. *Arch Intern Med*. 1996;156:49–53.

66. Donovan KD, Power BM, Hockings BE, Dobb GJ, Lee KY. Intravenous flecainide versus amiodarone for recent-onset atrial fibrillation. *Am J Cardiol*. 1995;75:693–697.

67. Hou ZY, Chang MS, Chen CY, Tu MS, Lin SL, Chiang HT, Woosley RL. Acute treatment of recent-onset atrial fibrillation and flutter with a tailored dosing regimen of intravenous amiodarone: a randomized, digoxin-controlled study [see comments]. *Eur Heart J*. 1995;16:521–528.

68. Di Biasi P, Scrofani R, Paje A, Cappiello E, Mangini A, Santoli C. Intravenous amiodarone vs propafenone for atrial fibrillation and flutter after cardiac operation [see comments]. *Eur J Cardiothorac Surg*. 1995;9:587–591.

69. Chapman MJ, Moran JL, O'Fathartaigh MS, Peisach AR, Cunningham DN. Management of atrial tachyarrhythmias in the critically ill: a comparison of intravenous procainamide and amiodarone. *Intensive Care Med*. 1993;19:48–52.

70. Horner SM. A comparison of cardioversion of atrial fibrillation using oral amiodarone, intravenous amiodarone and DC cardioversion [published erratum appears in *Acta Cardiol*. 1992;47:following table of contents]. *Acta Cardiol*. 1992;47:473–480.

71. Cowan JC, Gardiner P, Reid DS, Newell DJ, Campbell RW. A comparison of amiodarone and digoxin in the treatment of atrial fibrillation complicating suspected acute myocardial infarction. *J Cardiovasc Pharmacol*. 1986;8:252–256.

72. Strasberg B, Arditti A, Sclarovsky S, Lewin RF, Buimovici B, Agmon J. Efficacy of intravenous amiodarone in the management of paroxysmal or new atrial fibrillation with fast ventricular response. *Int J Cardiol*. 1985;7:47–58.

73. Faniel R, Schoenfeld P. Efficacy of i.v. amiodarone in converting rapid atrial fibrillation and flutter to sinus rhythm in intensive care patients. *Eur Heart J*. 1983;4:180–185.

74. Soult JA, Munoz M, Lopez JD, Romero A, Santos J, Tovaruela A. Efficacy and safety of intravenous amiodarone for short-term treatment of paroxysmal supraventricular tachycardia in children. *Pediatr Cardiol*. 1995;16:16–19.

75. Sagrista-Sauleda J, Permanyer-Miralda G, Soler-Soler J. Electrical cardioversion after amiodarone administration. *Am Heart J*. 1992;123:1536–1542.

76. Butler J, Harriss DR, Sinclair M, Westaby S. Amiodarone prophylaxis for tachycardias after coronary artery surgery: a randomised, double blind, placebo controlled trial. *Br Heart J*. 1993;70:56–60.

77. Holt AW. Hemodynamic responses to amiodarone in critically ill patients receiving catecholamine infusions. *Crit Care Med*. 1989;17:1270–1276.

78. Leak D. Intravenous amiodarone in the treatment of refractory life-threatening cardiac arrhythmias in the critically ill patient. *Am Heart J*. 1986;111:456–462.

79. Kuga K, Yamaguchi I, Sugishita Y. Effect of intravenous amiodarone on electrophysiologic variables and on the modes of termination of atrioventricular reciprocating tachycardia in Wolff-Parkinson-White syndrome. *Jpn Circ J*. 1999;63:189–195.

80. Kouvaras G, Cokkinos DV, Halal G, Chronopoulos G, Ioannou N. The effective treatment of multifocal atrial tachycardia with amiodarone. *Jpn Heart J*. 1989;30:301–312.

81. Figa FH, Gow RM, Hamilton RM, Freedom RM. Clinical efficacy and safety of intravenous amiodarone in infants and children. *Am J Cardiol*. 1994;74:573–577.

82. Mooss AN, Mohiuddin SM, Hee TT, Esterbrooks DJ, Hilleman DE, Rovang KS, Sketch MH Sr. Efficacy and tolerance of high-dose intravenous amiodarone for recurrent, refractory ventricular tachycardia. *Am J Cardiol*. 1990;65:609–614.

83. Schutzenberger W, Leisch F, Kerschner K, Harringer W, Herbinger W. Clinical efficacy of intravenous amiodarone in the short term treatment of recurrent sustained ventricular tachycardia and ventricular fibrillation. *Br Heart J*. 1989;62:367–371.

84. Helmy I, Herre JM, Gee G, Sharkey H, Malone P, Sauve MJ, Griffin JC, Scheinman MM. Use of intravenous amiodarone for emergency treatment of life-threatening ventricular arrhythmias. *J Am Coll Cardiol*. 1988;12:1015–1022.

85. Saksena S, Rothbart ST, Shah Y, Cappello G. Clinical efficacy and electropharmacology of continuous intravenous amiodarone infusion and chronic oral amiodarone in refractory ventricular tachycardia. *Am J Cardiol*. 1984;54:347–352.

86. Remme WJ, Van Hoogenhuyze DC, Krauss XH, Hofman A, Kruyssen DA, Storm CJ. Acute hemodynamic and antiischemic effects of intravenous amiodarone. *Am J Cardiol*. 1985;59:639–644.

87. Kowey PR, Levine JH, Herre JM, Pacifico A, Lindsay BD, Plumb VJ, Janosik DL, Kopelman HA, Scheinman MM, the Intravenous Amiodarone Multicenter Investigators Group. Randomized, double-blind comparison of intravenous amiodarone and bretylium in the treatment of patients with recurrent, hemodynamically destabilizing ventricular tachycardia or fibrillation [see comments]. *Circulation*. 1995;92:3255–3263.

88. Levine JH, Massumi A, Scheinman MM, Winkle RA, Platia EV, Chilson DA, Gomes A, Woosley RL, Intravenous Amiodarone Multicenter Trial Group. Intravenous amiodarone for recurrent sustained hypotensive ventricular tachyarrhythmias. *J Am Coll Cardiol*. 1996;27:67–75.

89. Scheinman MM, Levine JH, Cannom DS, Friehling T, Kopelman HA, Chilson DA, Platia EV, Wilber DJ, Kowey PR, the Intravenous Amiodarone Multicenter Investigators Group. Dose-ranging study of intravenous amiodarone in patients with life-threatening ventricular tachyarrhythmias [see comments]. *Circulation*. 1995;92:3264–3272.

90. Remme WJ, Kruyssen HA, Look MP, van Hoogenhuyze DC, Krauss XH. Hemodynamic effects and tolerability of intravenous amiodarone in patients with impaired left ventricular function. *Am Heart J*. 1991;122:96–103.

91. Kudenchuk PJ, Cobb LA, Copass MK, Cummins RO, Doherty AM, Fahrenbruch CE, Hallstrom AP, Murray WA, Olsufka M, Walsh T. Amiodarone for resuscitation after out-of-hospital cardiac arrest due to ventricular fibrillation. *N Engl J Med*. 1999;341:871–878.

92. Jawad-Kanber G, Sherrod TR. Effect of loading dose of procainamide on left ventricular performance in man. *Chest*. 1974;66:269–272.

93. Harrison DC, Sprouse JH, Morrow AG. The antiarrhythmic properties of lidocaine and procaine amide. *Circulation*. 1963;28:486–491.

94. Brady WJ, DeBehnke DJ, Laundrie D. Prevalence, therapeutic response, and outcome of ventricular tachycardia in the out-of-hospital setting: a comparison of monomorphic ventricular tachycardia, polymorphic ventricular tachycardia, and torsades de pointes. *Acad Emerg Med.* 1999; 6:609–617.

95. Totterman KJ, Turto H, Pellinen T. Overdrive pacing as treatment of sotalol-induced ventricular tachyarrhythmias (torsade de pointes). *Acta Med Scand Suppl.* 1982;668:28–33.

96. Inoue H, Matsuo H, Mashima S, Murao S. Effects of atrial pacing, isoprenaline and lignocaine on experimental polymorphous ventricular tachycardia. *Cardiovasc Res.* 1984;18:538–547.

97. Assimes TL, Malcolm I. Torsade de pointes with sotalol overdose treated successfully with lidocaine. *Can J Cardiol.* 1998;14:753–756.

98. Hondeghem LM. Selective depression of the ischemic and hypoxic myocardium by lidocaine. *Proc West Pharmacol Soc.* 1975;18:27–30.

99. Borer JS, Harrison LA, Kent KM, Levy R, Goldstein RE, Epstein SE. Beneficial effect of lidocaine on ventricular electrical stability and spontaneous ventricular fibrillation during experimental myocardial infarction. *Am J Cardiol.* 1976;37:860–863.

100. Spear JF, Moore EN, Gerstenblith G. Effect of lidocaine on the ventricular fibrillation threshold in the dog during acute ischemia and premature ventricular contractions. *Circulation.* 1972;46:65–73.

101. Carden NJ, Steinhaus JE. Lidocaine in cardiac resuscitation from ventricular fibrillation. *Circ Res.* 1956;4.

102. Lazzara R, el-Sherif N, Scherlag BJ. Electrophysiological properties of canine Purkinje cells in one-day-old myocardial infarction. *Circ Res.* 1973;33:722–734.

103. Lazzara R, Hope RR, El-Sherif N, Scherlag BJ. Effects of lidocaine on hypoxic and ischemic cardiac cells. *Am J Cardiol.* 1978;41:872–879.

104. Hanyok JJ, Chow MS, Kluger J, Fieldman A. Antifibrillatory effects of high dose bretylium and a lidocaine-bretylium combination during cardiopulmonary resuscitation. *Crit Care Med.* 1988;16:691–694.

105. Herlitz J, Ekstrom L, Wennerblom B, Axelsson A, Bang A, Lindkvist J, Persson NG, Holmberg S. Lidocaine in out-of-hospital ventricular fibrillation: does it improve survival? *Resuscitation.* 1997;33:199–205.

106. Harrison EE. Lidocaine in prehospital countershock refractory ventricular fibrillation. *Ann Emerg Med.* 1981;10:420–423.

107. Haynes RE, Chinn TL, Copass MK, Cobb LA. Comparison of bretylium tosylate and lidocaine in management of out of hospital ventricular fibrillation: a randomized clinical trial. *Am J Cardiol.* 1981;48:353–356.

108. Olson DW, Thompson BM, Darin JC, Milbrath MH. A randomized comparison study of bretylium tosylate and lidocaine in resuscitation of patients from out-of-hospital ventricular fibrillation in a paramedic system. *Ann Emerg Med.* 1984;13:807–810.

109. Kentsch M, Berkel H, Bleifeld W. Intravenose Amiodaron-Applikation bei therapierefraktarem Kammerflimmern. *Intensivmedizin.* 1988;25:70–74.

110. Weaver WD, Fahrenbruch CE, Johnson DD, Hallstrom AP, Cobb LA, Copass MK. Effect of epinephrine and lidocaine therapy on outcome after cardiac arrest due to ventricular fibrillation. *Circulation.* 1990;82: 2027–2034.

111. van Walraven C, Stiell IG, Wells GA, Hebert PC, Vandemheen K, the OTAC Study Group. Do advanced cardiac life support drugs increase resuscitation rates from in-hospital cardiac arrest? *Ann Emerg Med.* 1998;32:544–553.

112. Redding JS, Pearson JW. Resuscitation from ventricular fibrillation: drug therapy. *JAMA.* 1968;203:255–260.

113. Chow MS, Kluger J, Lawrence R, Fieldman A. The effect of lidocaine and bretylium on the defibrillation threshold during cardiac arrest and cardiopulmonary resuscitation. *Proc Soc Exp Biol Med.* 1986;182:63–67.

114. Babbs CF, Yim GK, Whistler SJ, Tacker WA, Geddes LA. Elevation of ventricular defibrillation threshold in dogs by antiarrhythmic drugs. *Am Heart J.* 1979;98:345–350.

115. Echt DS, Black JN, Barbey JT, Coxe DR, Cato E. Evaluation of antiarrhythmic drugs on defibrillation energy requirements in dogs: sodium channel block and action potential prolongation. *Circulation.* 1989;79: 1106–1117.

116. Dorian P, Fain ES, Davy JM, Winkle RA. Lidocaine causes a reversible, concentration-dependent increase in defibrillation energy requirements. *J Am Coll Cardiol.* 1986;8:327–332.

117. Kerber RE, Pandian NG, Jensen SR, Constantin L, Kieso RA, Melton J, Hunt M. Effect of lidocaine and bretylium on energy requirements for transthoracic defibrillation: experimental studies. *J Am Coll Cardiol.* 1986;7:397–405.

118. Vachiery JL, Reuse C, Blecic S, Contempre B, Vincent JL. Bretylium tosylate versus lidocaine in experimental cardiac arrest [see comments]. *Am J Emerg Med.* 1990;8:492–495.

119. Anastasiou-Nana MI, Nanas JN, Nanas SN, Rapti A, Poyadjis A, Stathaki S, Moulopoulos SD. Effects of amiodarone on refractory ventricular fibrillation in acute myocardial infarction: experimental study. *J Am Coll Cardiol.* 1994;23:253–258.

120. Stiell IG, Wells GA, Hebert PC, Laupacis A, Weitzman BN. Association of drug therapy with survival in cardiac arrest: limited role of advanced cardiac life support drugs. *Acad Emerg Med.* 1995;2:264–273.

121. Tzivoni D, Keren A, Cohen AM, Loebel H, Zahavi I, Chenzbraun A, Stern S. Magnesium therapy for torsades de pointes. *Am J Cardiol.* 1984;53:528–530.

122. Tzivoni D, Banai S, Schuger C, Benhorin J, Keren A, Gottlieb S, Stern S. Treatment of torsade de pointes with magnesium sulfate. *Circulation.* 1988;77:392–397.

123. Miller B, Craddock L, Hoffenberg S, Heinz S, Lefkowitz D, Callender ML, Battaglia C, Maines C, Masick D. Pilot study of intravenous magnesium sulfate in refractory cardiac arrest: safety data and recommendations for future studies. *Resuscitation.* 1995;30:3–14.

124. Thel MC, Armstrong AL, McNulty SE, Califf RM, O'Connor CM, Duke Internal Medicine Housestaff. Randomised trial of magnesium in in-hospital cardiac arrest [see comments]. *Lancet.* 1997;350:1272–1276.

125. Kudenchuk PD, Cobb L, Fahrenbruch C, Doherty A, Murray W, et al. The ARREST Trial. Randomized controlled trial of Amiodarone vs Placebo in the early treatment of refractory VF arrest in the out-of-hospital setting. *Circulation.* 1997;96:.

126. Moran JL, Gallagher J, Peake SL, Cunningham DN, Salagaras M, Leppard P. Parenteral magnesium sulfate versus amiodarone in the therapy of atrial tachyarrhythmias: a prospective, randomized study. *Crit Care Med.* 1995;23:1816–1824.

127. O'Nunain S, Garratt CJ, Linker NJ, Gill J, Ward DE, Camm AJ. A comparison of intravenous propafenone and flecainide in the treatment of tachycardias associated with the Wolff-Parkinson-White syndrome. *Pacing Clin Electrophysiol.* 1991;14:2028–2034.

128. Jordaens L, Gorgels A, Stroobandt R, Temmerman J, the Sotalol Versus Placebo Multicenter Study Group. Efficacy and safety of intravenous sotalol for termination of paroxysmal supraventricular tachycardia. *Am J Cardiol.* 1991;68:35–40.

129. Sung RJ, Tan HL, Karagounis L, Hanyok JJ, Falk R, Platia E, Das G, Hardy SA, Sotalol Multicenter Study Group. Intravenous sotalol for the termination of supraventricular tachycardia and atrial fibrillation and flutter: a multicenter, randomized, double-blind, placebo-controlled study. *Am Heart J.* 1995;129:739–748.

130. Echt DS, Liebson PR, Mitchell LB, Peters RW, Obias-Manno D, Barker AH, Arensberg D, Baker A, Friedman L, Greene HL, et al. Mortality and morbidity in patients receiving encainide, flecainide, or placebo: the Cardiac Arrhythmia Suppression Trial [see comments]. *N Engl J Med.* 1991;324:781–788.

131. Hellestrand KJ. Intravenous flecainide acetate for supraventricular tachycardias. *Am J Cardiol.* 1988;62:16D–22D.

132. Kuck KH, Kunze KP, Schluter M, Duckeck W. Encainide versus flecainide for chronic atrial and junctional ectopic tachycardia. *Am J Cardiol.* 1988;62:37L–44L.

133. Reimer A, Paul T, Kallfelz HC. Efficacy and safety of intravenous and oral propafenone in pediatric cardiac dysrhythmias. *Am J Cardiol.* 1991; 68:741–744.

134. Bauersfeld U, Gow RM, Hamilton RM, Izukawa T. Treatment of atrial ectopic tachycardia in infants < 6 months old. *Am Heart J.* 1995;129: 1145–1148.

135. Tommaso C, McDonough T, Parker M, Talano JV. Atrial fibrillation and flutter: immediate control and conversion with intravenously administered verapamil. *Arch Intern Med.* 1983;143:877–881.

136. Phillips BG, Gandhi AJ, Sanoski CA, Just VL, Bauman JL. Comparison of intravenous diltiazem and verapamil for the acute treatment of atrial fibrillation and atrial flutter. *Pharmacotherapy.* 1997;17:1238–1245.

137. Hwang MH, Danoviz J, Pacold I, Rad N, Loeb HS, Gunnar RM. Double-blind crossover randomized trial of intravenously administered verapamil: its use for atrial fibrillation and flutter following open heart surgery. *Arch Intern Med.* 1984;144:491–494.

138. Gray RJ, Conklin CM, Sethna DH, Mandel WJ, Matloff JM. Role of intravenous verapamil in supraventricular tachyarrhythmias after open-heart surgery. *Am Heart J.* 1982;104:799–802.

139. Gonzalez R, Scheinman MM. Treatment of supraventricular arrhythmias with intravenous and oral verapamil. *Chest.* 1981;80:465–470.

140. Aronow WS, Landa D, Plasencia G, Wong R, Karlsberg RP, Ferlinz J. Verapamil in atrial fibrillation and atrial flutter. *Clin Pharmacol Ther*. 1979;26:578–583.

141. Haynes BE, Niemann JT, Haynes KS. Supraventricular tachyarrhythmias and rate-related hypotension: cardiovascular effects and efficacy of intravenous verapamil [published erratum appears in *Ann Emerg Med*. 1991;20:671]. *Ann Emerg Med*. 1990;19:861–864.

142. Barnett JC, Touchon RC. Short-term control of supraventricular tachycardia with verapamil infusion and calcium pretreatment. *Chest*. 1990;97:1106–1109.

143. Heng MK, Singh BN, Roche AH, Norris RM, Mercer CJ. Effects of intravenous verapamil on cardiac arrhythmias and on the electrocardiogram. *Am Heart J*. 1975;90:487–498.

144. Schwartz M, Michelson EL, Sawin HS, MacVaugh H III. Esmolol: safety and efficacy in postoperative cardiothoracic patients with supraventricular tachyarrhythmias. *Chest*. 1988;93:705–711.

145. Shettigar UR, Toole JG, Appunn DO. Combined use of esmolol and digoxin in the acute treatment of atrial fibrillation or flutter. *Am Heart J*. 1993;126:368–374.

146. Gray RJ, Bateman TM, Czer LS, Conklin CM, Matloff JM. Esmolol: a new ultrashort-acting beta-adrenergic blocking agent for rapid control of heart rate in postoperative supraventricular tachyarrhythmias. *J Am Coll Cardiol*. 1985;5:1451–1456.

147. Byrd RC, Sung RJ, Marks J, Parmley WW. Safety and efficacy of esmolol (ASL-8052: an ultrashort-acting beta-adrenergic blocking agent) for control of ventricular rate in supraventricular tachycardias. *J Am Coll Cardiol*. 1984;3:394–399.

148. Amsterdam EA, Kulcyski J, Ridgeway MG. Efficacy of cardioselective beta-adrenergic blockade with intravenously administered metoprolol in the treatment of supraventricular tachyarrhythmias. *J Clin Pharmacol*. 1991;31:714–718.

149. Rehnqvist N. Clinical experience with intravenous metoprolol in supraventricular tachyarrhythmias: a multicentre study. *Ann Clin Res*. 1981;13(suppl 30):68–72.

150. Platia EV, Michelson EL, Porterfield JK, Das G. Esmolol versus verapamil in the acute treatment of atrial fibrillation or atrial flutter. *Am J Cardiol*. 1989;63:925–929.

151. Tisdale JE, Padhi ID, Goldberg AD, Silverman NA, Webb CR, Higgins RS, Paone G, Frank DM, Borzak S. A randomized, double-blind comparison of intravenous diltiazem and digoxin for atrial fibrillation after coronary artery bypass surgery. *Am Heart J*. 1998;135:739–747.

152. Schreck DM, Rivera AR, Tricarico VJ. Emergency management of atrial fibrillation and flutter: intravenous diltiazem versus intravenous digoxin [see comments]. *Ann Emerg Med*. 1997;29:135–140.

153. Boudonas G, Lefkos N, Efthymiadis AP, Styliadis IG, Tsapas G. Intravenous administration of diltiazem in the treatment of supraventricular tachyarrhythmias. *Acta Cardiol*. 1995;50:125–134.

154. Goldenberg IF, Lewis WR, Dias VC, Heywood JT, Pedersen WR. Intravenous diltiazem for the treatment of patients with atrial fibrillation or flutter and moderate to severe congestive heart failure [see comments]. *Am J Cardiol*. 1994;74:884–889.

155. Salerno DM, Dias VC, Kleiger RE, Tschida VH, Sung RJ, Sami M, Giorgi LV, the Diltiazem-Atrial Fibrillation/Flutter Study Group. Efficacy and safety of intravenous diltiazem for treatment of atrial fibrillation and atrial flutter. *Am J Cardiol*. 1989;63:1046–1051.

156. Millaire A, Leroy O, de Groote P, Santre C, Ducloux G. Usefulness of diltiazem in the acute management of supraventricular tachyarrhythmias in the elderly. *Cardiovasc Drugs Ther*. 1996;10:11–16.

157. Ellenbogen KA, Dias VC, Cardello FP, Strauss WE, Simonton CA, Pollak SJ, Wood MA, Stambler BS. Safety and efficacy of intravenous diltiazem in atrial fibrillation or atrial flutter. *Am J Cardiol*. 1995;75:45–49.

158. Jordaens L, Trouerbach J, Calle P, Tavernier R, Derycke E, Vertongen P, Bergez B, Vandekerckhove Y. Conversion of atrial fibrillation to sinus rhythm and rate control by digoxin in comparison to placebo [see comments]. *Eur Heart J*. 1997;18:643–648.

159. Heywood JT, Graham B, Marais GE, Jutzy KR. Effects of intravenous diltiazem on rapid atrial fibrillation accompanied by congestive heart failure. *Am J Cardiol*. 1991;67:1150–1152.

160. Cotter G, Blatt A, Kaluski E, Metzkor-Cotter E, Koren M, Litinski I, Simantov R, Moshkovitz Y, Zaidenstein R, Peleg E, Vered Z, Golik A. Conversion of recent onset paroxysmal atrial fibrillation to normal sinus rhythm: the effect of no treatment and high-dose amiodarone: a randomized, placebo-controlled study [see comments]. *Eur Heart J*. 1999; 20:1833–1842.

161. Touboul P, Atallah G, Kirkorian G, Lavaud P, Mathieu MP, Dellinger A. Effects of intravenous sotalol in patients with atrioventricular accessory pathways. *Am Heart J*. 1987;114:545–550.

162. Camm AJ, Garratt CJ. Adenosine and supraventricular tachycardia [see comments]. *N Engl J Med*. 1991;325:1621–1629.

163. Bersten AD, Holt AW. Vasoactive drugs and the importance of renal perfusion pressure. *New Horiz*. 1995;3:650–661.

164. Marik PE. Low-dose dopamine in critically ill oliguric patients: the influence of the renin-angiotensin system. *Heart Lung*. 1993;22:171–175.

165. Chertow GM, Sayegh MH, Allgren RL, Lazarus JM, Auriculin Anaritide Acute Renal Failure Study Group. Is the administration of dopamine associated with adverse or favorable outcomes in acute renal failure? [see comments]. *Am J Med*. 1996;101:49–53.

166. Thadani R, Pascual M, Bonventre J. Acute renal failure. *N Engl J Med*. 1996;334:1448–1460.

Section 6: Pharmacology II: Agents to Optimize Cardiac Output and Blood Pressure

Overview

This section presents drugs that affect 3 dimensions of the cardiovascular system:

- Peripheral vascular tone
- Inotropic state of the heart
- Chronotropic state of the heart

  Clinically these drugs are used in

- Acute ischemic heart disease
- Acute and chronic heart failure
- Shock (especially cardiogenic)
- Cardiac arrest

Epinephrine

Epinephrine hydrochloride produces beneficial effects in patients during cardiac arrest, primarily because of its α-adrenergic receptor–stimulating properties.[1] The adrenergic effects of epinephrine increase myocardial and cerebral blood flow during CPR.[2] The value and safety of the β-adrenergic effects of epinephrine are controversial because they may increase myocardial work and reduce subendocardial perfusion.[3]

Although epinephrine has been used universally in resuscitation, there is a paucity of evidence to show that it improves outcome in humans. For a number of years researchers and clinicians have also questioned the optimal dose of epinephrine. The "standard" dose of epinephrine (1.0 mg) is not based on body weight. Historically a standard dose of 1 mg epinephrine was used in surgical operating rooms for intracardiac injections.[4–6] Surgeons observed that 1 to 3 mg of intracardiac epinephrine was effective in restarting the arrested heart.[6,7] When these and other experts first produced resuscitation guidelines in the 1970s, they assumed that 1 mg of IV epinephrine would work in a similar manner as 1 mg of intracardiac epinephrine. Adult patients vary greatly in weight, yet clinicians continue to inject the same 1-mg dose of epinephrine for all body weights.

The dose-response curve of epinephrine was investigated in a series of animal experiments during the 1980s. This work showed that epinephrine produced its optimal response in the range of 0.045 to 0.20 mg/kg.[8–11] From these studies it seemed that higher doses of epinephrine were necessary to improve hemodynamics and achieve successful resuscitation, particularly as the interval from cardiac arrest increased. This work led many clinicians to use higher doses of epinephrine in humans, and optimistic case series and retrospective studies were published in the late 1980s and early 1990s.[12–14]

Results from 4 clinical trials then compared high-dose epinephrine with standard-dose epinephrine.[8,15–17] Overall the rate of return of spontaneous circulation (ROSC) was increased with higher doses of epinephrine (0.07 to 0.20 mg/kg); however, no statistically significant improvement in the rate of *survival to hospital discharge* occurred. On the positive side, these trials failed to detect any significant harm from administration of higher doses of epinephrine. On the basis of this information, in 1992 the guidelines recommended that the first epinephrine dose continue to be 1 mg IV. The 1992 guidelines also recommended that the interval between subsequent doses of epinephrine be every 3 to 5 minutes rather than every 5 minutes. If the 1 mg epinephrine every 3 to 5 minutes seemed to be ineffective, the 1992 guidelines accepted the use of higher doses of epinephrine in either escalating doses (1, 3, 5 mg), intermediate doses (5 mg per dose rather than 1 mg), or high doses based on body weight (0.1 mg/kg).

Both beneficial and toxic physiological effects of epinephrine administration during CPR have been shown in animal and human studies.[18–26] Initial or escalating high-dose epinephrine has occasionally improved initial ROSC and early survival. But 8 randomized clinical studies involving more than 9000 cardiac arrest patients have found no improvement in survival to hospital discharge or neurological outcome, even in subgroups with initial high-dose epinephrine, compared with standard doses.[15–17,27–31]

These trials largely addressed initial use of high-dose epinephrine and not escalating doses after an initial failure of a 1-mg dose. In these studies there was no evidence of a worse outcome with high-dose epinephrine. Retrospective studies, however, have suggested that high cumulative epinephrine dosage is associated with worse hemodynamic and neurological outcome, but they do not prove causal effect.[26,32] Careful laboratory studies corroborate both beneficial and harmful physiological effects and outcomes. High-dose epinephrine may improve coronary perfusion and increase vascular resistance to promote initial ROSC during CPR, but these same effects may lead to increased myocardial dysfunction and occasionally a severe toxic hyperadrenergic state in the postresuscitation period.[18,21,23,25] Target populations with increased risk and potential increased benefit (catecholamine-refractory conditions) need to be identified.

In summary, initial high-intravenous-dose epinephrine in cardiac arrest may increase coronary perfusion pressure and improve ROSC, but it may exacerbate postresuscitation myocardial dysfunction. Higher doses of epinephrine have not improved long-term survival and neurological outcome

Circulation. 2000;102(suppl I):I-129–I-135.
© 2000 American Heart Association, Inc.

Circulation is available at http://www.circulationaha.org

when used as initial therapy. Nor have higher doses definitively been shown to cause harm. Therefore, high-dose epinephrine is not recommended for *routine use* but can be considered if 1-mg doses fail (Class Indeterminate. Interpretation: acceptable but not recommended). There is conflicting evidence for and against the use of higher doses of epinephrine (up to 0.2 mg/kg) in cardiac arrest when 1-mg doses have failed (Class IIb: acceptable but not recommended; weak supporting evidence).

Epinephrine has good bioavailability following tracheal delivery if administered appropriately.[33] Although the optimal dose of epinephrine for tracheal delivery is unknown, a dose that is at least 2 to 2.5 times the peripheral IV dose may be needed.[34] Intracardiac administration should be used only during open cardiac massage or when other routes of administration are unavailable.[34] Intracardiac injections increase the risk of coronary artery laceration, cardiac tamponade, and pneumothorax. Intracardiac injections also cause interruption of external chest compression and ventilation.

The recommended dose of epinephrine hydrochloride is 1.0 mg (10 mL of a 1:10 000 solution) administered IV every 3 to 5 minutes during resuscitation.[35] Each dose given by peripheral injection should be followed by a 20-mL flush of IV fluid to ensure delivery of the drug into the central compartment.

Epinephrine can also be used as a vasopressor agent for patients who are not in cardiac arrest but who have other indications for a vasopressor. For example, epinephrine is considered Class IIb for symptomatic bradycardia (Class IIb: acceptable but not recommended; weak supporting evidence) after atropine and transcutaneous pacing fail.

Not in Cardiac Arrest

Epinephrine hydrochloride, 1 mg (1 mL of a 1:1000 solution), is added to 500 mL of normal saline or D_5W and administered by continuous infusion. The initial dose for adults is 1 μg/min titrated to the desired hemodynamic response (2 to 10 μg/min).

In Cardiac Arrest

During cardiac arrest epinephrine may be administered by continuous infusion. The dose should be comparable to the standard IV dose of epinephrine (1 mg every 3 to 5 minutes). This is accomplished by adding 1 mg of epinephrine hydrochloride to 250 mL of normal saline or D_5W to run at 1 μg/min and increased to 3 to 4 μg/min. Continuous infusions of epinephrine should be administered by central venous access to reduce the risk of extravasation and to ensure good bioavailability.

Vasopressin

Vasopressin is the naturally occurring antidiuretic hormone. In unnaturally high doses—much higher than those needed for antidiuretic hormone effects—vasopressin acts as a nonadrenergic peripheral vasoconstrictor. Vasopressin acts by direct stimulation of smooth muscle V_1 receptors. This smooth muscle constriction produces a variety of effects, including pallor of the skin, nausea, intestinal cramps, desire to defecate, bronchial constriction, and in women, uterine

contractions. Vasopressin, given intra-arterially, is an approved treatment for bleeding esophageal varices, because it causes vasoconstriction. Vasopressin also dispels bowel gas shadows during abdominal angiography by causing gastrointestinal smooth muscle constriction. It is usually not recommended for conscious patients with coronary artery disease because the increased peripheral vascular resistance may provoke angina pectoris. The half-life of vasopressin in animal models with an intact circulation is 10 to 20 minutes, which is longer than that of epinephrine during CPR.

Endogenous vasopressin levels in patients undergoing CPR are significantly higher in patients who survive than in patients who do not have ROSC.[36,37] This finding suggested that exogenous vasopressin might be beneficial during cardiac arrest. After a short duration of ventricular fibrillation, vasopressin during CPR increased coronary perfusion pressure,[38] vital organ blood flow,[39] ventricular fibrillation median frequency,[40] and cerebral oxygen delivery.[41] Similar results were found with prolonged cardiac arrest and pulseless electrical activity. Vasopressin did not result in bradycardia after ROSC.[39]

Interaction of vasopressin with V_1 receptors during CPR causes intense peripheral vasoconstriction of skin, skeletal muscle, intestine, and fat with relatively less constriction of coronary and renal vascular beds and vasodilatation of the cerebral vasculature.[42,43] Vasopressin produces no skeletal muscle vasodilatation or increased myocardial oxygen consumption during CPR because it has no β-adrenergic activity. A combination of vasopressin and epinephrine versus vasopressin alone resulted only in comparable left ventricular myocardial blood flow but significantly decreased cerebral perfusion.[44] Although vasopressin during CPR decreased catecholamine plasma levels in swine[45] and humans,[46] it remains to be determined whether it decreases myocardial oxygen consumption as well. Laboratory studies indicate that the same vasopressin dosage may be administered intravenously[47,48] and intraosseously.[49]

Repeated doses of vasopressin were more effective than epinephrine in maintaining coronary perfusion pressure above the critical threshold that correlates with successful ROSC.[45] In the postresuscitation period, vasopressin produces no increased myocardial oxygen demand because baroreceptor-mediated bradycardia in response to transient hypertension remains intact. A reduction in cardiac index in the postresuscitation phase is transient and fully reversible without administration of more drugs.[41] Although splanchnic blood flow is decreased after successful resuscitation with vasopressin, infusion of low-dose dopamine after CPR can return blood flow to baseline within 60 minutes.[50]

Clinically there is preliminary evidence that vasopressin may be effective in enhancing the probability of ROSC in humans with out-of-hospital ventricular fibrillation. In patients with cardiac arrest refractory to standard ACLS, vasopressin induced an increase in blood pressure, and in some cases, ROSC.[51] In a similar clinical evaluation after approximately 40 minutes of unsuccessful ACLS, 4 of 10 patients responded to vasopressin and had a mean increase in coronary perfusion pressure of 28 mm Hg.[46] In a small (n=40) investigation of patients with out-of-hospital ventricular fibrillation, a significantly larger proportion of patients initially treated with vasopressin (40 U IV) were successfully resuscitated and survived 24 hours compared with patients treated with epinephrine (1 mg IV). There was, however, no difference in survival to hospital discharge.[52] The unpublished manuscript of a larger (n=200), in-hospital clinical trial was reviewed at the time of the Guidelines 2000 Conference. Survival for 1 hour and to hospital discharge was not different whether initial pharmacological treatment was vasopressin or epinephrine (Ian Stiell, MD, oral communication). In this study, response times were short, indicating that CPR outcome achieved with both vasopressin and epinephrine in short-term cardiac arrest may be comparable. Animal and clinical studies as well as in vitro studies suggest that vasopressin may be especially useful when the duration of cardiac arrest is prolonged, because the adrenergic pressor response in severe acidosis is blunted. Vasopressin response in severe acidosis remains intact.[42,44] A large randomized controlled trial evaluating vasopressin versus epinephrine in out-of-hospital cardiac patients is in progress in Europe.

In summary, vasopressin is an effective vasopressor and can be used as an *alternative* to epinephrine for the treatment of adult shock-refractory VF (Class IIb: acceptable; fair supporting evidence). Vasopressin may be effective in patients with asystole or pulseless electrical activity as well. However, as of 2000 we lack sufficient data to support an active recommendation to use vasopressin (Class Indeterminate: not recommended; not forbidden). Vasopressin should be effective in patients who remain in cardiac arrest after treatment with epinephrine, but there is inadequate data to evaluate the efficacy and safety of vasopressin in these patients (Class Indeterminate).

Vasopressin may be useful for hemodynamic support in vasodilatory shock, such as septic shock and sepsis syndrome. Standard therapy of vasodilatory septic shock includes antibiotics, extracellular volume expansion, vasopressors, and drugs that increase myocardial contractility. Inotropic agents and vasoconstrictor drugs commonly used in this setting may have a diminished vasopressor action.[53,54] If standard therapy is inadequate, a continuous infusion of vasopressin may be beneficial (Class IIb).

Norepinephrine

Norepinephrine is a naturally occurring potent vasoconstrictor and inotropic agent. Cardiac output may increase or decrease in response to norepinephrine, depending on vascular resistance, the functional state of the left ventricle, and reflex responses, eg, those mediated by carotid baroreceptors. Norepinephrine usually induces renal and mesenteric vasoconstriction. It is indicated in patients with severe hypotension (systolic blood pressure <70 mm Hg) and a low total peripheral resistance. Norepinephrine is relatively contraindicated in patients with hypovolemia. Myocardial oxygen requirements may be increased, mandating cautious use of this agent in patients with ischemic heart disease. Ischemic necrosis and sloughing of superficial tissues may result from extravasation of norepinephrine.

Norepinephrine is administered by adding 4 mg of norepinephrine or 8 mg of norepinephrine bitartrate (2 mg of norepinephrine bitartrate is equivalent to 1 mg of norepinephrine) to 250 mL of D_5W with or without saline, resulting in a concentration of 16 μg/mL of norepinephrine or 32 μg/mL of norepinephrine bitartrate. The initial dose of norepinephrine is 0.5 to 1.0 μg/min titrated to effect. Patients with refractory shock may require 8 to 30 μg/min of norepinephrine. It should not be administered in the same IV line as alkaline solutions, which may inactivate it.

If extravasation occurs, 5 to 10 mg of phentolamine in 10 to 15 mL of saline solution should be infiltrated as soon as possible to prevent necrosis and sloughing.

Dopamine

Dopamine hydrochloride is a catecholamine-like agent and a chemical precursor of norepinephrine that has both α-receptor– and β-receptor–stimulating actions. In addition, there are receptors specific for this compound (DA_1, DA_2 dopaminergic receptors). Physiologically dopamine stimulates the heart through both α- and β-receptors. In the periphery, dopamine releases norepinephrine from stores in nerve endings, but the vasoconstricting effects of norepinephrine are countered by activity at the DA_2 receptors, producing vasodilation in physiological concentration.[55–57] In the central nervous system, dopamine is an important neurotransmitter. Pharmacologically dopamine is both a potent adrenergic receptor agonist and a strong peripheral dopamine receptor agonist. These effects are dose-dependent.

During resuscitation, treatment with dopamine is usually reserved for hypotension that occurs with symptomatic bradycardia or after ROSC. Dopamine in combination with other agents, including dobutamine, remains an option in the management of postresuscitation shock. If hypotension persists after filling pressure is optimized, inotropic (eg, dobutamine) or vasopressor (eg, norepinephrine) therapy is indicated. These therapies correct and maintain systemic perfusion and oxygen delivery.

Dopamine should not be mixed with sodium bicarbonate or other alkaline solutions in the IV line because some data indicates that it may be inactivated in alkaline solutions. Therapy should not be discontinued abruptly but tapered gradually.

The recommended dosage ranges from 5 to 20 μg/kg per minute. Doses in excess of 10 μg/kg per minute are associated with systemic and splanchnic vasoconstriction. Higher doses of dopamine, used as a single inotrope/vasoconstrictor, are associated with adverse effects on splanchnic perfusion in some patients.

In the dose range of 2 to 4 μg/kg per minute, dopamine is primarily a dopaminergic agonist with little inotropic effect and renosplanchnic perfusion augmentation. In doses of between 5 and 10 μg/kg per minute, β_1 and β_2 inotropy predominates. In addition, serotonin- and dopaminergic-mediated venoconstriction is noted in this dose range. In doses of 10 to 20 μg/kg per minute, α-receptor effects are noted with substantial systemic and splanchnic arteriolar vasoconstriction. Dobutamine, in contrast, is a predominantly β_1-selective ventricular inotrope that elicits decreased sympathetic nervous tone while augmenting cardiac output.

Dopamine in a dose of 2 to 4 μg/kg per minute has been advocated for acute oliguric renal failure. Although dopamine may occasionally promote diuresis, the increase in urine output does not reflect an improvement in renal glomerular filtration rate.[50,58,59] Consequently, low-dose dopamine (2 to 4 μg/kg per minute) is no longer recommended for the management of acute oliguric renal failure.

Dopamine is available in 5-mL ampules containing 400 mg of dopamine hydrochloride, which when mixed in 250 mL of D_5W produces a concentration of 1600 μg/mL.

Dobutamine

Dobutamine hydrochloride is a synthetic catecholamine and potent inotropic agent useful in the treatment of severe systolic heart failure. Dobutamine has predominant β-adrenergic receptor–stimulating effects that increase myocardial contractility in a dose-dependent manner, accompanied by a decrease in left ventricular filling pressures. An increase in stroke volume frequently induces reflex peripheral vasodilation (baroreceptor mediated) so that arterial pressure may remain unchanged. Hemodynamic end points rather than a specific dose should be employed to optimize the use of dobutamine. Hemodynamic monitoring should target the achievement of a normal cardiac output for optimal organ perfusion.

The usual dosage range is 5 to 20 μg/kg per minute. However, the individual inotropic and chronotropic responses can vary widely in critically ill patients. Elderly patients have a significantly decreased response to dobutamine. At doses >20 μg/kg per minute, increases in heart rate of >10% may induce or exacerbate myocardial ischemia. Doses of dobutamine as high as 40 μg/kg per minute have been used but may be toxic.

Amrinone and Milrinone

Amrinone and milrinone are phosphodiesterase III inhibitors that have inotropic and vasodilatory properties. Amrinone has a more significant effect on preload than catecholamines, and the hemodynamic effects are similar to those of dobutamine. Phosphodiesterase inhibitors are approved for use in severe heart failure or cardiogenic shock that is not adequately responsive to standard therapy. Patients who have not responded to catecholamine therapy and patients with tachyarrhythmias are candidates for such treatment. Amrinone may exacerbate myocardial ischemia or worsen ventricular ectopy. Optimal use requires hemodynamic monitoring. The drug is contraindicated with valvular obstructive disease.

Amrinone is administered as a dose of 0.75 mg/kg given initially over 2 to 3 minutes, followed by an infusion of 5 to 15 μg/kg per minute. An additional bolus may be given in 30 minutes.

Like amrinone, milrinone has a relatively long plasma half-life, which makes dose titration more difficult. Milrinone may also be combined with dobutamine at intermediate doses, enhancing the inotropic effects.

A slow intravenous loading dose (50 μg/kg over 10 minutes) is followed by an intravenous infusion at a rate of 375 to 750 ng/kg per minute for 2 to 3 days. In renal failure the dose should be adjusted.

Calcium

Although calcium ions play a critical role in myocardial contractile performance and impulse formation, retrospective and prospective studies in the cardiac arrest setting have not shown benefit from the use of calcium. In addition, there is concern on a theoretical basis that the high blood levels induced by calcium administration may be detrimental. When hyperkalemia, hypocalcemia (eg, after multiple blood transfusions), or calcium channel blocker toxicity is present, use of calcium is probably helpful (Class IIb). Otherwise, calcium should not be used (Class III).

When necessary, a 10% solution of calcium chloride can be given in a dose of 2 to 4 mg/kg and repeated as necessary at 10-minute intervals. (The 10% solution contains 1.36 mEq of calcium per 100 mg of salt per milliliter.) Calcium glucceptate can be given in a dose of 5 to 7 mL and calcium gluconate in a dose of 5 to 8 mL.

Digitalis

Digitalis preparations have limited use as inotropic agents in ECC. Digitalis decreases the ventricular rate in some patients with atrial flutter or fibrillation by slowing atrioventricular nodal conduction. The toxic-to-therapeutic ratio is narrow, especially when potassium depletion is present. Digitalis toxicity may cause serious ventricular arrhythmia and precipitate cardiac arrest. Digoxin-specific antibody is available for the treatment of serious toxicity (Digibind, Digitalis Antidote BM).

Digoxin provides safe and effective control of ventricular response rate in patients with chronic atrial fibrillation. Digoxin is less effective in patients with paroxysmal atrial fibrillation and in general does not provide adequate rate control in high adrenergic states (such as congestive heart failure, hyperthyroidism, or during exercise). Intravenous calcium channel blockers (diltiazem) or β-adrenergic blockers are now preferred for initial ventricular rate control of atrial fibrillation. In heightened adrenergic states, β-blockers may offer an advantage over calcium channel blockade.

Nitroglycerin

Nitrates have been used for their ability to relax vascular smooth muscle. Nitroglycerin is the initial treatment of choice for suspected ischemic-type pain or discomfort (see "Part 7: Acute Coronary Syndromes"). Sublingually administered nitroglycerin is readily absorbed and highly effective in relieving angina, typically within 1 to 2 minutes. The therapeutic effect may last up to 30 minutes. Nitroglycerin spray may also be used. If discomfort is not relieved with 3 tablets, the patient should seek emergency medical attention promptly by dialing the appropriate emergency number.

Intravenous nitroglycerin permits more controlled titration in patients with acute coronary syndromes, hypertensive urgencies, or congestive heart failure. Intravenous nitroglycerin is an effective adjunct in treatment of recurrent ischemia, hypertensive emergencies, or congestive heart failure associated with myocardial infarction (MI). Nitrates should be used cautiously in patients with inferior MI. Nitrates are contraindicated in patients who are preload-dependent with right ventricular infarction. The pharmacological effects of nitroglycerin are dependent primarily on intravascular volume status and to a lesser extent on the dose administered. Hypovolemia blunts the beneficial hemodynamic effects of nitroglycerin and increases the risk of hypotension. Hypotension may reduce coronary blood flow and exacerbate myocardial ischemia. Nitrate-induced hypotension responds to fluid replacement therapy. Other potential complications of IV nitroglycerin include tachycardia, paradoxical bradycardia, hypoxemia caused by increased pulmonary ventilation-perfusion mismatch, and headache. Nitroglycerin should be avoided with bradycardia and extreme tachycardia.

For suspected angina pectoris, 1 nitroglycerin tablet (0.3 or 0.4 mg) is administered sublingually and repeated at 3- to 5-minute intervals if discomfort is not relieved.

Nitroglycerin is administered by continuous infusion (nitroglycerin 50 or 100 mg in 250 mL of D_5W or 0.9% sodium chloride) at 10 to 20 μg/min and increased by 5 to 10 μg/min every 5 to 10 minutes until the desired hemodynamic or clinical response occurs.

Low doses (30 to 40 μg/min) predominantly produce venodilatation; high doses (150 to 500 μg/min) lead to arteriolar dilatation as well. Prolonged administration of nitroglycerin (>24 hours) may produce tolerance.

Sodium Nitroprusside

Sodium nitroprusside is a potent, rapid-acting direct peripheral vasodilator useful in the treatment of severe heart failure and hypertensive emergencies.[60] Direct venodilatation causes decreases in right and left ventricular filling (preload), resulting in relief of pulmonary congestion and reduced left ventricular volume and pressure. Arteriolar relaxation causes decreases in peripheral arterial resistance (afterload), resulting in enhanced systolic emptying with reduced left ventricular volume and wall stress and reduced myocardial oxygen consumption.

If intravascular volume is normal or high, reduction in peripheral vascular resistance is usually accompanied by an increased stroke volume, minimizing the fall in systemic blood pressure. In the presence of hypovolemia, nitroprusside is likely to cause excessive drop in blood pressure with reflex tachycardia. Hemodynamic monitoring is useful when nitroprusside is used. Left ventricular filling pressure should be optimized and maintained at 15 to 18 mm Hg.

Studies have reported improvement in clinical status in patients with low-output states and high systemic vascular resistance refractory to dopamine, although mortality was not reduced.[61] Nitroprusside has been reported as particularly useful in severe heart failure caused by the regurgitant valvular lesions of aortic insufficiency and mitral regurgitation.[62] Nitroprusside can decrease wall stress and myocardial work in patients with hypertension and acute ischemic heart disease. There is conflicting data about the effects of nitroprusside in patients with acute MI. Some studies indicate an adverse effect in patients treated early after onset,[63] contrasting with benefit in others during the same period.[64] Nitroglycerin is less likely to lower coronary perfusion pressure (produce coronary steal) and is more likely to increase blood supply to ischemic areas of the myocardium compared with nitroprusside.[65–67] Before the reperfusion era, nitroglycerin

reduced mortality in acute MI more than nitroprusside (45% versus 23%, relative reduction).[68] Nitroglycerin is the preferred vasodilator in acute MI, especially when infarction is complicated by congestive heart failure. Nitroprusside may be added when elevated blood pressures are present during acute MI and acute congestive heart failure if nitroglycerin fails to produce optimal levels. Nitroprusside has effects on the pulmonary arterial system. These effects may reverse hypoxic pulmonary vasoconstriction in patients with pulmonary disease (eg, pneumonia, adult respiratory distress syndrome). This may exacerbate intrapulmonary shunting, resulting in hypoxemia.

The major complication of nitroprusside is hypotension. Patients may also complain of headaches, nausea, vomiting, and abdominal cramps. Nitroprusside is rapidly metabolized to both cyanide and thiocyanate. Cyanide either is metabolized to thiocyanate in the liver or forms a complex with vitamin B_6. Thiocyanate undergoes renal elimination. Patients with hepatic or renal insufficiency and patients requiring >3 μg/kg per minute for more than 72 hours may accumulate cyanide or thiocyanate and should be monitored for signs of cyanide or thiocyanate toxic effects. Cyanide toxicity is detected by the development of metabolic acidosis. When levels exceed 12 mg/dL, thiocyanate toxicity is manifest as confusion, hyperreflexia, and convulsions. Treatment of elevated cyanide or thiocyanate levels includes immediate discontinuation of the infusion. If cyanide levels are extremely elevated and the patient is experiencing signs and symptoms of toxic effects, sodium nitrite and sodium thiosulfate should be administered.

Sodium nitroprusside is prepared by adding 50 or 100 mg to 250 mL of D_5W or saline. The solution and tubing should be wrapped in opaque material because nitroprusside deteriorates when exposed to light. Nitroprusside should be administered with an IV infusion pump.

The recommended dosing range for sodium nitroprusside is 0.1 to 5 μg/kg per minute, but higher doses (up to 10 μg/kg per minute) may be needed.

Sodium Bicarbonate

Adequate alveolar ventilation is central for control of acid-base balance during cardiac arrest and the postarrest period. Hyperventilation corrects respiratory acidosis by removing carbon dioxide, which is freely diffusible across cellular and organ membranes (eg, the brain). Little data indicates that therapy with buffers improves outcome. On the contrary, there is laboratory and clinical data indicating that bicarbonate (1) does not improve the ability to defibrillate or improve survival rates in animals; (2) can compromise coronary perfusion pressure; (3) may cause adverse effects due to extracellular alkalosis, including shifting the oxyhemoglobin saturation curve or inhibiting the release of oxygen; (4) may induce hyperosmolarity and hypernatremia; (5) produces carbon dioxide, which is freely diffusible into myocardial and cerebral cells and may paradoxically contribute to intracellular acidosis; (6) exacerbates central venous acidosis; and (7) may inactivate simultaneously administered catecholamines.

Tissue acidosis and resulting acidemia during cardiac arrest and resuscitation are dynamic processes resulting from low blood flow. These processes depend on the duration of cardiac arrest and the level of blood flow during CPR. Current understanding of acid-base pathophysiology during cardiac arrest and resuscitation indicates that carbon dioxide generated in tissues is poorly perfused during low-blood-flow conditions. Adequate alveolar ventilation and restoration of tissue perfusion, first with chest compressions, then with rapid restoration of spontaneous circulation, are the mainstays of control of acid-base balance during cardiac arrest. Laboratory and clinical data fails to conclusively show that low blood pH adversely affects ability to defibrillate, ability to restore spontaneous circulation, or short-term survival. Adrenergic responsiveness also appears to be unaffected by tissue acidosis.

In certain circumstances, such as patients with preexisting metabolic acidosis, hyperkalemia, or tricyclic or phenobarbitone overdose, bicarbonate can be beneficial. After protracted arrest or long resuscitative efforts, bicarbonate possibly benefits the patient. However, bicarbonate therapy should be considered only after the confirmed interventions, such as defibrillation, cardiac compression, intubation, ventilation, and vasopressor therapy, have been ineffective.

The recommendations for bicarbonate vary, depending on the clinical situation. (See Section 7, Figure 3: VF/VT algorithm; Figure 4: pulseless electrical activity algorithm; and Figure 5: asystole algorithm.) When bicarbonate is used, 1 mEq/kg should be given as the initial dose. Whenever possible, bicarbonate therapy should be guided by the bicarbonate concentration or calculated base deficit obtained from blood gas analysis or laboratory measurement. To minimize the risk of iatrogenically induced alkalosis, complete correction of the base deficit should be avoided.

Diuretics

Furosemide is a potent diuretic agent that inhibits reabsorption of sodium in the proximal and distal renal tubule and the loop of Henle. Furosemide also has a direct venodilating effect in patients with acute pulmonary edema, but it may have a transient vasoconstrictor effect when heart failure is chronic. The onset of vascular effects is within 5 minutes; however, diuresis occurs later. Furosemide may be useful in treatment of acute pulmonary edema.

Newer "loop" diuretics that act similarly to furosemide and have a similar profile of side effects include torsemide (1:2 relative potency to furosemide) and bumetanide (1:40 relative potency to furosemide). On occasion, in patients who do not respond to high doses of loop diuretics alone, a combination of such agents with "proximal tubule" thiazide diuretics (such as chlorthiazide or metolazone) may be given. Such combinations require close serial observation of serum electrolytes because profound potassium depletion can result from their use.

The initial dose of furosemide is 0.5 to 1.0 mg/kg IV injected slowly.

References

1. Yakaitis RW, Otto CW, Blitt CD. Relative importance of alpha and beta adrenergic receptors during resuscitation. *Crit Care Med.* 1979;7: 293–296.

2. Michael JR, Guerci AD, Koehler RC, Shi AY, Tsitlik J, Chandra N, Niedermeyer E, Rogers MC, Traystman RJ, Weisfeldt ML. Mechanisms by which epinephrine augments cerebral and myocardial perfusion during cardiopulmonary resuscitation in dogs. *Circulation.* 1984;69:822–835.

3. Ditchey RV, Lindenfeld J. Failure of epinephrine to improve the balance between myocardial oxygen supply and demand during closed-chest resuscitation in dogs. *Circulation.* 1988;78:382–389.

4. Beck C, Leighninger D. Reversal of death in good hearts. *J Cardiovasc Surg.* 1962;3:27–30.

5. Bodon C. The intracardiac injection of epinephrine. *Lancet.* 1923;1:586.

6. Beck C, Rand H III. Cardiac arrest during anesthesia and surgery. *JAMA.* 1949;1230–1233.

7. Gerbode F. The cardiac emergency. *Ann Surg.* 1952;135:431.

8. Lindner K, Ahnefeld F, Bowdler I. Comparison of different doses of epinephrine on myocardial perfusion and resuscitation success during cardiopulmonary resuscitation in a pig model. *Am J Emerg Med.* 1991; 9:27–31.

9. Brown C, Werman H, Davis E, et al. Effect of standard doses of epinephrine on myocardial oxygen delivery and utilization during CPR. *Crit Care Med.* 1988;16:536–539.

10. Brown C, Werman H, Davis E, Hobson J, Hamlin R. Comparative effect of graded doses of epinephrine on regional brain blood flow during CPR in a swine model. *Ann Emerg Med.* 1987;15:1138–1144.

11. Kosnik J, Jackson R, Keats S, Tworek R, Freeman S. Dose-related response of aortic diastolic pressure during closed-chest massage in dogs. *Ann Emerg Med.* 1985;14:204–208.

12. Callaham M. Epinephrine doses in cardiac arrest: is it time to outgrow the orthodoxy of ACLS? *Ann Emerg Med.* 1989;18:1011–1012.

13. Gonzalez ER, Ornato JP. The dose of epinephrine during cardiopulmonary resuscitation in humans: what should it be? *DICP.* 1991;25:773–777.

14. Otto CW, Yakaitis RW, Blitt CD. Mechanism of action of epinephrine in resuscitation from asphyxial arrest. *Crit Care Med.* 1981;9:364–365.

15. Brown CG, Martin DR, Pepe PE, Stueven H, Cummins RO, Gonzalez E, Jastremski M, The Multicenter High-Dose Epinephrine Study Group. A comparison of standard-dose and high-dose epinephrine in cardiac arrest outside the hospital [see comments]. *N Engl J Med.* 1992;327:1051–1055.

16. Stiell IG, Hebert PC, Weitzman BN, Wells GA, Raman S, Stark RM, Higginson LA, Ahuja J, Dickinson GE. High-dose epinephrine in adult cardiac arrest [see comments]. *N Engl J Med.* 1992;327:1045–1050.

17. Callaham M, Madsen CD, Barton CW, Saunders CE, Pointer J. A randomized clinical trial of high-dose epinephrine and norepinephrine vs standard-dose epinephrine in prehospital cardiac arrest [see comments]. *JAMA.* 1992;268:2667–2672.

18. Berg RA, Otto CW, Kern KB, Hilwig RW, Sanders AB, Henry CP, Ewy GA. A randomized, blinded trial of high-dose epinephrine versus standard-dose epinephrine in a swine model of pediatric asphyxial cardiac arrest. *Crit Care Med.* 1996;24:1695–1700.

19. Bleske BE, Rice TL, Warren EW, De Las Alas VR, Tait AR, Knight PR. The effect of sodium bicarbonate administration on the vasopressor effect of high-dose epinephrine during cardiopulmonary resuscitation in swine. *Am J Emerg Med.* 1993;11:439–443.

20. Hoekstra JW, Griffith R, Kelley R. Effect of standard-dose versus high-dose epinephrine on myocardial high-energy phosphates during ventricular fibrillation and closed chest. *CPR.* 1993;11:1385–1391.

21. Hornchen U, Lussi C, Schuttler J. Potential risks of high-dose epinephrine for resuscitation from ventricular fibrillation in a porcine model. *J Cardiothorac Vasc Anesth.* 1993;7:184–187.

22. Niemann JT, Cairns CB, Sharma J, Lewis RJ. Treatment of prolonged ventricular fibrillation: immediate countershock versus high-dose epinephrine and CPR preceding countershock. *Circulation.* 1992;85: 281–287.

23. Neumar RW, Bircher NG, Sim KM, Xiao F, Zadach KS, Radovsky A, Katz L, Ebmeyer E, Safar P. Epinephrine and sodium bicarbonate during CPR following asphyxial cardiac arrest in rats. *Resuscitation.* 1995;29: 249–263.

24. Tang W, Weil MH, Sun S, et al. Epinephrine increases the severity of postresuscitation myocardial dysfunction. *Circulation.* 1995;92: 3089–3093.

25. Schmitz B, Fischer M, Bockhorst K, Hoehn-Berlage M, Hossmann KA. Resuscitation from cardiac arrest in cats: influence of epinephrine dosage on brain recovery. *Resuscitation.* 1995;30:251–262.

26. Rivers E, Wortsman J, Rady M, Blake H, McGeorge F, Buderer N. The effect of the total cumulative epinephrine dose administered during human CPR on hemodynamic, oxygen transport, and utilization variables in the postresuscitation period. *Chest.* 1994;106:1499–1507.

27. Lindner KH, Ahnefeld FW, Prengel AW. Comparison of standard and high-dose adrenaline in the resuscitation of asystole and electromechanical dissociation. *Acta Anaesthesiol Scand.* 1991;35:253–256.

28. Lipman J, Wilson W, Kobilski S, Scribante J, Lee C, Kraus P, Cooper J, Barr J, Moyes D. High-dose adrenaline in adult in-hospital asystolic cardiopulmonary resuscitation: a double-blind randomised trial. *Anaesth Intensive Care.* 1993;21:192–196.

29. Choux C, Gueugniaud PY, Barbieux A, Pham E, Lae C, Dubien PY, Petit P. Standard doses versus repeated high doses of epinephrine in cardiac arrest outside the hospital. *Resuscitation.* 1995;29:3–9.

30. Sherman BW, Munger MA, Foulke GE, Rutherford WF, Panacek EA. High-dose versus standard-dose epinephrine treatment of cardiac arrest after failure of standard therapy. *Pharmacotherapy.* 1997;17:242–247.

31. Gueugniaud PY, Mols P, Goldstein P, Pham E, Dubien PY, Deweerdt C, Vergnion M, Petit P, Carli P, European Epinephrine Study Group. A comparison of repeated high doses and repeated standard doses of epinephrine for cardiac arrest outside the hospital [see comments]. *N Engl J Med.* 1998;339:1595–1601.

32. Behringer W, Kittler H, Sterz F, Domanovits H, Schoerkhuber W, Holzer M, Mullner M, Laggner AN. Cumulative epinephrine dose during cardiopulmonary resuscitation and neurologic outcome [see comments]. *Ann Intern Med.* 1998;129:450–456.

33. Roberts JR, Greenberg MI, Knaub MA, Kendrick ZV, Baskin SI. Blood levels following intravenous and endotracheal epinephrine administration. *J Am Coll Emerg Physicians.* 1979;8:53–56.

34. Aitkenhead AR. Drug administration during CPR: what route? *Resuscitation.* 1991;22:191–195.

35. Paradis N, Martin G, Rivers E, et al. Coronary perfusion pressure and the return of spontaneous circulation in human cardiopulmonary resuscitation. *JAMA.* 1987;263:1106–1113.

36. Lindner KH, Strohmenger HU, Endinger H. Stress hormone response during and after cardiopulmonary resuscitation. *Anesthesiology.* 1992;77:662–668.

37. Lindner KH, Haak T, Keller A, Bothner U, Lurie KG. Release of endogenous vasopressors during and after cardiopulmonary resuscitation. *Heart.* 1996;75:145–150.

38. Babar SI, Berg RA, Hilwig RW, Kern KB, Ewy GA. Vasopressin versus epinephrine during cardiopulmonary resuscitation: a randomized swine outcome study. *Resuscitation.* 1999;41:185–192.

39. Wenzel V, Lindner KH, Prengel AW, Maier C, Voelckel W, Lurie KG, Strohmenger HU. Vasopressin improves vital organ blood flow after prolonged cardiac arrest with postcountershock pulseless electrical activity in pigs [see comments]. *Crit Care Med.* 1999;27:486–492.

40. Strohmenger HU, Lindner KH, Prengel AW, Pfenninger EG, Bothner U, Lurie KG. Effects of epinephrine and vasopressin on median fibrillation frequency and defibrillation success in a porcine model of cardiopulmonary resuscitation. *Resuscitation.* 1996;31:65–73.

41. Prengel AW, Lindner KH, Keller A, Lurie KG. Cardiovascular function during the postresuscitation phase after cardiac arrest in pigs: a comparison of epinephrine versus vasopressin. *Crit Care Med.* 1996;24:2014–2019.

42. Fox AW, May RE, Mitch WE. Comparison of peptide and nonpeptide receptor-mediated responses in rat-tail artery. *J Cardiovasc Pharmacol.* 1992;20:282–289.

43. Oyama H, Suzuki Y, Satoh S. Role of nitric oxide in the cerebral vasodilatory responses to vasopressin and oxytocin in dogs. *J Cereb Blood Flow Metab.* 1993;13:285–290.

44. Wenzel V, Lindner KH, Augenstein S. Vasopressin combined with epinephrine decreases cerebral perfusion compared with vasopressin alone during CPR in pigs. *Stroke.* 1998;29:1467–1468.

45. Wenzel V, Lindner KH, Baubin MA. Vasopressin decreases endogenous catecholamine plasma levels during cardiopulmonary resuscitation in pigs. *Crit Care Med.* 2000;28:1096–1100.

46. Morris DC, Dereczyk BE, Grzybowski M. Vasopressin can increase coronary perfusion pressure during human cardiopulmonary resuscitation. *Acad Emerg Med.* 1997;20:609–614.

47. Lindner KH, Prengel AW, Pfenninger EG, Lindner IM, Strohmenger HU, Georgieff M, Lurie KG. Vasopressin improves vital organ blood flow during closed-chest cardiopulmonary resuscitation in pigs. *Circulation.* 1995;91:215–221.

48. Wenzel V, Lindner KH, Prengel AW. Endobronchial vasopressin improves survival during cardiopulmonary resuscitation in pigs. *Anesthesiology.* 1997;86:1375–1381.

49. Wenzel V, Lindner KH, Augenstein S. Intraosseous vasopressin improves coronary perfusion pressure rapidly during cardiopulmonary resuscitation in pigs. *Crit Care Med.* 1999;27:1565–1569.

50. Voelckel WG, Lindner KH, Wenzel V, Bonatti JO, Krismer AC, Miller EA, Lurie KG. Effect of small-dose dopamine on mesenteric blood flow and renal function in a pig model of cardiopulmonary resuscitation with vasopressin. *Anesth Analg.* 1999;89:1430–1436.

51. Lindner KH, Prengel AW, Brinkmann A, Strohmenger HU, Lindner IM, Lurie KG. Vasopressin administration in refractory cardiac arrest. *Ann Intern Med.* 1996;124:1061–1064.

52. Lindner KH, Dirks B, Strohmenger HU. Randomized comparison of epinephrine and vasopressin in patients with out-of-hospital ventricular fibrillation. *Lancet.* 1997;349:535–537.

53. Argenziano M, Chen JM, Cullinane S. Arginine vasopressin in the management of vasodilatory hypotension after cardiac transplantation. *J Heart Lung Transplant.* 1999;8:814–817.

54. Morales DL, Gregg D, Helman DN. Arginine vasopressin in the treatment of 50 patients with postcardiotomy vasodilatory shock. *Ann Thorac Surg.* 2000;69:102–106.

55. Farmer JB. Indirect sympathomimetic actions of dopamine. *J Pharm Pharmacol.* 1966;18:261–262.

56. Gonzalez ER, Ornato JP, Levine RL. Vasopressor effect of epinephrine with and without dopamine during cardiopulmonary resuscitation. *Drug Intell Clin Pharmacol.* 1988;22:868–872.

57. Leier CV, Heban PT, Huss P, Bush CA, Lewis RP. Comparative systemic and regional hemodynamic effects of dopamine and dobutamine in patients with cardiomyopathic heart failure. *Circulation.* 1978;58:466–475.

58. Marik PE. Low dose dopamine in critically ill oliguric patients: the influence of the renin-angiotensin system. *Heart Lung.* 1993;22:171–175.

59. Thompson B, Cockrill B. Renal-dose dopamine: a Siren song? *Lancet.* 1994;344:7–8.

60. Cummins RO, LoGerfo JP, Inui TS, Weiss NS. High-yield referral criteria for posttraumatic skull roentgenography: response of physicians and accuracy of criteria. *JAMA.* 1980;244:673–676.

61. Parmley WW, Chatterjee K, Charuzi Y, Swan HJ. Hemodynamic effects of noninvasive systolic unloading (nitroprusside) and diastolic augmentation (external counterpulsation) in patients with acute myocardial infarction. *Am J Cardiol.* 1974;33:819–825.

62. Durrer J, Lie K, van Capelle J, et al. Effect of sodium nitroprusside on mortality in acute myocardial infarction. *N Engl J Med.* 1982;306:1121–1128.

63. Cohn JN, Franciosa JA, Francis GS, Archibald D, Tristani F, Fletcher R, Montero A, Cintron G, Clarke J, Hager D, Saunders R, Cobb F, Smith R, Loeb H, Settle H. Effect of short-term infusion of sodium nitroprusside on mortality rate in acute myocardial infarction complicated by left ventricular failure: results of a Veterans Administration cooperative study. *N Engl J Med.* 1982;306:1129–1135.

64. Lie KI, Durrer JD, van Capelle FJ, Durrer D. Nitroprusside and heart failure complicating acute myocardial infarction. *Eur Heart J.* 1983;4(suppl A):209–210.

65. Chiariello M, Gold HK, Leinbach RC, Davis MA, Maroko PR. Comparison between the effects of nitroprusside and nitroglycerin on ischemic injury during acute myocardial infarction. *Circulation.* 1976;54:766–773.

66. Flaherty JT. Comparison of intravenous nitroglycerin and sodium nitroprusside in acute myocardial infarction. *Am J Med.* 1983;74:53–60.

67. Jaffe AS, Geltman EM, Tiefenbrunn AJ, Ambos HD, Strauss HD, Sobel BE, Roberts R. Reduction of infarct size in patients with inferior infarction with intravenous glyceryl trinitrate: a randomised study. *Br Heart J.* 1983;49:452–460.

68. Yusuf S, Wittes J, Friedman L. Overview of results of randomized clinical trials in heart disease, I: treatments following myocardial infarction. *JAMA.* 1988;260:2088–2093.

Section 7: Algorithm Approach to ACLS Emergencies
7A: Principles and Practice of ACLS

Key Principles in the Application of ACLS

The Importance of Time

The passage of time drives all aspects of ECC. The final outcomes are determined by the intervals between collapse or onset of the emergency and the delivery of basic and advanced interventions.[1,2] The probability of survival declines sharply with each passing minute of cardiopulmonary compromise. Some interventions, like basic CPR, slow the rate at which this decline in probability occurs. CPR makes this contribution by supplying some blood flow to the heart and brain. Some single interventions, such as tracheal intubation, clearing an obstructed airway, or defibrillating a heart in VF, are sufficient alone to restore a beating heart. For all of these interventions, independently sufficient or simply contributory, the longer it takes to administer these therapies, the lower the chances of benefit.

The "Periarrest" Period

Emergency cardiovascular care no longer focuses only on the patient in cardiac arrest. Emergency care providers cannot narrow their objectives to only the arrest state. They must recognize and treat effectively those patients "on their way to a cardiac arrest" and those recovering in the immediate postresuscitation period. Once these patients are identified, ECC personnel must be able to rapidly initiate appropriate therapy. If responders treat critical conditions properly in this "periarrest" or "prearrest" period, they can prevent a full cardiopulmonary arrest from occurring.

Consequently, the international ACLS recommendations present the science-based clinical guidelines and some educational material for these periarrest conditions:

- Acute coronary syndromes
- Acute pulmonary edema, hypotension, and shock
- Symptomatic bradycardias
- Stable and unstable tachycardias
- Acute ischemic stroke
- Impairments of rate, rhythm, or cardiac function in the postresuscitation period (by definition a periarrest/prearrest condition)

Other parts of the ECC and CPR guidelines present guidelines for more specific causes of cardiac arrest, such as electrolyte abnormalities, drug toxicity or overdoses, and toxic ingestions.

Never Forget the Patient

Resuscitation challenges care providers to make decisions quickly and under pressure. Providers must occasionally limit their focus for a brief time to a specific aspect of the resuscitative attempt: getting the IV infusion line started, placing the tracheal tube, identifying the rhythm, and remembering the "right" medication to order. But rescuers constantly must return to an overall view of each resuscitative attempt. The flow diagrams or algorithms focus the learner on the most important aspects of a resuscitative effort: airway and ventilation, basic CPR, defibrillation of VF, and medications suitable for a particular patient under specific conditions.

Code Organization: Using the Primary and Secondary ABCD Surveys

The International Perspective

Many approaches to code organization exist. The section that follows describes the approach taught in AHA courses for ACLS and pediatric resuscitation. This does not imply that methods of code organization used in other countries are incorrect or less successful.

Why Is Training in ACLS Intentionally Multidisciplinary?

An understandable tendency exists internationally to separate the highly trained professional from less skilled personnel during ACLS training. Such a practice, however, would jeopardize one of the most important objectives of resuscitation training. This objective is to have each member of the multidisciplinary response team know and understand the skills and roles of each of the other team members. An accomplished senior physician may claim, *"I already know the resuscitation guidelines and already possess the psychomotor skills. Why must I attend a learning session with less trained responders who are not authorized to perform tracheal intubation, start an IV drip, or order medications?"* An experienced instructor might respond in several ways, but the response should remind the expert that he or she must still work with the entire responding team. The expert must know what the other team members can and cannot perform so that attempted resuscitation proceeds smoothly, quietly, and effectively.

Of even greater importance, the ACLS team member who possesses the lowest level of professional training will attend future resuscitative attempts as a critical quality control agent. Nurses, for example, who work in critical care and emergency care areas may not perform intubation or defibrillation in some settings, but they can detect with surprising speed

Circulation. 2000;102(suppl I):I-136–I-139.
© 2000 American Heart Association, Inc.

Circulation is available at http://www.circulationaha.org

and accuracy when other team members attempt the procedure incorrectly! In American hospitals, particularly academic teaching centers, nurses prevent innumerable medical mishaps during resuscitative attempts. They gently (and sometimes not so gently) point out when the tracheal tube is misplaced, the IV line has become a subcutaneous line, CPR is inadequate, or the medication ordered was incorrect or wrongly dosed.

While emergency personnel are encouraged to know and experience the role of team leader, training should concentrate on the *team* aspects of resuscitative efforts. The course of resuscitative attempts may be complex and unpredictable. Indeed, a good resuscitation team has been likened to a fine symphony orchestra.[3] The team recognizes the team leader for broad skills of organization and performance. They recognize the individual team member for specific performance skills. Like an orchestra, all are performing the same piece, polished by practice and experience, with attention to both detail and outcome. There is no excuse for a disorganized and frenetic code scene.

The team leader should be decisive and composed. The team should stick to the ABCs (airway, breathing, and circulation) and keep the resuscitation room quiet so that all personnel can hear without repetitive commands. Team members should

- State the vital signs every 5 minutes or with any change in the monitored parameters
- State when procedures and medications are completed
- Request clarification of any orders
- Provide primary and secondary assessment information

The team leader should communicate her or his observations and should actively seek suggestions from team members. Evaluation of airway, breathing, and circulation should guide the efforts whenever the vital signs are unstable, when treatment appears to be failing, before procedures, and for periodic clinical updates.

The next section describes the Primary and Secondary ABCD Surveys. This aide-mémoire provides an easily remembered listing of the content and sequence of the specific assessment and management steps of a resuscitative attempt.

The Primary and Secondary ABCD Surveys

All who respond to cardiorespiratory emergencies should arrive well trained in a simple, easy-to-remember approach. The ACLS Provider Course teaches the *Primary and Secondary Survey Approach* to emergency cardiovascular care. This memory aid describes 2 sets of 4 steps: *A-B-C-D* (8 total steps). With each step the responder performs an *assessment* and then, if the assessment so indicates, a *management.*

Conduct the Primary ABCD Survey

The Primary ABCD Survey requires your hands (gloved!), a barrier device for CPR, and an AED for defibrillation. The Primary ABCD Survey assesses and manages most immediate life threats:

- Airway: *Assess and manage* the **A**irway with noninvasive techniques.

- Breathing: *Assess and manage* **B**reathing with positive-pressure ventilations.
- Circulation: *Assess and manage* the **C**irculation, performing CPR until an AED is brought to the scene.
- Defibrillation: *Assess and manage* **D**efibrillation, assessing the cardiac rhythm for VF/VT and providing defibrillatory shocks in a safe and effective manner if needed.

Conduct the Secondary ABCD Survey

This survey requires medically *advanced, invasive* techniques to again *assess and manage* the patient. The rescuer attempts to restore spontaneous respirations and circulation to the patient and when successful, continues to assess and manage the patient until relieved by appropriate emergency professionals. In brief: *resuscitate, stabilize,* and *transfer* to higher-level care.

- **A**irway: *Assess and manage.* Advanced rescuers manage a compromised airway by placing a tracheal tube.
- **B**reathing: *Assess and manage. Assess* adequacy of breathing and ventilation by checking tube placement and performance; correct all problems detected. *Manage* breathing by treating inadequate ventilation with positive-pressure ventilations through the tube.
- **C**irculation: *Assess and manage* the circulation of blood and delivery of medications by
  —Starting a peripheral IV line
  —Attaching ECG leads to examine the ECG for the most frequent cardiac arrest rhythms (VF, pulseless VT, asystole, and PEA)
  —Administering appropriate rhythm-based medications
- **D**ifferential **D**iagnosis: *Assess and manage* the differential diagnoses that you develop as you search for, find, and treat reversible causes.

The Resuscitation Attempt as a "Critical Incident": Code Critique and Debriefing

After any resuscitation attempt team members should perform a code critique. In busy emergency or casualty departments, carving out the necessary few minutes can be difficult. The lead physician, however, should assume responsibility to gather as many team members as possible for at least a pause to reflect. This debriefing provides feedback to prehospital and in-hospital personnel, gives a safe venue to express grieving, and provides an opportunity for education. Table 1 provides information on critical incident stress debriefing.

An alternative approach to critical stress debriefing is presented by Kenneth V. Iserson, MD, in his book *Pocket Protocols: Notifying Survivors About Sudden, Unexpected Deaths,*[4] from which the excerpt in Table 2 is adapted.

Family Presence in the Resuscitation Area

In a number of countries, hospitals have begun to allow family members and loved ones to remain in the resuscitation suite during procedures and actual resuscitative efforts. Evaluations of these programs, pioneered by critical care and emergency nurses, have confirmed a remarkable level of approval and gratitude by participating family members.

TABLE 1. Recommendations for Resuscitation Team Critique and Debriefing

Ask team members to assemble soon after the event. With few exceptions all team members should be present.

Gather the group in a private place if possible. Use the resuscitation room if available. State the purpose: "*We want to have a brief review (debriefing) of our resuscitative attempt.*"

Start with a review of the events and conduct of the code. "Let's start from the arrival of the paramedics. Could (nurse) review our sequence of interventions?"

State the algorithm or protocol that should have been followed; discuss what was actually done; discuss why there were any variations. "*So this was an out-of-hospital VF arrest treated by the medics. When we assumed care, what protocol was indicated? How well did we do?*"

Analyze the decisions and actions that were done correctly and effectively. Discuss decisions that may have been incorrect; discuss any actions that were performed less than optimally. Allow free discussion. "*When the patient's pulse was restored it seemed like everyone left the room. Only (nurse) was in the room when Mr. (patient) rearrested. Who wants to explain that delay?*"

All team members should share their feelings, anxieties, anger, and possible guilt. "I feel upset because when the admitting team arrived they were really obnoxious, demanding a lot of tests and x-rays. They made me feel that we had done a bad job."

Ask for recommendations or suggestions for future resuscitative attempts. "How can we do this better the next time?" (Nurse:) "I think we should not call the admitting team until the patient is completely stable and ready to go upstairs."

Inform team members unable to attend the debriefing of the process followed, the discussion generated, and the recommendations made. "*Chuck, we are going to implement that plan to allow family members in the code room during the resuscitation. I know you have been opposed to that. What if we designate our social worker to stay at the side of the family members the entire time they are near the resuscitation?*"

The team leader should encourage team members to contact him or her if questions arise later.

These evaluations, mostly in pediatric cases, have noted significant reduction in posttraumatic stress and self-reports of a greater sense of resolution and fulfillment. In the 2000 pediatric resuscitation guidelines, family presence in the resuscitation area has a Class IIb positive recommendation. Provision must be made for a professional to accompany the family members during these observed attempts, to direct positioning, to answer questions, and to explain procedures. In addition, the accompanying professional can observe for signs of acute discomfort in the family members and can end the observations.

We lack sufficient evidence about family presence during adult resuscitations, but this is simply due to an absence of research in adults. Success in such programs for adults is predictable, provided that the professionals involved demonstrate the same high level of care and concern as shown by nurses and social workers involved in pediatric resuscitative attempts.

Ethics and the Clinical Practice of BLS and ACLS: Do Resuscitation Efforts "Fail"?

Of major importance, but often neglected in the rush to learn all of advanced resuscitation training, we must not forget the

TABLE 2. Critical Incident Stress Debriefing of Professionals: A Simplified Protocol

There are 4 sequential aspects to critical incident stress debriefing (CISD). These are the on-scene debriefing, the initial defusing, the formal CISD, and the follow-up CISD. Not all 4 aspects are always used, however.

On-Scene or Near-Scene Debriefing

This is performed by an officer, chaplain, or health professional knowledgeable in both CISD and the operations of the team. This individual primarily watches for the development of any signs of acute stress reactions. Rather than a formal debriefing, it is mainly a period of aware observation.

Initial Defusing

Performed within a few hours of the incident, this is a situation in which participants have an opportunity to discuss their feelings and reactions in a positive and supportive atmosphere. This discussion may be led by a senior officer or health professional familiar with CISD who has good interpersonal skills, or it may have no leader at all and be a spontaneous interaction among team members. It is best done through a mandatory team meeting.

The key to success at this stage is to maintain a supportive rather than a critical atmosphere, to keep comments confidential, and to ban comments that are tough, insensitive, or could be construed as "gallows humor." If this is not done, it will quickly end any sharing feelings among team members.

Formal CISD

Typically led by a mental health professional familiar with CISD, these formal sessions are held within 24 to 48 hours after the incident. Specially trained public and private CISD teams now exist throughout the United States, Canada, and in many other countries. Many of these are associated with local or regional police or fire departments (who can also be contacted to locate other competent teams).

These sessions often follow a standard format by first laying out the noncritique and confidentiality ground rules. Then the participants are asked to describe themselves and key activities during the incident, their feelings during the incident and at present, and any unusual symptoms they experienced or are experiencing.

Participants may be asked to explore linkages between the event and past events, nonjudgmentally describe others' actions (to help describe their own actions), and describe their own and the group's successes during the incident. The facilitator then describes typical posttraumatic stress disorder (PTSD) symptoms and finally suggests an activity to help them regain a sense of purpose and unity (such as attending the memorial service for the victims). During this session, the leader also tries to identify those who may need more intensive counseling.

Follow-Up CISD

Not always or even frequently done, these sessions are held from several weeks to months after the incident. They can be held to resolve specific group issues or more often to help specific individuals. (When held on an individual basis, these are essentially psychological counseling sessions.)

Groups who will encounter events triggering PTSD in the course of their work must have this service available *before* it is needed. Individuals providing these counseling services may themselves be subject to PTSD, and, if so, should also undergo debriefing.

Additional Resources

For more information to assist professionals working with PTSD victims, contact the National Center of PTSD at telephone 802-296-5132, e-mail ptsd@dartmouth.edu, or website http://www.dartmouth.edu/dms/ptsd/Clinicians.htm or the Post Traumatic Stress Resources web page at http://www.long-beach-va-gov/ptsd/stress.htm.

From *Pocket Protocols—Notifying Survivors About Sudden, Unexpected Deaths*, pages 64–65. ©1999 by Kenneth V. Iserson, MD, and published by Galen Press, Ltd, Tucson, AZ, www.galenpress.com.

TABLE 3. Conveying News of a Sudden Death to Family Members

Call the family if they have not been notified. Explain that their relative has been admitted to the Emergency Department and that the situation is serious. Survivors should not be told of the death over the telephone.

Obtain as much information as possible about the patient and the circumstances surrounding the death. Carefully go over the events as they happened in the Emergency Department.

Ask someone to take family members to a private area. Walk in, introduce yourself, and sit down. Address the closest relative.

Briefly describe the circumstances leading to the death. Go over the sequence of events in the Emergency Department. Avoid euphemisms such as "he's passed on," "she's no longer with us," or "he's left us." Instead, use specific phrases and words such as "death," "dying," or "dead." "Your mother died quietly, without suffering. . . ." "Her death was quiet and peaceful. . . ."

Allow time for the shock to be absorbed. Make eye contact, touch, and share. Convey your feelings with a phrase such as "You have my (our) sincere sympathy" rather than "I (we) are sorry."

Allow as much time as necessary for questions and discussion. Go over the events several times to make sure everything is understood and to facilitate further questions.

Allow the family the opportunity to see their relative. If equipment is still connected, let the family know.

Know in advance what happens next and who will sign the death certificate. Physicians may impose burdens on staff and family if they fail to understand policies about death certification and disposition of the body. Know the answers to these questions before meeting the family.

Enlist the aid of a social worker or the clergy if not already present.

Offer to contact the patient's attending or family physician and to be available if there are further questions. Arrange for follow-up and continued support during the grieving period.

resuscitation team and team members, as well as the surviving friends and relatives. As soon as you declare death for the arrest victim, you immediately acquire a new set of patients—the family, friends, and loved ones of the person who dies (see Table 3).

Remember that when the heart or brain of a person in arrest cannot be restarted, do not use the word fail. The team did not *fail* to restore the heartbeat, nor did the heart itself *fail* to respond to the efforts. Instead think in terms of an attempt to restore a "*heart too good to die*"[5] rather than a "*heart too sick to live*."[6] At the start, however, the clinical reality is unknown; caregivers have no way of knowing the status of suddenly arrested hearts when they arrive on the scene of a cardiac emergency.

In the past we used the phrase "give a trial of CPR"; the only way to recognize "too good to die" versus "too sick to live" was to give the patient a rapid, aggressive evaluation period of BLS and ACLS. If spontaneous circulation did not return quickly, then we assumed that the verdict in the trial of CPR was "person at the end of his or her life." In such a situation continued resuscitative efforts are inappropriate, futile, undignified, and demeaning to both patient and rescuers. "Part 2: Ethical Aspects of CPR and ECC" provides an ethical framework with which to consider resuscitative efforts and presents specific recommendations for prehospital and in-hospital care providers.

References

1. Cummins RO, Chamberlain DA, Abramson NS, Allen M, Baskett P, Becker L, Bossaert L, Delooz H, Dick W, Eisenberg M, et al, Task Force of the American Heart Association, the European Resuscitation Council, the Heart and Stroke Foundation of Canada, and the Australian Resuscitation Council. Recommended guidelines for uniform reporting of data from out-of-hospital cardiac arrest: the Utstein Style [see comments]. *Ann Emerg Med*. 1991;20:861–874.
2. Cummins RO, Ornato JP, Thies WH, Pepe PE. Improving survival from sudden cardiac arrest: the "chain of survival" concept: a statement for health professionals from the Advanced Cardiac Life Support Subcommittee and the Emergency Cardiac Care Committee, American Heart Association. *Circulation*. 1991;83:1832–1847.
3. Burkle FM Jr, Rice MM. Code organization. *Am J Emerg Med*. 1987;5:235–239.
4. Iserson KV. *Pocket Protocols for Notifying Survivors About Sudden Unexpected Deaths*. Tuscon, Ariz: Galen Press, Ltd; 1999.
5. Beck C, Leighninger D. Reversal of death in good hearts. *J Cardiovasc Surg*. 1962;3:357–375.
6. Safar P, Bircher N. *Cardiopulmonary Cerebral Resuscitation: World Federation of Societies of Anaesthesiologists International CPCR Guidelines*. Philadelphia, Pa: WB Saunders Co; 1988.

7B: Understanding the Algorithm Approach to ACLS

Origin of the ACLS Algorithms

The first ACLS "algorithms" appeared in the 1986 ECC and CPR Guidelines.[1] These outlines of the 4 algorithms presented the interventions for the 4 arrest rhythms, using double-spaced lines of type connected by vertical arrows. Since those first primitive algorithms, diagrams have been a major tool to depict critical observations, critical actions, and critical decision points in resuscitation. Since 1986 similar algorithms have been published by the Resuscitation Councils of Europe (1992)[2,3] and in southern Africa (1995).[4-7] In the years since 1986 a variety of algorithmic approaches emerged. Differences have been in design and detail, not in science or clinical recommendations. Each set of ACLS algorithms contained information on the same general principles of resuscitation but presented it in a unique style with varying amounts of detail and very different target audiences.[4,5]

The Structure of the Algorithms

All resuscitation algorithms depict both *observation* and *action* steps. These steps typically alternate. The observation steps serve as a series of decision-making points or "decision nodes." You identify the problems present at the decision node and then select the proper action to take. The alternating *observation* and *decision* steps in the algorithms closely resemble the alternating "*assess-manage*" steps fundamental to emergency care and resuscitation.

In 2000 in this set of algorithms, we have given all *observational* boxes curved corners and all *action boxes* square corners. The treatment of every resuscitation emergency can be mapped into this assess-manage series of steps, with repeating loops and reassessment.

The Philosophy of the Algorithms

The algorithms have grown to mean different things to different resuscitation councils around the world. They mean different things to the training networks within those resuscitation councils. In some resuscitation councils the algorithms were designed to distill essential information about identification and treatment of a problem to its essence—such a concise display targets the novice practitioner and encourages the expert to provide his or her own detail or additional information. Such an approach was favored by Dr Walter Kloeck, National Chairman of the Resuscitation Councils of Southern Africa. Dr Kloeck's sparse, clean design aimed to depict the most common assessments and actions performed for the vast majority of patients. These algorithms were designed for the beginning or student learner of CPR, ECC, and ACLS. This elegantly simple style of teaching materials has come to dominate the teaching materials of many international resuscitation councils.[7]

At the same time, within the AHA the algorithms came to be used by instructors and experienced clinicians as teaching tools. The training network began to request inclusion of more and more detail to address a wider variety of clinical situations with more and more information for the clinician and for the ACLS instructor. These algorithms, although more complex, were thought to be more useful during actual resuscitations and more useful for teaching the scope of resuscitation practice.

Clearly, each approach—concise versus complex—has its merits. When the first international algorithms were developed for the ILCOR Advisory Statements, the differences in algorithmic approach became apparent.[8] Because the ILCOR advisory statements were evidence-based consensus documents, the algorithms that emerged there were spare. They were limited to those points of assessment and care on which there was absolute agreement.

The algorithms contained in the International Guidelines 2000 represent the second iteration of international algorithms, developed by science experts at the Evidence Evaluation Conference and at the Guidelines 2000 Conference. They represent a compromise between the concise approach of many international resuscitation councils and the detailed approach favored within the AHA. Details are provided within the text and in boxes pulled out of the main body of the algorithm.

Application of the Algorithms

These algorithms are designed to serve as an aide-mémoire, to remind the clinician of important aspects of assessment and therapy. They are *not* designed to be either comprehensive or limiting. The clinician should always determine whether the algorithm is appropriate for the patient and should be prepared to deviate from the algorithm if the patient's condition warrants. The algorithms should be thought of as a general recipe from a cherished grandmother—the general guiding principles are there, but the richness will be in the individual application. The algorithms may provide the recipe but they still require a "thinking cook" (see Table 4).

The algorithms are depicted in a sequential format. This is misleading, however, because in most resuscitation situations multiple care providers are present, and many assessments and interventions are accomplished simultaneously. Many of these algorithms contain notes on assessment and evaluation that should be considered throughout the resuscitation (eg, verify proper tracheal tube placement, identify and treat reversible causes).

Circulation. 2000;102(suppl I):I-140–I-141.
© 2000 American Heart Association, Inc.

Circulation is available at http://www.circulationaha.org

TABLE 4.   The Algorithm Approach to Emergency Cardiac Care

These guidelines use algorithms as an educational tool. They are an illustrative method to summarize information. Providers of emergency care should view algorithms as a summary and a memory aid. They provide a way to treat a broad range of patients. Algorithms, by nature, oversimplify. The effective teacher and care provider will use them wisely, not blindly. Some patients may require care not specified in the algorithms. When clinically appropriate, flexibility is accepted and encouraged. Many interventions and actions are listed as "considerations" to help providers think. These lists should not be considered endorsements or requirements or "standard of care" in a legal sense. Algorithms do not replace clinical understanding. Although the algorithms provide a good "cookbook," the patient always requires a "thinking cook."

The following clinical recommendations apply to all treatment algorithms:

- First, treat the patient, not the monitor.

Algorithms for cardiac arrest presume that the condition under discussion continually persists, that the patient remains in cardiac arrest, and that CPR is always performed.

- Apply different interventions whenever appropriate indications exist.
- The flow diagrams present mostly Class I (acceptable, definitely effective) recommendations. The footnotes present Class IIa (acceptable, probably effective), Class IIb (acceptable, possibly effective), and Class III (not indicated, may be harmful) recommendations.
- Adequate airway, ventilation, oxygenation, chest compressions, and defibrillation are more important than administration of medications and take precedence over initiating an intravenous line or injecting pharmacological agents.
- Several medications (epinephrine, lidocaine, and atropine) can be administered via the tracheal tube, but clinicians must use an endotracheal dose 2 to 2.5 times the intravenous dose.
- With a few exceptions, intravenous medications should always be administered rapidly, in bolus method.
- After each intravenous medication, give a 20- to 30-mL bolus of intravenous fluid and immediately elevate the extremity. This will enhance delivery of drugs to the central circulation, which may take 1 to 2 minutes.
- Last, treat the patient, not the monitor.

Learners and clinicians are not expected to memorize the algorithms in full detail. They are expected to consult the algorithms. It is hoped that copies of these algorithms will be available at courses and written evaluations for courses. The rationale for this approach is realistic and professional, based on established principles of adult education. The clinician should know where to find appropriate information and how to apply it. The algorithms are intended to lead the clinician along the path of assessment and intervention during the resuscitation experience.

References

1. American Heart Association. Standards and guidelines for cardiopulmonary resuscitation and emergency cardiac care, I: introduction. *JAMA.* 1986;255:2905–2914.
2. Holmberg S, Handley A, Bahr J, Baskett P, Bossaert L, et al. Guidelines for basic life support. *Resuscitation.* 1992;24:103–110.
3. Chamberlain D, Bossaert L, Carli P, Edgren E, Hapnes S, et al. Guidelines for adult advanced cardiac life support: a statement by the advanced life support working party of the European Resuscitation Council. *Resuscitation.* 1992;24:111–121.
4. Kloeck WG. A practical approach to the aetiology of pulseless electrical activity: a simple 10-step training mnemonic. *Resuscitation.* 1995;30:157–159.
5. Kloeck WG. Basic cardiopulmonary resuscitation techniques: national consensus achieved. *S Afr Med J.* 1990;77:259–261.
6. Kloeck WGJ. New recommendations for basic life support in adults, children and infants. *Trauma Emerg Med.* 1993;10:738–749.
7. Kloeck W. Advanced cardiac life support for adults and children. *Trauma Emerg Med.* 1993;10:757–773.
8. Cummins RO, Chamberlain DA. Advisory statements of the International Liaison Committee on Resuscitation. *Circulation.* 1997;95:2172–2173.

7C: A Guide to the International ACLS Algorithms

Summary/Overview

The ILCOR algorithm presents the actions to take and decisions to face for all people who appear to be in cardiac arrest—unconscious, unresponsive, without signs of life. The victim is not breathing normally, and no rescuer can feel a carotid pulse within 10 to 15 seconds. Since 1992 the resuscitation community has examined and reconfirmed the wisdom of most recommendations formulated by international groups through the 1990s. Sophisticated clinical trials provided high-level evidence on which to base several new drugs and interventions. Finally, we have learned that we should continue to place a strong emphasis after 2000 on building a base of critically appraised, international scientific evidence. Evidence-based review opened many eyes; only a small proportion of resuscitation care rests on a base of solid evidence.

Note: The numbers below, such as "1 (Figure 1)," match numbers in the algorithms.

Figure 1: ILCOR Universal/International ACLS Algorithm

Figure 1, the ILCOR Universal/International ACLS Algorithm, and Figure 2, the Comprehensive ECC Algorithm, are groundbreaking efforts to unify and simplify the essential information of adult ACLS. They demonstrate the integration of the steps of BLS, early defibrillation, and ACLS.

The ILCOR algorithm (Figure 1) shows how simply the overall approach can be presented, with minimum elaboration of separate steps. The Comprehensive ECC Algorithm (Figure 2) provides more details, particularly to support the AHA teaching approach based on the Primary and Secondary ABCD Surveys. Both algorithms depict many of the concepts and interventions that are new since 1992.

Notes to the ILCOR Universal/International ACLS Algorithm

1 (Figure 1)
BLS algorithm. The simple instruction "BLS algorithm" directs the rescuers to start the 6 basic steps of the international BLS algorithm:

1. Check responsiveness
2. Open the airway
3. Check breathing
4. Give 2 effective breaths
5. Assess circulation
6. Compress chest (no signs of circulation detected)

Note that step 6 does not use the term "pulse." In their 1998 BLS guidelines, the European Resuscitation Council and several ILCOR councils dropped a specific reference in their algorithms to "check the carotid pulse." They replaced the pulse check with a direction to "check for signs of circulation," namely, "look for any movement, including swallowing or breathing (more than an occasional gasp)." Their guidelines instruct rescuers to "check for the carotid pulse" as one of the "signs of circulation," but the pulse check does not receive the prominent emphasis that comes from inclusion in the algorithm. By 2000 many locations had confirmed the success of this European approach. Additional evidence had accumulated that the pulse check was not a good diagnostic test for the presence or absence of a beating heart. After international panels of experts reviewed the evidence at the Guidelines 2000 Conference, they also endorsed the approach of omitting the pulse check for lay responders from the International Guidelines 2000.

2 (Figure 1)
Attach defibrillator/monitor; assess rhythm. Once the responders start the BLS algorithm, they are directed to attach the defibrillator/monitor and assess the rhythm.

3 (Figure 1)
VF/pulseless VT. If they are using a conventional defibrillator and the monitor displays VF, the rescuers attempt defibrillation, up to 3 times as necessary. If using an AED, the rescuers follow the signal and voice prompts of the device, attempting defibrillation with up to 3 shocks. After 3 shocks they should immediately resume CPR for at least 1 minute. At the end of the minute, they should repeat rhythm assessment and shock when appropriate.

4 (Figure 1)
Non-VF rhythm. If the conventional defibrillator/monitor displays a non-VF tracing or the AED signals "no shock indicated," the responders should immediately check the pulse to determine whether the nonshockable rhythm is producing a spontaneous circulation. If not, then start CPR; continue CPR for approximately 3 minutes. With a non-VF rhythm the rescuer needs to return and recheck the rhythm for recurrent VF or for spontaneous return of an organized rhythm in a beating heart. At this point the algorithm enters the central column of comments.

5 (Figure 1)
During CPR: tracheal tube placement; IV access. In this period the rescuers have many tasks to accomplish. The central column includes the major interventions of ACLS: placing and confirming a tracheal tube, starting an IV, giving appropriate medications for the rhythm, and searching for and correcting reversible causes. Note that the ECC Comprehensive Algorithm (Figure 2) conveys this same approach using the memory aid of the Secondary ABCD

Circulation. **2000;102(suppl I):I-142–I-157.**
© 2000 American Heart Association, Inc.

Circulation is available at http://www.circulationaha.org

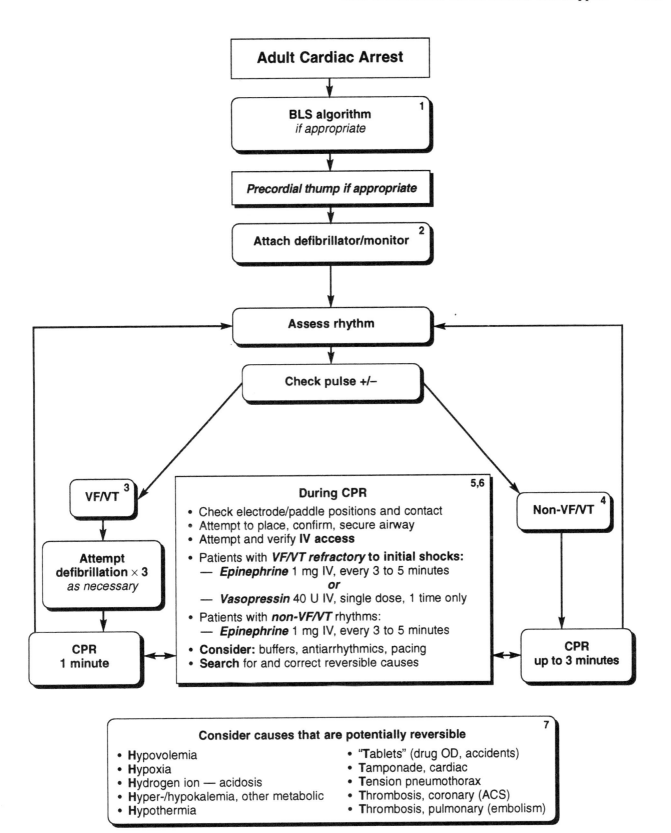

Figure 1. ILCOR Universal/International ACLS Algorithm.

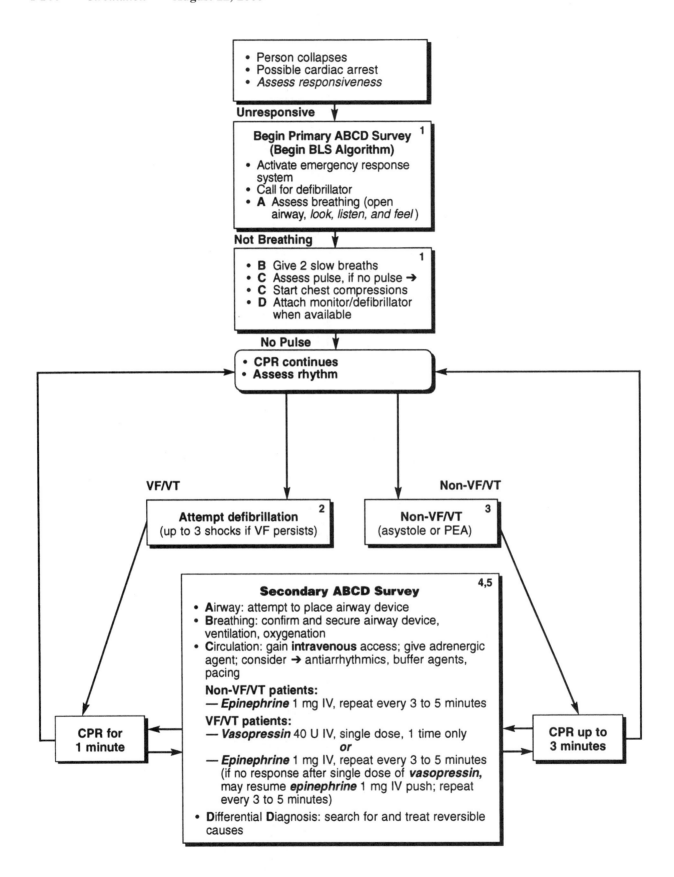

Figure 2. Comprehensive ECC Algorithm.

Survey. In this survey A=advanced airway (tracheal tube placement); B=confirmation of tube location, oxygenation, and ventilation; and C=circulation access via IV line and circulation medications.

6 (Figure 1)
VF/VT refractory to initial shocks: epinephrine or vasopressin. The ILCOR Universal Algorithm indicates that response personnel give all cardiac arrest patients a strong vasopressor, either epinephrine IV or vasopressin. This recommendation for vasopressin is one of the more interesting new guidelines. The discussions on adding amiodarone are detailed later in this section.

Consider buffers, antiarrhythmics, pacing, atropine; search for and correct reversible causes. This short phrase covers a multitude of interventions discussed and debated during the Evidence Evaluation Conference and the international Guidelines 2000 Conference: multiple antiarrhythmics, neutralization of acidosis, and transcutaneous pacing. The word "consider" has become an informal code in the resuscitation community interpreted to mean that we lack the evidence that establishes one intervention as superior to another. Whether this means that two interventions are equally effective or equally ineffective is a debate being waged constantly in resuscitation research.

7 (Figure 1)
Consider causes that are potentially reversible. This guideline applies primarily to non-VF/VT patients. For this group there is often a specific cause of the loss of an effective heartbeat. The International Guidelines 2000 take the innovative step of listing the 10 most common reversible causes of non-VF/VT arrest at the bottom of the algorithm. This is discussed in detail in the section on pulseless electrical activity.

End of Algorithm Notes

Figure 2: Comprehensive ECC Algorithm

Both the ILCOR Universal Algorithm and the Comprehensive ECC Algorithm (Figure 2) convey the concept that all cardiac arrest victims are in 1 of 2 "rhythms": VF/VT rhythms and non-VF rhythms.

- Non-VF comprises asystole and PEA, which are treated alike.
- Therefore, there is no critical need to separate the subjects into VF, pulseless VT, PEA, or asystole.

All cardiac arrest victims receive the same 4 treatments

- CPR
- Tracheal intubation
- Vasoconstrictors
- Antiarrhythmics

The only distinguishing treatment for arrest victims is that rescuers treat VF/VT patients with defibrillatory shocks.

The algorithms in Figures 1 and 2 demonstrate a simple concept. The ILCOR Universal Algorithm and the Comprehensive ECC Algorithm are the only teaching/learning displays rescuers will need because they treat everyone in cardiac arrest this way.

Notes to the Comprehensive ECC Algorithm
1 (Figure 2)
Begin Primary ABCD Survey. Unresponsive; not breathing. Boxes 1 and 2 cover the steps of the BLS Algorithm and cover the *Primary ABCD Survey*. The survey is a memory aid and conveys no therapeutic value as stated and displayed. The Primary and Secondary ABCD Surveys are simple mnemonics that assist initial learning. They also provide a useful mental "hook" for later review and recall. Listing more details within the algorithm provides easy review of the steps, especially when the learner has not participated routinely in actual resuscitation attempts.

2 (Figure 2)
VF/VT: attempt defibrillation (up to 3 shocks if VF persists). Rhythm assessment and continued CPR are at the center of the Comprehensive ECC Algorithm. The metaphor of a clock ticking away for a cardiac arrest victim in VF is overused but accurate. With each minute of persistent VF, the probability of survival declines. Two clocks are racing. One is the clock that measures the *therapeutic interval* (from collapse to arrival of the defibrillator). One is the clock that measures the *irreversible damage interval* (from cessation of blood flow to the brain to the start of permanent, irreversible brain death).

Here is an observation that will put the racing clocks into perspective. Several experts have observed that great amounts of time and money are spent on the development of new defibrillation waveforms, novel antiarrhythmics, innovative vasopressors, and fresh approaches to ventilation and oxygenation. The total combined effect on survival of these interventions is equivalent to nothing more than cutting the interval from collapse to defibrillatory shock by 2 minutes.[1]

3 (Figure 2)
Non-VF/VT. The ILCOR recommendation is to consider the non-VF/VT rhythms as one rhythm when the patient is in cardiac arrest. Consider non-VF/VT as either asystole or PEA. The treatment in the algorithm is the same for both: epinephrine, atropine, transcutaneous pacing. Electrical activity on the monitor screen is a more positive rhythm than asystole. Later in this discussion PEA and asystole are presented in much greater detail.

Both rhythms have a "differential diagnosis" in terms of what entities can produce a PEA and an asystolic rhythm. Responders must aggressively evaluate PEA victims to discover a potential reversible cause. There is a narrow diagnostic interval of just a few minutes at the discovery of PEA. Asystole, on the other hand, is rarely salvaged unless a reversible cause (eg, severe hyperkalemia, overdose of phenothiazine) is found. Only occasionally does asystole respond to epinephrine in higher doses, atropine, or pacing, because the patient is simply destined to die, given the nature of the original precipitating event.

4 (Figure 2)
Secondary ABCD Survey. Use of a vasopressor: epinephrine for non-VF/VT, vasopressin for refractory VF. This section of the algorithm makes the same points about persistent arrest from VF/VT and non-VF/VT as the ILCOR Universal Algorithm. The ECC Comprehensive Algorithm, however, uses the memory aid of the Secondary ABCD Survey, a device repeated in all the cardiac arrest algorithms. The algorithm notes expand on these concepts.

**Primary ABCD Survey
(Begin BLS Algorithm)**

Activate emergency response system

Call for defibrillator

A Airway: open airway; assess breathing (open airway, look, listen, feel)

B Breathing: give 2 slow breaths

C CPR: check pulse; if no pulse →

C Start **C**hest **C**ompressions

D Defibrillator: attach AED or monitor/defibrillator when available

Secondary ABCD Survey

A Intubate as soon as possible

B Confirm tube placement; use 2 methods to confirm

- Primary physical examination criteria *plus*
- Secondary confirmation device (qualitative and quantitative measures of end-tidal CO_2)

B Secure tracheal tube

- Prevent dislodgment; purpose-made tracheal tube holders recommended over tie-and-tape approaches

- If the patient is at risk for transport movement, cervical collar and backboard are recommended

B Confirm initial oxygenation and ventilation

- End-tidal CO_2 monitor
- Oxygen saturation monitor

C Oxygen, IV, monitor, fluids →
   rhythm appropriate medications

C Vital signs: temperature, blood pressure, heart rate, respirations

D Differential Diagnoses

Note: The primary and secondary ABCD action surveys above are slightly different from the surveys in other algorithms. In subsequent algorithms the wording of the Primary and Secondary ABCD Surveys is identical. The difference in wording between the first 2 algorithms and the later algorithms allows the learners to see that the overall concept is more important than "getting the algorithm exactly right." Review these 2 surveys for Figure 2. Notice the way in which the vocabulary of the survey changes but the overall content of the survey does not change. People learn in different styles and remember by different techniques. Understanding is more important than repetition.

5 (Figure 2)

Potentially reversible causes. Sudden VF/VT arrests are straightforward in their management. Management consists of early defibrillation, which can succeed independently of other interventions and independently of discovery of the cause of the arrhythmia. With non-VF/VT arrest, however, successful restoration of a spontaneous pulse depends almost entirely on recognizing and treating a potentially reversible cause. As an aide mémoire, Figure 1 places the following list, referred to as "the 5 H's and 5 T's," in the algorithm layout:

The "5 H's"

- Hypovolemia
- Hypoxia
- Hydrogen ion (acidosis)
- Hyperkalemia/hypokalemia and metabolic disorders
- Hypothermia/hyperthermia

The "5 T's"

- Toxins/tablets (drug overdose, illicit drugs)
- Tamponade, cardiac
- Tension pneumothorax
- Thrombosis, coronary
- Thrombosis, pulmonary

Figure 2, the Comprehensive ECC Algorithm, expands the table of reversible causes by listing possible therapeutic interventions next to each of the potential causes.

Consider: Is one of the following conditions playing a role?

Hypovolemia (volume infusion)

Hypoxia (oxygen, ventilation)

Hydrogen ion—acidosis (buffer, ventilation)

Hyperkalemia (CaCl plus others)

Hypothermia (see Hypothermia Algorithm in Part 8)

"Tablets" (drug overdoses, accidents)

Tamponade, cardiac (pericardiocentesis)

Tension pneumothorax (decompress—needle decompression)

Thrombosis, coronary (fibrinolytics)

Thrombosis, pulmonary (fibrinolytics, surgical evacuation)

End of Algorithm Notes

Newly Recommended Agent: Vasopressin for VF/VT

People knowledgeable about the ACLS recommendations during the 1990s will immediately notice that the recommendations for the requisite vasoconstrictor, epinephrine, have changed. The first 3 algorithms—the ILCOR Universal Algorithm, the Comprehensive ECC Algorithm, and Ventricular Fibrillation—each contain the same recommendation for vasopressin as an adrenergic agent equivalent to epinephrine for VF/VT cardiac arrest.

This is one of the most important new recommendations in the International Guidelines 2000. Vasopressin, the natural substance antidiuretic hormone, becomes a powerful vasoconstrictor when used at much higher doses than normally present in the body. Vasopressin possesses positive effects that duplicate the positive effects of epinephrine. Vasopressin does not duplicate the adverse effects of epinephrine. (See "Pharmacology II: Agents to Optimize Cardiac Output and Blood Pressure" for more detailed material on vasopressin.)

Vasopressin received a Class IIb recommendation (acceptable, not harmful, supported by fair evidence) from the panel of international experts on adrenergics. Notice that vasopressin is recommended as a single, 1-time dose in humans. Vasopressin requires less frequent administration because the 10- to 20-minute half-life of vasopressin is much greater than the 3- to 5-minute half-life of epinephrine.

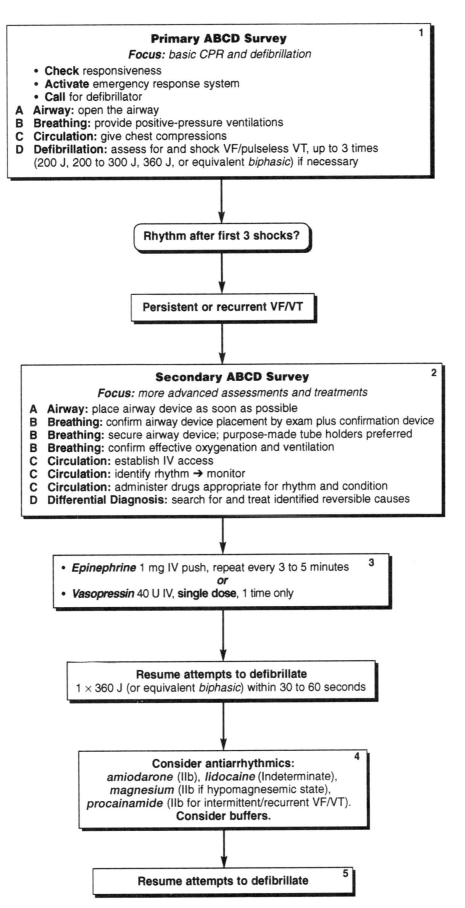

Figure 3. Ventricular Fibrillation/Pulseless VT Algorithm.

After the single dose of vasopressin, the algorithms allow a return to epinephrine if there is no clinical response to vasopressin. This return to epinephrine has no specific human evidence to provide support, although at least 1 clinical trial in Europe is under way. In an informal poll of the experts on the adrenergic panel, every person accepted this recommendation to return to epinephrine after 10 to 20 minutes. (The possibility of a second dose of vasopressin in 10 to 20 minutes was discussed and seems rational. However, this was listed as a Class Indeterminate recommendation because we lack research in humans that addresses this question.)

The rather imprecise time range between the dose of vasopressin and the administration of subsequent epinephrine allows flexibility in the decisions about when to give subsequent adrenergics. The dilemma is: give too soon and cause adverse effects from excessive vasopressin; give too late and the chances of a positive outcome vanish.

Primary and Secondary ABCD Surveys

In some locations, particularly in courses for ACLS providers, the learners are taught a memory aid called the Primary and Secondary ABCD Surveys. These 8 steps apply to all cardiovascular-cardiopulmonary emergencies. Course directors crafted the ABCD surveys to help ACLS providers remember the specific action steps. By memorizing the 2 surveys, ACLS students learn specific actions in a specific sequence. The surveys use the familiar mnemonic of the first 4 letters of the alphabet, and they maintain the traditional actions associated with those 4 letters:

A=Airway

B=Breathing

C=Circulation

D=Defibrillation (or Differential Diagnosis in the Secondary ABCD Survey)

Because repetition is a well-documented aid to learning, the elements of the Primary and Secondary ABCD Surveys are repeated in several other algorithms: VF/VT, PEA, and asystole.

Figure 3, VF/pulseless VT, conveys more details about the Secondary ABCD Survey:

A=Airway control with endotracheal intubation

B=Breathing effectively: verify with primary and secondary confirmation of proper tube placement

C=Circulation, which incorporates vital signs, ECG monitoring, access to the circulation via IV lines, and then administration of rhythm-appropriate medications

D=Differential Diagnosis

A directive to "consider the differential diagnoses" improves the resuscitation protocols, because this is a recommendation to stop and think: What caused this arrest? With the addition of this step, resuscitation teams will identify more cardiac arrests with reversible causes. Although we lack evidence that supports use of this memory aid, its use has the strong appeal of common sense.

The Secondary ABCD Survey in Figure 2 states perhaps the most important new recommendations for out-of-hospital care providers.

- We make stronger and more explicit recommendations to confirm tracheal tube placement.
- We recommend that resuscitation personnel take specific actions to prevent tube dislodgment after an initial correct placement.

During the years 1999 to 2000, publications about out-of-hospital pediatric resuscitation documented high rates of tube dislodgment. The researchers discovered that on arrival and evaluation in the Emergency Department, 8% to 12% of tracheal tubes were in the esophagus or hypopharynx. Given the study design, researchers were unable to determine whether these possibly lethal mishaps were due to incorrect initial tube placement or dislodgment after placement. This information has heightened concerns that ACLS providers may be committing undetected harm while performing our most critical interventions.

Figure 3: VF/Pulseless VT

Figure 3 covers the treatment of VF/pulseless VT in more depth than Figures 1 and 2. Figure 3 was created as a teaching aid to convey specific details about the Primary and Secondary ABCD Surveys. The treatments outlined in Figures 1, 2, and 3 are identical: CPR, defibrillation if VF/VT, advanced airway control, intravenous access, rhythm-appropriate medications.

Always Assume VF (Figures 1 Through 3)

Note that Figure 1, the ILCOR Universal ACLS Algorithm, Figure 2, the ECC Comprehensive Algorithm, and Figure 3, the Ventricular Fibrillation/Pulseless VT Algorithm, state this precept unequivocally: rescuers must assume that all *adult* sudden cardiac arrests are caused by VF/pulseless VT. All training efforts therefore place a strong emphasis on immediate recognition and treatment of VF/pulseless VT. Proper treatment with early defibrillatory shocks allows VF/pulseless VT to provide the majority of adult cardiac arrest survivors. Several mature EMS systems, such as Seattle/King County, Washington, USA, have collected data for >25 years. Year after year VF/VT contributes 85% to 95% of the survivors.

Energy Levels for Shock and Defibrillation Waveforms

The appearance of biphasic waveform defibrillators has generated great enthusiasm in the resuscitation community. Reaching EMS organizations in 1996, the first biphasic defibrillator approved for market shocked at only 1 energy level, approximately 170 J. Competitive market forces stirred up considerable controversy over the efficacy of biphasic waveform shocks in general and nonescalating energy levels in particular. This unseemly chapter in the history of medical device manufacturers has been reviewed in detail in a Medical Scientific Statement from the Senior Science Editors and the chairs of the ECC subcommittees.[1] Biphasic waveform defibrillators are *conditionally acceptable*—regardless of initial shock energy level and regardless of the energy level of subsequent shocks (nonescalating). The condition that must be met is clinical data that confirms equivalent or superior effectiveness to monophasic defibrillators when used in the same clinical context. For example, to meet this condition manufacturers cannot compare rescue defibrillatory shocks delivered to a fibrillating heart in the Electrophysiology Stimulation Laboratory versus defibrillatory shocks delivered to patients with 12-minute-old VF in the absence of CPR efforts from bystanders. (See "Defibrillation" in Part 6 for more detail on waveforms and energy levels.) The International Guidelines 2000 panel experts, the ILCOR representatives, and other delegates thought that the class of recommendation for biphasic shocks, nonescalating energy levels, should be upgraded from Class IIb in 1998 to Class IIa in 2000.

CPR, VF, and Defibrillation

After 3 unsuccessful attempts to achieve defibrillation, the first 3 algorithms instruct rescuers to provide approximately 1 minute of CPR. This produces some reoxygenation of the blood and some circulation of this blood to the heart and brain. The precise effect of this minute of CPR on refractory VF is unclear.

Stimulated by the 1999 publication of a retrospective analysis of out-of-hospital cardiac arrest data from the Seattle, Washington, EMS system, the Evidence Evaluation Conference (September 1999) included this topic on its agenda. The EMS personnel initially used a protocol in which arriving EMTs attached an AED and analyzed and shocked any VF rhythms as quickly as possible. Later the protocol directed the EMTs to perform 60 to 90 seconds of CPR before attaching the AED and shocking VF. The survival rates to hospital discharge were significantly higher during the period of prescribed preshock CPR. Other experts argued that a fibrillating myocardium suffers unrelenting deterioration as long as VF continues, CPR or no CPR. A minute or so of preshock CPR does not prevent this deterioration. This guideline recommendation was classed as Indeterminate because the quality and amount of evidence, on both sides of the question, were at lower levels: retrospective data (Level 5) and extrapolation of data from other sources (Level 7), particularly animal studies (Level 6).

Diminishing Roles for Drugs in VF Arrest

The ILCOR Universal Algorithm, the Comprehensive ECC Algorithm, and similar comments in Figure 3 relegate adrenergic agents, antiarrhythmic agents, and buffer therapy to secondary roles for both VF and non-VF patients. This secondary role applies to time-honored agents such as epinephrine, lidocaine, procainamide, and buffer agents and to newly available agents such as amiodarone. Meticulous, systematic review reveals that relevant, valid, and credible evidence to confirm a benefit due to these agents simply does not exist. This does not mean that resuscitation drugs were selected capriciously by the pioneers of resuscitation decades ago. They applied common sense,

rational conjecture, and extrapolations from animal studies to arrive at the antiarrhythmics used over the past decade. If an agent is shown in animal models to *raise* the *fibrillation threshold* and *lower the defibrillation threshold*, then a reasonable assumption would be that the drug would facilitate defibrillation of the human heart to a perfusing rhythm. This sort of rational conjecture produced the rather eclectic groups of drugs that have stocked resuscitation kits for more than a decade.

In addition, it was not until the 1990s that researchers discovered the dismal truth that antiarrhythmic drugs were acting more like proarrhythmic agents. Drugs given to prevent VF/VT arrest appear to generate VF/VT arrest. With critical reappraisal these disturbing discoveries undermined the validity and credibility of scores of excellently designed and executed studies. Through the use of critical appraisal, most researchers in this area realized that the only proper evaluation of new resuscitation agents had to be prospective, randomized clinical trials in which the only acceptable control group had to be placebo.

Designs of studies of new drugs versus standard therapy were unacceptable for the obvious reason—if both standard therapy and the new drug made cardiac arrest victims worse, we could never obtain valid results. The adverse effects would not be recognized unless one agent was significantly worse than the other. Ironically, the researchers would conclude that the less worse drug was actually a superior agent of positive benefit to patients. See "Pharmacology I: Agents for Arrhythmias" and "Pharmacology II: Agents to Optimize Cardiac Output and Blood Pressure" for more detailed material that supports these observations.

New Class of Recommendation for Epinephrine and Lidocaine: Indeterminate

An immense amount of animal research and lower-level human research exists on epinephrine in cardiac arrest. These projects are remarkable in the homogeneity of results—the findings are consistently and invariably *positive*. But almost no valid, consistent, and relevant human evidence exists to support epinephrine over placebo in human cardiac arrest. Clinical researchers have not conducted prospective, *placebo*-controlled, clinical trials in humans on this topic. Consequently, the international, evidence-based guidelines had to conclude that epinephrine was Class Indeterminate.

Similarly, no study has shown that lidocaine is effective as an agent to use in human arrest from refractory, shock-resistant VF. Our growing awareness of the *proarrhythmic* effects of *antiarrhythmics* now requires that researchers evaluate lidocaine and other antiarrhythmics against placebo, and not against some other antiarrhythmics. No clinical differences will be observed if 2 antiarrhythmics are equally ineffective or even equally harmful. At this time, therefore, lidocaine receives a Class Indeterminate recommendation.

Notes to Figure 3: VF/Pulseless VT Algorithm
Assume that VF/VT persists after each intervention.

1 (Figure 3)

Defibrillatory shock waveforms

- Use **monophasic shocks** at listed energy levels (300 J, 300 to 360 J, 360 J) or **biphasic shocks** at energy levels documented to be clinically equivalent (or superior) to the monophasic shocks.

2 (Figure 3)

2A Confirm tube placement with

- Primary physical examination criteria *plus*
- Secondary confirmation device (end-tidal CO_2, end-diastolic diameter) (Class IIa)

2B Secure tracheal tube

- To prevent dislodgment, especially in patients at risk for movement, use purpose-made (commercially available) tracheal tube holders, which are superior to tie-and-tape methods (Class IIb)
- Consider cervical collar and backboard for transport (Class Indeterminate)
- Consider continuous, quantitative end-tidal CO_2 monitor (Class IIa)

2C Confirm oxygenation and ventilation with

- End-tidal CO_2 monitor *and*
- Oxygen saturation monitor

3 (Figure 3)

3A *Epinephrine* (Class Indeterminate) 1 mg IV push every 3 to 5 minutes. If this fails, higher doses of epinephrine (up to 0.2 mg/kg) are acceptable but not recommended (there is growing evidence that it may be harmful).

3B *Vasopressin* is recommended only for VF/VT; there is no evidence to support its use in asystole or PEA. There is no evidence about the value of repeat vasopressin doses. There is no evidence about the best approach if there is no response after a single bolus of vasopressin. The following Class Indeterminate action is acceptable, but only on the basis of rational conjecture. If there is no response 5 to 10 minutes after a single IV dose of vasopressin, it is *acceptable* to resume epinephrine 1 mg IV push every 3 to 5 minutes.

4 (Figure 3)

4A *Antiarrhythmics* are indeterminate or Class IIb: acceptable; only fair evidence supports possible benefit of antiarrhythmics for shock-refractory VF/VT.

- *Amiodarone* (Class IIb) 300 mg IV push (cardiac arrest dose). If VF/pulseless VT recurs, consider administration of a second dose of 150 mg IV. Maximum cumulative dose: 2.2 g over 24 hours.
- *Lidocaine* (Class Indeterminate) 1.0 to 1.5 mg/kg IV push. Consider repeat in 3 to 5 minutes to a maximum cumulative

dose of 3 mg/kg. A single dose of 1.5 mg/kg in cardiac arrest is acceptable.

- *Magnesium sulfate* 1 to 2 g IV in polymorphic VT (torsades de pointes) and suspected hypomagnesemic state.
- *Procainamide* 30 mg/min in refractory VF (maximum total dose: 17 mg/kg) is acceptable but not recommended because prolonged administration time is unsuitable for cardiac arrest.

4B *Sodium bicarbonate* 1 mEq/kg IV is indicated for several conditions known to provoke sudden cardiac arrest. See Notes in the Asystole and PEA Algorithms for details.

5 (Figure 3)

Resume defibrillation attempts: use 360-J (or equivalent biphasic) shocks after each medication or after each minute of CPR. Acceptable patterns: CPR-drug-shock (repeat) or CPR-drug-shock-shock-shock (repeat).

End of Algorithm Notes

Figure 4: Pulseless Electrical Activity

The absence of a detectable pulse and the presence of some type of electrical activity other than VT or VF defines this group of arrhythmias. When electrical activity is organized and no pulse is detectable, clinicians traditionally have used the term *electromechanical dissociation (EMD)*. This term, however, is too specific and narrow. Strictly speaking, EMD means that organized electrical depolarization occurs throughout the myocardium, but no synchronous shortening of the myocardial fiber occurs and mechanical contractions are absent.

In the early 1990s the international resuscitation community began to adopt the summary term *pulseless electrical activity (PEA)*. PEA would more accurately embrace a heterogeneous group of rhythms that includes pseudo-EMD, idioventricular rhythms, ventricular escape rhythms, postdefibrillation idioventricular rhythms, and bradyasystolic rhythms. Additional research with cardiac ultrasonography and indwelling pressure catheters has confirmed that often a pulseless patient with electrical activity also has associated mechanical contractions. These contractions are too weak to produce a blood pressure detectable by the usual methods of palpation or sphygmomanometry. Of utmost importance, ACLS providers must know that PEA is often associated with specific clinical states that can be reversed when identified early and treated appropriately.

Notes to Figure 4: Pulseless Electrical Activity
Both VF/VT and PEA are "rhythms of survival." People in VF/VT can be resuscitated by timely arrival of a defibrillator, and people in PEA can be resuscitated if a reversible cause of PEA is identified and treated appropriately. The PEA algorithm puts great emphasis on searching for specific, reversible causes of PEA. The algorithm features a table of the top 10 causes of PEA, arranged as the "5 H's and 5 T's." If reversible causes are not considered, rescuers will have little chance of recognition and successful treatment. Sodium bicarbonate provides a good example of how the cause of the PEA relates to the therapy. Sodium bicarbonate can vary between being a Class I intervention and being a Class III intervention, depending on the cause.

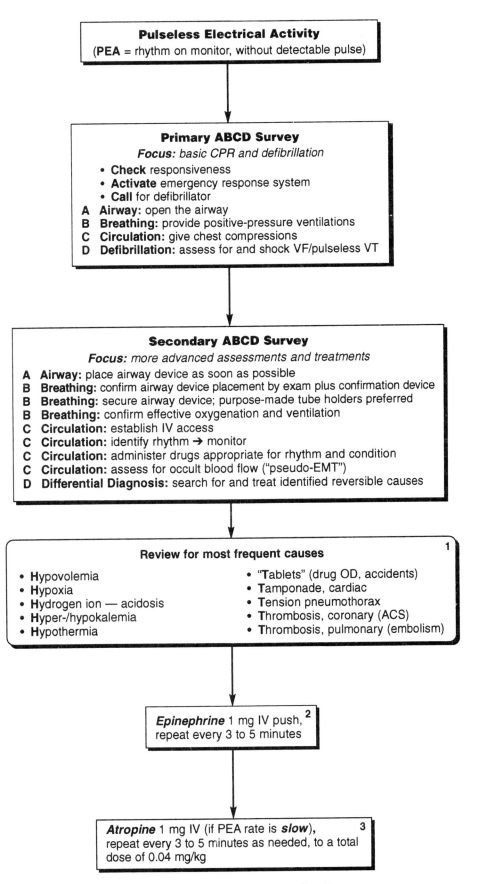

Figure 4. Pulseless Electrical Activity Algorithm.

1 (Figure 4)

Sodium bicarbonate 1 mEq/kg is used as follows:

Class I (acceptable, supported by definitive evidence)

- If patient has known, preexisting hyperkalemia

Class IIa (acceptable, good evidence supports)

- If known, preexisting bicarbonate-responsive acidosis
- In tricyclic antidepressant overdose
- To alkalinize urine in aspirin or other drug overdoses

Class IIb (acceptable, only fair evidence provides support)

- In intubated and ventilated patients with long arrest interval
- On return of circulation, after long arrest interval

May be harmful (Class III) in hypercarbic acidosis

2 (Figure 4)

Epinephrine: recommended dose is 1 mg IV push every 3 to 5 minutes (Class Indeterminate).

- If this approach fails, higher doses of epinephrine (up to 0.2 mg/kg) may be used but are not recommended.
- (Although one dose of vasopressin is acceptable for persistent or shock-refractory VF, we currently lack evidence to support routine use of vasopressin in victims of PEA or asystole.)

3 (Figure 4)

Atropine: the shorter atropine dose interval (every 3 to 5 minutes) is possibly helpful in cardiac arrest.

- ***Atropine*** 1 mg IV if electrical activity is *slow* (absolute bradycardia=rate <60 bpm) or
- ***Relatively slow*** (relative bradycardia=rate less than expected, relative to underlying condition)

End of Algorithm Notes

Other observed pulseless cardiac arrest arrhythmias are those in which the electrical activity (QRS complex) is wide versus narrow and fast versus slow. Most clinical studies have observed poor survival rates from PEA that is wide-complex and slow. These rhythms often indicate malfunction of the myocardium or the cardiac conduction system, such as occurs with massive AMI. These rhythms can represent the last electrical activity of a dying myocardium, or they may indicate specific critical rhythm disturbances. For example, severe hyperkalemia, hypothermia, hypoxia, preexisting acidosis, and a large variety of drug overdoses can be wide-complex PEAs. Overdoses of tricyclic antidepressants, β-blockers, calcium channel blockers, and digitalis will produce a slow, wide-complex PEA.

In contrast, a fast, narrow-complex PEA indicates a relatively normal heart responding exactly as it should for severe hypovolemia, infections, pulmonary emboli, or cardiac tamponade. These conditions have specific interventions.

The major action to take for a cardiac arrest victim in PEA is to search for possible causes. These rhythms are often a response to a specific condition, and helpful clues can appear if one simply looks at the electrical activity width and rate.

Hypovolemia is the most common cause of electrical activity without measurable blood pressure. Through prompt recognition and appropriate therapy, the many causes of hypovolemia can often be corrected, including hypovolemia from hemorrhage or from anaphylaxis-induced vasodilation. Other causes of PEA are cardiac tamponade, tension pneumothorax, and massive pulmonary embolism.

Nonspecific therapeutic interventions for PEA include epinephrine and (if the rate is slow) atropine, administered as presented in Figure 4. In addition, personnel should provide proper airway management and aggressive hyperventilation because hypoventilation and hypoxemia are frequent causes of PEA. Clinicians can give a fluid challenge because the PEA may be due to hypovolemia.

Immediate assessment of blood flow by Doppler ultrasound may reveal an actively contracting heart and significant blood flow. The blood pressure and flow, however, may fall below the threshold of detection by simple arterial palpation. Any PEA patient with a Doppler-detectable blood flow should be aggressively treated. These patients need volume expansion, norepinephrine, dopamine, or some combination of the three. They might benefit from early transcutaneous pacing because a healthy myocardium exists and only a temporarily disturbed cardiac conduction system stands between survival and death. Although in general PEA has poor outcomes, reversible causes should always be targeted and never missed when present.

Figure 5: Asystole: The Silent Heart Algorithm

Patients in cardiac arrest discovered on the defibrillator's monitor screen to be in asystole have a dismal rate of survival—usually as low as 1 or 2 people out of 100 cardiac arrests. During a resuscitation attempt, brief periods of an organized complex may appear on the monitor screen, but spontaneous circulation rarely emerges. As with PEA, the only hope for resuscitation of a person in asystole is to identify and treat a reversible cause.

Figure 5, the Asystole Algorithm, outlines an approach much more in keeping with our current understanding of the issues surrounding asystole. The Asystole Algorithm focuses on "not starting" and "when to stop." With prolonged, refractory asystole the patient is making the transition from life to death. ACLS providers who try to make that transition as sensitive and dignified as possible serve their patients well.

Notes to Figure 5: Asystole

1 (Figure 5)

Scene Survey: DNAR patient?

If Yes: do not start/attempt resuscitation. Any *objective* indicators of DNAR status? Bracelet? Anklet? Written documentation? Family statements? If Yes: do not start/attempt resuscitation.

- Any *clinical* indicators that resuscitation attempts are not indicated, eg, signs of death? If Yes: do not start/attempt resuscitation.

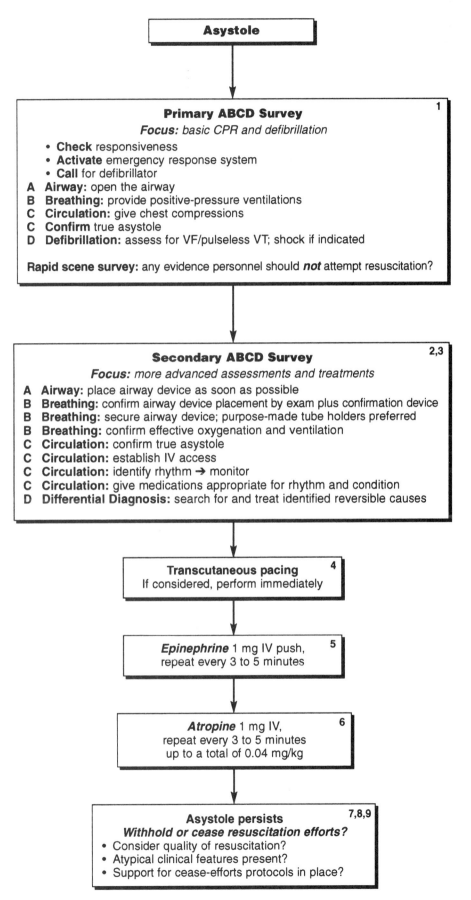

Figure 5. Asystole: The Silent Heart Algorithm.

2 (Figure 5)

Confirm true asystole

- Check lead and cable connections
- Monitor power on?
- Monitor gain up?
- Verify asystole in another lead?

3 (Figure 5)

Sodium bicarbonate 1 mEq/kg

- Indications for use include the following: overdose of tricyclic antidepressants; to alkalinize urine in overdoses; patients with tracheal intubation plus long arrest intervals; on return of spontaneous circulation if there is a long arrest interval.
- Ineffective or harmful in hypercarbic acidosis.

4 (Figure 5)

Transcutaneous pacing

- To be effective, must be performed early, combined with drug therapy. Evidence does not support routine use of transcutaneous pacing for asystole.

5 (Figure 5)

Epinephrine

- Recommended dose is 1 mg IV push every 3 to 5 minutes. If this approach fails, higher doses of epinephrine (up to 0.2 mg/kg) may be used but are not recommended.
- We currently lack evidence to support routine use of vasopressin in treatment of asystole.

6 (Figure 5)

Atropine

- Use the shorter dosing interval (every 3 to 5 minutes) in asystolic arrest.

7 (Figure 5)

Review the quality of the resuscitation attempt

- Was there an adequate trial of BLS? of ACLS? Has the team done the following:
- Achieved tracheal intubation?
- Performed effective ventilation?
- Shocked VF if present?
- Obtained IV access?
- Given epinephrine IV? atropine IV?
- Ruled out or corrected reversible causes?
- Continuously documented asystole >5 to 10 minutes after all of the above have been accomplished?

8 (Figure 5)

Reviewed for atypical clinical features?

- Not a victim of drowning or hypothermia?
- No reversible therapeutic or illicit drug overdose?
  - "Yes" to the questions in Notes 7 and 8 means the resuscitation team complies with recommended criteria to terminate resuscitative efforts where the patient lies (Class IIa)
  - If the response team and patient meet the above criteria, then withhold urgent field-to-hospital transport with continuing CPR=Class III (harmful; no benefit)

9 (Figure 5)

Withholding or stopping resuscitative efforts out-of-hospital

If criteria in 7 and 8 are fulfilled:

- Field personnel, in jurisdictions where authorized, should start protocols to cease resuscitative efforts or to pronounce death outside the hospital (Class IIa).
- In most US settings, the medical control official must give direct voice-to-voice or on-scene authorization.
- Advance planning for these protocols must occur. The planning should include specific directions for
  - Leaving the body at scene
  - Death certification
  - Transfer to funeral service
  - On-scene family advocate
  - Religious or nondenominational counseling

End of Algorithm Notes

Asystole most often represents a confirmation of death rather than a "rhythm" to be treated. Team leaders can cease efforts to resuscitate the patient from confirmed and persistent asystole when the resuscitation team has done the following:

- Provided suitable basic CPR
- Eliminated VF
- Achieved successful tracheal intubation with primary and secondary confirmation of tube placement
- Confirmed throughout the efforts that the tube was secure and had not been dislodged
- Monitored oxygen saturation and end-tidal CO_2 to ensure that the best possible oxygenation and ventilation were achieved
- Established successful IV access
- Maintained these interventions for $\geq$10 minutes, during which time the confirmed rhythm was asystole
- Administered all rhythm-appropriate medications
- Updated waiting family members, spouses, or available friends about the severity of the patient's condition and lack of response to interventions
- Discussed the concept of programs to support family presence during resuscitative attempts and offered that option to appropriate family members. Note that family presence at resuscitative efforts is not a spur-of-the-moment offer, extended or not extended at the whim of supervising physicians. Rather, family presence at resuscitative efforts requires a formal program, with advance planning, assigned roles, and even rehearsals.

When to Stop?

Is it possible to state a specific time interval beyond which rescuers have never resuscitated patients? Does every resuscitation attempt have to continue for that length of time to guarantee that every salvageable person will be identified and saved? As outlined in the algorithm notes, the resuscitation team must make a conscientious and competent effort to give patients "a trial of CPR and ACLS," provided that the person had not expressed a decision to forego resuscitative efforts. The final decision to stop efforts can never be as simple as an isolated time interval, but clinical judgment and a respect for human dignity must enter the decision making. Many people among the resuscitation community strongly believe that we have erred greatly in the tendency to try prolonged, excessive resuscitative efforts.

Emergency medical response systems should not require the field personnel to transport every victim of cardiac arrest back to a hospital or Emergency Department (ED). In European countries most out-of-hospital ALS care is provided by medical doctors, so decisions about stopping CPR, transportation back to the ED, and pronouncing death are handled by an authorized medical doctor in the field. Transportation with continuing CPR is justified if there are interventions available in the ED that cannot be performed in the field (such as central core rewarming equipment) or field interventions (such as tracheal intubation) that were unsuccessful in the field.

In the United States, outdated concepts of EMS care can linger for years. For example, many systems still dictate the practice of "scoop and run" on all major medical patients, not just major trauma. For nontraumatic cardiac arrest solid evidence confirms that ACLS care in the ED offers no advantage over ACLS care in the field. Stated succinctly—if ACLS care in the field cannot resuscitate the victim, neither will ED care. Civil rules, administrative concerns, medical insurance requirements, and even reimbursement enhancement have frequently led to requirements to transport all cardiac arrest victims back to a hospital or ED. If these are unselective requirements, they are inappropriate, futile, and ethically unacceptable. There should be no requirements for ambulance transport of *all* patients who suffer an out-of-hospital cardiac arrest. This is especially true when the patient is pulseless and CPR is continued during transport. Researchers and EMS experts continue to publish observational studies on this practice of transporting all field resuscitations back to an ED, most often for pronouncement of death. To have the resuscitation team succeed with one of these victims and then have the victim survive to hospital discharge is extremely rare—usually <1%.

Likewise, it is inappropriate for clinicians to apply routine "stopping rules" without thinking about the particular situation. "Part 2: Ethical Aspects of ECC and CPR" provides a more detailed discussion of these issues. Cessation of efforts in the prehospital setting, following system-specific criteria and under direct medical control, should be standard practice in all EMS systems.

Figure 6: Bradycardia

Notes to Figure 6: Bradycardia

1 (Figure 6)
If the patient has *serious signs or symptoms,* make sure they are related to the slow rate.

2 (Figure 6)
Clinical manifestations include

- Symptoms (chest pain, shortness of breath, decreased level of consciousness)
- Signs (low blood pressure, shock, pulmonary congestion, congestive heart failure)

3 (Figure 6)
If the patient is symptomatic, do not delay transcutaneous pacing while awaiting IV access or for *atropine* to take effect.

4 (Figure 6)
Denervated transplanted hearts will not respond to *atropine.* Go at once to pacing, *catecholamine* infusion, or both.

5 (Figure 6)
Atropine should be given in repeat doses every 3 to 5 minutes up to a total of 0.03 to 0.04 mg/kg. Use the shorter dosing interval (3 minutes) in severe clinical conditions.

6 (Figure 6)
Never treat the combination of *third-degree heart block* and *ventricular escape beats* with *lidocaine* (or any agent that suppresses ventricular escape rhythms).

7 (Figure 6)
Verify patient tolerance and mechanical capture. Use analgesia and sedation as needed.

End of Algorithm Notes

Transcutaneous pacing is a Class I intervention for all symptomatic bradycardias. If clinicians are concerned about the use of atropine in higher-level blocks, they should remember that transcutaneous pacing is always appropriate, although not as readily available as atropine. If the bradycardia is severe and the clinical condition is unstable, implement transcutaneous pacing immediately.

There are several other cautions to remember about treatment of symptomatic bradycardias. Lidocaine may be *lethal* if the bradycardia is a ventricular escape rhythm and unwary clinicians think they are treating preventricular contractions or slow VT. In addition, transcutaneous pacing can be painful and may fail to produce effective mechanical contractions. Sometimes the patient's "symptom" is not due to the bradycardia. For example, hypotension, associated with bradycardia, may be due to myocardial dysfunction or hypovolemia rather than to conducting system or autonomic problems.

Figure 6 lists interventions in a sequence based on the assumption of worsening clinical severity. Give patients who are "precardiac arrest," or moving in that direction, multiple interventions in rapid sequence. Begin preparations for *pacing, IV atropine,* and administration of an *epinephrine infusion.* If the patient displays only mild problems due to the bradycardia, then *atropine 0.5 to 1.0 mg IV* can be given in a repeat dose every 3 to 5 minutes, to a total of 0.03 mg/kg. (For severe bradycardia or asystole, a maximum dose of 0.04 mg/kg is advisable.) Selection of the dosing interval (3 to 5 minutes) requires judgment about the severity of the patient's symptoms. The provider should repeat atropine at shorter intervals for more distressed patients. *Dopamine* (at rates of 2

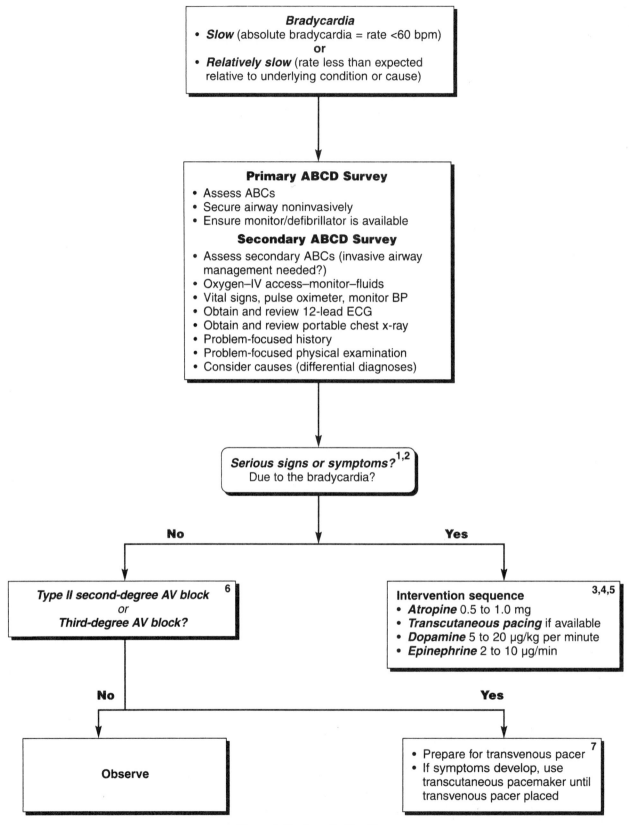

Figure 6. Bradycardia Algorithm.

to 5 μg/kg per minute) can be added and increased quickly to 5 to 20 μg/kg per minute if low blood pressure is associated with the bradycardia. If the patient displays severe symptoms, clinicians can go directly to an *epinephrine infusion.*

Transcutaneous pacing should be initiated quickly in patients who do not respond to atropine or who are severely symptomatic, especially when the block is at or below the His-Purkinje level. Newer defibrillator/monitors have the capability to perform transcutaneous pacing. This intervention, unlike insertion of transvenous pacemakers, is available to and can be performed by almost all ECC providers. This gives transcutaneous pacing enormous advantages over trans-venous pacing because transcutaneous pacing can be started quickly and conveniently at the bedside.

Reference

1. Cummins RO, Hazinski MF, Kerber RE, Kudenchuk P, Becker L, Nichol G, Malanga B, Aufderheide TP, Stapleton EM, Kern K, Ornato JP, Sanders A, Valenzuela T, Eisenberg M. Low-energy biphasic waveform defibrillation: evidence-based review applied to emergency cardiovascular care guidelines: a statement for healthcare professionals from the American Heart Association Committee on Emergency Cardiovascular Care and the Subcommittees on Basic Life Support, Advanced Cardiac Life Support, and Pediatric Resuscitation. *Circulation.* 1998;97:1654–1667.

7D: The Tachycardia Algorithms

Major New Concepts for the International Guidelines 2000

At the 1999 Evidence Evaluation Conference and the Guidelines 2000 Conference, experienced electrophysiologists, arrhythmia experts, and clinical cardiologists led the evidence review and discussions on the tachycardias (Figures 7, 8, and 9). They brought their expertise, their experience using new antiarrhythmics, and their knowledge of the incumbent tachycardia algorithm. The evidence reviews and discussions contributed many insights, revisions, and new medications. The tachycardia algorithm from the early 1990s forced an immediate decision in regard to "stable versus unstable." That same emphasis remains in 2000—the most important clinical decision to make when a rapid heart rate is noted is whether the patient is also experiencing signs and symptoms due to the rapid heart rate. In such situations the universal recommendation is immediate cardioversion rather than a trial of antiarrhythmics (see Figure 10, Electrical Cardioversion Algorithm).

For tachycardic patients not in need of immediate cardioversion, the International Guidelines 2000 place much more emphasis on 2 themes not previously highlighted:

- Making a specific rhythm diagnosis
- Recognizing those tachycardic patients who have significantly impaired cardiac function (ejection fraction <40%; overt signs of heart failure)

Emphasis on these themes has resulted in not just 1 complicated algorithm for tachycardias but 3 new algorithms and 1 table. The Guidelines 2000 Conference experts, clinicians, and teachers resisted any activity that would make ACLS training and learning more complicated. On learning of the background rationale, however, clinical leaders in resuscitation have accepted the need for more expansive algorithms, in return for providing better and safer acute care.

Specific Rhythm Diagnosis

Adenosine, first approved for marketing shortly before the publication of the 1992 guidelines, has been a highly successful agent for supraventricular arrhythmias. Teaching has emphasized its safety and its diagnostic capabilities. If a patient's monitor displayed a wide-complex tachycardia, clinicians became almost cavalier about pushing in higher and higher amounts of adenosine to see whether the rhythm converted out of a presumed supraventricular tachycardia with aberrancy. Most such patients are in VT with wide complexes. Faced with persistent wide-complex tachycardia, after 3 or 4 boluses of adenosine the clinician faced a dawning realization that treatment with adenosine or multiple calcium channel blockers for 30 to 45 minutes of persistent tachycardia was not helpful. This approach also exposes the patient to unpleasant side affects of adenosine, the possibility of worse rhythms, and a destabilization of heart rate and blood pressure. Consequently the International Guidelines 2000 attempt to avoid the simplistic approach of overuse of adenosine for diagnostic purposes. Instead, the clinicians are expected to devote more attention to making explicit diagnoses, within the scope of their available resources.

Antiarrhythmics or Proarrhythmics?

The other new concept that dominates the 2000 approach to tachycardias comes from continued evidence that antiarrhythmics are just as likely to be proarrhythmic agents as they are to be antiarrhythmic agents. Their tendency to induce arrhythmias becomes particularly acute in damaged or impaired hearts. In damaged hearts normal functional myocardium is interlaced with scarred and damaged tissue. These areas become the source of reentry arrhythmias, irritable foci, and blocked conduction.

Regardless of their Vaughn-Williams classification, all antiarrhythmics are capable of a proarrhythmic effect. When a second antiarrhythmic is added to this milieu the negative consequences escalate exponentially. Consequently—with rare exceptions—the International Guidelines 2000 recommend 1 and only 1 antiarrhythmic per patient. This should lead to far fewer events in which >1 antiarrhythmic causes significant worsening of the patient's condition and a much lower threshold to cardiovert patients nonurgently, before they become significantly more symptomatic.

Figure 7: The Tachycardia Overview Algorithm

The classic "chicken or egg" dilemma occurs often in symptomatic tachycardia events. Did the stress and discomfort of acute, severe, substernal chest pain lead to a cardiac response of tachycardia? or did the marginally compromised heart develop ischemia and chest pain as the sequelae of a paroxysmal tachycardia? The patients diagnosed as "unstable" will immediately be treated with urgent, electric, synchronized cardioversion.

Note: The numbers of notes, such as "Note 1," match numbers in the algorithms.

Circulation. 2000;102(suppl I):I-158–I-165.
© 2000 American Heart Association, Inc.

Circulation is available at http://www.circulationaha.org

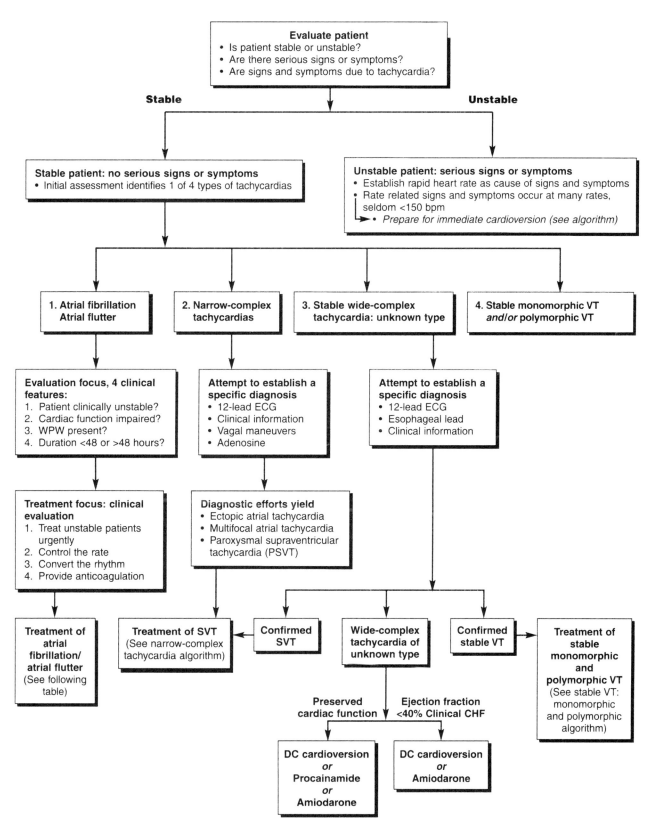

Figure 7. The Tachycardia Overview Algorithm.

Control of Rate and Rhythm (Continued From Tachycardia Overview)

Atrial fibrillation/ atrial flutter with • *Normal heart* • *Impaired heart* • *WPW*	1. Control Rate		2. Convert Rhythm	
	Heart Function Preserved	**Impaired Heart EF <40% or CHF**	**Duration <48 Hours**	**Duration >48 Hours or Unknown**
Normal cardiac function	**Note:** *If AF >48 hours' duration, use agents to convert rhythm with extreme caution in patients not receiving adequate anticoagulation because of possible embolic complications.* *Use only 1 of the following agents (see note below):* • Calcium channel blockers (Class I) • β-Blockers (Class I) • For additional drugs that are Class IIb recommendations, see Guidelines or ACLS text	*(Does not apply)*	**Consider** • DC cardioversion *Use only 1 of the following agents (see note below):* • Amiodarone (Class IIa) • Ibutilide (Class IIa) • Flecainide (Class IIa) • Propafenone (Class IIa) • Procainamide (Class IIa) • For additional drugs that are Class IIb recommendations, see Guidelines or ACLS text	• **NO DC cardioversion!** • **Note:** *Conversion of AF to NSR with drugs or shock may cause embolization of atrial thrombi unless patient has adequate anticoagulation.* • Use antiarrhythmic agents with extreme caution if AF >48 hours' duration *(see note above).* ***or*** ***Delayed cardioversion*** **Anticoagulation × 3 weeks at proper levels** • Cardioversion, *then* • Anticoagulation × 4 weeks more ***or*** ***Early cardioversion*** • Begin IV heparin at once • TEE to exclude atrial clot ***then*** • Cardioversion within 24 hours ***then*** • Anticoagulation × 4 more weeks
Impaired heart (EF <40% or CHF)	*(Does not apply)*	**Note:** *If AF >48 hours' duration, use agents to convert rhythm with extreme caution in patients not receiving adequate anticoagulation because of possible embolic complications.* *Use only 1 of the following agents (see note below):* • Digoxin (Class IIb) • Diltiazem (Class IIb) • Amiodarone (Class IIb)	**Consider** • DC cardioversion ***or*** • Amiodarone (Class IIb)	• **Anticoagulation** as described above, followed by • **DC cardioversion**

Note to Figure 7: The Tachycardia Overview Algorithm
Unstable condition must be related to the tachycardia. Signs and symptoms may include chest pain, shortness of breath, decreased level of consciousness, low blood pressure, shock, pulmonary congestion, congestive heart failure, and AMI.

End of Algorithm Note

The Tachycardia Overview Algorithm (Figure 7) divides tachycardias into 4 diagnostic categories. (In the algorithm the 4 columns have a number at the top to better orient the reader):

1. Atrial fibrillation/flutter
2. Narrow-complex tachycardias
3. Wide-complex tachycardias of unknown type
4. Stable monomorphic and polymorphic tachycardia

1. Atrial Fibrillation/Atrial Flutter (Column 1)

Figure 7 reminds the ACLS provider of the focus for evaluation:

1. Is the patient clinically unstable?
2. Is cardiac function impaired?
3. Is Wolff-Parkinson-White syndrome present?
4. Was the onset of the atrial fibrillation or atrial flutter clearly recognized by the patient? Has the atrial fibrillation/flutter been present for more than or less than 48 hours?

The treatment focus for atrial fibrillation/flutter is on 4 areas as well:

1. Unstable versus stable? Treat urgently.
2. Control rate with agents that reduce the rate of conduction across the AV node.
3. Convert the rhythm with either medications or cardioversion when indications are present and urgent.
4. Provide anticoagulation if indicated.

See "Section 5: Pharmacology I" and "Section 6: Pharmacology II" for more detailed presentations on these topics.

The table accompanying Figure 7 provides treatment details for atrial fibrillation and flutter. The table displays the

Control of Rate and Rhythm (Continued From Tachycardia Overview)

Atrial fibrillation/ atrial flutter with • Normal heart • Impaired heart • WPW	1. Control Rate		2. Convert Rhythm	
	Heart Function Preserved	Impaired Heart EF <40% or CHF	Duration <48 Hours	Duration >48 Hours or Unknown

WPW	**Note:** *If AF >48 hours' duration, use agents to convert rhythm with extreme caution in patients not receiving adequate anticoagulation because of possible embolic complications.*
	
	• DC cardioversion
	
	or
	
	• **Primary anti-arrhythmic agents** *Use only 1 of the following agents (see note below):*
	  • Amiodarone (Class IIb)
	  • Flecainide (Class IIb)
	  • Procainamide (Class IIb)
	  • Propafenone (Class IIb)
	  • Sotalol (Class IIb)
	
	--- 	
	Class III *(can be harmful)*
	• Adenosine
	• β-Blockers
	• Calcium blockers
	• Digoxin
		Note: *If AF >48 hours' duration, use agents to convert rhythm with extreme caution in patients not receiving adequate anticoagulation because of possible embolic complications.*
		
		• DC cardioversion
		
		or
		
		• Amiodarone (Class IIb)
			• DC cardioversion
			
			or
			
			• **Primary anti-arrhythmic agents** *Use only 1 of the following agents (see note below**):*
			  • Amiodarone (Class IIb)
			  • Flecainide (Class IIb)
			  • Procainamide (Class IIb)
			  • Propafenone (Class IIb)
			  • Sotalol (Class IIb)
			
			--- 	
			Class III *(can be harmful)*
			• Adenosine
			• β-Blockers
			• Calcium blockers
			• Digoxin
				• **Anticoagulation** as described above, followed by
				• **DC cardioversion**

WPW indicates Wolff-Parkinson-White syndrome; AF, atrial fibrillation; NSR, normal sinus rhythm; TEE, transesophageal echocardiogram; and EF, ejection fraction.

Note: Occasionally 2 of the named antiarrhythmic agents may be used, but use of these agents in combination may have proarrhythmic potential. The classes listed represent the Class of Recommendation rather than the Vaughn-Williams classification of antiarrhythmics.

major questions to ask and factors to consider when formulating a treatment plan for atrial fibrillation/flutter:

- What is the cardiac status? normal? impaired?
- Does the person have Wolff-Parkinson-White syndrome?
- What is the duration of the atrial fibrillation? Can you date and time the onset unequivocally? Is the duration less than or more than 48 hours? Is anticoagulation indicated? Electrical cardioversion?
- Would pharmacological conversion pose higher risk of emboli?
- Is the rate too high?

2. Tachycardia (Atrial Fibrillation and Flutter)
See the table accompanying Figure 7.

Narrow-Complex Tachycardias
The ACLS provider needs to move from the end of column 2, Narrow-Complex Tachycardias (Figure 7), to Figure 8: Narrow-Complex Supraventricular Tachycardia.

Figure 7, under Narrow-Complex Tachycardias, demonstrates the emphasis in 2000 on establishing a specific diagnosis first by close ECG analysis, then by consulting cardiology specialists if available. The consultants may choose to use esophageal-lead ECGs or echocardiograms as well as serial 12-lead ECGs. In narrow-complex, stable supraventricular tachycardias, the algorithm recommends diagnostic use of vagal maneuvers and adenosine. These diagnostic efforts should yield a diagnosis such as PSVT, ectopic atrial tachycardia, or MAT.

The overview algorithm then directs the clinician to Figure 8, Narrow-Complex Supraventricular Tachycardia. Here clinicians make the clinical assessment of cardiac function, with ejection fractions <40% qualifying as enough compromise to alter the therapeutic approach.

Figure 8: Narrow-Complex Supraventricular Tachycardia
In general, narrow-complex supraventricular tachycardias can be treated with amiodarone, β-blockers, or calcium channel blockers if cardiac function is preserved. (This list is in alphabetical order and does not imply that 1 of these 3 is better than another.) If cardiac function is compro-

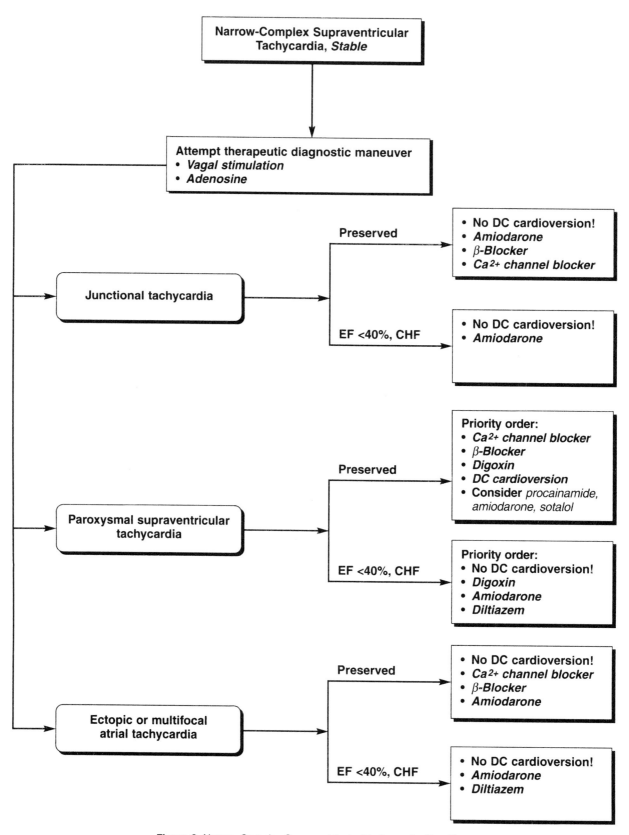

Figure 8. Narrow-Complex Supraventricular Tachycardia Algorithm.

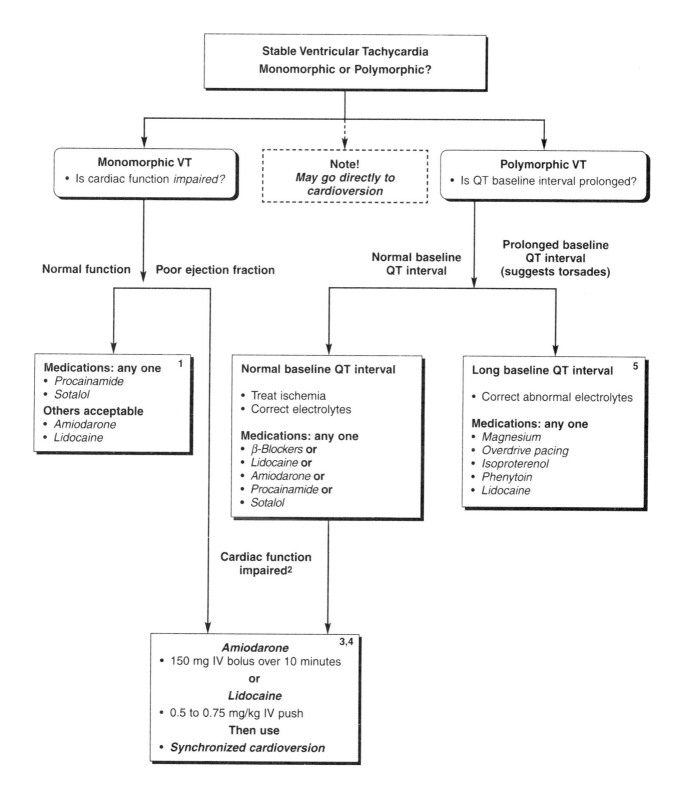

Figure 9. Stable Ventricular Tachycardia (Monomorphic or Polymorphic) Algorithm.

mised, then the drug options narrow to only amiodarone, the agent with the best balance between side effects and effectiveness in heart failure patients. Note the prohibition to DC cardioversion in all patients with impaired cardiac function.

3. Stable Wide-Complex Tachycardias: Unknown Type

Figure 7, Column 3, recommends the same diagnostic/therapeutic approach as recommended for narrow-complex tachycardias. After a series of diagnostic efforts clinicians

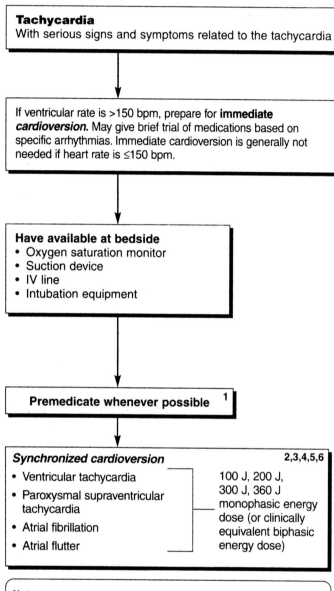

Tachycardia
With serious signs and symptoms related to the tachycardia

If ventricular rate is >150 bpm, prepare for **immediate cardioversion.** May give brief trial of medications based on specific arrhythmias. Immediate cardioversion is generally not needed if heart rate is ≤150 bpm.

Have available at bedside
- Oxygen saturation monitor
- Suction device
- IV line
- Intubation equipment

Premedicate whenever possible 1

Synchronized cardioversion   2,3,4,5,6
- Ventricular tachycardia
- Paroxysmal supraventricular tachycardia
- Atrial fibrillation
- Atrial flutter

100 J, 200 J, 300 J, 360 J monophasic energy dose (or clinically equivalent biphasic energy dose)

Notes:
1. Effective regimens have included a sedative (eg, **diazepam, midazolam, barbiturates, etomidate, ketamine, methohexital)** with or without an analgesic agent (eg, **fentanyl, morphine, meperidine).** Many experts recommend anesthesia if service is readily available.
2. Both monophasic and biphasic waveforms are acceptable if documented as clinically equivalent to reports of monophasic shock success.
3. Note possible need to resynchronize after each cardioversion.
4. If delays in synchronization occur and clinical condition is critical, go immediately to unsynchronized shocks.
5. Treat polymorphic ventricular tachycardia (irregular form and rate) like ventricular fibrillation: see ventricular fibrillation/pulseless ventricular tachycardia algorithm.
6. Paroxysmal supraventricular tachycardia and atrial flutter often respond to lower energy levels (start with 50 J).

**Steps for
Synchronized Cardioversion**

1. Consider sedation.
2. Turn on defibrillator (monophasic or biphasic).
3. Attach monitor leads to the patient ("white to right, red to ribs, what's left over to the left shoulder") and ensure proper display of the patient's rhythm.
4. Engage the synchronization mode by pressing the "sync" control button.
5. Look for markers on R waves indicating sync mode.
6. If necessary, adjust monitor gain until sync markers occur with each R wave.
7. Select appropriate energy level.
8. Position conductor pads on patient (or apply gel to paddles).
9. Position paddle on patient (sternum-apex).
10. Announce to team members: *"Charging defibrillator—stand clear!"*
11. Press "charge" button on apex paddle (right hand).
12. When the defibrillator is charged, begin the final clearing chant. State firmly in a forceful voice the following chant before each shock:
    - *"I am going to shock on three. One, I'm clear."* (Check to make sure you are clear of contact with the patient, the stretcher, and the equipment.)
    - *"Two, you are clear."* (Make a visual check to ensure that no one continues to touch the patient or stretcher. In particular, do not forget about the person providing ventilations. That person's hands should not be touching the ventilatory adjuncts, including the tracheal tube!)
    - *"Three, everybody's clear."* (Check yourself one more time before pressing the "shock" buttons.)
13. Apply 25 lb pressure on both paddles.
14. Press the "discharge" buttons simultaneously.
15. Check the monitor. If tachycardia persists, increase the joules according to the electrical cardioversion algorithm.
16. **Reset the sync mode after each synchronized cardioversion because most defibrillators default back to unsynchronized mode.** This default allows an immediate defibrillation if the cardioversion produces VF.

Figure 10. Synchronized Cardioversion Algorithm.

should be able to establish into which of 3 arrhythmic categories the wide-complex tachycardia belongs:

1. Narrow-complex tachycardia with aberrancy obscuring the narrow QRS (subsequently these patients are referred to Figure 8: Narrow-Complex Supraventricular Tachycardia)
2. Stable monomorphic or polymorphic VT (subsequently these patients are referred to Figure 9: Stable VT: Monomorphic or Polymorphic)
3. Stable wide-complex tachycardia: if this is the most likely rhythm diagnosis for you and your patient, proceed to evaluate the cardiac functional status. Figure 7 shows that DC cardioversion and amiodarone are recommended treatments for those tachycardic patients who have clinical heart failure. Be careful with adding anything else to the treatment for these patients. For the patient with well-preserved cardiac function, choose either DC cardioversion (Figure 10) or procainamide or amiodarone. Most experts choose DC cardioversion as their first treatment and treatment of choice for all wide-complex tachycardias regardless of cardiac function. That way they can easily add another antiarrhythmic if the cardioversion fails; however, the converse (use cardioversion if antiarrhythmic fails) does not always hold true.

Figure 9: Stable Ventricular Tachycardia: Monomorphic or Polymorphic?

4. Monomorphic and Polymorphic VT

Figure 7, Column 4, directs the clinician to Figure 9 for more details on the treatment of those stable VTs that fall into 2 subsets: monomorphic VT and polymorphic VT. If the polymorphic VT has a prolonged QT interval, it becomes a question of whether the patient is suffering from torsades de pointes. With such an exotic name it is only right that the rhythm of polymorphic VT looks distinctive and unusual, with the entire rhythm tracing resembling an up-and-down, thick-and-thin pattern characterized as a "spindle and node" pattern.

Polymorphic VT merits special attention because it is a common arrest rhythm suffered by drug overdose patients and toxin patients from exposures to nonmedicinal drugs.

Figure 9 provides directions for the immediate treatment of these arrhythmias, with the cardiac function status of primary importance. Notice that amiodarone is becoming the only antiarrhythmic agent acceptable for the elderly and those with progressive decline in cardiac function.

See the callout notes for stable VTs for more details.

Notes to Figure 9: Stable VT: Monomorphic or Polymorphic?

1 (Figure 9)

Monomorphic VF with normal cardiac function

Use just 1 agent (to avoid proarrhythmic effects of combination therapy).

This reduces adverse side effects. Choose 1 agent from these lists:

Top agents

- Procainamide (IIa)
- Sotalol (IIa)

Others acceptable

- Amiodarone (IIb)
- Lidocaine (IIb)

2 (Figure 9)

Monomorphic or polymorphic VT with impaired cardiac function

If clinical signs are suggestive of impaired LV function (ejection fraction <40% or congestive heart failure) in either long- or normal-QRS tachycardias, use

- Amiodarone (IIb)
- Lidocaine (IIb)

then use

- Synchronized cardioversion

3 (Figure 9)

Detailed dosing of amiodarone (Class IIb) in patients with impaired cardiac function

- 150 mg IV bolus over 10 minutes (international dose: 5 mg/kg)
- Repeat 150 mg IV (over 10 minutes) every 10 to 15 minutes as needed
- Alternative infusion: 360 mg over 6 hours (1 mg/min over 6 hours), then 540 mg over the remaining 18 hours (0.5 mg/min)
- Maximum total dose: 2.2 g in 24 hours. This means that *all* doses (including those used in resuscitation) should be added together, so the total cumulative dose per 24 hours is limited to 2.2 g
- See guidelines or ECC Handbook Drug Table

4 (Figure 9)

Detailed dosing of lidocaine (Class Indeterminate) in patients with impaired cardiac function

- 0.5 to 0.75 mg/kg IV push
- Repeat every 5 to 10 minutes
- Then infuse 1 to 4 mg/min
- Maximum total dose: 3 mg/kg (over 1 hour)

5 (Figure 9)

If rhythm is suggestive of torsades de pointes

- Stop/avoid treatments that prolong QT
- Identify and treat abnormal electrolytes

Medications (all Class Indeterminate):

- Magnesium
- Overdrive pacing (with or without β-blocker)
- Isoproterenol (as temporizing measure to overdrive pacing)
- Phenytoin or lidocaine

End of Algorithm Notes

Section 8: Postresuscitation Care

Return of Spontaneous Circulation After a No-Flow Cardiac Arrest

Cardiovascular and hemodynamic derangements are common when spontaneous circulation returns (ROSC) after a cardiac arrest. These abnormalities include hypovolemic shock, cardiogenic shock, and the vasodilatory shock associated with the systemic inflammatory response syndrome (SIRS).

Multiple pathogenic factors contribute to the postresuscitation syndrome:

- Reperfusion failure
- Reperfusion injury
- Cerebral intoxication from ischemic metabolites
- Coagulopathy[1,1a–1d]

After restoration of circulation, 4 phases of the postresuscitation syndrome occur, dependent on the degree and duration of organ ischemia.[2]

1. Almost one-half of postresuscitation syndrome deaths that occur take place within 24 hours of the event. In the hours after the ROSC, cardiovascular dysfunction is present to a variable degree, with a tendency to normalize over 12 to 24 hours. Microcirculatory dysfunction from the multifocal hypoxia leads to rapid release of toxic enzymes and free radicals into the cerebrospinal fluid and blood. Cerebral and microvascular abnormalities persist as metabolic disorders progress.
2. Over 1 to 3 days cardiac function and systemic function improve but intestinal permeability increases, predisposing to sepsis syndrome. Several organs have progressive dysfunction, particularly the liver, pancreas, and kidneys, leading to the multiple organ dysfunction syndrome (MODS).
3. Finally, days after the cardiac arrest serious infection occurs and the patient declines rapidly.
4. Death occurs.

The principal objective of the postresuscitation phase is the complete reestablishment of regional organ and tissue perfusion. Simple restoration of blood pressure alone and improvement in tissue gas exchange do not necessarily improve survival. Notably, these end points fail to indicate appropriate resuscitation of peripheral organ systems and their blood supply, particularly the splanchnic and renal circulation, which contribute importantly to MODS after hypoxic-ischemic arrest.[3–5]

In most cases the acidemia associated with cardiac arrest improves spontaneously when adequate ventilation and perfusion have been restored. Persistent unrecognized splanchnic hypoperfusion will be identified only with specific monitoring and requires targeted therapy.[6,7] In addition to invasive hemodynamic monitoring with pulmonary artery catheters, which remains controversial,[8–10] splanchnic resuscitation should be directed by quantitative gastric tonometric measurement of the systemic:gastric mucosal Pco_2 gradient. Targeted correction of systemic:gastric mucosal Pco_2 gradient may be an important adjunct to invasive hemodynamic monitoring in the ICU but is presently unproven and is not widely available.[11,11a,12] The purpose is to maximize splanchnic perfusion in the early postresuscitation phase and avoid progression to MODS.

These 2000 ACLS guidelines incorporate our evolving understanding of the hemodynamic abnormalities encountered in patients who survive resuscitation. Recommendations are generally based on data derived from studies of posttraumatic and medical SIRS. Very few clinical randomized studies have been published dealing specifically with hemodynamic support after neurocerebral resuscitation for cardiac arrest.

The immediate goals of postresuscitation care are to

- Provide cardiorespiratory support to optimize tissue perfusion, especially to the brain
- Transport the prehospital cardiac arrest patient to the hospital Emergency Department and then to an appropriately equipped critical care unit
- Attempt to identify the precipitating causes of the arrest
- Institute measures such as antiarrhythmic therapy to prevent recurrence

Immediately after resuscitation, patients may exhibit a wide spectrum of physiological states. Patients may recover fully with normal hemodynamic and cerebral function. At the other end of the spectrum, patients remain comatose with cardiorespiratory abnormalities. All patients require careful, repeated assessments to establish the status of their cardiovascular, respiratory, and neurological systems. Clinicians should identify complications, such as rib fracture, hemopneumothorax, pericardial tamponade, intra-abdominal trauma, and misplaced tracheal tube.

Optimal Response to Resuscitation

In the optimal situation after resuscitation, the patient is awake, responsive, and breathing spontaneously. Apply ECG monitor leads and provide supplemental oxygen. If not already done during resuscitation, start an IV infusion with normal saline. Glucose administration is reserved for patients with documented hypoglycemia. Change peripheral or central intravenous lines placed without proper sterile technique or those maintained inadequately. If the arrest rhythm was VF or VT and no antiarrhythmic treatment was given, consider use

Circulation. 2000;102(suppl I):I-166–I-171.
© 2000 American Heart Association, Inc.

Circulation is available at http://www.circulationaha.org

of a lidocaine bolus followed by maintenance infusion unless contraindicated (ie, in patients with ventricular escape rhythm) and continue the infusion for several hours while primary ventricular fibrillation secondary to an acute coronary syndrome is excluded and other correctable causes are assessed.

Clinicians should consider the precipitating cause of the cardiac arrest, particularly an AMI, electrolyte disturbances, or primary arrhythmias. If an antiarrhythmic agent was used successfully during the resuscitation, administer a continuous infusion of that agent. If hemodynamically significant bradycardia is present, initiate therapy as described in the guidelines section on bradycardia. Consider fibrinolytic therapy for patients who survive resuscitations of short duration and with minimal trauma with evidence of acute ST-segment elevation MI on their postresuscitation 12-lead ECG and who have no contraindications to fibrinolytic therapy. Patients with contraindications to fibrinolytic therapy should be considered for urgent coronary angiography and appropriate intervention.[14] Consider the patient's neurological status, but coma should not preclude indicated interventions. Acute coronary syndromes must be evaluated with serial ECG and cardiac markers in all patients. Assess the hemodynamic status, vital signs, and urine output.

Perform laboratory investigations, including a 12-lead ECG; portable chest x-ray; determination of arterial blood gases, electrolyte, glucose, serum creatinine, blood urea nitrogen, magnesium, and calcium levels; and other appropriate chemical analyses. Treat aberrations in potassium, magnesium, calcium, and sodium levels aggressively. In candidates for fibrinolytic therapy, perform arterial punctures only if less invasive assessments of oxygenation (pulse oximetry), ventilation (expired CO_2), and acid-base status (venous sample) are unavailable and clinically relevant information is unavailable by other noninvasive methods. Prearrest status must be reviewed carefully, particularly if the patient was receiving drug therapy. After completion of these steps, transfer the patient with oxygen and ECG monitoring to a special care unit for observation, continuous monitoring, and further therapeutic intervention. Resuscitation equipment and an adequate number of trained personnel must accompany the patient in transport.

Temperature Regulation

Regional cerebral metabolic rate determines the regional blood flow requirements of the brain. The cerebral metabolic rate increases approximately 8% per degree Celsius (2 degrees Fahrenheit) of body temperature elevation. After resuscitation, temperature elevation above normal can create a significant imbalance between oxygen supply and demand and impair brain recovery. Treat fever aggressively in the postischemic period.

Hypothermia

Hypothermia, in contrast, is an effective method to suppress cerebral metabolic activity. Although previously used widely during cardiovascular surgery, hypothermia has significant detrimental effects that might adversely affect the post–cardiac arrest patient, including increased blood viscosity,

decreased cardiac output, and increased susceptibility to infection. Many reports indicate benefit after brain ischemia, although some document detrimental effects or lack of improvement. Recent evidence indicates that mild levels of hypothermia (eg, 34°C [93°F]) are effective in mitigating postischemic brain damage without detrimental side effects.[15–21] In the normal brain, a 7% reduction in the cerebral metabolic rate occurs with every 1°C (2°F) reduction in brain temperature.[22]

After cardiac arrest, hypermetabolism may cause fever and disrupt the balance between cerebral oxygen supply and demand. This suggests a possible clinical role for induced mild hypothermia.[17]

Interest in hypothermia as a treatment modality for brain injury was rekindled in the late 1980s and early 1990s when experiments performed in carefully controlled rodent models of brain ischemia (by cerebral vascular occlusion techniques) and dog experiments of cardiac arrest showed that even *mild intraischemic* hypothermia could be neuroprotective. The ability to improve neurological outcomes by cooling brain-injured humans quickly and safely was demonstrated by Marion et al[17] in a randomized, controlled trial comparing the effects of moderate hypothermia (32°C to 33°C [89.5°F to 91.5°F] for 24 hours) with normothermia in 82 patients with severe closed-head injuries. As of early 2000 there was an active, randomized European multicenter trial of resuscitative hypothermia after cardiac arrest. The investigators anticipate an enrollment of 500 patients.

Side effects of hypothermia include coagulopathy, cardiac dysrhythmias, impaired cardiac function, and increased susceptibility to infection. The prevalence and severity of these side effects is proportional to the depth and duration of hypothermia. Investigations inducing mild to moderate hypothermia in humans after cardiac arrest (minimum temperature ≥32°C [89.5°F]) for 24 to 36 hours have reported hypothermia-related side effects.

In summary, hemodynamically stable patients who develop a mild degree of hypothermia (>33°C [91.5°F]) *spontaneously* after cardiac arrest should not be actively warmed. Mild hypothermia may be beneficial to neurological outcome and is likely to be well tolerated (Class IIb). However, hypothermia should not be induced actively after resuscitation from cardiac arrest (Class Indeterminate).

Hyperthermia

There are many studies in animal models of brain injury that show exacerbation of injury if body/brain temperature is increased during (intraischemic) or after cardiac arrest. Moreover, several studies have documented worse neurological outcome in humans who have fever after ischemic brain injury. Closely monitor temperature after resuscitation from cardiac arrest, and treat fever aggressively (Class IIa).

Single- or Multiple-Organ System Failure: Requires Total or Near-Total Support

After ROSC, patients may remain comatose for a variable period of time. Spontaneous breathing may be absent, and a period of mechanical ventilation via tracheal tube may be required. The hemodynamic status may be unstable with abnormalities of cardiac rate, rhythm, systemic blood pressure, and organ perfusion. Hypoxemia and hypotension exacerbate brain injury and must be avoided. The patient may be in a coma or show decreased responsiveness. The baseline postarrest status of each organ system must be defined and monitored and appropriate interventions instituted. With adequate ventilation and reperfusion, the acidemia of arrest will normally improve spontaneously in most cases without the need for buffer administration.

During transportation of the patient to a critical care unit, mechanical ventilation and oxygenation must be maintained along with ECG monitoring. Assessment of circulatory status in transport with physical palpation of carotid or femoral pulses, continuous intra-arterial pressure monitoring, or pulse oximetry will allow for immediate initiation of CPR should another arrest occur. Equipment and personnel to accomplish immediate defibrillation and drug therapy must accompany the patient in transport.

Respiratory System

After ROSC, patients may exhibit various degrees of respiratory dysfunction. Some patients will remain dependent on mechanical ventilation and will need supplementary oxygen. Perform a complete clinical examination and review the chest x-ray. Pay special attention to potential complications of resuscitation, such as pneumothorax and misplacement of the tracheal tube. The level of mechanical ventilatory support is determined by the blood gas values, respiratory rate, and perceived work of breathing. As spontaneous ventilation becomes more efficient, the level of respiratory support can be decreased until respiration is entirely spontaneous (decreasing intermittent mandatory ventilation rates). If high oxygen concentrations are needed, it is important to establish whether the cause is pulmonary or cardiac dysfunction. Positive end-expiratory pressure (PEEP) may be helpful in the patient with pulmonary dysfunction complicated by left ventricular failure if the patient is hemodynamically stable. If cardiac dysfunction is present, support of the failing myocardium is important. Adjust inspired oxygen concentration, PEEP, and minute ventilation based on sequential arterial blood gas analyses and/or noninvasive monitoring, such as pulse oximetry and capnography. To facilitate repeated arterial blood sampling, an arterial cannula may be necessary. The systemic blood pressure can also be accurately and continuously monitored from this arterial line.

Ventilatory Parameters

Recent evidence supports the theory that sustained hypocapnea (low Pco_2) may worsen cerebral ischemia.[23–25] After cardiac arrest, restoration of blood flow results in an initial hyperemic blood flow response lasting 10 to 30 minutes, which is followed by a more prolonged period of low blood flow. During this period of delayed hypoperfusion a mismatch between blood flow (oxygen delivery) and oxygen metabolism may occur. If the patient is hyperventilated at this stage, the additional cerebral vasoconstriction resulting from a low Pco_2 may further decrease cerebral blood flow and worsen cerebral ischemia. There is no evidence that hyperventilation protects vital organs from further ischemic damage after cardiac arrest. The potential risk for further brain ischemia is real, and hyperventilation after cardiac arrest should be avoided. Safar et al[26] also showed indirectly that hyperventilation results in worse neurological outcome. After cardiac arrest, dogs treated with mild hypothermia enhanced by hypertension and ventilated to normocarbia had improved outcome with this clinical management.

Hyperventilation may generate airway pressures and auto-PEEP, leading to an increase in cerebral venous and intracranial pressures.[27,28] The increase in cerebral vascular pressure results in a decreased cerebral blood flow and a further worsening of brain ischemia. This mechanism is independent of the effects of Pco_2 or pH on cerebral vessel reactivity.

In summary, after either cardiac arrest or head trauma, ventilate the comatose patient to achieve normocarbia (Class IIa). *Routine* hyperventilation may be detrimental and should be avoided (Class III). In specific situations hyperventilation to achieve hypocarbia may be beneficial. Treat cerebral herniation syndrome with hyperventilation (Class IIa). Hyperventilation may also have a role when pulmonary hypertension is the cause of arrest (Class IIa). With restoration of cardiac output, metabolic acidosis usually corrects over time, and hyperventilation should not be used as a primary treatment modality. The use of buffer therapy is also not indicated and should be used for specific indications only (see above).[29,30]

Cardiovascular System

Evaluation must include a complete vascular examination and review of serial vital signs and urine output. Compare a 12-lead ECG with previous tracings if available. Assess the chest x-ray; serum electrolyte levels, including calcium and magnesium; and cardiac marker levels. Review current and previous drug therapy. Serum cardiac marker levels may be elevated because of resuscitative efforts alone as global ischemia occurs during arrested or low-flow states. If the patient's condition is hemodynamically unstable, assess both circulating fluid volume and ventricular function. Avoid even mild hypotension because it can impair recovery of cerebral function. Noninvasive assessment of blood pressure may be inaccurate in patients with low cardiac output and peripheral vasoconstriction. Intra-arterial assessment of blood pressure is usually more accurate in these patients and allows better titration of potentially dangerous catecholamine infusions. In the presence of severe vasoconstriction, blood pressure measurement from the radial artery may be inaccurate, and a femoral artery catheter may be considered.

In the critically ill patient, invasive hemodynamic monitoring is often undertaken with a pulmonary artery catheter. The use of these devices is controversial.[8–10] Obtain pressure measurements of the pulmonary circulation using a pulmonary artery flow–directed catheter. These catheters also permit cardiac output measurements using the thermodilution technique. If both cardiac output and pulmonary artery occlusive pressures are low, fluid challenge with reassessment of pressures and cardiac output is indicated. In the patient with an AMI, ventricular compliance may be reduced and filling pressures elevated. The precise level of pulmonary occlusive pressure needed to achieve optimal cardiac output will vary, but it is often 18 mm Hg, which is higher than normal and may vary depending on patient and pathological conditions. If hypotension or hypoperfusion persists after filling pressure is optimized, inotropic (dobutamine), vasopressor (dopamine or norepinephrine), or vasodilator (nitroprusside or nitroglycerin) therapy may be indicated. The use of these agents is outlined in the algorithm for acute pulmonary edema, hypotension, and shock (Part 7, Section 1) and is discussed in the related text.

Renal System

The bladder must be catheterized so that urine output can be measured hourly and an accurate volume can be established (output includes suctioned gastric secretions, diarrheal fluid, and vomitus as well as urine). In the oliguric patient, measurement of pulmonary artery occlusive pressures and cardiac output along with evaluation of the urine sediment, electrolyte values, and measurement of the fractional excretion of filtered sodium may be helpful in differentiating prerenal from renal failure. Furosemide may maintain urine output despite developing renal failure. Dopamine at low doses (1 to 3 μg/kg per minute) does not improve splanchnic blood flow or provide specific renal protection and is no longer indicated in acute oliguric renal failure.[31-36] Nephrotoxic drugs and drugs eliminated via the kidneys should be used with caution and monitored appropriately, and doses should be adjusted. Progressive renal failure is indicated by a steadily rising serum urea nitrogen and creatinine, usually with hyperkalemia, and mortality and comorbidity are high in these patients, who often require dialysis.

Central Nervous System

A healthy brain and a functional patient are the primary goal of cardiopulmonary-cerebral resuscitation. Brain-oriented intensive care is essential. Cessation of circulation for 10 seconds results in a deficiency of oxygen supply to the brain that causes unconsciousness. After 2 to 4 minutes, glucose and glycogen stores of the brain are depleted, and after 4 to 5 minutes ATP is exhausted. Autoregulation of cerebral blood flow is lost after extended hypoxemia or hypercarbia, or both, and cerebral blood flow becomes dependent on cerebral perfusion pressure. The cerebral perfusion pressure is equal to mean arterial pressure minus intracranial pressure (CPP=MAP−ICP). Following ROSC, after a brief initial period of hyperemia, cerebral blood flow is reduced (the "no-reflow phenomenon") as a result of microvascular dysfunction. This reduction occurs even when cerebral perfusion pressure is normal. Any elevation of intracranial pressure or reduction in systemic mean arterial pressure may reduce cerebral perfusion pressure and further compromise cerebral blood flow.

Therapy for the unresponsive patient should include measures to optimize cerebral perfusion pressure by maintaining a normal or slightly elevated mean arterial pressure and reducing intracranial pressure if it is increased. Because hyperthermia and seizures increase the oxygen requirements of the brain, normothermia should be maintained and seizure activity controlled with phenobarbital, phenytoin, or diazepam or barbiturate. The head should be elevated to approxi-

mately 30° and maintained in a midline position to increase cerebral venous drainage. Care should be observed during tracheal suctioning because of the increase in intracranial pressure during this procedure. Preoxygenation with 100% oxygen helps prevent hypoxemia during suctioning. Although there is exciting experimental data on preserving central nervous system function, no treatment is sufficiently established at present to warrant its routine use after resuscitation. Nonetheless, vigilant attention to the details of oxygenation and perfusion of the brain after resuscitation can significantly reduce the possibility of secondary neurological injury and maximize the chances of full neurological recovery.

Gastrointestinal System

A nasogastric tube should be inserted if bowel sounds are absent and in those patients with a reduced level of consciousness who are mechanically ventilated. Start enteric feeding as soon as possible. If enteric feeding is not tolerated, administer histamine H_2-receptor blockers or sucralfate to reduce the risk of stress ulceration and gastrointestinal bleeding.

SIRS and Septic Shock

SIRS is a complex process that may be triggered by a variety of initial insults, such as trauma, burn, or infection.[37-39] The inflammatory response results in tissue damage and initiates a self-perpetuating process that results in local tissue damage and MODS. Signs of a systemic inflammatory response (fever and leukocytosis) may also occur after prolonged CPR. When infection is the cause, the resulting clinical syndrome is by definition sepsis.[40] Patients with septic shock have MODS usually combined with vasodilatory shock, resulting in a relative and absolute hypovolemia.

The goal of hemodynamic management is normal tissue oxygen uptake. Initial management consists of volume replacement. Following volume replacement, an inotrope or vasopressin is usually required.[41-43] Dobutamine and norepinephrine may be useful in severe septic shock.[44-47] Improved outcome, however, has not been shown with the use of volume expansion and inotropic support. When sepsis is suspected, empirical antibiotic therapy is indicated and should be directed at common and usual organisms.

The use of glucocorticoid therapy in septic shock has been the subject of unresolved debates in critical care for almost half a century. The predominant controversies focus on the normal adrenal responses to sepsis, "normal" cortisol levels in the stressed state, exacerbation of active infectious processes, and significant metabolic derangements.

Relative hypoadrenalism occurs in septic shock even in the presence of normal and high cortisol levels. Methylprednisolone was found to have no mortality benefit and, in fact, in patients taking methylprednisolone there was a slight increase in mortality. No significant differences were found in the prevention of shock, the reversal of shock, or overall mortality. Patients treated with methylprednisolone experienced more deaths from secondary infection than the control group.[48]

Studies using lower, "supraphysiological" corticosteroid doses have been published.[49-51] These studies have concluded that methylprednisolone shortens the pressor-dependent phase of shock and reduces the amount of organ system dysfunction. At present there is no evidence that corticosteroids improve survival rates.

Supraphysiological doses of corticosteroids may be beneficial for patients with persistent vasopressor-resistant shock maximally treated with broad-spectrum or organism-specific antimicrobial therapy (Class IIb).

In summary, care of the patient after resuscitation from cardiac arrest involves a careful assessment of the many organs subjected to an anoxic-hypoxic insult. Information in the patient with the postresuscitation syndrome is continuing to evolve as pathophysiological mechanisms of the SIRS and MODS are elucidated. The splanchnic circulation and gut are assuming increased importance for targeted therapy in long-term outcome and survival.[6] Physicians should be skilled and knowledgeable in all aspects of care in these complicated survivors of cardiac arrest and shock syndromes.

References

1. Hamvas A, Palazzo R, Kaiser L, Cooper J, Shuman T, Velazquez M, Freeman B, Schuster DP. Inflammation and oxygen free radical formation during pulmonary ischemia-reperfusion injury. *J Appl Physiol.* 1992;72: 621–628.

1a. Lafont A, Marwick TH, Chisolm GM, Van Lente F, Vaska KJ, Whitlow PL. Decreased free radical scavengers with reperfusion after coronary angioplasty in patients with acute myocardial infarction. *Am Heart J.* 1996;131:219–223.

1b. Lonn E, Factor SM, Van Hoeven KH, Wen WH, Zhao M, Dawood F, Liu P. Effects of oxygen free radicals and scavengers on the cardiac extracellular collagen matrix during ischemia-reperfusion. *Can J Cardiol.* 1994;10:203–213.

1c. Tan S, Yokoyama Y, Wang Z, Zhou F, Nielsen V, Murdoch AD, Adams C, Parks DA. Hypoxia-reoxygenation is as damaging as ischemia-reperfusion in the rat liver [see comments]. *Crit Care Med.* 1998;26: 1089–1095.

1d. Zimmerman BJ, Granger DN. Mechanisms of reperfusion injury. *Am J Med Sci.* 1994;307:284–292.

2. Negrovsky VA. The second step in resuscitation: the treatment of post-resuscitation disease. *Resuscitation.* 1972;1:1–7.

3. Homer-Vanniasinkam S, Crinnion JN, Gough MJ. Post-ischaemic organ dysfunction: a review. *Eur J Vasc Endovasc Surg.* 1997;14:195–203.

4. Nielsen VG, Tan S, Baird MS, McCammon AT, Parks DA. Gastric intramucosal pH and multiple organ injury: impact of ischemia-reperfusion and xanthine oxidase. *Crit Care Med.* 1996;248:1339–1344.

5. Weinbroum AA, Hochhauser E, Rudick V, Kluger Y, Sorkine P, Karchevsky E, Graf E, Boher P, Flaishon R, Fjodorov D, Niv D, Vidne BA. Direct induction of acute lung and myocardial dysfunction by liver ischemia and reperfusion. *J Trauma.* 1997;43:627–633; discussion 633–635.

6. Marik PE. Total splanchnic resuscitation, SIRS, and MODS [editorial; comment]. *Crit Care Med.* 1999;27:257–258.

7. Maynard N, Bihari D, Beale R, Smithies M, Baldock G, Mason R, McColl I. Assessment of splanchnic oxygenation by gastric tonometry in patients with acute circulatory failure [see comments]. *JAMA.* 1993;270: 1203–1210.

8. Bernard GR, Sopko G, Cerra F, Demling R, Edmunds H, Kaplan S, Kessler L, Masur H, Parsons P, Shure D, Webb C, Weidemann H, Weinmann G, Williams D. Pulmonary artery catheterization and clinical outcomes: National Heart, Lung, and Blood Institute and Food and Drug Administration workshop report. *JAMA.* 2000;283:2568–2572.

9. Mimoz O, Rauss A, Rekik N, Brun-Buisson C, Lemaire F, Brochard L. Pulmonary artery catheterization in critically ill patients: a prospective analysis of outcome changes associated with catheter-prompted changes in therapy [see comments]. *Crit Care Med.* 1994;22:573–579.

10. Vincent JL, Dhainaut JF, Perret C, Suter P. Is the pulmonary artery catheter misused? A European view [see comments]. *Crit Care Med.* 1998;26:1283–1287.

11. Doglio GR, Pusajo JF, Egurrola MA, Bonfigli GC, Parra C, Vetere L, Hernandez MS, Fernandez S, Palizas F, Gutierrez G. Gastric mucosal pH as a prognostic index of mortality in critically ill patients [see comments]. *Crit Care Med.* 1991;19:1037–1040.

11a. Gutierrez G, Palizas F, Doglio G, Wainsztein N, Gallesio A, Pacin J, Dubin A, Schiavi E, Jorge M, Pusajo J, et al. Gastric intramucosal pH as a therapeutic index of tissue oxygenation in critically ill patients [see comments]. *Lancet.* 1992;339:195–199.

12. Gys T, Hubens A, Neels H, Lauwers LF, Peeters R. Prognostic value of gastric intramural pH in surgical intensive care patients. *Crit Care Med.* 1988;16:1222–1224.

13. Nielsen VG, Tan S, Baird MS, McCammon AT, Parks DA. Gastric intramucosal pH and multiple organ injury: impact of ischemia-reperfusion and xanthine oxidase. *Crit Care Med.* 1996;24:1339–1344.

14. Spaulding CM, Joly LM, Rosenberg A, Monchi M, Weber SN, Dhainaut JF, Carli P. Immediate coronary angiography in survivors of out-of-hospital cardiac arrest [see comments]. *N Engl J Med.* 1997;336: 1629–1633.

15. Holzer M, Behringer W, Schorkhuber W, Zeiner A, Sterz F, Laggner AN, Frass M, Siostrozonek P, Ratheiser K, Kaff A, Hypothermia for Cardiac Arrest (HACA) Study Group. Mild hypothermia and outcome after CPR. *Acta Anaesthesiol Scand Suppl.* 1997;111:55–58.

16. Leonov Y, Sterz F, Safar P, Radovsky A, Oku K, Tisherman S, Stezoski SW. Mild cerebral hypothermia during and after cardiac arrest improves neurologic outcome in dogs. *J Cereb Blood Flow Metab.* 1990;10:57–70.

17. Marion DW, Leonov Y, Ginsberg M, Katz LM, Kochanek PM, Lechleuthner A, Nemoto EM, Obrist W, Safar P, Sterz F, Tisherman SA, White RJ, Xiao F, Zar H. Resuscitative hypothermia. *Crit Care Med.* 1996;24:S81–S89.

18. Schwab S, Schwarz S, Spranger M, Keller E, Bertram M, Hacke W. Moderate hypothermia in the treatment of patients with severe middle cerebral artery infarction [see comments]. *Stroke.* 1998;29:2461–2466.

19. Steinman AM. Cardiopulmonary resuscitation and hypothermia. *Circulation.* 1986;74(suppl IV):IV-29–IV-32.

20. Sterz F, Safar P, Tisherman S, Radovsky A, Kuboyama K, Oku K. Mild hypothermic cardiopulmonary resuscitation improves outcome after prolonged cardiac arrest in dogs [see comments]. *Crit Care Med.* 1991;19: 379–389.

21. Sterz F, Zeiner A, Kurkciyan I, Janata K, Mullner M, Domanovits H, Safar P. Mild resuscitative hypothermia and outcome after cardiopulmonary resuscitation. *J Neurosurg Anesthesiol.* 1996;8:88–96.

22. Rosomoff HL, Holaday DA. Cerebral blood flow and cerebral oxygen consumption during hypothermia. *Am J Physiol.* 1954;179:85–88.

23. Ausina A, Baguena M, Nadal M, Manrique S, Ferrer A, Sahuquillo J, Garnacho A. Cerebral hemodynamic changes during sustained hypocapnia in severe head injury: can hyperventilation cause cerebral ischemia? *Acta Neurochir Suppl.* 1998;71:1–4.

24. Diringer MN, Yundt K, Videen TO, Adams RE, Zazulia AR, Deibert E, Aiyagari V, Dacey RG Jr, Grubb RL Jr, Powers WJ. No reduction in cerebral metabolism as a result of early moderate hyperventilation following severe traumatic brain injury. *J Neurosurg.* 2000;92:7–13.

25. Yundt KD, Diringer MN. The use of hyperventilation and its impact on cerebral ischemia in the treatment of traumatic brain injury. *Crit Care Clin.* 1997;13:163–184.

26. Safar P, Xiao F, Radovsky A, Tanigawa K, Ebmeyer U, Bircher N, Alexander H, Stezoski SW. Improved cerebral resuscitation from cardiac arrest in dogs with mild hypothermia plus blood flow promotion. *Stroke.* 1996;27:105–113.

27. Gottfried SB, Rossi A, Milic-Emili J. Dynamic hyperinflation, intrinsic PEEP, and the mechanically ventilated patient. *Crit Care Digest.* 1986; 5:30–33.

28. Ligas JR, Mosiehi F, Epstein MAF. Occult positive end-expiratory pressure with different types of mechanical ventilators. *J Crit Care.* 1990;52:95–100.

29. Dybvik T, Strand T, Steen PA. Buffer therapy during out-of-hospital cardiopulmonary resuscitation [see comments]. *Resuscitation.* 1995;29: 89–95.

30. Kette F, Weil MH, Gazmuri RJ. Buffer solutions may compromise cardiac resuscitation by reducing coronary perfusion pressure [published erratum appears in *JAMA.* 1991;266:3286] [see comments]. *JAMA.* 1991; 266:2121–2126.

31. Bersten AD, Holt AW. Vasoactive drugs and the importance of renal perfusion pressure. *New Horiz.* 1995;3:650–661.

32. Marik PE. Low-dose dopamine in critically ill oliguric patients: the influence of the renin-angiotensin system. *Heart Lung.* 1993;22:171–175.

33. Marik PE, Iglesias J, NORASEPT II Study Investigators. Low-dose dopamine does not prevent acute renal failure in patients with septic shock and oliguria. *Am J Med.* 1999;107:387–390.

34. Chertow GM, Sayegh MH, Allgren RL, Lazarus JM, Auriculin Anaritide Acute Renal Failure Study Group. Is the administration of dopamine associated with adverse or favorable outcomes in acute renal failure? *Am J Med*. 1996;101:49–53.

35. Denton MD, Chertow GM, Brady HR. Renal-dose dopamine for the treatment of acute renal failure: scientific rationale, experimental studies and clinical trials. *Kidney Int*. 1996;50:4–14.

36. Thompson BT, Cockrill BA. Renal-dose dopamine: a siren song? *Lancet*. 1994;344:7–8.

37. Baue AE, Durham R, Faist E. Systemic inflammatory response syndrome (SIRS), multiple organ dysfunction syndrome (MODS), multiple organ failure (MOF): are we winning the battle? [see comments]. *Shock*. 1998;10:79–89.

38. Goris RJ. MODS/SIRS: result of an overwhelming inflammatory response? [see comments]. *World J Surg*. 1996;20:418–421.

39. Rangel-Frausto MS, Pittet D, Costigan M, Hwang T, Davis CS, Wenzel RP. The natural history of the systemic inflammatory response syndrome (SIRS): a prospective study [see comments]. *JAMA*. 1995;273:117–123.

40. Muckart DJ, Bhagwanjee S. American College of Chest Physicians/Society of Critical Care Medicine Consensus Conference definitions of the systemic inflammatory response syndrome and allied disorders in relation to critically injured patients [see comments]. *Crit Care Med*. 1997;25:1789–1795.

41. Landry DW, Levin HR, Gallant EM, Ashton RC Jr, Seo S, D'Alessandro D, Oz MC, Oliver JA. Vasopressin deficiency contributes to the vasodilation of septic shock [see comments]. *Circulation*. 1997;95:1122–1125.

42. Malay MB, Ashton RC Jr, Landry DW, Townsend RN. Low-dose vasopressin in the treatment of vasodilatory septic shock. *J Trauma*. 1999;47:699–703; discussion 703–705.

43. Reid IA. Role of vasopressin deficiency in the vasodilation of septic shock [editorial; comment]. *Circulation*. 1997;95:1108–1110.

44. Rhodes A, Lamb FJ, Malagon I, Newman PJ, Grounds RM, Bennett ED. A prospective study of the use of a dobutamine stress test to identify outcome in patients with sepsis, severe sepsis, or septic shock [see comments]. *Crit Care Med*. 1999;27:2361–2366.

45. Lherm T, Troche G, Rossignol M, Bordes P, Zazzo JF. Renal effects of low-dose dopamine in patients with sepsis syndrome or septic shock treated with catecholamines. *Intensive Care Med*. 1996;22:213–219.

46. Marik PE, Mohedin M. The contrasting effects of dopamine and norepinephrine on systemic and splanchnic oxygen utilization in hyperdynamic sepsis. *JAMA*. 1994;272:1354–1357.

47. Duke GJ, Briedis JH, Weaver RA. Renal support in critically ill patients: low-dose dopamine or low-dose dobutamine? [see comments]. *Crit Care Med*. 1994;22:1919–1925.

48. Bone RC, Fisher CJ Jr, Clemmer TP, Slotman GJ, Metz CA, Balk RA. A controlled clinical trial of high-dose methylprednisolone in the treatment of severe sepsis and septic shock. *N Engl J Med*. 1987;317:653–658.

49. Briegel J, Forst H, Haller M, Schelling G, Kilger E, Kuprat G, Hemmer B, Hummel T, Lenhart A, Heyduck M, Stoll C, Peter K. Stress doses of hydrocortisone reverse hyperdynamic septic shock: a prospective, randomized, double-blind, single-center study [see comments]. *Crit Care Med*. 1999;27:723–732.

50. Schelling G, Stoll C, Kapfhammer HP, Rothenhausler HB, Krauseneck T, Durst K, Haller M, Briegel J. The effect of stress doses of hydrocortisone during septic shock on posttraumatic stress disorder and health-related quality of life in survivors. *Crit Care Med*. 1999;27:2678–2683.

51. Bollaert PE, Charpentier C, Levy B, Debouverie M, Audibert G, Larcan A. Reversal of late septic shock with supraphysiologic doses of hydrocortisone [see comments]. *Crit Care Med*. 1998;26:645–650.

Part 7: The Era of Reperfusion
Section 1: Acute Coronary Syndromes (Acute Myocardial Infarction)

Major Guidelines Recommendations

Prehospital Care

- Implementation of out-of-hospital 12-lead ECG diagnostic programs is recommended in urban and suburban paramedic systems (Class I).
- Out-of-hospital fibrinolytic therapy is recommended when a physician is present or out-of-hospital transport time is ≥60 minutes (Class IIa).
- When possible, patients at high risk for mortality or severe left ventricular (LV) dysfunction with signs of shock, pulmonary congestion, heart rate >100 beats per minute (bpm), plus systolic blood pressure (SBP) <100 mm Hg should be triaged to facilities capable of performing cardiac catheterization and rapid revascularization (PCI or coronary artery bypass graft surgery [CABG]). For patients <75 years of age, this is a Class I recommendation.

Reperfusion Therapies

- Many clinical trials have established early fibrinolytic therapy as a standard of care for acute ST-segment elevation myocardial infarction (MI) (Class I for patients <75 years old and Class IIa for patients >75 years old).
- Percutaneous coronary intervention (PCI), including angioplasty/stent, is a Class I recommendation for patients <75 years of age with acute coronary syndromes (ACS) and signs of shock.
- Patients in whom fibrinolytic therapy is contraindicated should be considered for transfer to interventional facilities when potential benefit from reperfusion exists (Class IIa).
- Heparin is currently recommended for patients receiving selective fibrinolytic agents (tissue plasminogen activator [tPA]/reteplase [rPA]) (Class IIa).
- Heparin dosing with fibrinolytics is changed to reduce the incidence of intracerebral hemorrhage (ICH) and minimize reocclusion. Give heparin in a 60-U/kg bolus followed by a maintenance infusion of 12 U/kg per hour (with a maximum of 4000 U bolus and 1000 U/h infusion for patients weighing >70 kg). The activated partial thromboplastin time should be maintained at 50 to 70 seconds for 48 hours.

New Therapy for Unstable Angina/Non–Q-Wave MI

- Glycoprotein (GP) IIb/IIIa inhibitors are recommended for patients with non–ST-segment elevation MI or high-risk unstable angina (Class IIa).

- GP IIb/IIIa inhibitors have incremental benefit in addition to conventional therapy with unfractionated heparin (UFH) and aspirin (Class IIa).
- Low-molecular-weight heparin (LMWH) is an alternative to UFH for the treatment of non–Q-wave MI and unstable angina.
- Troponin-positive patients are at risk for major adverse cardiac events (MACE) and should be considered for aggressive therapy.

Introduction

Evidence-based data for the management of acute myocardial infarction (AMI) has evolved dramatically in the past decade. AMI and unstable angina are now recognized as part of a spectrum of clinical disease collectively identified as *acute coronary syndromes,* which have in common a ruptured or eroded atheromatous plaque.[1–5] These syndromes include unstable angina, non–Q-wave MI, and Q-wave MI. The ECG presentation of ACS encompasses ST-segment elevation infarction, ST-segment depression (including non–Q-wave MI and unstable angina), and nondiagnostic ST-segment and T-wave abnormalities. The majority of patients with ST-segment elevation will develop Q-wave MI. Only a minority of patients with ischemic chest discomfort at rest who do not have ST-segment elevation will develop Q-wave MI and will eventually be diagnosed as non–Q-wave MI or unstable angina. A significant portion of patients with an initial diagnosis of angina will not have ischemic coronary disease. Sudden cardiac death may occur with each of these syndromes. ACS is the proximate cause of sudden cardiac death in most adult patients.[6–10]

The primary goals of therapy for patients with ACS are

- Reduction of myocardial necrosis in patients with ongoing infarction
- Prevention of major adverse cardiac events (death, nonfatal MI, and need for urgent revascularization)
- Rapid defibrillation when ventricular fibrillation (VF) occurs

To date >750 000 patients with ACS have been studied worldwide in randomized clinical trials, producing an abundance of outcome-based data for healthcare providers. Several consensus panels,[11–17] including the American College of Cardiology (ACC)/American Heart Association (AHA) Guidelines Committees for the Management of Acute Myocardial Infarction and Unstable Angina[11–14,16] and the European Society of Cardiology and European Resuscitation

Circulation. 2000;102(suppl I):I-172–I-203.
© 2000 American Heart Association, Inc.

Circulation is available at http://www.circulationaha.org

Council,[15,17] have considered the clinical impact of this data and have published guidelines for the management of ACS. The guidelines that follow are a refinement of these international guidelines for healthcare providers who treat patients with ACS within the first several hours after onset of symptoms. These guidelines address out-of-hospital, emergency department (ED), and critical-care issues. Regional practices vary as a result of differences in out-of-hospital and in-hospital resources, availability of healthcare professionals, expertise, and skill. Therefore, these guidelines are designed to provide general directions for care.

Pathogenesis

Understanding the principles of management of ACS requires a knowledge of developing concepts of thrombus initiation and coronary plaque pathobiology.[1,18,19] Patients with coronary atherosclerosis in whom these clinical syndromes develop have various degrees of coronary artery occlusion. Typically ACS is caused by rupture of a lipid-laden plaque with a thin cap.[1,3,5] Most of these plaques are not hemodynamically significant before rupture.[20,21] However, an inflammatory component present in the subendothelial area further weakens the plaque and predisposes it to rupture.[22] Blood flow velocity and turbulence as well as vessel anatomy may also be important contributing factors to plaque disruption. Superficial erosion of a plaque occurs in approximately 25% of patients who also manifest increased systemic markers of inflammation.[23] The degree and duration of occlusion, as well as the presence or absence of collateral vessels, determine the type of infarction that occurs.

After plaque rupture or erosion, a monolayer of platelets covers the surface of the ruptured plaque (platelet adhesion). Additional platelets are recruited (platelet aggregation) and activated. Fibrinogen cross-links platelets, and the coagulation system is further activated by thrombin generation. A partially occluding thrombus produces symptoms of ischemia that may be prolonged and may occur at rest. At this stage the thrombus is platelet-rich. Therapy with antiplatelet agents, such as aspirin and GP IIb/IIIa receptor inhibitors, is most effective at this time. Fibrinolytic therapy is *not* effective and paradoxically may accelerate occlusion by causing the release of clot-bound thrombin, which further activates platelets.[24,25]

An intermittently occlusive thrombus may cause distal myocyte necrosis in the region supplied by the culprit artery, producing non–Q-wave MI. As the clot enlarges, microemboli originating in the thrombus may embolize and lodge in the coronary microvasculature, causing small elevations of cardiac troponins, new sensitive cardiac markers.[10,19,26,27] Microvascular dysfunction is now understood to be an additional determinant of myocardial dysfunction in patients with ACS and those treated with PCI.[27–30] Patients with such a thrombus are at highest risk for progression to MI. This process is known as minimal myocardial damage. Other mechanisms for myocardial ischemia and minimal necrosis include intermittent dynamic occlusion and spasm at the thrombus site.[31] If the thrombus occludes the coronary vessel for a prolonged period of time, Q-wave MI occurs. The clot causing Q-wave MI is rich in thrombin and fibrin.[32] In these patients, fibrinolysis or PCI (eg, angioplasty/stent) may limit

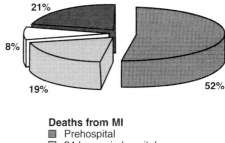

Figure 1. Distribution of mortality in patients with AMI who die during the first 30 days. Slightly more than 50% of patients who die will do so before reaching the hospital. An additional 25% of deaths will occur within the next 48 hours. The leading cause of early and late mortality after AMI is LV dysfunction with congestive heart failure; 10% of patients have cardiac rupture. Data is derived from a combination of AHA statistical data and Kleinman NS, White HD, Ohman EM, et al, GUSTO-I Investigators, Global Utilization of Streptokinase and Tissue Plasminogen Activator for Occluded Coronary Arteries. Mortality within 24 hours of thrombolysis for myocardial infarction: the importance of early reperfusion. *Circulation.* 1994;90:2658–2665.

the size of the infarct if performed sufficiently early in the course.

Out-of-Hospital Management

Early Defibrillation

Half of the patients who die of AMI do so early, before reaching a hospital (see Figure 1). In most of these deaths the presenting rhythm is ventricular tachycardia (VT)/VF.[33–35] The major risk of VF occurs during the first 4 hours after onset of symptoms.[36,37,37a] VF that occurs during the acute phase (usually within the first few hours) of an MI is called "primary VF"; it occurs in 4% to 18% of patients with infarction.[37a,38,39]

Once the patient is admitted to the hospital, the incidence of in-hospital VF is approximately 5%.[40] VF incidence appears to be declining even further in the modern era of reperfusion. Investigators in the Gruppo Italiano per lo Studio della Streptochinasi nell'Infarto Miocardico Study (GISSI) found a 3.6% incidence of early VF and a 0.6% incidence of late VF. Fibrinolytic therapy reduced the occurrence of VF primarily within the first 3 hours; the occurrence of VF did not predict reperfusion.[41,42] The presence of primary VF increases in-hospital mortality and complications[41,43] but does not appear to increase long-term mortality.[44]

All emergency medical services (EMS) and dispatch systems should have a trained and dedicated staff to respond to cardiac emergencies. Because the incidence of VF is highest out of hospital, every emergency vehicle that responds to cardiac emergencies should carry a defibrillator with staff skilled in its use. The AHA, the European Resuscitation Council, and the International Liaison Council on Resuscitation endorse the position that all emergency personnel, including first responders both in-hospital and in the field, should be trained to operate a defibrillator.[45,46]

Automated external defibrillators (AEDs) have been used safely and effectively by first responders with minimal training.[47–51] Whether greater availability of AEDs and access to them will increase survival is the subject of ongoing evaluation.[52–54] The AHA public health initiative *public access defibrillation* proposes to achieve more widespread early defibrillation through placement of AEDs throughout the community, making them available to a large number of trained lay community and nontraditional emergency responders. (See "Part 4: The Automated External Defibrillator.")

Ideally an EMS system should have enough trained personnel that a first responder can be at a victim's side anywhere in the system within 5 minutes. Early access is promoted by an emergency phone system with a dedicated number for that area (or region or country), with dispatchers trained to prioritize responses to these calls (see "Part 3: Adult Basic Life Support," Emergency Medical Dispatchers). Because patients with AMI have a high risk of sudden cardiac death during the first hour after onset of symptoms, an *out-of-hospital EMS system that can provide immediate defibrillation is mandatory. Every ambulance that transports cardiac patients should be equipped with a defibrillator and personnel proficient in its use.* If VF occurs under observation and immediate defibrillation is available, many patients will survive (see Figure 1).

When patients with ACS, including MI and other ischemic syndromes, reach the ED and hospital critical care unit (CCU), their risk of sudden cardiac death due to lethal arrhythmias falls dramatically.[40] This decline in risk stems from a combination of early reperfusion, administration of β-blockers, and other adjunctive agents used in the reperfusion era.[55,56] The deaths that do occur during this period are due to VF/VT, LV power failure with congestive heart failure (CHF) and cardiogenic shock, reocclusion with extension of the infarct, or mechanical complications of cardiac rupture and structural damage (Figure 1). For these reasons, healthcare professionals should focus on limiting the size of the infarct, treating arrhythmias, and preserving LV function.

Patient Education and Delays in Therapy

Delays in therapy after the onset of symptoms for ACS occur during 3 periods: during the interval from onset of symptoms to patient recognition, during out-of-hospital transport, and during in-hospital evaluation. Potential delay during the in-hospital evaluation period may occur from *d*oor to *d*ata, from data (ECG) to *d*ecision, and from decision to *d*rug; these 4 major points of in-hospital therapy are commonly referred to as the "4 D's."[57]

Because myocardial salvage is time dependent, with the greatest potential benefit in the first few hours of ACS, it is imperative that patients arrive at the treating hospital and receive evaluation and therapy as quickly as possible. Delay by patients, EMS personnel, and hospitals significantly prolongs the time to reperfusion therapy,[58,59] reducing the effectiveness of fibrinolytic therapy and increasing mortality.

Patient delay to symptom recognition constitutes the longest period of delay to treatment. Prodromal symptoms are common among patients with ACS,[60] but these symptoms are frequently denied or misinterpreted. The elderly, women, persons with diabetes, and hypertensive patients are most likely to delay, partly because they tend to have atypical symptoms or unusual presentations.[61–64] In the US Rapid Early Action for Coronary Treatment (REACT) trial, the median out-of-hospital delay was ≥2 hours in non-Hispanic blacks, the elderly and disabled, homemakers, and Medicaid recipients. The decision to use an ambulance was an important variable that reduced out-of-hospital delay and persisted after correction for variables associated with severity of symptoms.[65] Other factors that have an impact on the patient's arrival at the hospital include time of day, location (eg, work or home), and the presence of a family member.[66a,69] The REACT trial also found that community members recognized the value of EMS systems and warning signs of heart attack when they were involved as bystanders but often failed to act on their own behalf when having similar symptoms.[66a]

Out-of-hospital transport time constitutes only 5% of delay to treatment time, whereas in-hospital evaluation constitutes 25% to 33% of delay to treatment.[67,68] EMS systems, hospitals, and communities should educate patients about symptoms of cardiac ischemia, rapidly triage patients to appropriate care, and provide rapid defibrillation and medical care to patients with ischemic-type chest discomfort.

Education of patients is the primary intervention to reduce denial or misinterpretation of symptoms. The physician and family members of patients with known coronary disease should reinforce the need to seek medical attention when symptoms recur, because these patients paradoxically present later than patients with no known disease. Public education campaigns have been effective in increasing public awareness and knowledge of the symptoms and signs of heart attack.[69] The results of these campaigns, however, have been transient and unrewarding. An educational program emphasizing early recognition of symptoms and reasons for misinterpretation or denial of symptoms is important. Physicians should also educate their patients about the local EMS system and encourage early activation for appropriate symptoms.[70] Physicians should discuss prompt and appropriate use of nitroglycerin (glyceryl trinitrate in Europe) and aspirin, EMS activation, and location of the nearest hospital that offers 24-hour emergency cardiac care.

Out-of-Hospital Fibrinolysis

Clinical trials have shown the benefit of initiating fibrinolysis as soon as possible after onset of ischemic-type chest pain. Because the potential for myocardial salvage is greatest very early in AMI, a number of researchers have studied administration of fibrinolytics during the out-of-hospital period. Several studies demonstrated the feasibility and safety of out-of-hospital fibrinolytic administration,[71,72] but early small trials yielded conflicting results about the efficiency and efficacy of this strategy.[73–78]

Physicians in the Grampian Region Early Anistreplase Trial (GREAT) administered fibrinolytic therapy to patients at home 130 minutes earlier than to patients at the hospital and noted a 50% reduction in mortality in those treated earlier.[77] At the 5-year follow-up examination, investigators found that fewer patients (25%) in the out-of-hospital treatment group had died compared with a greater number (36%)

in the hospital treatment group (log-rank test, $P<0.025$).[79] Delaying fibrinolytic treatment by 30 minutes reduced average life expectancy by approximately 1 year. Delaying fibrinolytic treatment by 1 hour increased the hazard ratio of death by 20%, which is equivalent to the loss of 43 lives per 1000 patients within the next 5 years.

The European Myocardial Infarction Project group (EMIP) found that patients in the out-of-hospital treatment group received fibrinolytic therapy a median of 55 minutes earlier than those in the in-hospital treatment group.[72,77] Death due to cardiac causes was significantly less common in the group treated out of hospital than in the group treated in-hospital (8.3% versus 9.8%; reduction in risk, 16%; 95% CI, 0% to 29%; $P=0.049$). Only a nonsignificant reduction in overall mortality was observed at 30 days in the out-of-hospital group (9.7% versus 11.1% in the hospital group; reduction in risk 13%; 95% CI, −1% to 26%; $P=0.08$).

In the Myocardial Infarction Triage and Intervention (MITI) trial,[71] no significant difference in mortality between out-of-hospital and in-hospital fibrinolysis was observed. In a retrospective analysis, however, researchers noted that any patient treated within a median time of 70 minutes, whether before or after hospital arrival, had a significantly improved outcome. A confounding variable in this trial was advance notification of hospital staff and the shortening of hospital treatment times compared with historic controls.[80]

A meta-analysis of out-of-hospital fibrinolytic trials summarized by the EMIP group found a 17% relative improvement in outcome associated with out-of-hospital fibrinolytic therapy. The greatest improvement was observed when therapy was initiated 60 to 90 minutes earlier than in the hospital.[81] More recently a meta-analysis evaluated time to therapy and impact of prehospital fibrinolysis on all-cause mortality. Pooled results of 6 randomized trials with >6000 patients found a significant 58-minute reduction in time to administration ($P=0.007$) and decreased all-cause hospital mortality (OR 0.83; CI 0.70 to 0.98).[82] Although fibrinolytic therapy initiated out of hospital results in earlier treatment, the time savings can be offset in most instances by an improved hospital triage with a door-to-needle time ≤30 minutes.

In summary, administration of fibrinolytics during the out-of-hospital period appears to reduce mortality when transport times are long (Figure 2). The 1996 ACC/AHA Task Force on Practice Guidelines recommended that out-of-hospital systems focus on early diagnosis and that fibrinolytics be administered in the field when a physician is present or transport time is >90 minutes.[12] The European Society of Cardiology and the European Resuscitation Council recommend out-of-hospital fibrinolysis when transport time is >30 minutes or hospital door-to-needle time (beginning infusion of a fibrinolytic agent) is expected to be >60 minutes.[17] The AHA Committee on Emergency Cardiovascular Care, the Evidence Evaluation Conference, and the international Guidelines 2000 Conference expert panelists evaluated these recommendations and recent data and practice. We recommend out-of-hospital fibrinolytic therapy only when a physician is present or out-of-hospital transport time is ≥60 minutes (Class IIa). Observations from trials of out-of-

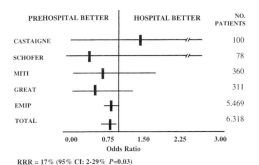

Figure 2. Results of a meta-analysis of prehospital fibrinolysis trials. RRR=17% (95% CI, 2% to 29%, $P=0.03$). Modified from Table 5 in The European Myocardial Infarction Project Group. Prehospital thrombolytic therapy in patients with suspected acute myocardial infarction. *N Engl J Med.* 1993;329:383–389.

hospital fibrinolysis suggest that most EMS systems should focus on early diagnosis and rapid transport instead of delivery of therapy.

Out-of-Hospital ECGs

Out-of-hospital performance of electrocardiography and transmission of the ECG to the ED speeds the care of patients with AMI. Multiple studies have shown the feasibility of obtaining a 12-lead ECG during the out-of-hospital period.[71,83–91] Diagnostic-quality ECGs can be successfully transmitted for approximately 85% of patients with chest pain who are eligible for 12-lead ECGs.[84] Recording an ECG increases the time spent at the scene of an emergency by only 0 to 4 minutes.[71,84,87,92] In addition, there is no difference between the quality of information collected out-of-hospital and that received by cellular transmission at the base station.[83] A diagnosis of AMI can be made sooner when the 12-lead ECG is obtained before the patient arrives in the hospital than if the ECG is performed after arrival.

The use of out-of-hospital ECGs and a chest pain evaluation form leads to more rapid initiation of reperfusion therapy without substantially delaying out-of-hospital time. A 12-lead ECG transmitted to the hospital speeds diagnosis and shortens time to fibrinolysis.[85,86,93,94] Many studies have shown significant reductions in hospital-based time to treatment with fibrinolytic therapy in patients with AMI identified before arrival by a 12-lead ECG.[87–89,95] Time savings in these studies ranged from 20 to 55 minutes.[87–89] Patients with an AMI identified by an out-of-hospital 12-lead ECG were more frequently treated in the ED than the CCU, and a trend toward more rapid ED and CCU treatment was demonstrated.[96] The US National Heart Attack Alert Program recommends that EMS systems provide out-of-hospital 12-lead ECGs to facilitate early identification of AMI and that all advanced lifesaving vehicles be able to transmit a 12-lead ECG to the hospital.[97]

A retrospective study of the US National Registry of Myocardial Infarction database showed a mortality benefit (reduction in mortality) for patients with AMI identified by an out-of-hospital 12-lead ECG.[98] Canto et al evaluated the treatment and outcome of patients with and without an out-of-hospital 12-lead ECG. Although the median time from onset of infarction to arrival at the hospital was longer among patients in the out-of-hospital ECG group, the median time to initiation of fibrinolysis or primary angioplasty was significantly shorter. The out-of-hospital ECG group was also significantly more likely to receive fibrinolytic therapy, primary angioplasty, or CABG. The in-hospital mortality rate was 8% among patients with an out-of-hospital ECG and 12% among those without an out-of-hospital ECG (*P*<0.001).[98]

By implementing the 12-lead ECG as a diagnostic procedure, the EMS system can expand its role in coordinating the community response to patients with signs and symptoms of ACS. Paramedics trained and equipped to obtain 12-lead ECGs in the field can provide the ED with a definitive diagnosis, allowing the administration of fibrinolytic agents (or primary angioplasty) soon after the patient's arrival. The safety, feasibility, and practicality of obtaining out-of-hospital 12-lead ECGs are well documented.

In summary, earlier diagnosis and faster treatment of AMI with fibrinolytic drugs is possible when a 12-lead ECG is obtained in the field and transmitted to the receiving emergency physician. Even shorter hospital delays have been observed in patients whose out-of-hospital identification by history and ECG was obtained as part of a protocol-driven out-of-hospital diagnostic strategy (out-of-hospital identification of fibrinolytic candidates) and whose out-of-hospital information was effectively communicated to the receiving physician before arrival at the hospital. Advances in computer interpretation of ECGs and development of predictive instruments have the potential to improve diagnostic sensitivity and enhance out-of-hospital evaluation of patients. Evidence supports the contention that out-of-hospital 12-lead ECG diagnostic programs are cost-effective and may be underused. We recommend implementation of out-of-hospital 12-lead ECG diagnostic programs in urban and suburban paramedic systems (Class I).

Cardiogenic Shock and Out-of-Hospital Facility Triage

Controversy continues over whether fibrinolytic therapy or PCI is the best method of reperfusion (see below). Mortality among patients with cardiogenic shock is high in reported studies.[99–102] In recent years an increasing body of evidence has suggested that early hemodynamic stabilization is beneficial and reduces mortality in certain patients. The Global Utilization of Streptokinase and Tissue Plasminogen Activator for Occluded Coronary Arteries (GUSTO-I) investigators retrospectively evaluated patients with cardiogenic shock after MI. The incidence of cardiogenic shock in the study was 11%, and an aggressive strategy (PCI) was associated with a lower mortality than that associated with fibrinolytic therapy.[103] The use of early invasive interventions is more common in the United States than in other countries, but patients who underwent revascularization had better survival in all countries.[104] In the Second National US Registry of Myocardial Infarction, the mortality rate in patients with AMI and shock was lower in those treated with PCI as a primary strategy than in those treated with fibrinolysis.[105] In a large registry of patients with shock, mortality was also lower in

AMI patients who received early revascularization with either PCI or CABG.[106]

A recently completed randomized trial found reduced mortality among patients with cardiogenic shock treated aggressively with intra-aortic balloon pulsation (IABP) and mechanical or surgical revascularization. In the SHOCK trial 152 patients were randomly assigned to an early revascularization strategy (ERV) and 150 patients were assigned to a strategy of initial medical stabilization (IMS).[106a] The initial medical management strategy was aggressive for both the ERV and IMS groups; intra-aortic balloon pump (IABP) support was used in 86% of both groups. Sixty-three percent of the IMS group received fibrinolytic agents, and 25% underwent delayed revascularization. Of the ERV group of patients who underwent emergency early revascularization, >60% received PCI and 40% had surgical revascularization. The 30-day mortality rate for ERV patients was lower but not significantly lower than those with IMS. A secondary end point, mortality rate at 6 months, was significantly lower in the ERV group (50.3% versus 63.1%, *P*=0.027). In this study a prespecified subgroup analysis was performed for patients <75 *years old*. The analysis showed a 15.4% reduction in 30-day mortality with early revascularization (IMS group, 56.8% versus ERV group, 41.4%, *P*<0.01). Outcome for patients >75 *years old was worse* for the ERV group. These results were thought to mirror those in the SHOCK registry.[107]

The 1999 update of the ACC/AHA Guidelines for the Management of Patients With Myocardial Infarction was revised to indicate a Class I recommendation for PCI in patients with shock who are <75 years of age. These recommendations were supported at the Guidelines 2000 Conference.[13] Use of IABP followed by diagnostic cardiac catheterization and, where anatomically appropriate, coronary revascularization with either PCI or CABG may reduce mortality.[108–112]

When possible, transfer patients at high risk for mortality or severe LV dysfunction with signs of shock, pulmonary congestion, heart rate >100 bpm, *and* SBP <100 mm Hg to facilities capable of cardiac catheterization and rapid revascularization (PCI or CABG) (for patients <75 years old, Class I). An out-of-hospital checklist can also identify patients who have contraindications to fibrinolytic therapy. Patients with contraindications to fibrinolytic therapy should be considered for transfer to interventional facilities when benefit from reperfusion exists (Class IIa).

Initial General Measures

Immediately begin continuous cardiac monitoring for patients with suspected ischemic-type chest pain and obtain intravenous access. Administer morphine, oxygen, nitroglycerin, and aspirin ("MONA") to patients without contraindications. Determine the immediate treatment necessary, rapidly assess reperfusion eligibility, and administer necessary adjunctive treatments (Table 1 and Figure 3).

Oxygen

Administer oxygen to all patients complaining of ischemic-type chest discomfort. Also administer oxygen, usually by

TABLE 1. Assessments and Treatments to Consider for Patients Who Present With ACS

Initial assessment

- Targeted history, including AMI inclusions, fibrinolytic exclusions
- Vital signs and focused physical examination
- 12-lead ECG; serial ECGs as indicated (postlytic evaluation of ST-segment resolution; recurrent discomfort)
- Chest x-ray (preferably upright)
- ECG monitoring

Initial general treatment (memory aid: "MONA")

- Morphine, 2 to 4 mg repeated every 5 to 10 min to provide adequate analgesia (diamorphine may be used instead of morphine in some countries)
- Oxygen, 4 L/min; continue if arterial oxygen saturation <90%
- Nitroglycerin, sublingual or spray, followed by IV for persistent or recurrent discomfort
- Aspirin, 160 to 325 mg (chew and swallow)

Specific treatments

- Target times for *reperfusion therapy*

  Fibrinolytic agents: door-to-needle time <30 min

  Primary PCI: door-to-dilation time 90±30 min
- *Conjunctive therapy* (combined with fibrinolytic agents)

  Aspirin

  Heparin (especially with fibrin-specific lytics)
- *Adjunctive therapies*

  β-Blocker if no contraindications

  IV nitroglycerin (for recurrent ischemia, large anterior MI, heart failure, antihypertensive effects)
- ACE inhibitor (especially large anterior wall MI, heart failure without hypotension [SBP >100 mm Hg], previous MI)

Patients with ST-segment elevation or new or presumably new bundle-branch block are candidates for reperfusion therapy.

nasal cannula, to all patients with suspected ACS. Experimental evidence suggests that breathing supplemental oxygen may limit ischemic myocardial injury. There is also evidence that oxygen reduces the amount of ST-segment elevation, although it is not known whether this therapy reduces morbidity or mortality among patients with AMI. Results of early experimental studies aimed at reducing the size of the infarct suggested that oxygen might be beneficial. In addition, oxygen can reduce ST-segment elevation among patients with anterior infarction.[113,114]

If a patient has overt pulmonary congestion or if oxygen saturation is <90%, continue oxygen therapy until the patient's condition has stabilized. If hypoxemia is persistent and respiratory muscle fatigue develops, consider early intubation with assisted mechanical ventilation and a higher fraction of inspired oxygen (Fio_2). Hypoxemia and respiratory insufficiency can tax a marginal cardiac output substantially, leading to increased infarct size and cardiovascular collapse. No clinical studies, however, have shown a reduction in morbidity or mortality with the routine use of supplemental oxygen and current treatment regimens. In the absence of compelling indications in uncomplicated cases, there is little justification for continued use of oxygen beyond 2 to 3 hours.

Nitroglycerin (or Glyceryl Trinitrate)

Nitroglycerin (glyceryl trinitrate in Europe) is an effective analgesic for ischemic-type chest discomfort. Nitrates also have beneficial hemodynamic effects, including dilation of the coronary arteries (particularly in the region of plaque disruption) and the peripheral arterial bed and venous capacitance vessels. Administer sublingual or aerosol nitroglycerin; repeat twice at 5-minute intervals until pain is relieved or low blood pressure limits its use. Initially administer nitrates to all patients with suspected ischemic-type pain unless SBP is <90 mm Hg.

The most significant potential complication of nitroglycerin therapy is systemic hypotension; this complication should be avoided when possible. Also avoid use of nitroglycerin in patients with extreme bradycardia (<50 bpm) or tachycardia. Administer nitrates with extreme caution, if at all, to patients with suspected right ventricular (RV) infarction.

Routine use of nitroglycerin has not been shown to be beneficial in AMI. In trials conducted before the fibrinolytic era, intravenous nitrates reduced infarct size. An analysis of subgroups in the largest of these studies showed that most of this benefit was in large anterior wall infarcts,[115] and a meta-analysis concluded that nitroglycerin was effective in reducing mortality.[116] In the Fourth International Study of Infarct Survival (ISIS-4) and GISSI-3, no conclusive evidence was presented to recommend routine use of oral or topical nitrate therapy in patients with AMI.[117]

Nitroglycerin is indicated for the initial management of pain and ischemia with AMI without hypotension (SBP <90 mm Hg), except in patients with RV infarction. Nitroglycerin should be used cautiously in patients with inferior wall MI with possible RV involvement (see below). Evidence does not support the routine administration of nitroglycerin in patients with uncomplicated AMI. In patients with recurrent ischemia, nitrates are indicated in the first 24 to 48 hours. They may be useful in patients with hypertension, CHF, and large anterior wall MI. In the absence of these indications, use of nitrates should be carefully considered, especially when lower blood pressure precludes the use of other agents shown to be effective in reducing morbidity and mortality, eg, β-blockers and angiotensin-converting enzyme (ACE) inhibitors (ACEIs). The continued use of nitroglycerin beyond 48 hours is indicated for patients with recurrent angina or persistent pulmonary congestion. Initially avoid the use of long-acting nitrates, including topical preparations whose absorption may be altered as skin blood flow changes in response to neurohumoral alterations during the peri-infarction period. Instead use intravenous preparations, which can be controlled more precisely during periods of hemodynamic lability.

Morphine

Although nitroglycerin effectively relieves ischemic-type chest discomfort due to ACS, it should not be used as a substitute for narcotic analgesia, which is often necessary to relieve pain associated with MI. Morphine is indicated for continuing pain unresponsive to nitrates. Morphine is also effective in patients with vascular congestion complicating AMI because of its favorable hemodynamic effects. Mor-

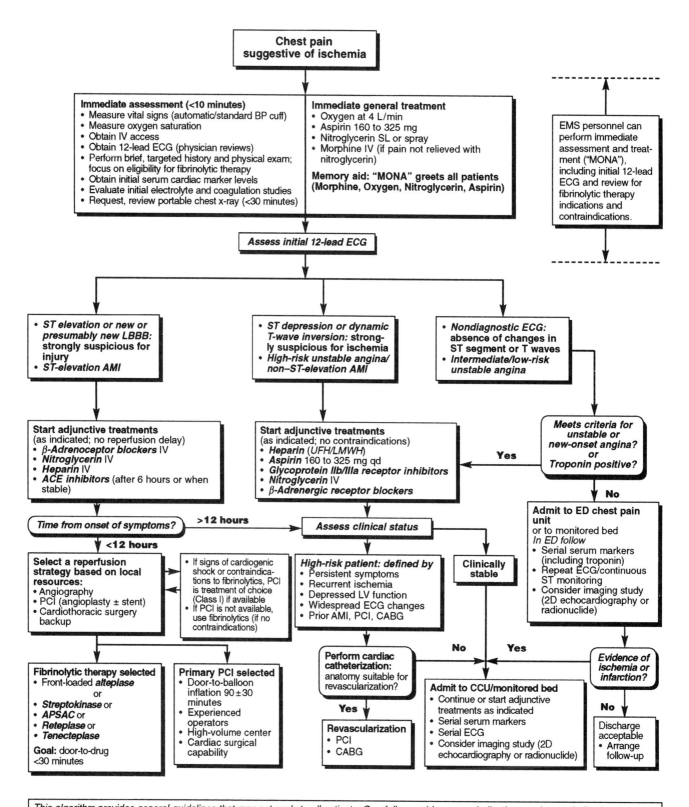

Figure 3. Acute ischemic chest pain protocol. Although local evaluation, diagnosis, and treatment may vary, core concepts involve the prompt treatment of ischemic-type chest pain with oxygen, nitrates, and morphine. The ECG is central to the initial triage of patients and allows identification of patients at high, intermediate, or low risk, who may then be further evaluated. Patients with ST-segment elevation should be rapidly assessed for reperfusion therapy (fibrinolytic; PCI). ST-segment depression identifies a group of patients at high short-term risk for cardiac events, and aggressive antiplatelet therapy is indicated whether a medical or invasive strategy is chosen. Some patients at increased risk also have nondiagnostic or normal ECGs, and the use of cardiac markers, C-reactive protein, and functional studies allows additional risk stratification.

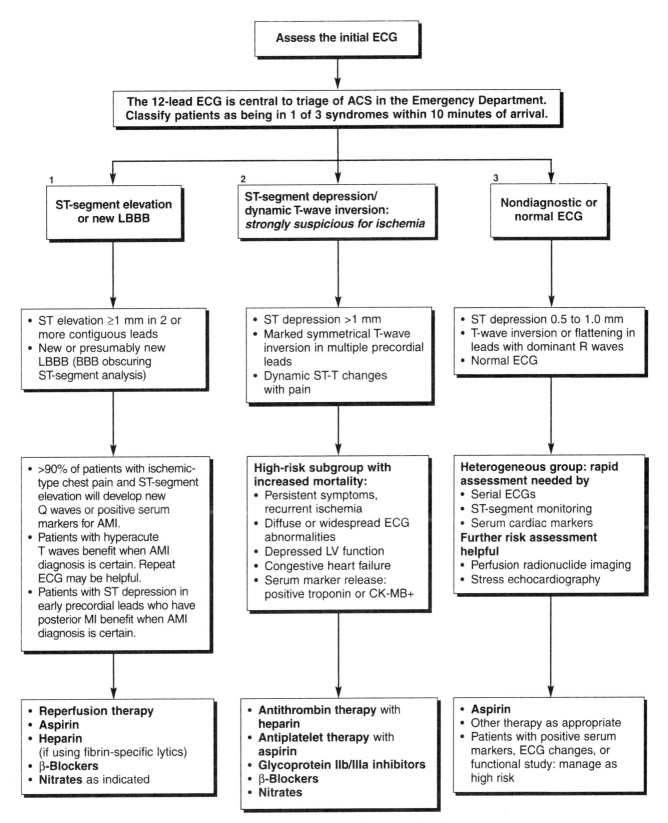

Figure 4. The Acute Coronary Syndromes Algorithm.

phine reduces ventricular preload and oxygen requirements primarily by venodilation. For this reason it should not be used in patients who may have hypovolemia. If hypotension develops, elevation of the patient's legs and volume infusion with saline will usually reverse adverse hemodynamics. Pain associated with MI may be due to continuing ischemia of viable myocardium in the evolving infarct region. β-Adrenergic receptor blocking agents are effective anti-ischemic agents that often also reduce or control the pain of infarction.

Aspirin

Although a time-dependent effect of aspirin is not supported by evidence, aspirin should be given as soon as possible to all patients with suspected ACS unless the patient is allergic to it. A dose of 160 to 325 mg causes rapid and near-total inhibition of thromboxane A_2 production. This inhibition reduces coronary reocclusion and recurrent events after fibrinolytic therapy. Aspirin alone reduced death from MI in the Second International Study of Infarct Survival (ISIS-2), and its effect was additive to that of streptokinase.[118] In a review of 145 trials involving aspirin, the Antiplatelet Trialists Collaboration reported a reduction in vascular events from 14% to 10% in patients with MI. In high-risk patients, aspirin reduced nonfatal MI by 30% and vascular death by 17%.[119] Aspirin is also effective in patients with unstable angina. For this reason, aspirin should be part of the early treatment of all patients with suspected ACS. Aspirin is relatively contraindicated for patients with active peptic ulcer disease and a history of asthma.

Chewable aspirin is absorbed more quickly than swallowed tablets in the early hours after infarction, particularly if morphine has been given. Aspirin suppositories (325 mg) are safe and recommended for patients with severe nausea, vomiting, or disorders of the upper gastrointestinal tract.

Risk Stratification, Initial Therapy, and Evaluation for Reperfusion in the ED

The Ischemic Chest Pain Algorithm (Figure 3) provides an overview of the recommended approach to patients presenting with ACS. Such an organized and interdisciplinary protocol is essential for efficient, effective treatment of these patients. The initial clinical history and ECG are used to triage patients into risk categories and choose a treatment strategy. Patients with ischemic-type chest discomfort and ST-segment elevation should be rapidly identified and considered for reperfusion therapy. If an ECG was not obtained during the out-of-hospital period, one should be obtained and reviewed by the senior physician treating the patient within 10 minutes of the patient's arrival in the ED.[120] If the patient meets the criteria for reperfusion therapy, a door-to-needle time (beginning of infusion of a fibrinolytic agent) of ≤30 minutes is consistent with the urgent need for reperfusion.

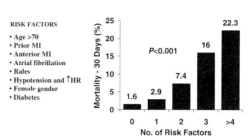

Risk Stratification

Prediction of Mortality at 30 Days

Figure 5. The TIMI investigators found that baseline characteristics, including age, sex, previous or anterior MI, indicators of LV dysfunction such as rales and hypotension/tachycardia, atrial fibrillation, or diabetes were predictive of mortality at 30 days. Mortality increased from 1.4% with no risk factors to >22% when ≥4 risk factors were present. From Cannon CP, et al. *J Am Coll Cardiol.* 1999;33(suppl A):396A.

The first physician who encounters a patient with MI should be able to determine the need for fibrinolysis and direct its administration. Protocols for rapid evaluation and treatment should be available. Consultation with a cardiologist or the patient's personal physician delays therapy, is associated with increased hospital mortality, and is recommended only in equivocal or uncertain cases.[121] Patients with ST-segment elevation and new or presumably new left bundle-branch block should be quickly screened for indications and contraindications to fibrinolytic therapy. See Figure 4, The Acute Coronary Syndromes.

Risk Stratification With the First 12-Lead ECG

Use the 12-lead ECG to triage patients into 1 of 3 groups:

1. ST-segment elevation
2. ST-segment depression (≥1 mm)
3. Nondiagnostic or normal ECG

Patients with ischemic-type pain but normal or nondiagnostic ECGs or ECGs consistent with ischemia (ST-segment depression only) do not benefit from fibrinolytic therapy. These patients are not candidates for fibrinolytic agents. In

TABLE 2.   Patients With Chest Pain Suggestive of Ischemia: Probability of Significant CAD Based on Clinical Features and Presenting ECG

High Risk (≥1 of the Following Features)	Intermediate Risk (No High-Risk Features Plus 1 of the Following)	Low Risk (No High- or Intermediate-Risk Features Plus 1 of the Following)
Prior MI or life-threatening arrhythmia episode	Definite clinical angina in young age	Possible angina
Known CAD		
Definite clinical angina	Probable angina in older age	1 risk factor, not diabetes
Dynamic ST-segment changes with chest symptoms	Possible angina	T-wave inversion <1 mm
	Diabetes	
	3 other risk factors	
Marked T-wave changes in anterior precordial leads	ST-segment depression ≤1 mm	Normal ECG
	T-wave inversion ≥1 mm (leads with dominant R waves)	

CAD indicates coronary artery disease. Modified from Reference 14.

TABLE 3.   Patients With Chest Pain Suggestive of Ischemia: Short-Term Risk of Death and Nonfatal MI

High Risk of Death or Nonfatal AMI (≥1 of the Following)	Intermediate Risk of Death or Nonfatal AMI (No High-Risk Features Plus 1 of the Following)	Low Risk of Death or Nonfatal AMI (No High- or Intermediate-Risk Features Plus 1 of the Following)
Prolonged continuing pain not relieved by rest (>20 min)	Prolonged angina (>20 min) but resolved at time of evaluation; moderately high likelihood of CAD	Angina increased in frequency, severity, or duration
Pulmonary edema related to ischemia	Rest angina >20 min or relieved with nitroglycerin	Lower activity threshold before angina
S_3 or rales		1 risk factor, not diabetes
Hypotension with angina	Age >65 y	New-onset angina >2 wk to 2 mo before presentation
Rest angina with dynamic ST-segment changes >1 mm	Dynamic T-wave changes and angina	Normal or unchanged ECG
Elevated serum troponin T or I	Pathological Q waves or ST-segment depression <1 mm multiple-lead groups	

Modified from Reference 14 and from Antman E, Fox K. Guidelines for the diagnosis and management of unstable angina and non–Q-wave myocardial infarction: proposed revisions. International Cardiology Forum. *Am Heart J.* 2000;139:461–475.

fact, treatment with fibrinolytic agents presents a risk of harm. The Thrombolysis in Myocardial Infarction (TIMI-IIIB) study specifically addressed the use of tPA in patients with unstable angina or non–Q-wave infarction and found no benefit of fibrinolytic therapy and a possible risk of harm.[25]

Although the ECG is nondiagnostic in approximately 50% of patients with chest discomfort, it is central and helpful in risk stratification of patients with suspected ACS. The terms *transmural MI* and *subendocardial MI* have been replaced by *Q-wave MI* and *non–Q-wave MI*. However, physicians in the ED will not be able to determine whether an infarction will evolve into a Q-wave or non–Q-wave MI. Initial triage and reperfusion decisions are therefore based on the presence of *ST-segment elevation, ST-segment depression,* and *nondiagnostic ST-segment and T-wave abnormalities* on the ECG.

Patients with ischemic-type chest pain and ST-segment elevation ≥1 mm in 2 contiguous leads have a 45% sensitivity but a 98% specificity for AMI. In the TIMI IIIB registry of patients with unstable angina/non–Q-wave MI, the ECG ancillary study found that 60% of patients with ischemic pain had no ECG changes.[122] Patients traditionally thought to be at high risk with >1 mm ST-segment depression constituted 12.4% of patients and had an 11% 1-year rate of death or nonfatal MI. However, patients with 0.5-mm ST-segment depression were also found to be at high risk, and death or MI occurred in 16.3% at 1 year, suggesting that the more traditional use of 1 mm ST-segment depression warrants review. T-wave inversion did not add to the clinical history or significantly increase the 1-year event rate. Although patients presenting with left bundle-branch block had a low hospital event rate (1%), with no significant coronary disease in >34%, they had the highest 1-year mortality rate and more heart failure. Careful follow-up and more intensive medical therapy are appropriate.[122]

Patients with normal or nondiagnostic ECGs should be reevaluated for the cause of their symptoms. Coronary angiographic studies have shown that as many as 20% of patients with unstable angina will have normal or nonsignificant coronary artery disease. In the Women's Ischemia Symptom Evaluation (WISE) trial, 70% of women had

normal arteries or no significant obstructive disease (<50% closed).[123]

A prior ECG for comparison is useful when the initial ECG is consistent with ischemia or infarction. Diagnostic accuracy and triage decisions are improved by reducing the admission of patients without ACS (increased specificity) without reducing the admission of patients with these diagnoses (unchanged sensitivity).[124] A repeat ECG with pain or after initial assessment may be helpful when the initial ECG is normal or nondiagnostic and should be obtained approximately 1 hour after admission or sooner if clinically indicated.

The presence of Q waves does not preclude the use of reperfusion therapy but predicts a worse outcome.[125] In fact, Q waves may develop quite early in ACS. In 1 study,[126] 53% of patients presenting within 1 hour of onset of symptoms already displayed abnormal Q waves. This early development of Q waves appears to predict the size of the infarct but may not negate beneficial effects of fibrinolytic therapy on mortality or myocardial salvage.

Failure of reperfusion with fibrinolytics has been difficult to evaluate with clinical parameters.[127] More recently, studies evaluating resolution of ST-segment elevation following fibrinolysis have shown a strong correlation with infarct patency and therapeutic efficacy.[128–132]

Risk Stratification and Clinical Variables

When combined with clinical information, the ECG helps triage patients into treatment and risk profile groups. The TIMI-II and TIMI-9 studies found that clinical risk factors, including age, female sex, history of MI, anterior MI, rales, hypotension and increased heart rate, diabetes, and atrial fibrillation, were incremental and predicted mortality at 30 days (Figure 5). The hospital mortality rate was 1.6% in patients with no risk factors and 22.3% in those with >4 risk factors. Clinical variables can be used to assess the probability of coronary artery disease (Table 2) and the risk of a major adverse cardiac event in the presence of unstable angina (Table 3).[14] Patients with unstable angina can be placed into high-, intermediate-, and low-risk groups for more aggressive treatment strategies and newer therapies in a cost-effective manner. Most recently, the Platelet Glycoprotein IIb/IIIa in Unstable Angina: Receptor Suppression Using Integrilin Therapy (PURSUIT) investigators[133] have also found that, in addition to age, ST-segment depression and signs of heart failure, and positive cardiac markers predicted mortality or myocardial (re)infarction.

New cardiac markers more sensitive than the myocardial muscle creatine kinase isoenzyme are useful in risk stratification and determination of prognosis. An elevated level of *troponin* correlates with an increased risk of death, and greater elevations predict greater risk.[134] An elevated level of troponin also has incremental value beyond that of the ECG and clinical variables.[135] In addition, elevated troponin levels have predicted the benefits of newer treatment therapies, including GP IIb/IIIa inhibitors and LMWH.[136–138] Patients with increased troponin levels have increased thrombus burden and microvascular embolization. In the absence of troponin elevation, inflammatory markers help identify chest pain patients with unstable plaques and active inflammation. C-reactive protein has independent prognostic utility and is incremental when troponin levels are considered.[139,140] C-reaction protein appears to predict 6-month but not short-term major cardiac events in ACS. More clinical studies are needed to determine whether C-reactive protein can identify patients who will benefit from aggressive medical treatment strategies or early coronary intervention.

ST-Segment Elevation MI

Patients with ST-segment elevation should be rapidly evaluated for reperfusion therapy. Strategies for reperfusion include the administration of fibrinolytics and primary PCI.

Reperfusion Therapy: Fibrinolytics

Perhaps the most significant advance in treatment of cardiovascular disease in the last decade is reperfusion therapy for AMI. Many clinical trials have established early fibrinolytic therapy as a standard of care (Class I for persons <75 years of age and Class IIa for persons >75 years of age) for acute ST-segment elevation MI.[24,141–143] In addition, the era of reperfusion has enriched our understanding of MI and other ACS.

The first megatrial to show a reduction in mortality associated with fibrinolytic therapy was the GISSI-1 trial, which randomly assigned 11 721 patients to streptokinase or placebo and found a significant reduction in 21-day mortality in the streptokinase-treated group.[145] This effect on mortality has recently been documented to persist for up to 10 years.[144] The GISSI-1 trial also found the greatest benefit when treatment occurred during the first 3 hours after onset of symptoms. This trial predicted a maximum reduction in mortality of 47% for patients treated in the first hour.[145] The landmark ISIS-2 study convincingly showed that antiplatelet therapy with aspirin (OR 23%) or fibrinolytic therapy with streptokinase (OR 25%) alone reduced mortality in patients with MI (see Figure 6). The effect of combining these 2 treatments was additive; mortality was reduced by 42%. Most of this reduction (53%) occurred if therapy was provided during the first 4 hours after the onset of symptoms.[118] An overview of all available randomized trials in 1990 noted a

reduction in short-term mortality of 24% (treated 12.8%; placebo 10%; *P*<0.0001) with a maintained benefit in the 2 largest trials. The reperfusion era had come of age.

The major determinants of myocardial salvage and long-term prognosis are

- Short time to reperfusion[24,145]
- Early and sustained patency of the infarct-related artery with normal flow (TIMI grade 3)[147,148]
- Normal microvascular perfusion[26,130,149,150]

Early studies in laboratory animals suggested that the infarct was substantially complete within 6 hours.[151] Results of early fibrinolytic trials in humans were similar: Most reduction in mortality occurred when therapy was initiated in the first few hours after infarction. In GISSI-1 a 50% reduction in mortality was found in patients treated within the first hour.[145] Results of the Myocardial Infarction Triage and Intervention (MITI) trial supported this finding and showed that patients treated within the first 70 minutes of onset of symptoms had a >50% reduction in infarct size and a reduction in mortality from 8.7% to 1.2%.[80] These studies led to the initial US recommendation that all patients with ST-segment elevation infarction within 6 hours of onset of symptoms be considered candidates for fibrinolytic therapy.[12]

Additional studies have suggested that the benefit of treatment may extend up to 12 hours.[152,153] Reduction in mortality was confirmed in a large meta-analysis, which showed an 18% *proportional* reduction (*P*<0.00001) in mortality, leading to a reduction in mortality of 18 deaths per 1000 patients treated.[24] Subsequent recommendations have expanded treatment indications and increased the time window for patients in whom the risk-benefit ratio is favorable.[12] The early benefit results from myocardial salvage. This "saving of muscle" is due to early rapid patency and complete restoration of normal flow ("time is muscle").[154,155] An additional late benefit of infarct-artery patency is the mortality benefit, which occurs independent of ventricular function.[156,157] This late benefit appears to come from a reduction of scar formation and from attenuation of ventricular dilation and infarct remodeling. Attenuation of remodeling of the infarcted myocardium reduces the development of CHF, promotes electrical stability of the infarct substrate, and increases the likelihood of recovery of watershed ("penum-

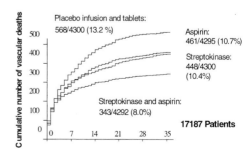

Figure 6. Results from the ISIS-2 trial comparing aspirin and streptokinase alone and in combination in patients with AMI. Aspirin was effective in reducing mortality alone and was additive when given with streptokinase. From ISIS-2 Collaborative Group. *Lancet.* 1988;2:349–360.

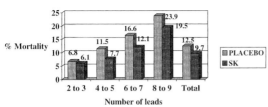

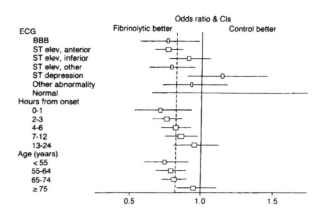

Figure 7. Patients in the GISSI trial demonstrated increasing mortality with the number of leads showing ST-segment elevation. Patients in each category, except those with ST-segment elevation in 2 or 3 leads, benefited from fibrinolytic therapy with a significant reduction in mortality. Of patients with inferior and lateral wall MI, 92% and 61%, respectively, had ST-segment elevation in only 2 to 3 leads.[160]

bra") areas of ischemia. This is particularly true for areas of the myocardium that depend on collateral circulation.[157]

Risk/Benefit of Fibrinolytic Therapy

Physicians who administer fibrinolytic agents should be aware of the indications, contraindications, benefits, and major risks of administration. Most of the reluctance to administer fibrinolytic agents is related to the risks of hemorrhage and intracranial bleeding. In addition, a number of patients are considered marginal, which makes it difficult to apply eligibility criteria. Familiarity with these risk/benefit principles will allow the physician at the bedside to weigh the net clinical benefit for each patient.[158,159]

A large body of evidence confirms that patients who present with ischemic pain and ST-segment elevation (>0.1 mV in ≥2 contiguous leads) within 12 hours of onset of persistent pain receive the greatest benefit from fibrinolytic therapy. The initial ECG can be prognostic as well as diagnostic, with useful information for the clinician evaluating the patient for risk and benefit. The GISSI investigators found that stratification of patients by both infarct site (inferior, anterior, lateral, multiple) and the number of leads with ST-segment elevation predicted both benefit from fibrinolysis and mortality. Mortality was almost linearly related to the number of leads with ST-segment elevation[160] (Figure 7).

The Fibrinolytic Therapy Trialists' (FTT) Collaborative Group[24] evaluated 9 major randomized trials with >1000 patients each (45 000 total patients) to determine the safety and benefit of fibrinolytic therapy in a wide variety of patient subgroups (Figure 8). Treatment was helpful regardless of patients' sex, presenting blood pressure (if SBP was <180 mm Hg), previous MI, or diabetes. Although cardiogenic shock was not specifically identified, patients with low blood pressure and tachycardia also benefited. Therapeutic benefit was seen for up to 12 hours but was greatest when fibrinolytics were administered in the first 3 hours. The benefits were less impressive in inferior wall infarction, except when it was associated with RV infarction (ST-segment elevation in lead V_4R or anterior ST-segment depression). Older patients had a higher absolute risk of death, but absolute benefit in older patients was similar to that in younger patients. Fewer numbers of older patients (>75 years

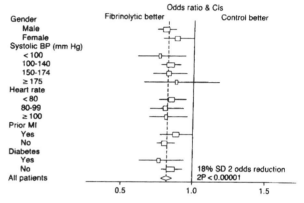

Figure 8. Proportional effects of fibrinolytic therapy and mortality rates in the Fibrinolytic Therapy Trialists' Collaborative Group meta-analysis,[24] subdivided by presentation features. Line of identity indicates a neutral treatment effect with no benefit. Characteristics to the left of the line of identity indicate survival advantage attributable to fibrinolytic therapy; those to the right indicate a higher mortality rate attributable to fibrinolytic therapy.

old) were included in the analysis, however, and most patients had been treated with streptokinase.

Although age is not a contraindication to fibrinolytic therapy and absolute benefit remains, the incidence of stroke increases with advancing age,[161,162] and the relative benefit of fibrinolytic therapy is reduced. Older age is the most important baseline variable predicting nonhemorrhagic stroke.[161] Investigators from the Global Utilization of Streptokinase and t-PA for Occluded Arteries (GUSTO-I) trial recently reported lower mortality and net clinical benefit with accelerated administration of tPA in patients <85 years old; this treatment also resulted in lower mortality at 1 year.[162a] Too few patients >85 years old were included in the clinical trial for analysis. A recent retrospective analysis of the US Medicare database of patients >75 years of age treated with fibrinolytic therapy found no specific survival advantage and possible risk for patients >75 years old.[164] Additional studies are needed to clarify risk-benefit parameters in the elderly. A careful review of associated risks and potential benefits in the elderly is needed, and recent clinical trials with larger numbers of elderly subjects have recorded an increased incidence of stroke.[142,143] Elderly patients should be carefully assessed.

One method for expressing the time-dependent benefit of fibrinolytic therapy is the concept of "lives saved per 1000

TABLE 4. Comparison of Fibrinolytic Therapy With Standard Therapy

Fibrinolytics Started	Additional Lives Saved per 1000 Patients Treated
In the first hour	65
In the second hour	37
In the third hour	29
Between hours 3 and 6	26
Between hours 6 and 12	18
Between hours 12 and 24	9

patients treated."[165] The method assumes 1000 patients treated with fibrinolytics and 1000 patients treated with standard care that does not include fibrinolytics. The analysis calculates the number of additional lives saved (or the number of deaths) per 1000 people. This recent study pooled findings from 22 randomized, controlled trials of fibrinolytic therapy published from 1983 to 1993. The study results are summarized in Table 4.

Intracerebral Hemorrhage

Fibrinolytic therapy is associated with a small but definite increase in the risk of hemorrhagic stroke, which contributes to the early hazard of therapy in the first day (increased mortality).[24] More intensive fibrinolytic regimens using tPA (alteplase) and heparin pose a greater risk than streptokinase and aspirin.[166,167] Clinical risk factors that may help risk-stratify patients at the time of presentation are age (>65 years), low body weight (<70 kg), initial hypertension (180/110 mm Hg), and use of tPA. The number of risk factors can be used to estimate the frequency of stroke, which ranges from 0.25% with no risk factors to 2.5% with 3 risk factors.[159]

Fibrinolytic therapy is not recommended if >12 hours has passed since the onset of symptoms. In patients who present >12 hours after onset of symptoms with extensive infarction and ongoing ischemic pain, however, fibrinolytic therapy may be considered (Class IIb). Fibrinolytic therapy is contraindicated and may be harmful when continuous, persistent pain has been present for >24 hours, even in the presence of ST-segment elevation. There is only a small trend for benefit after a delay of 12 to 24 hours since symptom onset.

The presence of high blood pressure (SBP >175 mm Hg) at presentation to the ED increases the risk of stroke.[168] Current clinical practice is directed at lowering blood pressure before administration of fibrinolytic agents, although this has not been proved to reduce the risk of stroke.[168] Fibrinolytic treatment of patients who present with an SBP >180 mm Hg or a diastolic blood pressure >110 mm Hg is relatively contraindicated. The risk-benefit ratio should be carefully considered. Patients with AMI precipitated by cocaine use can be safely treated with fibrinolytics.[169]

Patients with ST-segment depression are a heterogeneous population with a high mortality rate who do not benefit from fibrinolytic treatment.[170] Whether a subgroup of these patients could benefit from therapy was a question raised by a retrospective analysis of the Late Assessment of Thrombolytic Efficacy (LATE) trial.[171] More precise selection of patients based on new diagnostic strategies (eg, cardiac markers) will be the subject of future prospective trials. Fibrinolytic therapy for patients with ST-segment depression and ischemic pain at rest (unstable angina or non–Q-wave infarction) is currently not recommended.[12]

Treatment Regimens

Initial trials demonstrated the efficacy of currently approved fibrinolytic agents: streptokinase,[118,145,172] anistreplase,[173,174] alteplase,[175,176] reteplase,[177,178] and tenectaplase.[143,179] These trials differed in enrollment, time to treatment, patient demographics, and conjunctive therapy, particularly use of heparin. The GUSTO trial subsequently tested 4 fibrinolytic regimens in >40 000 patients.[166] Thirty-day mortality was lowest with the alteplase and intravenous heparin regimen, but a small increase in the number of hemorrhagic strokes occurred in patients treated with this accelerated protocol. Nevertheless, an overall net benefit of 9 fewer deaths per 1000 patients treated was achieved. The GUSTO-I angiographic substudy found differences in early (90-minute) patency among the 4 subgroups that closely predicted survival, suggesting that earlier reperfusion was the physiological mechanism responsible for outcome.[155]

Studies have shown that complete restoration of arterial flow (TIMI grade 3) rather than partial restoration of flow (TIMI grade 1 and 2) correlates with improved outcome.[180] The accelerated alteplase regimen used in GUSTO currently appears to provide the earliest and most complete reperfusion, supporting the treatment goal of very early and complete restoration of vessel patency. Recent findings also stress the importance of microvascular dysfunction, which limits myocardial function and recovery, and the numerous factors involved in optimal myocardial function.[181]

A paradoxical effect of fibrinolytic administration is platelet activation. Newer regimens that include more effective platelet inhibitors, such as direct GP IIb/IIIa receptor inhibitors, increase the incidence and speed of reperfusion.[182–184] Large clinical trials are now evaluating the newer fibrinolytic agents[143,185,186] and combination therapies for AMI. Novel fibrinolytic regimens can be expected for both AMI and unstable angina.[187,188]

After GUSTO-I several clinical applications of the risk-benefit ratio have attempted to compare the cost-benefit ratio, risk of ICH, and mortality benefits in subgroups of patients. Alteplase (tPA) appears to have the greatest benefit in patients with large infarctions and appears to pose a low risk of ICH in younger patients who present early. Streptokinase appears to provide greater benefit in older patients with a smaller amount of myocardium at risk who present later and those with a greater risk of ICH. In addition, streptokinase appears to be most effective in the first 3 hours before the clot organizes. In EDs these facts should lead to a careful evaluation of risk and benefit.

Reperfusion Therapy: PCI

Clinical trials support the finding that direct coronary angioplasty is potentially superior to fibrinolytic therapy in the restoration of infarct patency (Figure 9).[189,190] Coronary angioplasty provides higher rates of TIMI grade 3 flow, is successful in >90% of patients, and is associated with lower

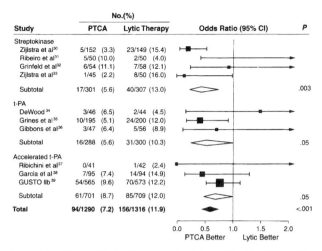

	No.(%)			
Study	PTCA	Lytic Therapy	Odds Ratio (95% CI)	P
Streptokinase				
Zijlstra et al[30]	5/152 (3.3)	23/149 (15.4)		
Ribeiro et al[31]	5/50 (10.0)	2/50 (4.0)		
Grinfeld et al[32]	6/54 (11.1)	7/58 (12.1)		
Zijlstra et al[33]	1/45 (2.2)	8/50 (16.0)		
Subtotal	17/301 (5.6)	40/307 (13.0)		.003
t-PA				
DeWood[34]	3/46 (6.5)	2/44 (4.5)		
Grines et al[35]	10/195 (5.1)	24/200 (12.0)		
Gibbons et al[36]	3/47 (6.4)	5/56 (8.9)		
Subtotal	16/288 (5.6)	31/300 (10.3)		.05
Accelerated t-PA				
Ribichini et al[37]	0/41	1/42 (2.4)		
Garcia et al[38]	7/95 (7.4)	14/94 (14.9)		
GUSTO IIb[39]	54/565 (9.6)	70/573 (12.2)		
Subtotal	61/701 (8.7)	85/709 (12.0)		.05
Total	94/1290 (7.2)	156/1316 (11.9)		<.001

0.0   0.5   1.0   1.5   2.0
PTCA Better   Lytic Better

Figure 9. Fibrinolytic therapy versus angioplasty. Mortality and nonfatal reinfarction rates for randomized trials comparing primary angioplasty with fibrinolytic therapy. Data displayed as odds ratio of 95% CI for each study, each fibrinolytic regimen, and combined trials. Reprinted from Gersh BJ. Current issues in reperfusion therapy. *Am J Cardiol.* 1998;82:3P–11P. With permission of Excerpta Medica, Inc.

rates of reocclusion and postinfarction ischemia than fibrinolytic therapy. Early randomized trials were small, but researchers found a reduction in short-term (6-week) mortality (OR 0.53; 95% CI 0.33 to 0.94) and in the combined outcome of short-term mortality and nonfatal reinfarction (OR 0.53; 95% CI 0.35 to 0.80). These positive results are particularly notable because they were performed during the early developmental stages of angioplasty. A meta-analysis including more recent trials found a 34% reduction (6.5% versus 4.4%) in 30-day mortality favoring angioplasty (OR 0.66; 95% CI 0.46 to 0.94). More impressively, the rate of reduction of the combined end point of death and nonfatal reinfarction was 40% (OR 0.58; 95% CI 0.44 to 0.76; $P<0.001$) and that of hemorrhagic stroke was 90% (0.1% versus 1.1%; $P<0.001$).

The majority of trials reported through 1996 had short-term follow-up, including the relatively large GUSTO-IIB angiographic substudy. The Cochrane database evaluated 10 trials involving 2573 patients and noted that a meta-analysis found superior short-term results for angioplasty and 66% fewer strokes, but long-term outcome and superiority were less certain.[191] Long-term results from the Primary Angioplasty in Myocardial Infarction trial[192] were recently reported. At 2 years patients undergoing primary angioplasty had less recurrent ischemia and lower rates of reintervention and hospital readmission than those treated with fibrinolysis. The combined end point of death or reinfarction was 14.9% in patients treated with angioplasty and 23% in those treated with tPA. The GUSTO-IIb investigators recently reported that the benefits of angioplasty extend equally to the elderly, a group at increased risk for ICH.[193]

Primary stenting for MI is being evaluated in ongoing studies. Results from these studies confirm the superiority of a strategy of angioplasty and stent, which has resulted in higher patency rates and reduced rates of postinfarction ischemia and repeated revascularization.[194–198] Interestingly mortality rates have not declined as expected, consistent with

a patent artery hypothesis. This may be due to microvascular abnormalities, which appear to improve with concomitant use of GP IIb/IIIa inhibitors.[130]

A major criticism of primary angioplasty is the need for on-site catheterization facilities and experienced operators. Triage by EMS personnel of patients with large anterior infarction and those with severe LV dysfunction may attenuate this problem. Door-to-balloon times are suboptimal, but experienced centers can reduce this delay so that reperfusion times may be comparable to those of fibrinolytic therapy.

When possible, triage patients at high risk for mortality or severe LV dysfunction with signs of shock, pulmonary congestion, heart rate >100 bpm, and SBP <100 mm Hg to facilities capable of performing cardiac catheterization and rapid revascularization (PCI or CABG). For patients <75 years of age, this is a Class I recommendation. When available without delay, consider primary PCI for patients who are reperfusion candidates but have a risk of bleeding that contraindicates use of fibrinolytic therapy (Class IIa).

ST-Segment Depression: Non–Q-Wave MI/High-Risk Unstable Angina

Non–Q-wave MI and unstable angina presenting with ST-segment depression constitute a pathological process on the continuum between chronic stable angina and typical Q-wave MI. These patients with ST-segment depression on presentation constitute a high-risk subgroup. In some patients non–Q-wave MI will evolve. Recent registries suggest that the incidence of non–Q-wave MI is increasing as the population of older patients with more advanced disease increases. The widespread use of fibrinolytics, aspirin, and β-blockers may also contribute to this increase.

Despite the relatively high mortality rate among patients with ST-segment depression, fibrinolytic therapy provides no benefit. The available data does not support routine use of fibrinolytic therapy as a treatment option in patients with ST-segment depression or nondiagnostic ECGs with elevated cardiac markers.

Treat patients with ST-segment depression or T-wave inversion with ischemic-type chest pain with aspirin and heparin (see Figure 10). Administer nitrates for recurrent angina. Initiate or optimize β-blockade. If patients have persistent symptoms despite adequate β-blockade or cannot tolerate this therapy, add a calcium antagonist. Consider coronary angiography for high-risk patients with recurrent ischemia, depressed LV function, widespread changes on the ECG, or prior MI. Consider revascularization with PCI or CABG for patients with a suitable anatomy. Continue medical therapy in patients who are clinically stable. Further stratify risk with stress tests when appropriate.

Aggressive medical therapy is indicated for patients at high risk for major adverse cardiac events. The TIMI-III investigators have defined high-risk clinical indicators.[199] TIMI III evaluated clinically useful predictors to help distinguish patients with non–Q-wave MI from those with unstable angina at the time of presentation. *Four baseline characteristics independently predict non–Q-wave MI:*

ST-Segment Depression, Dynamic T-Wave Changes: Non–Q-Wave Infarction — Unstable Angina

Recommendations for Initial Management and Therapy

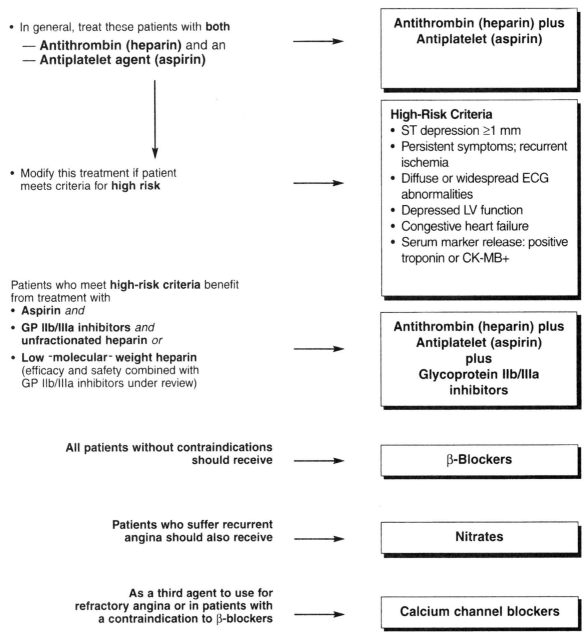

Figure 10. Recommendations for initial management and therapy of ST-segment depression, dynamic T-wave changes, non–Q-wave infarction, and unstable angina.

1. Absence of prior coronary angioplasty (OR 3.3; $P<0.001$)
2. Duration of pain $\geq$60 minutes (OR 2.9; $P<0.001$)
3. ST-segment deviation on the admission ECG (OR 2.0; $P<0.001$)
4. Recent-onset angina (OR 1.7; $P=0.002$)

Non–Q-wave AMI developed in 7.0%, 19.6%, 24.4%, 49.9%, and 70.6% of patients with 0, 1, 2, 3, and 4 risk factors,

respectively ($P<0.001$). Aggressive medical therapy is indicated in high-risk patients; such therapy includes use of heparin, aspirin, nitrates (administered intravenously), β-blockers, and GP IIb/IIIa inhibitors. Whether patients benefit most from a conservative or initially invasive strategy is the subject of recent studies and continuing discussion.[200–202] Many clinicians will elect to perform angiography in higher-risk patients, especially those with recurrent or persistent symptoms on medical therapy.[203]

GP IIb/IIIa Inhibitors in PCI and ACS

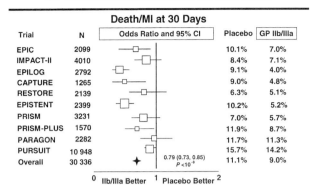

Figure 11. Results of a meta-analysis of the recent trials of GP IIb/IIIa inhibitor therapy. Meta-analysis notes homogeneity of effect for GP IIb/IIIa agents. From Topol et al. *Lancet.* 1999;353:227–231.

Optimal medical management of unstable angina and non–ST-segment elevation MI is rapidly evolving. Fibrinolysis releases thrombin and, paradoxically, increases the tendency toward thrombosis, a possible explanation for fibrinolytic failure in patients with non–Q-wave MI/unstable angina. Patients with a clot composed predominantly of platelets require antithrombin and antiplatelet therapy. New drugs and treatment strategies have focused on this pathogenesis, and new therapies have evolved.

GP IIb/IIIa Inhibitors

After plaque rupture in the coronary artery, tissue factor in the lipid-rich core is exposed and forms complexes with factor VIIa, promoting generation of factor Xa. In the coagulation cascade, relatively low concentrations of factor Xa lead to production of large amounts of thrombin, with deposition of fibrin strands and activation of platelets. Platelet adhesion, activation, and aggregation may result in formation of an arterial thrombus and are pivotal in the pathogenesis of ACS. The integrin GP IIb/IIIa receptor is considered the final common pathway to platelet aggregation, leading to binding of circulating adhesive macromolecules such as fibrinogen and von Willebrand factor, which cross-link on adjacent platelets, allowing platelet aggregation. Administration of a GP IIb/IIIa receptor antagonist (inhibitor) is one method of reducing acute ischemic complications after plaque fissure or rupture.

More than 30 000 patients with ACS without ST-segment elevation have been studied in clinical trials evaluating multiple therapeutic agents to block the GP IIb/IIIa receptor.[204] Although GP IIb/IIIa inhibitors have an impressive ability to reduce adverse cardiac events such as MI and death (see Figure 11), another class of drugs, LMWH, has also been shown to reduce death and nonfatal MI in patients with unstable angina or non–ST-segment elevation AMI (see LMWH later in this section).

The PURSUIT trial enrolled 10 948 patients in a multicenter, randomized, placebo-controlled trial of GP IIb/IIIa inhibition.[205] The primary end point was death from any cause or nonfatal MI at 30 days. Patients were enrolled a median of 11 hours after onset of symptoms, and eptifibatide

was infused for a median of 72 hours. Treatment with eptifibatide for 72 hours or until discharge significantly reduced the incidence of death and MI at each time point. There was a 1.5% absolute reduction in the frequency of the combined end point by 96 hours; this reduction was maintained for 30 days. The early divergence of the Kaplan-Meier curves was maintained throughout the study. PCI was used in 23.3% of patients in the eptifibatide group and 24.8% of patients in the placebo group.

The Platelet Receptor Inhibition in Ischemic Syndrome Management (PRISM) and Platelet Receptor Inhibition in Ischemic Syndrome Management in Patients Limited by Unstable Signs and Symptoms (PRISM-PLUS) trials both used tirofiban (another GP IIb/IIIa inhibitor) to manage unstable angina and non–ST-segment elevation MI.[206] In the PRISM trial, researchers hypothesized that inhibition of the final common pathway for platelet aggregation with tirofiban, a nonpeptide GP IIb/IIIa receptor antagonist, would improve clinical outcome in patients with unstable angina or non–ST-segment elevation MI. A total of 3232 patients were randomly assigned to receive tirofiban, aspirin, and placebo heparin, or aspirin and heparin. The primary end point was death, MI, or refractory ischemia at 7 days. The rate of death, MI, or refractory ischemia at 7 days was 10.3% in the tirofiban group and 11.2% in the heparin group; the difference between the groups was nonsignificant. Although the difference was nonsignificant at 7 days, Kaplan-Meier curves showed an early divergence of and a significant difference in mortality at 30 days. A reduction in the combined end point was observed during early (48-hour) administration of tirofiban. This reduction was not maintained at 7 or 30 days.

The PRISM-PLUS trial continued to evaluate tirofiban, generally in the treatment of higher-risk patients with unstable angina or non–Q-wave MI. A total of 1915 patients were enrolled to evaluate tirofiban, heparin, or the combination of tirofiban and heparin. The primary end point was death due to any cause, new MI, or refractory ischemia within 7 days after randomization. The study of tirofiban without heparin was discontinued early because of excess mortality at 7 days. Tirofiban provided additional benefit when added to standard therapy (heparin and aspirin) at 7 days. Kaplan-Meier curves showed early divergence at 48 hours before PCI in many patients.

A meta-analysis of clinical trials evaluating GP IIb/IIIa receptor antagonists included 32 134 patients.[204] The meta-analysis reviewed death, MI, and revascularization in 16 controlled trials of GP IIb/IIIa inhibitors in which a Bayesian random-effects model was used to describe combined outcomes. For the combined end point of death or nonfatal MI, there was a highly significant benefit of use of GP IIb/IIIa inhibitors at every time point (48 to 96 hours, 30 days, and 6 months). Use of GP IIb/IIIa inhibitors in the ACS trials resulted in no significant differences in mortality at any end point, but a significant benefit of GP IIb/IIIa inhibitors was observed for the combined end point early and at 30 days. For the combined end point of death, MI, or revascularization in the ACS trials, a highly significant benefit favoring GP IIb/IIIa inhibitors was noted at all time points (48 to 96 hours, 30 days, and 6 months).

Inclusion criteria and end point definitions in the GP IIb/IIIa inhibitor trials vary widely. For example, there are differences in definitions of high-risk unstable angina, ECG inclusion criteria, definitions of abnormal cardiac marker results, timing of randomization from 12 to 24 hours after the index event, and definitions of recurrent and new MI and refractory ischemia. Aspirin was administered during all trials, but administration of heparin, heparin dosing, and activated partial thromboplastin times (aPTTs) varied among trials. None of these trials used troponin as a predictor of high risk during risk stratification. Risk stratification of patients with unstable angina also varied among trials.

GP IIb/IIIa inhibitors provide additional benefit in reducing adverse events over aspirin and heparin. There has been a slight increase in bleeding when GP IIb/IIIa inhibitors have been used. Most bleeding has been at vascular access sites, and attention to early vascular sheath withdrawal and heparin dosing had reduced this observation in early clinical trials with these agents. There has been no increase in ICH, as seen with fibrinolytic therapies. Kaplan-Meier curves showed early divergence of the GP IIb/IIIa groups in the PRISM, PURSUIT, and PRISM-PLUS trials. These results suggest an additional benefit of early treatment with GP IIb/IIIa inhibitors in the high-risk ACS population. Direct comparisons among GP IIb/IIIa inhibitors are unavailable, and the specific choice of agent remains speculative. The TARGET trial (Tirofiban and Abciximab for Revascularization Give Equivalent Outcomes) is currently comparing the efficacy of abciximab and tirofiban in several subsets of patients.

On the basis of this new evidence, we recommend the use of GP IIb/IIIa inhibitors for patients with non–ST-segment elevation MI or high-risk unstable angina (Class IIa). GP IIb/IIIa inhibitors have incremental benefit in addition to conventional therapy with UFH and aspirin (Class IIa). LMWH is an *equivalent alternative* for UFH in patients with non–ST-segment elevation MI or unstable angina. However, GP IIb/IIIa inhibitor therapy should be used with UFH until the results of safety and efficacy trials with LMWH are reported. The combination of GP IIb/IIIa inhibitor with LMWH appears promising.[207]

Low-Molecular-Weight Heparin

In addition to platelet activation, plaque disruption activates the extrinsic coagulation system by exposing tissue factor to plasma proteins. Heparin, an indirect inhibitor of thrombin, has been widely used as adjunctive therapy for fibrin-specific lytics and, in combination with aspirin, for the treatment of unstable angina. New antithrombins have been studied, including LMWH. UFH is a heterogeneous mixture of sulfated glycosaminoglycans with varying chain lengths. UFH has several disadvantages, including an unpredictable anticoagulant response in individual patients, the need for intravenous administration, and the requirement for frequent monitoring of aPTT. Also, heparin can stimulate platelet activation, be inhibited by platelet factor 4, and cause thrombocytopenia,[208] which can be serious or fatal in a small percentage of patients.

Three LMWHs have been compared with heparin: enoxaparin (Lovenox, Clexane),[209,210] dalteparin (Fragmin),[210a] and nadroparin (Fraxiparin, Fraxaparine).[210b] The TIMI-11B

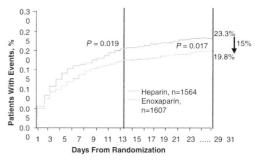

Figure 12. Results of the ESSENCE trial showing a 3.5% absolute reduction in end point of death, MI, and recurrent angina. UA indicates unstable angina; NQWMI, non–Q-wave MI. From Cohen et al. *N Engl J Med.* 1997;337:447–452.

trial studied enoxaparin in 3910 patients with high-risk unstable angina or non–Q-wave MI.[210] After 1800 patients were enrolled, inclusion criteria were modified to focus on higher-risk patients; the new criteria required either ST-segment deviation or positive cardiac markers. The primary end point was all-cause mortality, recurrent MI, or urgent revascularization at 8 days (43 days for those receiving tPA therapy). At 8 days the primary end point was observed in 14.5% of patients receiving UFH and in 12.4% of patients receiving enoxaparin (OR 0.83; 95% CI 0.69 to 1.00; $P=0.048$). Death or MI was reduced from 5.9% in the UFH group and 4.6% in the enoxaparin group ($P=NS$). Kaplan-Meier plots remained parallel, suggesting no further relative benefit of an additional 35 days of enoxaparin therapy.

The ESSENCE study (see Figure 12) was a prospective, randomized, double-blind, parallel-group, multicenter trial.[209] A total of 3171 patients were enrolled in this study, which included recent-onset angina occurring within 24 hours before randomization. The primary end point was death, MI, or recurrent angina at 14 days. The risk of death, MI, or recurrent angina was significantly lower in the enoxaparin group than in the UFH group (16.6% versus 19.8%, OR 0.80, 95% CI 0.67 to 0.96, $P=0.019$). This benefit was maintained over 30 days.

The Fragmin and Fast Revascularization during InStability In Coronary disease (FRISC II) trial evaluated >2000 patients with unstable coronary disease and administered subcutaneous dalteparin twice daily for 3 months. At 30 days and at 3 months there was a significant reduction in the primary end points of death and nonfatal MI, but this advantage was lost at the 6-month follow-up.[211] This study also compared an invasive strategy with conservative medical management. Patients in the invasive arm underwent coronary angiography before 7 days and revascularization before 10 days. Patients who underwent early angiography with indicated revascularization had a significantly decreased incidence of MI. There was also a nonsignificant trend toward reduction in mortality. Angina and recurrent admissions were halved by the invasive strategy.[202]

Nondiagnostic ECG

Screening of patients with nondiagnostic ECGs and ischemic or atypical chest pain in the ED is an area of clinical, legal,

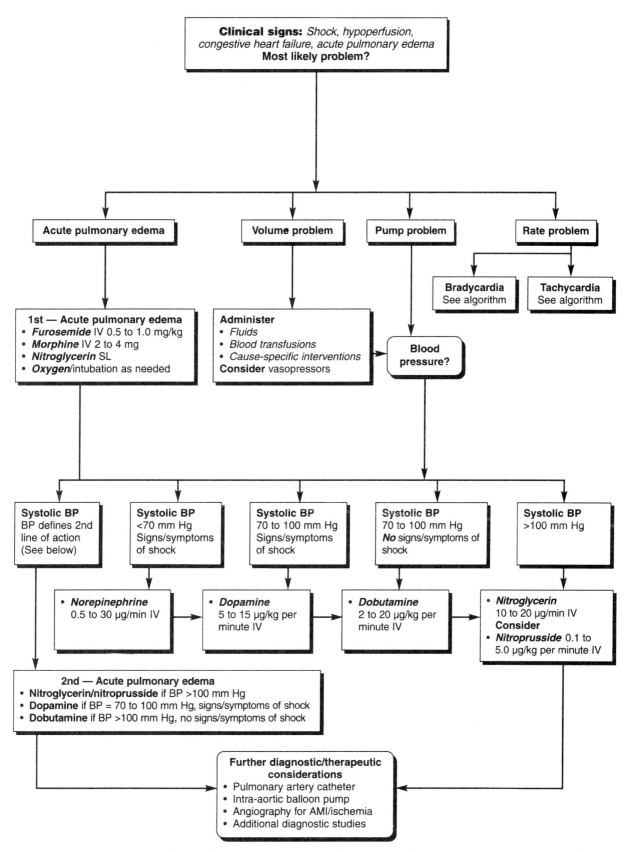

Figure 13. The Acute Pulmonary Edema, Hypotension, and Shock Algorithm.

and economic significance. Special protocols, rapid determination of cardiac markers, 2D echocardiographic screening for regional wall motion abnormalities, myocardial perfusion imaging, and computer-based diagnostic aids are of greatest importance in these patients. Use of new cardiac markers, echocardiography, and perfusion imaging continues to be evaluated.

Patients with a nondiagnostic ECG who have an indeterminate or a low risk of MI should receive aspirin and other therapy as clinically indicated while undergoing serial cardiac studies to assess ongoing cardiac necrosis or unstable coronary syndromes. It is important to examine serial ECG tracings during evaluation in the ED, chest pain unit, or CCU for the development of ST-segment deviation or dynamic T-wave changes with pain, events that may also be detected by systems with continuous ST-segment monitoring capabilities. Patients in whom myocardial necrosis is excluded should then undergo a functional study based on clinical assessment, facility capabilities, and physician expertise.

Complicated AMI

Cardiogenic Shock, LV Power Failure, and CHF
Infarction of 40% of the LV myocardium usually results in cardiogenic shock and death. Despite recent advances in therapy, from 1975 to 1988 the incidence of cardiogenic shock remained relatively constant (approximately 7.5%).[100] Although the incidence of cardiogenic shock has decreased in recent trials, mortality is still high, averaging 50% to 70%.[101,143,212] There also are differences between patients with ST-segment elevation and ST-segment depression. Of those who developed shock,[213] patients without ST-segment elevation developed shock significantly later than patients with ST-segment elevation. Patients without ST-segment elevation are older, more frequently have diabetes mellitus, and have more 3-vessel disease. Mortality was high for both groups: 63% among patients with ST-segment elevation and 73% in those without ST-segment elevation. Nondiagnostic ECGs are more common in the elderly and patients with previous MI.

Severe but lesser degrees of infarction may result in hemodynamic instability and CHF. The ejection fraction of the heart falls when the amount of blood pumped with each heart beat (stroke volume) decreases. The ventricle dilates with an increase in end-diastolic volume. These changes may increase myocardial oxygen consumption, increase ischemia in viable or distant myocardium, and extend infarction. Progressive dysfunction may be manifested by increasing heart rate (sinus tachycardia) as the failing ventricle attempts to compensate for decreased stroke volume. Patients then develop pulmonary congestion and edema as LV filling pressures rise, and they develop hypotension as cardiac output falls. The combination of hypotension and pulmonary edema constitutes clinical cardiogenic shock. Hemodynamically the patient with LV dysfunction often has a cardiac index (cardiac output corrected for body weight) <2.5 L · min^{-1} · m^{-2}, an elevated pulmonary capillary wedge pressure >18 to 20 mm Hg, and SBP <100 mm Hg. When the cardiac index falls to 2.2 L · min^{-1} · m^{-2} and SBP falls to 90 mm Hg, frank signs of poor peripheral perfusion are usually present.

Initial therapy for LV dysfunction includes intravenous diuresis and preload and afterload reduction with intravenous administration of nitrates (see Figure 13). Use an initial low nitrate dose (approximately 5 μg/kg) and gradually increase the dose until mean SBP falls by 10% to 15%, being careful to avoid hypotension (SBP <90 mm Hg). If the patient becomes markedly hypotensive, administer norepinephrine intravenously until SBP is 80 mm Hg, and then try dopamine. When SBP reaches 90 mm Hg, add dobutamine to reduce the requirement for dopamine (see "Part 6, Section 6: Agents to Optimize Cardiac Output and Blood Pressure"). Consider using intra-aortic balloon counterpulsation if available, or transfer the patient to a cardiac interventional facility. Results from the GUSTO-I trial[104] and SHOCK trial[212] suggest that an aggressive, invasive approach increases survival and that use of these resources reduces mortality.

Fibrinolytic therapy has not been shown to consistently improve outcome in patients with cardiogenic shock, and it may have several limitations.[214,219] The small number of patients in clinical trials has limited outcome data and recommendations. In early clinical trials hospital survival rates of 20% to 50% were reported after treatment with fibrinolytic therapy. The only placebo-controlled trial of fibrinolytics compared streptokinase without adjunctive aspirin. A mortality rate of 70% was found for both treated and control patients. The FTT trial did not specifically identify patients with shock but found that patients with sinus tachycardia and low blood pressure benefited from reperfusion therapy.[24] This finding implies inclusion of a group with cardiogenic shock. In the GUSTO trial, fewer deaths occurred in patients who presented with shock and were treated with streptokinase, and shock developed in fewer patients treated with tPA.[213] Primary PCI has been advocated for patients in shock.[215,216] In nonrandomized trials, survival rates as high as 70% have been reported,[217,218] but in 1 trial the mortality rate was 80% in patients in whom patency was not achieved.[106] Current randomized trials are further defining the role of PCI in patients with shock.[107] In the GUSTO trial the mortality rate at 30 days and 1 year was lower in patients treated with aggressive medical therapy and with PCI.[104,213] Early revascularization benefited patients in shock who were <75 years of age (see above).[212]

When possible, triage high-risk patients with cardiogenic shock or refer them to cardiovascular facilities with interventional specialists. Consider triage or transfer for patients with a large anterior wall infarct and for patients with CHF or pulmonary edema. Cardiogenic shock is not a contraindication to fibrinolysis, but defer fibrinolytic therapy when interventional procedures are rapidly available as an alternative (balloon inflation time of 60 minutes). In hospitals without such facilities, rapidly administer a fibrinolytic agent and transfer the patient to a tertiary care facility in which adjunct PCI can be performed if low-output syndromes or ischemia continues.[219]

RV Infarction
RV ischemia or infarction (ST-segment elevation in lead V_4R) may occur in up to 50% of patients with inferior wall

MI. RV infarction is clinically manifested by jugular venous distention, Kussmaul's sign, and various degrees of hypotension. These clinical findings develop in 10% to 15% of patients with inferior MI.[220,221] Suspect RV infarction in patients with inferior wall infarction, hypotension, and clear lung fields. In patients with inferior wall infarction, obtain an ECG of the right side of the heart by using precordial leads. ST-segment elevation in lead V_4R is sensitive (90%) and a strong predictor of in-hospital complications and mortality.[222] A right atrial pressure ≥ 10 mm Hg or 80% of the pulmonary capillary wedge pressure indicates RV dysfunction. The in-hospital mortality rate of patients with RV dysfunction is 25% to 30%. Routinely consider reperfusion therapy for these patients. Fibrinolytic therapy reduces the incidence of RV dysfunction.[223] PCI is indicated for patients in shock.

It is important to recognize that patients with RV dysfunction and acute infarction are very dependent on maintenance of RV filling pressures to maintain cardiac output.[224] Avoid use of agents that reduce preload, such as nitrates and diuretics, because severe hypotension may develop. If hypotension develops in patients with inferior wall infarction who were treated with sublingual nitrates, evaluate for RV infarction. Initial therapy consists of volume loading with a 500-mL intravenous bolus of normal saline, up to 1 to 2 L. Perform serial assessments for pulmonary congestion. Depending on the coronary anatomy, various degrees of LV infarction and dysfunction may develop, and pulmonary edema may be a complication, particularly in patients with previous MI. If blood pressure does not improve after fluid loading, give dobutamine for inotropic support of the right ventricle. For refractory hypotension, consider augmentation of the systemic pressure by means of an IABP to allow reduction of RV afterload and combination therapy with arterial vasodilators.

Adjunctive Therapy for ACS

Heparin
The Fifth American College of Chest Physicians Consensus Conference on Antithrombotic Therapy recommended administration of heparin to all patients with diagnosed AMI.[225] Use of heparin in patients receiving fibrinolytic therapy is controversial, and some issues have yet to be resolved. Randomized trials performed before the reperfusion era documented a 17% reduction in mortality and a 22% reduction in the risk of reinfarction with heparin therapy. A recent meta-analysis of anticoagulant therapy for patients with suspected MI found only a 6% reduction in mortality when heparin was used in the presence of aspirin.[226] There is little data to suggest an additional benefit of heparin administration when patients are treated with aspirin, β-blockers, nitrates, and ACEIs. Use of heparin with nonselective fibrinolytic agents has been equivocal at best, and subcutaneous heparin appeared to be as beneficial as intravenous heparin when benefit was shown.

In angiographic trials heparin has been shown to increase patency of the infarcted artery when tPA is used,[155,227] but the effects of heparin on overall clinical outcomes have not been as impressive. Heparin is currently recommended in patients

TABLE 5. Heparin and ST-Segment Elevation MI

- *Class I (supported by definitive evidence):* all patients undergoing PCI

- *Class IIa (evidence strongly supports use):* IV heparin in patients receiving selective fibrinolytic agents (alteplase, reteplase, tenectaplase); heparin in patients treated with nonselective fibrinolytic agents (streptokinase, APSAC) who are at increased risk for systemic emboli (large anterior MI, atrial fibrillation, known LV thrombus, or previous embolic event)

- *Class IIb (supported by less definitive evidence):* subcutaneously (7500 U twice daily) for pulmonary embolism prophylaxis until fully ambulatory, particularly in the presence of CHF

- *Class III (not beneficial, possibly harmful):* routine IV heparin within 6 hours to patients receiving a nonselective fibrinolytic agent (streptokinase, APSAC) who are not at high risk for systemic emboli

APSAC indicates anisoylated plasminogen streptokinase activator complex.

receiving selective fibrinolytic agents (tPA/retaplase/tenectaplase) (Class IIa).[13]

To reduce the incidence of ICH, the 1999 update to the ACC/AHA Guidelines for the Management of Myocardial Infarction recommends a lower dose of heparin than was previously recommended. The current recommendations now call for a bolus dose of 60 U/kg followed by infusion at a rate of 12 U/kg per hour (a maximum bolus of 4000 U/kg and infusion of 1000 U/h for patients weighing <70 kg).[13] An aPTT of 50 to 70 seconds is considered optimal. Increased rates of bleeding and ICH have been related to more intensive heparin therapy and higher aPTTs (>70 seconds). The incidence of stroke is increased in patients with a large anterior wall infarction and thrombus,[228] significant LV dysfunction,[229] atrial fibrillation, and a previous embolic event. Treat these high-risk patients with heparin for an extended period; warfarin therapy may be initiated in some.

The indications for heparin use in some clinical situations remain controversial. The following recommendations, however, are consistent with data from randomized trials and expert consensus opinion for use in ST-segment elevation acute MI (Table 5) and non–Q-wave MI/unstable angina (Table 6).

β-Adrenergic Receptor Blockers
β-Blockers reduce the size of the infarct in patients who do not receive fibrinolytic therapy.[55,230,231] They also reduce the incidence of ventricular ectopy and fibrillation.[232,233] In patients who receive fibrinolytic agents, β-blockers decrease postinfarction ischemia and nonfatal MI. A small but significant decrease in death and nonfatal infarction has been

TABLE 6. Heparin and ST-Segment Depression and Non–Q-Wave MI/Unstable Angina

- IV heparin therapy for 3 to 5 days is standard for high-risk and some intermediate-risk patients. The ACC/AHA Practice Guidelines recommend treatment for 48 hours, then individualized therapy.

- LMWH is an acceptable alternative to IV UFH (see above). Enoxaparin is preferable to UFH.

- UFH is recommended for use with GP IIb/IIIa inhibitors until data on safety and efficacy regarding combination with LMWH is available.

- All unstable angina patients should receive 325 mg of aspirin per day.

TABLE 7.   Absolute Contraindications to β-Blocker Therapy

- Severe LV failure and pulmonary edema
- Bradycardia (heart rate <60 bpm)
- Hypotension (SBP <100 mm Hg)
- Signs of poor peripheral perfusion
- Second- or third-degree heart block

observed in patients treated with β-blockers very soon after infarction.[234]

Start β-blockers within 12 hours of onset of infarction; they are usually administered intravenously in the ED unless contraindications are present (see Table 7). β-Blockers are also indicated for recurrent or continuing ischemia. They are particularly useful as an adjunct to morphine and to help control ventricular response in atrial fibrillation. Their use in non–Q-wave infarction is controversial.

Nitroglycerin (or Glyceryl Trinitrate)
In trials conducted before the era of fibrinolytics, intravenous nitrate therapy (nitroglycerin; glyceryl trinitrate in Europe) was shown to reduce the size of infarcts. An analysis of subgroups in the largest of these studies showed that most of this benefit occurred in patients with large anterior wall infarcts,[115] and a meta-analysis[116] concluded that nitroglycerin effectively reduced mortality. Evidence from ISIS-4 and GISSI-3 was insufficiently conclusive to recommend routine administration in AMI.[117,235]

The totality of evidence does not support routine administration of nitroglycerin. Nitroglycerin is indicated for the initial management of pain and ischemia in patients with AMI, except in those with RV infarction.[236] Nitrates are indicated during the first 24 to 48 hours in patients with recurrent ischemia. They may be useful in patients with hypertension, CHF, and large anterior wall MI. Use nitrates if these indications are present, but discontinue nitrates if low blood pressure precludes use of other agents known to be effective in reducing mortality and morbidity (β-blockers and ACEIs).

Calcium Channel Blockers
Calcium channel blockers have been previously recommended for use in patients with non–Q-wave MI with preserved ejection fraction and no heart failure. However, trials have not demonstrated a reduction in mortality or combined cardiovascular end points. The totality of evidence and current recommendations call for β-blockers as first-line agents unless contraindicated. Calcium channel blocking agents may be added as an alternative or additional therapy if β-blockers are contraindicated or the maximum dose has been achieved.

The ACC/AHA guidelines for the management of patients with AMI[12] make the following comment about calcium channel blockers:

Calcium channel blocking agents have not been shown to reduce mortality after acute MI, and in certain patients with cardiovascular disease there is data to suggest that they are harmful. It is the consensus of the ACC/AHA AMI Guidelines Committee that these agents are still used too frequently

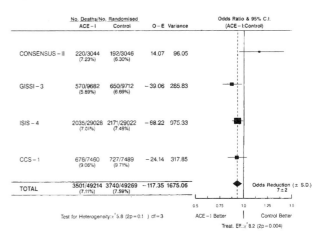

Figure 14. Meta-analysis of ACEI therapy administered to patients with AMI. Results represent the proportional effects of therapy on 30-day mortality. From ACE Inhibitor Myocardial Infarction Collaborative Group. *Circulation.* 1998;97:2202–2212.

in patients with acute MI and that β-adrenergic receptor blocking agents are a more appropriate choice across a broad spectrum of patients with MI (with exceptions as noted).

Immediate-release nifedipine does not reduce the incidence of reinfarction or mortality when given early or late after MI. Nifedipine may be harmful, particularly in patients with hypotension or tachycardia.[237] Verapamil may reduce reinfarction or death when initiated several days after MI, provided that LV function is well preserved and there is no evidence of clinical heart failure.[238] Some data suggests that diltiazem may benefit patients with non–Q-wave MI or those with Q-wave MI, preserved LV function, and no evidence of clinical failure.[239] This data, however, was obtained during the early reperfusion era and may be confounded by concomitant treatment with β-blockers in 50% of patients. A more recent trial (Incomplete Infarction Trial of European Research Collaborators Evaluating Prognosis post-Thrombolysis; INTERCEPT) found that diltiazem was not effective in reducing the cumulative occurrence of death, nonfatal MI, or refractory ischemia in patients who first received fibrinolytic therapy. The need for revascularization was reduced at 6 months.[240] In general, give calcium antagonists only when β-blockers are contraindicated or have been given at maximum clinical doses.

ACEI Therapy
Inhibition of ACE has improved survival in patients with AMI.[117,241–244] The reduction in mortality is seen early after onset of AMI. Proposed mechanisms include an early effect on limitation of infarct expansion, attenuation of the remodeling process, reduction of the neurohumoral impact on the heart, and increases in collateral flow to the peri-infarct ischemic area.

The larger trials have consistently demonstrated a survival advantage for ACEI therapy started early during the acute phase of MI. An overview of 4 trials with nearly 100 000 patients evaluated data on patients who received ACEI (Figure 14). Overall, a reduction of 5 deaths per 1000 patients treated was observed, and most of this benefit occurred early in the first week. Selection of higher-risk patients amplified the modest 7% proportional reduction in mortality; patients with evidence of LV dysfunction and anterior wall MI benefited most.[245] The Cooperative New Scandinavian Enalapril Survival Study II (CONSENSUS II) trial was terminated early—a controversial decision—when it was thought that a high probability of a beneficial effect would be lacking. Concern was also raised because of an early hypotensive effect observed in the elderly treated with ACEI. The study used an intravenous preparation of enalapril, enalaprilat.[246] Largely based on this trial, IV ACEI therapy is not recommended. Oral ACEI therapy is initiated after 6 hours when the patient is stable and other initial treatments have been started (lytics, β-blockers, nitrates).

The data supports the 2 strategies currently used: ACEI administration to a general group of AMI patients with subsequent reassessment of the need for continued treatment (eg, LV ejection fraction <0.35) at 4 to 6 weeks (Class IIa) or selective administration to higher-risk patients with clinical heart failure or large AMI (Class I). Give ACEI therapy early within the first day after MI when the patient is stable and after reperfusion, initial measures, and other therapies have been started. Avoid its use in the presence of hypotension (SBP <100 mm Hg), clinically relevant renal failure, bilateral renal artery stenosis, or documented allergy.

Magnesium

The routine use of magnesium in AMI was proposed after a meta-analysis of 7 small randomized trials found an impressive reduction in mortality of 55% associated with administration of magnesium.[247] The mechanism of effect was thought to be a reduction in ventricular arrhythmias and VF. The Second Leicester Intravenous Magnesium Interventional Trial (LIMIT-2) subsequently reported a 24% reduction in mortality, but this reduction was not due to a reduction in arrhythmia.[248] Post hoc analyses suggested that the reduction in mortality was associated with a reduction in CHF. This finding led to a reconsideration of the importance of the cellular protective effects that magnesium had against calcium ion influx in ischemia.[248]

No reduction in mortality was found in the large ISIS-4 trial,[117] and a possibility of slight harm was noted in association with magnesium administration. Relatively late administration of magnesium, after administration of the fibrinolytic, was suggested as one possible reason for the negative outcome.[249] A small randomized trial conducted in patients ineligible for fibrinolytic therapy found a significant reduction in mortality due to a decreased incidence of CHF and cardiogenic shock. ISIS investigators performed a retrospective review and compared patients treated early and late with magnesium but still found no benefit or difference in mortality.

To further address this issue, the Magnesium in Coronary Disease (MAGIC) trial will evaluate the role of magnesium in AMI, particularly early administration before fibrinolytic therapy in high-risk patients, including the elderly and patients not eligible for fibrinolytic therapy.[250] Currently there is no routine indication for administration of magnesium to patients with MI.

Metabolic Manipulation of the Infarct: Glucose-Insulin-Potassium

Metabolic modulation of the acute myocardial infarct was first proposed by Sodi-Pallares et al in 1962 and brought to clinical trial in 1969.[251] Early experimental and clinical studies were promising and demonstrated a reduction in infarct size, heart failure, and mortality.[252-255] Initial enthusiasm fell dormant until a meta-analysis revived interest in this simple and inexpensive therapy[256] after the Diabetes Insulin-Glucose in Acute Myocardial Infarction (DIGAMI) study group reported favorable results in diabetic patients with AMI.[257] The trials and meta-analysis provided the impetus for a prospective randomized clinical trial.[258] Two clinical trials recently reported conflicting results, and a large clinical trial is essential to determine the magnitude of benefit and subgroups who may particularly benefit.[259,260]

Glucose-insulin-potassium (GIK) therapy may reduce mortality during AMI by several mechanisms. GIK has anti–free fatty acid (FFA) activity. FFAs are toxic to the ischemic myocardium, and GIK reduces circulating FFAs and myocardial uptake. GIK also antagonizes the effects of catecholamines and heparin on increased FFAs. A relatively small increase in ischemic glycolytic adenosine triphosphate may be beneficial in the low-flow myocardium.

A meta-analysis performed in patients before the era of fibrinolytic therapy found a reduction in mortality of 28% to 48% associated with GIK therapy, depending on the dose and timing of administration.[256] Researchers in the DIGAMI trial also found an impressive 29% to 58% decrease in relative mortality, depending on the subgroup evaluated.[261] The Estudios Cardiologicos Latinoamerica (ECLA) Collaborative Group, which conducted a large prospective randomized trial during the era of fibrinolytic therapy, reported an impressive 66% relative reduction (15.2% to 5.2% absolute reduction) in mortality.[259] Only the recently reported Pol-GIK trial failed to find a reduction in mortality with a nonsignificant hazard in treated patients.[260] The difference between these 2 trials may be attributable to patient selection, because patients in the ECLA trial were sicker than those in the Pol-GIK trial and were treated with higher doses of GIK.

In summary, GIK therapy for patients with AMI may be helpful; it is easily administered and associated with few adverse effects. Administration through a peripheral vein is associated with a 2% incidence of significant phlebitis but no serious metabolic consequences, even in diabetic patients. Before GIK is widely recommended, larger clinical trials are needed to further evaluate its efficacy in a broad patient group with AMI and to identify patient subgroups for which it may be particularly beneficial (Class Indeterminate).

Arrhythmias Associated With Ischemia, Infarction, and Reperfusion

Cardiac rhythm abnormalities and the clinical pharmacology of agents used to treat them are discussed in "Part 6: Advanced Cardiovascular Life Support." This section discusses management of these arrhythmias during acute ischemia and infarction.

Ventricular Rhythm Disturbances

Treatment of ventricular arrhythmias after MI has been a controversial topic for 2 decades. Similarly, management of ventricular arrhythmias during the acute phase of MI continues to evolve as treatment strategies are reviewed in the context of new information and changing epidemiological data during the era of adjunctive medical and reperfusion therapy.

Primary VF accounts for the majority of early deaths during AMI. The incidence of primary VF is highest (3% to 5%) during the first 4 hours after coronary occlusion and then declines markedly. VF is an important contributor to mortality during the first 24 hours. Primary VF should be distinguished from secondary VF occurring in the setting of CHF or cardiogenic shock. Epidemiological data suggests that the incidence of primary VF may be decreasing. Although prophylaxis with lidocaine reduced the incidence of VF by approximately one third, a meta-analysis of randomized trials suggests that this decrease was offset by an increased incidence of total mortality by the same degree. *However, too few events and limited follow-up precluded any conclusion regarding harm or efficacy.*[262] Thus, the practice of routine prophylactic administration of lidocaine has been largely abandoned.

Routine intravenous administration of β-blockers to patients without hemodynamic or electrical contraindications, however, is associated with a reduced incidence of primary VF. Low serum levels of potassium but not magnesium have been associated with ventricular arrhythmia. It is prudent clinical practice to maintain serum potassium levels >4.0 mEq/L and magnesium levels >2.0 mEq/L. Routine administration of magnesium to patients with MI has no significant clinical mortality benefit, particularly in patients receiving fibrinolytic therapy. As noted above, a mortality benefit may be seen in high-risk patients, provided that magnesium is administered soon after the onset of symptoms. Continuing trials will evaluate use of magnesium in these patients.

Ventricular rhythm abnormalities observed during acute ischemia and infarction include premature ventricular complexes, VT, and VF. The use of the external defibrillator and the proliferation of CCUs reduced hospital mortality by half after the introduction of defibrillation by trained staff. Lidocaine was then shown to be effective in reducing the incidence of VF and complex ventricular rhythm disturbances. It was logical to propose prophylactic use of lidocaine to prevent VF and treat "warning arrhythmias." Neither of these tenets has withstood the tests of multiple clinical studies. Serious ventricular arrhythmias are absent in almost 50% of patients who experience early VF. Also, the incidence of VF has declined and is low in the fibrinolytic era, in which adjunctive therapy with β-blockers is common. An analysis of data from ISIS-3 showed a reduction in VF in patients treated with lidocaine but a trend toward increased mortality, possibly and inferentially because of an increased incidence of asystole. A subsequent meta-analysis and recent clinical data supported this trend toward increased mortality and increased incidence of asystole, negating the benefit of reduction in primary VF.[262] At present we do not recommend prophylactic treatment of arrhythmias or treatment of asymptomatic warning arrhythmias. Current ACLS protocols recommend lidocaine for the treatment of hemodynamically stable VT and prevention of recurrent VF.

There is no conclusive data to support the use of lidocaine or any particular strategy for preventing recurrent VF. If lidocaine is used, continue it for a short time after MI but no more than 24 hours unless symptomatic VT persists. Identify and correct exacerbating or modulating factors. Hypokalemia is a risk factor for ventricular ectopy and VF. Correct hypoxemia and treat heart failure aggressively. The evidence for magnesium is less clear. Nevertheless, we recommend maintaining serum potassium levels >4.0 mEq/L and magnesium levels >2.0 mEq/L.

Management of ventricular rhythm disturbances is discussed in "Part 6: Advanced Cardiovascular Life Support."

Bradycardia and Heart Block: Indications for Pacing During AMI

Approximately one third of patients with AMI develop sinus bradycardia. Because of increased vagal tone, it is often seen in patients with inferior wall infarcts secondary to occlusion of the right coronary artery when that artery supplies the sinus or atrioventricular (AV) nodes. Sinus bradycardia may also occur with reperfusion of the right coronary artery. Atropine-resistant bradycardia and heart block may occur; accumulation of adenosine in ischemic nodal tissue may be responsible.[263–265] Initial treatment with atropine is indicated only when serious signs and symptoms are related to the decreased rate.

Second- or third-degree AV block complicates approximately 20% of myocardial infarcts. Heart block is present on admission in 42% of patients and within the first 24 hours in two thirds.[220] Heart block is present in 12% of patients who receive fibrinolytic therapy and is associated with increased hospital mortality in these patients. This mortality is usually due to extensive MI with cardiac dysfunction. Only rarely will a patient die of heart block. Heart block is not an independent predictor of mortality, and it is a poor predictor of mortality in patients who survive to discharge. Prognosis is related to the site of infarction (anterior or inferior), level of block in the AV node (infranodal or intranodal), escape rhythm, and degree of hemodynamic compromise.

In general, treatment of first- or second-degree AV block with atropine is not required. When serious rate-related signs and symptoms occur, administer 0.5 to 1.0 mg of atropine every 3 minutes up to a total dose of 0.03 to 0.04 mg/kg. Treatment of patients with symptomatic type I second-degree AV block is occasionally required.

Atropine may be particularly inappropriate for treatment of bradycardia in some patients. For example, patients who have had a heart transplant have denervated hearts and will not respond to atropine. Atropine should not be used to treat some forms of heart block. Avoid administering atropine in type II second-degree AV block. Atropine usually has no effect on AV conduction (infranodal block), and a resulting increase in sinus rate may actually enhance the block or precipitate third-degree AV block. Atropine may be helpful for treating third-degree AV block occurring at the AV node (narrow-complex QRS), because it may improve AV block or accel-

TABLE 8. Indications for Transcutaneous Patches/Pacing

- Hemodynamically unstable bradycardia (<50 bpm)
- Mobitz type II second-degree AV block
- Third-degree heart block
- Bilateral BBB (alternating BBB or RBBB and alternating LBBB)
- Left anterior fascicular block
- Newly acquired or age-indeterminate LBBB
- RBBB or LBBB and first-degree AV block

RBBB, LBBB indicate right and left bundle-branch block, respectively.

erate the escape rhythm. However, *do not* use atropine for third-degree AV block with a new wide-QRS complex presumed to be due to AMI. *Administration of lidocaine to these patients may also have the effect of suppressing a slow escape rhythm and in this setting may result in ventricular standstill.*

The availability of transcutaneous pacing and the need to avoid venipuncture in noncompressible vessels in patients who may receive or have received fibrinolytic therapy have significantly changed the approach to emergency pacing. Transcutaneous pacing should be used as an emergency bridge to temporary transvenous pacing performed by experts, preferably under fluoroscopic guidance, for appropriate indications (Table 8).

Consider placement of transcutaneous patches with provision for immediate pacing for stable bradycardia, new or age-indeterminate right bundle-branch block, and new or age-indeterminate first-degree AV block.

Atrial Fibrillation Complicating AMI

New-onset atrial fibrillation complicating MI occurs in 10% to 15% of patients.[266–268] It is usually transient and often self-limited, requiring no therapy. It is associated with increasing age, large infarcts, LV hypertrophy, and CHF.[269] Atrial fibrillation may also be a result of atrial infarction,[270] which occurs with occlusion of the right coronary artery before the sinus node branch or with occlusion of the circumflex coronary artery before the left atrial circumflex branch.[271] Later in the hospital course, pericarditis may precipitate atrial fibrillation.[272]

Fibrinolytic therapy with tPA or streptokinase reduces the incidence of atrial fibrillation.[273] Episodes of atrial fibrillation that are brief and transient or have ventricular response rates <110 bpm require no immediate therapy. Attempt to identify and treat any underlying causes or aggravating conditions (hypoxia, CHF, or an electrolyte abnormality).

When atrial fibrillation produces a rapid ventricular rate resulting in ischemic symptoms or hemodynamic compromise, immediate cardioversion is indicated. In stable patients, β-adrenergic receptor blocking agents may be used to effectively slow the ventricular rate if severe CHF, asthma, and other contraindications are absent. Intravenous administration of diltiazem is often used if β-blockers are contraindicated. Verapamil should be used with caution—if at all—in patients with clinical heart failure or depressed ejection fraction. Calcium channel blockers are not recommended as first-line

therapy because of their negative inotropic effect and recent concerns about their use in AMI.

Rapid digitalization may occasionally be effective, but rate control is achieved more slowly, and toxicity is a significant concern, particularly in the setting of acute ischemia.

Mortality is increased when atrial fibrillation develops in the setting of AMI. The risk of stroke is increased with atrial fibrillation. Systemic embolization is 3 times more common in patients with atrial fibrillation, with 50% of episodes occurring within the first 24 hours after onset of the arrhythmia.[274] Echocardiography is recommended to assess the possibility of LV mural thrombi with large anterior wall and apical MIs. If atrial fibrillation develops, administer heparin and maintain aPTT between 50 and 70 seconds.

ACS at the Dawn of a New Millennium

Significant progress has been made in the identification, urgent treatment, and long-term care of patients with ACS. The reperfusion era ushered in a period of rapid progress in our understanding of coronary artery disease, plaque instability, and the myriad of clinical symptoms and scenarios that are possible. The next decade will certainly focus on the role of the platelet and optimal management in different stages of the ACS spectrum. Intense investigation of the role of inflammation and its prognostic and treatment potential is now unfolding. The focus on the epicardial artery and patency will continue as new treatment strategies are developed and tested to initiate and maintain patency with ACS. A new focus on the microvasculature as an important contributor to myocardial salvage and preservation is beginning, and the target of microvascular dysfunction will add another perspective to our understanding and therapeutic options in the near future.

References

1. Chesebro JH, Rauch U, Fuster V, Badimon JJ. Pathogenesis of thrombosis in coronary artery disease. *Haemostasis.* 1997;27(suppl 1): 12–18.
2. Fuster V. Elucidation of the role of plaque instability and rupture in acute coronary events. *Am J Cardiol.* 1995;76:24C–33C.
3. Fuster V, Badimon L, Badimon JJ, Chesebro JH. The pathogenesis of coronary artery disease and the acute coronary syndromes (1). *N Engl J Med.* 1992;326:242–250.
4. Fuster V, Badimon L, Badimon JJ, Chesebro JH. The pathogenesis of coronary artery disease and the acute coronary syndromes (2). *N Engl J Med.* 1992;326:310–318.
5. Fuster V, Fallon JT, Badimon JJ, Nemerson Y. The unstable atherosclerotic plaque: clinical significance and therapeutic intervention. *Thromb Haemost.* 1997;78:247–255.
6. Davies MJ. Anatomic features in victims of sudden coronary death: coronary artery pathology. *Circulation.* 1992;85(suppl I):I-19–I-24.
7. Burke AP, Farb A, Malcom GT, Liang Y, Smialek JE, Virmani R. Plaque rupture and sudden death related to exertion in men with coronary artery disease. *JAMA.* 1999;281:921–926.
8. Farb A, Tang AL, Burke AP, Sessums L, Liang Y, Virmani R. Sudden coronary death: frequency of active coronary lesions, inactive coronary lesions, and myocardial infarction. *Circulation.* 1995;92:1701–1709.
9. Virmani R, Burke AP, Farb A. Plaque morphology in sudden coronary death. *Cardiologia.* 1998;43:267–271.
10. Falk E. Unstable angina with fatal outcome: dynamic coronary thrombosis leading to infarction and/or sudden death: autopsy evidence of recurrent mural thrombosis with peripheral embolization culminating in total vascular occlusion. *Circulation.* 1985;71:699–708.

11. Gunnar R, Bourdillon P, Dixon D, Fuster V, Karp R, Kennedy J, et al. ACC/AHA Guidelines for the Early Management of Patients with Acute Myocardial Infarction. *Circulation.* 1990;82:664–707.

12. Ryan TJ, Anderson JL, Antman EM, Braniff BA, Brooks NH, Califf RM, Hillis LD, Hiratzka LF, Rapaport E, Riegel BJ, Russell RO, Smith EE III, Weaver WD. ACC/AHA guidelines for the management of patients with acute myocardial infarction: executive summary: a report of the American College of Cardiology/American Heart Association Task Force on Practice Guidelines (Committee on Management of Acute Myocardial Infarction). *Circulation.* 1996;94:2341–2345.

13. Ryan T. Update: guidelines for the management of patients with acute myocardial infarction. *J Am Coll Cardiol.* 1999;34:890–911.

14. Braunwald E, Jones RH, Mark DB, Brown J, Brown L, Cheitlin MD, Concannon CA, Cowan M, Edwards C, Fuster V, et al. Diagnosing and managing unstable angina: Agency for Health Care Policy and Research. *Circulation.* 1994;90:613–622.

15. Task Force on the Management of Acute Myocardial Infarction of the European Society of Cardiology. Acute myocardial infarction: pre-hospital and in-hospital management. *Eur Heart J.* 1996;17:43–63.

16. ACC/AHA guidelines for the management of unstable angina. *Circulation.* In press.

17. The pre-hospital management of acute heart attacks: recommendations of a task force of the European Society of Cardiology and the European Resuscitation Council. *Eur Heart J.* 1998;19:1140–1164.

18. Ridker PM, Antman EM. Pathogenesis and pathology of coronary heart disease syndromes. *J Thromb Thrombolysis.* 1999;8:167–189.

19. Davies MJ. The pathophysiology of acute coronary syndromes. *Heart.* 2000;83:361–366.

20. Ambrose JA, Fuster V. Can we predict future acute coronary events in patients with stable coronary artery disease? [editorial; comment]. *JAMA.* 1997;277:343–344.

21. Ambrose JA, Winters SL, Arora RR, Haft JI, Goldstein J, Rentrop KP, Gorlin R, Fuster V. Coronary angiographic morphology in myocardial infarction: a link between the pathogenesis of unstable angina and myocardial infarction. *J Am Coll Cardiol.* 1985;6:1233–1238.

22. Azar R, Waters D. The inflammatory etiology of unstable angina. *Am Heart J.* 1996;132:1101–1106.

23. Anderson JL, Carlquist JF, Muhlestein JB, Horne BD, Elmer SP. Evaluation of C-reactive protein, an inflammatory marker, and infectious serology as risk factors for coronary artery disease and myocardial infarction. *J Am Coll Cardiol.* 1998;32:35–41.

24. Fibrinolytic Trialists Collaborative Group. Indications for fibrinolytic therapy in suspected acute myocardial infarction: collaborative overview of early mortality and major morbidity results from all randomised trials of more than 1000 patients. Fibrinolytic Therapy Trialists' (FTT) Collaborative Group [published erratum appears in *Lancet.* 1994;343:742] [see comments]. *Lancet.* 1994;343:311–322.

25. TIMI investigators. Effects of tissue plasminogen activator and a comparison of early invasive and conservative strategies in unstable angina and non–Q-wave myocardial infarction: results of the TIMI IIIB Trial. Thrombolysis in Myocardial Ischemia [see comments]. *Circulation.* 1994;89:1545–1556.

26. Topol EJ. Inflammation and embolization in ischemic heart disease. *J Invasive Cardiol.* 2000;12(suppl B):2B–7B [MEDLINE record in process].

27. Erbel R, Heusch G. Coronary microembolization: its role in acute coronary syndromes and interventions. *Herz.* 1999;24:558–575.

28. Saber RS, Edwards WD, Bailey KR, McGovern TW, Schwartz RS, Holmes DR Jr. Coronary embolization after balloon angioplasty or thrombolytic therapy: an autopsy study of 32 cases. *J Am Coll Cardiol.* 1993;22:1283–1288.

29. Topol EJ, Yadav JS. Recognition of the importance of embolization in atherosclerotic vascular disease. *Circulation.* 2000;101:570–580.

30. Ravkilde J, Nissen H, Mickley H, Andersen PE, Thayssen P, Horder M. Cardiac troponin T and CK-MB mass release after visually successful percutaneous transluminal coronary angioplasty in stable angina pectoris. *Am Heart J.* 1994;127:13–20.

31. Maseri A, L'Abbate A, Baroldi G, Chierchia S, Marzilli M, Ballestra AM, Severi S, Parodi O, Biagini A, Distante A, Pesola A. Coronary vasospasm as a possible cause of myocardial infarction: a conclusion derived from the study of "preinfarction" angina. *N Engl J Med.* 1978;299:1271–1277.

32. Sinapius D. Relationship between coronary-artery thrombosis and myocardial infarction [in German]. *Dtsch Med Wochenschr.* 1972;97:443–448.

33. Pantridge JF, Geddes JS. A mobile intensive-care unit in the management of myocardial infarction. *Lancet.* 1967;2:271–273.

34. Cohen MC, Rohtla KM, Lavery CE, Muller JE, Mittleman MA. Meta-analysis of the morning excess of acute myocardial infarction and sudden cardiac death [published erratum appears in *Am J Cardiol.* 1998;81:260]. *Am J Cardiol.* 1997;79:1512–1516.

35. Colquhoun MC, Julien DG. Sudden death in the community: the arrhythmia causing cardiac arrest and results of immediate resuscitation. *Resuscitation.* 1992;24:177A.

36. Rose LB. The Oregon Coronary Ambulance Project: an experiment. *Heart Lung.* 1974;3:753–755.

37. Campbell RW, Murray A, Julian DG. Ventricular arrhythmias in first 12 hours of acute myocardial infarction: natural history study. *Br Heart J.* 1981;46:351–357.

37a. O'Doherty M, Taylor DI, Quinn E, Vincent R, Chamberlain DA. Five hundred patients with myocardial infarction monitored within one hour of symptoms. *Br Med J.* 1983;286:1405–1408.

38. Lie KI, Wellens HJ, Downar E, Durrer D. Observations on patients with primary ventricular fibrillation complicating acute myocardial infarction. *Circulation.* 1975;52:755–759.

39. El-Sherif N, Myerburg RJ, Scherlag BJ, Befeler B, Aranda JM, Castellanos A, Lazzara R. Electrocardiographic antecedents of primary ventricular fibrillation: value of the R-on-T phenomenon in myocardial infarction. *Br Heart J.* 1976;38:415–422.

40. Chiriboga D, Yarzebski J, Goldberg RJ, Gore JM, Alpert JS. Temporal trends (1975 through 1990) in the incidence and case-fatality rates of primary ventricular fibrillation complicating acute myocardial infarction: a communitywide perspective [see comments]. *Circulation.* 1994;89:998–1003.

41. Volpi A, Cavalli A, Franzosi MG, Maggioni A, Mauri F, Santoro E, Tognoni G, GISSI (Gruppo Italiano per lo Studio della Streptochinasi nell'Infarto Miocardico) investigators. One-year prognosis of primary ventricular fibrillation complicating acute myocardial infarction. *Am J Cardiol.* 1989;63:1174–1178.

42. Volpi A, De Vita C, Franzosi MG, Geraci E, Maggioni AP, Mauri F, Negri E, Santoro E, Tavazzi L, Tognoni G, ad hoc Working Group of the Gruppo Italiano per lo Studio della Sopravvivenza nell'Infarto Miocardico (GISSI)-2 Data Base. Determinants of 6-month mortality in survivors of myocardial infarction after thrombolysis: results of the GISSI-2 data base. *Circulation.* 1993;88:416–429.

43. Nicod P, Gilpin E, Dittrich H, Wright M, Engler R, Rittlemeyer J, Henning H, Ross J Jr. Late clinical outcome in patients with early ventricular fibrillation after myocardial infarction. *J Am Coll Cardiol.* 1988;11:464–470.

44. Behar S, Goldbourt U, Reicher-Reiss H, Kaplinsky E, principal investigators of the SPRINT study. Prognosis of acute myocardial infarction complicated by primary ventricular fibrillation. *Am J Cardiol.* 1990;66:1208–1211.

45. Kerber R, Members of Emergency Cardiac Care Committee. Statement on early defibrillation from the American Heart Association. *Circulation.* 1991;83:2233.

46. Kloeck W, Cummins RO, Chamberlain D, Bossaert L, Callanan V, Carli P, Christenson J, Connolly B, Ornato JP, Sanders A, Steen P. Early defibrillation: an advisory statement from the Advanced Life Support Working Group of the International Liaison Committee on Resuscitation. *Circulation.* 1997;95:2183–2184.

47. Stults K, Brown D, Kerber R. Efficacy of an automated external defibrillator in the management of out-of-hospital cardiac arrest: validations of the diagnostic algorithm and initial experience in a rural environment. *Circulation.* 1986;73:701–709.

48. Eisenberg MS, Cummins RO. Defibrillation performed by the emergency medical technician. *Circulation.* 1986;74(suppl IV):IV-9–IV-12.

49. Olson D, LaRochelle J, Fark D, Aprahamian C, Aufderheide T, Mateer J, Hartgarten K, Stueven H. EMT-defibrillation: the Wisconsin experience. *Ann Emerg Med.* 1990;19:613–614.

50. Cummins RO, Eisenberg MS, Litwin PE, Graves JR, Hearne TR, Hallstrom AP. Automatic external defibrillators used by emergency medical technicians: a controlled clinical trial. *JAMA.* 1987;257:1605–1610.

51. Mols P, Beaucarne E, Bruyninx J, Labruyere JP, De Myttenaere L, Naeije N, Watteeuw G, Verset D, Flamand JP. Early defibrillation by EMTs: the Brussels experience. *Resuscitation.* 1994;27:129–136.

52. Weisfeldt ML, Kerber RE, McGoldrick RP, Moss AJ, Nichol G, Ornato JP, Palmer DG, Riegel B, Smith SC Jr. Public access defibrillation: a statement for healthcare professionals from the American Heart Asso-

ciation Task Force on Automatic External Defibrillation. *Circulation.* 1995;92:2763.

53. Weisfeldt ML, Kerber RE, McGoldrick RP, Moss AJ, Nichol G, Ornato JP, Palmer DG, Riegel B, Smith SC Jr, Automatic External Defibrillation Task Force. American Heart Association report on the Public Access Defibrillation Conference December 8–10, 1994 [see comments]. *Circulation.* 1995;92:2740–2747.

54. Kern KB. Public access defibrillation: a review. *Heart.* 1998;80: 402–404.

55. Hjalmarson A, Herlitz J, Holmberg S, Ryden L, Swedberg K, Vedin A, Waagstein F, Waldenstrom A, Waldenstrom J, Wedel H, Wilhelmsen L, Wilhelmsson C. The Goteborg metoprolol trial: effects on mortality and morbidity in acute myocardial infarction. *Circulation.* 1983;67(suppl I):I-26–I-32.

56. Risenfors M, Herlitz J, Berg CH, Dellborg M, Gustavsson G, Gottfridsson C, Lomsky M, Swedberg K, Hjalmarsson A. Early treatment with thrombolysis and beta-blockade in suspected acute myocardial infarction: results from the TEAHAT Study. *J Intern Med Suppl.* 1991;734:35–42.

57. Lambrew CT, Bowlby LJ, Rogers WJ, Chandra NC, Weaver WD. Factors influencing the time to thrombolysis in acute myocardial infarction: Time to Thrombolysis Substudy of the National Registry of Myocardial Infarction-1. *Arch Intern Med.* 1997;157:2577–2582.

58. Kereiakes DJ, Weaver WD, Anderson JL, Feldman T, Gibler B, Aufderheide T, Williams DO, Martin LH, Anderson LC, Martin JS, et al. Time delays in the diagnosis and treatment of acute myocardial infarction: a tale of eight cities: report from the Pre-hospital Study Group and the Cincinnati Heart Project. *Am Heart J.* 1990;120:773–780.

59. Weaver WD. Time to thrombolytic treatment: factors affecting delay and their influence on outcome. *J Am Coll Cardiol.* 1995;25:3S–9S.

60. Hofgren C, Karlson BW, Herlitz J. Prodromal symptoms in subsets of patients hospitalized for suspected acute myocardial infarction. *Heart Lung.* 1995;24:3–10.

61. Dempsey SJ, Dracup K, Moser DK. Women's decision to seek care for symptoms of acute myocardial infarction. *Heart Lung.* 1995;24: 444–456.

62. Solomon CG, Lee TH, Cook EF, Weisberg MC, Brand DA, Rouan GW, Goldman L. Comparison of clinical presentation of acute myocardial infarction in patients older than 65 years of age to younger patients: the Multicenter Chest Pain Study experience. *Am J Cardiol.* 1989;63: 772–776.

63. Peberdy M, Ornato J. Coronary artery disease in women. *Heart Dis Stroke.* 1992;1:315–319.

64. Douglas PS, Ginsburg GS. The evaluation of chest pain in women. *N Engl J Med.* 1996;334:1311–1315.

65. Goff DC Jr, Feldman HA, McGovern PG, Goldberg RJ, Simons-Morton DG, Cornell CE, Osganian SK, Cooper LS, Hedges JR, Rapid Early Action for Coronary Treatment (REACT) Study Group. Prehospital delay in patients hospitalized with heart attack symptoms in the United States: the REACT trial [see comments]. *Am Heart J.* 1999;138: 1046–1057.

66. Berglin Blohm M, Hartford M, Karlsson T, Herlitz J. Factors associated with pre-hospital and in-hospital delay time in acute myocardial infarction: a 6-year experience. *J Intern Med.* 1998;243:243–250.

66a.Brown AL, Mann NC, Daya M, Goldberg R, Meischke H, Taylor J, Smith K, Osganian S, Cooper L. Demographic, belief, and situational factors influencing the decision to utilize emergency medical services among chest pain patients. *Circulation.* 2000;102:173–178.

67. Bleeker JK, Simoons ML, Erdman RA, Leenders CM, Kruyssen HA, Lamers LM, van der Does E. Patient and doctor delay in acute myocardial infarction: a study in Rotterdam, The Netherlands. *Br J Gen Pract.* 1995;45:181–184.

68. Goldberg RJ, McGovern PG, Guggina T, Savageau J, Rosamond WD, Luepker RV. Prehospital delay in patients with acute coronary heart disease: concordance between patient interviews and medical records. *Am Heart J.* 1998;135:293–299.

69. Blohm M, Herlitz J, Schroder U, Hartford M, Karlson BW, Risenfors M, Larsson E, Luepker R, Wennerblom B, Holmberg S. Reaction to a media campaign focusing on delay in acute myocardial infarction. *Heart Lung.* 1991;20:661–666.

70. Dracup K, Alonzo AA, Atkins JM, Bennett NM, Braslow A, Clark LT, Eisenberg M, Ferdinand KC, Frye R, Green L, Hill MN, Kennedy JW, Kline-Rogers E, Moser DK, Ornato JP, Pitt B, Scott JD, Selker HP, Silva SJ, Thies W, Weaver WD, Wenger NK, White SK, Working Group on Educational Strategies to Prevent Prehospital Delay in Patients

at High Risk for Acute Myocardial Infarction. The physician's role in minimizing prehospital delay in patients at high risk for acute myocardial infarction: recommendations from the National Heart Attack Alert Program. *Ann Intern Med.* 1997;126:645–651.

71. Weaver WD, Cerqueira M, Hallstrom AP, Litwin PE, Martin JS, Kudenchuk PJ, Eisenberg M. Prehospital-initiated vs hospital-initiated thrombolytic therapy: the Myocardial Infarction Triage and Intervention Trial [see comments]. *JAMA.* 1993;270:1211–1216.

72. EMIP Investigators, European Myocardial Infarction Project Group. Prehospital thrombolytic therapy in patients with suspected acute myocardial infarction [see comments]. *N Engl J Med.* 1993;329:383–389.

73. Schofer J, Buttner J, Geng G, Gutschmidt K, Herden HN, Mathey DG, Moecke HP, Polster P, Raftopoulo A, Sheehan FH, et al. Prehospital thrombolysis in acute myocardial infarction. *Am J Cardiol.* 1990;66: 1429–1433.

74. Gibler WB, Kereiakes DJ, Dean EN, Martin L, Anderson L, Abbottsmith CW, Blanton J, Blanton D, Morris JA Jr, Gibler CD, et al. Prehospital diagnosis and treatment of acute myocardial infarction: a north-south perspective: the Cincinnati Heart Project and the Nashville Prehospital TPA Trial. *Am Heart J.* 1991;121:1–11.

75. Linderer T, Schroder R, Arntz R, Heineking ML, Wunderlich W, Kohl K, Forycki F, Henzgen R, Wagner J. Prehospital thrombolysis: beneficial effects of very early treatment on infarct size and left ventricular function. *J Am Coll Cardiol.* 1993;22:1304–1310.

76. Rozenman Y, Gotsman M, Weiss T, Lotan C, Mosseri M, Sapoznikov D, Welber S, Nassar H, Hasin Y, Gilon D. Very early thrombolysis in acute myocardial infarction: a light at the end of the tunnel. *Isr J Med Sci.* 1994;30:99–107.

77. Rawles J. Halving of mortality at 1 year by domiciliary thrombolysis in the Grampian Region Early Anistreplase Trial (GREAT). *J Am Coll Cardiol.* 1994;23:1–5.

78. Rawles JM. Myocardial salvage with early anistreplase treatment. *Clin Cardiol.* 1997;20:III-6–III-10.

79. Rawles JM. Quantification of the benefit of earlier thrombolytic therapy: five-year results of the Grampian Region Early Anistreplase Trial (GREAT). *J Am Coll Cardiol.* 1997;30:1181–1186.

80. Brouwer MA, Martin JS, Maynard C, Wirkus M, Litwin PE, Verheugt FW, Weaver WD, MITI Project Investigators. Influence of early prehospital thrombolysis on mortality and event-free survival (the Myocardial Infarction Triage and Intervention [MITI] Randomized Trial). *Am J Cardiol.* 1996;78:497–502.

81. The European Myocardial Infarction Project Group. Prehospital thrombolytic therapy in patients with suspected acute myocardial infarction [see comments]. *N Engl J Med.* 1993;329:383–389.

82. Morrison LJ, Verbeek PR, McDonald AC, Sawadsky BV, Cook DJ. Mortality and prehospital thrombolysis for acute myocardial infarction: a meta-analysis. *JAMA.* 2000;283:2686–2692.

83. National Heart Attack Alert Program Coordinating Committee. Access to timely and optimal care of patients with acute coronary syndromes-community planning considerations: a report by the National Heart Attack Alert Program. *J Thromb Thrombolysis.* 1998;6:19–47.

84. National Heart Attack Alert Program Coordinating Committee Access to Care Subcommittee. Staffing and equipping emergency medical services system: rapid identification and treatment of acute myocardial infarction. *Am J Emerg Med.* 1995;13:58–66.

85. Kereiakes DJ, Gibler WB, Martin LH, Pieper KS, Anderson LC. Relative importance of emergency medical system transport and the prehospital electrocardiogram on reducing hospital time delay to therapy for acute myocardial infarction: a preliminary report from the Cincinnati Heart Project. *Am Heart J.* 1992;123:835–840.

86. Karagounis L, Ipsen SK, Jessop MR, Gilmore KM, Valenti DA, Clawson JJ, Teichman S, Anderson JL. Impact of field-transmitted electrocardiography on time to in-hospital thrombolytic therapy in acute myocardial infarction. *Am J Cardiol.* 1990;66:786–791.

87. Foster DB, Dufendach JH, Barkdoll CM, Mitchell BK. Prehospital recognition of AMI using independent nurse/paramedic 12-lead ECG evaluation: impact on in-hospital times to thrombolysis in a rural community hospital. *Am J Emerg Med.* 1994;12:25–31.

88. Aufderheide TP, Kereiakes DJ, Weaver WD, Gibler WB, Simoons ML. Planning, implementation, and process monitoring for prehospital 12-lead ECG diagnostic programs. *Prehospital Disaster Med.* 1996;11: 162–171.

89. Aufderheide TP, Hendley GE, Woo J, Lawrence S, Valley V, Teichman SL. A prospective evaluation of prehospital 12-lead ECG application in chest pain patients. *J Electrocardiol.* 1992;24(suppl):8–13.

90. Aufderheide TP, Haselow WC, Hendley GE, Robinson NA, Armaganian L, Hargarten KM, Olson DW, Valley VT, Stueven HA. Feasibility of prehospital r-TPA therapy in chest pain patients. *Ann Emerg Med.* 1992;21:379–383.

91. Aufderheide TP, Keelan MH, Hendley GE, Robinson NA, Hastings TE, Lewin RF, Hewes HF, Daniel A, Engle D, Gimbel BK, et al. Milwaukee Prehospital Chest Pain Project: phase I: feasibility and accuracy of prehospital thrombolytic candidate selection. *Am J Cardiol.* 1992;69:991–996.

92. Pantridge JF, Adgey AA, Webb SW. The first hour after the onset of acute myocardial infarction. In: Yu PN, Goodwin JF. *Progress in Cardiology.* Philadelphia, Pa: Lea & Febiger; 1975:173–178.

93. Grim P, Feldman T, Martin M, Donovan R, Nevins V, Childers RW. Cellular telephone transmission of 12-lead electrocardiograms from ambulance to hospital. *Am J Cardiol.* 1987;60:715–720.

94. Kudenchuck PJ, Ho MT, Litwin P, Martin JS, Weaver WD, for the MITI Project Investigators. Accuracy of cardiologist vs computerized ECG analysis in selecting patients for out-of-hospital thrombolytic therapy. *Circulation.* 1989;80(suppl II):II-354.

95. BEPS Collaborative Group. Prehospital thrombolysis in acute myocardial infarction. *Eur Heart J.* 1991;12:965–967.

96. Weaver W, Cerqueira M, Hallstrom A, Litwin P, Martin J, Kudenchuk P, Eisenberg M. Prehospital-initiated vs hospital-initiated thrombolytic therapy: the Myocardial Infarction Triage and Intervention Trial (MITI). *JAMA.* 1993;270:1203–1210.

97. National Heart Attack Alert Program Coordinating Committee Access to Care Subcommittee. Staffing and equipping emergency medical services systems: rapid identification and treatment of acute myocardial infarction. *Am J Emerg Med.* 1995;13:58–66.

98. Canto JG, Rogers WJ, Bowlby LJ, French WJ, Pearce DJ, Weaver WD, National Registry of Myocardial Infarction 2 Investigators. The prehospital electrocardiogram in acute myocardial infarction: is its full potential being realized? *J Am Coll Cardiol.* 1997;29:498–505.

99. Bengtson JR, Kaplan AJ, Pieper KS, Wildermann NM, Mark DB, Pryor DB, Phillips HR III, Califf RM. Prognosis in cardiogenic shock after acute myocardial infarction in the interventional era. *J Am Coll Cardiol.* 1992;20:1482–1489.

100. Goldberg RJ, Gore JM, Alpert JS, Osganian V, de Groot J, Bade J, Chen Z, Frid D, Dalen JE. Cardiogenic shock after acute myocardial infarction: incidence and mortality from a community-wide perspective, 1975 to 1988 [see comments]. *N Engl J Med.* 1991;325:1117–1122.

101. Hasdai D, Holmes DR Jr, Topol EJ, Berger PB, Criger DA, Hochman JS, Bates ER, Vahanian A, Armstrong PW, Wilcox R, Ohman EM, Califf RM. Frequency and clinical outcome of cardiogenic shock during acute myocardial infarction among patients receiving reteplase or alteplase: results from GUSTO-III: Global Use of Strategies to Open Occluded Coronary Arteries [see comments]. *Eur Heart J.* 1999;20:128–135.

102. Itoh T, Fukami K, Oriso S, Umemura J, Nakajima J, Obonai H, Hiramori K. Survival following cardiogenic shock caused by acute left main coronary artery total occlusion: a case report and review of the literature. *Angiology.* 1997;48:163–171.

103. Berger PB, Holmes DR Jr, Stebbins AL, Bates ER, Califf RM, Topol EJ. Impact of an aggressive invasive catheterization and revascularization strategy on survival in patients with cardiogenic shock in the Global Utilization of Streptokinase and Tissue Plasminogen Activator for Occluded Coronary Arteries (GUSTO-I) trial: an observational study. *Circulation.* 1997;96:122–127.

104. Holmes DR Jr, Califf RM, Van de Werf F, Berger PB, Bates ER, Simoons ML, White HD, Thompson TD, Topol EJ. Difference in countries' use of resources and clinical outcome for patients with cardiogenic shock after myocardial infarction: results from the GUSTO trial [see comments]. *Lancet.* 1997;349:75–78.

105. Tiefenbrunn AJ, Chandra NC, French WJ, Gore JM, Rogers WJ. Clinical experience with primary percutaneous transluminal coronary angioplasty compared with alteplase (recombinant tissue-type plasminogen activator) in patients with acute myocardial infarction: a report from the Second National Registry of Myocardial Infarction (NRMI-2). *J Am Coll Cardiol.* 1998;31:1240–1245.

106. Lee L, Erbel R, Brown TM, Laufer N, Meyer J, O'Neill WW. Multicenter registry of angioplasty therapy of cardiogenic shock: initial and long-term survival. *J Am Coll Cardiol.* 1991;17:599–603.

106a. Hochman JS, Sleeper LA, Webb JG, Sanborn TA, White HD, Talley JD, Buller CE, Jacobs AK, Slater JN, Col J, McKinlay SM, LeJemtel TH. Early revascularization in acute myocardial infarction complicated by

107. Hochman JS, Boland J, Sleeper LA, Porway M, Brinker J, Col J, Jacobs A, Slater J, Miller D, Wasserman H, et al, SHOCK Registry Investigators. Current spectrum of cardiogenic shock and effect of early revascularization on mortality: results of an International Registry [see comments]. *Circulation.* 1995;91:873–881.

108. Grines CL. Aggressive intervention for myocardial infarction: angioplasty, stents, and intra-aortic balloon pumping. *Am J Cardiol.* 1996;78:29–34.

109. Ishihara M, Sato H, Tateishi H, Kawagoe T, Shimatani Y, Kurisu S, Sakai K. Intraaortic balloon pumping as adjunctive therapy to rescue coronary angioplasty after failed thrombolysis in anterior wall acute myocardial infarction. *Am J Cardiol.* 1995;76:73–75.

110. Nanas JN, Nanas SN, Kontoyannis DA, Moussoutzani KS, Hatzigeorgiou JP, Heras PB, Makaritsis KP, Agapitos EB, Moulopoulos SD. Myocardial salvage by the use of reperfusion and intraaortic balloon pump: experimental study. *Ann Thorac Surg.* 1996;61:629–634.

111. Ohman EM, Califf RM, George BS, Quigley PJ, Kereiakes DJ, Harrelson-Woodlief L, Candela RJ, Flanagan C, Stack RS, Topol EJ, Thrombolysis and Angioplasty in Myocardial Infarction (TAMI) Study Group. The use of intraaortic balloon pumping as an adjunct to reperfusion therapy in acute myocardial infarction [see comments]. *Am Heart J.* 1991;121:895–901.

112. Talley JD, Ohman EM, Mark DB, George BS, Leimberger JD, Berdan LG, Davidson-Ray L, Rawert M, Lam LC, Phillips HR, Califf RM, Randomized IABP Study Group. Economic implications of the prophylactic use of intraaortic balloon counterpulsation in the setting of acute myocardial infarction: intraaortic balloon pump. *Am J Cardiol.* 1997;79:590–594.

113. Madias JE, Madias NE, Hood WB Jr. Precordial ST-segment mapping, II: effects of oxygen inhalation on ischemic injury in patients with acute myocardial infarction. *Circulation.* 1976;53:411–417.

114. Maroko PR, Radvany P, Braunwald E, Hale SL. Reduction of infarct size by oxygen inhalation following acute coronary occlusion. *Circulation.* 1975;52:360–368.

115. Jugdutt BI, Warnica JW. Intravenous nitroglycerin therapy to limit myocardial infarct size, expansion, and complications: effect of timing, dosage, and infarct location [published erratum appears in *Circulation.* 1989;79:1151]. *Circulation.* 1988;78:906–919.

116. Yusuf S, MacMahon S, Collins R, Peto R. Effect of intravenous nitrates on mortality in acute myocardial infarction: an overview of the randomised trials. *Lancet.* 1988;1:1088–1092.

117. ISIS-4 (Fourth International Study of Infarct Survival) Collaborative Group. ISIS-4: a randomised factorial trial assessing early oral captopril, oral mononitrate, and intravenous magnesium sulphate in 58,050 patients with suspected acute myocardial infarction [see comments]. *Lancet.* 1995;345:669–685.

118. ISIS-2 (Second International Study of Infarct Survival) Collaborative Group. Randomized trial of intravenous streptokinase, oral aspirin, both or neither among 17,187 cases of suspected acute myocardial infarction: ISIS-2. *Lancet.* 1988;2:349–360.

119. Antiplatelet Trialists' Collaboration. Collaborative overview of randomised trials of antiplatelet therapy, I: prevention of death, myocardial infarction, and stroke by prolonged antiplatelet therapy in various categories of patients [see comments] [published erratum appears in *BMJ.* 1994;308:1540]. *BMJ.* 1994;308:81–106.

120. National Heart Attack Alert Program Coordinating Committee 60 Minutes to Treatment Working Group. Emergency department: rapid identification and treatment of patients with acute myocardial infarction. *Ann Emerg Med.* 1994;23:311–329.

121. Al-Mubarak N, Rogers WJ, Lambrew CT, Bowlby LJ, French WJ, Second National Registry of Myocardial Infarction (NRMI 2) Investigators. Consultation before thrombolytic therapy in acute myocardial infarction. *Am J Cardiol.* 1999;83:89–93, A8.

122. Cannon CP, McCabe CH, Stone PH, Rogers WJ, Schactman M, Thompson BW, Pearce DJ, Diver DJ, Kells C, Feldman T, Williams M, Gibson RS, Kronenberg MW, Ganz LI, Anderson HV, Braunwald E. The electrocardiogram predicts one-year outcome of patients with unstable angina and non-Q wave myocardial infarction: results of the TIMI III Registry ECG Ancillary Study: Thrombolysis in Myocardial Ischemia. *J Am Coll Cardiol.* 1997;30:133–140.

123. Merz CN, Kelsey SF, Pepine CJ, Reichek N, Reis SE, Rogers WJ, Sharaf BL, Sopko G. The Women's Ischemia Syndrome Evaluation

(WISE) study: protocol design, methodology and feasibility report. *J Am Coll Cardiol.* 1999;33:1453–1461.

124. Lee TH, Cook EF, Weisberg MC, Rouan GW, Brand DA, Goldman L. Impact of the availability of a prior electrocardiogram on the triage of the patient with acute chest pain [see comments]. *J Gen Intern Med.* 1990;5:381–388.

125. Bar FW, Vermeer F, de Zwaan C, Ramentol M, Braat S, Simoons ML, Hermens WT, van der Laarse A, Verheugt FW, Krauss XH, et al. Value of admission electrocardiogram in predicting outcome of thrombolytic therapy in acute myocardial infarction: a randomized trial conducted by The Netherlands Interuniversity Cardiology Institute. *Am J Cardiol.* 1987;59:6–13.

126. Bar FW, Volders PG, Hoppener P, Vermeer F, Meyer J, Wellens HJ. Development of ST-segment elevation and Q- and R-wave changes in acute myocardial infarction and the influence of thrombolytic therapy. *Am J Cardiol.* 1996;77:337–343.

127. Califf RM, O'Neil W, Stack RS, Aronson L, Mark DB, Mantell S, George BS, Candela RJ, Kereiakes DJ, Abbottsmith C, et al. Failure of simple clinical measurements to predict perfusion status after intravenous thrombolysis. *Ann Intern Med.* 1988;108:658–662.

128. Krucoff MW, Croll MA, Pope JE, Granger CB, O'Connor CM, Sigmon KN, Wagner BL, Ryan JA, Lee KL, Kereiakes DJ, et al. Continuous 12-lead ST-segment recovery analysis in the TAMI 7 study: performance of a noninvasive method for real-time detection of failed myocardial reperfusion. *Circulation.* 1993;88:437–446.

129. Krucoff MW, Croll MA, Pope JE, Pieper KS, Kanani PM, Granger CB, Veldkamp RF, Wagner BL, Sawchak ST, Califf RM. Continuously updated 12-lead ST-segment recovery analysis for myocardial infarct artery patency assessment and its correlation with multiple simultaneous early angiographic observations. *Am J Cardiol.* 1993;71:145–151.

130. de Lemos JA, Antman EM, Gibson CM, McCabe CH, Giugliano RP, Murphy SA, Coulter SA, Anderson K, Scherer J, Frey MJ, Van Der Wieken R, Van De Werf F, Braunwald E. Abciximab improves both epicardial flow and myocardial reperfusion in ST-elevation myocardial infarction: observations from the TIMI 14 trial. *Circulation.* 2000;101: 239–243.

131. Shah A, Wagner GS, Granger CB, O'Connor CM, Green CL, Trollinger KM, Califf RM, Krucoff MW. Prognostic implications of TIMI flow grade in the infarct related artery compared with continuous 12-lead ST-segment resolution analysis: reexamining the "gold standard" for myocardial reperfusion assessment. *J Am Coll Cardiol.* 2000;35: 666–672.

132. Schroder R, Zeymer U, Wegscheider K, Neuhaus KL. Comparison of the predictive value of ST segment elevation resolution at 90 and 180 min after start of streptokinase in acute myocardial infarction: a substudy of the hirudin for improvement of thrombolysis (HIT)-4 study. *Eur Heart J.* 1999;20:1563–1571.

133. Boersma E, Pieper KS, Steyerberg EW, Wilcox RG, Chang WC, Lee KL, Akkerhuis KM, Harrington RA, Deckers JW, Armstrong PW, Lincoff AM, Califf RM, Topol EJ, Simoons ML, for the PURSUIT Investigators. Predictors of outcome in patients with acute coronary syndromes without persistent ST-segment elevation: results from an international trial of 9461 patients. *Circulation.* 2000;101:2557–2567.

134. Antman EM, Tanasijevic MJ, Thompson B, Schactman M, McCabe CH, Cannon CP, Fischer GA, Fung AY, Thompson C, Wybenga D, Braunwald E. Cardiac-specific troponin I levels to predict the risk of mortality in patients with acute coronary syndromes [see comments]. *N Engl J Med.* 1996;335:1342–1349.

135. Tanasijevic MJ, Cannon CP, Antman EM. The role of cardiac troponin-I (cTnI) in risk stratification of patients with unstable coronary artery disease. *Clin Cardiol.* 1999;22:13–16.

136. Heeschen C, Hamm CW, Goldmann B, Deu A, Langenbrink L, White HD, Platelet Receptor Inhibition in Ischemic Syndrome Management (PRISM) Study Investigators. Troponin concentrations for stratification of patients with acute coronary syndromes in relation to therapeutic efficacy of tirofiban. *Lancet.* 1999;354:1757–1762.

137. Lindahl B, Venge P, Wallentin L, Fragmin in Unstable Coronary Artery Disease (FRISC) Study Group. Troponin T identifies patients with unstable coronary artery disease who benefit from long-term antithrombotic protection. *J Am Coll Cardiol.* 1997;29:43–48.

138. Hamm CW, Heeschen C, Goldmann B, Vahanian A, Adgey J, Miguel CM, Rutsch W, Berger J, Kootstra J, Simoons ML, c7E3 Fab Antiplatelet Therapy in Unstable Refractory Angina (CAPTURE) Study Investigators. Benefit of abciximab in patients with refractory unstable angina

in relation to serum troponin T levels. *N Engl J Med.* 1999;340: 1623–1629.

139. Morrow DA, Rifai N, Antman EM, Weiner DL, McCabe CH, Cannon CP, Braunwald E. C-reactive protein is a potent predictor of mortality independently of and in combination with troponin T in acute coronary syndromes: a TIMI 11A substudy. Thrombolysis in Myocardial Infarction. *J Am Coll Cardiol.* 1998;31:1460–1465.

140. Rebuzzi AG, Quaranta G, Liuzzo G, Caligiuri G, Lanza GA, Gallimore JR, Grillo RL, Cianflone D, Biasucci LM, Maseri A. Incremental prognostic value of serum levels of troponin T and C-reactive protein on admission in patients with unstable angina pectoris. *Am J Cardiol.* 1998;82:715–719.

141. Deleted in proof.

142. Global Use of Strategies to Open Occluded Coronary Arteries (GUSTO III) Investigators. A comparison of reteplase with alteplase for acute myocardial infarction [see comments]. *N Engl J Med.* 1997;337: 1118–1123.

143. Assessment of the Safety and Efficacy of a New Thrombolytic (ASSENT) Investigators. Single-bolus tenecteplase compared with front-loaded alteplase in acute myocardial infarction: the ASSENT-2 double-blind randomised trial [see comments]. *Lancet.* 1999;354: 716–722.

144. Franzosi MG, Santoro E, De Vita C, Geraci E, Lotto A, Maggioni AP, Mauri F, Rovelli F, Santoro L, Tavazzi L, Tognoni G, GISSI Investigators. Ten-year follow-up of the first megatrial testing thrombolytic therapy in patients with acute myocardial infarction: results of the Gruppo Italiano per lo Studio della Sopravvivenza nell'Infarto-1 study [see comments]. *Circulation.* 1998;98:2659–2665.

145. Gruppo Italiano per lo Studio della Streptochinasi nell'Infarto Miocardico (GISSI). Effectiveness of intravenous thrombolytic treatment in acute myocardial infarction. *Lancet.* 1986;1:397–402.

146. Deleted in proof.

147. Brodie BR, Stuckey TD, Kissling G, Hansen CJ, Weintraub RA, Kelly TA. Importance of infarct-related artery patency for recovery of left ventricular function and late survival after primary angioplasty for acute myocardial infarction. *J Am Coll Cardiol.* 1996;28:319–325.

148. Puma JA, Sketch MH Jr, Thompson TD, Simes RJ, Morris DC, White HD, Topol EJ, Califf RM. Support for the open-artery hypothesis in survivors of acute myocardial infarction: analysis of 11,228 patients treated with thrombolytic therapy. *Am J Cardiol.* 1999;83:482–487.

149. Claeys MJ, Bosmans J, Veenstra L, Jorens P, De Raedt H, Vrints CJ. Determinants and prognostic implications of persistent ST-segment elevation after primary angioplasty for acute myocardial infarction: importance of microvascular reperfusion injury on clinical outcome. *Circulation.* 1999;99:1972–1977.

150. Gibson CM, Murphy SA, Rizzo MJ, Ryan KA, Marble SJ, McCabe CH, Cannon CP, Van de Werf F, Braunwald E, Thrombolysis In Myocardial Infarction (TIMI) Study Group. Relationship between TIMI frame count and clinical outcomes after thrombolytic administration. *Circulation.* 1999;99:1945–1950.

151. Reimer KA, Lowe JE, Rasmussen MM, Jennings RB. The wavefront phenomenon of ischemic cell death, I: myocardial infarct size vs duration of coronary occlusion in dogs. *Circulation.* 1977;56:786–794.

152. EMERAS (Estudio Multicentrico Estreptoquinasa Republicas de America del Sur) Collaborative Group. Randomised trial of late thrombolysis in patients with suspected acute myocardial infarction [see comments]. *Lancet.* 1993;342:767–772.

153. Late Assessment of Thrombolytic Efficacy (LATE) study with alteplase 6–24 hours after onset of acute myocardial infarction [see comments]. *Lancet.* 1993;342:759–766.

154. Simes RJ, Topol EJ, Holmes DR Jr, White HD, Rutsch WR, Vahanian A, Simoons ML, Morris D, Betriu A, Califf RM, et al, GUSTO-I Investigators. Link between the angiographic substudy and mortality outcomes in a large randomized trial of myocardial reperfusion: importance of early and complete infarct artery reperfusion [see comments]. *Circulation.* 1995;91:1923–1928.

155. GUSTO Angiographic Investigators. The effects of tissue plasminogen activator, streptokinase, or both on coronary-artery patency, ventricular function, and survival after acute myocardial infarction [see comments] [published erratum appears in *N Engl J Med.* 1994;330:516]. *N Engl J Med.* 1993;329:1615–1622.

156. Lamas GA, Flaker GC, Mitchell G, Smith SC Jr, Gersh BJ, Wun CC, Moye L, Rouleau JL, Rutherford JD, Pfeffer MA, et al, Survival and Ventricular Enlargement Investigators. Effect of infarct artery patency

on prognosis after acute myocardial infarction. *Circulation*. 1995;92: 1101–1109.

157. Kim CB, Braunwald E. Potential benefits of late reperfusion of infarcted myocardium: the open artery hypothesis. *Circulation*. 1993;88: 2426–2436.

158. Hillis LD, Forman S, Braunwald E, Thrombolysis in Myocardial Infarction (TIMI) Phase II Co-Investigators. Risk stratification before thrombolytic therapy in patients with acute myocardial infarction. *J Am Coll Cardiol*. 1990;16:313–315.

159. Simoons ML, Maggioni AP, Knatterud G, Leimberger JD, de Jaegere P, van Domburg R, Boersma E, Franzosi MG, Califf R, Schroder R, et al. Individual risk assessment for intracranial haemorrhage during thrombolytic therapy. *Lancet*. 1993;342:1523–1528.

160. Mauri F, Gasparini M, Barbonaglia L, Santoro E, Grazia Franzosi M, Tognoni G, Rovelli F. Prognostic significance of the extent of myocardial injury in acute myocardial infarction treated by streptokinase (the GISSI trial). *Am J Cardiol*. 1989;63:1291–1295.

161. Mahaffey KW, Granger CB, Sloan MA, Thompson TD, Gore JM, Weaver WD, White HD, Simoons ML, Barbash GI, Topol EJ, Califf RM. Risk factors for in-hospital nonhemorrhagic stroke in patients with acute myocardial infarction treated with thrombolysis: results from GUSTO-I. *Circulation*. 1998;97:757–764.

162. Gore JM, Granger CB, Simoons ML, Sloan MA, Weaver WD, White HD, Barbash GI, Van de Werf F, Aylward PE, Topol EJ, et al. Stroke after thrombolysis: mortality and functional outcomes in the GUSTO-I trial. Global Use of Strategies to Open Occluded Coronary Arteries [see comments]. *Circulation*. 1995;92:2811–2818.

162a.White HD, Barbash GI, Califf RM, Simes RJ, Granger CB, Weaver WD, Kleiman NS, Aylward PE, Gore JM, Vahanian A, Lee KL, Ross AM, Topol EJ. Age and outcome with contemporary thrombolytic therapy: results from the GUSTO-I trial. Global Utilization of Streptokinase and TPA for Occluded Coronary Arteries Trial. *Circulation*. 1996;94: 1826–1833.

163. Maggioni AP, Franzosi MG, Santoro E, White H, Van de Werf F, Tognoni G, Gruppo Italiano per lo Studio della Sopravvivenza nell'Infarto Miocardico II (GISSI-2) and The International Study Group. The risk of stroke in patients with acute myocardial infarction after thrombolytic and antithrombotic treatment [see comments]. *N Engl J Med*. 1992;327:1–6.

164. Thiemann DR, Coresh J, Schulman SP, Gerstenblith G, Oetgen WJ, Powe NR. Lack of benefit for intravenous thrombolysis in patients with myocardial infarction who are older than 75 years. *Circulation*. 2000; 101:2239–2246.

165. Boersma E, Maas AC, Deckers JW, Simoons ML. Early thrombolytic treatment in acute myocardial infarction: reappraisal of the golden hour. *Lancet*. 1996;348:771–775.

166. GUSTO Investigators. An international randomized trial comparing four thrombolytic strategies for acute myocardial infarction [see comments]. *N Engl J Med*. 1993;329:673–682.

167. Collins R, Peto R, Parish S, Sleight P. ISIS-3 and GISSI-2: no survival advantage with tissue plasminogen activator over streptokinase, but a significant excess of strokes with tissue plasminogen activator in both trials [letter]. *Am J Cardiol*. 1993;71:1127–1130.

168. Aylward PE, Wilcox RG, Horgan JH, White HD, Granger CB, Califf RM, Topol EJ, GUSTO-I Investigators. Relation of increased arterial blood pressure to mortality and stroke in the context of contemporary thrombolytic therapy for acute myocardial infarction: a randomized trial. *Ann Intern Med*. 1996;125:891–900.

169. Hollander JE, Burstein JL, Hoffman RS, Shih RD, Wilson LD, Cocaine-Associated Myocardial Infarction (CAMI) Study Group. Cocaine-associated myocardial infarction: clinical safety of thrombolytic therapy. *Chest*. 1995;107:1237–1241.

170. Anderson HV, Cannon CP, Stone PH, Williams DO, McCabe CH, Knatterud GL, Thompson B, Willerson JT, Braunwald E. One-year results of the Thrombolysis in Myocardial Infarction (TIMI) IIIB clinical trial: a randomized comparison of tissue-type plasminogen activator versus placebo and early invasive versus early conservative strategies in unstable angina and non-Q wave myocardial infarction. *J Am Coll Cardiol*. 1995;26:1643–1650.

171. Langer A, Goodman SG, Topol EJ, Charlesworth A, Skene AM, Wilcox RG, Armstrong PW, LATE Study Investigators. Late assessment of thrombolytic efficacy (LATE) study: prognosis in patients with non-Q wave myocardial infarction [see comments]. *J Am Coll Cardiol*. 1996; 27:1327–1332.

172. Kennedy JW, Martin GV, Davis KB, Maynard C, Stadius M, Sheehan FH, Ritchie JL. The Western Washington Intravenous Streptokinase in Acute Myocardial Infarction Randomized Trial [published erratum appears in *Circulation*. 1988;77:1037]. *Circulation*. 1988;77:345–352.

173. AIMS Trial Study Group. Effect of intravenous APSAC on mortality after acute myocardial infarction: preliminary report of a placebo-controlled clinical trial. *Lancet*. 1988;1:545–549.

174. Timmis AD, Griffin B, Crick JC, Sowton E. Anisoylated plasminogen streptokinase activator complex in acute myocardial infarction: a placebo-controlled arteriographic coronary recanalization study. *J Am Coll Cardiol*. 1987;10:205–210.

175. Verstraete M, Bernard R, Bory M, Brower RW, Collen D, de Bono DP, Erbel R, Huhmann W, Lennane RJ, Lubsen J, et al. Randomised trial of intravenous recombinant tissue-type plasminogen activator versus intravenous streptokinase in acute myocardial infarction: report from the European Cooperative Study Group for Recombinant Tissue-type Plasminogen Activator. *Lancet*. 1985;1:842–847.

176. Wilcox RG, von der Lippe G, Olsson CG, Jensen G, Skene AM, Hampton JR. Trial of tissue plasminogen activator for mortality reduction in acute myocardial infarction: Anglo-Scandinavian Study of Early Thrombolysis (ASSET). *Lancet*. 1988;2:525–530.

177. Bode C, Smalling RW, Berg G, Burnett C, Lorch G, Kalbfleisch JM, Chernoff R, Christie LG, Feldman RL, Seals AA, Weaver WD, RAPID II Investigators. Randomized comparison of coronary thrombolysis achieved with double-bolus reteplase (recombinant plasminogen activator) and front-loaded, accelerated alteplase (recombinant tissue plasminogen activator) in patients with acute myocardial infarction. *Circulation*. 1996;94:891–898.

178. Randomised, double-blind comparison of reteplase double-bolus administration with streptokinase in acute myocardial infarction (INJECT): trial to investigate equivalence: International Joint Efficacy Comparison of Thrombolytics [see comments] [published erratum appears in *Lancet*. 1995;346:980]. *Lancet*. 1995;346:329–336.

179. Van de Werf F, Cannon CP, Luyten A, Houbracken K, McCabe CH, Berioli S, Bluhmki E, Sarelin H, Wang-Clow F, Fox NL, Braunwald E, ASSENT-1 Investigators. Safety assessment of single-bolus administration of TNK tissue-plasminogen activator in acute myocardial infarction: the ASSENT-1 trial. *Am Heart J*. 1999;137:786–791.

180. Anderson JL, Karagounis LA, Becker LC, Sorensen SG, Menlove RL. TIMI perfusion grade 3 but not grade 2 results in improved outcome after thrombolysis for myocardial infarction: ventriculographic, enzymatic, and electrocardiographic evidence from the TEAM-3 Study. *Circulation*. 1993;87:1829–1839.

181. Lincoff AM, Topol EJ. Illusion of reperfusion: does anyone achieve optimal reperfusion during acute myocardial infarction? [corrected and republished article originally printed in *Circulation*. 1993;87: 1792–1805]. *Circulation*. 1993;88:1361–1374.

182. Ohman EM, Kleiman NS, Gacioch G, Worley SJ, Navetta FI, Talley JD, Anderson HV, Ellis SG, Cohen MD, Spriggs D, Miller M, Kereiakes D, Yakubov S, Kitt MM, Sigmon KN, Califf RM, Krucoff MW, Topol EJ, IMPACT-AMI Investigators. Combined accelerated tissue-plasminogen activator and platelet glycoprotein IIb/IIIa integrin receptor blockade with Integrilin in acute myocardial infarction: results of a randomized, placebo-controlled, dose-ranging trial [see comments]. *Circulation*. 1997;95:846–854.

183. Chaitman BR, Thompson BW, Kern MJ, Vandormael MG, Cohen MB, Ruocco NA, Solomon RE, Braunwald E, TIMI Investigators. Tissue plasminogen activator followed by percutaneous transluminal coronary angioplasty: one-year TIMI phase II pilot results [published erratum appears in *Am Heart J*. 1990;120(6 pt 1):1486]. *Am Heart J*. 1990;119: 213–223.

184. van den Merkhof LF, Zijlstra F, Olsson H, Grip L, Veen G, Bar FW, van den Brand MJ, Simoons ML, Verheugt FW. Abciximab in the treatment of acute myocardial infarction eligible for primary percutaneous transluminal coronary angioplasty: results of the Glycoprotein Receptor Antagonist Patency Evaluation (GRAPE) pilot study. *J Am Coll Cardiol*. 1999;33:1528–1532.

185. den Heijer P, Vermeer F, Ambrosioni E, Sadowski Z, Lopez-Sendon JL, von Essen R, Beaufils P, Thadani U, Adgey J, Pierard L, Brinker J, Davies RF, Smalling RW, Wallentin L, Caspi A, Pangerl A, Trickett L, Hauck C, Henry D, Chew P. Evaluation of a weight-adjusted single-bolus plasminogen activator in patients with myocardial infarction: a double-blind, randomized angiographic trial of lanoteplase versus alteplase. *Circulation*. 1998;98:2117–2125.

186. Nordt TK, Moser M, Kohler B, Kubler W, Bode C. Pharmacokinetics and pharmacodynamics of lanoteplase (n-PA). *Thromb Haemost*. 1999; 82(suppl 1):121–123.

187. Califf RM. Glycoprotein IIb/IIIa blockade and thrombolytics: early lessons from the SPEED and GUSTO IV trials. *Am Heart J*. 1999;138: S12–S15.

188. Antman EM, Giugliano RP, Gibson CM, McCabe CH, Coussement P, Kleiman NS, Vahanian A, Adgey AA, Menown I, Rupprecht HJ, Van der Wieken R, Ducas J, Scherer J, Anderson K, Van de Werf F, Braunwald E, TIMI 14 Investigators. Abciximab facilitates the rate and extent of thrombolysis: results of the Thrombolysis in Myocardial Infarction (TIMI) 14 trial. *Circulation*. 1999;99:2720–2732.

189. Michels KB, Yusuf S. Does PTCA in acute myocardial infarction affect mortality and reinfarction rates? A quantitative overview (meta-analysis) of the randomized clinical trials [see comments]. *Circulation*. 1995; 91:476–485.

190. Every NR, Parsons LS, Hlatky M, Martin JS, Weaver WD, Myocardial Infarction Triage and Intervention Investigators. A comparison of thrombolytic therapy with primary coronary angioplasty for acute myocardial infarction [see comments]. *N Engl J Med*. 1996;335:1253–1260.

191. Cucherat M, Bonnefoy E, Tremeau G. Primary angioplasty versus intravenous thrombolysis for acute myocardial infarction. *Cochrane Database Syst Rev*. 2000;2:CD001560.

192. Nunn CM, O'Neill WW, Rothbaum D, Stone GW, O'Keefe J, Overlie P, Donohue B, Grines L, Browne KF, Vlietstra RE, Catlin T, Grines CL. Long-term outcome after primary angioplasty: report from the primary angioplasty in myocardial infarction (PAMI-I) trial. *J Am Coll Cardiol*. 1999;33:640–646.

193. Holmes DR Jr, White HD, Pieper KS, Ellis SG, Califf RM, Topol EJ. Effect of age on outcome with primary angioplasty versus thrombolysis. *J Am Coll Cardiol*. 1999;33:412–419.

194. Stone GW, Brodie BR, Griffin JJ, Costantini C, Morice MC, St Goar FG, Overlie PA, Popma JJ, McDonnell J, Jones D, O'Neill WW, Grines CL. Clinical and angiographic follow-up after primary stenting in acute myocardial infarction: the Primary Angioplasty in Myocardial Infarction (PAMI) stent pilot trial. *Circulation*. 1999;99:1548–1554.

195. Antoniucci D, Santoro GM, Bolognese L, Valenti R, Trapani M, Fazzini PF. A clinical trial comparing primary stenting of the infarct-related artery with optimal primary angioplasty for acute myocardial infarction: results from the Florence Randomized Elective Stenting in Acute Coronary Occlusions (FRESCO) trial. *J Am Coll Cardiol*. 1998;31: 1234–1239.

196. Antoniucci D, Valenti R, Buonamici P, Santoro GM, Leoncini M, Bolognese L, Fazzini PF. Direct angioplasty and stenting of the infarct-related artery in acute myocardial infarction. *Am J Cardiol*. 1996;78: 568–571.

197. Cannon AD, Roubin GS, Macander PJ, Agrawal SK. Intracoronary stenting as an adjunct to angioplasty in acute myocardial infarction. *J Invasive Cardiol*. 1991;3:255–258.

198. Stone GW, Brodie BR, Griffin JJ, Morice MC, Costantini C, St Goar FG, Overlie PA, Popma JJ, McDonnell J, Jones D, O'Neill WW, Grines CL, Primary Angioplasty in Myocardial Infarction Stent Pilot Trial Investigators. Prospective, multicenter study of the safety and feasibility of primary stenting in acute myocardial infarction: in-hospital and 30-day results of the PAMI stent pilot trial. *J Am Coll Cardiol*. 1998; 31:23–30.

199. Cannon CP, Thompson B, McCabe CH, Mueller HS, Kirshenbaum JM, Herson S, Nasmith JB, Chaitman BR, Braunwald E. Predictors of non-Q-wave acute myocardial infarction in patients with acute ischemic syndromes: an analysis from the Thrombolysis in Myocardial Ischemia (TIMI) III trials [see comments]. *Am J Cardiol*. 1995;75:977–981.

200. Boden WE, O'Rourke RA, Crawford MH, Blaustein AS, Deedwania PC, Zoble RG, Wexler LF, Kleiger RE, Pepine CJ, Ferry DR, Chow BK, Lavori PW, Veterans Affairs Non-Q-Wave Infarction Strategies in Hospital (VANQWISH) Trial Investigators. Outcomes in patients with acute non-Q-wave myocardial infarction randomly assigned to an invasive as compared with a conservative management strategy [see comments]. *N Engl J Med*. 1998;338:1785–1792.

201. Yusuf S, Flather M, Pogue J, Hunt D, Varigos J, Piegas L, Avezum A, Anderson J, Keltai M, Budaj A, Fox K, Ceremuzynski L, OASIS (Organisation to Assess Strategies for Ischaemic Syndromes) Registry Investigators. Variations between countries in invasive cardiac procedures and outcomes in patients with suspected unstable angina or myocardial infarction without initial ST elevation [see comments]. *Lancet*. 1998;352:507–514.

202. FRagmin and Fast Revascularisation during InStability in Coronary artery disease Investigators. Invasive compared with non-invasive treatment in unstable coronary-artery disease: FRISC II prospective randomised multicentre study [see comments]. *Lancet*. 1999;354: 708–715.

203. Armstrong PW, Fu Y, Chang WC, Topol EJ, Granger CB, Betriu A, Van de Werf F, Lee KL, Califf RM, GUSTO-IIb Investigators. Acute coronary syndromes in the GUSTO-IIb trial: prognostic insights and impact of recurrent ischemia. *Circulation*. 1998;98:1860–1868.

204. Kong DF, Califf RM, Miller DP, Moliterno DJ, White HD, Harrington RA, Tcheng JE, Lincoff AM, Hasselblad V, Topol EJ. Clinical outcomes of therapeutic agents that block the platelet glycoprotein IIb/IIIa integrin in ischemic heart disease. *Circulation*. 1998;98:2829–2835.

205. The Platelet Glycoprotein IIb/IIIa in Unstable Angina: Receptor Suppression Using Integrilin Therapy (PURSUIT) Trial Investigators. Inhibition of platelet glycoprotein IIb/IIIa with eptifibatide in patients with acute coronary syndromes [see comments]. *N Engl J Med*. 1998;339: 436–443.

206. Platelet Receptor Inhibition in Ischemic Syndrome Management in Patients Limited by Unstable Signs and Symptoms (PRISM-PLUS) Study Investigators. Inhibition of the platelet glycoprotein IIb/IIIa receptor with tirofiban in unstable angina and non-Q-wave myocardial infarction [see comments] [published erratum appears in *N Engl J Med*. 1998;339:415]. *N Engl J Med*. 1998;338:1488–1497.

207. Kereiakes D, Grines C, Fry E, Barr L, Matthai W, Broderick T, Lengerich R, Cohen M, Esente P. Abciximab-enoxaparin interaction during percutaneous coronary intervention: results of the NICE-1 and NICE-2 Trials. *J Am Coll Cardiol*. 2000;35:92A.

208. Brieger DB, Mak KH, Kottke-Marchant K, Topol EJ. Heparin-induced thrombocytopenia. *J Am Coll Cardiol*. 1998;31:1449–1459.

209. Cohen M, Demers C, Gurfinkel EP, Turpie AG, Fromell GJ, Goodman S, Langer A, Califf RM, Fox KA, Premmereur J, Bigonzi F, Efficacy and Safety of Subcutaneous Enoxaparin in Non-Q-Wave Coronary Events Study Group. A comparison of low-molecular-weight heparin with unfractionated heparin for unstable coronary artery disease [see comments]. *N Engl J Med*. 1997;337:447–452.

210. Antman EM, McCabe CH, Gurfinkel EP, Turpie AG, Bernink PJ, Salein D, Bayes De Luna A, Fox K, Lablanche JM, Radley D, Premmereur J, Braunwald E. Enoxaparin prevents death and cardiac ischemic events in unstable angina/non-Q-wave myocardial infarction: results of the Thrombolysis in Myocardial Infarction (TIMI) 11B trial. *Circulation*. 1999;100:1593–1601.

210a. Klein W, Buchwald A, Hillis SE, Monrad S, Sanz G, Turpie AG, van der Meer J, Olaisson E, Undeland S, Ludwig K. Comparison of low-molecular-weight heparin with unfractionated heparin acutely and with placebo for 6 weeks in the management of unstable coronary artery disease: Fragmin in Unstable Coronary Artery Disease Study. *Circulation*. 1997;96:61–68.

210b. Fraxis Study Group. Comparison of two treatment durations (6 days and 14 days) of a low molecular weight heparin with a 6-day treatment of unfractionated heparin in the initial management of unstable angina or non-Q wave myocardial infarction: FRAX.I.S. *Eur Heart J*. 1999;20: 1553–1562.

211. FRagmin and Fast Revascularisation during InStability in Coronary artery disease Investigators. Long-term low-molecular-mass heparin in unstable coronary-artery disease: FRISC II prospective randomised multicentre study [see comments] [published erratum appears in *Lancet*. 1999;354:1478]. *Lancet*. 1999;354:701–707.

212. Hochman JS, Sleeper LA, Webb JG, Sanborn TA, White HD, Talley JD, Buller CE, Jacobs AK, Slater JN, Col J, McKinlay SM, LeJemtel TH, for the Should We Emergently Revascularize Occluded Coronaries for Cardiogenic Shock (SHOCK) Investigators. Early revascularization in acute myocardial infarction complicated by cardiogenic shock [see comments]. *N Engl J Med*. 1999;341:625–634.

213. Holmes DR Jr, Bates ER, Kleiman NS, Sadowski Z, Horgan JH, Morris DC, Califf RM, Berger PB, Topol EJ, Global Utilization of Streptokinase and Tissue Plasminogen Activator for Occluded Coronary Arteries (GUSTO-I) Investigators. Contemporary reperfusion therapy for cardiogenic shock: the GUSTO-I trial experience. *J Am Coll Cardiol*. 1995;26:668–674.

214. Bates ER, Topol EJ. Limitations of thrombolytic therapy for acute myocardial infarction complicated by congestive heart failure and cardiogenic shock. *J Am Coll Cardiol*. 1991;18:1077–1084.

215. Ellis SG, O'Neill WW, Bates ER, Walton JA Jr, Nabel EG, Werns SW, Topol EJ. Implications for patient triage from survival and left ventric-

ular functional recovery analyses in 500 patients treated with coronary angioplasty for acute myocardial infarction. *J Am Coll Cardiol*. 1989; 13:1251–1259.

216. Moosvi AR, Khaja F, Villanueva L, Gheorghiade M, Douthat L, Goldstein S. Early revascularization improves survival in cardiogenic shock complicating acute myocardial infarction [see comments]. *J Am Coll Cardiol*. 1992;19:907–914.

217. Lee L, Bates ER, Pitt B, Walton JA, Laufer N, O'Neill WW. Percutaneous transluminal coronary angioplasty improves survival in acute myocardial infarction complicated by cardiogenic shock. *Circulation*. 1988;78:1345–1351.

218. Verna E, Repetto S, Boscarini M, Ghezzi I, Binaghi G. Emergency coronary angioplasty in patients with severe left ventricular dysfunction or cardiogenic shock after acute myocardial infarction. *Eur Heart J*. 1989;10:958–966.

219. Califf RM, Bengtson JR. Cardiogenic shock. *N Engl J Med*. 1994;330: 1724–1730.

220. Berger PB, Ryan TJ. Inferior myocardial infarction: high-risk subgroups. *Circulation*. 1990;81:401–411.

221. Kinch JW, Ryan TJ. Right ventricular infarction [see comments]. *N Engl J Med*. 1994;330:1211–1217.

222. Zehender M, Kasper W, Kauder E, Schonthaler M, Geibel A, Olschewski M, Just H. Right ventricular infarction as an independent predictor of prognosis after acute inferior myocardial infarction [see comments]. *N Engl J Med*. 1993;328:981–988.

223. Berger PB, Ruocco NA Jr, Ryan TJ, Jacobs AK, Zaret BL, Wackers FJ, Frederick MM, Faxon DP, TIMI Research Group. Frequency and significance of right ventricular dysfunction during inferior wall left ventricular myocardial infarction treated with thrombolytic therapy (results from the Thrombolysis In Myocardial Infarction [TIMI] II trial). *Am J Cardiol*. 1993;71:1148–1152.

224. Goldstein JA, Barzilai B, Rosamond TL, Eisenberg PR, Jaffe AS. Determinants of hemodynamic compromise with severe right ventricular infarction. *Circulation*. 1990;82:359–368.

225. Dalen J, Hirsch J. Fifth ACCP Consensus Conference on Antithrombotic Therapy. *Chest*. 1998;114(5 suppl):439S–769S.

226. Collins R, MacMahon S, Flather M, Baigent C, Remvig L, Mortensen S, Appleby P, Godwin J, Yusuf S, Peto R. Clinical effects of anticoagulant therapy in suspected acute myocardial infarction: systematic overview of randomised trials. *BMJ*. 1996;313:652–659.

227. Hsia J, Hamilton WP, Kleiman N, Roberts R, Chaitman BR, Ross AM, Heparin-Aspirin Reperfusion Trial (HART) Investigators. A comparison between heparin and low-dose aspirin as adjunctive therapy with tissue plasminogen activator for acute myocardial infarction [see comments]. *N Engl J Med*. 1990;323:1433–1437.

228. Tanne D, Reicher-Reiss H, Boyko V, Behar S, Secondary Prevention Reinfarction Israeli Nifedipine Trial (SPRINT) Study Group. Stroke risk after anterior wall acute myocardial infarction. *Am J Cardiol*. 1995;76: 825–826.

229. Loh E, Sutton MS, Wun CC, Rouleau JL, Flaker GC, Gottlieb SS, Lamas GA, Moye LA, Goldhaber SZ, Pfeffer MA. Ventricular dysfunction and the risk of stroke after myocardial infarction. *N Engl J Med*. 1997;336:251–257.

230. MIAMI Trial Research Group. Metoprolol in acute myocardial infarction (MIAMI): a randomised placebo-controlled international trial. *Eur Heart J*. 1985;6:199–226.

231. First International Study of Infarct Survival Collaborative Group. Randomised trial of intravenous atenolol among 16 027 cases of suspected acute myocardial infarction: ISIS-1. *Lancet*. 1986;2:57–66.

232. Rehnqvist N, Olsson G, Erhardt L, Ekman AM. Metoprolol in acute myocardial infarction reduces ventricular arrhythmias both in the early stage and after the acute event. *Int J Cardiol*. 1987;15:301–308.

233. Herlitz J, Edvardsson N, Holmberg S, Ryden L, Waagstein F, Waldenstrom A, Swedberg K, Hjalmarson A. Goteborg Metoprolol Trial: effects on arrhythmias. *Am J Cardiol*. 1984;53:27D–31D.

234. Roberts R, Rogers WJ, Mueller HS, Lambrew CT, Diver DJ, Smith HC, Willerson JT, Knatterud GL, Forman S, Passamani E, et al. Immediate versus deferred β-blockade following thrombolytic therapy in patients with acute myocardial infarction: results of the Thrombolysis in Myocardial Infarction (TIMI) II-B Study [see comments]. *Circulation*. 1991; 83:422–437.

235. Gruppo Italiano per lo Studio della Sopravvivenza nell'Infarto Miocardico. Six-month effects of early treatment with lisinopril and transdermal glyceryl trinitrate singly and together withdrawn six weeks after

acute myocardial infarction: the GISSI-3 trial [see comments]. *J Am Coll Cardiol*. 1996;27:337–344.

236. Ferguson JJ, Diver DJ, Boldt M, Pasternak RC. Significance of nitroglycerin-induced hypotension with inferior wall acute myocardial infarction. *Am J Cardiol*. 1989;64:311–314.

237. Muller JE, Morrison J, Stone PH, Rude RE, Rosner B, Roberts R, Pearle DL, Turi ZG, Schneider JF, Serfas DH, et al. Nifedipine therapy for patients with threatened and acute myocardial infarction: a randomized, double-blind, placebo-controlled comparison. *Circulation*. 1984;69: 740–747.

238. Effect of verapamil on mortality and major events after acute myocardial infarction (the Danish Verapamil Infarction Trial II–DAVIT II) [see comments]. *Am J Cardiol*. 1990;66:779–785.

239. Multicenter Diltiazem Postinfarction Trial Research Group. The effect of diltiazem on mortality and reinfarction after myocardial infarction. *N Engl J Med*. 1988;319:385–392.

240. Boden WE, van Gilst WH, Scheldewaert RG, Starkey IR, Carlier MF, Julian DG, Whitehead A, Bertrand ME, Col JJ, Pedersen OL, Lie KI, Santoni JP, Fox KM. Diltiazem in acute myocardial infarction treated with thrombolytic agents: a randomised placebo-controlled trial: Incomplete Infarction Trial of European Research Collaborators Evaluating Prognosis post-Thrombolysis (INTERCEPT). *Lancet*. 2000;355: 1751–1756.

241. Gruppo Italiano per lo Studio della Sopravvivenza nell'infarto Miocardico (GISSI-3). Effects of lisinopril and transdermal glyceryl trinitrate singly and together on 6-week mortality and ventricular function after acute myocardial infarction [see comments]. *Lancet*. 1994;343:1115–1122.

242. Chinese Cardiac Study (CCS-1) Collaborative Group. Oral captopril versus placebo among 14,962 patients with suspected acute myocardial infarction: a multicenter, randomized, double-blind, placebo controlled clinical trial. *Chin Med J*. 1997;110:834–838.

243. Ambrosioni E, Borghi C, Magnani B, Survival of Myocardial Infarction Long-Term Evaluation (SMILE) Study Investigators. The effect of the angiotensin-converting-enzyme inhibitor zofenopril on mortality and morbidity after anterior myocardial infarction [see comments]. *N Engl J Med*. 1995;332:80–85.

244. Borghi C, Marino P, Zardini P, Magnani B, Collatina S, Ambrosioni E, FAMIS Working Party. Short- and long-term effects of early fosinopril administration in patients with acute anterior myocardial infarction undergoing intravenous thrombolysis: results from the Fosinopril in Acute Myocardial Infarction Study. *Am Heart J*. 1998;136:213–225.

245. ACE Inhibitor Myocardial Infarction Collaborative Group. Indications for ACE inhibitors in the early treatment of acute myocardial infarction: systematic overview of individual data from 100 000 patients in randomized trials [see comments]. *Circulation*. 1998;97:2202–2212.

246. Swedberg K, Held P, Kjekshus J, Rasmussen K, Ryden L, Wedel H. Effects of the early administration of enalapril on mortality in patients with acute myocardial infarction: results of the Cooperative New Scandinavian Enalapril Survival Study II (CONSENSUS II) [see comments]. *N Engl J Med*. 1992;327:678–684.

247. Teo KK, Yusuf S, Collins R, Held PH, Peto R. Effects of intravenous magnesium in suspected acute myocardial infarction: overview of randomised trials [see comments]. *BMJ*. 1991;303:1499–1503.

248. Woods KL, Fletcher S, Roffe C, Haider Y. Intravenous magnesium sulphate in suspected acute myocardial infarction: results of the second Leicester Intravenous Magnesium Intervention Trial (LIMIT-2) [see comments]. *Lancet*. 1992;339:1553–1558.

249. Antman EM. Magnesium in acute myocardial infarction: overview of available evidence. *Am Heart J*. 1996;132:487–495; discussion 496–502.

250. The MAGIC Steering Committee. Rationale and design of the Magnesium in Coronaries (MAGIC) study: a clinical trial to reevaluate the efficacy of early administration of magnesium in acute myocardial infarction. *Am Heart J*. 2000;139:10–14.

251. Sodi-Pallares D, Ponce de Leon J, Bisteni A, Medrano GA. Potassium, glucose, and insulin in myocardial infarction. *Lancet*. 1969;1: 1315–1316.

252. Maroko PR, Libby P, Sobel BE, Bloor CM, Sybers HD, Shell WE, Covell JW, Braunwald E. Effect of glucose-insulin-potassium infusion on myocardial infarction following experimental coronary artery occlusion. *Circulation*. 1972;45:1160–1175.

253. Opie LH. Myocardial infarct size, II: comparison of anti-infarct effects of beta-blockade, glucose-insulin-potassium, nitrates, and hyaluronidase. *Am Heart J*. 1980;100:531–552.

254. Rackley CE, Russell RO Jr, Rogers WJ, Mantle JA, McDaniel HG, Papapietro SE. Clinical experience with glucose-insulin-potassium therapy in acute myocardial infarction. *Am Heart J.* 1981;102:1038–1049.

255. Rogers WJ, Stanley AW Jr, Breinig JB, Prather JW, McDaniel HG, Moraski RE, Mantle JA, Russell RO Jr, Rackley CE. Reduction of hospital mortality rate of acute myocardial infarction with glucose-insulin-potassium infusion. *Am Heart J.* 1976;92:441–454.

256. Fath-Ordoubadi F, Beatt KJ. Glucose-insulin-potassium therapy for treatment of acute myocardial infarction: an overview of randomized placebo-controlled trials [see comments]. *Circulation.* 1997;96: 1152–1156.

257. Diabetes Insulin-Glucose in Acute Myocardial Infarction (DIGAMI) Study Group. Malmberg K, Ryden L, Hamsten A, Herlitz J, Waldenstrom A, Wedel H. Effects of insulin treatment on cause-specific one-year mortality and morbidity in diabetic patients with acute myocardial infarction [see comments]. *Eur Heart J.* 1996;17:1337–1344.

258. Apstein CS, Taegtmeyer H. Glucose-insulin-potassium in acute myocardial infarction: the time has come for a large, prospective trial [editorial; comment]. *Circulation.* 1997;96:1074–1077.

259. The ECLA (Estudios Cardiologicos Latinoamerica) Collaborative Group. Diaz R, Paolasso EA, Piegas LS, Tajer CD, Moreno MG, Corvalan R, Isea JE, Romero G. Metabolic modulation of acute myocardial infarction. *Circulation.* 1998;98:2227–2234.

260. Ceremuzynski L, Budaj A, Czepiel A, Burzykowski T, Achremczyk P, Smielak-Korombel W, Maciejewicz J, Dziubinska J, Nartowicz E, Kawka-Urbanek T, Piotrowski W, Hanzlik J, Cieslinski A, Kawecka-Jaszcz K, Gessek J, Wrabec K. Low-dose glucose-insulin-potassium is ineffective in acute myocardial infarction: results of a randomized multicenter Pol-GIK trial. *Cardiovasc Drugs Ther.* 1999;13:191–200.

261. Malmberg K, DIGAMI (Diabetes Mellitus, Insulin Glucose Infusion in Acute Myocardial Infarction) Study Group. Prospective randomised study of intensive insulin treatment on long term survival after acute myocardial infarction in patients with diabetes mellitus [see comments]. *BMJ.* 1997;314:1512–1515.

262. MacMahon S, Collins R, Peto R, Koster RW, Yusuf S. Effects of prophylactic lidocaine in suspected acute myocardial infarction: an overview of results from the randomized, controlled trials. *JAMA.* 1988; 260:1910–1916.

263. Belardinelli L, Shryock J, West GA, Clemo HF, DiMarco JP, Berne RM. Effects of adenosine and adenine nucleotides on the atrioventricular node of isolated guinea pig hearts. *Circulation.* 1984;70:1083–1091.

264. Feigl D, Ashkenazy J, Kishon Y. Early and late atrioventricular block in acute inferior myocardial infarction. *J Am Coll Cardiol.* 1984;4:35–38.

265. Shah PK, Nalos P, Peter T. Atropine resistant post infarction complete AV block: possible role of adenosine and improvement with aminophylline. *Am Heart J.* 1987;113:194–195.

266. Goldberg RJ, Seeley D, Becker RC, Brady P, Chen ZY, Osganian V, Gore JM, Alpert JS, Dalen JE. Impact of atrial fibrillation on the in-hospital and long-term survival of patients with acute myocardial infarction: a community-wide perspective. *Am Heart J.* 1990;119: 996–1001.

267. Behar S, Reicher-Reiss H, Abinader E, Agmon J, Barzilai J, Friedman Y, Kaplinsky E, Kauli N, Kishon Y, Palant A, et al, SPRINT Study Group. Long-term prognosis after acute myocardial infarction in patients with left ventricular hypertrophy on the electrocardiogram. *Am J Cardiol.* 1992;69:985–990.

268. Eldar M, Canetti M, Rotstein Z, Boyko V, Gottlieb S, Kaplinsky E, Behar S, SPRINT and Thrombolytic Survey Groups. Significance of paroxysmal atrial fibrillation complicating acute myocardial infarction in the thrombolytic era. *Circulation.* 1998;97:965–970.

269. Madias JE, Patel DC, Singh D. Atrial fibrillation in acute myocardial infarction: a prospective study based on data from a consecutive series of patients admitted to the coronary care unit. *Clin Cardiol.* 1996;19: 180–186.

270. Nielsen FE, Andersen HH, Gram-Hansen P, Sorensen HT, Klausen IC. The relationship between ECG signs of atrial infarction and the development of supraventricular arrhythmias in patients with acute myocardial infarction. *Am Heart J.* 1992;123:69–72.

271. Hod H, Lew AS, Keltai M, Cercek B, Geft IL, Shah PK, Ganz W. Early atrial fibrillation during evolving myocardial infarction: a consequence of impaired left atrial perfusion. *Circulation.* 1987;75:146–150.

272. Widimsky P, Gregor P. Recent atrial fibrillation in acute myocardial infarction: a sign of pericarditis. *Cor Vasa.* 1993;35:230–232.

273. Nielsen FE, Sorensen HT, Christensen JH, Ravn L, Rasmussen SE. Reduced occurrence of atrial fibrillation in acute myocardial infarction treated with streptokinase. *Eur Heart J.* 1991;12:1081–1083.

274. Behar S, Zahavi Z, Goldbourt U, Reicher-Reiss H, SPRINT Study Group. Long-term prognosis of patients with paroxysmal atrial fibrillation complicating acute myocardial infarction. *Eur Heart J.* 1992;13: 45–50.

Part 7: The Era of Reperfusion
Section 2: Acute Stroke

Major Guidelines Changes

- Intravenous administration of tissue-type plasminogen activator (tPA) for patients with acute ischemic stroke and no contraindications is recommended:
  - —Within 3 hours of onset of stroke symptoms (Class I)
  - —Between 3 and 6 hours of onset of stroke symptoms (Class Indeterminate)
- Intra-arterial fibrinolysis within 3 to 6 hours after the onset of symptoms may be beneficial in patients with occlusion of the middle cerebral artery (Class IIb).

Introduction

A stroke is a disruption in blood supply to a region of the brain that causes neurological impairment. Stroke is ranked among the top 3 leading causes of death in most countries and is the leading cause of brain injury in adults. Internationally millions of people have a new or recurrent stroke each year, and nearly a quarter of these people die.[1] The stroke rate is declining in most western and northern European countries, but there is a large and increasing rate in Russia, possibly attributable to a higher prevalence of hypertension.[2] Although stroke mortality and attack rates are falling in many countries, the gain achieved by prevention has been counterbalanced by a growth in the aging population (more people at risk).[3,4]

Strokes can be classified into 2 major categories, ischemic and hemorrhagic. Approximately 85% of all strokes are ischemic.[5] Ischemic strokes occur primarily because a blood vessel supplying the brain is occluded, usually by a thrombus or embolism. Hemorrhagic strokes are the result of rupture of a cerebral artery. Associated spasm of the artery and various degrees of bleeding occur. Until recently, care of the stroke patient was largely supportive, focusing on prevention and treatment of respiratory and cardiovascular complications. No specific therapy was available to alter the course and extent of the evolving stroke. Therefore, little emphasis or need was placed on rapid transport or intervention.

Fibrinolytic therapy now offers healthcare providers an opportunity to possibly limit the extent of neurological damage and to improve outcome in stroke patients. A time-dependent benefit similar to that observed in patients with acute myocardial infarction (AMI) is possible. The time available for treatment, however, is limited.[6] Early recognition of stroke and rapid triage, evaluation in the Emergency Department (ED), and definitive management are essential.[7–9]

Early Recognition

Early treatment of stroke depends strongly on recognition of the event by the patient, family members, or bystanders.[10] Common symptoms of transient ischemic attack (TIA) and stroke are described in Table 1.

Role of EMS in Stroke Care

Rapid activation of the EMS system is essential to optimize care of the patient with stroke. Stroke patients who use the EMS system arrive at the hospital faster than those who do not, a major advantage for time-critical treatment.[11–18] Furthermore, emergency dispatchers can send the appropriate emergency team with a priority dispatch response and provide instructions for care of the patient until arrival of EMS personnel.[19–21] EMS personnel can then quickly transport the patient to a stroke center and notify the facility before arrival to ensure rapid hospital-based evaluation and treatment. Initial contact of the family physician and transport of the patient by car have been shown to delay patient arrival and initial evaluation at the hospital. Such delays may render the patient ineligible for fibrinolytic therapy.[11,15,19]

Only half of stroke patients currently use the EMS system for transport to the hospital.[11,22] Strokes that occur when the patient is alone or sleeping may further delay prompt recognition and action.[23] Eighty-five percent of strokes occur at home.[22] As a result, public education programs have appropriately focused their efforts on persons at risk for stroke and their friends and family members. Public education has reduced the time to arrival at the ED.[8,12]

The 7 "D's" of Stroke Management

Key points in the management of stroke can be remembered by using the mnemonic of the 7 D's: Detection, Dispatch, Delivery, Door, Data, Decision, and Drug (see algorithm for suspected stroke).[24] Delay may occur at any point, so the response at each point must be skilled and efficient. The first 3 D's (detection, dispatch, and delivery) are the responsibility of BLS providers in the community, including the lay public and EMS responders. Detection occurs when a patient, family member, or bystander recognizes the signs and symptoms of a stroke or TIA and activates the EMS system (by phoning 911 or other emergency response number). EMS dispatchers must prioritize the call for a suspected stroke patient as they would for a victim of AMI or serious trauma and dispatch the appropriate EMS team with high transport priority. EMS providers must respond rapidly, confirm the signs and symptoms of stroke, and transport the patient (delivery) to a stroke center (a hospital that can provide fibrino-

Circulation. 2000;102(suppl I):I-204–I-216.
© 2000 American Heart Association, Inc.

Circulation is available at http://www.circulationaha.org

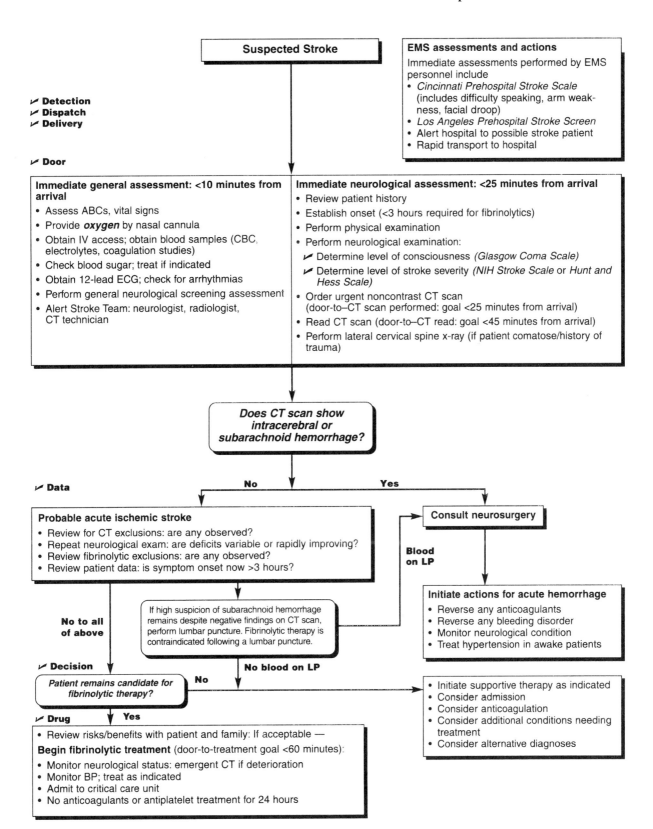

Figure. Algorithm for suspected stroke.

lytic therapy within 1 hour after arrival at the ED *door*). The remaining 3 D's are performed in the hospital: *d*ata includes obtaining a computed tomography (CT) scan, *d*ecision is made in identifying candidates eligible for fibrinolytic therapy, and *d*rug includes treating eligible patients with fibrinolytic therapy.

Airway and Ventilation

Airway obstruction may be a major problem in acute stroke, particularly if the patient loses consciousness. Hypoxia and hypercarbia can occur as the result of inadequate ventilation, contributing to cardiac and respiratory instability. Aspiration

TABLE 1. Common Signs and Symptoms of Transient Ischemic Attack (TIA) and Stroke

Unilateral paralysis—Weakness, clumsiness, or heaviness, usually involving 1 side of the body

Unilateral numbness—Sensory loss, tingling, or abnormal sensation, usually involving 1 side of the body

Language disturbance—Trouble understanding or speaking (*aphasia*) or slurred speech (*dysarthria*)

Monocular blindness—Painless visual loss in one eye, often described as a curtain dropping

Vertigo—Sense of spinning or whirling that persists at rest. Isolated vertigo is also a common symptom of many nonvascular diseases; therefore, at least one other symptom of TIA or stroke should also be present.

Ataxia—Poor balance, stumbling gait, staggering, incoordination of one side of the body

of secretions or gastric contents is a serious complication associated with considerable morbidity and mortality. EMS providers must ensure that the patient has an adequate airway. Assisted ventilation or tracheal intubation may be required.

Vital Signs

Check vital signs (pulse, respirations, blood pressure, and temperature) frequently to detect abnormalities and changes. Abnormal respirations are particularly prevalent in comatose stroke patients and usually reflect serious brain dysfunction. Hypertension often occurs after a stroke and may be caused by underlying hypertension, a stress reaction to the neurological event, or a physiological response to decreased brain perfusion. Blood pressure often returns to normal without antihypertensive treatment.[25]

A variety of cardiovascular problems may be present in the patient with stroke. Cardiac arrhythmias may contribute to the cerebral thromboembolism, or they may be the consequence of brain injury. In particular, episodes of paroxysmal atrial fibrillation, severe symptomatic bradycardia, or high-degree atrioventricular block may point to cardiac rhythm disturbances as causative or contributory. In the elderly and in patients with diabetes, AMI with atypical or undetectable symptoms can occur.[26,27] Obtain a 12-lead ECG and attempt to rule out left ventricular mural emboli if an acute or recent MI is suspected. Life-threatening cardiac arrhythmias are a potential early complication of stroke, particularly of intracranial hemorrhages.[28-30] Continuous monitoring of cardiac rhythm and systemic perfusion is part of the early management of a stroke patient.

General Medical Assessment

Examine the patient for evidence of injury to the head or neck, because trauma is an important consideration in the differential diagnosis of stroke. Blood pressure in both upper extremities should be measured. A difference of >10 mm Hg should raise consideration of aortic dissection and compromise of brain blood supply. Perform diagnostic studies such as CT or angiography if indicated by history or clinical findings. Cardiac murmur, arterial bruit, absent pulse, or other abnormalities should be sought during the cardiovascu-

lar examination. The presence of an ocular hemorrhage may allow early identification of intracranial bleeding.

Brief Emergency Neurological Evaluation

The emergency neurological evaluation for stroke should include 6 key elements:

- Stroke screen or scale
- Time of onset of stroke signs
- Level of consciousness
- Type of stroke (hemorrhagic versus nonhemorrhagic)
- Location of stroke (carotid versus vertebrobasilar)
- Severity of stroke

Stroke Screen or Scale

Performing an extensive neurological examination outside the hospital is impractical because it delays transport of the patient to the ED. To conduct an out-of-hospital neurological evaluation, use a validated tool such as the Cincinnati Prehospital Stroke Scale (Table 2) or the Los Angeles Prehospital Stroke Screen (LAPSS)[16] (Table 3).[31,32] The Cincinnati scale is used to elicit any of the 3 major physical findings suggestive of stroke: facial droop, arm drift, and abnormal speech.[31] LAPSS requires the examiner to rule out other causes of altered level of consciousness (eg, history of seizures or severe hyperglycemia or hypoglycemia) and then identify asymmetry (right versus left) in facial smile/grimace, grip, or arm strength. Asymmetry in any category indicates a possible stroke.[18,32] These two scales are sensitive and specific in identifying stroke patients.[18,31,32] Either evaluation can be performed quickly.

Ambulance personnel can identify stroke patients with reasonable sensitivity and specificity. Once a stroke is suspected, minimize time in the field and immediately transport the patient to a stroke center.

Clinical signs and symptoms of acute stroke often fluctuate. Deterioration or improvement can be detected by frequent and repeated focal neurological examinations. Repeated examinations need not be exhaustive. The Glasgow Coma Scale tests eye opening, verbal response, and motor

TABLE 2. Cincinnati Prehospital Stroke Scale

Try to elicit one of the following signs (abnormality in any *one* is strongly suggestive of stroke):

Facial droop (have patient show teeth or smile):

Normal: both sides of face move equally well

Abnormal: one side of face does not move as well as the other side

Arm drift (have patient close eyes and hold both arms straight out for 10 seconds):

Normal: both arms move the same or both arms do not move at all (other findings, such as pronator grip, may be helpful)

Abnormal: one arm does not move or one arm drifts down

Abnormal speech (have the patient say "you can't teach an old dog new tricks"):

Normal: patient uses correct words with no slurring

Abnormal: patient slurs words, uses the wrong words, or is unable to speak

From Reference 31.

TABLE 3.   Los Angeles Prehospital Stroke Screen (LAPSS)

For evaluation of acute, noncomatose, nontraumatic neurological complaint: If items 1 through 6 are **ALL checked "yes"** (or "unknown"), notify the receiving hospital before arrival of the potential stroke patient. If any are checked "no," follow appropriate treatment protocol.

Interpretation: Ninety-three percent of patients with stroke will have positive findings (all items checked "yes" or "unknown") on the LAPSS (sensitivity=93%), and 97% of those with positive findings will have a stroke (specificity=97%). The patient may still be having a stroke if LAPSS criteria are not met.

Criteria	Yes	Unknown	No
1. Age >45 years	[]	[]	[]
2. History of seizures or epilepsy **absent**	[]	[]	[]
3. Symptom duration <24 hours	[]	[]	[]
4. At baseline, patient is **not** wheelchair bound or bedridden	[]	[]	[]
5. Blood glucose between 60 and 400	[]	[]	[]
6. *Obvious asymmetry* (right vs left) in *any* of the following 3 categories (*must be unilateral*)	[]	[]	[]

	Equal	R Weak	L Weak
Facial smile/grimace	[]	[] Droop	[] Droop
Grip	[]	[] Weak grip	[] Weak grip
	[]	[] No grip	[] No grip
Arm strength	[]	[] Drifts down	[] Drifts down
	[]	[] Falls rapidly	[] Falls rapidly

From References 18 and 32.

response.[33] It is useful for assessing the initial severity of neurological injury in patients with altered consciousness, especially in cases of injury caused by intracerebral hemorrhage.

Obtain the following information en route to or at the hospital. (*Do not delay transport to complete a more detailed evaluation.* Rapid transport is essential.)

Time of Onset of Symptoms
If stroke symptoms started within 6 hours of the arrival of EMS personnel, immediately notify the receiving hospital. Prearrival notification of the receiving hospital shortens the time to definitive hospital-based evaluation and intervention. *Provide results of the stroke scale or screen, the Glasgow Coma Scale score, and the estimated time of symptom onset* in addition to standard information. This allows the ED or Casualty Service time to prepare and coordinate the patient's time-sensitive therapy. The receiving hospital should have a written plan to begin therapy as quickly as possible.

Level of Consciousness
Determining the stroke patient's level of consciousness is crucial. Depressed consciousness within hours of the onset of symptoms implies severe brain injury with increased intracranial pressure (ICP), usually due to an intracerebral or subarachnoid hemorrhage. Coma, the lack of any purposeful response to external stimuli, is the result of damage to both cerebral hemispheres or the brain stem. Coma usually implies massive hemorrhage, occlusion of the basilar artery, or cardiac arrest with global brain ischemia. Massive ischemic stroke with cerebral edema may cause coma but is rare. Do not overlook concurrent metabolic problems. Consider drug overdose, sepsis, or severe metabolic abnormalities.

Type of Stroke (Ischemic Versus Hemorrhagic)
The history and physical findings of hemorrhagic and ischemic stroke overlap (see Table 4). Do not depend solely on clinical presentation for diagnosis. *In most cases, noncontrast CT is the definitive test for differentiating ischemic and hemorrhagic stroke.* (CT is discussed in "Emergency Diagnostic Studies.")

Location of Stroke
Higher cortical, language, visual, cranial nerve, motor, and sensory functions should be assessed in alert patients with brain infarction. Neurological signs help distinguish infarction of the carotid territory from infarction with a vertebrobasilar distribution. Crossed (cranial nerve palsy with contralateral motor or sensory deficit) or bilateral neurological signs suggest that the infarct is located in the brain stem. Specific patterns of deficit, such as pure sensory stroke or dysarthria with a clumsy hand, may be present. Such deficits suggest a subcortical or lacunar infarct caused by small-vessel disease. The specificity of clinical signs such as pure motor deficit, however, is low. Distinguishing between lacunar and nonlacunar infarcts on the basis of clinical features is often difficult, especially within hours of the onset of stroke.

Severity of Stroke
The National Institutes of Health Stroke Scale (NIHSS) measures neurological function, and scores on this scale are correlated with the severity of stroke and long-term outcome in patients with ischemic stroke.[25,34,35] The scale provides a reliable, valid, and

TABLE 4.   Presenting Clinical Features of Hemorrhagic and Nonhemorrhagic Stroke

	Headache	Decreased Level of Consciousness	Focal Deficit
Infarction	++	+	+++
Intracerebral hemorrhage	+++	+++	+++
Subarachnoid hemorrhage	+++	++	+

+ indicates mild; ++, moderate; and +++, severe.

easy-to-perform alternative to the standard neurological evaluation for patients with ischemic stroke, and it has been used for triage of patients to different treatment protocols.[36,37] The NIHSS total score ranges from 0 (normal) to 42 points, evaluating 5 major areas of functioning:

1. Level of consciousness
2. Visual function
3. Motor function
4. Sensation and neglect
5. Cerebellar function

The NIHSS is not a comprehensive neurological examination (eg, it does not record gait or all cranial nerve deficits), and more detailed neurological assessment may be required in certain cases.

The Scandinavian Stroke Scale was used in the European Cooperative Acute Stroke Study and has been shown to identify predictors of early and late progression in stroke patients.[38,39]

The Hunt and Hess Scale (see Table 5) is often used to grade the severity of stroke in patients with subarachnoid hemorrhage.[40] The Hunt and Hess grade is correlated with survival after subarachnoid hemorrhage and the risk of complications such as vasospasm. The scale may be used to guide the timing of aneurysm clipping or coiling.

Differential Diagnosis

Very few nonvascular neurological diseases will cause *sudden onset of focal brain dysfunction, the hallmark of stroke.* The list of potential diagnoses (see Table 6) is longer if the patient is comatose and the medical history is unavailable. If the patient's condition gradually worsens over several days, a nonvascular neurological disease may be present.

Prehospital Transport

EMS systems should develop protocols that provide for priority dispatch, treatment, and transport of patients with signs and symptoms of acute ischemic stroke. These protocols should convey the same urgency as those for patients with signs and symptoms of AMI or major trauma (Class IIb). Give highest priority to patients with a suspected stroke and airway compromise or an altered level of consciousness.

In addition, triage and transport patients with acute onset of stroke symptoms to a facility that can begin fibrinolytic therapy within 1 hour of arrival, unless that facility is >30 minutes away by ground ambulance (Class IIb).

ED Triage and Treatment

The ED must be prepared for the arrival of the stroke patient so that triage and therapy can begin immediately. Maximum

TABLE 5.   Hunt and Hess Scale for Subarachnoid Hemorrhage

Grade	Neurological Status
1	Asymptomatic
2	Severe headache or nuchal rigidity; no neurological deficit
3	Drowsy; minimal neurological deficit
4	Stuporous; moderate to severe hemiparesis
5	Deep coma; decerebrate posturing

From Reference 40.

TABLE 6.   Differential Diagnosis of Stroke

Hemorrhagic stroke
Ischemic stroke
Craniocerebral/cervical trauma
Meningitis/encephalitis
Hypertensive encephalopathy
Intracranial mass
Tumor
Subdural/epidural hematoma
Seizure with persistent neurological signs (Todd's paralysis)
Migraine with persistent neurological signs
Metabolic disturbances
Hyperglycemia (nonketotic hyperosmolar coma)
Hypoglycemia
Postcardiac arrest ischemia
Toxicological cause
Endocrine disorder (myxedema)
Uremia
Psychiatric syndromes
Shock and CNS hypoperfusion

CNS indicates central nervous system.

time intervals for completion of diagnostic studies of candidates for fibrinolytic therapy are listed in Table 7.

Emergency Diagnostic Studies

Emergency diagnostic studies are used to establish stroke as the cause of the patient's symptoms, to differentiate between brain infarction and brain hemorrhage, and to determine the most likely cause of the stroke. Protocols may prioritize and streamline the order of these tests.

CT is the most important diagnostic test for differentiating between infarction and hemorrhage or other intracranial masses.[41] To avoid confusing blood and contrast medium, perform CT *without contrast* enhancement. Withhold anticoagulants and fibrinolytics until brain hemorrhage is ruled out.

The CT scan of almost all patients with a recent intracerebral hemorrhage will show increased density at the site of bleeding.[42] Findings in patients with subarachnoid hemorrhage, however, may be subtle (eg, the scan may show only a thin, white layer adjacent to the brain). Approximately 5% of patients with subarachnoid hemorrhage will have normal findings on the CT scan.[43,44] Such patients usually have a small subarachnoid hemorrhage and are alert with no focal neurological deficits (Hunt and Hess grade 1). If clinical suspicion of subarachnoid hemorrhage remains despite negative findings on the CT scan, perform lumbar puncture.

Magnetic resonance imaging (MRI) is not part of the routine evaluation of acute stroke. MRI is very sensitive and will detect some lesions missed by CT. Although MRI can detect early hemorrhage,[45,46] it is not superior to CT. MRI is also time consuming and may hamper continuous observation of acutely ill patients. New MRI techniques such as magnetic resonance angiography and diffusion- and perfusion-weighted MRI may help delineate the site of occlusion or the region of the brain at risk for infarction.[47,48] These techniques

TABLE 7. NINDS-Recommended Stroke Evaluation Targets for Potential Fibrinolytic Candidates*

	Time Target
Door to doctor	10 Minutes
Door to CT completion	25 Minutes
Door to CT read	45 Minutes
Door to treatment	60 Minutes
Access to neurological expertise†	15 Minutes
Access to neurosurgical expertise†	2 Hours
Admission to monitored bed	3 Hours

NINDS indicates National Institute of Neurological Disorders and Stroke; CT, computed tomography.

*Target times will not be achieved in all cases, but they represent a reasonable goal.

†By phone or in person.

are being evaluated for use in clinical practice. Diffusion-weighted MRI has been approved for use in stroke patients by the US Food and Drug Administration (Class Indeterminate).

Emergency cerebral angiography is performed in many patients with subarachnoid hemorrhage in anticipation of aneurysm clipping. Neurointerventional procedures such as aneurysm coiling, angioplasty, and intra-arterial thrombolysis also require emergency angiography in certain patients. Many other studies, including echocardiography, ultrasonography of the carotid artery, and transcranial Doppler, can be performed electively.

Emergency Management

Rapidly identify, evaluate, and treat all patients with signs and symptoms of acute stroke. Stroke protocols and pathways may assist in the rapid assessment of these patients. Clinicians may find the use of a checklist helpful to identify contraindications to tPA therapy.[49] Target times for in-hospital evaluation and treatment are given in Table 7.[50]

General Emergency Therapy

Establish intravenous access en route to the hospital or in the ED (see Table 8). Administer normal saline or lactated Ringer's solution at a rate of 50 mL/h. Unless the patient is hypotensive, avoid rapid infusions, which increase the risk of cerebral edema. Do not administer dextrose in water unless hypoglycemia is strongly suspected; this solution is hypotonic and may increase cerebral edema.[51–57] Correct hyperglycemia and hyperthermia (Class IIa). Do not routinely administer supplemental oxygen to *nonhypoxic* (oxygen saturation >90%) stroke victims with minor or moderate strokes. Oxygen may be beneficial, however, to patients with severe strokes, but additional research is needed.[58]

Management of Elevated Blood Pressure

Management of blood pressure after acute ischemic or hemorrhagic stroke is controversial. Many patients have hypertension after an ischemic or hemorrhagic stroke, but few require emergency treatment. Elevated blood pressure after a stroke is not a hypertensive emergency unless there are other medical problems (eg, AMI or aortic dissection).[59] In most patients, blood pressure will spontaneously decline as pain, agitation, vomiting, and increased ICP are controlled.[25]

TABLE 8. General Management of Acute Stroke

1. Intravenous fluids	Avoid D₅W and excessive fluid loading
2. Blood sugar	Determine immediately. Bolus of 50% dextrose if hypoglycemic; insulin if >300 mg%
3. Thiamine	100 mg if malnourished, alcoholic
4. Oxygen	Pulse oximetry. Supplement if So₂ <90%
5. Acetaminophen	If febrile
6. NPO	If at risk for aspiration
7. Cardiac monitor	

D₅W indicates 5% dextrose in water; So₂, oxygen saturation.

Antihypertensive treatment is reserved for patients with markedly elevated blood pressures or specific medical indications. Current recommendations are based on the type of stroke (hemorrhagic or ischemic) and whether the patient with ischemic stroke is a candidate for fibrinolytic therapy. In response to requests for general guidance regarding the management of hypertension in stroke patients, a table of suggested antihypertensive therapy approaches is provided (see Table 9). It is important to note, however, that these suggestions were based on consensus opinion and are not evidence-based.

Antihypertensive therapy can be harmful. Antihypertensive therapy can lower the cerebral perfusion pressure and lead to worsening of the stroke.[59] In addition, the response of stroke patients to antihypertensive therapy can be exaggerated. Use of short-acting nifedipine is contraindicated.[59] For patients with an arterial occlusion, maintenance of adequate collateral flow is of paramount importance.

In candidates for fibrinolytic therapy, however, strict control of blood pressure is required to reduce the potential for bleeding. Fibrinolytic therapy is not recommended for patients who have a systolic blood pressure >185 mm Hg or a diastolic blood pressure >110 mm Hg at the time of treatment (see Table 9).[60,61] Simple measures often can lower blood pressure below this level. If more aggressive measures are required, do not use fibrinolytics.

Management of Seizures

Recurrent seizures are a potentially life-threatening complication of stroke. They can worsen the stroke and should be controlled. Administration of anticonvulsant medications to prevent recurrent seizures is strongly recommended, but prophylactic administration is not indicated.[59] Protection of the airway, administration of supplementary oxygen, and maintenance of normothermia are part of supportive care.

Benzodiazepines are first-line agents for treating seizures. Intravenous diazepam (5 mg over 2 minutes to a maximum of 10 mg) or lorazepam (1 to 4 mg over 2 to 10 minutes) usually will stop seizures but may produce respiratory depression. Lorazepam, which has a short half-life, may be the superior agent. Administration of these agents can be repeated, but they should be followed by a longer-acting anticonvulsant such as phenytoin, fosphenytoin, or phenobarbital.

Management of Increased ICP

Death during the first week after stroke commonly is caused by brain edema and increased ICP. Fortunately only 10% to 20% of

TABLE 9.   Suggested Antihypertensive Therapy for Patients With Acute Stroke

Blood Pressure*	Treatment
Patients ineligible for fibrinolytic therapy	
1. DBP >140 mm Hg	Sodium nitroprusside (0.5 μg/kg per minute).
	Aim for 10% to 20% reduction in DBP.
2. SBP >220, DBP 121 to 140, or MAP† >130 mm Hg	10 to 20 mg labetalol‡ IV push over 1 to 2 minutes. May repeat or double labetalol every 20 minutes to a maximum dose of 150 mg.
3. SBP <220, DBP ≤120, or MAP† <130 mm Hg	Emergency antihypertensive therapy is deferred in the absence of aortic dissection, AMI, severe CHF, or hypertensive encephalopathy.
Candidates for fibrinolytic therapy	
Pretreatment	
1. SBP >185 or DBP >110 mm Hg	1 to 2 inches of nitropaste or 1 to 2 doses of 10 to 20 mg labetalol‡ IV push. If BP is not reduced to and maintained at <185/110 mm Hg, do not administer fibrinolytics.
During and after treatment	
1. Monitor BP	Check BP every 15 minutes for 2 hours, then every 30 minutes for 6 hours, and then every 1 hour for 16 hours.
2. DBP >140 mm Hg	Sodium nitroprusside (0.5 μg/kg per minute)
3. SBP >230 or DBP 121 to 140 mm Hg	(1) 10 mg labetalol‡ IV push over 1 to 2 minutes. May repeat or double labetalol every 10 minutes to a maximum dose of 150 mg, or give the initial labetalol bolus and then start a labetalol drip at 2 to 8 mg/min.
	(2) If BP is not controlled by labetalol, consider sodium nitroprusside.
4. SBP 180 to 230 or DBP 105 to 120 mm Hg	10 mg labetalol‡ IV push. May repeat or double labetalol every 10 to 20 minutes to a maximum dose of 150 mg, or give initial labetalol bolus and then start a labetalol drip at 2 to 8 mg/min.

(Note: These suggestions are consensus rather than evidence-based and should be individualized, with consideration given to clinical status and baseline blood pressure.)

DBP indicates diastolic blood pressure; SBP, systolic blood pressure; MAP, mean arterial pressure; BP, blood pressure; IV, intravenous; AMI, acute myocardial infarction; and CHF, congestive heart failure.

*Before treatment, all initial blood pressures should be verified by repeating reading in 5 minutes.

†As estimated by one third the sum of SBP and double DBP.

‡Avoid labetalol in patients with asthma, cardiac failure, or severe abnormalities in cardiac conduction. For patients with refractory hypertension, consider alternative therapy with sodium nitroprusside or enalapril.

stroke patients develop brain edema sufficient to cause clinical deterioration. When brain edema is clinically suspect, modest fluid restriction, elevation of the head of the bed (20° to 30°), support of oxygenation and ventilation (avoidance of hypoxemia and hypoventilation), and control of agitation and pain will help lower increased ICP. Goals of therapy are (1) reduction of increased ICP, (2) maintenance of cerebral perfusion to prevent worsening of ischemia, and (3) prevention of brain herniation.

Reduction of the partial pressure of CO_2 in arterial gas ($PaCO_2$) through intubation and hyperventilation is the most rapid means of lowering ICP in cases of impending brain herniation. Optimal $PaCO_2$ is 30 to 35 mm Hg.[62] $PaCO_2$ values ≤25 mm Hg are occasionally acceptable in rapidly deteriorating patients, but if such values are sustained, ischemia of the brain may occur.[62] Aggressive tracheal suctioning increases ICP and should be avoided, with suctioning reduced in frequency and duration to that necessary to maintain tracheal tube patency.

Hyperosmolar therapy with mannitol is used to reduce the mass effect on diencephalic structures or to maximize cerebral perfusion pressure. Mannitol can be given as a bolus (0.25 to 0.5 g/kg per dose given over 20 minutes rapidly) and repeated every 6 hours to a maximum dose of 2 g/kg daily.[59] High initial doses are given in emergencies. The effect on ICP usually occurs about 20 minutes after administration. Lower doses (25 to 50 g every 4 hours) given as intermittent boluses are used to manage ICP

over longer periods. Furosemide, hypertonic saline, and acetazolamide may also help lower ICP.

High doses of barbiturates (eg, thiopental 1 to 5 mg/kg) rapidly lower ICP and suppress electrical brain activity. Because high doses of barbiturates suppress respiratory activity and may produce vasodilation and myocardial depression, they should be administered in conjunction with mechanical ventilatory support and careful blood pressure monitoring. ICP must be monitored when a barbiturate coma is induced, because the barbiturates obliterate the clinical response. The ICP is used to evaluate response to therapy.

Routine measurement of ICP is not indicated, and the value of ICP measurement has not been shown. ICP measurement, however, may be helpful in deteriorating patients, can guide therapy, and can serve as an indicator of prognosis and outcome.[59]

Neurosurgical decompression can be lifesaving in some patients with high ICP and intracranial hemorrhage, edema after stroke, or other mass effects on brain tissue. Surgery for cerebellar hemorrhage or edema after stroke can produce remarkable improvement. Pharmacological and ventilatory measures for controlling ICP are much less effective than surgery in patients with cerebellar lesions. Corticosteroids are not effective and should not be used.[63] Cerebellar edema or hemorrhage frequently causes obstructive hydrocephalus, necessitating ventricular drainage. Closely monitor patients with cerebellar lesions for neurological deterioration.

Pharmacological and Interventional Therapies

Ischemic Stroke

Fibrinolytic Therapy

Use of intra-arterial and intravenous fibrinolytic agents such as tPA, streptokinase, ancrod, urokinase, and prourokinase in stroke patients has been evaluated in several clinical trials.[39,64–72] The Cochrane Stroke Review group[73] evaluated 17 trials with >5000 patients in which >50% of patients received tPA. Fibrinolytic therapy significantly increased the odds ratio of death within the first 10 days and at follow-up, mainly because of fatal intracerebral hemorrhage. Patients treated within 3 hours, however, had reduced death and dependency compared with patients treated within 3 to 6 hours. Overall, the proportion of patients with death or disability was reduced. It is difficult to draw conclusions from this review because there was significant heterogeneity among the comparison trials.[73] In the clinical trials reviewed, many different agents were administered, with many different time intervals between onset of stroke symptoms and drug administration.

The National Institute of Neurological Disorders and Stroke rtPA Stroke Trial[64] evaluated a single agent administered within 3 hours of symptom onset in a prospective, blinded, randomized, controlled clinical trial. Intravenous tPA was administered in a dose of 0.9 mg given as a 10% bolus over 1 minute, followed by a 1-hour infusion versus a placebo. In this trial, patients treated with tPA within 3 hours of onset of symptoms were at least 30% more likely to have minimal or no disability at 3 months compared with those treated with placebo. The risk of fatal intracranial hemorrhage, however, was 10 times greater in the tPA-treated group (3% versus 0.3%). A similar increase in the frequency of all symptomatic hemorrhages (6.4% versus 0.6%) was also observed in this group. This increase in symptomatic hemorrhage did not lead to an overall increase in mortality in the treated group.

Based on the results of parts I and II of the National Institute of Neurological Disorders and Stroke study, intravenous administration of tPA is recommended for carefully selected patients with acute ischemic stroke if they have no contraindications to fibrinolytic therapy and if the drug can be administered within 3 hours of the onset of stroke symptoms (Class I). Contraindications to tPA are listed in Table 10.

Investigators have tried to extend the time for treatment beyond 3 hours by using various fibrinolytic agents and new approaches to administration (eg, intra-arterial therapy).[39,65–67,69–72] Evidence suggested that use of intravenous tPA 3 to 6 hours after the onset of symptoms may be beneficial in certain patients,[73] but recent studies have been discouraging. The ATLANTIS Trial found no significant differences in 90-day efficacy end points in patients treated between 3 and 5 hours.[65] The Thrombolytic Therapy in Acute Ischemic Stroke Study enrolled 142 patients at 42 sites in North America and found a small but significant benefit of tPA in patients treated after 3 hours when assessed at 1 day; this benefit was not maintained at

30 days.[74] In both of these trials, the rate of symptomatic intracerebral hemorrhage was increased. At this time routine use of *intravenous tPA >3 hours* after the onset of symptoms is not recommended (Class Indeterminate).

Results of a recent, randomized trial of *intra-arterial* prourokinase suggest that use of intra-arterial fibrinolytic agents 3 to 6 hours after the onset of symptoms may be beneficial in patients with occlusion of the middle cerebral artery (Class IIb).[71]

Three large, randomized trials of streptokinase in patients with stroke have been reported.[69,70,75] All 3 studies were suspended because of increased hemorrhage and mortality in the group treated with streptokinase. Do not use streptokinase in patients who have had a stroke except in clinical studies approved by the appropriate institutional review board.

Anticoagulant Therapy

The efficacy of anticoagulants in acute stroke has not been established. Heparin is frequently administered to patients with acute ischemic stroke, but its value is unproved.[76,77] Heparin may help prevent recurrent embolism or propagation of a thrombus, but it may lead to bleeding complications, including brain hemorrhage. There is no consensus on when heparin therapy should be started or on the dose and duration of therapy. Emergency physicians should consult the attending neurologist about the use of heparin in specific patients (Class IIb). Low-molecular-weight anticoagulants have several advantages not provided by unfractionated heparin.[71] Use of low-molecular-weight anticoagulants in the management of stroke is being evaluated.

Aspirin, warfarin, and ticlopidine reduce the risk of subsequent stroke in patients with TIA.[78–81] These antiplatelet agents should be started within the first few days after a TIA. When started within 48 hours of the onset of ischemic stroke, aspirin produces a small but definite net benefit in patients who are ineligible for fibrinolytic

TABLE 10.   Contraindications to tPA Therapy for Acute Ischemic Stroke

Evidence of intracranial hemorrhage on pretreatment evaluation

Suspicion of subarachnoid hemorrhage on pretreatment evaluation

Recent (within 3 months) intracranial or intraspinal surgery, serious head trauma, or previous stroke

History of intracranial hemorrhage

Uncontrolled hypertension at time of treatment (see "Management of High Blood Pressure")

Seizure at stroke onset

Active internal bleeding

Intracranial neoplasm, arteriovenous malformation, or aneurysm

Known bleeding diathesis, including but not limited to

—Current use of oral anticoagulants (eg, warfarin sodium), an international normalized ratio >1.7, or a prothrombin time >15 seconds

—Administration of heparin within 48 hours preceding the onset of stroke and an elevated activated partial thromboplastin time at presentation

—Platelet count <100 000/mm³

tPA indicates tissue plasminogen activator.

therapy.[82,83] Antiplatelet therapy with aspirin 160 to 300 mg daily within 48 hours of onset of presumed ischemic stroke reduces the risk of early recurrent ischemic stroke without a major risk of early hemorrhagic complications and improves long-term outcome.[84]

The Cochrane Stroke Group completed a comprehensive review of anticoagulants in 21 trials involving 23 427 patients. A number of anticoagulants were used in clinical trials: standard unfractionated heparin, low-molecular-weight heparins, heparinoids, oral anticoagulants, and thrombin inhibitors. The conclusion of the Cochrane group was that immediate anticoagulant therapy in patients with acute ischemic stroke is not associated with net gain for either short- or long-term benefit. Routine use of any type of anticoagulant in acute ischemic stroke is not recommended.[85]

Other Treatments

Calcium channel–blocking drugs, volume expansion, hemodilution, and low-molecular-weight dextran have not been shown to improve clinical outcome after ischemic stroke. A number of cytoprotective agents are being investigated for use in patients with acute ischemic or hemorrhagic stroke. Many of these agents have been shown to provide no benefit in humans, even though benefit was shown in animal models.[86]

Hemorrhagic Stroke

Subarachnoid Hemorrhage

Patients with subarachnoid hemorrhage often require emergency arteriography. If a saccular aneurysm is detected, early intracranial surgery with clipping (or coiling) of the aneurysm is usually advised.[87] The calcium channel–blocking drug nimodipine (60 mg orally every 4 hours, 0.35 mg/kg) improves outcome after subarachnoid hemorrhage.[88–92] Correction of hyponatremia and water loss is also important. Avoid strict fluid restriction, however, which may stimulate inappropriate secretion of antidiuretic hormone.

Intracerebral Hemorrhage

Hemorrhage into the brain can be devastating. Death may occur because of compression or distortion of vital deep-brain structures or increased ICP. Mortality is a function of the volume and location of the intracerebral bleeding. Optimal management requires prevention of continued bleeding, appropriate management of ICP, and timely neurosurgical decompression when warranted. Large intracerebral or cerebellar hematomas often require surgical intervention. A CT scan is required for differential diagnosis. Placement of a ventriculostomy tube through a burr hole can be lifesaving if hydrocephalus is the cause of coma.

Appendix A: NIH Stroke Scale
"Quick and Easy" Version

Category	Description	Score	Baseline Date/Time	Date/Time
1a. Level of consciousness (LOC) *(Alert, drowsy, etc)*	Alert	0		
	Drowsy	1		
	Stuporous	2		
	Coma	3		
1b. LOC questions *(Month, age)*	Answers both correctly	0		
	Answers 1 correctly	1		
	Incorrect	2		
1c. LOC commands *(Open, close eyes, make fist, let go)*	Obeys both correctly	0		
	Obeys 1 correctly	1		
	Incorrect	2		
2. Best gaze *(Eyes open—patient follows examiner's finger or face)*	Normal	0		
	Partial gaze palsy	1		
	Forced deviation	2		
3. Visual *(Introduce visual stimulus/threat to patient's visual field quadrants)*	No visual loss	0		
	Partial hemianopia	1		
	Complete hemianopia	2		
	Bilateral hemianopia	3		
4. Facial palsy *(Show teeth, raise eyebrows, and squeeze eyes shut)*	Normal	0		
	Minor	1		
	Partial	2		
	Complete	3		

Appendix A: Continued

Category	Description	Score	Baseline Date/Time	Date/Time
5a. Motor arm—left *(Elevate extremity to 90° and score drift/movement)*	No drift	0		
	Drift	1		
	Can't resist gravity	2		
	No effort against gravity	3		
	No movement	4		
	Amputation, joint fusion (explain)	9		
5b. Motor arm—right *(Elevate extremity to 90° and score drift/movement)*	No drift	0		
	Drift	1		
	Can't resist gravity	2		
	No effort against gravity	3		
	No movement	4		
	Amputation, joint fusion (explain)	9		
6a. Motor leg—left *(Elevate extremity to 30° and score drift/movement)*	No drift	0		
	Drift	1		
	Can't resist gravity	2		
	No effort against gravity	3		
	No movement	4		
	Amputation, joint fusion (explain)	9		
6b. Motor leg—right *(Elevate extremity to 30° and score drift/movement)*	No drift	0		
	Drift	1		
	Can't resist gravity	2		
	No effort against gravity	3		
	No movement	4		
	Amputation, joint fusion (explain)	9		
7. Limb ataxia *(Finger–nose, heel down shin)*	Absent	0		
	Present in 1 limb	1		
	Present in 2 limbs	2		
8. Sensory *(Pin prick to face, arm, trunk, and leg—compare side to side)*	Normal	0		
	Partial loss	1		
	Severe loss	2		
9. Best language *(Name items, describe a picture, and read sentences)*	No aphasia	0		
	Mild to moderate aphasia	1		
	Severe aphasia	2		
	Mute	3		
10. Dysarthria *(Evaluate speech clarity by patient repeating listed words)*	Normal articulation	0		
	Mild to moderate dysarthria	1		
	Near to unintelligible or worse	2		
	Intubated or other physical barrier	9		
11. Extinction and inattention *(Use information from prior testing to identify neglect or double simultaneous stimuli testing)*	No neglect	0		
	Partial neglect	1		
	Complete neglect	2		

Individual Administering Scale:

Adapted with permission from Spilker J, Kongable G. The NIH Stroke Scale: its importance and practical application in the clinical setting. *Stroke Intervent.* 2000;2:7–14. For further information, please refer to the website *http://www.stroke-site.org.*

Appendix B: Scandinavian Stroke Scale (Scandinavian Stroke Study Group, 1985)

1. Consciousness

   Fully conscious–6

   Somnolent, can be awakened to full consciousness–4

   Reacts to verbal command but is not fully conscious–2

   Stupor (reacts to pain only)–0

   Coma–0

2. Orientation

   Correct for time, place, and person–6

   Two of these (time, place, person)–4

   One of these–2

   Completely disoriented–0

3. Speech

   No aphasia–10

   Impairment of comprehension or expression disability–6

   More than yes/no but not longer sentences–3

   Only yes/no or less–0

4. Eye movement

   No gaze palsy–4

   Gaze palsy present–2

   Forced lateral gaze–0

5. Facial palsy

   None/dubious/slight–2

   Present–0

6. Gait

   Walks at least 5 m without aids–12

   Walks with aids–9

   Walks with help of another person–6

   Sits without support–3

   Bedridden/wheelchair–0

7. Arm, motor power (assessed only on affected side)

   Raises arm with normal strength–6

   Raises arm with reduced strength–5

   Raises arm with flexion in elbow–4

   Can move but not against gravity–2

   Paralysis–0

8. Hand, motor power (assessed only on affected side)

   Normal strength–6

   Reduced strength in full range–4

   Some movement, fingertips do not reach palm–2

   Paralysis–0

9. Leg, motor power (assessed only on affected side)

   Normal strength–6

   Raises straight leg against resistance with reduced strength–5

   Raises leg with flexion of knee against gravity–4

   Can move but not against gravity–2

   Paralysis–0

10. Foot paresis

    None–2

    Present–0

References

1. Broderick JP, Brott T, Tomsick T, Huster G, Miller R. The risk of subarachnoid and intracerebral hemorrhages in blacks as compared with whites. *N Engl J Med.* 1992;326:733–736.

2. Stegmayr B, Vinogradova T, Malyutina S, Peltonen M, Nikitin Y, Asplund K. Widening gap of stroke between east and west: eight-year trends in occurrence and risk factors in Russia and Sweden. *Stroke.* 2000;31:2–8.

3. Thorvaldsen P, Davidsen M, Bronnum-Hansen H, Schroll M. Stable stroke occurrence despite incidence reduction in an aging population: stroke trends in the Danish monitoring trends and determinants in cardiovascular disease (MONICA) population. *Stroke.* 1999;30:2529–2534.

4. Thorvaldsen P, Kuulasmaa K, Rajakangas AM, Rastenyte D, Sarti C, Wilhelmsen L. Stroke trends in the WHO MONICA project. *Stroke.* 1997;28:500–506.

5. Williams GR, Jiang JG, Matchar DB, Samsa GP. Incidence and occurrence of total (first-ever and recurrent) stroke. *Stroke.* 1999;30: 2523–2528.

6. Grotta JC. The importance of time. In: *Proceedings of a National Symposium on Rapid Identification and Treatment of Acute Stroke.* Bethesda, Md: National Institute of Neurological Disorders and Stroke; 1997:5–9.

7. Pepe PE. Overview: the initial links in the chain of recovery for brain attack: access, prehospital care, notification, and treatment. In: *Proceedings of a National Symposium on Rapid Identification and Treatment of Acute Stroke.* Bethesda, Md: National Institute of Neurological Disorders and Stroke; 1997:17–28.

8. Spilker JA. Overview: the importance of patient and public education in acute ischemic stroke. In: *Proceedings of a National Symposium on Rapid Identification and Treatment of Acute Stroke.* Bethesda, Md: National Institute of Neurological Disorders and Stroke; 1997:119–126.

9. Sayre MR, Swor RA, Honeycutt LK. Prehospital identification and treatment. In: *Proceedings of a National Symposium on Rapid Identification and Treatment of Acute Stroke.* Bethesda, Md: National Institute of Neurological Disorders and Stroke; 1997:35–44.

10. Kothari R, Sauerbeck L, Jauch E, Broderick J, Brott T, Khoury J, Liu T. Patients' awareness of stroke signs, symptoms, and risk factors. *Stroke.* 1997;28:1871–1875.

11. Barsan WG, Brott TG, Broderick JP, Haley EC, Levy DE, Marler JR. Time of hospital presentation in patients with acute stroke. *Arch Intern Med.* 1993;153:2558–2561.

12. Alberts MJ, Perry A, Dawson DV, Bertels C. Effects of public and professional education on reducing the delay in presentation and referral of stroke patients. *Stroke.* 1992;23:352–356.

13. The National Institute of Neurological Disorders and Stroke (NINDS) rt-PA Stroke Study Group. A systems approach to immediate evaluation and management of hyperacute stroke. Experience at eight centers and implications for community practice and patient care. *Stroke.* 1997;28: 1530–1540.

14. Crocco TJ, Kothari RU, Sayre MR, Liu T. A nationwide prehospital stroke survey. *Prehosp Emerg Care.* 1999;3:201–206.

15. Ferro JM, Melo TP, Oliveira V, Crespo M, Canhao P, Pinto AN. An analysis of the admission delay of acute strokes. *Cerebrovasc Dis.* 1994; 4:72–75.

16. Kothari R, Jauch E, Broderick J, Brott T, Sauerbeck L, Khoury J, Liu T. Acute stroke: delays to presentation and emergency department evaluation. *Ann Emerg Med.* 1999;33:3–8.

17. Morris DL, Rosamond WD, Hinn AR, Gorton RA. Time delays in accessing stroke care in the emergency department. *Acad Emerg Med.* 1999;6:218–223.

18. Kidwell CS, Saver JL, Schubert GB, Eckstein M, Starkman S. Design and retrospective analysis of the Los Angeles Prehospital Stroke Screen (LAPSS). *Prehosp Emerg Care.* 1998;2:267–273.

19. Kothari R, Barsan W, Brott T, Broderick J, Ashbrock S. Frequency and accuracy of prehospital diagnosis of acute stroke. *Stroke.* 1995;26: 937–941.

20. Zachariah B, Dunford J, Van Cott CC. Dispatch life support and the acute stroke patient: making the right call. In: *Proceedings of a National Symposium on Rapid Identification and Treatment of Acute Stroke.* Bethesda, Md: National Institute of Neurological Disorders and Stroke; 1997:29–34.

21. Davalos A, Castillo J, Martinez-Vila E, Cerebrovascular Diseases Study Group of the Spanish Society of Neurology. Delay in neurological attention and stroke outcome.. *Stroke.* 1995;26:2233–2237.

22. Lyden PD, Rapp K, Babcock T, Rothcock J. Ultra-rapid identification, triage, and enrollment of stroke patients into clinical trials. *J Stroke Cerebrovasc Dis.* 1994;4:106–107.

23. Bornstein NM, Gur AY, Fainshtein P, Korczyn AD. Stroke during sleep: epidemiological and clinical features. *Cerebrovasc Dis.* 1999;9:320–322.

24. Hazinski MF. Demystifying recognition and management of stroke. *Curr Emerg Card Care.* 1996;7:8–9.

25. Broderick J, Brott T, Barsan W. Blood pressure during the first minutes of focal cerebral ischemia. *Ann Emerg Med.* 1993;22:1438–1443.

26. Maggioni AP, Franzosi MG, Farina ML, Santoro E, Celani MG, Ricci S, Tognoni G, Gruppo Italiano per lo Studio della Streptochinasi nell'Infarto Miocardico (GISSI). Cerebrovascular events after myocardial infarction: analysis of the GISSI trial. *BMJ.* 1991;302:1428–1431.

27. Mooe T, Eriksson P, Stegmayr B. Ischemic stroke after acute myocardial infarction: a population based study. *Stroke.* 1997;28:762–767.

28. Silver FL, Norris JW, Lewis AL. Early mortality following stroke: a prospective review. *Stroke.* 1984;45:492–496.

29. Tokgozoglu SL, Batur MK, Topcuoglu MA. Effects of stroke localization on cardiac autonomic balance and sudden death. *Stroke.* 1999;30:1307–1311.

30. Korpelainen JT, Sotaniemi KA, Makikallio A. Dynamic behavior of heart rate in ischemic stroke. *Stroke.* 1999;30:1008–1013.

31. Kothari RU, Pancioli A, Liu T, Brott T, Broderick J. Cincinnati Prehospital Stroke Scale: reproducibility and validity [see comments]. *Ann Emerg Med.* 1999;33:373–378.

32. Kidwell CS, Starkman S, Eckstein M, Weems K, Saver JL. Identifying stroke in the field: prospective validation of the Los Angeles Prehospital Stroke Screen (LAPSS). *Stroke.* 2000;31:71–76.

33. Teasdale G, Jennett B. Assessment of coma and impaired consciousness: a practical scale. *Lancet.* 1974;2:81–84.

34. Brott G, Adams HP Jr, Olinger CP, et al. Measurements of acute cerebral infarction: a clinical examination scale. *Stroke.* 1989;20:864–870.

35. Lyden P, Lu M, Jackson C, Marler J, Kothari R, Brott T, Zivin J, NINDS tPA Stroke Trial Investigators. Underlying structure of the National Institutes of Health Stroke Scale: results of a factor analysis. *Stroke.* 1999;30:2347–2354.

36. Lewandowski CA, Frankel M, Tomsick TA, Broderick J, Frey J, Clark W, Starkman S, Grotta J, Spilker J, Khoury J, Brott T, and the Emergency Management of Stroke (EMS) Bridging Trial Investigators. Combined intravenous and intra-arterial r-TPA versus intra-arterial therapy of acute ischemic stroke. *Stroke.* 1999;30:2598–2609.

37. DeGraba TJ, Hallenbeck JM, Pettirew KD. Progression in acute stroke: value of the initial NIH Stroke Scale score on patient stratification in future trials. *Stroke.* 1999;30:1208–1212.

38. Davalos A, Toni D, Iweins F, Lesaffre E, Bastianello S, Castillo J. Neurological deterioration in acute ischemic stroke: potential predictors and associated factors in the European Cooperative Acute Stroke Study (ECASS) I. *Stroke.* 1999;30:2631–2636.

39. Hacke W, Kaste M, Fieschi C, Toni D, Lesaffre E, von Kummer R, Boysen G, Bluhmki E, Hoxter G, Mahagne MH, et al. Intravenous thrombolysis with recombinant tissue plasminogen activator for acute hemispheric stroke: the European Cooperative Acute Stroke Study (ECASS). *JAMA.* 1995;274:1017–1025.

40. Hunt WE, Hess RM. Surgical risk as related to time of intervention in the repair of intracranial aneurysms. *J Neurosurg.* 1968;28:14–20.

41. Gilman S. Imaging the brain. *N Engl J Med.* 1998;338:812–820, 889–896.

42. Davis KR, Ackerman RH, Kistler JP. Computed tomography of cerebral infarction: hemorrhagic, contrast enhancement, and time of appearance. *Comput Tomogr.* 1977;1:71–86.

43. Sames TA, Storrow AB, Finkelstein JA, Magoon MR. Sensitivity of new-generation computer tomography in subarachnoid hemorrhage. *Acad Emerg Med.* 1996;3:16–20.

44. Adams HP Jr, Kassell NF, Torner JC, Sahs AL. CT and clinical correlations in recent aneurysmal subarachnoid hemorrhage: a preliminary report of the Cooperative Aneurysm Study. *Neurology.* 1983;33:981–988.

45. Linfante I, Llinas RH, Caplan LR. MRI features of intracerebral hemorrhage within 2 hours from symptom onset. *Stroke.* 1999;30:2263–2267.

46. Schellinger PD, Jansen O, Fiebach JB. A standardized MRI stroke protocol: comparison with CT in hyperacute intracerebral hemorrhage. *Stroke.* 1999;30:765–768.

47. Baird AE, Benfield A, Schlaug G. Enlargement of human cerebral ischemic lesion volumes measured by diffusion-weighted magnetic resonance imaging. *Ann Neurol.* 1997;41:581–589.

48. Tong DC, Yenari MA, Albers GW. Correlation of perfusion and diffusion weighted MRI with NIHSS score in acute (<6.5 hour) ischemic stroke. *Neurology.* 1998;50:864–870.

49. Hazinski MF, Cummins RO, Field JM. *2000 Handbook of Emergency Cardiovascular Care for Healthcare Providers.* Dallas, Tex: American Heart Association; 2000.

50. Barsan WG. Overview: emergency department management of stroke. In: *Proceedings of a National Symposium on Rapid Identification and Treatment of Acute Stroke.* Bethesda, Md: National Institute of Neurological Disorders and Stroke; 1997:49–54.

51. Weir CJ, Murray GD, Dyker AG. Is hyperglycemia an independent predictor of poor outcome after acute stroke? results of a long-term follow-up study. *BMJ.* 1997;314:1303–1306.

52. Helgasun CM. Blood glucose and stroke. *Stroke.* 1988;19:1049–1053.

53. De Courten-Myers GM, Kleinholz M, Hulm P, et al. Hemorrhagic infarct conversion in experimental stroke. *Ann Emerg Med.* 1992;21:210–215.

54. Broderick JP, Hagen T, Brott T. Hyperglycemia and hemorrhagic transformation of cerebral infarcts. *Stroke.* 1995;26:4848–4887.

55. Yip PK, He YY, Hsu CY et al. Effect of plasma glucose on infarct size in focal cerebral ischemia reperfusion. *Neurology.* 1991;41:899–905.

56. Chew W, Kucharczky J, Moseley M. Hyperglycemia augments ischemic brain injury: in vivo MR imaging spectroscopic study with nicardipine in cats with occluded middle cerebral arteries. *Am J Neuroradiol.* 1991;12:603–609.

57. Vazquez-Cruz J, Marti-Vilata JT, Ferrer L. Progressing cerebral infarction in relation to plasma glucose in gerbils. *Stroke.* 1990;21:1621–1642.

58. Ronning OM, Guldvog B. Should stroke victims routinely receive supplemental oxygen? a quasi-randomized controlled trial. *Stroke.* 1999;30:2033–2037.

59. Adams HJ, Brott T, Crowell R, Furlan A, Gomez C, Grotta J, Helgason C, Marler J, Woolson R, Zivin J, Feinberg W, Mayberg M. Guidelines for the management of patients with acute ischemic stroke: a statement for healthcare professionals from a special writing group of the Stroke Council, American Heart Association. *Stroke.* 1994;25:1901–1914.

60. Brott T, Lu M, Kothari R, Fagan SC, Frankel M, Grotta JC, Broderick J, Kwiatkowski T, Lewandowski C, Haley EC, Marler JR, Tilley BC. Hypertension and its treatment in the NINDS rt-PA Stroke Trial. *Stroke.* 1998;29:1504–1509.

61. Adams HJ, Brott T, Furlan A, Gomez C, Grotta J, Helgason C, Kiatkowski T, Lyden P, Marler J, Torner J, Feinberg W, Mayberg M, Thies W. Guidelines for Thrombolytic Therapy for Acute Stroke: a supplement to the guidelines for the management of patients with acute ischemic stroke. *Circulation.* 1996;94:1167–1174.

62. Broderick JP, Adams HP, Barsan W, Feinberg W, Feldmann E, Grotta J, Kase C, Krieger D, Mayberg M, Tilley B, Zabramski JM, Zuccarello M. Guidelines for the management of spontaneous intracerebral hemorrhage: a statement for healthcare professionals from a special writing group of the Stroke Council, American Heart Association. *Stroke.* 1999;30:905–915.

63. Qizilbash N, Lewington SL, Lopez-Arrieta JM. Corticosteroids for acute ischaemic stroke. *Cochrane Database Syst Rev.* 2000;2:CD000064.

64. The National Institute of Neurological Disorders and Stroke rt-PA Stroke Study Group. Tissue plasminogen activator for acute ischemic stroke. [see comments]. *N Engl J Med.* 1995;333:1581–1587.

65. Clark W, Wissman S, Albers GW, Jhamanda JH, Madden KP, Hamilton S, for the ATLANTIS Stroke Study Investigators. Recombinant tissue-type plasminogen activator (Alteplase) for ischemic stroke 3 to 5 hours after symptom onset: the ALANTIS study: a randomized controlled trial. *JAMA.* 1999;282:2019–2026.

66. Andreotti F, Pasceri V, Hackett DR, Davies GJ, Haider AW, Maseri A. Preinfarction angina as a predictor of more rapid coronary thrombolysis in patients with acute myocardial infarction. *N Engl J Med.* 1996;334:7–12.

67. The MAST-I Collaborative Group. Thrombolytic and antithrombolytic therapy in acute ischemic stroke: Multicenter Acute Stroke Trial—Italy (MAST-I). In: del Zoppo GJ, Mori E, Hacke W, eds. *Thrombolytic Therapy in Acute Ischemic Stroke.* New York, NY: Springer-Verlag; 1993:86–94.

68. Hacke W, Kaste M, Fieschi C, von Kummer R, Davalos A, Meier D, Larrue V, Bluhmki E, Davis S, Donnan G, Schneider D, Diez-Tejedor E, Trouillas P, Second European-Australasian Acute Stroke Study Investigators. Randomised double-blind placebo-controlled trial of thrombolytic therapy with intravenous alteplase in acute ischaemic stroke (ECASS II) [see comments]. *Lancet.* 1998;352:1245–1251.

69. Multicentre Acute Stroke Trial-Italy (MAST-I) Group. Randomised controlled trial of streptokinase, aspirin, and combination of both in treatment of acute ischaemic stroke. *Lancet.* 1995;346:1509–1514.

70. Shahar E, McGovern PG. Trials of streptokinase in severe acute ischaemic stroke [letter]. *Lancet.* 1995;345:578.

71. del Zoppo GJ, Higashida RT, Furlan AJ, Pessin MS, Rowley HA, Gent M, Prolyse in Acute Cerebral Thromboembolism (PROACT) Investigators. PROACT: a phase II randomized trial of recombinant pro-urokinase by direct arterial delivery in acute middle cerebral artery stroke [see comments]. *Stroke.* 1998;29:4–11.

72. Furlan A, Higashida R, Wechsler L, Gent M, Rowley H, Kase C PM, Ahuja A, Callahan F, Clark WM, Silver F, Rivera F, for the PROACT investigators. Intra-arterial prourokinase for acute ischemic stroke: the PROACT II Study: a randomized controlled trial. *JAMA.* 1999;282:2003–2011.

73. Wardlaw JM, del Zoppo G, Yamaguchi T. Thrombolysis for acute ischaemic stroke. *Cochrane Database Syst Rev.* 2000;2:CD000213.

74. Clark WM, Albers GW, Madden KP, Hamilton S, thrombolytic therapy in acute ischemic stroke study investigators. The rtPA (alteplase) 0- to 6-hour acute stroke trial, part A (A0276g): results of a double-blind, placebo-controlled, multicenter study. *Stroke.* 2000;31:811–816.

75. ISIS (Second International Study of Infarct Survival) Collaborative Group. Randomized trial of intravenous streptokinase, oral aspirin, both or neither among 17,187 cases of suspected acute myocardial infarction: ISIS-2. *Lancet.* 1988;2:349–360.

76. Gilles Geraud AB. Is anticoagulant therapy too frequently used in ischemic stroke? *Cerebrovasc Dis.* 1991;1(suppl 1):120–123.

77. Marsh EE III, Adams HP Jr, Biller J. Use of antithrombotic drugs in the treatment of acute ischemic stroke: a survey of neurologists in practice in the United States. *Neurology.* 1989;39:1631–1634.

78. Antiplatelet Trialists' Collaboration. Secondary prevention of vascular disease by prolonged antiplatelet treatment. *BMJ.* 1988;296:320–331.

79. The Dutch TIA Trial Study Group. A comparison of two doses of aspirin (30 mg vs 283 mg a day) in patients after a transient ischemic attack or minor ischemic stroke. *N Engl J Med.* 1991;325:1261–1266.

80. Barnett HJ. Aspirin in stroke prevention: an overview. *Stroke.* 1990;21(suppl IV):IV-40–IV-43.

81. Hass WK, Easton JD, Adams HP Jr, Ticlopidine Aspirin Stroke Study Group. A randomized trial comparing ticlopidine hydrochloride with aspirin for the prevention of stroke in high-risk patients. *N Engl J Med.* 1989;321:501–507.

82. International Stroke Trial Collaborative Group. The International Stroke Trial (IST): a randomized trial of aspirin, subcutaneous heparin, both, or neither among 19,435 patients with acute ischaemic stroke. *Lancet.* 1997;349:1569–1581.

83. Chinese Acute Stroke Trial Collaborative Group. CAST: randomized placebo-controlled trial of early aspirin use in 20,000 patients with acute ischaemic stroke. *Lancet.* 1997;349:1641–1649.

84. Gubitz G, Sandercock P, Counsell C. Antiplatelet therapy for acute ischaemic stroke. *Cochrane Database Syst Rev.* 2000;2:CD000029.

85. Gubitz G, Counsell C, Sandercock P, Signorini D. Anticoagulants for acute ischaemic stroke. *Cochrane Database Syst Rev.* 2000;2:CD000024.

86. Clark WM, Williams BJ, Sacco KA, Zweifler RM, Sabounjian LA, Gamman RE, for the Citicoline Stroke Study Group. A randomized efficacy trial of citicoline in patients with acute ischemic stroke. *Stroke.* 1999;31:2592–2597.

87. Mayberg MR, Batjer HH, Dacey R, Diringer M, Haley EC, Heros RC, Sternau LL, Torner J, Adams HP Jr, Feinberg W, et al. Guidelines for the management of aneurysmal subarachnoid hemorrhage: a statement for healthcare professionals from a special writing group of the Stroke Council, American Heart Association. *Stroke.* 1994;25:2315–2328.

88. Allen GS, Ahn HS, Preziosi TJ, Battye R, Boone SC, Boone SC, Chou SN, Kelly DL, Weir BK, Crabbe RA, Lavik PJ, Rosenbloom SB, Dorsey FC, Ingram CR, Mellits DE, Bertsch LA, Boisvert DP, Hundley MB, Johnson RK, Strom JA, Transou CR. Cerebral arterial spasm: a controlled trial of nimodipine in patients with subarachnoid hemorrhage. *N Engl J Med.* 1983;308:619–624.

89. Neil-Dwyer G, Mee E, Dorrance D, Lowe D. Early intervention with nimodipine in subarachnoid haemorrhage. *Eur Heart J.* 1987;8(suppl K):41–47.

90. Peturk KC, West M, Mohr G, et al. Nimodipine treatment in poor-grade aneurysm patients: results of a multi-center double-blind placebo-controlled trial. *J Neursorug.* 1988;68:505–517.

91. Philippon J, Grob R, Dagreeou F. Prevention of vasospasm in subarachnoid haemorrhage: a controlled study with nimodipine. *Acta Neurochir (Wien).* 1986;82:110–114.

92. Pickard JD, Murray GD, Illingworth R. Effect of oral nimodipine on cerebral infarction and outcome after subarachnoid haemorrhage: British aneurysm nimodipine trial. *BMJ.* 1989;298:636–642.

Part 8: Advanced Challenges in Resuscitation
Section 1: Life-Threatening Electrolyte Abnormalities

Introduction

Electrolyte abnormalities are commonly associated with cardiovascular emergencies. These abnormalities may cause or contribute to cardiac arrest and may hinder resuscitative efforts. It is important to identify clinical situations in which electrolyte problems may be expected. In some cases therapy for life-threatening electrolyte disorders should be initiated even before laboratory results become available.

Potassium

The magnitude of the potassium gradient across cell membranes determines excitability of nerve and muscle cells, including the myocardium. Minor changes in serum potassium concentration can have major effects on cardiac rhythm and function. Of all the electrolytes, rapid changes in potassium concentration can cause the most immediate life-threatening consequences.

Evaluation of serum potassium must consider the effects of changes in serum pH. When serum pH falls, serum potassium rises because potassium shifts from the cellular to the vascular space. When serum pH rises, serum potassium falls because potassium shifts intracellularly. *In general, serum K^+ decreases by approximately 0.3 mEq/L for every 0.1 U increase in pH above normal.* Effects of pH changes on serum potassium should be anticipated during evaluation and therapy for hyperkalemia or hypokalemia. Correction of an alkalotic pH will produce an increase in serum potassium even without administration of additional potassium. If serum potassium is "normal" in the face of acidosis, a fall in serum potassium should be anticipated when the acidosis is corrected, and potassium administration should be planned.

Hyperkalemia

Hyperkalemia is defined as serum potassium concentration above the normal range of 3.5 to 5.0 mEq/L. Hyperkalemia is most frequently caused by increased K^+ release from cells or by impaired excretion by the kidneys (see Table 1). The most common clinical presentation of severe hyperkalemia involves patients with end-stage renal failure. These patients may present with severe weakness or arrhythmias.

Medications may also contribute to development of hyperkalemia, particularly in the presence of impaired renal function. Not surprisingly, potassium supplements commonly prescribed to prevent hypokalemia may lead to potassium overload. Potassium-sparing diuretics such as spironolactone, triamterene, and amiloride are well-recognized causes of hyperkalemia. Use of angiotensin-converting enzyme (ACE) inhibitors (eg, captopril) can also lead to elevation of serum potassium, particularly when combined with oral potassium supplements. Nonsteroidal anti-inflammatory medicines (eg, ibuprofen) can cause hyperkalemia through direct effects on the kidney. Identification of potential causes of hyperkalemia will contribute to rapid identification and treatment of patients who may be experiencing hyperkalemic cardiac arrhythmias.[1–3]

Changes in pH inversely affect serum potassium. Acidosis (low pH) leads to an extracellular shift of potassium, thus raising serum potassium. Conversely, high pH (alkalosis) shifts potassium back into the cell, lowering serum potassium.

Physical symptoms of hyperkalemia include ECG changes, weakness, ascending paralysis, and respiratory failure. ECG changes suggestive of hyperkalemia include

- Peaked T waves (tenting)
- Flattened P waves
- Prolonged PR interval (first-degree heart block)
- Widened QRS complex
- Deepened S waves and merging of S and T waves
- Idioventricular rhythm
- Sine-wave formation
- VF and cardiac arrest

Tenting of T waves is one of the prominent early ECG changes. If untreated, hyperkalemia causes progressive heart dysfunction, leading to sine waves and finally to asystole. Aggressive therapy should begin as soon as possible to improve outcome.

Treatment of Hyperkalemia

Treatment of hyperkalemia depends on level of severity and the patient's clinical condition:

- *Mild elevation* (5 to 6 mEq/L): Remove potassium from the body

  1. Diuretics—furosemide 1 mg/kg IV slowly
  2. Resins—Kayexalate 15 to 30 g in 50 to 100 mL of 20% sorbitol either orally or by retention enema (50 g of Kayexalate)
  3. Dialysis—peritoneal or hemodialysis

- *Moderate elevation* (6 to 7 mEq/L): Also shift potassium intracellularly by using

Circulation. 2000;102(suppl I):I-217–I-222.
© 2000 American Heart Association, Inc.

Circulation is available at http://www.circulationaha.org

TABLE 1. Causes of Hyperkalemia

Drugs (K^+-sparing diuretics, ACE inhibitors, NSAIDs, potassium supplements)
End-stage renal disease
Muscle breakdown (rhabdomyolysis)
Metabolic acidosis
Pseudohyperkalemia
Hemolysis
Tumor lysis syndrome
Diet (rarely sole cause)
Hypoaldosteronism (Addison disease, hyporeninemia)
Type 4 renal tubular acidosis
Other: hyperkalemic periodic paralysis

1. Sodium bicarbonate—50 mEq IV over 5 minutes
2. Glucose plus insulin—mix 50 g glucose and 10 U regular insulin and give IV over 15 to 30 minutes
3. Nebulized albuterol 10 to 20 mg nebulized over 15 minutes

- *Severe elevation* (>7 mEq/L with toxic ECG changes)

1. Calcium chloride—10% 5 to 10 mL IV over 2 to 5 minutes to antagonize the toxic effects of potassium at the myocardial cell membrane (lowers risk of ventricular fibrillation [VF]).
2. Sodium bicarbonate—50 mEq IV over 5 minutes (may be less effective for patients with end-stage renal disease)[4-6]
3. Glucose plus insulin—mix 50 g glucose and 10 U regular insulin and give IV over 15 to 30 minutes
4. Nebulized albuterol—10 to 20 mg nebulized over 15 minutes
5. Diuresis (furosemide—40 to 80 mg IV)
6. Kayexalate enema
7. Dialysis

Hypokalemia

Hypokalemia is defined as a serum potassium level <3.5 mEq/L. As with hyperkalemia, nerves and muscles (including the heart) are most affected by hypokalemia, particularly if the patient has other, preexisting disease (such as coronary artery disease).

Hypokalemia results from one or more of the following: decreased dietary intake, shift into cells, or increased net loss from the body. The most common causes of low serum potassium include gastrointestinal loss (diarrhea, laxatives), renal loss (hyperaldosteronism, potassium-losing diuretics, carbenicillin, sodium penicillin, amphotericin B), intracellular shift (alkalosis or a rise in pH), and malnutrition. Symptoms of hypokalemia include weakness, fatigue, paralysis, respiratory difficulty, muscle breakdown (rhabdomyolysis), constipation, paralytic ileus, and leg cramps.

Hypokalemia is suggested by changes in the ECG, including

- U waves
- T-wave flattening
- ST-segment changes

- Arrhythmias (especially if the patient is taking digoxin)
- Pulseless electrical activity (PEA) or asystole

Hypokalemia exacerbates digitalis toxicity. Thus, hypokalemia should be avoided or treated promptly in patients receiving digitalis derivatives.

Treatment of Hypokalemia

The treatment of hypokalemia includes minimizing further potassium loss and giving potassium replacement. IV administration of potassium is indicated when arrhythmias are present or hypokalemia is severe (K^+ <2.5 mEq/L).

Acute potassium administration may be empirical in emergent conditions. When indicated, maximum IV K^+ replacement should be 10 to 20 mEq/h with continuous ECG monitoring during infusion. Central or peripheral IV sites may be used. A more concentrated solution of potassium may be infused if a central line is used, but the catheter tip should not extend into the right atrium.

If cardiac arrest from hypokalemia is imminent (ie, malignant ventricular arrhythmias), rapid replacement of potassium is required. Give an initial infusion of 2 mEq/min, followed by another 10 mEq IV over 5 to 10 minutes. *In the patient's chart, document that rapid infusion is intentional in response to life-threatening hypokalemia.* Once the patient is stabilized, reduce the infusion to continue potassium replacement more gradually.

Estimates of total body deficit of potassium range from 150 to 400 mEq for every 1-mEq decrease in serum potassium. The lower range of the estimate would be appropriate for an elderly woman with low muscle mass and the higher range for a young, muscular man. Gradual correction of hypokalemia is preferable to rapid correction unless the patient is clinically unstable.

Sodium

Sodium is the major positively charged ion in the extracellular space and the major intravascular ion that influences serum osmolality. An acute increase in serum sodium will produce an acute increase in serum osmolality; an acute decrease in serum sodium will produce an acute fall in serum osmolality.

Under normal conditions sodium concentration and osmolality equilibrate across the vascular membrane. *Acute* changes in serum sodium will produce acute free water shifts into and out of the vascular space until osmolality equilibrates in these compartments. An acute fall in serum sodium and an acute fluid shift into the interstitial space may cause cerebral edema.[7,8] An acute rise in serum sodium will produce an acute shift of free water from the interstitial to the vascular space. Rapid correction of hyponatremia has been associated with development of pontine myelinolysis and cerebral bleeding.[9-11] For these reasons, monitor neurological function closely in the patient with hypernatremia or hyponatremia and during correction of these conditions. Whenever possible, correct serum sodium slowly, carefully controlling the absolute magnitude of change in serum sodium over 48 hours and avoiding overcorrection.[12,13]

Hypernatremia

Hypernatremia is defined as a serum sodium concentration above the normal range of 135 to 145 mEq/L. Hypernatremia may be caused by a primary Na^+ gain or excess water loss. A common cause of hypernatremia is free water loss in excess of sodium loss, such as that which occurs with diabetes insipidus or hypernatremic dehydration.

Hypernatremia produces a free water shift from the interstitial to the vascular space. Hypernatremia also causes water to shift out of cells, leading to decreased intracellular volume. In the brain, decreased nerve cell volume can cause neurological symptoms, including altered mental status, weakness, irritability, focal neurological deficits, and even coma or seizures.

The hypernatremic patient usually complains of excessive thirst. The severity of symptoms depends on how acute and how great the increase in serum sodium is. If the sodium rises quickly or to a very high level, signs and symptoms will be more severe.

Treatment of Hypernatremia

To treat hypernatremia, it is important to stop ongoing water losses (by treating the underlying cause) while correcting the water deficit. In hypovolemic patients the extracellular fluid (ECF) volume must be restored with normal saline.

The quantity of water needed to correct hypernatremia can be calculated by the following equation:

Water deficit =

$$\frac{\text{plasma } Na^+ \text{ concentration} - 140}{140} \times \text{total body water.}$$

Total body water is approximately 50% of lean body weight in men and 40% in women. For example, if a 70-kg man had a serum Na^+ level of 160 mmol/L, the estimated free water deficit would be

$$\frac{160 - 140}{140} \times (0.5 \times 70) = 5 \text{ L.}$$

Once the free water deficit is calculated, administer fluid to lower serum sodium at a rate of 0.5 to 1.0 mEq/h with a decrease of no more than 12 mmol in the first 24 hours. Total correction should be achieved over 48 to 72 hours. The method of replacement of free water depends on the patient's clinical status. For stable, asymptomatic patients, replacement of fluid by mouth or through a nasogastric tube is effective and safe. If this is not possible or if the patient's clinical status demands more aggressive treatment, 5% dextrose in half-normal saline may be given IV. Check the patient's serum sodium and neurological function frequently to avoid overly rapid correction.

Hyponatremia

Hyponatremia is defined as a serum sodium concentration below the normal range of 135 to 145 mEq/L. It is caused by an excess of water relative to sodium. Most cases of hyponatremia are caused by reduced renal excretion of water with continued water intake. Impairment of renal water excretion may be due to

- Use of thiazide diuretics
- Renal failure
- ECF depletion (eg, vomiting with continued water intake)
- Syndrome of inappropriate antidiuretic hormone secretion (SIADH)
- Edematous states (congestive heart failure, cirrhosis with ascites, etc)
- Hypothyroidism
- Adrenal insufficiency
- "Tea and toast diet" or excessive beer drinking (diminished solute intake)

Most cases of hyponatremia are associated with low serum osmolality (so-called hypo-osmolar hyponatremia). The one common exception to this is in uncontrolled diabetes, in which hyperglycemia leads to a hyperosmolar state, whereas serum sodium is below normal (hyperosmolar hyponatremia).

Hyponatremia is usually asymptomatic unless it is acute or severe (<120 mEq/L). An abrupt fall in serum sodium produces a free water shift from the vascular to the interstitial space that can cause cerebral edema. In this case the patient may present with nausea, vomiting, headache, irritability, lethargy, seizures, coma, or even death.

SIADH is an important cause of potentially life-threatening hyponatremia. It can occur in a wide variety of clinical situations. SIADH can complicate a variety of conditions common to ACLS patients, including trauma, increased intracranial pressure, cancer, and respiratory failure.

Treatment of Hyponatremia

Treatment of hyponatremia involves administration of sodium and elimination of intravascular free water. If SIADH is present, the treatment is strict restriction of fluid intake to 50% to 66% of maintenance fluids.

Correction of asymptomatic hyponatremia should be gradual: usually an increase in Na^+ of 0.5 mEq/L per hour to a maximum change of 10 to 15 mEq/L in the first 24 hours. Rapid correction of hyponatremia can cause *pontine myelinolysis*, a lethal disorder thought to be caused by rapid fluid shifts in the brain.[9-11]

If the patient demonstrates neurological compromise, urgent administration of 3% saline IV at a rate of 1 mEq/L per hour is necessary to correct hyponatremia until neurological symptoms are controlled. Thereafter, continued correction should be at a rate of 0.5 mEq/L per hour to raise serum sodium.

Ultimate correction of serum sodium requires calculation of the sodium deficit. The following formula may be used:

Na^+ deficit =

(desired $[Na^+]$ − current $[Na^+]$) $\times$ 0.6* $\times$ body wt (kg)
(*Use 0.6 for men, 0.5 for women.)

Once the deficit is estimated, determine the volume of 3% saline (513 mEq Na^+/L) necessary to correct the deficit (divide the deficit by 513 mEq/L). Plan to increase the sodium by 1 mEq/L per hour over 4 hours. Check serum sodium frequently and monitor neurological status closely.

Magnesium

Magnesium is the fourth most common mineral in the human body, but it is also the most frequently overlooked clinically. One third of extracellular magnesium is bound to serum albumin. Therefore, serum magnesium levels are not reliable predictors of total body magnesium stores. Magnesium is required for the action of many important enzymes and hormones. It is necessary for the movement of sodium, potassium, and calcium into and out of cells. In fact, when a patient is hypomagnesemic, it is impossible to correct intracellular potassium deficiency. Magnesium is also important in stabilizing excitable membranes and useful for atrial and ventricular arrhythmias.[14]

Hypermagnesemia

Hypermagnesemia is defined as a serum magnesium concentration above the normal range of 1.3 to 2.2 mEq/L. Magnesium balance is influenced by many of the same regulatory systems that control calcium balance. In addition, magnesium balance is influenced by diseases and factors that control serum potassium. As a result, magnesium balance is closely tied to both calcium and potassium balance.

The most common cause of hypermagnesemia is renal failure. Hypermagnesemia may also be iatrogenic (caused by overuse of magnesium) or caused by a perforated viscus with continued intake of food and use of laxatives/antacids containing magnesium (an important cause in the elderly).

Neurological symptoms of hypermagnesemia include muscular weakness, paralysis, ataxia, drowsiness, and confusion. Gastrointestinal symptoms include nausea and vomiting. Moderate hypermagnesemia can produce vasodilation, and severe hypermagnesemia can produce hypotension. Extremely high serum magnesium levels may produce a depressed level of consciousness, bradycardia, hypoventilation, and cardiorespiratory arrest.[14]

ECG changes of hypermagnesemia include

- Increased PR and QT intervals
- Increased QRS duration
- Variable decrease in P-wave voltage
- Variable degree of T-wave peaking
- Complete AV block, asystole

Treatment of Hypermagnesemia

Hypermagnesemia is treated by antagonizing magnesium with calcium, removing magnesium from serum, and eliminating sources of ongoing magnesium intake. Cardiorespiratory support may be needed until magnesium levels are reduced. Administration of calcium chloride (5 to 10 mEq IV) will often correct lethal arrhythmias. This dose may be repeated if needed.

Dialysis is the treatment of choice for treatment of hypermagnesemia. Until that can be done, if renal function is normal and cardiovascular function adequate, IV saline diuresis (IV normal saline and furosemide [1 mEq/kg]) can be used to hasten elimination of magnesium from the body. However, this diuresis can also increase calcium excretion; the development of hypocalcemia will make signs and symptoms of hypermagnesemia worse. While treatment continues, the patient may require cardiorespiratory support.

TABLE 2. Causes of Hypomagnesemia

GI loss: bowel resection, pancreatitis, diarrhea
Renal disease
Starvation
Drugs: diuretics, pentamidine, gentamicin, digoxin
Alcohol
Hypothermia
Hypercalcemia
Diabetic ketoacidosis
Hyperthyroidism/hypothyroidism
Phosphate deficiency
Burns
Sepsis
Lactation

GI indicates gastrointestinal.

Hypomagnesemia

Hypomagnesemia is far more common clinically than hypermagnesemia. Defined as a serum magnesium concentration below the normal range of 1.3 to 2.2 mEq/L, hypomagnesemia usually results from decreased absorption or increased loss, either from the kidneys or intestines (diarrhea). Alterations in parathyroid hormone and certain medications (eg, pentamidine, diuretics, alcohol) can also induce hypomagnesemia. Lactating women are at higher risk of developing hypomagnesemia.[15]

The various causes of hypomagnesemia are listed in Table 2.

The principal signs of hypomagnesemia are neurological, although interesting research has tied together the neurological and cardiac effects of magnesium.[16] Hypomagnesemia interferes with the effects of parathyroid hormone, resulting in hypocalcemia. It may also cause hypokalemia. Symptoms of low serum magnesium include muscular tremors and fasciculations, ocular nystagmus, tetany, and altered mentation. Other possible symptoms include ataxia, vertigo, seizures, and dysphagia. A number of ECG abnormalities occur with low magnesium levels, including

- Prolonged QT and PR intervals
- ST-segment depression
- T-wave inversion
- Flattening or inversion of precordial P waves
- Widening of QRS
- Torsades de pointes
- Treatment-resistant VF (and other arrhythmias)
- Worsening of digitalis toxicity[17]

Treatment of Hypomagnesemia

Treatment of hypomagnesemia depends on its severity and the patient's clinical status. For severe or symptomatic hypomagnesemia, administer 1 to 2 g IV $MgSO_4$ over 15 minutes. If torsades de pointes are present, administer 2 g of $MgSO_4$ over 1 to 2 minutes. If seizures are present, administer 2 g IV $MgSO_4$ over 10 minutes. Calcium gluconate administration (1 g) is usually appropriate because most patients with hypomagnesemia are also hypocalcemic.[18]

Replace magnesium cautiously in patients with renal insufficiency because there is a real danger of causing life-threatening hypermagnesemia.

Calcium

Calcium is the most abundant mineral in the body. It is essential for bone strength and neuromuscular function and plays a major role in myocardial contraction. Half of all calcium in the ECF is bound to albumin; the other half is in the biologically active, ionized form. The ionized form is most active.

The serum ionized calcium level must be evaluated in light of serum pH and serum albumin. The concentration of ionized calcium is pH-dependent. Alkalosis increases the binding of calcium to albumin and thus reduces ionized calcium. Conversely, the development of acidosis will produce an increase in the ionized calcium level.

Total serum calcium is dependent on serum albumin concentration. Serum calcium changes in the same direction as a change in albumin (adjust total serum calcium by 0.8 mg/dL for every 1 g/dL change in serum albumin). Although total serum albumin is directly related to total serum calcium, the ionized calcium is inversely related to serum albumin. The lower the serum albumin, the higher the ionized calcium. In the presence of hypoalbuminemia, although total calcium level may be low, the ionized calcium level may be normal.

Calcium antagonizes the effects of both potassium and magnesium at the cell membrane. Therefore, it is extremely useful for treating the effects of hyperkalemia and hypermagnesemia.

Calcium concentration is normally closely regulated by PTH and vitamin D. When such control fails, a wide variety of clinical problems occur.

Hypercalcemia

Hypercalcemia is defined as a serum calcium concentration above the normal range of 8.5 to 10.5 mEq/L (or an elevation in ionized calcium above 4.2 to 4.8 mg/dL). Primary hyperparathyroidism and malignancy account for >90% of reported cases.[19] In these and most forms of hypercalcemia, calcium release from the bone and intestines is increased, and renal clearance may be compromised.

Symptoms of hypercalcemia usually develop when the total scrum calcium concentration reaches or exceeds 12 to 15 mg/dL. Neurological symptoms include depression, weakness, fatigue, and confusion at lower levels. At higher levels patients may exhibit hallucinations, disorientation, hypotonicity, and coma. Hypercalcemia interferes with renal concentration of urine, causing dehydration to develop.

Cardiovascular symptoms of elevated calcium levels are variable. Myocardial contractility may initially increase until the calcium level reaches 15 to 20 mg/dL. Above this level myocardial depression occurs. Automaticity is decreased and ventricular systole is shortened. Arrhythmias occur because the refractory period is shortened. Digitalis toxicity is worsened. Hypertension is common. In addition, many patients with hypercalcemia develop hypokalemia; these conditions both contribute to cardiac arrhythmias.[20]

ECG changes of hypercalcemia include

- Shortened QT interval (usually when Ca^{2+} is >13 mg/dL)
- Prolonged PR and QRS intervals
- Increased QRS voltage
- T-wave flattening and widening
- Notching of QRS
- AV block: progresses to complete heart block, then to cardiac arrest when serum calcium is >15 to 20 mg/dL

Gastrointestinal symptoms of hypercalcemia include dysphagia, constipation, peptic ulcers, and pancreatitis. Effects on the kidney include diminished ability to concentrate urine; diuresis, leading to loss of sodium, potassium, magnesium, and phosphate; and a vicious circle of calcium reabsorption that further worsens hypercalcemia.

Treatment of Hypercalcemia

If hypercalcemia is due to malignancy, careful consideration of the patient's prognosis and wishes is needed. If the patient is in the last stages of death, hypercalcemia need not be treated. In all other cases, however, treatment should be rapid and aggressive.

Treatment for hypercalcemia is required if the patient is symptomatic (typically a concentration of approximately 12 mg/dL). Treatment is instituted at a level >15 mg/dL regardless of symptoms. Immediate therapy is directed at promoting calcium excretion in the urine. This is accomplished in patients with adequate cardiovascular and renal function with infusion of 0.9% saline at 300 to 500 mL/h until any fluid deficit is replaced and diuresis occurs (urine output ≥200 to 300 mL/h). Once adequate rehydration has occurred, the saline infusion rate is reduced to 100 to 200 mL/h. This diuresis will further reduce serum potassium and magnesium concentrations, which may increase the arrhythmogenic potential of the hypercalcemia. Thus, potassium and magnesium concentrations should be closely monitored and maintained.

Hemodialysis is the treatment of choice to rapidly decrease serum calcium in patients with heart failure or renal insufficiency.[21] Chelating agents may be used for extreme conditions (eg, 50 mmol PO_4 over 8 to 12 hours or EDTA 10 to 50 mg/kg over 4 hours).

Use of furosemide (1 mg/kg IV) during treatment of hypercalcemia is controversial. In the presence of heart failure, furosemide administration is required, but it can actually foster reuptake of calcium from bone, thus worsening hypercalcemia. Calcium may also be lowered by drugs that reduce bone resorption (eg, calcitonin, glucocorticoids). A discussion of this therapy is beyond the scope of these guidelines.

Hypocalcemia

Hypocalcemia is defined as a serum calcium concentration below the normal range of 8.5 to 10.5 mg/dL (or an ionized calcium below the range of 4.2 to 4.8 mg/dL). Hypocalcemia may develop with toxic shock syndrome, abnormalities in serum magnesium, and tumor lysis syndrome (rapid cell turnover with resultant hyperkalemia, hyperphosphatemia, and hypocalcemia). Calcium exchange is dependent on concentrations of potassium and magnesium, so treatment depends on replacing all 3 electrolytes.

Symptoms of hypocalcemia usually occur when ionized levels fall below 2.5 mg/dL. Symptoms include paraesthesias of the extremities and face, followed by muscle cramps, carpopedal spasm, stridor, tetany, and seizures. Hypocalcemic patients demonstrate hyperreflexia and positive Chvostek and Trousseau signs. Cardiac symptoms include decreased contractility and heart failure. ECG changes of hypocalcemia include

- QT-interval prolongation
- Terminal T-wave inversion
- Heart blocks
- Ventricular fibrillation

Hypocalcemia can exacerbate digitalis toxicity.

Treatment of Hypocalcemia

Treatment of hypocalcemia requires administration of calcium. Treat acute, symptomatic hypocalcemia with 10% calcium gluconate, 90 to 180 mg of elemental calcium IV over 10 minutes. Follow this with an IV drip of 540 to 720 mg of elemental calcium in 500 to 1000 mL D_5W at 0.5 to 2.0 mg/kg per hour (10 to 15 mg/kg). Measure serum calcium every 4 to 6 hours. Aim to maintain the total serum calcium concentration between 7 and 9 mg/dL. Abnormalities in magnesium, potassium, and pH must be corrected simultaneously. Note that untreated hypomagnesemia will make hypocalcemia refractory to therapy.

Summary

Electrolyte abnormalities are among the most common reasons for patients to develop cardiac arrhythmias. Of all the electrolyte abnormalities, hyperkalemia is most rapidly fatal. A high degree of clinical suspicion and aggressive treatment of underlying electrolyte abnormalities can prevent many patients from progressing to cardiac arrest.

References

1. Jackson MA, Lodwick R, Hutchinson SG. Hyperkalaemic cardiac arrest successfully treated with peritoneal dialysis [see comments]. *BMJ*. 1996; 312:1289–1290.
2. Voelckel W, Kroesen G. Unexpected return of cardiac action after termination of cardiopulmonary resuscitation. *Resuscitation*. 1996;32: 27–29.
3. Niemann JT, Cairns CB. Hyperkalemia and ionized hypocalcemia during cardiac arrest and resuscitation: possible culprits for postcountershock arrhythmias? *Ann Emerg Med*. 1999;34:1–7.
4. Lin JL, Lim PS, Leu ML, Huang CC. Outcomes of severe hyperkalemia in cardiopulmonary resuscitation with concomitant hemodialysis. *Intensive Care Med*. 1994;20:287–290.
5. Allon M. Hyperkalemia in end-stage renal disease: mechanisms and management [editorial]. *J Am Soc Nephrol*. 1995;6:1134–1142.
6. Allon M, Shanklin N. Effect of bicarbonate administration on plasma potassium in dialysis patients: interactions with insulin and albuterol. *Am J Kidney Dis*. 1996;28:508–514.
7. Adrogue HJ, Madias NE. Aiding fluid prescription for the dysnatremias. *Intensive Care Med*. 1997;23:309–316.
8. Fraser CL, Arieff AI. Epidemiology, pathophysiology, and management of hyponatremic encephalopathy. *Am J Med*. 1997;102:67–77.
9. Laureno R, Karp BI. Myelinolysis after correction of hyponatremia [see comments]. *Ann Intern Med*. 1997;126:57–62.
10. Gross P, Reimann D, Neidel J, Doke C, Prospert F, Decaux G, Verbalis J, Schrier RW. The treatment of severe hyponatremia. *Kidney Int Suppl*. 1998;64:S6–S11.
11. Soupart A, Decaux G. Therapeutic recommendations for management of severe hyponatremia: current concepts on pathogenesis and prevention of neurologic complications. *Clin Nephrol*. 1996;46:149–169.
12. Brunner JE, Redmond JM, Haggar AM, Kruger DF, Elias SB. Central pontine myelinolysis and pontine lesions after rapid correction of hyponatremia: a prospective magnetic resonance imaging study. *Ann Neurol*. 1990;27:61–66.
13. Ayus JC, Krothapalli RK, Arieff AI. Treatment of symptomatic hyponatremia and its relation to brain damage: a prospective study. *N Engl J Med*. 1987;317:1190–1195.
14. Higham PD, Adams PC, Murray A, Campbell RW. Plasma potassium, serum magnesium and ventricular fibrillation: a prospective study. *Q J Med*. 1993;86:609–617.
15. Navarro-Gonzalez JF. Magnesium in dialysis patients: serum levels and clinical implications. *Clin Nephrol*. 1998;49:373–378.
16. Fiset C, Kargacin ME, Kondo CS, Lester WM, Duff HJ. Hypomagnesemia: characterization of a model of sudden cardiac death. *J Am Coll Cardiol*. 1996;27:1771–1776.
17. Leier CV, Dei Cas L, Metra M. Clinical relevance and management of the major electrolyte abnormalities in congestive heart failure: hyponatremia, hypokalemia, and hypomagnesemia. *Am Heart J*. 1994;128:564–574.
18. al-Ghamdi SM, Cameron EC, Sutton RA. Magnesium deficiency: pathophysiologic and clinical overview [see comments]. *Am J Kidney Dis*. 1994;24:737–752.
19. Barri YM, Knochel JP. Hypercalemia and electrolyte disturbances in malignancy. *Hematol Oncol Clin North Am*. 1996;10:775–790.
20. Aldinger KA, Samaan NA. Hypokalemia with hypercalcemia: prevalence and significance in treatment. *Ann Intern Med*. 1977;87:571–573.
21. Edelson GW, Kleerekoper M. Hypercalcemic crisis. *Med Clin North Am*. 1995;79:79–92.

Section 2: Toxicology in ECC

General Considerations

Poisoning is the third leading cause (11%) of injury-related mortality in the United States and is among the top 3 causes in most other countries. In the United States in 1995 there were an estimated 2.4 million exposures to poison and 1 million visits to the Emergency Department (1% of all visits), 215 000 admissions to the hospital, and 18 549 deaths due to poisoning.[1–3] Although exposure to poison is common, life-threatening or fatal poisoning is not. Poisoning is a relatively infrequent cause of cardiac arrest overall but is a leading cause in victims <40 years old. The long-term survival rate among victims of cardiac arrest due to poisoning is good, averaging 24% in 6 studies.

The relatively small number of life-threatening poisonings and the lack of a prehospital triage protocol for severe poisonings in the United States are major obstacles to the performance of high-quality clinical research. Because the research in this area consists primarily of small case series (level of evidence [LOE] 5), animal studies (LOE 6), and case reports, the American Heart Association (AHA) class of recommendation for most recommendations for treating victims of poisoning is IIb. The following evidence- and consensus-based guidelines were developed by a toxicology work group of the AHA Advanced Cardiovascular Life Support (ACLS) Committee to provide guidance in the management of severe poisoning when standard ECC guidelines may not be optimal or appropriate. In addition to these guidelines we recommend consultation with a medical toxicologist or certified regional poison information center and use of a poison treatment center for unusual cases of poisoning.[4,5] See Tables 1 and 2.

Drug-Induced Emergencies: Prearrest

Airway and Respiratory Management

Because poisoned patients can deteriorate rapidly, frequently assess their ability to protect their airway and breathe adequately. International guidelines recommend gastric lavage only for patients who have ingested a potentially lethal amount of drug or toxin and present within 1 hour of ingestion.[6] In obtunded or comatose patients, perform rapid-sequence intubation before gastric lavage to prevent aspiration pneumonia. Because reversal of benzodiazepine intoxication with flumazenil is hazardous, we do not recommend routine inclusion of this practice in "coma cocktail" protocols.

Opiate Poisoning

If a patient suspected of overdosing on an opiate has a pulse, try to reverse respiratory insufficiency with naloxone, an opiate antagonist, before inserting an endotracheal tube. Do not withhold naloxone until artificial ventilation is initiated. Heroin is the opiate taken in most cases of opiate overdose treated in emergency settings. Severe complications after opiate reversal are uncommon (<2%). Although the effects of naloxone do not last as long as those of heroin (45 to 70 minutes compared with 4 to 5 hours), naloxone is the preferred agent for reversal. Some EMS systems allow selected patients aroused with naloxone to refuse transport to the hospital against medical advice. Allowing selected patients to refuse observation against medical advice rarely leads to serious consequences such as severe renarcotization or delayed pulmonary edema.[7,8] Naloxone can be administered intramuscularly, subcutaneously, or intravenously. The IM and SC routes theoretically provide greater ease of administration, less risk of needle puncture, and less risk of severe withdrawal in patients addicted to opiates than the IV route.

The desired end points of opiate reversal are adequate airway reflexes and ventilations, not complete arousal. Acute, abrupt withdrawal from opiates may increase the frequency of severe complications such as pulmonary edema, ventricular arrhythmia, and severe agitation. In 2 studies of opiate reversal with naloxone, only small doses were required for opiate reversal. In emergency settings the recommended initial dose of naloxone is 0.4 to 0.8 mg IV or 0.8 mg IM or SC. In communities in which abuse of naloxone-resistant opiates is prevalent, larger initial doses of naloxone may be needed. When opiate overdose is strongly suspected or in areas where abuse of "China white" is prevalent, titration to a total naloxone dose of 6 to 10 mg is recommended if needed.

Drug-Induced Hemodynamically Significant Bradycardia

In cases of drug-induced hemodynamically significant bradycardia (HSB), atropine is seldom helpful but is acceptable to administer because it is not harmful. The major exception is acute organophosphate or carbamate poisoning, in which case atropine may be lifesaving. The recommended starting dose of atropine for adults with insecticide poisoning is 2 to 4 mg. Avoid use of isoproterenol, which may induce or aggravate hypotension and ventricular arrhythmias.

In cases of massive β-blocker poisoning, however, isoproterenol given in very high doses is reportedly effective. Digoxin-specific Fab antibody fragments are extremely effective therapy for life-threatening ventricular arrhythmias or heart block due to poisoning with digoxin or cardiac glycosides.[9] Electrical cardiac pacing is often effective in cases of mild to moderate drug-

Circulation. **2000;102(suppl I):I-223–I-228.**
© 2000 American Heart Association, Inc.

Circulation is available at http://www.circulationaha.org

TABLE 1. Sympathomimetic and Cardiotoxic Drugs

Drug Class	Cardiovascular Signs of Toxicity*	Therapy to Consider
Stimulants, sympathomimetic		
Amphetamines	Tachycardia	α-Blockers
Methamphetamine	Supraventricular and ventricular arrhythmias	Benzodiazepines
Cocaine	Impaired conduction	Lidocaine
Phencyclidine (PCP)	Hypertensive emergencies	Sodium bicarbonate
	Acute coronary syndromes	
	Shock, cardiac arrest	
Calcium channel blockers		
Verapamil	Bradycardia	Mixed α-/β-agonists
Nifedipine	Impaired conduction	Pacemakers
Diltiazem	Shock	Calcium infusions
	Cardiac arrest	Insulin euglycemia
β-Adrenergic receptor antagonists		
Propranolol	Bradycardia	Pacemakers
Atenolol	Impaired conduction	Mixed α-/β-agonists
	Shock	Glucagon, insulin
	Cardiac arrest	Insulin euglycemia
Tricyclic antidepressants		
Amitriptyline	Tachycardia	Sodium bicarbonate
Desipramine	Bradycardia	Mixed α-/β-agonists or α-agonists
Nortriptyline	Ventricular arrhythmia	Lidocaine
	Impaired conduction	Procainamide is contraindicated
	Shock, cardiac arrest	
Cardiac glycosides		
Digoxin	Bradycardia	Digoxin-specific Fab fragments
Digitoxin	Supraventricular and ventricular arrhythmias	(Digibind)
Foxglove	Impaired conduction	Magnesium
Oleander	Shock, cardiac arrest	Pacemakers
Anticholinergics		
Diphenhydramine	Tachycardia	Physostigmine
Doxylamine	Supraventricular and ventricular arrhythmias	
	Impaired conduction	
	Shock	
	Cardiac arrest	
Cholinergics		
Carbamates	Bradycardia	Atropine
Nerve agents	Ventricular arrhythmias	Decontamination
Organophosphates	Impaired conduction, shock	Pralidoxime
	Pulmonary edema, bronchospasm	Obidoxime
	Cardiac arrest	
Opiates		
Heroin	Hypoventilation (slow, shallow respirations)	Naloxone
Fentanyl	Bradycardia, hypotension	Nalmefene
Methadone		
Isoniazid	Lactic acidosis with or without seizures	Pyridoxine (vitamin B_6)
	Tachycardia or bradycardia	
	Shock, cardiac arrest	
Sodium channel blockers		
Type 1_A antiarrhythmics, propranolol, verapamil, TCAs	Impaired conduction	Sodium bicarbonates
	Bradycardia	Pacemakers
	Ventricular arrhythmias	α-/β-Agonists, high dose if necessary
	Seizures	Hypertonic saline
	Shock, cardiac arrest	

*Unless stated otherwise, assume that all altered vital signs (bradycardia, tachycardia, tachypnea) are "hemodynamically significant."

induced HSB. If external pacing is poorly tolerated or electrical capture is difficult to maintain, use transvenous pacing. When transcutaneous pacing is used, prophylactic transvenous placement of the pacer wire is not recommended because the tip of the catheter may trigger ventricular arrhythmias when the myocardium is irritable. In cases of very severe poisoning, capture may not occur despite proper location of the wire and use of the highest voltage settings. If HSB is resistant to atropine and

TABLE 2. Drug-Induced Cardiovascular Emergencies and Altered Vital Signs

Drug-Induced Emergency	Therapy	
	Indicated	Contraindicated
Bradycardia*	Pacemaker (TC, IV) Mixed α-/β-agonists For OD of calcium channel blocker: calcium For OD of β-blocker: glucagon or β-agonist	Isoproterenol if hypotensive Prophylactic TV pacing
Tachycardia	Benzodiazepines Selective β_1-blockers Mixed α-/β-blockers	Cardioversion Adenosine, verapamil, diltiazem For OD of TCA: physostigmine
Impaired conduction, ventricular arrhythmias	Sodium bicarbonate Lidocaine	For OD of TCA: type I$_A$ antiarrhythmics (procainamide)
Hypertensive emergency	Benzodiazepines Mixed α-/β-blockers Nitroprusside	Nonselective β-blocker (propranolol)
Acute coronary syndrome	Benzodiazepines Nitroglycerin α-Blocker	Nonselective β-blockers (propranolol)
Shock	Mixed α-/β-agonists (high dose if necessary) For OD of calcium channel blocker: calcium, insulin† For OD of β-blocker: glucagon, insulin† If refractory to *maximal* medical therapy: circulatory assist devices	Isoproterenol
Acute cholinergic syndrome	Atropine Pralidoxime/obidoxime	Succinylcholine
Acute anticholinergic syndrome	Physostigmine	Antipsychotics or other anticholinergics
Opiate poisoning	Naloxone Nalmefene	

TC indicates transcutaneous; IV, intravenous; TV, transvenous; and OD, overdose.

*Unless stated otherwise, assume all altered vital signs (bradycardia, tachycardia, tachypnea) are "hemodynamically significant."

†Administer to achieve euglycemia.

pacing, use vasopressors with greater β-agonist activity. Management of more resistant drug-induced HSB is discussed in Drug-Induced Shock.

Drug-Induced Hemodynamically Significant Tachycardia

Drug-induced hemodynamically significant tachycardia (HST) may induce myocardial ischemia, myocardial infarction, or ventricular arrhythmias and lead to high-output heart failure and shock. Avoid use of routine measures such as adenosine therapy and synchronized cardioversion in patients with drug-induced HST because the tachycardia is likely to recur or to be refractory. In patients with borderline hypotension, diltiazem and verapamil are relatively contraindicated because they may precipitate more severe shock. Pharmacological measures are preferred when rate control is necessary.

Benzodiazepines such as diazepam or lorazepam are generally safe and effective in patients with drug-induced HST. Avoid using benzodiazepines in amounts that depress the level of consciousness and create the need for respiratory assistance. Physostigmine is a specific antidote that may be preferable for drug-induced HST and central anticholinergic syndrome due to *pure* anticholinergic poisoning. Very cautious use of a nonselective β-blocker such as propranolol may be effective in patients with drug-induced HST due to sympathomimetic poisoning.

Drug-Induced Hypertensive Emergencies

A drug-induced hypertensive emergency is often short-lived, and aggressive therapy is not needed. This is an important caution because hypotension may occur later in cases of severe stimulant poisoning. Benzodiazepines are first-line therapy. In patients with a drug-induced hypertensive emergency refractory to benzodiazepines, use short-acting antihypertensive agents, such as nitroprusside, as second-line therapy. Labetalol (a nonselective β-blocker, α-blocker, and β_2-agonist) in carefully titrated doses is a third-line agent, effective at times for drug-induced hypertensive emergencies associated with sympathomimetic poisoning. Propranolol (a nonselective β-blocker) is contraindicated because it may block the β_2-receptors, leaving α-adrenergic stimulation unopposed and worsening hypertension.[10]

Drug-Induced Acute Coronary Syndromes

Treatment of drug-induced acute coronary syndromes is similar to the treatment recommended for drug-induced hypertensive emergencies. Catheterization studies have shown that nitroglycerin and phentolamine (an α-blocker) reverse cocaine-induced vasoconstriction, that labetalol has no significant effect, and that propranolol worsens it.[11–14] Therefore, benzodiazepines and nitroglycerin are first-line agents, phentolamine is a second-line agent, and propranolol is contraindicated. Although labetalol has been reported to be effective in isolated cases, use of this agent is controversial because it is a nonselective β-blocker.[15,16] Esmolol and metoprolol are selective β-blockers (β_1 but not β_2) that will not aggravate hypertension, but these agents can induce hypotension.[17] Because esmolol has a very short half-life, the adverse effects of this agent should disappear a few minutes after the infusion is stopped.

Intracoronary administration of thrombolytics or coronary vasodilators is preferred to blind peripheral administration in cases of a drug-induced acute coronary syndrome resistant to the treatments described here. Thrombolytics are contraindicated if an uncontrolled, severe drug-induced hypertensive emergency is present.

Drug-Induced VT and VF

Drug-induced ventricular tachycardia (VT) may be difficult to distinguish from drug-induced impaired conduction (wide complex). When sudden conversion to a wider-complex rhythm occurs with hypotension, drug-induced VT is likely and cardioversion is indicated. Use of antiarrhythmics is indicated in cases of hemodynamically stable drug-induced VT, but there is scant evidence to guide the choice of agent. Procainamide is contraindicated in cases of poisoning with tricyclic antidepressants (TCAs) or poisonings with other drugs that have similar antiarrhythmic properties. In theory lidocaine should be contraindicated in cases of cocaine poisoning. The current consensus, however, based on extensive clinical experience, is that lidocaine is safe and effective.[18]

In the past phenytoin was recommended for TCA-induced VT, but more recently the efficacy and safety of this agent have been questioned.[19,20] There is no acceptable published data on the use of bretylium tosylate for drug-induced VT or VF. Although magnesium has beneficial effects in certain cases of drug-induced VT, it may also aggravate drug-induced hypotension.[21,22] In most cases of drug-induced monomorphic VT or VF, lidocaine is the antiarrhythmic of choice.

Torsades de pointes can occur with exposure to many drugs, either therapeutic or toxic. Correctable factors that increase the risk of torsades de pointes include hypoxemia, hypokalemia, and hypomagnesemia. Treatment of drug-induced torsades de pointes includes correction of risk factors and electrical and pharmacological therapy:

- Magnesium supplementation is recommended for patients with torsades de pointes even if the serum concentration is normal.
- Lidocaine has produced mixed results in studies of torsades de pointes and is Class Indeterminate.
- Electrical overdrive pacing at rates of 100 to 120 beats per minute will usually terminate torsades de pointes.
- Pharmacological overdrive pacing with isoproterenol has also been recommended.
- Some toxicologists recommend potassium supplementation even if the serum concentration is normal.

The safety and efficacy of these recommended therapies for drug-induced polymorphic VT has not been established by higher levels of research. From the perspective of evidence-based guidelines, we have only lower-level publications of case reports, case series, and extrapolated data. These recommendations, therefore, are Class Indeterminate. This class neither prohibits nor encourages clinical use. It merely acknowledges that many toxicology approaches are "best guesses."

Drug-Induced Impaired Conduction

Poisoning with membrane-stabilizing agents prolongs ventricular conduction (increases QRS interval). This predisposes the heart to monomorphic VT. Hypertonic saline and systemic alkalinization often reverse the adverse electrophysiological effects. This prevents or terminates VT secondary to poisoning from many types of sodium channel blocking agents.[23] Hypertonic sodium bicarbonate is particularly valuable because it both provides hypertonic saline and induces systemic alkalinization. This appears to benefit several types of poisonings caused by sodium channel blockers (eg, TCA). When hypertonic sodium bicarbonate is used to treat severe poisoning, the goal is an arterial pH of 7.50 to 7.55. Respiratory alkalosis can be used as a temporary measure until the appropriate degree of metabolic alkalosis can be attained with sodium bicarbonate. Establish systemic alkalinization to the target arterial pH with repetitive boluses of 1 to 2 mEq/kg sodium bicarbonate. Maintain the alkalinization via a titrated infusion of an alkaline solution consisting of 3 ampules of sodium bicarbonate (150 mEq) and KCl (30 mEq) in 850 mL of D_5W.

Drug-Induced Shock

Drug-induced shock usually results when the drug induces decreases in intravascular volume, falls in systemic vascular resistance (SVR), diminished myocardial contractility, or a combination of these factors.

Drug-Induced Hypovolemic Shock

Initial treatment of drug-induced shock usually includes a fluid challenge to correct hypovolemia and to optimize preload. If the offending agent is cardiotoxic, it will reduce the patient's ability to tolerate a high intravascular volume and may lead to iatrogenic congestive heart failure. If shock persists after an adequate fluid challenge, start a vasopressor. Evidence supports dopamine as the most effective pressor agent in mild to moderate poisoning.[24] Most patients with drug-induced shock have decreased contractility and low SVR. Empirical treatment of dopamine-resistant shock with more potent vasopressors is based on the assumption that decreased SVR is present.

When drug-induced shock is unresponsive to volume loading and conventional doses of vasopressors, high-dose vasopressors are indicated. If possible, establish central hemodynamic monitoring using a Swan-Ganz catheter before starting high-dose vasopressors. But do not delay vasopressor therapy to have a central monitoring line in place. Optimize cardiac preload quickly. Then use cardiac output (CO) and SVR to guide vasopressor and inotrope selection.

Drug-Induced Distributive Shock

When CO is normal or high and SVR is low (distributive shock), more potent vasoconstriction (ie, a greater α-adrenergic effect as produced by norepinephrine or phenylephrine) is needed. Dobutamine and isoproterenol decrease SVR and are contraindicated. The dose of an α-adrenergic–selective vasopressor should be increased until the shock is adequately treated or adverse effects such as ventricular arrhythmias are observed. Some patients require doses of vasopressors far above the usual doses. Use of powerful vasoconstrictors such as vasopressin or endothelin in cases of severe poisoning has not been well studied but may be considered if ventricular arrhythmia develops before the shock is adequately treated.

Drug-Induced Cardiogenic Shock

In cases of drug-induced shock characterized by low CO and high SVR (cardiogenic shock) or low SVR (typical drug-induced shock), inotropic agents are often required. Agents to choose from include calcium, amrinone, glucagon, insulin, isoproterenol, and dobutamine. Sometimes more than one agent is necessary.[25,26] Although these agents may increase contractility and CO, they may also decrease SVR. A concomitant vasopressor is often required.[27]

Drug-Induced Cardiac Arrest

Cardioversion/Defibrillation

Electrical cardioversion or defibrillation is appropriate for pulseless patients with drug-induced VT or VF. In cases of sympathomimetic poisoning with refractory VF, the cost-benefit ratio of epinephrine in management is unknown. If epinephrine is used in such cases, increase the interval between doses and use only standard dose amounts (1 mg IV). Avoid high-dose epinephrine. Furthermore, propranolol is contraindicated in sympathomimetic poisoning, on the basis of limited human studies in the cardiac catheterization suite and limited animal survival studies.

Prolonged CPR and Resuscitation

In ACLS, cardiac resuscitation is usually terminated after 20 to 30 minutes unless there are signs that the central nervous system is viable. More prolonged CPR and resuscitation are warranted in poisoned patients. Cerebral blood flow drops dramatically with prolonged CPR in animal models of cardiac arrest. Nevertheless, in cases of severe poisoning, recovery with good neurological outcomes has occasionally been reported in patients who received prolonged CPR, sometimes for up to 3 to 5 hours.[28,29] The marked vasodilatation associated with many types of severe poisonings may explain these observations.

Circulatory Assist Devices

Intra-aortic balloon pumps and cardiopulmonary bypass circuits are circulatory assist devices that have been used successfully in cases of critical poisoning. Because these techniques are expensive, personnel intensive, and associated with significant morbidity, they should be used only in cases refractory to *maximal* medical care. A disadvantage of the intra-aortic balloon pump is the need for an intrinsic cardiac rhythm for synchronization and diastolic augmentation.

Emergency cardiopulmonary bypass does not require an intrinsic rhythm. Recent technological advances have made rapid application through peripheral vessels possible. To be effective, circulatory assist devices must be used rapidly (ie, before the irreversible effects of severe shock occur).

Brain Death and Organ Donation Criteria

Electroencephalographic and neurological criteria for brain death are not valid during acute toxic encephalopathy and can be applied only when drug concentrations are no longer toxic. In the presence of toxic drug concentrations the only valid criterion for brain death is the absence of cerebral blood flow. Successful transplantation of organs from victims of fatal poisoning with acetaminophen, cyanide, methanol, and carbon monoxide has been reported.[30] Transplantation of organs from victims poisoned with agents capable of severe end-organ damage (eg, carbon monoxide, cocaine, and iron) is controversial but may be appropriate if the donor is thoroughly evaluated.

Summary

Use of standard ACLS protocols for all patients who are critically poisoned may not result in an optimal outcome. Care of severely poisoned patients can be enhanced by urgent consultation with a medical toxicologist. Alternative approaches required in severely poisoned patients include

- Higher doses than usual
- Drugs that are rarely used to treat cardiac arrest (amrinone, calcium, esmolol, glucagon, insulin, labetalol, phenylephrine, physostigmine, and sodium bicarbonate)
- Heroic measures, such as prolonged CPR and use of circulatory assist devices

When resuscitation is unsuccessful, organ donation may still be an option.

References

1. Litovitz TL, Felberg L, White S, et al. 1995 Annual Report of the American Association of Poison Control Centers Toxic Exposure Surveillance System. *Am J Emerg Med.* 1996;14:487–537.
2. McCaig LF, Burt CW. Poisoning-related visits to emergency departments in the United States, 1993–1996. *J Toxicol Clin Toxicol.* 1999;37:817–826.
3. Fingerhut LA, Cox CS. Poisoning mortality, 1985–1995. *Public Health Rep.* 1998;113:221–235.
4. American Academy of Clinical Toxicology. Facility assessment guidelines for regional toxicology treatment centers. *J Toxicol Clin Toxicol.* 1993;31:211–217.
5. American College of Emergency Physicians. Poison information and treatment systems. *Ann Emerg Med.* 1996;28:384.
6. Vale JA, for the American Academy of Clinical Toxicology; European Association of Poisons Centres and Clinical Toxicologists. Position statement: gastric lavage. *J Toxicol Clin Toxicol.* 1997;35:711–719.
7. Moss ST, Chan TC, Buchanan J, et al. Outcome study of prehospital patients signed out against medical advice by field paramedics. *Ann Emerg Med.* 1998;31:247–250.
8. Vilke GM, Buchanan J, Dunford JV, et al. Are heroin overdose deaths related to patient release after prehospital treatment with naloxone? *Prehosp Emerg Care.* 1999;3:183–186.
9. Antman EM, Wenger TL, Butler VP Jr, et al. Treatment of 150 cases of life-threatening digitalis intoxication with digoxin-specific Fab antibody fragments: final report of a multicenter study. *Circulation.* 1990;81:1744–1752.
10. Ramoska E, Sacchetti AD. Propranolol-induced hypertension in treatment of cocaine intoxication. *Ann Emerg Med.* 1985;14:1112–1113.

11. Brogan WC, Lange RA, Kim AS, et al. Alleviation of cocaine-induced coronary vasoconstriction by nitroglycerin. *J Am Coll Cardiol.* 1991;18: 581–586.

12. Lange RA, Cigarroa RG, Clyde WY, et al. Cocaine-induced coronary-artery vasoconstriction. *N Engl J Med.* 1989;321:1557–1562.

13. Boehrer JD, Moliterno DJ, Willard JE, et al. Influence of labetalol on cocaine-induced coronary vasoconstriction in humans. *Am J Med.* 1993; 94:608–610.

14. Lange RA, Cigarroa RG, Flores ED, et al. Potentiation of cocaine-induced coronary vasoconstriction by beta-adrenergic blockade. *Ann Intern Med.* 1990;112:897–903.

15. Gay GR, Loper KA. The use of labetalol in the management of cocaine crisis. *Ann Emerg Med.* 1988;17:282–283.

16. Dusenberry SJ, Hicks MJ, Mariani PJ. Labetalol treatment of cocaine toxicity. *Ann Emerg Med.* 1987;16:235.

17. Sand C, Brody SL, Wrenn KD, et al. Experience with esmolol for the treatment of cocaine-associated cardiovascular complications. *Am J Emerg Med.* 1991;9:161–163.

18. Shih RD, Hollander JE, Burstein JL, et al. Clinical safety of lidocaine in patients with cocaine-associated myocardial infarction. *Ann Emerg Med.* 1995;26:702–706.

19. Mayron R, Ruiz E. Phenytoin: does it reverse tricyclic-antidepressant-induced cardiac conduction abnormalities? *Ann Emerg Med.* 1986;15: 876–880.

20. Callaham M, Schumaker H, Pentel P. Phenytoin prophylaxis of cardiotoxicity in experimental amitriptyline poisoning. *J Pharmacol Exp Ther.* 1988;245:216–220.

21. Knudsen K, Abrahamsson J. Effects of magnesium sulfate and lidocaine in the treatment of ventricular arrhythmias in experimental amitriptyline poisoning in the rat. *Crit Care Med.* 1994;22:494–498.

22. Kline JA, DeStefano AA, Schroeder JD, et al. Magnesium potentiates imipramine toxicity in the isolated rat heart. *Ann Emerg Med.* 1994;24: 224–232.

23. Brown TCK. Tricyclic antidepressant overdosage: experimental studies on the management of circulatory complications. *Clin Toxicol.* 1976;9: 255–272.

24. Vernon DD, Banner W Jr, Garrett JS. Efficacy of dopamine and norepinephrine for treatment of hemodynamic compromise in amitriptyline intoxication. *Crit Care Med.* 1991;19:544–549.

25. Love JN, Leasure JA, Mundt DJ. A comparison of combined amrinone and glucagon therapy to glucagon alone for cardiovascular depression associated with propranolol toxicity in a canine model. *Am J Emerg Med.* 1993;11:360–363.

26. Wolf LR, Spadafora MP, Otten EJ. Use of amrinone and glucagon in a case of calcium channel blocker overdose. *Ann Emerg Med.* 1993;22: 1225–1228.

27. Kollef MH. Labetalol overdose successfully treated with amrinone and alpha-adrenergic receptor agonists. *Chest.* 1994;105:626–627.

28. Ramsay ID. Survival after imipramine poisoning. *Lancet.* 1967;2: 1308–1309.

29. Southall DR, Kilpatrick SM. Imipramine poisoning: survival of a child after prolonged cardiac massage. *BMJ.* 1974;4:508.

30. Hebert MJ, Boucher A, Beaugage G, et al. Transplantation of kidneys from donor with carbon monoxide poisoning. *N Engl J Med.* 1992;326:1571.

Section 3: Special Challenges in ECC

Hypothermia

Definition/Background

Severe hypothermia (body temperature below 30°C [86°F]) is associated with marked depression of cerebral blood flow and oxygen requirement, reduced cardiac output, and decreased arterial pressure.[1] Victims can appear to be clinically dead because of marked depression of brain function.[1,2]

Hypothermia may exert a protective effect on the brain and organs in cardiac arrest.[3,4] If the victim cools rapidly without hypoxemia, decreased oxygen consumption and metabolism may precede the arrest and reduce organ ischemia.[5] Although rare, full resuscitation with intact neurological recovery may be possible after hypothermic cardiac arrest.[1,6] .

The victim's pulses and respiratory efforts may be difficult to detect, but do not withhold lifesaving procedures on the basis of clinical presentation.[1] Transport victims as soon as possible to a center where monitored rewarming is possible.

Severe unintentional hypothermia is a serious and preventable health problem. Hypothermia in inner-city areas has a high association with mental illness, poverty, and use of drugs and alcohol.[7,8] In some rural areas >90% of hypothermic deaths are associated with elevated blood alcohol levels.[9] Successful treatment of hypothermia requires optimal training of emergency personnel and appropriate resuscitation methods at each institution.

The Figure presents a recommended hypothermia treatment algorithm with recommended actions that should be taken for all possible victims of hypothermia.

Prevention of Arrest in Victims of Hypothermia: General Care for All Victims of Hypothermia

When the victim is extremely cold but has maintained a perfusing rhythm, interventions focus on prevention of further heat loss, careful transport, and rewarming:

- Prevent additional evaporative heat loss by removing wet garments, insulating the victim, and shielding the victim from wind.
- Carefully transport the victim to the hospital, taking care to avoid rough movement and activity, because these can precipitate VF.
- Monitor core temperature and cardiac rhythm. If the victim's skin is extremely cold, it may not be possible to obtain an ECG or monitor cardiac rhythm by use of adhesive electrodes. If necessary, needle electrodes may be used.

- Do not delay urgently needed procedures such as intubation or insertion of vascular catheters, but perform them gently and monitor cardiac rhythm closely.

Rewarm patients with a core temperature of <34°C (<93°F). Passive rewarming can be achieved with blankets and a warm room. This form of rewarming will not be effective for a patient in cardiopulmonary arrest or with severe hypothermia.[5]

Active external rewarming uses heating devices (radiant heat, forced hot air, or warm bath water) or heated devices (warm packs). These devices require careful monitoring of patient and device and should be used with caution, if at all. Some researchers think that active external rewarming contributes to "afterdrop" (continued drop in core temperature when cold blood from the periphery is mobilized). In addition, topical application of warm devices may result in tissue injury. If they are used, heated packs should be applied and only to truncal areas (neck, armpits, or groin).

Active internal rewarming techniques typically are reserved for patients with a core body temperature <30°C (86°F). They may include the administration of warmed (42°C to 46°C [108°F to 115°F]) humidified oxygen, use of extracorporeal membrane oxygenators, peritoneal lavage, intravenous administration of warmed (42°C to 44°C [108°F to 111°F]) saline, and esophageal rewarming tubes. No randomized, controlled clinical trials have been reported comparing the efficacy of these methods.[5]

Modifications of BLS for Hypothermia

When the victim is hypothermic, pulse and respiratory rates will be slow, breathing will be shallow, and peripheral vasoconstriction will make pulses difficult to feel. For these reasons the BLS rescuer should assess breathing and, later, pulse for a period of 30 to 45 seconds to confirm respiratory arrest, pulseless cardiac arrest, or bradycardia profound enough to require CPR.[2] If the victim is not breathing, initiate rescue breathing immediately. If possible, administer warmed (42°C to 46°C [108°F to 115°F]) humidified oxygen during bag-mask ventilation. If the victim is pulseless with no detectable signs of circulation, start chest compressions immediately. Do not withhold BLS until the victim is rewarmed.

To prevent further core heat loss from the victim, remove wet garments from the victim; insulate or shield the victim from wind, heat, or cold; and if possible ventilate with warm, humidified oxygen.[1,2,10] Avoid rough movement and do not apply external rewarming devices in the field. As soon as possible, carefully prepare the patient for transport to a

Circulation. 2000;102(suppl I):I-229–I-232.
© 2000 American Heart Association, Inc.

Circulation is available at http://www.circulationaha.org

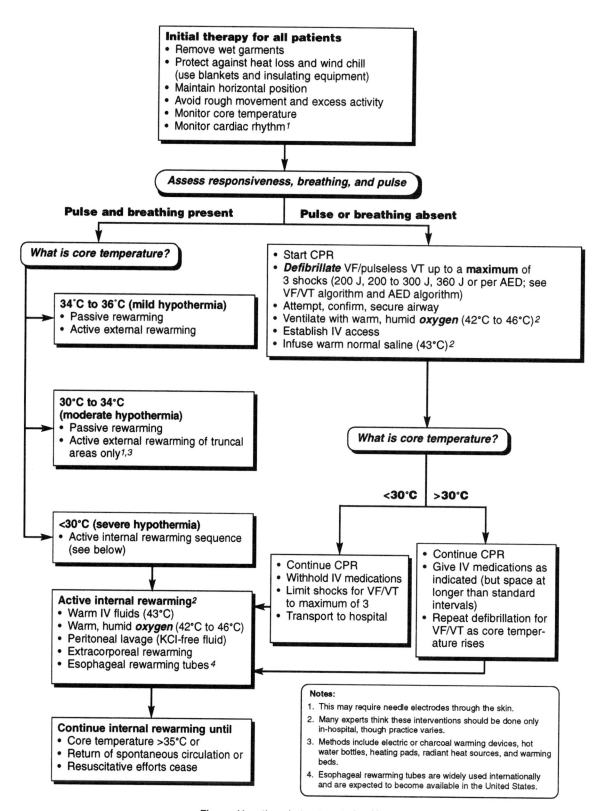

Figure. Hypothermia treatment algorithm.

hospital. All other field interventions require ACLS capability.

Treatment of severe hypothermia (temperature <30°C [86°F]) in the field remains controversial. Many providers do not have the equipment or time to assess core body temperature adequately or to institute rewarming with warm, humid-

ified oxygen or warm fluids, although these methods should be initiated when available to help prevent temperature afterdrop.[1,10–12] We recommend core temperature determinations in the field with either tympanic membrane sensors or rectal probes (for EMS systems so equipped), but these should not delay transfer. To prevent VF, avoid rough movement and excess activity. Transport the patient in the horizontal position to avoid aggravating hypotension.

If the hypothermic victim is in cardiac arrest, the general approach to BLS management still targets airway, breathing, and circulation, but some modifications in approach are required. If VT or VF is present, attempt defibrillation. Automated external defibrillators (AEDs) should be available on virtually all BLS rescue units, and if VF is detected, emergency personnel should be allowed to deliver up to 3 shocks to determine fibrillation responsiveness.[2] If VF persists after 3 shocks, further defibrillation attempts should be deferred. Emergency personnel should immediately begin CPR and rewarming (administer warmed, humidified oxygen and warmed intravenous saline) and attempt to stabilize the victim for transportation. If core temperature is <30°C (86°F), successful conversion to normal sinus rhythm may not be possible until rewarming is accomplished.[13]

Some clinicians believe that patients who appear dead after prolonged exposure to cold temperatures should not be considered dead until they are near normal core temperature and are still unresponsive to CPR.[2,13] Hypothermia may exert a protective effect on the brain and organs if the hypothermia develops rapidly in victims of cardiac arrest. When a victim of hypothermia is discovered, however, it may be impossible to separate primary from secondary hypothermia. If the victim is found in arrest in an extremely cold environment and the event was unwitnessed, emergency personnel and hospital providers will not know whether the arrest was due to hypothermia or whether hypothermia was a sequel to a normothermic arrest (eg, a man experiencing cardiac arrest while shoveling snow will develop hypothermia only after the arrest). In addition, the patient may have sustained additional organ insult. For example, successful resuscitation may be more difficult if drowning preceded hypothermia. When it is clinically impossible to know whether the arrest or the hypothermia occurred first, rescuers should attempt to stabilize the patient with CPR. If hypothermia is documented, initiate basic maneuvers to limit heat loss and begin rewarming. Physicians in the hospital should use their clinical judgment to decide when resuscitative efforts should cease in a hypothermic arrest victim.

Modifications of ACLS for Hypothermia

If the hypothermic victim has not yet developed cardiac arrest, focus attention on assessment and support of oxygenation and ventilation, assessment and support of circulation, warming, and prevention of further heat loss. Handle the victim gently for all procedures; many physical manipulations (including endotracheal or nasogastric intubation, temporary pacing, or insertion of a pulmonary artery catheter) have been reported to precipitate VF.[1,12] When specifically and urgently indicated, however, do not withhold such procedures. In a prospective multicenter study of hypothermia victims, careful endotracheal intubation did not result in a single incident of VF.[14] In fact, the fear of precipitating VF during endotracheal intubation may be exaggerated,[5] and it should not prevent or delay performance of careful intubation.

Endotracheal intubation is required if the hypothermic victim is unconscious or if ventilation is inadequate. The intubation will serve 2 purposes: it will enable provision of effective ventilation with warm, humidified oxygen, and it can isolate the airway to reduce the likelihood of aspiration. We recommend ventilation with 100% oxygen via bag-mask before any intubation attempt.

Conscious victims who are cold with only mild symptoms of hypothermia may be rewarmed with external active and passive rewarming techniques (eg, warm packs, warmed sleeping bags, and warm baths).

ACLS management of cardiac arrest due to hypothermia is quite different from management of normothermic arrest. Active core rewarming techniques are the primary therapeutic modality in hypothermic victims in cardiac arrest or unconscious with a slow heart rate. The hypothermic heart may be unresponsive to cardioactive drugs, pacemaker stimulation, and defibrillation,[12] and drug metabolism is reduced. Although administration of epinephrine and vasopressin has been shown to improve coronary artery perfusion pressure in animals,[15] there is concern that administered medications, including epinephrine, lidocaine, and procainamide, can accumulate to toxic levels in the peripheral circulation if they are administered repeatedly in the severely hypothermic victim. For these reasons intravenous drugs are often withheld if the victim's core body temperature is <30°C (86°F). If the victim's core body temperature is >30°C (86°F), intravenous medications may be administered but with increased intervals between doses.

The temperature at which defibrillation should first be attempted and how often it should be tried in the severely hypothermic patient have not been firmly established. In general, an attempt at defibrillation is appropriate if VT/VF is present. If the patient fails to respond to 3 initial defibrillation attempts or initial drug therapy, subsequent defibrillation attempts or additional boluses of medication should be deferred until the core temperature rises above 30°C (86°F).[16] Bradycardia may be physiological in severe hypothermia, and cardiac pacing is usually not indicated unless bradycardia persists after rewarming.

Treatment of severely hypothermic victims (core temperature <30°C [86°F]) in cardiac arrest in the hospital should be directed at rapid core rewarming. Techniques that can be used for in-hospital controlled rewarming include

- Administration of warmed, humidified oxygen (42°C to 46°C [108°F to 115°F])
- Administration of warmed intravenous fluids (normal saline) at 43°C (109°F) infused centrally at rates of approximately 150 to 200 mL/h (to avoid overhydration)
- Peritoneal lavage with warmed (43°C [109°F]) potassium-free fluid administered 2 L at a time

Note the following:

- Extracorporeal blood warming with partial bypass is the preferred method of active internal rewarming because it ensures adequate support of oxygenation and ventilation while the core body temperature is gradually rewarmed.[1,10,12,17,18]

- The use of esophageal rewarming tubes in the United States has not been reported, although they have been used extensively and successfully in Europe.[19]
- Pleural lavage with warm saline instilled through a chest tube has also been used successfully.[14]

During rewarming, patients who have been hypothermic for >45 to 60 minutes are likely to require volume administration because their vascular space expands with vasodilation. Careful monitoring of heart rate and hemodynamic monitoring are important at this time. The routine administration of steroids, barbiturates, or antibiotics has not been documented to help increase survival or decrease postresuscitative damage.[20,21]

During rewarming, significant hyperkalemia may develop. Extreme hyperkalemia has been reported in avalanche victims who sustained crushing injuries and hypothermia.[5] Severe hyperkalemia has also been reported among hypothermic patients in North America who did not sustain crushing injuries.[22] In fact, severity of hyperkalemia has been linked with mortality. Management of hyperkalemia should include the traditional ACLS approach, with administration of calcium chloride, sodium bicarbonate, glucose plus insulin, and Kayexalate enema. More aggressive measures to reduce extremely high serum potassium may include dialysis or exchange transfusion.

If drowning preceded the victim's hypothermia, successful resuscitation will be rare. Because severe hypothermia is frequently preceded by other disorders (eg, drug overdose, alcohol use, or trauma), the clinician must look for and treat these underlying conditions while simultaneously treating the hypothermia. If the victim appears malnourished or has a history of chronic alcoholism, administer thiamine (100 mg IV) early during the rewarming procedures.

Withholding and Cessation of Resuscitative Efforts

In the field, resuscitation may be withheld if the victim has obvious lethal injuries or if the body is frozen so completely that chest compression is impossible and the nose and mouth are blocked with ice.[22]

Physicians in the hospital should use their clinical judgment to decide when resuscitative efforts should cease in a hypothermic arrest victim. Complete rewarming is not indicated for all victims. Predictors of outcome may be unreliable in the face of injury or other complicating factors. A high (nonhemolyzed) serum potassium has been associated with a poor outcome, but these results will be unreliable in the presence of crushing injuries, hemolysis, or succinylcholine administration.[5]

References

1. Schneider SM. Hypothermia: from recognition to rewarming. *Emerg Med Rep.* 1992;13:1–20.
2. Steinman AM. Cardiopulmonary resuscitation and hypothermia. *Circulation.* 1986;74(suppl IV):IV-29–IV-32.
3. Holzer M, Behringer W, Schorkhuber W, Zeiner A, Sterz F, Laggner AN, Frass M, Siostrozonek P, Ratheiser K, Kaff A, Hypothermia for Cardiac Arrest (HACA) Study Group. Mild hypothermia and outcome after CPR. *Acta Anaesthesiol Scand Suppl.* 1997;111:55–58.
4. Sterz F, Safar P, Tisherman S, Radovsky A, Kuboyama K, Oku K. Mild hypothermic cardiopulmonary resuscitation improves outcome after prolonged cardiac arrest in dogs [see comments]. *Crit Care Med.* 1991;19:379–389.
5. Larach MG. Accidental hypothermia [see comments]. *Lancet.* 1995;345:493–498.
6. Gilbert M, Busund R, Skagseth A, Nilsen PA, Solbo JP. Resuscitation from accidental hypothermia of 13.7 degrees C with circulatory arrest. *Lancet.* 2000;355:375–376. Letter.
7. Woodhouse P, Keatinge WR, Coleshaw SR. Factors associated with hypothermia in patients admitted to a group of inner city hospitals [see comments]. *Lancet.* 1989;2:1201–1205.
8. Danzl DF, Pozos RS, Auerbach PS, Glazer S, Goetz W, Johnson E, Jui J, Lilja P, Marx JA, Miller J, et al. Multicenter hypothermia survey. *Ann Emerg Med.* 1987;16:1042–1055.
9. Gallaher MM, Fleming DW, Berger LR, Sewell CM. Pedestrian and hypothermia deaths among Native Americans in New Mexico: between bar and home [published erratum appears in *JAMA.* 1992;268:2378] [see comments]. *JAMA.* 1992;267:1345–1348.
10. Weinberg AD, Hamlet MP, Paturas JL, White RD, McAninch GW. *Cold Weather Emergencies: Principles of Patient Management.* Branford, Conn: American Medical Publishing Co; 1990:10–30.
11. Romet TT. Mechanism of afterdrop after cold water immersion. *J Appl Physiol.* 1988;65:1535–1538.
12. Reuler JB. Hypothermia: pathophysiology, clinical settings, and management. *Ann Intern Med.* 1978;89:519–527.
13. Southwick FS, Dalglish PH Jr. Recovery after prolonged asystolic cardiac arrest in profound hypothermia: a case report and literature review. *JAMA.* 1980;243:1250–1253.
14. Hall KN, Syverud SA. Closed thoracic cavity lavage in the treatment of severe hypothermia in human beings [see comments]. *Ann Emerg Med.* 1990;19:204–206.
15. Krismer AC, Lindner KH, Kornberger R, Wenzel V, Mueller G, Hund W, Oroszy S, Lurie KG, Mair P. Cardiopulmonary resuscitation during severe hypothermia in pigs: does epinephrine or vasopressin increase coronary perfusion pressure? *Anesth Analg.* 2000;90:69–73.
16. Reuler JB. Hypothermia: pathophysiology, clinical settings, and management. *Ann Intern Med.* 1978;89:519–527.
17. Zell SC, Kurtz KJ. Severe exposure hypothermia: a resuscitation protocol. *Ann Emerg Med.* 1985;14:339–345.
18. Althaus U, Aeberhard P, Schupbach P, Nachbur BH, Muhlemann W. Management of profound accidental hypothermia with cardiorespiratory arrest. *Ann Surg.* 1982;195:492–495.
19. Kristensen G, Drenck NE, Jordening H. Simple system for central rewarming of hypothermic patients. *Lancet.* 1986;2:1467–1468. Letter.
20. Moss J. Accidental severe hypothermia. *Surg Gynecol Obstet.* 1986;162:501–513.
21. Safar P. Cerebral resuscitation after cardiac arrest: research initiatives and future directions [published erratum appears in *Ann Emerg Med.* 1993;22:759] [see comments]. *Ann Emerg Med.* 1993;22:324–349.
22. Danzl DF, Pozos RS, Auerbach PS, Glazer S, Goetz W, Johnson E, Jui J, Lilja P, Marx JA, Miller J, et al. Multicenter hypothermia survey. *Ann Emerg Med.* 1987;16:1042–1055.

Submersion or Near-Drowning

Submersion: Overview

The most important and detrimental consequence of submersion without ventilation is hypoxia. The duration of hypoxia is the critical factor in determining the victim's outcome. Therefore, oxygenation, ventilation, and perfusion should be restored as rapidly as possible. Immediate resuscitation at the scene is essential for survival and neurological recovery after submersion. This will require bystander provision of CPR plus immediate activation of the EMS system. Victims who have spontaneous circulation and breathing when they reach the hospital usually recover with good outcomes.

Hypoxia can produce multisystem insult and complications, including hypoxic encephalopathy and acute respiratory distress syndrome (ARDS). These complications are relevant to the care of the victim after resuscitation and will not be addressed here.

Victims of submersion may develop primary or secondary hypothermia. If the submersion occurs in icy water ($<5°C$ [41°F]), hypothermia may develop rapidly and provide some protection against hypoxia. Such effects, however, have typically been reported only after submersion of *small* victims in *icy* water.[1] Hypothermia may also develop as a secondary complication of the submersion and subsequent heat loss through evaporation during attempted resuscitation. In these victims the hypothermia is not protective (see Hypothermia earlier in this section).

All victims of submersion who require resuscitation should be transported to the hospital for evaluation and monitoring. The hypoxic insult can produce an increase in pulmonary capillary permeability with resultant pulmonary edema.

Definitions, Classifications, and Prognostic Indicators

A number of terms are used to describe submersion. Clinicians and others who report about submersion often apply the misunderstood term *drowning* to victims *who die within 24 hours of a submersion episode*. They apply the term *near-drowning* to submersion victims who survive >24 hours after the episode if the victim also requires active intervention for one or more submersion complications. Complications can include pneumonia, ARDS, or neurological sequelae. Rescuers and emergency personnel find these definitions irrelevant, because the drowning versus near-drowning distinction often cannot be made for 24 hours.

Pending the future recommendations of an ILCOR Task Force revising the Utstein Guidelines, the Guidelines 2000 Conference recommends these terms:

Water rescue: a person who is alert but experiences some distress while swimming. The victim may receive some help from others and displays minimal, transient symptoms, such as coughing, that clear quickly. In general the person is left on shore and is not transported for further evaluation and care.

Submersion: a person who experiences some swimming-related distress that is sufficient to require support in the field plus transportation to an emergency facility for further observation and treatment.

Drowning: this is a "mortal" event; this refers to submersion events in which the victim is pronounced dead at the scene of the attempted resuscitation, in the Emergency Department (ED), or in the hospital. With drowning, the victim suffers cardiopulmonary arrest and cannot be resuscitated. Death can be pronounced at the scene, in the ED, or within 24 hours of the event. If death occurs after 24 hours, the term *drowning* is still used as in "drowning-related death." Up until the time of drowning-related death, refer to the victim as a *submersion victim*.

We recommend that the term *near-drowning* no longer be used.

We recommend that clinicians, managers, and research teams stop the classification of submersion victims by submersion fluid (salt water versus fresh water). Although there are theoretical differences between the effects of salt-water and fresh-water submersion in the laboratory, these differences are not clinically significant. The single most important factor that determines outcome of submersion is the duration of the submersion and the duration and severity of the hypoxia.

Although survival is uncommon in victims who have undergone prolonged submersion and require prolonged resuscitation,[2,3] successful resuscitation with full neurological recovery has occasionally occurred in near-drowning victims with prolonged submersion in extremely cold water.[4–6] Therefore, resuscitation should be initiated by rescuers at the scene unless there is obvious physical evidence of death, such as putrefaction, dependent lividity, or rigor mortis. The victim should be transported with continued CPR to an emergency facility. In many European countries a physician will be available on scene as part of the EMS team.

Prognostic indicators after submersion in children and adolescents (up to 20 years of age) include 3 factors associated with 100% mortality in one study[1]:

- Submersion duration >25 minutes
- Resuscitation duration >25 minutes
- Pulseless cardiac arrest on arrival in the ED

Additional factors associated with poor prognosis in the same study[1] included

- Presence of VT/VF on initial ECG (93% mortality)
- Fixed pupils noted in the ED (89% mortality)
- Severe acidosis (89% mortality) in the ED
- Respiratory arrest (87% mortality) in the ED
- In a more recent study of adults and children from the same investigators, level of consciousness and responsiveness correlated with survival. Deaths occurred only among victims who remained comatose at the scene and comatose on arrival at the hospital. No deaths occurred among victims who were alert or lethargic but responsive either at the scene or in the hospital.[7]
- A number of classification systems have been proposed to link clinical findings with outcome of submersion victims.[8,9] In a

Circulation. 2000;102(suppl I):I-233–I-236.
© 2000 American Heart Association, Inc.

Circulation is available at http://www.circulationaha.org

TABLE. Clinical Factors Associated With Submersion Mortality

Classification Grade	Definition	Mortality, %[9]
1	Normal pulmonary auscultation, with coughing	0
2	Abnormal pulmonary auscultation, with rales in some fields	0.6
3	Pulmonary auscultation=acute pulmonary edema; no arterial hypotension	5.2
4	Acute pulmonary edema with arterial hypotension	19.4
5	Isolated respiratory arrest	44
6	Cardiopulmonary arrest	93

recent analysis of 1831 submersion episodes from the beaches of Brazil, mortality was related to severity of cardiopulmonary involvement as assessed by an on-scene physician with the drowning response team needing only 4 variables: coughing (yes or no), auscultation, blood pressure, and heart rate. Unlike other researchers in this area, Szpilman[9] did not start with an implicitly derived classification scheme into which he forces each case. Instead, the classification grades were derived retrospectively by asking what simple list of criteria had the best association with severe pulmonary compromise. As displayed in the Table, increasing mortality correlated with ascending grades of clinical severity.[9]

- Auscultation of breath sounds will not be applicable to the BLS provider. For the ACLS provider, however, auscultatory findings provide a helpful classification of the severity of cardiopulmonary failure after submersion. The algorithm we have developed (Figure) is largely a translation of Szpilman's results and an algorithm he derived in a manner that can be used by epidemiologists to support a prospective database of submersion victims.

- Any prognostic approach should consider the temperature of the submersion fluid (icy versus nonicy) and the size and age of the victim. Aggressive attempts at resuscitation in the hospital may be continued for the small victim of icy-water submersion and hypothermia.

Modifications to Guidelines for BLS for Resuscitation From Submersion

No modification of standard BLS sequencing is necessary. There are, however, cautions and emphasis that should be considered when beginning CPR for the submersion victim.

Recovery From the Water

When attempting to rescue a near-drowning victim, the rescuer should get to the victim as quickly as possible, preferably by some conveyance (boat, raft, surfboard, or flotation device). The rescuer must always be aware of personal safety and should minimize the danger to the rescuer and the victim. Treat all victims as potential victims of spinal cord injury, and immobilize the cervical and thoracic spine. Spinal injury is particularly likely after submersion associated with diving or involving recreational equipment, but it should be suspected if the submersion episode was not witnessed.

If first-responding rescuers suspect a spinal cord injury, they should use their hands to stabilize the victim's neck in a neutral position (without flexion or extension). They should float the victim, supine, onto a horizontal back support device before removing the victim from the water. The rescue from the water should be done quickly to ensure timely application of CPR if required. If the victim

must be turned, align and support the head, neck, chest, and body. Carefully log-roll the victim to a horizontal and supine position. Provide rescue breathing while maintaining the head in a neutral position, using the jaw thrust without head tilt or chin lift to open the airway.

Rescue breathing should begin as quickly as possible (see below). Provision of chest compression typically will have to wait until the victim has been removed from the water. External chest compressions cannot be performed in the water unless the victim is extremely small and can be supported on the rescuer's forearm or unless flotation devices are used. Proper use of in-water resuscitation flotation devices requires training.

Rescue Breathing

The first and most important treatment of the near-drowning victim is provision of immediate mouth-to-mouth ventilation. Prompt initiation of rescue breathing has a positive association with survival.[10]

Start rescue breathing as soon as the victim's airway can be opened and the rescuer's safety ensured. This is usually achieved when the victim is in shallow water or out of the water. If it is difficult for the rescuer to pinch the victim's nose and support the head and open the airway in the water, mouth-to-nose ventilation may be used as an alternative to mouth-to-mouth ventilation.

Appliances (such as a snorkel for the mouth-to-snorkel technique or buoyancy aids) may permit specially trained rescuers to perform rescue breathing in deep water. But rescue breathing should not be delayed for lack of such equipment if it can otherwise be provided safely. Untrained rescuers should not attempt to use such adjuncts.

Management of the airway and breathing of the submersion victim is similar to that of any victim with potential trauma in cardiopulmonary arrest. The airway can be managed with adjuncts in the near-drowning victim.[2,11]

There is no need to clear the airway of aspirated water.[12] Some victims aspirate nothing because of laryngospasm or breath-holding.[3,8,13] At most only a modest amount of water is aspirated by the majority of drowning victims, and it is rapidly absorbed into the central circulation.[3] An attempt to remove water from the breathing passages by any means other than suction is unnecessary and dangerous. Abdominal thrusts, for example, cause regurgitation of gastric contents and subsequent aspiration and have been associated with other injuries.[12] Do not routinely perform the Heimlich maneuver for resuscitation of submersion victims. It delays the initiation of ventilation and produces complications.[12] Use of the Heimlich maneuver as the first step in resuscitation of submersion victims is not evidence-based. Use the Heimlich maneuver *only* if the rescuer suspects foreign-body airway obstruction.[11,12,14,15] If

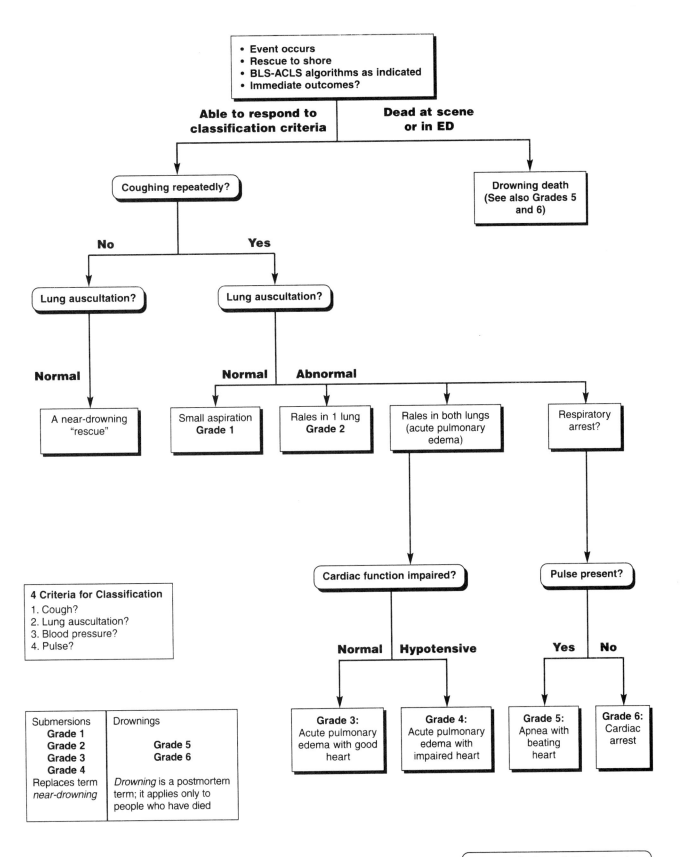

- Event occurs
- Rescue to shore
- BLS-ACLS algorithms as indicated
- Immediate outcomes?

Able to respond to classification criteria

Dead at scene or in ED

Coughing repeatedly?

Drowning death
(See also Grades 5 and 6)

No   **Yes**

Lung auscultation?   **Lung auscultation?**

Normal   **Normal**   **Abnormal**

A near-drowning "rescue"

Small aspiration
Grade 1

Rales in 1 lung
Grade 2

Rales in both lungs
(acute pulmonary edema)

Respiratory arrest?

4 Criteria for Classification
1. Cough?
2. Lung auscultation?
3. Blood pressure?
4. Pulse?

Cardiac function impaired?   **Pulse present?**

Normal   **Hypotensive**   **Yes**   **No**

Submersions	Drownings
Grade 1	
Grade 2	**Grade 5**
Grade 3	**Grade 6**
Grade 4	
Replaces term *near-drowning*	*Drowning* is a postmortem term; it applies only to people who have died

Grade 3:
Acute pulmonary edema with good heart

Grade 4:
Acute pulmonary edema with impaired heart

Grade 5:
Apnea with beating heart

Grade 6:
Cardiac arrest

Based on Szpilman D. Near-drowning and drowning classification; proposal to stratify mortality based on 1,831 cases. *Chest*. 1997;112:660-665.

Figure. Uniform reporting of submersion episodes.

foreign-body airway obstruction is suspected, consider chest compressions rather than the Heimlich maneuver. There is recent evidence that chest compressions are superior to the Heimlich maneuver in generating increases in intrathoracic pressure to assist with the expulsion of foreign material.[16]

Chest Compressions

As soon as the victim is removed from the water, check for signs of circulation. The lay rescuer will look for general signs of circulation (breathing, coughing, or movement in response to the rescue breaths). The healthcare provider will look for signs of circulation, including the presence of a central pulse. The pulse may be difficult to appreciate in a near-drowning victim, particularly if the victim is cold. If signs of circulation (including a pulse, if appropriate) are not present, start chest compressions at once. Chest compressions should not be attempted in the water.

If there are no signs of circulation, an AED should be used to evaluate rhythm for victims older than 8 years of age. Attempt defibrillation if a shockable rhythm is identified. If hypothermia is present in a victim of VF and the victim's core body temperature is ≤30°C (86°F), give a maximum of 3 defibrillation attempts (shocks). If a total of 3 defibrillation attempts are unsuccessful, return to BLS and ACLS care until the core body temperature rises above 30°C (86°F).

Vomiting During Resuscitation

Vomiting is likely to occur when chest compressions or rescue breathing is performed, and it will complicate efforts to maintain a patent airway. In fact, in a 10-year study in Australia, vomiting occurred in half of submersion victims who required no interventions after removal from the water. Vomiting occurred in two thirds of victims who received rescue breathing and 86% of victims who required compression and ventilation.[17] If vomiting occurs, turn the victim's mouth to the side and remove the vomitus with the finger sweep or use a cloth to wipe the mouth or use suction. If spinal cord injury is possible, log-roll the victim so that the head, neck, and torso are turned as a unit to remove the vomitus.

Modifications to Guidelines for ACLS for Arrest After Submersion

The submersion victim in cardiac arrest requires ACLS including intubation without delay. Every submersion victim, even one who requires only minimal resuscitation and regains consciousness at the scene, should be transferred to a medical facility for follow-up care. Monitoring of life support measures must be continued en route with oxygen administered in the transport vehicle.

Victims in cardiac arrest may present with asystole, pulseless electrical activity, or pulseless VT/VF. PALS and ACLS guidelines should be followed for the treatment of these rhythms. If severe hypothermia is present (core body temperature ≤30°C [86°F]), defibrillation attempts are typically limited to 3, and intravenous medications are withheld until the core body temperature rises above these levels. If moderate hypothermia is present, intravenous medications are spaced at longer than standard intervals (see Hypothermia earlier in this section). In children and adolescents, VT/VF on initial ECG is an extremely poor prognostic sign.[1]

Attempts have been made to improve neurological outcome in the intensive care unit with the use of barbiturates, intracranial pressure (ICP) monitoring, induced hypothermia, and steroid administration. None of these interventions has been shown to alter outcome. In fact, signs of ICP serve as a symptom of significant neurological hypoxic injury, and there is no evidence that attempts to alter the ICP will affect outcome.

References

1. Quan L, Kinder D. Pediatric submersions: prehospital predictors of outcome [see comments]. *Pediatrics.* 1992;90:909–913.
2. Quan L, Wentz KR, Gore EJ, Copass MK. Outcome and predictors of outcome in pediatric submersion victims receiving prehospital care in King County, Washington [see comments]. *Pediatrics.* 1990;86:586–593.
3. Modell JH, Davis JH. Electrolyte changes in human drowning victims. *Anesthesiology.* 1969;30:414–420.
4. Southwick FS, Dalglish PH Jr. Recovery after prolonged asystolic cardiac arrest in profound hypothermia: a case report and literature review. *JAMA.* 1980;243:1250–1253.
5. Siebke H, Rod T, Breivik H, Link B. Survival after 40 minutes; submersion without cerebral sequelae. *Lancet.* 1975;1:1275–1277.
6. Bolte RG, Black PG, Bowers RS, Thorne JK, Corneli HM. The use of extracorporeal rewarming in a child submerged for 66 minutes. *JAMA.* 1988;260:377–379.
7. Cummings P, Quan L. Trends in unintentional drowning: the role of alcohol and medical care [see comments]. *JAMA.* 1999;281:2198–2202.
8. Modell J. Drowning. *N Engl J Med.* 1993;328:253–256.
9. Szpilman D. Near-drowning and drowning classification: a proposal to stratify mortality based on the analysis of 1,831 cases. *Chest.* 1997;112:660–665.
10. Kyriacou DN, Arcinue EL, Peek C, Kraus JF. Effect of immediate resuscitation on children with submersion injury. *Pediatrics.* 1994;94:137–142.
11. Heimlich HJ. Subdiaphragmatic pressure to expel water from the lungs of drowning persons. *Ann Emerg Med.* 1981;10:476–480.
12. Rosen P, Stoto M, Harley J. The use of the Heimlich maneuver in near drowning: Institute of Medicine report. *J Emerg Med.* 1995;13:397–405.
13. Deleted in proof.
14. Patrick EA. A case report: The Heimlich maneuver. *Emergency.* 1981;13:45–47.
15. Heimlich HJ. The Heimlich maneuver: first treatment for drowning victims. *Emerg Med Serv.* 1981;10:27–30.
16. Langhelle A, Sunde K, Wik L, Steen PA. Airway pressure with chest compressions versus Heimlich manoeuvre in recently dead adults with complete airway obstruction. *Resuscitation.* 2000;44:105–108.
17. Manolios N, Mackie I. Drowning and near-drowning on Australian beaches patrolled by life-savers: a 10-year study, 1973–1983. *Med J Aust.* 1988;148:165–167, 170–171.

Near-Fatal Asthma

Introduction

This section of the International Guidelines 2000 focuses on near-fatal asthma. The recommendations deviate immediately from routine asthma care and address the sequence of action steps needed to prevent death. Some recommendations, such as use of aminophylline, permissive hypercarbia, and early tracheal intubation, do not reflect routine asthma attacks. Nevertheless, in the desperate race to prevent cardiopulmonary arrest, heroic measures must be considered and considered early.

Severe exacerbation of asthma can lead to several forms of sudden death. One classification scheme categorizes asthma on the basis of the onset of symptoms. Signs of rapid-onset asthma develop in <2.5 hours, signs and symptoms of slow-onset asthma develop over several days.[1] Cardiac arrest in patients with severe asthma has been linked to

- Severe bronchospasm and mucous plugging leading to asphyxia[2] (this condition causes the vast majority of asthma-related deaths).
- Cardiac arrhythmias due to hypoxia, which is the common cause of asthma-related arrhythmia. In addition, arrhythmias are caused by use of β-adrenergic agonists. (In rare instances these arrhythmias may be due to prolongation of the QT interval resulting from β-adrenergic agonists[3–5] or toxicity caused by medications such as theophylline.)
- Auto-PEEP (positive end-expiratory pressure) occurs in some patients who are intubated and mechanically ventilated. Patients fail to expire as much air as they took in; gradual buildup of pressure occurs and reduces blood flow and blood pressure. Auto-PEEP is secondary to air trapping and "breath stacking" (breathed air entering and being unable to escape).
- Tension pneumothorax (often bilateral)

Most asthma-related deaths occur outside the hospital. The number of patients with severe attacks of asthma who present to the Emergency Department at night is 10 times greater than the number presenting during the day.[6] Multiple factors affect the outcome of therapy in asthmatic patients. Constantly review these issues during evaluation and treatment:

- Determine whether the patient has true acute asthma. When a patient presents with dyspnea in extremis you may not be able to obtain the recent history.
- Depending on the patient's history and medication use, other conditions may be present. These include
  —Cardiac disease (congestive heart failure, myocarditis), pulmonary disease (emphysema, pneumonia, upper-airway obstruction—structural or psychogenic), acute allergic bronchospasm or anaphylaxis (aspirin, foods, or idiopathic), pulmonary embolism, or vasculitis (Churg-Strauss syndrome).[7]
  —Medications and drugs of abuse: bronchospasm as sequelae to medications (β-blockers)[8] or drugs of abuse (cocaine and opiates).[9,10]
  —Discontinuation of corticosteroids. Patients who have used corticosteroids for a long time may have relative adrenal insufficiency. With the stress of discontinuation of the steroids and the adrenal insufficiency, these patients may present with near-fatal asthma.

Key Interventions to Prevent Arrest

The major clinical action is to treat the severe asthmatic crisis aggressively, before deterioration to full arrest. The specific agents and the treatment sequence will vary according to local practice. Emergency treatment will include some combination of the agents and interventions discussed below. The challenge of most concern for the ALS provider is the patient who deteriorates progressively, unresponsive to multiple therapeutic efforts.

Oxygen

Use a concentration of inspired oxygen to achieve a PaO_2 of ≥ 92 mm Hg. High-flow oxygen by mask is sometimes necessary. In patients with an asthmatic crisis, the following signs indicate that the need for rapid tracheal intubation is imminent:

- Findings of obtundation
- Profuse diaphoresis
- Poor ("floppy") muscle tone (clinical signs of hypercarbia)
- Findings of severe agitation, confusion, and fighting against the oxygen mask (clinical signs of hypoxemia)[11]
- Elevation of the PCO_2 by itself is not indicative of a need for tracheal intubation. Elevated PCO_2 does indicate severity of the episode. Reserve intubation for patients with the clinical findings mentioned above or a clearly rising PCO_2. *Treat the patient, not the numbers.*

Nebulized β_2-Agonists

Albuterol (salbutamol) is the cornerstone of therapy for acute asthma in most of the world. Standard practice in Emergency Departments is a dose of 2.5 to 5.0 mg every 15 to 20 minutes given up to 3 times in 1 hour (total dose of 7.5 to 15 mg/h). Patients who do not respond to albuterol may respond well to subcutaneous epinephrine or terbutaline.[12]

Intravenous Corticosteroids

By 2000 it became a common practice in accident and emergency departments to begin corticosteroid therapy early (in the first 30 minutes) for patients with life-threatening asthma. Corticosteroids should be started early, but oxygen and β-agonists always have priority as the initial agents.

Circulation. 2000;102(suppl I):I-237–I-240.
© 2000 American Heart Association, Inc.

Circulation is available at http://www.circulationaha.org

Clinicians typically use 125 mg of methylprednisolone (or equivalent hydrocortisone 200 mg IV) as a starting dose in cases of severe asthma.[13–15] Doses can range as low as 40 mg to as high as 250 mg IV or its equivalent.

Nebulized Anticholinergics

Use ipratropium, an inhaled anticholinergic agent, as a moist nebulizing agent in combination with albuterol at a dose of 0.5 mg.[16] Unlike β_2-agonists, which have an immediate onset of action, nebulized anticholinergic agents have a delayed onset of approximately 20 minutes.

Intravenous Aminophylline

Aminophylline, now used as secondary therapy after β_2-agonists and corticosteroids, can enhance the effects of those agents. As a bronchodilator aminophylline is approximately one third as potent as β_2-agonists. Clinicians use aminophylline much more frequently in children than in adults. A loading dose of 5 mg/kg is given over 30 to 45 minutes followed by an infusion of 0.5 to 0.7 mg/kg per hour, but this loading dose is not advised in people already taking theophylline, who should receive either half loading doses or maintenance doses. Addition of this agent to high doses of β_2-agonists is thought to increase side effects more than it increases bronchodilation. This is most evident in patients already taking theophyllines. The risk-benefit ratio may be different in patients not taking theophyllines.[17]

Intravenous Magnesium Sulfate

A number of authors have reported success with magnesium sulfate in patients refractory to inhaled adrenergic agents and corticosteroids. Although not consistently effective, magnesium is widely available and can be administered with few if any side effects at a dose of 2 to 3 g IV at rates as fast as 1 g/min (1 g magnesium sulfate=98 mg of elemental magnesium).[18,19]

Parenteral or Subcutaneous or Intramuscular Epinephrine or Terbutaline

Subcutaneous administration of epinephrine or terbutaline may prevent the need for artificial ventilation in cases of life-threatening asthma, especially in patients who do not respond to inhaled β_2-agonists. The total epinephrine dose (at a concentration of 1:1000) is 0.01 mg/kg, usually divided into 3 doses at 20-minute intervals. For convenience and easy recall a non–weight-based dose of 0.3 mg usually is given to adults. This dose of epinephrine (0.3 mg) can be repeated twice at 20-minute intervals to a total of 3 injections.

The dose of terbutaline is 0.25 mg SC every 30 minutes; up to 3 doses may be given. At this time there is no good evidence of advantages for IV β-agonists over inhaled bronchodilators.[20] The value of IV bronchodilators, however, compared with that of inhaled bronchodilators merits further study.

Ketamine

Ketamine is a parenteral dissociative anesthetic that has been found to be a useful bronchodilator. Most experts think that ketamine is the anesthetic agent of choice for intubation of severe asthmatics. Ketamine potentiates catecholamines and directly induces relaxation of smooth muscle. It also increases bronchial secretions and can cause emergent reactions. Because of the effect of ketamine on bronchial secretions, atropine (0.01 mg/kg, minimum dose of 0.1 mg) also should be administered if this agent is used. Benzodiazepines help to minimize emergent reactions, although hallucinations may occur after the patient awakes. The initial dose of ketamine is 0.1 to 0.2 mg/kg followed by an infusion of 0.5 mg/kg per hour. In intubated patients or in those being prepared for intubation, the usual dose of ketamine is a bolus of 0.5 to 1.5 mg/kg, repeated 20 minutes later, or infusion of 1 to 5 mg/kg per hour.[21]

Heliox

Heliox is a mixture of helium and oxygen (usually 70:30) that may delay the need for intubation by decreasing the work of breathing while the other medications are beginning to take effect.[22]

Bilevel Positive Airway Pressure

Bilevel positive airway pressure intermittently provides assisted ventilation. Like a combination of positive-pressure ventilation and PEEP, bilevel airway pressure helps to delay or abort the need for tracheal intubation. This ventilation counteracts the effects of auto-PEEP, thereby reducing the work of breathing. Begin with an inspiratory positive airway pressure of 8 to 10 cm H_2O and an expiratory positive airway pressure of 3 to 5 cm H_2O.[23]

Tracheal Intubation With Artificial Ventilation

In some patients oxygenation and ventilation can be achieved only after sedation, general anesthesia, muscle paralysis, and tracheal intubation. Patients with severe asthma experience some obstruction of inspiration and marked obstruction of expiration. This results in auto-PEEP, which is secondary to air trapping and "breath stacking" (breathed air entering and being unable to escape).

The following critical points relate to tracheal intubation for life-threatening asthma:

- Provide adequate sedation with ketamine, a benzodiazepine, or a barbiturate.
- Paralyze the patient with succinylcholine or vecuronium.
- Once intubated some patients may need permissive hypercarbia with elective hypoventilation.[24]
- Inhaled volatile anesthetics, although no longer widely used or available outside the operating room, are powerful relaxants of bronchial smooth muscle. Agents such as halothane, isoflurane, enflurane, and ether have been used to reverse status asthmaticus refractory to all other treatments.[25] Use these agents with extreme caution because (except for ether) they are also vasodilators and myocardial depressants. Some anesthetics sensitize the myocardium to catecholamines, leading to life-threatening arrhythmias.
- Extracorporeal membrane oxygenation has been used as a lifesaving measure for severe refractory asthma when all else has failed, but this technique is not generally available.

- For most experts ketamine is the intravenous anesthetic of choice for patients with status asthmaticus. In titrated doses ketamine has a mild bronchodilator effect and does not cause vasodilatation, circulatory collapse, or myocardial depression.

Steps to Take Immediately After Intubation

Tracheal intubation only provides more external mechanical power to the patient's failing ventilation efforts; it does not solve the problem. Patients with severe asthma may be extremely difficult to preoxygenate manually before intubation and even once the tube is in place.

Because breathing efforts may be uncoordinated, the patient may not have inhaled an adequate amount of β_2-agonist before intubation. Immediately after intubation inject 2.5 to 5.0 mg of albuterol directly into the tracheal tube. Confirm correct placement of the tracheal tube by the following newly recommended sequence:

- *Primary tracheal tube confirmation.* Visualize the tube past the vocal cords; perform 5-point auscultation; watch chest rise; condensation in tube. Auscultation can be misleading because poor ventilation and air movement may result in inaudible breath sounds in patients with severe refractory asthma.
- *Secondary confirmation of tube placement.* Qualitative end-tidal CO_2 detectors; esophageal detector device; dynamic pulse oximetry readings; quantitative and continuous CO_2 measurements using capnometers or capnographs.

Ventilate the patient with 100% oxygen.

The absence of any significant obstruction to airflow immediately after intubation suggests that the diagnosis of acute asthma may have been incorrect, and the problem may have been more in the upper airway (eg, vocal cord dysfunction, tumor, or a foreign body). The person who performs manual ventilation after intubation should be instructed *beforehand* to ventilate at a rate of only 8 to 10 breaths per minute to avoid auto-PEEP and its consequences (eg, sudden severe hypotension). The drop in blood pressure with hyperventilation may be extremely sudden. Prevention of this problem is clearly better than treatment of it.

Acute asthma can be confused with exacerbation of emphysema, especially in the elderly. For different reasons hyperventilation immediately after intubation can cause dire consequences in elderly patients with emphysema. (See the textbook *Advanced Cardiovascular Life Support* for an in-depth discussion of this topic.)

Intubated, Critically Ill Asthmatic: Ventilator-Dependent

Permissive Hypercapnia

Adequately sedate and paralyze the patient to allow a "passive" ventilator-patient interaction. Allow PCO_2 to rise (permissive hypercapnia) to values as high as 80 mm Hg. The ensuing drop in pH can be controlled with bicarbonate if needed.

To set the ventilator for permissive hypercapnia:

- Rate: provide mechanical ventilation, 8 to 10 breaths per minute
- Volume: tidal volume, 5 to 7 mL/kg
- Peak flow: 60 L/min with a decelerating pattern
- Inspired oxygen: FIO_2, 1.0 (ie, 100%)

If the patient's airway is extremely difficult to ventilate, perform the following procedures *in order* until ventilation is adequate:

1. Ensure that the patient is adequately sedated or paralyzed so that there is passive patient-ventilator interaction.
2. Check the patency of the tube for obstructions caused by kinking, mucous plugging, or biting. Aspirate the tube as needed.
3. To ensure that the patient is receiving adequate tidal volume, increase the time for exhalation, decrease the time for inhalation, and increase the peak pressure.
4. Reduce the respiratory rate to 6 to 8 breaths per minute to reduce auto-PEEP to ≤15 mm Hg.
5. Reduce the tidal volume to 3 to 5 mL/kg to reduce auto-PEEP to ≤15 mm Hg.
6. Increase peak flow to >60 L/min (90 to 120 L/min is commonly used) to further shorten inspiratory time and increase the ratio of inspired to expired air (I:E).[26]

Troubleshooting: Hypotension or Desaturation Immediately After Intubation[26]

Ensure that the tracheal tube is in the correct position. The tube should be inserted to 21 to 23 cm (measured at the incisors) in most men and to 20 cm in most women. These values may need to be reduced in a small person.

Incorrect placement of the tube must be addressed *immediately*. Do not take the time to obtain a chest x-ray, although an x-ray of the chest after intubation is always appropriate. The immediate consequences of insertion of the tube incorrectly in a patient with severe refractory asthma may be fatal.

If the patient is difficult to ventilate, check the patency of the tube for obstructions caused by kinking, mucous plugging, or biting. Aspirate the tube.

The differential diagnosis of hypotension or desaturation immediately after intubation, once tube position is confirmed, includes tension pneumothorax and massive auto-PEEP buildup. In patients with severe refractory asthma the chest often is silent to auscultation because of poor airflow and hyperinflation of the chest wall.

Tension Pneumothorax

Evidence of a tension pneumothorax includes unilateral expansion of the chest wall, shifting of the trachea, and subcutaneous emphysema. The lifesaving action is to release air from the pleural space with needle decompression. Slowly insert a 16-gauge cannula in the second intercostal space along the midclavicular line, being careful to avoid direct puncture of the lung. If air is emitted, insert a chest tube.

Caution! Insertion of a chest tube in a patient with severe refractory asthma without pneumothorax will have dire consequences because the visceral pleura of the hyperinflated lung could be punctured, iatrogenically producing pneumothorax. The person inserting the tube would not realize that this has occurred because puncture of the lung would cause a release of air under pressure through the needle catheter or thoracostomy tube, just as would occur with relief of tension pneumothorax. Because of the high pressures experienced by the contralateral mechanically ventilated lung and coexisting auto-PEEP, contralateral pneumothorax would be generated, most likely under tension.

Massive Auto-PEEP Buildup

The most common cause of profound hypotension after intubation is a massive buildup of auto-PEEP. Stop ventilating the patient for a brief period (<1 minute) and allow the auto-PEEP to dissipate. At the same time observe the patient's oxygenation.

Hypotension may also be due to the intubation sedatives, which should respond to volume infusion.

If high auto-PEEP is not present, reconsider alternative explanations.

- Obtain an ECG: Exclude myocardial ischemia or infarction as a consequence of acute respiratory failure (ie, hypoxemia, intubation, and medications).[27,28]
- Request emergency consultation from a pulmonologist.
- Request emergency consultation from an anesthesiologist.
- Admit the patient to the Critical Care Unit.

References

1. Wasserfallen J, Schaller M, Feihl F, et al. Sudden asphyxic asthma: a distinct entity? *Am Rev Respir Dis.* 1990;142:108–111.
2. Molfino NA, Nannini AN, Matelli A, et al. Respiratory arrest in near-fatal asthma. *N Engl J Med.* 1991;99:358–362.
3. Robin ED, Lewiston N. Unexpected, unexplained sudden death in young asthmatic subjects. *Chest.* 1989;96:790–793.
4. Robin ED, McCauley R. Sudden cardiac death in bronchial asthma and inhaled β-adrenergic agonists. *Chest.* 1992;101:1699–1702.
5. Rosero SZ, Zareba W, Moss AJ, Robinson, Hajj ARH, Locati EH, et al. Asthma and the risk of cardiac events in the long QT syndrome. *Am J Cardiol.* 1999;84:1406–1411.
6. Brenner BE, Chavda K, Karakurum M, Camargo CA Jr. Circadian differences among 4096 patients presenting to the emergency department with acute asthma. *Acad Emerg Med.* 1999;6:523.
7. Brenner BE, Tyndall JA, Crain EF. The clinical presentation of acute asthma in adults and children. In: Brenner BE, ed. *Emergency Asthma.* New York, NY: Marcel-Dekker; 1999:201–232.
8. Odeh M, Oliven A, Bassan H. Timolol eye-drop-induced fatal bronchospasm in an asthmatic patient. *J Fam Pract.* 1991;32:97–98.
9. Weitzman JB, Kanarek NF, Smialek JE. Medical examiner asthma death autopsies: a distinct group of asthma deaths with implications for public health strategies. *Arch Pathol Lab Med.* 1998;122:691–699.
10. Levenson T, Greenberger PA, Donoghue ER, Lifschultz BD. Asthma deaths confounded by substance abuse: an assessment of fatal asthma. *Chest.* 1996;110:604–610.
11. Brenner BE, Abraham E, Simon RR. Position and diaphoresis in acute asthma. *Am J Med.* 1983;74:1005–1009.
12. Appel D, Karpel JP, Sherman M. Epinephrine improves expiratory flow rates in patients with asthma who do not respond to inhaled metaproterenol sulfate. *J Allergy Clin Immunol.* 1989;84:90–98.
13. Rowe BH. Effectiveness of steroid therapy in acute exacerbations of asthma: a meta-analysis. *Am J Emerg Med.* 1992;10:301–310.
14. McFadden ER Jr. Dosages of corticosteroids in asthma. *Am Rev Respir Dis.* 1993;147:1306–1312.
15. Rowe BH, Spooner CH, Ducharme FM, Bretzlaff JA, Bota GW. Early emergency department treatment of acute asthma with systemic corticosteroids (Cochrane Review). Cochrane Library, Issue 2, 2000. Oxford: Update Software.
16. Karpel JP, Schacter EN, Fanta C, Levey D, Spiro P, Aldrich TK, Menjjoge SS, Witek T. A comparison of ipratropium and albuterol vs albuterol alone for the treatment of acute asthma. *Chest.* 1996;110:611–616.
17. Littenberg B. Aminophylline treatment in severe, acute asthma: a meta-analysis. *JAMA.* 1988;259:1678–1684.
18. Schiermeyer RP, Finkelstein JA. Rapid infusion of magnesium sulfate obviates need for intubation in status asthmaticus. *Am J Emerg Med.* 1994;12:164–166.
19. Rowe BH, Bretzlaff JA, Bourdon C, Bota GW, Camargo CA. Systematic review of magnesium sulfate in the treatment of acute asthma (Cochrane Review). Cochrane Library, Issue 4, 1998. Oxford: Update Software.
20. Gibbs NA, Camargo CA Jr, Rowe BH, Silverman RA. State of the art: therapeutic controversies in severe acute asthma. *Acad Emerg Med.* 2000;7:800–815.
21. Hemmingsen C, Kielsen P, Ordorico J. Ketamine in the treatment of bronchospasm during mechanical ventilation. *Am J Emerg Med.* 1994;12:417–420.
22. Kass JE, Terregino CA. The effect of Heliox in acute severe asthma: a randomized controlled trial. *Chest.* 1999;116:296–300.
23. Panacek EA, Pollack C. Medical management of severe asthma. In: Brenner BE, ed. *Emergency Asthma.* New York, NY: Marcel-Dekker; 1999:395–417.
24. Tuxen DV. Permissive hypercapnic ventilation. *Am J Respir Crit Care Med.* 1994;150:870–874.
25. Saulnier FF, Durocher AV, Deturck RA, et al. Respiratory and hemodynamic effects of halothane in status asthmaticus. *Intensive Care Med.* 1990;16:104–107.
26. Mayo P, Radeos MS. The severe asthmatic: intubated and difficult to ventilate. In: Brenner BE, ed. *Emergency Asthma.* New York, NY: Marcel-Dekker; 1999:469–487.
27. Bashir R, Padder F, Khan FA. Myocardial stunning following respiratory arrest. *Chest.* 1995;108:1459–1460.
28. Hurford WE, Favorito F. Association of myocardial ischemia with failure to wean from mechanical ventilation. *Crit Care Med.* 1995;23:1475–1480.

Anaphylaxis

Background

Anaphylactic and anaphylactoid reactions lack universally accepted definitions.

- The term anaphylaxis is typically applied to hypersensitivity reactions mediated by the IgE and IgG4 subclass of antibodies. Some may be mediated by complement (eg, allergic reactions to blood products). Signs of an anaphylactic reaction develop after reexposure to a sensitizing antigen within minutes.
- *Anaphylactoid reactions* look exactly the same, but they are not mediated by an antigen-antibody reaction.
- The manifestations and management of anaphylactic and anaphylactoid reactions are similar so that the distinction is unimportant in relation to treatment of an acute attack.

Incidence

The annual incidence of anaphylaxis is unknown. Recent US estimates have averaged 30 per 100 000.[1] A study in the United Kingdom has reported a frequency of 1 of every 2300 attendees at a hospital Emergency Department.[2] The annual international incidence of fatal anaphylactic reactions seems to be 154 per 1 million hospitalized patients per year.[3]

Etiology

Insect stings, drugs, contrast media, and some foods (milk, eggs, fish, and shellfish) are the most common causes of anaphylaxis. When hypersensitivity to insect stings is present, 35% to 60% of affected patients will experience anaphylaxis to a subsequent sting.[4] Peanut and tree nut (Brazil, almond, hazel, and macadamia nuts) allergies have recently been recognized as particularly dangerous.[5] Aspirin and other nonsteroidal anti-inflammatory agents, parenteral penicillins, many other drugs and toxins, vaccines, and beer have become notorious causes of anaphylaxis. Latex-associated anaphylaxis has become a major problem in medical centers. An exercise-induced anaphylaxis (especially after ingestion of certain foods) has been reported. Anaphylaxis may even be idiopathic, typically managed with long-term use of oral steroids. β-Blockers may increase the incidence and severity of anaphylaxis and can produce a paradoxical response to epinephrine.

Signs and Symptoms

The manifestations of anaphylaxis are related to release of chemical mediators from mast cells. The most important mediators of anaphylaxis are histamines, leukotrienes, prostaglandins, thromboxanes, and bradykinins. These mediators contribute to vasodilation, increased capillary permeability, and airway constriction and produce the clinical signs of hypotension, bronchospasm, and angioedema.

The location and concentration of mast cells determine the organ(s) affected. Typically 2 or more of the following systems are involved: cutaneous, respiratory, cardiovascular, and gastrointestinal. The sooner the reaction occurs after exposure, the more likely it is to be severe.

- Upper airway (laryngeal) edema, lower airway edema (asthma), or both may develop acutely and become life-threatening.
- *Cardiovascular collapse* is the most common periarrest manifestation. It is caused by an absolute and a relative hypovolemia. Vasodilation produces a relative hypovolemia, and the intravascular volume loss associated with increased capillary permeability contributes to the absolute volume loss. Cardiac dysfunction is due principally to hypotension but may be complicated by presence of underlying disease or development of myocardial ischemia from epinephrine administration.
- Other symptoms include urticaria, rhinitis, conjunctivitis, abdominal pain, vomiting, diarrhea, and a sense of impending doom.
- The patient may appear either flushed or pale.

Differential Diagnosis

The diagnosis of anaphylaxis is challenging because there is a wide variety of presentations, and no single finding is pathognomonic. Many conditions, including vasovagal reactions (from parenteral injections), functional vocal cord dysfunction, and panic attacks, have been misdiagnosed as anaphylaxis, whereas patients with genuine anaphylaxis do not always receive appropriate therapy.

Angioedema (diffuse soft-tissue swelling) is often present in anaphylaxis. It is typically associated with urticaria, with small to even giant-sized lesions observed. There are, however, many other potential causes of angioedema and urticaria that should be considered.

Scombroid poisoning, which often develops within 30 minutes of eating spoiled tuna, mackerel, or dolphin (mahi-mahi), typically presents with urticaria, nausea, vomiting, diarrhea, and headache. It is treated with antihistamines.

Hereditary angioedema (in which there is a family history of angioedema) presents with no urticaria, but gastrointestinal mucosal edema produces severe abdominal pain, and respiratory mucosal edema produces airway compromise. This form of angioedema is treated with fresh-frozen plasma.

ACE inhibitors are associated with a reactive angioedema predominantly of the upper airway. This reaction can develop days or years after ACE inhibitor therapy is begun. The best medical treatment of this form of angioedema is unclear, but aggressive early airway management is critical.[6]

Circulation. 2000;102(suppl I):I-241–I-243.
© 2000 American Heart Association, Inc.

Circulation is available at http://www.circulationaha.org

Finally, in some forms of *panic disorder,* functional stridor develops as a result of forced adduction of the vocal cords. In a panic attack there is no urticaria, angioedema, or hypotension.

Key Interventions to Prevent Arrest[7]

The approach to therapy is difficult to standardize because etiology, clinical presentation (including severity and course), and organ involvement vary widely. Few randomized trials of treatment approaches have been reported. The following recommendations are commonly used and widely accepted but are based more on consensus than on evidence:

- **Position.** Place victims in a position of comfort. If hypotension is present, elevate the legs until replacement fluids and vasopressors restore the blood pressure.
- **Oxygen.** Administer oxygen at high flow rates.
- **Epinephrine.** Administer epinephrine to all patients with clinical signs of shock, airway swelling, or definite breathing difficulty. Administer intravenous epinephrine if anaphylaxis is profound and life-threatening and vascular access is available. If vascular access is not available or if anaphylaxis is not profound and life-threatening, administer epinephrine by intramuscular injection. Subcutaneous administration may be used but absorption and subsequent achievement of maximum plasma concentration may be delayed with shock.[8]
  —The IM dose of 0.3 to 0.5 mg (1:1000; 1 mL) may be repeated after 5 to 10 minutes if no clinical improvement.
  —Intravenous epinephrine (1:10 000; 10 mL) 1 to 5 mL or 0.1 to 0.5 mg over 5 minutes should be used only for profound, immediately life-threatening manifestations and when there are no delays in intravenous access. Epinephrine may be diluted to a 1:10 000 solution before infusion. An intravenous infusion (1 mg in 250 mL D$_5$W [4 μg/mL]) at rates of 1 to 4 μg/min may avoid frequent repeat epinephrine injections.[9]
- **Antihistamines.** Administer antihistamines slowly intravenously or intramuscularly (eg, 25 mg of diphenhydramine).
- **H$_2$ blockers.** Administer H$_2$ blockers, such as cimetidine (300 mg PO, IM, or IV).[10]
- **Isotonic solutions.** Give isotonic crystalloid (normal saline) if hypotension is present and does not respond rapidly to epinephrine. A rapid infusion of 1 to 2 L or even 4 L may be needed initially.
- **Inhaled β-adrenergic agents.** Provide inhaled albuterol if bronchospasm is a major feature. If hypotension is present, administer parenteral epinephrine before inhaled albuterol to prevent a possible further decrease in blood pressure. Inhaled ipratropium may be especially useful for treatment of bronchospasm in patients on β-blockers.
- **Corticosteroids.** Infuse high-dose intravenous corticosteroids slowly or administer intramuscularly after severe attacks, especially for asthmatic patients and those already receiving steroids. The beneficial effects are delayed at least 4 to 6 hours.
- **Envenomation.** Rarely insect envenomation by bees, but not wasps, leaves a venom sac. Immediately scrape away any insect parts at the site of the sting.[11] Squeezing is alleged to increase envenomation. Judicious local application of ice may also slow antigen absorption. The application of papain (available in meat tenderizers) to the stinger site is a common home remedy that appears to have no therapeutic value.[12]
- **Glucagon.** For patients unresponsive to epinephrine, especially those receiving β-blockers, glucagon may be effective. This agent is short-acting (1 to 2 mg every 5 minutes IM or IV). Nausea, vomiting, and hyperglycemia are common side effects.
- **Observation.** Observe closely up to 24 hours. Many patients do not respond promptly to therapy, and symptoms may recur in some patients (up to 20%) within 1 to 8 hours despite an intervening asymptomatic period.[13–15]

Special Considerations

Rapid Progression to Lethal Airway Obstruction

Close observation is required during conventional therapy (see above). Early, elective intubation is indicated for patients with hoarseness, lingual edema, and posterior or oropharyngeal swelling. If respiratory function deteriorates, perform semielective (awake, sedated) tracheal intubation without paralytic agents.

Angioedema. Patients with angioedema pose a particularly worrisome problem because they are at high risk for rapid deterioration. Most will present with some degree of labial or facial swelling. Patients with hoarseness, lingual edema, and posterior or oropharyngeal swelling are at particular risk for respiratory compromise.

Early tracheal intubation. If intubation is delayed, patients can deteriorate over a brief period of time (0.5 to 3 hours), with development of progressive stridor, severe dysphonia or aphonia, laryngeal edema, massive lingual swelling, facial and neck swelling, and hypoxemia. At this point both tracheal intubation and cricothyrotomy may be difficult or impossible. Attempts at tracheal intubation may only further increase laryngeal edema or compromise the airway with bleeding into the oropharynx and narrow glottic opening. The patient may become agitated as a result of hypoxia and may be uncooperative with oxygen therapy.

Paralysis followed by an attempt at tracheal intubation may prove lethal, because the glottic opening is narrow and difficult to see because of the lingual and oropharyngeal edema and the patient is iatrogenically apneic. If tracheal intubation is not successful, even bag-mask ventilation may be impossible, because laryngeal edema will prevent air entry and facial edema will prevent creation of an effective seal between the face and bag mask. Pharmacological paralysis at this point may deprive the patient of the sole mechanism for ventilation, ie, spontaneous breathing attempts.

During Arrest: Key Interventions and Modifications of BLS/ALS Therapy

Death from anaphylaxis may be associated with profound vasodilation, intravascular collapse, tissue hypoxia, and asystole. No data is available on how cardiac arrest procedures should be modified, but difficulties in achieving adequate volume replacement and ventilation are frequent. Reasonable recommendations can be based on experience with nonfatal cases.

Airway, Oxygenation, and Ventilation

Death may result from angioedema and upper or lower airway obstruction. Bag-mask ventilation and tracheal intubation may fail. Cricothyrotomy may be difficult or impossible because severe swelling will obliterate landmarks. In these desperate circumstances, consider the following airway techniques:

- Fiberoptic tracheal intubation
- Digital tracheal intubation, in which the fingers are used to guide insertion of a small ($\leq$7 mm) tracheal tube
- Needle cricothyrotomy followed by transtracheal ventilation
- Cricothyrotomy as described for the patient with massive neck swelling[16]

Support of Circulation

Support of circulation requires rapid volume resuscitation and administration of vasopressors to support blood pressure. Epinephrine is the drug of choice for treatment of both vasodilation/hypotension and cardiac arrest.

- **Rapid volume expansion** is an absolute requirement.
  —When anaphylaxis occurs, it can produce profound vasodilation that significantly increases intravascular capacity. Very large volumes should be administered over very short periods; typically 2 to 4 L of isotonic crystalloid should be given.
- **High-dose epinephrine IV** (ie, rapid progression to high dose) should be used without hesitation in patients in full cardiac arrest.
  —A commonly used sequence: 1 to 3 mg IV (3 minutes), 3 to 5 mg IV (3 minutes), then 4 to 10 μg/min.
- **Antihistamines IV.** There is little data about the value of antihistamines in anaphylactic cardiac arrest, but it is reasonable to assume that little additional harm could result.
- **Steroid therapy.** Although steroids should have no effect if given during a cardiac arrest, they may be of value in the postresuscitation period.
- **Asystole/PEA Algorithms.** Because the arrest rhythm in anaphylaxis is often PEA or asystole, the ILCOR panel recommended adding the other steps in the Asystole and PEA Algorithms. These include
  —Administration of atropine
  —Transcutaneous pacing

- **Prolonged CPR.** Cardiac arrest associated with anaphylaxis may respond to longer therapy than usual.
  —In these circumstances the patient is often a young person with a healthy heart and cardiovascular system. Rapid correction of vasodilation and low blood volume is required.
  —Effective CPR may maintain sufficient oxygen delivery until the catastrophic effects of the anaphylactic reaction resolve.

Summary

The management of anaphylaxis includes early recognition, anticipation of deterioration, and aggressive support of airway, oxygenation, ventilation, and circulation. Prompt, aggressive therapy may be successful even if cardiac arrest develops.

References

1. Yocum MW, Butterfield JH, Klein JS, et al. Epidemiology of anaphylaxis in Olmsted County: a population based study. *J Allergy Clin Immunol.* 1999;104:454–466.
2. Stewart AG, Ewan PG. The incidence, aetiology and management of anaphylaxis presenting to an accident and emergency department. *Q J Med.* 1996;89:859–864.
3. The International Collaborative Study of Severe Anaphylaxis. An epidemiologic study of severe anaphylactic and anaphylactoid reactions among hospital patients: methods and overall risks. *Epidemiology.* 1998;9:141–146.
4. Hauk P, Friedl K, Kaufmehl K, et al. Subsequent insect stings in children with hypersensitivity to *Hymenoptera. J Pediatr.* 1995;126:185–190.
5. Ewan PW. Clinical study of peanut and nut allergy in 6 consecutive patients: new features and associations. *BMJ.* 1996;312:1074–1078.
6. Ishoo E, Shah UK, Grillone GA, et al. Predicting airway risk in angioedema: staging system based on presentation. *Otolaryngol Head Neck Surg.* 1999;121:263–268.
7. Project Team of the Resuscitation Council. Emergency medical treatment of anaphylactic reactions. *J Accid Emerg Med.* 1999;16:243–247.
8. Simons FE, Robert JR, Gu X, Simons KJ. Epinephrine absorption in children with a history of anaphylaxis. *J Allergy Clin Immunol.* 1998;101:33–37.
9. Barach EM, Nowak RM, Lee TG, Tomlanovich MC. Epinephrine for treatment of anaphylactic shock. *JAMA.* 1984;251:2118–2122.
10. Runge JW, Martinez JC, Caravati EM, et al. Histamine antagonists in the treatment of allergic reactions. *Ann Emerg Med.* 1992;21:237–242.
11. Visscher PK, Vetter RS, Camazine S. Removing bee stings. *Lancet.* 1996;348:301–2.
12. Ross EV, Badame AJ, Dale SE. Meat tenderizer in the acute treatment of imported fire ant stings. *J Am Acad Dermatol.* 1987;16:1189–1192.
13. Stark BJ, Sullivan TJ. Biphasic and protracted anaphylaxis. *J Allergy Clin Immunol.* 1986;78:76–83.
14. Smith PL, Kagey-Sobotka A, Bleecker E, et al. Physiologic manifestations of human anaphylaxis. *J Clin Invest.* 1980;66:1072–1080.
15. Brazil E, MacNamara AF. "Not so immediate" hypersensitivity: the danger of biphasic anaphylactic reactions. *J Accid Emerg Med.* 1998;15:252–253.
16. Simon RR, Brenner BE. Emergency procedures and techniques. In: *Airway Procedures.* Baltimore, Md: Williams & Wilkins; 1994:79.

Cardiac Arrest Associated With Trauma

Introduction

Survival from out-of-hospital cardiac arrest secondary to blunt trauma is uniformly low in children and adults.[1–3] In some out-of-hospital and Emergency Department settings, resuscitative efforts are withheld when patients with blunt trauma are found in asystole or agonal electrical cardiac activity. Survival after cardiac arrest resulting from penetrating trauma is only slightly better; rapid transport to a trauma center is associated with better outcome than resuscitation attempts in the field.[4]

BLS and ALS for the trauma patient are fundamentally the same as the care of the patient with a primary cardiac or respiratory arrest. In trauma resuscitation, a "Primary Survey" is performed, with rapid evaluation and stabilization of airway, breathing, and circulation. The trauma rescuer must anticipate, rapidly identify, and immediately treat life-threatening conditions that will interfere with establishing effective airway, oxygenation, ventilation, and circulation.

Cardiopulmonary deterioration associated with trauma has several possible causes, and the management plan may vary for each. Potential causes of cardiopulmonary deterioration and arrest include

1. Severe central neurological injury with secondary cardiovascular collapse
2. Hypoxia secondary to respiratory arrest resulting from neurological injury, airway obstruction, large open pneumothorax, or severe tracheobronchial laceration or crush
3. Direct and severe injury to vital structures, such as the heart, aorta, or pulmonary arteries
4. Underlying medical problems or other conditions that led to the injury, such as sudden VF in the driver of a motor vehicle or the victim of an electric shock
5. Severely diminished cardiac output from tension pneumothorax or pericardial tamponade
6. Exsanguination leading to hypovolemia and severely diminished oxygen delivery
7. Injuries in a cold environment (eg, fractured leg) complicated by secondary severe hypothermia

In cases of cardiac arrest associated with uncontrolled internal hemorrhage or pericardial tamponade, a favorable outcome requires that the victim be rapidly transported to an emergency facility with immediate operative capabilities.[4,5] Despite a rapid and effective out-of-hospital and trauma center response, patients with out-of-hospital cardiopulmonary arrest due to multiple-organ hemorrhage (as commonly seen with blunt trauma) will rarely survive neurologically intact.[5–8]

Patients who survive out-of-hospital cardiopulmonary arrest associated with trauma generally are young, have penetrating injuries, have received early (out-of-hospital) endotracheal intubation, and undergo prompt transport by highly skilled paramedics to a definitive care facility.[7–10]

Extrication and Initial Evaluation

When resuscitative efforts will be attempted, the victim should be rapidly extricated, with protection of the cervical spine. Immediate BLS and ALS interventions will ensure adequate airway, oxygenation, ventilation, and circulation. As soon as the victim is stabilized (and even during stabilization), prepare the victim for rapid evacuation to a facility that provides definitive trauma care. Use lateral neck supports, strapping, and backboards throughout transport to minimize exacerbation of an occult neck and spinal cord injury.[5]

When multiple patients receive serious injuries, emergency personnel must establish priorities for care. When the number of patients with critical injuries exceeds the capability of the EMS system, those without a pulse should be considered the lowest priority for care and triage. Most EMS systems have developed guidelines that permit the out-of-hospital pronouncement of death or withholding of cardiac resuscitative efforts when there are multiple patients with critical injuries or when there are injuries incompatible with life. EMS personnel therefore should work within such guidelines when available.

BLS for Cardiac Arrest Associated With Trauma

Provision of BLS requires assessment of responsiveness, establishment of a patent airway, assessment of breathing, support of oxygenation and ventilation if indicated, and assessment and support of circulation.

Establish Unresponsiveness

Head trauma or shock may produce loss of consciousness. If spinal cord injury is present the victim may be conscious but unable to move. Throughout initial assessment and stabilization, the rescuer should monitor patient responsiveness; deterioration could indicate either neurological compromise or cardiorespiratory failure.

Airway

When multisystem trauma is present, or trauma isolated to the head and neck, the spine must be immobilized throughout BLS maneuvers. A jaw thrust is used instead of a head tilt–chin lift to open the airway. If at all possible, a second rescuer should be responsible for immobilizing the head and neck during BLS and until spinal immobilization equipment is applied.

Once the airway is anatomically open, the mouth should be cleared of blood, vomitus, and other secretions. Remove this

Circulation. 2000;102(suppl I):I-244–I-246.
© 2000 American Heart Association, Inc.

Circulation is available at http://www.circulationaha.org

material with a (gloved) finger sweep or use gauze or a towel to wipe out the mouth. It may also be cleared with suction.

Breathing/Ventilation
Once a patent airway is established, the rescuer should assess for breathing. If breathing is absent or grossly inadequate (eg, agonal or slow and extremely shallow), ventilation is needed. When ventilation is provided with a barrier device, a pocket mask, or a bag-mask system, the cervical spine should be immobilized. If the chest does not expand during ventilation despite repeated attempts to open the airway with a jaw thrust, a tension pneumothorax or hemothorax may be present and should be ruled out or treated by ACLS personnel.

Deliver breaths slowly to reduce the development of gastric inflation and possible regurgitation.

Circulation
If the victim has no signs of circulation (no breathing, coughing, or movement) in response to the rescue breaths and if the healthcare provider detects no carotid pulse, chest compressions should be provided. If an AED is available, it is applied when absence of circulation is detected. The purpose is to check whether VF/VT occurred *first*, causing loss of consciousness, then the trauma. The AED will evaluate the victim's cardiac rhythm and advise shock delivery if appropriate.

Apply external compression to stop external hemorrhage.

Disability
Throughout all interventions, assess the victim's response. The Glasgow Coma Scale is useful and can be assessed in seconds. Monitor closely for signs of deterioration.

Exposure
The victim may lose heat to the environment through evaporation. Such heat loss will be exacerbated if the victim's clothes are removed or the victim is covered in blood. When possible, keep the victim warm.

ACLS for Cardiac Arrest Associated With Trauma
ALS includes continued assessment and support of airway, oxygenation and ventilation (breathing), and circulation.

Airway
Indications for intubation in the injured patient include

- Respiratory arrest or apnea
- Respiratory failure, including severe hypoventilation, hypoxemia despite oxygen therapy, or respiratory acidosis
- Shock
- Severe head injury
- Inability to protect upper airway (eg, loss of gag reflex, depressed level of consciousness, coma)
- Thoracic injuries (eg, flail chest, pulmonary contusion, penetrating trauma)
- Signs of airway obstruction
- Injuries associated with potential airway obstruction (eg, crushing facial or neck injuries)
- Anticipation of the need for mechanical ventilatory support

Endotracheal intubation is performed with cervical spine outside the trachea. Generally orotracheal intubation is performed. Avoid nasotracheal intubation in the presence of severe maxillofacial injuries, because the tube may migrate outside the trachea during placement. Proper tube placement should be confirmed by clinical examination and use of oximetry and exhaled CO_2 monitor immediately after intubation, during transport, and after any transfer of the patient (eg, from ambulance to hospital gurney).

Unsuccessful tracheal intubation for the patient with massive facial injury and edema is an indication for cricothyrotomy. Cricothyrotomy will provide an emergent, secure airway that supports oxygenation, although ventilation will be suboptimal.

Once a tracheal tube is inserted, simultaneous ventilations and compressions may result in a tension pneumothorax in an already damaged lung, especially if fractured ribs or a fractured sternum is present. Synchronized ventilations and compressions in a ratio of 1 to 5 may be required in the presence of a damaged thoracic cage.

Unless severe maxillofacial injuries are present, a gastric tube can be inserted to decompress the stomach. In the presence of severe maxillofacial injuries, inserted gastric tubes can migrate intracranially. They should be placed with caution under these conditions, with confirmation of placement into the stomach.

Ventilation
High concentrations of oxygen should be provided even if the victim's oxygenation appears adequate. Once a patent airway is ensured, assess breath sounds and chest expansion. A unilateral decrease in breath sounds associated with inadequate chest expansion during positive-pressure ventilation should be presumed to be caused by *tension pneumothorax* until that complication can be ruled out. Perform needle decompression of the pneumothorax immediately, followed by chest tube insertion. In the absence of an immediate hemodynamic response to thoracic decompression or alternatively in the presence of a penetrating thoracic wound, surgical exploration is warranted.[9]

Rescuers should look for and seal any significant open pneumothorax. Tension pneumothorax may develop after sealing of an open pneumothorax, so decompression may be needed.[5]

Hemothorax may also interfere with ventilation and chest expansion; treat hemothorax with blood replacement and chest tube insertion. If hemorrhage is severe and continues, surgical exploration may be required.

If the victim has a significant *flail chest*, spontaneous ventilation likely will be inadequate to maintain oxygenation. Treat flail chest with positive-pressure ventilation.

Circulation
Once airway, oxygenation, and ventilation are adequate, circulation is evaluated and supported. As noted above, if pulseless arrest develops, outcome is poor unless a reversible cause can be immediately identified and treated (eg, tension pneumothorax). Successful trauma resuscitation is often dependent on restoration of an adequate circulating blood volume.

The most common terminal cardiac rhythms observed in trauma victims are PEA, bradyasystolic rhythms, and occasionally VT/VF. Treatment of PEA requires identification and treatment of reversible causes, such as severe hypovolemia, hypothermia, cardiac tamponade, or tension pneumothorax.[11] Development of bradyasystolic rhythms often indicates the presence of severe hypovolemia, severe hypoxemia, or cardio-respiratory failure. VF/VT is of course treated with defibrillation. Although epinephrine is typically administered during the ACLS treatment of these arrhythmias, it may be ineffective in the presence of uncorrected severe hypovolemia.

Open thoracotomy does not improve outcome from out-of-hospital blunt trauma arrest, but open thoracotomy can be lifesaving for patients with penetrating chest trauma, particularly penetrating wounds of the heart.[6,8] During concurrent volume resuscitation for penetrating trauma, prompt emergency thoracotomy will permit direct massage of the heart and indicated surgical procedures. Such procedures may involve relief of cardiac tamponade, control of thoracic and extrathoracic hemorrhage, and aortic cross-clamping.[6,8]

Penetrating cardiac injury should be suspected whenever penetrating trauma to the left chest occurs and whenever penetrating injury is associated with low cardiac output or signs of tamponade (distended neck veins, hypotension, and decreased heart tones). Although pericardiocentesis theoretically is useful, efforts to relieve pericardial tamponade due to penetrating injury should be undertaken only in the hospital.

Cardiac contusions causing significant arrhythmias or impairing cardiac function are present in approximately 10% to 20% of victims of severe, blunt chest trauma.[12] Myocardial contusion should be suspected if the trauma victim demonstrates extreme tachycardia, arrhythmias, and ST-T–wave changes. Serum creatinine phosphokines are often elevated in the patient with blunt chest trauma. An MB fraction >5% has been used historically to diagnose cardiac contusion, but this is not a sensitive indicator of myocardial contusion.[13] The diagnosis of myocardial contusion is confirmed by echocardiography or radionuclide angiography.

Volume resuscitation is an important but controversial part of trauma resuscitation. In the field, bolus administration of isotonic crystalloid is indicated to treat hypovolemic shock. Adequate and aggressive volume replacement may be necessary to obtain adequate perfusing pressures.

For patients with penetrating chest trauma who are located a short distance from the trauma center, aggressive fluid resuscitation in the field can increase transport time and has been associated with lower survival than rapid transport with less aggressive fluid resuscitation.[4] When massive penetrating trauma or severe hemorrhage is present, immediate surgical exploration is required. Aggressive volume resuscitation in the field will delay arrival at the trauma center, delay surgical interventions to close off bleeding vessels, increase the blood pressure, and consequently accelerate the rate of blood loss.[4,14] Replacement of blood loss in the hospital is accomplished with a combination of packed red blood cells and isotonic crystalloids.

Bleeding must be controlled as soon as possible by whatever appropriate means to maintain adequate blood volume and oxygen-carrying capacity. If external pressure does not stop bleeding or internal bleeding continues, surgical exploration is required.

Indications for Surgical Exploration

Resuscitation may be impossible in the presence of severe, uncontrolled hemorrhage or in the presence of some cardiac, thoracic, or abdominal injuries. In these cases surgical intervention is required. Urgent surgical exploration is indicated for the following conditions:

- Hemodynamic instability despite volume resuscitation
- Excessive chest tube drainage (1.5 to 2.0 L or more total, or >300 mL/h for 3 or more hours)
- Significant hemothorax on chest x-ray
- Suspected cardiac trauma
- Gunshot wounds to the abdomen
- Penetrating torso trauma, particularly if associated with peritoneal perforation
- Positive diagnostic peritoneal lavage (particularly with evidence of ongoing hemorrhage)
- Significant solid-organ or bowel injury

References

1. Rosemurgy AS, Norris PA, Olson SM, Hurst JM, Albrink MH. Prehospital traumatic cardiac arrest: the cost of futility. *J Trauma*. 1993;35: 468–73; discussion 473–474.
2. Bouillon B, Walther T, Kramer M, Neugebauer E. Trauma and circulatory arrest: 224 preclinical resuscitations in Cologne in 1987–1990 [in German]. *Anaesthesist*. 1994;43:786–790.
3. Hazinski MF, Chahine AA, Holcomb GW III, Morris JA Jr. Outcome of cardiovascular collapse in pediatric blunt trauma. *Ann Emerg Med*. 1994;23: 1229–1235.
4. Bickell WH, Wall MJ Jr, Pepe PE, Martin RR, Ginger VF, Allen MK, Mattox KL. Immediate versus delayed fluid resuscitation for hypotensive patients with penetrating torso injuries. *N Engl J Med*. 1994;331:1105–1109.
5. Pepe PE. Emergency medical services systems and prehospital management of patients requiring critical care. In: Carlson R, Geheb M, eds. *Principles and Practice of Medical Intensive Care*. Philadelphia, Pa: Saunders; 1993:9–24.
6. Rozycki G, Adams C, Champion HR, Kihn R. Resuscitative thoracotomy: trends in outcome. *Ann Emerg Med*. 1990;19:462.
7. Copass MK, Oreskovich MR, Bladergroen MR, Carrico CJ. Prehospital cardiopulmonary resuscitation of the critically injured patient. *Am J Surg*. 1984;148:20–26.
8. Durham LA III, Richardson RJ, Wall MJ Jr, Pepe PE, Mattox KL. Emergency center thoracotomy: impact of prehospital resuscitation. *J Trauma*. 1992;32:775–779.
9. Kloeck WGJ, Kramer EB. Prehospital advanced CPR in the trauma patient. *Trauma Emerg Med*. 1993;10:772–776.
10. Schmidt U, Frame SB, Nerlich ML, Rowe DW, Enderson BL, Maull KI, Tscherne H. On-scene helicopter transport of patients with multiple injuries: comparison of a German and an American system [see comments]. *J Trauma*. 1992;33:548–553; discussion 553–555.
11. Kloeck WG. A practical approach to the aetiology of pulseless electrical activity: a simple 10-step training mnemonic. *Resuscitation*. 1995;30: 157–159.
12. McLean RF, Devitt JH, Dubbin J, McLellan BA. Incidence of abnormal RNA studies and dysrhythmias in patients with blunt chest trauma. *J Trauma*. 1991;31:968–970.
13. Paone RF, Peacock JB, Smith DL. Diagnosis of myocardial contusion. *South Med J*. 1993;86:867–870.
14. Solomonov E, Hirsh M, Yahiya A, Krausz MM. The effect of vigorous fluid resuscitation in uncontrolled hemorrhagic shock after massive splenic injury [see comments]. *Crit Care Med*. 2000;28:749–754.

Cardiac Arrest Associated With Pregnancy

Background

Most pregnant women have little interest in thinking about the prospect of death. Mortality related to the pregnancy itself is rare, occurring in an estimated 1 of every 30 000 deliveries.[1]

A cardiovascular emergency in a pregnant woman creates a special situation—the involvement of a second person, the in utero child. The child must always be considered when an adverse cardiovascular event occurs in a pregnant woman. The decision of whether to perform an emergency cesarean section must be made quickly. Emergency cesarean section has the highest chance of improving the outcome for both mother and child.[2]

Significant physiological changes occur in a woman during pregnancy. For example, cardiac output, blood volume, minute ventilation, and oxygen consumption all increase. Furthermore, the gravid uterus may cause significant compression of iliac and abdominal vessels when the mother is in the supine position, resulting in reduced cardiac output and hypotension.

Causes of Cardiac Arrest Associated With Pregnancy

There are many different causes of cardiac arrest in pregnant women. Cardiac arrest in the mother is most commonly related to changes and events that occur at the time of delivery, such as

- Amniotic fluid embolism
- Eclampsia
- Drug toxicity (eg, due to magnesium sulfate or epidural anesthetics)

It may also be related to the complex physiological changes associated with the pregnancy itself, such as

- Congestive cardiomyopathy
- Aortic dissection
- Pulmonary embolism
- Hemorrhage due to a pregnancy-related pathological condition

Finally, and tragically, pregnant women suffer the same problems of motor vehicle accidents, falls, assault, attempted suicide, and penetrating trauma (eg, stabbings and gunshot wounds) as the rest of modern society.[3] Regrettably, this daily stream of violence and trauma causes many dramatic events that require heroic interventions. Our response has been to craft harsh phrases to guide emergency care, such as "postmortem C-section," "perimortem delivery," "sacrifice mother or child or save mother or child," "harvest the fetus," and "empty the uterus." We walk a thin line between aiding our memory and demeaning our patients. These guidelines will not repeat such phrases.[4]

Key Interventions to Prevent Arrest

In an emergency the simplest action may be the most often ignored action. Many cardiovascular problems associated with pregnancy are due to nothing more than anatomy interacting with gravity. The pregnant woman's uterus, great with child, may press down against the inferior vena cava, reducing or blocking blood flow. The ensuing failure of venous blood return can produce hypotension and even shock.[5,6]

To treat a distressed or compromised pregnant patient:

- Place the patient in the left lateral position or *manually and gently* displace the uterus to the left.
- Give 100% oxygen.
- Give a fluid bolus.
- Immediately reevaluate the need for any drugs being administered.

Modifications to BLS Guidelines for Arrest

Do not forget the simple BLS actions you can take:

- Relieve aortocaval compression by manually displacing the gravid uterus.
- You can also use wedge-shaped cushions, multiple pillows, overturned chairs, a rescuer's thighs, or commercially available foam-cushion wedges (eg, the Cardiff wedge) to displace the uterus.[7]
- Generally perform chest compressions higher on the sternum to adjust for the shifting of pelvic and abdominal contents toward the head. We lack clear guidelines on how far the compression point should be shifted. Use the pulse check during chest compressions to adjust the sternal compression point.
- Address the need for left-lateral tilt of the torso to prevent compression or blockage of the vena cava. Foam-cushion wedges work best because they provide a wide, firm, angled surface to support the tilted torso during chest compressions. In the usual circumstances surrounding a suddenly pulseless, gravid woman, however, such single-purpose equipment will not be available.
- Two alternative means of support are the angled backs of several chairs and the angled thighs of several rescuers.

Circulation. 2000;102(suppl I):I-247–I-249.
© 2000 American Heart Association, Inc.

Circulation is available at http://www.circulationaha.org

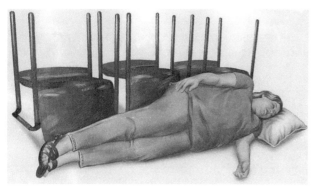

Figure. Left lateral position for pregnant woman.

Overturn a 4-legged chair so that the top of the chair back touches the floor. Align 1 or 2 more overturned chairs on either side of the first so that all are tilted in the same manner. Place the woman on her left side, align her torso parallel with the chair backs, and begin chest compressions (see Figure).

Modifications to ACLS Guidelines for Arrest

There are ***no*** changes to the standard ACLS algorithms for medications, intubation, and defibrillation. Assess and treat the pregnant woman who has a sudden cardiac arrest by using the Primary and Secondary ABCD Surveys of ACLS as modified for the pregnant woman (Table 1).

Consider a wide variety of possible causes of arrest such as amniotic fluid embolism, magnesium sulfate toxicity, mishap in patients who received spinal anesthesia, drug overdose, drug abuse, medication toxicity, and iatrogenic events.

Should You Perform an Emergency Cesarean Section to Reduce the Size and Weight of the Gravid Uterus?

When Standard BLS and ACLS Fail

If standard application of BLS and ACLS fail and there is some chance that the fetus is viable, consider immediate perimortem cesarean section. The goal is to deliver the fetus within 4 to 5 minutes after the onset of arrest. If at all possible involve obstetric and neonatal personnel.[8]

Why Reduce the Size and Weight of the Uterus?

With the mother in cardiac arrest, the blood supply to the fetus rapidly becomes hypoxic and acidotic, causing adverse effects in the fetus. Return of blood to the mother's heart, blocked by the uterus pressing against the inferior vena cava, must be restored. Consequently *the key to resuscitation of the child is resuscitation of the mother.* The mother cannot be resuscitated until blood flow to her right ventricle is restored.

This results in the familiar admonition to immediately begin cesarean section and remove the baby and placenta when arrest occurs in a near-term pregnant woman. That single act allows access to the infant so that newborn

TABLE 1. Primary and Secondary ABCD Surveys: Modifications for Pregnant Women

ACLS Approach	Modifications to Standard BLS and ACLS Guidelines
Primary ABCD Survey	**A**irway No modifications.
	Breathing No modifications.
	Circulation Chest compressions are ineffective when a woman in her last trimester lies on her back because the gravid uterus blocks the return of blood from the inferior vena cava. Start chest compressions after you place the woman on her left side with her back angled 30° to 45° from the floor. *or* Start chest compressions after you place a wedge under the woman's right side (so that she lies on her left side). *or* Have 1 rescuer kneel next to the woman on her left side and gently pull the gravid uterus laterally to relieve pressure on the inferior vena cava.
	Defibrillation No modifications. Defibrillatory shocks transfer no significant current to the fetus in utero.
Secondary ABCD Survey	**A**irway No modifications to intubation techniques.
	Breathing No modifications to secondary confirmation of successful intubation. A gravid uterus is known to push up the diaphragm and therefore decrease ventilatory volumes and make positive-pressure ventilation difficult.
	Circulation Follow standard ACLS recommendations for administration of all resuscitation medications.
	Differential Diagnosis and Decisions Decide whether to perform emergency cesarean section (see Table 2).

resuscitation can be started. Cesarean section also immediately corrects much of the abnormal physiology of the full-term mother. The critical point to remember is that *you will lose both mother and infant if you cannot restore blood flow to the mother's heart.*[9]

Advance Preparation

Table 2 lists the multiple factors that must be considered in a very short time during an emotionally dramatic event. All Emergency Departments should rehearse their plan of action for this type of event, including location of supplies, sources of extra equipment, and best methods for obtaining subspecialty assistance.

TABLE 2. The C-Section Decision: Factors to Consider in the Decision to Perform Emergency Cesarean Section During Arrest

Factors to Consider	Comments
Arrest factors to consider	**Arrest factors**
Has >3 or 4 minutes passed since the onset of arrest?	Almost no time passes before the clinican must decide whether to perform a C-section. The optimal chance for survival of mother and child depends on rapid delivery of the child.
Has the mother responded to appropriate BLS and ACLS care?	
CPR performed at the proper angle?	This decision must be made within 4 to 5 minutes of the maternal arrest.
Proper placement of the endotracheal tube?	We purposely omit recommending a maximum time to allow before making the decision. Such a "standard" is of interest only to those involved in disputes over proper care during the arrest. There are many legitimate reasons for additional minutes of delay.
IV medications?	
	Ensure that the mother has received superior resuscitative efforts. You cannot declare her "refractory" to CPR and ACLS unless all interventions have been implemented and implemented well.
Mother-child factors	**Mother-child factors**
Has the mother suffered an inevitably fatal injury? Is the only issue whether the child is old enough to have a good chance of meaningful survival?	Do not lose sight of the goal of this dramatic event: to yield a live, neurologically intact infant and mother.
Is the fetus so small or young that survival is unlikely? Is the only issue whether the mother would benefit from C-section?	Carefully consider the future before pushing the margins of survivability.
Removing the fetus and placenta can be beneficial to the mother even when the fetus is too small to compress the inferior vena cava.	Even if the fetus's chances of survival are extremely low, the mother may benefit from emergency C-section.
Has too much time passed between the mother's collapse and removal of the fetus? Is meaningful survival of either mother or infant highly unlikely or impossible?	Some obstetric experts argue for empirical postarrest C-section on any pregnant woman who has a cardiac arrest regardless of the cause.
Setting and personnel	
Are appropriate supplies and equipment available?	
Is C-section within the rescuer's "comfort zone" of skill?	
Are skilled pediatric support personnel available to care for the infant, especially if it is not at full term?	
Are obstetric personnel immediately available to support the mother after C-section?	
In both in-hospital and out-of-hospital settings, is there staff support and approval? In out-of-hospital settings, is bystander support available?	
Differential diagnosis	
Consider whether persistent arrest is due to an immediately reversible problem (eg, excess anesthesia, reaction to analgesia, or severe bronchospasm). If it is, do not perform C-section.	
Consider whether persistent arrest is due to a fatal, untreatable problem (eg, massive amniotic fluid embolism). If it is, quickly perform C-section to save the child, considering the viability of the child.	

References

1. Wolcomir M, ed. *Advanced Life Support for Obstetrics.* Kansas City, Mo: American Academy of Family Physicians; 1996.
2. Katz VL, Wells SR, Kuller JA, Hansen WF, McMahon MJ, Bowes WA Jr. Cesarean delivery: a reconsideration of terminology. *Obstet Gynecol.* 1995;86:152–153.
3. Kupas DF, Harter SC, Vosk A. Out-of-hospital perimortem cesarean section. *Prehosp Emerg Care.* 1998;2:206–208.
4. Kam CW. Perimortem caesarean sections (PMCS). *J Accid Emerg Med.* 1994;11:57–58.
5. Page-Rodriguez A, Gonzalez-Sanchez JA. Perimortem cesarean section of twin pregnancy: case report and review of the literature. *Acad Emerg Med.* 1999;6:1072–1074.
6. Cardosi RJ, Porter KB. Cesarean delivery of twins during maternal cardiopulmonary arrest. *Obstet Gynecol.* 1998;92:695–697.
7. Goodwin AP, Pearce AJ. The human wedge: a manoeuvre to relieve aortocaval compression in resuscitation during late pregnancy. *Anaesthesia.* 1992;47:433–434.
8. Whitten M, Irvine LM. Postmortem and perimortem caesarean section: what are the indications? *J R Soc Med.* 2000;93:6–9.
9. Lanoix R, Akkapeddi V, Goldfeder B. Perimortem cesarean section: case reports and recommendations. *Acad Emerg Med.* 1995;2:1063–1067.

Electric Shock and Lightning Strikes

Background

Electric Shock

Most electric shock injuries to adults occur in the occupational setting.[1] Pediatric electric shock injuries occur most commonly in the home, when the child bites electrical wires, places an object in an electrical socket, contacts an exposed low-voltage wire or appliance, or touches a high-voltage wire outdoors.[2]

Electric shock injuries result from the direct effects of current on cell membranes and vascular smooth muscle and from the conversion of electric energy into heat energy as current passes through body tissues. Factors that determine the nature and severity of electric trauma include the magnitude of energy delivered, voltage, resistance to current flow, type of current, duration of contact with the current source, and current pathway. Victims of electric shock can sustain a wide variety of injuries, ranging from a transient unpleasant sensation caused by low-intensity current to instantaneous cardiac arrest caused by exposure to high voltage or high current.

High-tension current generally causes the most serious injuries, although fatal electrocutions may occur with household current (110 V in the United States and Canada, 220 V in Europe, Australia, Asia, and many other localities).[3] Bone and skin are most resistant to the passage of electric current; muscle, blood vessels, and nerves conduct with least resistance.[4] Skin resistance, the most important factor impeding current flow, can be reduced substantially by moisture, thereby converting what ordinarily might be a minor injury into a life-threatening shock.[5] Skin resistance can be overcome with increased duration of exposure to current flow. Contact with alternating current at 60 cycles per second (the frequency used in most household and commercial sources of electricity) may cause tetanic skeletal muscle contractions and prevent self-release from the source of the electricity, thereby leading to prolonged duration of exposure. The repetitive frequency of alternating current also increases the likelihood of current flow through the heart during the vulnerable recovery period of the cardiac cycle. This exposure can precipitate VF, analogous to the R-on-T phenomenon.[6]

Transthoracic current flow (eg, a hand-to-hand pathway) is more likely to be fatal than a vertical (hand-to-foot) or straddle (foot-to-foot) current path.[7] The vertical pathway, however, often causes myocardial injury, which has been attributed to the direct effects of current and coronary artery spasm.[8–10]

Lightning Strike

Lightning strike kills hundreds of people internationally every year and injures many times that number. Lightning injuries have a 30% mortality rate, and up to 70% of survivors sustain significant morbidity.[11–13]

The presentation of lightning strike injuries varies widely, even among groups of people struck at the same time.[14] In some victims symptoms are mild and may not require hospitalization, whereas others die from the injury.[15,16]

The primary cause of death in lightning-strike victims is cardiac arrest, which may be associated with primary VF or asystole.[15–18] Lightning acts as an instantaneous, massive direct current countershock, simultaneously depolarizing the entire myocardium.[16,19] In many cases cardiac automaticity may restore organized cardiac activity, and a perfusing rhythm may return spontaneously. However, concomitant respiratory arrest due to thoracic muscle spasm and suppression of the respiratory center may continue after return of spontaneous circulation. Thus, unless ventilatory assistance is provided, a secondary hypoxic cardiac arrest may occur.[20]

Lightning can also produce widespread effects on the cardiovascular system, producing extensive catecholamine release or autonomic stimulation. If cardiac arrest does not occur, the victim may develop hypertension, tachycardia, nonspecific ECG changes (including prolongation of the QT interval and transient T-wave inversion), and myocardial necrosis with release of creatine kinase-MB fraction. Right and left ventricular ejection fractions may also be depressed, but this injury appears to be reversible.[18]

Lightning can produce a wide spectrum of neurological injuries. Injuries may be primary, resulting from the effects on the brain. Effects may also be secondary, as a complication of cardiac arrest and hypoxia.[12] The current can produce brain hemorrhages, edema, and small-vessel and neuronal injury. Hypoxic encephalopathy can result from cardiac arrest. Effects of a lightning strike on the peripheral nervous system include myelin damage.[12]

Patients most likely to die of lightning injury if no treatment is forthcoming are those who suffer immediate cardiac arrest. Patients who do not suffer cardiac arrest and those who respond to immediate treatment have an excellent chance of recovery because subsequent arrest is uncommon. Therefore, when multiple victims are struck simultaneously by lightning, rescuers should give highest priority to patients in respiratory or cardiac arrest.

For victims in cardiopulmonary arrest, BLS and ACLS should be instituted immediately. The goal is to oxygenate the heart and brain adequately until cardiac activity is restored. Victims with respiratory arrest may require only ventilation and oxygenation to avoid secondary hypoxic cardiac arrest. Resuscitative attempts may have higher success rates in lightning victims than in patients with cardiac arrest from

Circulation. 2000;102(suppl I):I-250–I-252.
© 2000 American Heart Association, Inc.

Circulation is available at http://www.circulationaha.org

other causes, and efforts may be effective even when the interval before the resuscitative attempt is prolonged.[20]

Clinical Effects

Immediately after electrocution or lightning strike, the victim's respiratory function, circulation, or both, may fail. The patient may be apneic, mottled, unconscious, and in cardiac arrest from VF or asystole.

Respiratory arrest may be caused by a variety of mechanisms:

- Electric current passing through the brain and causing inhibition of medullary respiratory center function
- Tetanic contraction of the diaphragm and chest wall musculature during current exposure
- Prolonged paralysis of respiratory muscles, which may continue for minutes after the electric shock has terminated

If respiratory arrest persists, hypoxic cardiac arrest may occur.

Cardiopulmonary arrest is the primary cause of immediate death due to electrical injury.[21] VF or ventricular asystole may occur as a direct result of electric shock. Other serious cardiac arrhythmias, including VT that may progress to VF, may result from exposure to low- or high-voltage current.[22]

Modifications of BLS Actions for Arrest Caused by Electric Shock or Lightning Strike

The rescuer must be certain that rescue efforts will not put him or her in danger of electric shock. After the power is turned off by authorized personnel or the energized source is safely cleared from the victim, determine the victim's cardiorespiratory status. Immediately after electrocution, respiration or circulation or both may fail. The patient may be apneic, mottled, unconscious, and in circulatory collapse with VF or asystole.

Vigorous resuscitative measures are indicated, even for those who appear dead on initial evaluation. The prognosis for recovery from electric shock or lightning strike is not readily predictable because the amplitude and duration of the charge usually are unknown. However, because many victims are young and without preexisting cardiopulmonary disease, they have a reasonable chance for survival if immediate support of cardiopulmonary function is provided.

If spontaneous respiration or circulation is absent, initiate the ABCD techniques outlined in parts 3 and 4 of these guidelines, including EMS system activation, prompt CPR, and use of the AED. The presenting cardiac ECG rhythm may be asystole or VF.[23]

As soon as possible, secure the airway and provide ventilation and supplemental oxygen. When electric shock occurs in a location not readily accessible, such as on a utility pole, rescuers must lower the victim to the ground as quickly as possible. Note: Actions that involve rescuer proximity to live current must be performed only by specially trained rescuers who know how to execute this task. If the victim remains unresponsive, rescuers should start the standard ABCD protocols, including AED use by lay responders.

If the victim has no signs of circulation, start chest compressions as soon as feasible. In addition, use the AED to identify and treat VT or VF.

Maintain spinal protection and immobilization during extrication and treatment if there is any likelihood of head or neck trauma.[23,24] Electrical injuries often cause related trauma, including injury to the spine[24] and muscular strains and fractures due to the tetanic response of skeletal muscles. Remove smoldering clothing, shoes, and belts to prevent further thermal damage.

Modification of ACLS Support for Arrest Caused by Electric Shock or Lightning Strike

Treat VF, asystole, and other serious arrhythmias with ACLS techniques outlined in these guidelines. Quickly attempt defibrillation, if needed, at the scene.

Establishing an airway may be difficult for patients with electric burns of the face, mouth, or anterior neck. Extensive soft-tissue swelling may develop rapidly and complicate airway control measures, such as endotracheal intubation. For these reasons, intubation should be accomplished on an elective basis before signs of airway obstruction become severe.

For victims with hypovolemic shock or significant tissue destruction, rapid intravenous fluid administration is indicated to counteract shock and correct ongoing fluid losses. Fluid administration should be adequate to maintain diuresis to facilitate excretion of myoglobin, potassium, and other by-products of tissue destruction.[19] Increased capillary permeability may develop in association with tissue injury, so local tissue edema may develop at the site of injury. Because electrothermal burns and underlying tissue injury may require surgical attention, we encourage early consultation with a physician skilled in treatment of electrical injury.

References

1. Cooper MA. Electrical and lightning injuries. *Emerg Med Clin North Am*. 1984;2:489–501.
2. Kobernick M. Electrical injuries: pathophysiology and emergency management. *Ann Emerg Med*. 1982;11:633–638.
3. Budnick LD. Bathtub-related electrocutions in the United States, 1979 to 1982. *JAMA*. 1984;252:918–920.
4. Browne BJ, Gaasch WR. Electrical injuries and lightning. *Emerg Med Clin North Am*. 1992;10:211–229.
5. Wallace JF. Electrical injuries. In: *Harrison's Principles of Internal Medicine*. 12th ed. New York, NY: McGraw-Hill, Health Professions Division; 1991:various pagings.
6. Geddes LA, Bourland JD, Ford G. The mechanism underlying sudden death from electric shock. *Med Instrum*. 1986;20:303–315.
7. Thompson JC, Ashwal S. Electrical injuries in children. *Am J Dis Child*. 1983;137:231–235.
8. Chandra NC, Siu CO, Munster AM. Clinical predictors of myocardial damage after high voltage electrical injury. *Crit Care Med*. 1990;18:293–297.
9. Ku CS, Lin SL, Hsu TL, Wang SP, Chang MS. Myocardial damage associated with electrical injury. *Am Heart J*. 1989;118:621–624.
10. Xenopoulos N, Movahed A, Hudson P, Reeves WC. Myocardial injury in electrocution. *Am Heart J*. 1991;122:1481–1484.
11. Cooper MA. Lightning injuries: prognostic signs for death. *Ann Emerg Med*. 1980;9:134–138.
12. Kleinschmidt-DeMasters BK. Neuropathology of lightning-strike injuries. *Semin Neurol*. 1995;15:323–328.

13. Stewart CE. When lightning strikes. *Emerg Med Serv*. 2000;29:57–67; quiz 103.

14. Fahmy FS, Brinsden MD, Smith J, Frame JD. Lightning: the multisystem group injuries. *J Trauma*. 1999;46:937–940.

15. Patten BM. Lightning and electrical injuries. *Neurol Clin*. 1992;10: 1047–1058.

16. Browne BJ, Gaasch WR. Electrical injuries and lightning. *Emerg Med Clin North Am*. 1992;10:211–229.

17. Kleiner JP, Wilkin JH. Cardiac effects of lightning stroke. *JAMA*. 1978; 240:2757–2759.

18. Lichtenberg R, Dries D, Ward K, Marshall W, Scanlon P. Cardiovascular effects of lightning strikes. *J Am Coll Cardiol*. 1993;21:531–536.

19. Cooper MA. Emergent care of lightning and electrical injuries. *Semin Neurol*. 1995;15:268–278.

20. Milzman DP, Moskowitz L, Hardel M. Lightning strikes at a mass gathering. *South Med J*. 1999;92:708–710.

21. Homma S, Gillam LD, Weyman AE. Echocardiographic observations in survivors of acute electrical injury. *Chest*. 1990;97:103–105.

22. Jensen PJ, Thomsen PE, Bagger JP, Norgaard A, Baandrup U. Electrical injury causing ventricular arrhythmias. *Br Heart J*. 1987;57:279–283.

23. Duclos PJ, Sanderson LM. An epidemiological description of lightning-related deaths in the United States. *Int J Epidemiol*. 1990;19:673–679.

24. Epperly TD, Stewart JR. The physical effects of lightning injury. *J Fam Pract*. 1989;29:267–272.

Part 9: Pediatric Basic Life Support

Major Guidelines Changes

Changes in the pediatric section of the International Guidelines 2000 generally represent qualifications and refinements rather than major paradigm shifts from the 1992 Guidelines.[1] The new guidelines continue to emphasize prevention of cardiac arrest. Pediatric BLS guidelines detail specific modifications of adult techniques necessary to address anatomic, physiological, etiologic, and psychosocial issues for infants and children. The initial sequence of BLS interventions in the pediatric Chain of Survival continues to be based on the most common etiology of arrest for a given age group, with modifications encouraged for special resuscitation circumstances.

Multiple studies have documented poor skills retention by participants of traditional BLS courses and improved skills retention when course information is simplified. As a result, all potential science changes were evaluated with respect to their effect on the complexity of teaching. Changes expected to simplify CPR teaching were encouraged.

Highlights of the pediatric resuscitation section of the International Guidelines 2000 are as follows:

Chain of Survival

- An etiology-based sequence for resuscitation was considered, but the age-based sequence ("phone fast" for infants and children, "phone first" for children >8 years old and adults) was retained (Class Indeterminate).
- Lay rescuers should be taught exceptions to the age-based sequence of resuscitation, which may include the following:
  —Lone rescuers should "phone fast" (provide immediate rescue breathing and other steps of CPR before phoning the EMS system) when submersion victims of any age are rescued from the water.
  —Lone rescuers should "phone first" (phone EMS before beginning CPR) after the sudden collapse of a child with a known history of heart disease.
- There is a need for more and better data regarding the epidemiology, treatment, and outcome of pediatric cardiopulmonary arrest.[2] There is insufficient data to guide recommendations for pediatric resuscitation. Data collection efforts should use consistent terminology and record important time intervals. Critical elements for data collection have been described by an international consensus process, the Pediatric Utstein Guidelines for Reporting Outcome of Pediatric Cardiopulmonary Arrest.[3]
- Teaching of cardiopulmonary resuscitation skills must be simplified, and courses must be skill-based and outcome driven.

Basic Life Support Sequence

Pulse Check

- All rescuers are instructed to assess for *signs of circulation* before beginning chest compressions:
  —Lay rescuers are instructed to assess for signs of circulation rather than attempt to check a pulse (Class IIa).
  —Healthcare providers are instructed to assess for signs of circulation, including a pulse check.

Rescue Breathing and Bag-Mask Ventilation

Education in bag-mask ventilation should be included in all BLS curricula for the healthcare provider (Class IIa).

Bag-mask ventilation can provide lifesaving support for infants and children in both the out-of-hospital and in-hospital settings and is a skill that BLS providers should master (Class IIa).

Chest Compressions and Use of Automated External Defibrillators

- If 2 or more suitably trained healthcare providers are present, the 2 thumb–encircling hands chest compression technique is preferred over the 2-finger compression technique for infants when technically feasible. This technique is not taught to lay rescuers.
- If the victim of out-of-hospital cardiac arrest is ≥8 years old (approximately >25 kg body weight), use of automated external defibrillators (AEDs) is encouraged (Class IIb), although data regarding the use of AEDs in this age group is limited.

Relief of Foreign-Body Airway Obstruction

- The extremely complex skills sequence for *lay rescuer* relief of foreign-body airway obstruction (FBAO) in the unconscious victim has been simplified. The sequence for healthcare provider relief of FBAO in the unconscious victim remains unchanged (Class IIb).

Introduction

Pediatric BLS refers to the provision of CPR, with no devices or with bag-mask ventilation or barrier devices, until advanced life support (ALS) can be provided. The population addressed in this chapter includes infants from birth to 1 year of age and children from 1 to 8 years of age.

CPR and life support in the pediatric age group should be part of a community-wide Chain of Survival that links the child to the best hope of survival following emergencies. The Chain of Survival integrates education in prevention of cardiopulmonary arrest, BLS, early access to EMS systems prepared for children's needs, early and effective pediatric

Circulation. 2000;102(suppl I):I-253–I-290.
© 2000 American Heart Association, Inc.

Circulation is available at http://www.circulationaha.org

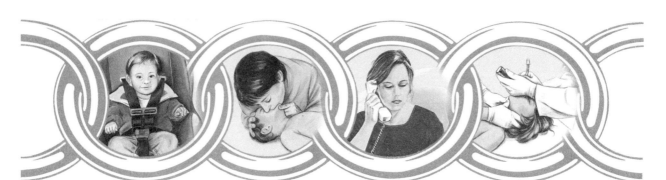

Figure 1. Pediatric Chain of Survival.

ALS, and pediatric postresuscitation and rehabilitative care (Figure 1).

Sudden cardiopulmonary arrest in infants and children is much less common than sudden cardiac arrest in adults.[4] In contrast to cardiac arrest in adults, cardiac arrest in infants and children is rarely a sudden event, and *non*-cardiac causes predominate.[4] The etiology of cardiac arrest in infants and children varies by age, setting, and the underlying health of the child. For these reasons, the sequence of CPR for infants and children requires a different approach from that used for adult victims.

Cardiac arrest in the under-21-year-old age group occurs most commonly at either end of the age spectrum: under 1 year of age and during the teenage years. In the newly born infant, respiratory failure is the most common cause of cardiopulmonary deterioration and arrest. During infancy the most common causes of arrest include sudden infant death syndrome (SIDS), respiratory diseases, airway obstruction (including foreign-body aspiration), submersion, sepsis, and neurological disease.[5–11] Beyond 1 year of age, injuries are the leading cause of death.[12–14]

Cardiac arrest in children typically represents the terminal event of progressive shock or respiratory failure. Either shock or respiratory failure may include a compensated state from which children can rapidly deteriorate to a decompensated condition with progression to respiratory or cardiac arrest. Therefore, rescuers must detect and promptly treat early signs of respiratory and circulatory failure to prevent cardiac arrest. In children, early effective bystander CPR has been associated with successful return of spontaneous circulation and neurologically intact survival.[15,16] BLS courses should be offered to target populations such as expectant parents, child care providers, teachers, sports supervisors, and others who regularly care for children. Parents and child care providers of children with underlying conditions that predispose them to cardiopulmonary failure should be particularly targeted for these courses.

These guidelines are based on a review and analysis of clinical and experimental evidence.[17] Because this evidence varies widely in quality and quantity, each new guideline recommendation includes information about the strength of the scientific data on which it was based. In addition, a summary class of recommendation is indicated. For more information on the evidence evaluation process, see Evidence-Based Evaluation in "Part 1: Introduction."

Throughout these Guidelines, the following definitions of classes of recommendations are used:

- **Class I** recommendations are always acceptable. They are proven safe and definitely useful, and they are supported by excellent evidence from at least 1 prospective, randomized controlled clinical trial.
- **Class IIa** recommendations are considered acceptable and useful with good to very good evidence providing support. The weight of evidence and expert opinions strongly favor these interventions.
- **Class IIb** recommendations are considered acceptable and useful with weak or only fair evidence providing support. The weight of evidence and expert opinion are not strongly in favor of the intervention.
- **Class III** refers to interventions that are unacceptable. These interventions lack any evidence of benefit, and often the evidence suggests or confirms harm.
- **Class Indeterminate** refers to an intervention that is promising, but the evidence is insufficient in quantity and/or quality to support a definitive class of recommendation. The Indeterminate Class was added to indicate interventions that are considered safe and perhaps effective and are recommended by expert consensus. However, the available evidence supporting the recommendation is either too weak or too limited at present to make a definite recommendation based on the published data.

Levels of evidence and classes of recommendations are fully defined in "Part 1: Introduction." Ideally, treatments of choice are supported by excellent evidence and are Class I recommendations. Unfortunately the limited depth or quality of published pediatric cardiac arrest and resuscitation data often limited the strength of recommendations included in these guidelines to Class IIa or IIb.

International Guidelines: International Liaison Committee on Resuscitation Advisory Statements

Following the implementation of the 1992 guidelines,[1] the representatives of 7 of the world's resuscitation councils formed the International Liaison Committee on Resuscitation (ILCOR). For the next 8 years, members of ILCOR developed advisory statements containing consensus recommendations based on existing resuscitation guidelines, practical experience, and informal interpretation. During this time an ILCOR task force met to address issues regarding resuscitation of the newly born, infant, and child; these meetings produced 2 ILCOR advisory statements.[18,19]

A high degree of uniformity exists in current guidelines for resuscitation of the newly born, neonates, infants, and young children endorsed by the resuscitation councils in developed countries around the world. Differences are largely the result of local and regional preferences or customs, training networks, and equipment/medication availability rather than differences in interpretation of scientific evidence.

To develop the pediatric resuscitation section of the International Guidelines 2000, the Subcommittee on Pediatric Resuscitation of the American Heart Association and other pediatric representatives from ILCOR identified issues or new developments worthy of further in-depth evaluation. From this list, areas of active research and evolving controversy were identified. Evidence-based evaluation of each of these areas was conducted and debated, culminating in assignment of consensus-defined levels of evidence for specific Guidelines questions. After identification and careful review of this evidence, the Pediatric Working Group of ILCOR and the AHA Pediatric Resuscitation Subcommittee updated the Pediatric guidelines and objectively attempted to link the class of recommendation to the identified level of evidence.

During these discussions the authors recognized the need to make recommendations for important interventions and treatment even when the only level of evidence was poor or absent. In the absence of specific pediatric data (outcome validity), recommendations were made on the basis of common sense (face validity) or ease of teaching or skills retention (construct validity).

To reduce confusion and simplify education, pediatric recommendations are consistent with the adult and neonatal BLS and ALS algorithms and guidelines whenever possible and appropriate. Areas of departure from the adult algorithms and interventions are noted with the rationale. Ultimately the practicality of implementing recommendations must be considered in the context of local resources (technology and personnel) and customs. No resuscitation protocol or guideline can be expected to appropriately anticipate all potential scenarios. These guidelines and treatment algorithms should serve as a guiding template to provide most critically ill children with appropriate support while thoughtful and appropriate etiology-based interventions are assembled and implemented.

The ILCOR advisory statements targeted existing and developing national resuscitation councils. The pediatric section of the International Guidelines 2000 attempts to apply the ILCOR advisory statements and updated international review of evidence to create advisory guidelines for local and regional EMS systems and organizations that care for children. Individual systems must adapt these guidelines to fit the needs and resources of their community, especially in regions in which EMS systems are not well developed. The principles and mechanics of resuscitation presented here should apply to all children, but application and methodology of a specific Chain of Survival is largely dependent on EMS systems and availability of resources. Specific training materials are necessary to target individual instructors and resuscitation providers in a given community.

Response to Cardiovascular Emergencies During Infancy and Childhood

Definition of Newly Born, Neonate, Infant, Child, and Adult

The term "neonate" is applied to infants in the first 28 days (month) of life.[5] The term "newly born" is used in these guidelines to refer specifically to the neonate in the first minutes to hours after birth. This term is used to focus attention on the needs of the infant *at* and *immediately after birth* (including the first hours of life). The terms newborn or neonate were previously used but did not clearly refer to the first hours—rather than month—of life. The term "infant" includes the neonatal period and extends to the age of 1 year (12 months). For the purposes of these guidelines, the term "child" refers to ages 1 to 8 years. The term "adult" applies to victims ≥8 years of age through adult years.

Pediatric BLS and ALS interventions tend to "blur at the margins" of the age definitions of infant, child, and adult because no single anatomic or physiological characteristic consistently distinguishes the infant from the child from the adult victim of cardiac arrest. Furthermore, new technologies such as AEDs and airway and vascular access adjuncts that can be implemented with minimal advanced training create the need to re-examine previous age-based recommendations for therapies. The child's developing anatomy and physiology and the most common causes of cardiopulmonary arrest should be considered in the development and use of resuscitation guidelines for children of different ages.

For the purposes of BLS, the term "infant" is defined by the approximate size of the young child who can receive effective chest compression given with 2 fingers or 2 thumbs with encircling hands. By consensus, the age cut-off for infants is 1 year. Note, however, that this definition is not based on physiological differences between infants and children. For example, the differences between an 11-month-old "infant" and a 17-month-old "child" are smaller than the differences in anatomy and physiology between a 1-week-old and a 10-month-old infant.

Historically the use of the term "child" in the ECC guidelines has been limited to age 8 years to simplify BLS education. Cardiac compression can generally be accomplished with 1 hand for victims between the ages of 1 and 8 years. However, variability in the size of the victim or the size and strength of the rescuer can require use of the 2-finger or 2 thumb–encircling hands technique for chest compression in a small toddler or 2-handed "adult" compression technique for chest compression in a large child who is 6 to 7 years old.[20,21]

Anatomic and Physiological Differences Affecting Cardiac Arrest and Resuscitation

Respiratory failure or arrest is a common cause of cardiac arrest during infancy and childhood. These guidelines emphasize immediate provision of bystander CPR—including opening of the airway and delivery of rescue breathing—

before activation of the local EMS system. This emphasis on immediate support of oxygenation and ventilation is based on knowledge of the important role of respiratory failure in cardiac arrest. Optimal application of early oxygenation and ventilation requires an understanding of airway anatomy and physiology.

Airway Anatomy and Physiology

For many reasons, the infant and child are at risk for the development of airway obstruction and respiratory failure.[22,23] The upper and lower airways of the infant and child are much smaller than the upper and lower airways of the adult. As a result, modest airway obstruction from edema, mucous plugs, or a foreign body can significantly reduce pediatric airway diameter and increase resistance to air flow and work of breathing.

1. The infant tongue is proportionately large in relation to the size of the oropharynx. As a result, posterior displacement of the tongue occurs readily and may cause severe airway obstruction in the infant.
2. In the infant and child the subglottic airway is smaller and more compliant and the supporting cartilage less developed than in the adult. As a result, this portion of the airway can easily become obstructed by mucus, blood, pus, edema, active constriction, external compression, or pressure differences created during spontaneous respiratory effort in the presence of airway obstruction. The pediatric airway is very compliant and may collapse during spontaneous respiratory effort in the face of airway obstruction.
3. The ribs and sternum normally contribute to maintenance of lung volume. In infants these ribs are very compliant and may fail to maintain lung volume, particularly when the elastic recoil of the lungs is increased and/or lung compliance is decreased. As a result, functional residual capacity is reduced when respiratory effort is diminished or absent. In addition, the limited support of lung volume expansion by the ribs makes the infant more dependent on diaphragm movement to generate a tidal volume. Anything that interferes with diaphragm movement (eg, gastric distention, acute abdomen) may produce respiratory insufficiency.
4. Infants and children have limited oxygen reserve. Physiological collapse of the small airways at or below lung functional residual capacity and an interval of hypoxemia and hypercarbia preceding arrest often influence oxygen reserve and arrest metabolic conditions.[24]

Cardiac Output, Oxygen Delivery, and Oxygen Demand

Cardiac output is the product of heart rate and stroke volume. Although the pediatric heart is capable of increasing stroke volume, cardiac output during infancy and childhood is largely dependent on maintenance of an adequate heart rate. Bradycardia may be associated with a rapid fall in cardiac output, leading to rapid deterioration in systemic perfusion. In fact, bradycardia is one of the most common terminal rhythms observed in children. For this reason, lay rescuers are taught to provide chest compressions when there are no observed signs of circulation. Healthcare providers are taught to provide chest compressions when there are no observed signs of circulation (including absence of a pulse) or when

severe bradycardia (heart rate <60 beats per minute [bpm]) develops in the presence of poor systemic perfusion.

Epidemiology of Cardiopulmonary Arrest: "Phone Fast" (Infant, Child)/"Phone First" (Adult)

In adults, most sudden, nontraumatic cardiopulmonary arrest is *cardiac* in origin, and the most common terminal cardiac rhythm is ventricular fibrillation (VF).[25] In research studies the "gold standard" type of out-of-hospital adult arrest used to compare outcomes is *nontraumatic, witnessed arrest with a presenting rhythm of VF or pulseless ventricular tachycardia.*[26] For these victims, the time from collapse to defibrillation is the single greatest determinant of survival.[27–32] In addition, bystander CPR increases survival after sudden, witnessed adult cardiopulmonary arrest (relative odds of survival=2.6; 95% CI=2.0 to 3.4).[33,34]

In children, the incidence, precise etiology, and outcome of cardiac arrest and resuscitation are difficult to ascertain because most reports contain insufficient patient numbers or use exclusion criteria or inconsistent definitions that prohibit broad generalization to all children.[18] The causes of pediatric cardiopulmonary arrest are heterogeneous, including SIDS, asphyxia, near-drowning, trauma, and sepsis.[5,35–40] Therefore, there is no single gold standard pediatric cardiac arrest stereotype for research or single accepted gold standard resuscitation outcome.[41] Reported successful "outcomes" from arrest may include change in cardiac rhythm, improved hemodynamics during CPR, return of spontaneous circulation, survival to hospital admission, survival to hospital discharge, short- or long-term survival, or neurologically intact survival. Selection of the appropriate outcome variable and its specific relation to a single resuscitation intervention is often difficult.

In the pediatric age group, resuscitation is most frequently required at the time of birth. Approximately 5% to 10% of newly born infants require some degree of active resuscitation at birth, including stimulation to breathe,[42] and approximately 1% to 10% born in the hospital may require assisted ventilation.[43] Worldwide, >5 million neonatal deaths occur annually, with asphyxia at birth responsible for approximately 19% of these deaths.[44] Implementation of relatively simple resuscitation techniques could save an estimated 1 million infants per year.[19] For further information about resuscitation at the time of birth, see "Part 11: Neonatal Resuscitation."

Throughout infancy and childhood, most out-of-hospital cardiac arrest occurs in or around the home, where children are under the supervision of parents and child care providers. In this setting, conditions such as SIDS, trauma, drowning, poisoning, choking, severe asthma, and pneumonia are the most common causes of arrest. In industrialized nations, trauma is the leading cause of death from the age of 6 months through young adulthood.[13] In general, pediatric out-of-hospital arrest is characterized by a progression from hypoxia and hypercarbia to respiratory arrest and bradycardia and then asystolic cardiac arrest.[4,37,40] Ventricular tachycardia or fibrillation has been reported in ≤15% of pediatric victims of out-of-hospital arrest,[16,45,46] even when rhythm is assessed by first responders.[47,48] Survival after out-of-hospital cardiopulmonary arrest ranges from 3% to 17% in most studies,* and survivors are often neurologically devastated. Neurologically intact survival rates ≥50% have been reported for resuscitation of children with respiratory arrest alone.[9,55] Prompt, effective chest compressions and rescue breathing have been shown to improve return of spontaneous circulation and increase neurologically intact survival in children with cardiac arrest[16,40]; however, no other intervention has been definitively shown to improve survival or neurological outcome.

Organized rapid delivery of out-of-hospital BLS and ALS has improved the outcome of drowning victims in cardiac arrest, perhaps the best-studied scenario of out-of-hospital cardiac arrest.[15,57] Because most pediatric arrests are secondary to progressive respiratory failure and/or shock and because VF is relatively uncommon, immediate CPR ("phone fast") is recommended for pediatric victims of cardiopulmonary arrest in the out-of-hospital setting rather than the adult approach, immediate EMS activation ("phone first") and/or defibrillation. Effective BLS should be provided for infants and children as quickly as possible.

There are some circumstances in which primary arrhythmic cardiac arrest (ie, VF or pulseless ventricular tachycardia) is more likely; in these circumstances the lay rescuer may be instructed to activate the EMS system before beginning CPR. Examples include the sudden collapse of children with underlying cardiac disease or a history of arrhythmias. Families of children with *identified* risk for sudden cardiac arrest should be taught the "phone first" or adult sequence of CPR: if the child collapses suddenly, a lone bystander should *first* activate the local emergency medical response system and then return to the victim to begin CPR. Of course, whenever multiple rescuers are present for the victim of any age, one rescuer should remain with the victim to begin CPR while the other activates the emergency medical response system.

A *sudden* witnessed collapse in a previously healthy child or adolescent suggests that the arrest is cardiac in origin, and immediate activation of the EMS system may be beneficial, even if the victim is <8 years of age. Potential causes of sudden collapse in children with no known history of heart disease include prolonged-QT syndrome, hypertrophic cardiomyopathy, and drug-induced cardiac arrest.[36,58,59] Drug-induced arrest is most likely to occur in the adolescent age group related to a drug overdose.

Although it may be ideal to ask rescuers to individualize each resuscitation sequence on the basis of the most likely etiology of the victim's cardiac arrest, this approach is impractical. Education of the lay rescuer is most effective if the message is simple and can be applied in a wide variety of situations. The more complex the teaching sequence or message, the less likely it is that the rescuer will remember what to do and do it.[60,61] Therefore, a simple, consistent message for lone lay rescuers of most infants and children is to "phone fast"—provide approximately 1 minute of CPR and then activate (phone) the EMS system.

In victims ≥8 years of age in the out-of-hospital setting, the adult Chain of Survival and resuscitation sequence is recommended. If the victim is unresponsive, the lone rescuer should immediately activate the EMS response system and retrieve the AED, if available. The "phone first" approach is particularly appropriate if the victim has experienced a sudden arrest. Again, exceptions to this rule should be noted. If the victim's arrest is secondary to submersion (near-drowning), a "phone fast" approach is appropriate. For near-drowning victims of all ages, immediate CPR should begin while the victim is still in the water. Immediate bystander CPR is associated with improved early return of spontaneous circulation and neurologically intact survival for submersion victims of all ages.[15,62] Other victims ≥8 years of age who may benefit from immediate CPR include those with respiratory or cardiac arrest caused by trauma and those with respiratory or cardiac arrest caused by drug overdose.

In the hospital setting the most common causes of cardiac arrest include sepsis, respiratory failure, drug toxicity, metabolic disorders, and arrhythmia. These in-hospital causes of arrest are often complicated by underlying (premorbid) conditions. The emergency department represents a transition from the out-of-hospital to hospital location; therefore, cardiac arrest may develop in children with underlying conditions typical for the hospital setting and in children with conditions seen more often in the out-of-hospital setting.

BLS for Children With Special Needs

Children with special health care needs have chronic physical, developmental, behavioral, or emotional conditions and require health and related services of a type or amount not usually required by typically developing children.[63–65] These children may need emergency care for acute, life-threatening complications that are unique to their chronic conditions,[65] such as obstruction of a tracheostomy, failure of support technology (eg, ventilator failure), or progression of underlying respiratory failure or neurological disease. However, approximately half of EMS responses to children with special health care needs are unrelated to the child's special needs and may include traditional causes of EMS calls, such as trauma,[66] which require no treatment beyond the normal EMS standard of care.

Emergency care of children with special health care needs, however, can be complicated by lack of specific medical information about the child's baseline condition, medical plan of care, current medications, and any "do not attempt to resuscitate" orders. Certainly the best source of information about a chronically ill child is the person who cares for the child on a daily basis. However, if that person is unavailable or incapacitated (eg, following an automobile crash), some means is needed to access important information. A wide variety of methods have been developed to make this information immediately accessible, including the use of standard forms, containers kept in a standard place in the home (eg, the refrigerator), window stickers, wallet cards, and medical alert bracelets. No single method of communicating information has proved to be superior. A standardized form, the Emergency Information Form (EIF), was developed by the American Academy of Pediatrics and the American College of

---

*References 4, 6, 8, 9, 16, 18, 35, 40, 46, 47, 49–56.

Emergency Physicians[65] and is available on the Worldwide Web (http://www.pediatrics.org/cgi/content/full/104/4/e53). Parents and child care providers should keep essential medical information at home, with the child, and at the child's school or child care facility. Child care providers should have access to this information and should be familiar with signs of deterioration in the child and any existing advance directives.[66,67]

If the physician, parents, and child (as appropriate) have made a decision to limit resuscitation efforts or withhold attempts at resuscitation, a physician order indicating the limits of resuscitative efforts must be written for use in the in-hospital setting; in most countries, a separate order must be written for the out-of-hospital setting. Legal issues and regulations regarding requirements for these out-of-hospital no-CPR directives vary from country to country and, in the United States, from state to state. However, it is always important for families to inform the local EMS system when such directives are established for out-of-hospital care. For further information about ethical issues of resuscitation, see "Part 2: Ethical Aspects of CPR and ECC."

Whenever a child with a chronic or life-threatening condition is discharged from the hospital, parents, school nurses, and any home healthcare providers should be informed about possible complications that the child may experience and anticipated signs of deterioration and their cause. Specific instructions should be given regarding CPR and other interventions that the child may require, as well as instructions about who to contact and why.[67]

If the child has a tracheostomy, anyone responsible for the child's care (including parents, school nurses, and home healthcare providers) should be taught to assess airway patency, clear the airway, and provide CPR with the artificial airway. If CPR is required, rescue breathing and bag-mask ventilation are performed through the tracheostomy tube. As with any form of rescue breathing, effective ventilation is judged by adequate bilateral chest expansion. If the tracheostomy tube becomes obstructed and impossible to use, even after attempts to clear the tube with suctioning, the tube should be replaced. If a clean tube is not available, provide ventilations at the tracheostomy stoma until an artificial airway can be placed. If the upper airway is patent, it may be possible to provide effective conventional bag-mask ventilation through the nose and mouth while occluding the superficial tracheal stoma site.

Out-of-Hospital (EMS) Care

EMS systems were initially created for adults in developed nations. EMS equipment, training, experience, and expertise are often less well developed to meet the needs of children. In the United States death rates are higher in children than in adults treated in the EMS system, especially in areas where tertiary pediatric care is unavailable.[68–75] To improve pediatric out-of-hospital care, EMS personnel should be optimally trained and equipped to care for pediatric victims (see "Part 10: Pediatric Advanced Life Support"), medical dispatchers should use emergency protocols appropriate for children, and emergency departments caring for children should be appropriately staffed and equipped. Emergency departments that care for acutely ill or injured children should have an ongoing agreement with a pediatric tertiary service through which patients can receive postresuscitation care in a pediatric intensive care unit (ICU) under the supervision of trained personnel.

Prevention of Cardiopulmonary Arrest in Infants and Children

Prevention of Sudden Infant Death Syndrome

SIDS is the sudden death of an infant, typically between the ages of 1 month and 1 year, that is unexpected from history and unexplained by other causes when a postmortem examination is performed. SIDS probably represents a variety of conditions, all of which result in death while sleeping. It is probably caused by several mechanisms, including rebreathing asphyxia, with a decreased arousal and possible blunted response to hypoxemia or hypercarbia.[76] The peak incidence of SIDS occurs in infants 2 to 4 months of age; 70% to 90% of SIDS deaths are reported in the first 6 months of life.[76] Many characteristics are associated with increased risk of SIDS, including prone sleeping position, the winter months, infants of lower-income families, males, siblings of SIDS victims, infants of mothers who smoke cigarettes, infants who have survived severe apparent life-threatening events, infants of mothers who are drug addicts, and low birthweight infants.

One of the most successful public health initiatives to reduce infant mortality was based on the observation that the risk of SIDS is associated with the prone (on the stomach) sleeping position. Infants who sleep prone have a much higher frequency of SIDS than infants who sleep supine (on the back) or on their sides.[77–79] The prone position, particularly on a soft surface, is thought to contribute to rebreathing asphyxia.[76] Australia, New Zealand, and several European countries have documented a significant reduction in the incidence of SIDS when parents and child care providers are taught to place healthy infants to sleep supine or on their sides.[80] This "Back to Sleep" public education campaign was introduced in the United States in 1992, when approximately 7000 infants died of SIDS. In 1997, 2991 infants died of SIDS in the United States.[5]

Recent reports from New Zealand[80] and England[81] have documented a slightly greater risk of SIDS when infants are placed on their sides than when they are placed supine for sleep. Either side or supine position, however, continues to be associated with a much lower risk of SIDS than the prone position.

All parents and those responsible for the care of children should be aware of the need to place healthy infants supine for sleeping. The supine sleeping position has not been associated with an increase in any significant adverse events, such as vomiting or aspiration.[77] A side position may be used as an alternative, but infants in this position should be propped and positioned to prevent them from rolling to the prone position. In addition, the infant should not sleep on soft surfaces, such as lambswool, fluffy comforters, or other objects that might trap exhaled air near the infant's face.

Injury: The Magnitude of the Problem

In the United States, injury is the leading cause of death in children and adults aged 1 to 44 years and is responsible for more childhood deaths than all other causes combined.[12,14] Internationally, injury death rates are highest for children 1 to 14 years of age and young adults 15 to 24 years of age, relative to other causes of death.[13,82] The term *injury* is emphasized rather than the term *accident* because the injury is often preventable, and the term accident implies that nothing can be done to prevent the episode.

The Science of Injury Control

Injury control attempts to prevent injury or minimize its effects on the child and family in 3 phases: prevention, minimization of injury damage, and postinjury care. In planning of injury prevention strategies, 3 principles deserve emphasis. First, passive injury prevention strategies are generally preferred because they are more likely to be used than active strategies, which require repeated, conscious effort. Second, specific instructions (eg, keep the water heater temperature <120°F to 130°F or 48.9°C to 54.4°C) are more likely to be followed than general advice (eg, reduce the maximum temperature of home tap hot water). Third, individual education reinforced by community-wide educational programs is more effective than isolated educational sessions.[83,84] Although current prevention efforts can be directed to those groups with the highest incidence and cost estimates (eg, males, adolescents, and low-income background), more specific strategies will need to be developed with more cause-specific injury morbidity data.[82]

Epidemiology and Prevention of Common Childhood and Adolescent Injuries

Injury prevention will have the greatest effect by focusing on injuries that are frequent and for which effective strategies are available. The leading causes of death internationally in children 1 to 14 years of age are depicted in Figure 2. The 6 most common types of fatal childhood injuries amenable to injury prevention strategies are motor vehicle passenger injuries, pedestrian injuries, bicycle injuries, submersion, burns, and firearm injuries.[12,13,83,85]

Prevention of these common fatal injuries would substantially reduce childhood deaths and disability internationally. For this reason, information regarding injury prevention is included with information about infant/child resuscitation. In an attempt to make this information relevant to the largest possible segment of the pediatric population over many years, the following section addresses prevention of injuries in infants, children, and adolescents.

Motor Vehicle Injuries

Motor vehicle–related trauma accounts for nearly half of all pediatric injuries and deaths in the United States and 40% of injury mortality in children 1 to 14 years of age internationally.[12,13,57] Motor vehicle traffic death rates for children are lowest in England and Wales, Norway, The Netherlands, and Australia and highest in New Zealand.[13] Contributing factors include failure to use proper passenger restraints, inexperi-

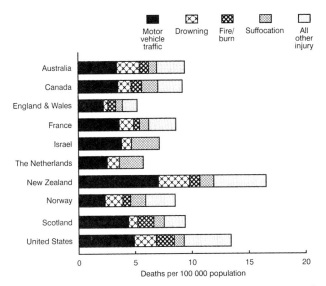

Figure 2. International injury deaths for children 1 to 14 years of age. Reproduced from Fingerhut LA, Cox CS, Warner M. International comparative analysis of injury mortality: findings from the International Collaborative Effort (ICE) on injury statistics. Vital and Health Statistics, Centers for Disease Control and Prevention, National Center for Health Statistics, No. 303, October 7, 1998.

enced adolescent drivers, and alcohol abuse. Each of these should be addressed by injury prevention programs.

Proper use of child seat restraints and lap-shoulder harnesses will prevent an estimated 65% to 75% of serious injuries and fatalities to passengers <4 years of age and 45% to 55% of all pediatric motor vehicle passenger injuries and deaths.[12,86] The American Academy of Pediatrics, the Centers for Disease Control and Prevention, and the National Highway Traffic Safety Administration have made the following child passenger safety recommendations:

1. Children should ride in rear-facing infant seats until they are at least 20 pounds (9 kg) *and* at least 1 year of age, with good head control. These seats should be secured in the *back* seat of the automobile.
   - A rear-facing safety seat must *never* be placed in the front passenger seat of a car with a passenger-side airbag.
   - Convertible seats can be used for children <1 year of age and <20 pounds (9 kg) if they are used in the reclined and rear-facing position.
2. A child who is >1 year old *and* weighs 20 to 40 pounds (9 to 18 kg) should be placed in a convertible car safety seat used in the upright and forward-facing position as long as he or she fits well in the seat. The harness straps should be positioned at or above the child's shoulders. These seats should also be placed in the *back* seat of the automobile.
3. Belt-positioning booster seats should be used for children weighing 40 to 80 pounds (18 to 36 kg) until they are at least 58 to 60 inches (148 cm) in height. These belt-positioning seats ensure that the lap and shoulder belts restrain the child over bones rather than soft tissues.
4. Children may be restrained in automobile lap and shoulder belts when they weigh 40 to 80 pounds (18 to

36 kg) and are at least 58 inches (148 cm) tall. A properly fitting lap-shoulder belt should lie low across the child's hips while the shoulder belt lies flat across the shoulder and sternum, away from the neck and face.

5. Children approximately 12 years old and younger should not sit in the front seat of cars equipped with passenger-side air bags.[87,88]

Parents should be taught the proper use of automobile safety restraints. Children should also learn about the importance of safety restraints during their early primary school education.[89] Parents should be taught to check the installation of child passenger safety seats and follow the manufacturer's instructions carefully. If the safety seat is properly installed, it should not move more than 1/2 inch (1 cm) front to back or side to side when pushed.

Further development of passive restraint devices, including adjustable shoulder harnesses, automatic lap and shoulder belts, and air bags, is needed. The benefits of air bags continue to far outweigh the risks, saving approximately 2663 lives in the United States alone from 1987 to 1997. The vast majority of the 74 US children with fatal airbag-related injuries reported through April 1999 were improperly restrained for their age or not restrained at all. They included infants restrained in rear-facing infant seats placed in the front passenger seats of cars with passenger-side airbags, children <4 years of age restrained by lap and shoulder belts, and children who were not restrained at all. To prevent airbag and most other occupant injuries, children <12 years of age should be properly restrained for age and size in the back seat of cars. When a child is old enough (>12 years) and large enough to sit in the front seat of an automobile with a passenger-side airbag, the child should be properly restrained for age and size, and the automobile seat should be moved as far back and away from the airbag cover as possible. The development of "smart" airbags that adjust inflation time and force according to the weight of the passenger should further reduce injuries related to airbags.

Adolescent drivers are responsible for a disproportionate number of motor vehicle–related injuries. Surprisingly, adolescent driver education classes have increased the number of adolescent drivers at risk with no improvement in safety.[90–93] Approximately 50% of motor vehicle fatalities involving adolescents also involve alcohol. In fact, a large proportion of all pediatric motor vehicle occupant deaths occur in vehicles operated by inebriated drivers.[94–97] Although intoxication rates decreased for drivers of all age groups from 1987 to 1999, drunk drivers are still responsible for a large portion of all motor vehicle crashes and pose significant risk to children.[12,98]

Pedestrian Injuries
Pedestrian injuries are a leading cause of death among children 5 to 9 years of age in the United States.[57,83] Internationally, childhood pedestrian injuries are highest in New Zealand, the United States, and Australia.[13] Pedestrian injuries typically occur when a child darts out into the street, crossing between intersections.[12] Although educational programs aimed at improving children's street-related behavior hold promise, roadway interventions, including adequate lighting, construction of sidewalks, and roadway barriers, must also be pursued in areas of high pedestrian traffic.

Bicycle Injuries
Bicycle crashes are responsible for approximately 200 000 injuries and >600 deaths to children and adolescents in the United States every year.[57,99] Head injuries are the cause of most bicycle injury–related morbidity and mortality. In fact, bicycle-related trauma is a leading cause of severe pediatric closed-head injuries.[100] Bicycle helmets can prevent an estimated 85% of head injuries and 88% of brain injuries. Yet many parents are unaware of the need for helmets, and children may be reluctant to wear them.[100,101] A successful bicycle helmet education program includes an ongoing community-wide multidisciplinary approach that provides focused information about the protection afforded by a helmet. Such programs should ensure the acceptability, accessibility, and affordability of helmets.[99,101]

Submersion/Drowning
Internationally, drowning is responsible for approximately 15% of injury deaths to children 1 to 14 years of age.[13] It is a significant cause of death and disability in children <4 years old and is a leading cause of death in this age group in the United States.[12,57,83,102] Drowning constitutes 1 of the top 3 mechanisms of injury death in the 1- to 14-year-old age group in New Zealand, Australia, the United States, France, Canada, The Netherlands, and Israel. New Zealand has the highest rate of childhood drowning.[13] For every death due to submersion, 6 children are hospitalized, and approximately 20% of hospitalized survivors are severely brain damaged.[57,103]

Parents should be aware of the dangers to young children posed by any body of water. Young children and children with seizure disorders should never be left unattended in bathtubs or near swimming pools, ponds, or beaches. Some drownings in swimming pools may be prevented by completely surrounding the pool with appropriate fencing, including gates with secure latching mechanisms.[102,104] The house will not serve as an effective barrier to the pool if it has a door opening onto the pool area.

Children >5 years of age should learn how to swim. No one should ever swim alone, and even supervised children should wear personal flotation devices when playing in rivers, streams, or lakes.

Alcohol appears to be a significant risk factor in adolescent drowning. As a result, adolescent education, limiting access to alcohol, and the use of personal flotation devices on waterways should be encouraged.

Burns
Fires, burns, and suffocation are a leading cause of injury death worldwide and are higher in the United States and Scotland than in the other countries surveyed.[13] Approximately 80% of fire- and burn-related deaths result from house fires, with associated smoke inhalation injury.[86,105–108] Most fire-related deaths occur in private residences, usually in homes without working smoke detectors.[86,105,106,109] From 1995 to 1996 nearly 15% of total US fatalities related to home fires were children <5 years old.[12] Nonfatal burns and burn

complications, including smoke inhalation, scalds, and contact and electric burns are especially likely to affect children.

Socioeconomic factors such as overcrowding, single-parent families, scarce financial resources, inadequate child care/supervision, and distance from fire department all contribute to increased risk for burn injury. *Smoke detectors are one of the most effective interventions for preventing deaths from burns and smoke inhalation.* When used correctly, they can reduce fire-related death and severe injury by 86% to 88%.[106,109] Smoke detectors should be placed near or on the ceilings outside the doors to sleeping or napping rooms and on each floor at the top of the stairway. Parents should be aware of the effectiveness of these devices and the need to change device batteries every 6 months. Families and schools should develop and practice a fire evacuation plan. Continued improvements in flammability standards for furniture, bedding, and home builders' materials should further reduce the incidence of fire-related injuries and deaths. Child-resistant ignition products are also under investigation. School-based fire-safety programs should be continued and evaluated.

Firearm Injuries

Firearms, particularly handguns, are responsible for a large number of injuries and deaths to infants, children, and adolescents, particularly in the United States, Norway, Israel, and France. Firearm-related deaths may be labeled as unintentional, homicide, or suicide.[5] The United States has the highest firearm-related injury rate of any industrialized nation—more than twice that of any other country.[13,110]

Although firearm-related deaths have declined from 1995 to 1997 compared with previous years,[5] firearm homicide remains the leading cause of death among African-American adolescents and young adults and the second-highest cause of death among all adolescents and young adults in the United States, Norway, Israel, and France.[13,110,111] Firearms have been used in an increasing proportion of child and adolescent suicides. Mortality from firearm injuries is highest in young children, whether the firearm injury is unintentional or related to homicide or suicide.[112]

Most guns used in childhood unintentional shootings, school shootings, and suicides are found in the home. Many firearm owners admit to storing guns loaded and in readily accessible locations.[113] Thirty-four percent of high school students surveyed reported easy access to guns, and an increasing number of children carry guns to school.[114–116]

If guns are present in homes in which children and adolescents live and visit, it is likely that the children and adolescents will find and handle the guns. The mere presence of a gun in the home is associated with an increased likelihood of adolescent suicide[117,118] as well as an increased incidence of adult suicide or homicide.[119–121] Every gun owner, potential gun purchaser, and parent must be made aware of the risks of unsecured firearms and the need to ensure that weapons in the home are inaccessible to unsupervised children and adolescents.[122–124] Guns should be stored locked and unloaded, with ammunition stored separately from the gun. The consistent use of trigger locks may not only reduce the incidence of unintentional injury and suicide among children and young adolescents but will most likely reduce the number of gun homicides. In addition, locked guns obtained during burglaries would be useless. "Smart" guns, which can only be fired by the gun owner, are expected to reduce the frequency of unintentional injuries and suicides among children and young adolescents and limit the usefulness of guns obtained during burglaries.[125]

Prevention of Choking (Foreign-Body Airway Obstruction)

More than 90% of deaths from foreign-body aspiration in children occur in those younger than 5 years; 65% of victims are infants. With the development of consumer product safety standards regulating the minimum size of toys and toy parts for young children,[126] the incidence of foreign-body aspiration has decreased significantly. However, toys, balloons, small objects, and foods (eg, hot dogs, round candies, nuts, and grapes) may still produce FBAO[127,128] and should be kept away from infants and small children.

Sequence of Pediatric BLS: The ABCs of CPR

The BLS sequence (see Figure 3) described below refers to both infants (neonate outside the delivery room setting to 1 year of age) and children (1 to 8 years of age) unless specified. For information on newly born infants (resuscitation immediately after birth), see "Part 11: Neonatal Resuscitation." For BLS for children >8 years of age, see "Part 3: Adult Basic Life Support."

Resuscitation Sequence

To maximize survival and neurologically intact outcome following life-threatening cardiovascular emergencies, each link in the Chain of Survival must be strong, including prevention of arrest, early and effective bystander CPR, rapid activation of the EMS system, and early and effective ALS (including rapid stabilization and transport to definitive care and rehabilitation). When a child develops respiratory or cardiac arrest, immediate bystander CPR is crucial to survival. In both adult[28,33,34] and pediatric[15,16,40] studies, bystander CPR is linked to improved return of spontaneous circulation and neurologically intact survival. The greatest impact of bystander CPR will probably be on children with noncardiac (respiratory) causes of out-of-hospital arrest.[129] Two studies report on the outcome of series of children who were successfully resuscitated before EMS arrival solely by bystander CPR.[16,40] The true frequency of this type of resuscitation is unknown, but it is likely to be underestimated, because victims successfully resuscitated by bystanders are often excluded from studies of out-of-hospital cardiac arrest. Unfortunately, bystander CPR is provided for only approximately 30% of out-of-hospital pediatric arrests.[4,40]

BLS guidelines delineate a series of skills performed sequentially to assess and support or restore effective ventilation and circulation to the child with respiratory or cardiorespiratory arrest. Pediatric resuscitation requires a process of observation, evaluation, interventions, and assessments that is difficult to capture in a sequential description of CPR. You should initially assess the victim's responsiveness and then continuously monitor the victim's response to intervention (appearance, movement, breathing, etc). Evaluation and intervention are often

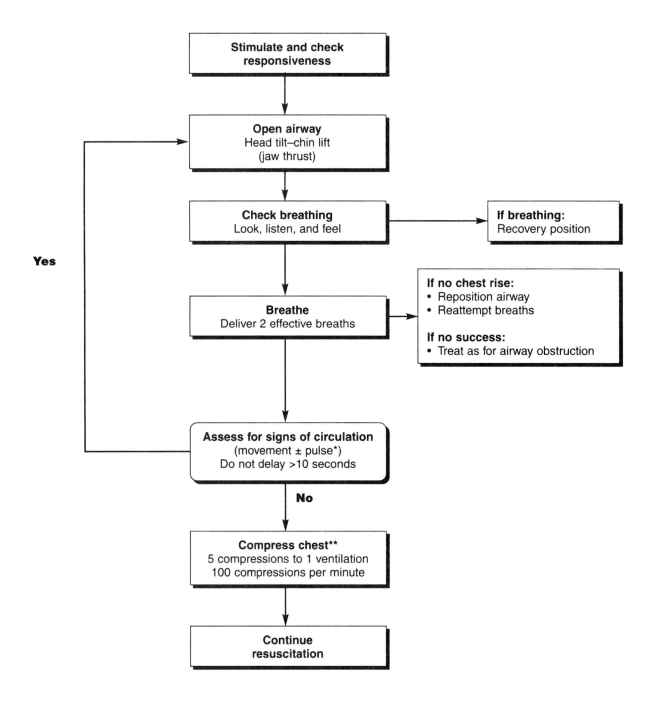

Figure 3. Pediatric BLS algorithm.

simultaneous processes, especially when more than 1 trained provider is present. Although this process is taught as a *sequence* of distinct steps to enhance skills retention, several actions may be accomplished *simultaneously* (eg, begin CPR and phone EMS) if multiple rescuers are present. The appropriate BLS actions also depend on the interval since the arrest, how the victim responded to previous resuscitative interventions, and whether special resuscitation circumstances exist.

Ensure the Safety of Rescuer and Victim
When CPR is provided in the out-of-hospital setting, the rescuer should first verify the safety of the scene. If resusci-

tation is needed near a burning building, in water, or in proximity to electrical wires, the rescuer must first ensure that both the victim and rescuer are in a safe location. In the case of trauma, the victim should not be moved unless it is necessary to ensure the victim's or the rescuer's safety.

Although rescuer exposure during CPR carries a theoretical risk of infectious disease transmission, the risk is very low.[130] Most out-of-hospital cardiac arrests in infants and children occur at home. If the victim has an infectious disease, it is likely that family members have already been exposed to that disease or are aware of the disease and appropriate barrier devices are available. Surveys of family members indicate that risk of infection is not a concern that would prevent delivery of CPR to a loved one.[131]

When CPR is provided in the workplace, the rescuer is advised to use a barrier device or mask with 1-way valve to deliver ventilation. These protective devices should be available in the workplace.

Healthcare providers are required to treat all fluids from patients as potentially infectious, particularly in the hospital setting. Healthcare providers should wear gloves and protective shields during procedures that are likely to expose them to droplets of blood, saliva, or other body fluids.

Assess Responsiveness

Gently stimulate the child and ask loudly, "Are you all right?" Quickly assess the presence or extent of injury and determine whether the child is *responsive*. Do not move or shake the victim who has sustained head or neck trauma, because such handling may aggravate a spinal cord injury. If the child is responsive, he or she will answer your questions or move on command. If the child responds but is injured or needs medical assistance, you may leave the child in the position found to summon help (phone the EMS system, if needed). Return to the child as quickly as possible and recheck the child's condition frequently. Responsive children with respiratory distress will often assume a position that maintains airway patency and optimizes ventilation; they should be allowed to remain in the position that is most comfortable to them.

If the child is *unresponsive* and you are the only rescuer present, be prepared to provide BLS, if necessary, for approximately 1 minute before leaving the child to activate the EMS system. As soon as you determine that the child is unresponsive, shout for help. If trauma has not occurred and the child is small, you may consider moving the child near a telephone so that you can contact the EMS system more quickly. The EMS medical dispatcher may then guide you through CPR. The child must be moved if he or she is in a dangerous location (eg, a burning building) or if CPR cannot be performed where the child was found.

If a second rescuer is present during the initial assessment of the child, that rescuer should activate the EMS system as soon as the emergency is recognized. If trauma is suspected, the second rescuer should activate the EMS system and then may assist in immobilizing the child's cervical spine, preventing movement of the neck (extension, flexion, and rotation) and torso. If the child must be positioned for

resuscitation or moved for safety reasons, support the head and body and turn as a unit.

Activate EMS System if Second Rescuer Is Available

Because all of the links in the Chain of Survival are connected, it is difficult to evaluate the effect of EMS system activation or specific EMS interventions in isolation. In addition, local EMS response intervals, dispatcher training, and EMS protocols may dictate the most appropriate sequence of EMS activation and early life support interventions for a given situation.

Current AHA guidelines instruct the rescuer to provide approximately 1 minute of CPR before activating the EMS system in out-of-hospital arrest for infants and children up to the age of 8 years.[1] *In the International Guidelines 2000 the "phone first" sequence of resuscitation continues to be recommended for children ≥8 years of age and adults. The "phone fast" sequence of resuscitation continues to be recommended for children <8 years of age on the basis of face and construct validity (Class Indeterminate).*

The AHA Subcommittees on Pediatric Resuscitation and BLS and a panel addressing the citizen's response in the Chain of Survival debated a proposal to teach lay rescuers to tailor the CPR sequence and EMS activation to the likely cause of the victim's arrest rather than the victim's age. This proposed approach would teach lone lay rescuers to provide 1 minute of CPR before activating the EMS system if a victim of any age collapses with what is thought to be a probable breathing/respiratory problem. Lone lay rescuers would also be taught to activate the EMS system immediately if a victim of any age collapses suddenly (presumed sudden cardiac arrest). Although the proposal has appeal when considered for an individual victim, it was rejected for several reasons. First, no data was presented that indicated that a change to an etiology-based triage method for all age groups would improve survival for victims of out-of-hospital cardiac arrest. Second, the proposal would probably complicate the education of lay rescuers. CPR instruction must remain simple for lay rescuers. Retention of CPR skills and knowledge is already suboptimal. The addition of complex instructions to existing CPR guidelines would most likely make them more difficult to teach, learn, remember, and perform.[132–138]

It is important to note that the "phone first" or "phone fast" sequence is applicable only to the lone rescuer. When multiple rescuers are present, 1 rescuer remains with the victim of any age to begin CPR while another rescuer goes to activate the EMS system. It is unknown how frequently 2 or more lay responders are present during initial evaluation of a pediatric cardiopulmonary emergency.

Sophisticated healthcare providers, family members, and potential rescuers of infants and children at high risk for cardiopulmonary emergencies should be taught a sequence of rescue actions tailored to the potential victim's specific high-risk condition.[139] For example, parents and child care providers of children with congenital heart disease who are known to be at risk for arrhythmias should be instructed to "phone first" (activate the EMS system before beginning CPR) if they are alone and the child suddenly collapses.

Alternatively, there may be exceptions to the "phone first" approach for victims ≥8 years of age, including adults. Parents of children ≥8 years of age who are at high risk for apnea or respiratory failure should be instructed to provide 1 minute of CPR before activating the EMS system if they are alone and find the child unresponsive. Submersion (near-drowning) victims of all ages who are unresponsive when pulled from the water should receive approximately 1 minute of BLS support (opening of the airway and rescue breathing and chest compressions, if needed) before the lone rescuer leaves to phone the local EMS system. Trauma victims or those with a drug overdose or apparent respiratory arrest of any age may also benefit from 1 minute of CPR before the EMS system is contacted. Knowledgeable and experienced providers should use common sense and "phone first" for any apparent sudden cardiac arrest (eg, sudden collapse at any age) and "phone fast" in other circumstances in which breathing difficulties are documented or likely to be present (eg, trauma or an apparent choking event).

The rescuer calling the EMS system should be prepared to provide the following information:

1. Location of the emergency, including address and names of streets or landmarks
2. Telephone number from which the call is being made
3. What happened, eg, auto accident, submersion
4. Number of victims
5. Condition of victim(s)
6. Nature of aid being given
7. Any other information requested

The caller should hang up *only* when instructed to do so by the dispatcher, and then caller should report back to rescuer doing CPR.

Hospitals and medical facilities and many businesses and building complexes have established emergency medical response systems that provide a first response or early response on-site. Such a response system notifies rescuers of the location of an emergency and the type of response needed. If the cardiopulmonary emergency occurs in a facility with an established medical response system, that system should be notified, because it can respond more quickly than EMS personnel arriving from outside the facility. For rescuers in these facilities, the emergency medical response system should replace the EMS system in the sequences below.

Airway

Position the Victim
If the child is unresponsive, move the child as a unit to the supine (face up) position, and place the child supine on a flat, hard surface, such as a sturdy table, the floor, or the ground. If head or neck trauma is present or suspected, move the child only if necessary and turn the head and torso as a unit. If the victim is an infant, and no trauma is suspected, carry the child supported by your forearm (your forearm should support the long axis of the infant's torso, with the infant's legs straddling your elbow and your hand supporting the infant's head). It may be possible to carry the infant to the phone in this manner while beginning the steps of CPR.

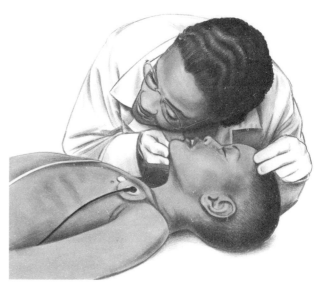

Figure 4. Head tilt–chin lift for child victim.

Open the Airway
The most common cause of airway obstruction in the unresponsive pediatric victim is the tongue.[140–143] Therefore, once the child is found to be unresponsive, open the airway using a maneuver designed to lift the tongue away from the back of the pharynx, creating an open airway.[144]

Head Tilt–Chin Lift Maneuver
If the victim is unresponsive *and trauma is not suspected*, open the child's airway by tilting the head back and lifting the chin (Figure 4). Place one hand on the child's forehead and gently tilt the head back. At the same time place the fingertips of your other hand on the bony part of the child's lower jaw, near the point of the chin, and lift the chin to open the airway. Do not push on the soft tissues under the chin as this may block the airway. *If injury to the head or neck is suspected, use the jaw-thrust maneuver to open the airway; do not use the head tilt–chin lift maneuver.*

Jaw-Thrust Maneuver
If head or neck injury is suspected, use only the *jaw-thrust* method of opening the airway. Place 2 or 3 fingers under each side of the lower jaw at its angle, and lift the jaw upward and outward (Figure 5). Your elbows may rest on the surface on which the victim is lying. If a second rescuer is present, that rescuer should immobilize the cervical spine (see "BLS in Trauma" below) after the EMS system is activated.

Foreign-Body Airway Obstruction
If the victim becomes unresponsive with an FBAO or if an FBAO is suspected, open the airway wide and look for an object in the pharynx. If an object is present, remove it carefully (under vision). Healthcare providers should perform a tongue-jaw lift to look for obstructing objects (see next section), but this maneuver will not be taught to lay rescuers.

Techniques for Healthcare Providers
Hypoxia and respiratory arrest may cause or contribute to acute deterioration and cardiopulmonary arrest. Thus, maintenance of a patent airway and support of adequate ventilation are essential. Both the head tilt–chin lift and jaw-thrust

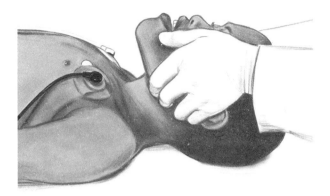

Figure 5. Jaw thrust for child victim.

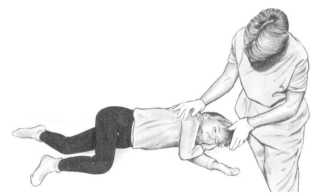

Figure 6. Recovery position.

techniques should be taught to lay rescuers. Healthcare providers should also learn additional maneuvers, such as the tongue-jaw lift, for use in unresponsive victims of FBAO. Healthcare providers are taught a sequence of actions to attempt to relieve FBAO in the unresponsive victim. If FBAO is suspected, open the airway using a tongue-jaw lift and look for the foreign body before attempting ventilation. If you see the foreign body, remove it carefully (under vision).

Breathing

Assessment: Check for Breathing
Hold the victim's airway open and look for signs that the victim is breathing. *Look* for the rise and fall of the chest and abdomen, *listen* at the child's nose and mouth for exhaled breath sounds, and *feel* for air movement from the child's mouth on your cheek for no more than 10 seconds.

It may be difficult to determine whether the victim is breathing.[145,146] Care must be taken to differentiate ineffective, gasping, or obstructed breathing efforts from effective breathing.[147,148] If you are not confident that respirations are adequate, proceed with rescue breathing.

If the child is breathing spontaneously and effectively and there is no evidence of trauma, turn the child to the side in a *recovery position* (Figure 6). This position should help maintain a patent airway. Although many recovery positions are used in the management of pediatric patients,[149–152] no single recovery position can be universally endorsed on the basis of scientific studies of children. There is consensus that an ideal recovery position should be a stable position that enables the following: maintenance of a patent airway, maintenance of cervical spine stability, minimization of risk for aspiration, limitation of pressure on bony prominences and peripheral nerves, visualization of the child's respiratory effort and appearance (including color), and access to the patient for interventions.

Provide Rescue Breathing
If no spontaneous breathing is detected, maintain a patent airway by head tilt–chin lift or jaw thrust. Carefully (under vision) remove any obvious airway obstruction, take a deep breath, and deliver rescue breaths. With each rescue breath, provide a volume sufficient for you to see the child's chest rise. Provide 2 slow breaths (1 to 1½ seconds per breath) to the victim, pausing after the first breath to take a breath to maximize oxygen content and minimize carbon dioxide

concentration in the delivered breaths. Your exhaled air can provide oxygen to the victim, but the rescue breathing pattern you use will affect the amount of oxygen and carbon dioxide delivered to the victim.[153,154] When ventilation adjuncts and oxygen are available (eg, bag-mask) to assist with ventilation, provide high flow oxygen to all unresponsive victims or victims in respiratory distress.

The 1992 guidelines[1] recommended that 2 initial breaths be delivered. The current ILCOR recommendations suggest that between 2 and 5 rescue breaths should be delivered initially to ensure that at least 2 effective ventilations are provided.[18,155] *There is no data to support the choice of any single number of initial breaths to be delivered to the unresponsive, nonbreathing victim.* Most pediatric victims of cardiac arrest are both hypoxic and hypercarbic. If the rescuer is unable to establish effective ventilation with 2 rescue breaths, additional breaths may be beneficial in improving oxygenation and restoring an adequate heart rate for an apneic, bradycardic infant or child. *There is inadequate data to recommend changing the number of initial ventilations delivered during CPR at this time. Therefore, lay rescuers and healthcare providers should administer 2 initial* **effective** *breaths to the unresponsive, nonbreathing infant or child (Class Indeterminate).* The rescuer should ensure that at least 2 breaths delivered are effective and produce visible chest rise.

Mouth-to-Mouth-and-Nose and Mouth-to-Mouth Breathing
If the victim is an infant (<1 year old), place your mouth over the infant's mouth and nose to create a seal (Figure 7). Blow into the infant's nose and mouth (pausing to inhale between breaths), attempting to make the chest rise with each breath. A variety of techniques can be used to provide rescue breathing for infants. A rescuer with a small mouth may have difficulty covering both the nose and open mouth of a large infant.[156–165] Under these conditions, mouth-to-nose ventilation may be adequate.[156,158] There is no convincing data to justify a change from the recommendation that the rescuer attempt *mouth-to-mouth-and-nose ventilation* for infants up to 1 year of age. During rescue breathing attempts you must maintain good head position for the infant (head tilt–chin lift to maintain a patent airway) and create an airtight seal over the airway.

The *mouth-to-nose* rescue breathing technique is a reasonable adjunctive or alternative method of providing rescue breathing for an infant (Class IIb). The mouth-to-nose breath-

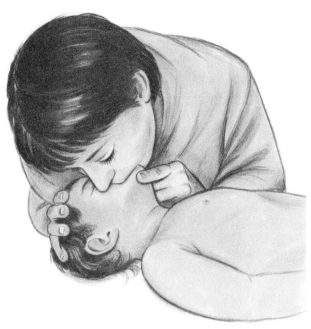

Figure 7. Mouth-to-mouth-and-nose breathing for small infant victim.

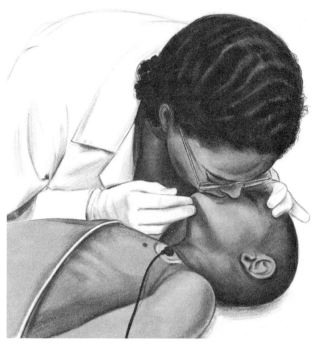

Figure 8. Mouth-to-mouth breathing for child victim.

ing technique may be particularly useful if you have difficulty with the mouth-to-mouth-and-nose technique. To perform mouth-to-nose ventilation, place your mouth over the infant's nose and proceed with rescue breathing. It may be necessary to close the infant's mouth during rescue breathing to prevent the rescue breaths from escaping through the infant's mouth. A chin lift will help maintain airway patency by moving the tongue forward and may help keep the mouth closed.

If the victim is a large infant or a child (1 to 8 years of age), provide *mouth-to-mouth* rescue breathing. Maintain a head tilt–chin lift or jaw thrust (to keep the airway patent), and pinch the victim's nose tightly with thumb and forefinger. Make a mouth-to-mouth seal and provide 2 rescue breaths, making sure that the child's chest rises visibly with each breath (Figure 8). Inhale between rescue breaths.

Evaluation of Effectiveness of Breaths Delivered
Rescue breaths provide essential support for a nonbreathing infant or child. Because children vary widely in size and lung compliance, it is impossible to make precise recommendations about the pressure or volume of breaths to be delivered during rescue breathing. Although the goal of assisted ventilation is delivery of adequate oxygen and removal of carbon dioxide with the smallest risk of iatrogenic injury, measurement of oxygen and CO_2 levels during pediatric BLS is often not practical. Therefore, *the volume of each rescue breath should be sufficient to cause the chest to visibly rise* without causing excessive gastric distention.[166] *If the child's chest does not rise during rescue breathing, ventilation is not effective.* Because the small airway of the infant or child may provide high resistance to air flow, particularly in the presence of large or small airway obstruction, a relatively high pressure may be required to deliver an adequate volume of air to ensure chest expansion. The correct volume for each breath is the volume that causes the chest to rise.

If air enters freely and the chest rises, the airway is clear. If air does not enter freely (if the chest does not rise), either the airway is obstructed or greater volume or pressure is needed to provide adequate rescue breaths. Improper opening of the airway is the most common cause of airway obstruction and inadequate ventilation during resuscitation. As a result, if air does not enter freely and the chest does not rise during initial ventilation attempts, reposition the airway and reattempt ventilation.[155] It may be necessary to move the child's head through a range of positions to obtain optimal airway patency and effective rescue breathing. The head should not be moved if neck or spine trauma is suspected; the jaw thrust should be used to open the airway in these victims. If rescue breathing fails to produce chest expansion despite repeated attempts at opening the airway, an FBAO may be present (see "Foreign-Body Airway Obstruction" below).

The ideal ventilation rate during CPR and low circulatory flow states is unknown. Current recommended ventilation (rescue breathing) rates are derived from normal respiratory rates for age, with some adjustments for the time needed to coordinate rescue breathing with chest compressions to ensure that ventilation is adequate.

Cricoid Pressure
Rescue breathing, especially if performed rapidly, may cause gastric distention.[167–171] Excessive gastric distention can interfere with rescue breathing by elevating the diaphragm and decreasing lung volume, and it may result in regurgitation of gastric contents.[166] Gastric distention may be minimized if rescue breaths are delivered slowly during rescue breathing, because slow breaths will enable delivery of effective tidal volume at low inspiratory pressure. Deliver initial breaths slowly, over 1 to 1½ seconds, with a force sufficient to make the chest visibly rise. Firm but gentle pressure on the cricoid cartilage during ventilation may help compress the esophagus

and decrease the amount of air transmitted to the stomach.[172,173] Healthcare providers may insert a nasogastric or orogastric tube to decompress the stomach if gastric distention develops during resuscitation. Ideally this is done after tracheal intubation.

Ventilation With Barrier Devices
Mouth-to-mouth rescue breathing is a safe and effective technique that has saved many lives. Despite decades of experience indicating its safety for victims and rescuers alike, some potential rescuers may hesitate to perform mouth-to-mouth rescue breathing because of concerns about transmission of infectious diseases. Most children who require resuscitation outside the hospital arrest at home, and the primary child care provider is aware of the child's infectious status. Adults who work with children (particularly infants and preschool children) are exposed to pediatric infectious agents daily and often may experience the consequent illnesses. In contrast, the exposure of rescuers to victims is brief, and infections after mouth-to-mouth rescue breathing are extremely rare.[130]

Although healthcare providers typically have access to barrier devices, in most lay rescue situations these devices are not immediately available. If the child is unresponsive and apneic, immediate provision of mouth-to-mouth rescue breathing may be lifesaving. Rescue breathing should not be delayed while the rescuer searches for a barrier device or tries to learn how to use it.

If an infection control barrier device is readily available, some rescuers may prefer to provide rescue breathing with such a device (Class Indeterminate). Barrier devices may improve esthetics for the rescuer but have not been shown to reduce the risk of disease transmission.[130,174] In addition, barrier devices may increase resistance to gas flow.[175,176] Rescuers with a duty to respond and those who respond in the work place should have a supply of barrier devices readily available for use during any attempted resuscitation and should be trained in their use.

Two broad categories of barrier devices are available: masks and face shields. Most masks have a 1-way valve, which prevents the victim's exhaled air from entering the rescuer's mouth. When barrier devices are used in resuscitation of infants and children, they are used in the same manner as in resuscitation of adults (see "Part 3: Adult BLS").

Bag-Mask Ventilation
Healthcare providers who provide BLS for infants and children should be trained to deliver effective oxygenation and ventilation with a manual resuscitator bag and mask (Class IIa). Ventilation with a bag-mask device requires more skill than mouth-to-mouth or mouth-to-mask ventilation and should be used only by personnel who have received proper training. Training should focus on selection of an appropriately sized mask and bag, opening the airway and securing the mask to the face, delivering adequate ventilation, and assessing the effectiveness of ventilation. Periodic demonstration of proficiency is recommended.

Types of Ventilation Bags (Manual Resuscitators). There are 2 basic types of manual resuscitators (ventilation bags): self-inflating and flow-inflating resuscitators. Ventilation bags should be self-inflating and available in child and adult sizes suitable for the entire pediatric age range.

Flow-inflating bags (also called *anesthesia bags*) refill only with oxygen inflow, and the inflow must be individually regulated. Since flow-inflating manual resuscitators are more difficult to use, they should be used only by trained personnel.[177] Flow-inflating bags permit continuous delivery of supplemental oxygen to a spontaneously breathing victim. In contrast, self-inflating bag-mask systems that contain a fish-mouth or leaf-flap outlet valve *cannot* be used to provide continuous supplemental oxygen during spontaneous ventilation. When the bag is not squeezed, the child's inspiratory effort may be insufficient to open the valve. In such a case the child will receive inadequate oxygen flow (a negligible flow of oxygen escapes through the outlet valve) and will rebreathe the exhaled gases contained in the mask.

Neonatal-size (250 mL) ventilation bags may be inadequate to support effective tidal volume and the longer inspiratory times required by full-term neonates and infants.[178,179] For this reason, resuscitation bags used for ventilation of full-term newly born infants, infants, and children should have a minimum volume of 450 to 500 mL. Studies involving infant manikins demonstrated that effective infant ventilation can be achieved with pediatric (and larger) resuscitation bags.[165]

Regardless of the size of the manual resuscitator used, *the rescuer should use only the force and tidal volume necessary to cause the chest to rise visibly.* Excessive ventilation volumes and airway pressures may have harmful effects. They may compromise cardiac output by raising intrathoracic pressure, distending alveoli and/or the stomach, impeding ventilation, and increasing the risk of regurgitation and aspiration.[180] In patients with small-airway obstructions (eg, asthma and bronchiolitis), excessive tidal volume and ventilation rate can result in air trapping, barotrauma, air leak, and severely compromised cardiac output. In the patient with a head injury or cardiac arrest, excessive ventilation volume and rate may result in hyperventilation with potentially adverse effects on neurological outcome. Therefore, the goal of ventilation with a bag and mask should be to approximate normal ventilation and achieve physiological oxygen and carbon dioxide levels while minimizing risk of iatrogenic injury (Class IIa).

Ideally, bag-mask systems used for resuscitation should either have no pressure-relief valve or have a valve with an override feature to permit use of high pressures, if necessary, to achieve visible chest expansion.[180] High pressures may be required during bag-mask ventilation of patients with upper or lower airway obstruction or poor lung compliance. In these patients a pressure-relief valve may prevent delivery of sufficient tidal volume.[181]

The self-inflating bag delivers only room air (21% oxygen) unless the bag is joined to an oxygen source. At an oxygen inflow of 10 L/min, pediatric bag-valve devices without oxygen reservoirs deliver from 30% to 80% oxygen to the patient.[181] The actual concentration of oxygen delivered is unpredictable because a variable amount of room air is pulled into the bag to replace some of the gas mixture delivered to the patient. To deliver consistently higher oxygen concentra-

A

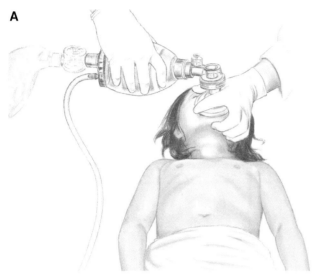

B

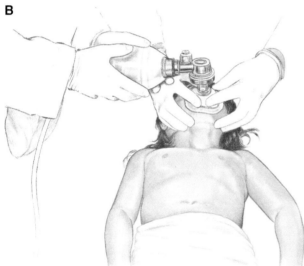

Figure 9. Bag-mask ventilation for child victim. A, 1 rescuer; B, 2 rescuers.

tions (60% to 95%), all bag-valve devices used for resuscitation should be equipped with an oxygen reservoir. At least 10 to 15 L/min of oxygen flow is required to maintain an adequate oxygen volume in the reservoir of a pediatric manual resuscitator, and this should be considered the minimum flow rate.[181] The larger adult manual resuscitators require ≥15 L/min of oxygen flow to reliably deliver high oxygen concentrations.

Technique. To provide bag-mask ventilation, select a bag and mask of appropriate size. The mask must be able to completely cover the victim's mouth and nose without covering the eyes or overlapping the chin. Once the bag and mask are selected and connected to an oxygen supply, open the victim's airway and seal the mask to the face.

If no signs of trauma are present, tilt the victim's head back to help open the airway. If trauma is suspected, do not move the head. To open the airway of the victim with trauma, lift the jaw, using the last 3 fingers (fingers 3, 4, and 5) of one hand. Position these 3 fingers under the angle of the mandible to lift the jaw up and forward. Do not put pressure on the soft

tissues under the jaw, because this may compress the airway. When lifting the jaw, you also lift the tongue off the posterior pharynx, preventing the tongue from obstructing the pharynx. Place your thumb and forefinger in a "C" shape over the mask and exert downward pressure on the mask. This hand position uses the thumb and forefinger to squeeze the mask onto the face while the remaining fingers of the same hand lift the jaw, pulling the face toward the mask. This should create a tight seal between the mask and the victim's face (Figure 9A). This technique of opening the airway and sealing the mask to the face is called the "E-C clamp" technique. Fingers 3, 4, and 5 form an E positioned under the jaw to provide a chin lift; the thumb and index finger form a C and hold the mask on the child's face. Once you successfully apply the mask with one hand, compress the ventilation bag with the other hand until the chest visibly rises.

Superior bag-mask ventilation can be achieved with 2 rescuers, and 2 rescuers may be required when the victim has significant airway obstruction or poor lung compliance (Figure 9B). One rescuer uses both hands to open the airway and maintain a tight mask-to-face seal while the other rescuer compresses the ventilation bag (see "Part 3: Adult BLS," 2-rescuer technique for bag-mask ventilation).[182] Both rescuers should observe the chest to ensure that it rises visibly with each breath.

Gastric Inflation. Gastric inflation in unresponsive or obtunded patients can be minimized by increasing inspiratory time so the necessary tidal volume can be delivered at low peak inspiratory pressures. Pace the ventilation rate and ensure adequate time for exhalation. To reduce gastric inflation, a second trained provider can apply cricoid pressure, but only with an unconscious victim.[173] Cricoid pressure may also prevent regurgitation (and possible aspiration) of gastric contents.[183,184] Do not use excessive pressure on the cricoid cartilage, because it may produce tracheal compression and obstruction or distortion of the upper airway anatomy.[185] Gastric distention after prolonged bag-mask ventilation can limit effective ventilation.[166] If gastric distention develops, healthcare providers should decompress the stomach with an orogastric or a nasogastric tube. If tracheal intubation is planned, you ideally defer gastric intubation until after tracheal intubation is accomplished. This will reduce the risk of vomiting and laryngospasm.

Ventilation Through a Tracheostomy or Stoma

Anyone responsible for the care of a child with a tracheostomy (including parents, school nurses, and home healthcare providers) should be taught to ensure that the airway is patent and to provide CPR by using the artificial airway. If CPR is required, perform rescue breathing and bag-mask ventilation through the tracheostomy. As with any form of rescue breathing, the key sign of effective ventilation is adequate chest expansion bilaterally. If the tracheostomy becomes obstructed and ventilation cannot be provided through it, remove and replace the tracheostomy tube. If a clean tube is not available, provide ventilation at the tracheostomy stoma until the site can be intubated with a tracheostomy or tracheal tube. If the child's upper airway is patent, it may be possible to provide bag-mask ventilation through the nose and mouth using a conventional bag and mask while occluding the superficial tracheal stoma site.

Oxygen
Healthcare providers should administer oxygen to all seriously ill or injured patients with respiratory insufficiency, shock, or trauma as soon as it is available. In these patients inadequate pulmonary gas exchange and/or inadequate cardiac output limits tissue oxygen delivery.

During cardiac arrest a number of factors contribute to severe progressive tissue hypoxia and the need for supplementary oxygen administration. At best, mouth-to-mouth ventilation provides 16% to 17% oxygen with a maximal alveolar oxygen tension of 80 mm Hg.[153] Because even optimal external chest compressions provide only a fraction of the normal cardiac output, blood flow to the brain and body and tissue oxygen delivery are markedly diminished. In addition, CPR is associated with right-to-left pulmonary shunting due to ventilation-perfusion mismatch. Preexisting expiratory conditions may further compromise oxygenation. The combination of low blood flow and low oxygenation contributes to metabolic acidosis and organ failure. For these reasons, oxygen should be administered to children with demonstrated cardiopulmonary arrest or compromise, even if measured arterial oxygen tension is high. Whenever possible, administered oxygen should be humidified to prevent drying and thickening of pulmonary secretions; dried secretions may contribute to obstruction of natural or artificial airways.

Occasionally an infant may require *reduced* inspired oxygen concentration or manipulation of oxygenation and ventilation to control pulmonary blood flow (eg, the neonate with single ventricle). A review of these unique situations is beyond the scope of this document.

Oxygen may be administered during bag-mask ventilation. In addition, if the victim is breathing spontaneously, oxygen may be delivered by nasal cannula, simple face masks, and nonrebreathing masks (for further information, see "Part 10: Pediatric Advanced Life Support").[186–190] The concentration of oxygen delivered depends on the oxygen flow rate, the type of mask being used, and the patient's minute ventilation. As long as the flow of oxygen exceeds the maximal inspiratory flow rate, the prescribed concentration of oxygen will be delivered. If the inspiratory flow rate exceeds the oxygen flow rate, room air is entrained, reducing the oxygen concentration delivered to the patient.

Circulation

Assessment: No Pulse Check for Lay Rescuers
When you have opened the airway and provided 2 effective rescue breaths, determine whether the victim is in cardiac arrest and requires chest compressions. Cardiac arrest results in the absence of *signs of circulation*, including the absence of a pulse. The pulse check has been the "gold standard" usually relied on by professional rescuers to evaluate circulation. The carotid artery is palpated for the pulse check in adults and children[191]; brachial artery palpation is recommended in infants.[192] In the previous guidelines the pulse check was used to identify pulseless patients in cardiac arrest who required chest compression. If the rescuer failed to detect

a pulse in 5 to 10 seconds in an unresponsive nonbreathing victim, cardiac arrest was presumed to be present and chest compressions were initiated.

Since 1992 several published studies have questioned the validity of the pulse check as a test for cardiac arrest, particularly when used by laypersons.[191,193–205] Previous guidelines de-emphasized the pulse check for infant-child CPR for 2 reasons. First, 3 small studies suggested that parents had difficulty finding and counting the pulse even in healthy infants.[192,203,206] Second, the reported complication rate from chest compressions in infants and children is low.[207–214]

After publication of the 1992 ECC Guidelines, additional investigators evaluated the reliability of the pulse check with adult manikin simulation[198] in unconscious adult patients undergoing cardiopulmonary bypass,[202] unconscious mechanically ventilated adult patients,[199] and conscious adult "test persons."[194,201] These studies concluded that as a diagnostic test for cardiac arrest, the pulse check has serious limitations in accuracy, sensitivity, and specificity.

When lay rescuers check the pulse, they often spend a long time deciding whether or not a pulse is present; then they may fail 1 time out of 10 to recognize the absence of a pulse or cardiac arrest (poor sensitivity). When assessing unresponsive victims who do have a pulse, lay rescuers miss the pulse 4 times out of 10 (poor specificity). Details of the published studies include the following conclusions[197]:

1. Rescuers take far too much time to check the pulse: most rescue groups, including laypersons, medical students, paramedics, and physicians, take much longer than the recommended period of 5 to 10 seconds to check for the carotid pulse in adult victims. In 1 study half of the rescuers required >24 seconds to decide whether a pulse was present. Only 15% of the participants correctly confirmed the presence of a pulse within 10 seconds, the maximum time allotted for the pulse check.
2. When used as a diagnostic test, the pulse check is extremely inaccurate. In the most comprehensive study documented,[202] the accuracy of the pulse check was described as follows[197]:
   a. Sensitivity (ability to correctly identify victims who have no pulse and *are* in cardiac arrest) is only 90%. When subjects were pulseless, rescuers thought a pulse was present approximately 10% of the time. By mistakenly thinking a pulse *is* present when it is not, rescuers fail to provide chest compressions for 10 of every 100 victims of cardiac arrest. Without a resuscitation attempt, the consequence of such errors would be death for 10 of every 100 victims of cardiac arrest.
   b. Specificity (ability to correctly recognize victims who *have* a pulse and *are not* in cardiac arrest) is only 60%. When the pulse was present, rescuers assessed the pulse as being absent approximately 40% of the time. By erroneously thinking a pulse is absent, rescuers provide chest compressions for approximately 4 of 10 victims who do not need them.
   c. Overall accuracy was 65%, leaving an error rate of 35%.

Data is limited regarding the specificity and sensitivity of the pulse check in pediatric victims of cardiac arrest.[216] Three studies have documented the inability of lay rescuers to find and count a pulse in healthy infants.[192,203,206] Healthcare providers may also have difficulty reliably separating venous from arterial pulsation during CPR.[217]

On a review of this and other data, the experts and delegates at the 1999 Evidence Evaluation Conference and the International Guidelines 2000 Conference concluded that the pulse check could not be recommended as a tool for lay rescuers to use in the CPR sequence to identify victims of cardiac arrest. If rescuers use the pulse check to identify victims of cardiac arrest, they will "miss" true cardiac arrest at least 10 of 100 times. In addition, rescuers will provide unnecessary chest compressions for many victims who are not in cardiac arrest and do not require such an intervention. This error is less serious but still undesirable. Clearly more worrisome is the potential failure to intervene for a substantial number of victims of cardiac arrest who require immediate intervention to survive.

Therefore, the lay rescuer should not rely on the pulse check to determine the need for chest compressions. Lay rescuers should not perform the pulse check and will not be taught the pulse check in CPR courses (Class IIa). Instead laypersons will be taught to look for *signs of circulation* (normal breathing, coughing, or movement) in response to rescue breaths. This recommendation applies to victims of any age. Healthcare providers should continue to use the pulse check as one of several signs of circulation. Other signs of circulation include breathing, coughing, or movement in response to rescue breaths. It is anticipated that this guideline change will result in more rapid and accurate identification of cardiac arrest. More importantly, it should reduce the number of missed opportunities to provide CPR (and early defibrillation using an AED for victims ≥8 years of age) for victims of cardiac arrest.

Assessment: Check for Signs of Circulation

The International Guidelines 2000 refer to assessment of signs of circulation. For the lay rescuer, this means the following: deliver initial rescue breaths and evaluate the victim for normal breathing, coughing, or movement in response to rescue breaths. The lay rescuer will look, listen, and feel for breathing while scanning the victim for other signs of movement. Lay rescuers will look for "normal" breathing to minimize confusion with agonal respirations.

In practice, lay rescuers should assess the victim for signs of circulation as follows:

1. Provide initial rescue breaths to the unresponsive, nonbreathing victim.
2. Look for signs of circulation:
   a. With your ear next to the victim's mouth, look, listen, and feel for normal breathing or coughing.
   b. Quickly scan the victim for any signs of movement.
3. If the victim is not breathing normally, coughing, or moving, immediately begin chest compressions.

Healthcare professionals should assess signs of circulation by performing a pulse check while simultaneously evaluating the victim for breathing, coughing, or movement after deliv-

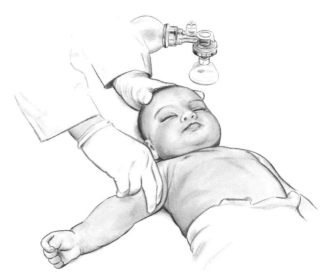

Figure 10. Brachial pulse check in infant.

ering rescue breaths. Healthcare providers should look for breathing because they are trained to distinguish between agonal breathing and other forms of ventilation not associated with cardiac arrest. This assessment should take no more than 10 seconds. If you do not confidently detect a pulse or other signs of circulation or if the heart rate is <60 bpm with signs of poor perfusion, provide chest compressions. It is important to note that unresponsive, nonbreathing infants and children are very likely to have a slow heart rate or no heart rate at all. Therefore, do not delay the initiation of chest compressions to locate a pulse.

Healthcare providers should learn to palpate the brachial pulse in infants and the carotid pulse in children 1 to 8 years of age. The short, chubby neck of children <1 year of age makes rapid location of the carotid artery difficult. In addition, it is easy to compress the airway while attempting to palpate a carotid pulse in the infant's neck. For these reasons, the healthcare provider should attempt to palpate the brachial artery when performing the pulse check in infants.[192] The brachial pulse is on the inside of the upper arm, between the infant's elbow and shoulder. Press the index and middle fingers gently on the inside of the upper arm for no more than 10 seconds, in an attempt to feel the pulse (Figure 10).

Healthcare providers should learn to locate and palpate the child's carotid artery on the side of the neck. It is the most accessible central artery in children and adults. The carotid artery lies on the side of the neck between the trachea and the strap (sternocleidomastoid) muscles. To feel the artery, locate the victim's thyroid cartilage (Adam's apple) with 2 or 3 fingers of one hand while maintaining head tilt with the other hand. Then slide the fingers into the groove on the side closer to the rescuer, between the trachea and the sternocleidomastoid muscles, and gently palpate the area over the artery (Figure 11) for no more than 10 seconds.

If signs of circulation are present but spontaneous breathing is absent, provide rescue breathing at a rate of 20 breaths per minute (once every 3 seconds) until spontaneous breathing resumes. After provision of approximately 20 breaths (slighty longer than 1 minute), the lone rescuer should

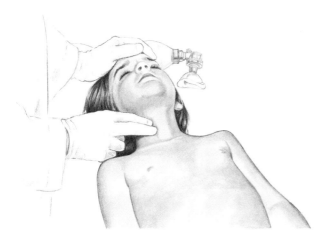

Figure 11. Carotid pulse check in child.

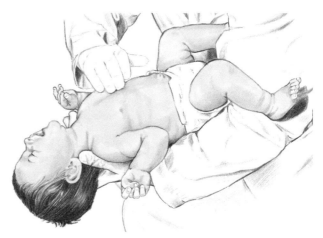

Figure 12. One-rescuer infant CPR while carrying victim, with infant supported on rescuer's forearm.

activate EMS. If adequate breathing resumes and there is no suspicion of neck trauma, turn the child onto the side into a recovery position.

If signs of circulation are absent (or, for the healthcare provider, the heart rate is <60 bpm with signs of poor perfusion), begin chest compressions. This will include a series of compressions coordinated with ventilations. If there are no signs of circulation, the victim is ≥8 years of age, and an AED is available in the out-of-hospital setting, use the AED. A weight of 25 kg corresponds to a body length of approximately 50 inches (128 cm) using the Broselow color-coded tape.[217a] For information about use of AEDs for victims ≥8 years of age, see "Part 4: The Automated External Defibrillator."

Provide Chest Compressions

Chest compressions are serial, rhythmic compressions of the chest that cause blood to flow to the vital organs (heart, lungs, and brain) in an attempt to keep them viable until ALS can be provided. Chest compressions provide circulation as a result of changes in intrathoracic pressure and/or direct compression of the heart.[218–222] Chest compressions for infants and children should be provided with ventilations.[223,224]

Compress the lower half of sternum to a relative depth of approximately one third to one half the anterior/posterior diameter of the chest at a rate of at least 100 compressions per minute for the infant and approximately 100 compressions per minute for the child victim. Be sure to avoid compression of the xiphoid. This depth of compression differs slightly from that recommended for the newly born. The neonatal resuscitation guidelines call for compression to approximately one third the depth of the chest. The wider range of recommended compression depth and potentially deeper compressions in infants and children is not evidence based but consensus based. Chest compressions must be adequate to produce a palpable pulse during resuscitation. Lay rescuers will not attempt to feel a pulse, so they should be taught a compression technique that will most likely result in delivery of effective compressions.

Healthcare providers should evaluate the effectiveness of compressions during CPR. If effective compressions are provided, they should all produce palpable pulses in a central

artery (eg, the carotid, brachial, or femoral artery). Although pulses palpated during chest compression may actually represent venous pulsations rather than arterial pulses,[217] pulse assessment by the healthcare provider during CPR remains the most practical quick assessment of chest compression efficacy.

Exhaled carbon dioxide detectors and displayed arterial pressure waveforms (if invasive arterial monitoring is in place) can assist the healthcare provider in evaluating the effectiveness of chest compressions. If chest compressions produce inadequate cardiac output and pulmonary blood flow, exhaled carbon dioxide will remain extremely low throughout resuscitation. If an arterial catheter is in place during resuscitation (eg, during chest compressions provided to a patient in the ICU with an arterial monitor in place), chest compressions can be guided by the displayed arterial waveform.

To facilitate optimal chest compressions, the child should be supine on a hard, flat surface. CPR should be performed where the victim is found. If cardiac arrest occurs in a hospital bed, place firm support (a resuscitation board) beneath the patient's back. Optimal support is provided by a resuscitation board that extends from the shoulders to the waist and across the full width of the bed. The use of a wide board is particularly important when providing chest compressions to larger children. If the board is too small, it will be pushed deep into the mattress during compressions, dispersing the force of each compression. Spine boards, preferably with head wells, can be used in ambulances and mobile life support units.[225,226] They provide a firm surface for CPR in the emergency vehicle or on a wheeled stretcher and may also be useful for extricating and immobilizing victims.

Infants with no signs of head or neck trauma may be successfully carried during resuscitation on the rescuer's forearm. The palm of one hand can support the infant's back while the fingers of the other hand compress the sternum. This maneuver effectively lowers the infant's head, allowing the head to tilt back slightly into a neutral position that maintains airway patency. If the infant is carried during CPR, the hard surface is created by the rescuer's forearm, which

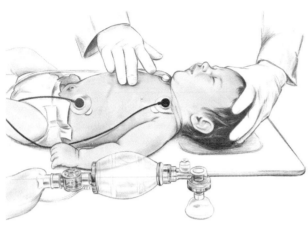

Figure 13. Two-finger chest compression technique in infant (1 rescuer).

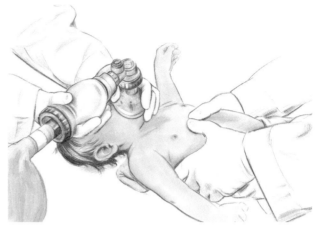

Figure 14. Two thumb–encircling hands chest compression technique in infant (2 rescuers).

supports the length of the infant's torso, while the infant's head and neck are supported by the rescuer's hand. Take care to keep the infant's head no higher than the rest of the body. Use the other hand to perform chest compressions. You can lift the infant to provide ventilation (Figure 12).

Indications for Chest Compressions
Lay rescuers should provide chest compressions if the infant or child shows no signs of circulation (normal breathing, coughing, or movement) after delivery of rescue breaths. Healthcare providers should provide chest compressions if the infant or child shows no signs of circulation (breathing, coughing, movement, or pulse) or if the heart rate/pulse is <60 bpm with signs of poor perfusion after delivery of rescue breaths. Profound bradycardia in the presence of poor perfusion is an indication for chest compressions because cardiac output in infancy and childhood is largely dependent on heart rate, and an inadequate heart rate with poor perfusion indicates that cardiac arrest is imminent. No scientific data has identified an absolute heart rate at which chest compressions should be initiated; the recommendation to provide cardiac compression for a heart rate <60 bpm with signs of poor perfusion is based on ease of teaching and skills retention.

Chest Compression in the Infant (<1 Year of Age) (Figures 13 and 14)
Two-finger technique (the preferred technique for laypersons and lone rescuers):

1. Place the 2 fingers of one hand over the lower half of the sternum[227–230] approximately 1 finger's width below the intermammary line, ensuring that you are not on or near the xiphoid process.[20] The intermammary line is an imaginary line located between the nipples, over the breastbone. An alternative method of locating compression position is to run 1 finger along the lower costal margin to locate the bony end of the sternum and place 1 finger over the end of the sternum; this will mark the xiphoid process. Then place 2 fingers of your other hand above the finger (moving up the sternum toward the head). The 2 fingers will now be in the appropriate position for chest compressions, avoiding the xiphoid.[20] You may place your other hand under the infant's chest to create a compression surface and slightly elevate the

chest so that the neck is neither flexed nor hyperextended and the airway will be maintained in a neutral position.

2. Press down on the sternum to depress it approximately one third to one half the depth of the infant's chest. This will correspond to a depth of about ½ to 1 inch (1½ to 2½ cm), but these measurements are not precise. After each compression, completely release the pressure on the sternum and allow the sternum to return to its normal position without lifting your fingers off the chest wall.

3. Deliver compressions in a smooth fashion, with equal time in the compression and relaxation phases. A somewhat shorter time in the compression phase offers theoretical advantages for blood flow in a very young infant animal model of CPR [231] and is reviewed in the neonatal guidelines. As a practical matter, with compression rates ≥100 per minute (nearly 2 compressions per second), it is unrealistic to think that rescuers will be able to judge or manipulate compression and relaxation phases. In addition, details about such manipulation would increase the complexity of CPR instruction. For these reasons, provide compressions in approximately equal compression and relaxation phases for infants and children.

4. Compress the sternum at *a rate of at least 100 times per minute* (this corresponds to a rate that is slightly less than 2 compressions per second during the groups of 5 compressions). The compression *rate* refers to the *speed* of compressions, not the actual number of compressions delivered per minute. Note that this compression rate will actually result in provision of <100 compressions each minute, because you will pause to provide 1 ventilation after every fifth compression. The actual number of compressions delivered per minute will vary from rescuer to rescuer and will be influenced by the compression rate and the speed with which you can position the head, open the airway, and deliver ventilation.[136,232]

5. After 5 compressions, open the airway with a head tilt–chin lift (or, if trauma is present, use the jaw thrust) and give 1 effective breath. Be sure that the chest rises with the breath. Coordinate compressions and ventilations to avoid simultaneous delivery and ensure adequate ventilation and chest expansion, especially when

the airway is unprotected.[233] You may use your other hand (the one not compressing the chest) to maintain the infant's head in a neutral position during the 5 chest compressions. (Again see Figure 3.) This may help you provide ventilation without the need to reposition the head after each set of 5 compressions. Alternatively, to maintain a neutral head position, place your other hand behind the infant's chest (this will elevate the chest, ensuring that the head is in neutral position relative to the chest). If there *are* signs of head or neck trauma, you can place your other hand on the infant's forehead to maintain stability (do not tilt head).

Continue compressions and breaths in a ratio of 5:1 (for 1 or 2 rescuers). Note that this differs from the recommended ratio of 3:1 (compressions to ventilations) for the newly born or premature infant in the neonatal ICU. (See "Part 11: Neonatal Resuscitation.") This difference is based on ease of teaching and skills retention for specifically trained providers in the delivery room setting, with increased emphasis on effective and frequent ventilation for the newly born infant.

Two thumb–encircling hands technique (this is the preferred 2-rescuer technique for healthcare providers when physically feasible; see Figure 14):

1. Place both thumbs side by side over the lower half of the infant's sternum, ensuring that the thumbs do not compress on or near the xiphoid process.[20,227–230] Encircle the infant's chest and support the infant's back with the fingers of both hands. Place both thumbs on the lower half of the infant's sternum, approximately 1 finger's width below the intermammary line. The intermammary line is an imaginary line located between the nipples, over the breastbone.

2. With your hands encircling the chest, use both thumbs to depress the sternum approximately one third to one half the depth of the child's chest. This will correspond to a depth of approximately ½ to 1 inch, but these measurements are not precise. After each compression, completely release the pressure on the sternum and allow the sternum to return to its normal position without lifting your thumbs off the chest wall.

3. Deliver compressions in a smooth fashion, with equal time in the compression and relaxation phases. A somewhat shorter time in the compression than relaxation phase offers theoretical advantages for blood flow in a very young infant animal model of CPR[231] and is discussed in the neonatal guidelines. As a practical matter, with compression rates of at least 100 per minute (nearly 2 compressions per second), it is unrealistic to think that rescuers will be able to judge or manipulate compression and relaxation phases. In addition, details regarding such manipulation would increase the complexity of CPR instruction. For these reasons, provide compressions in approximately equal compression and relaxation phases for infants and children.

4. Compress the sternum at *a rate of at least 100 times per minute* (this corresponds to a rate that is slightly less than 2 compressions per second during the groups of 5 compressions). The compression *rate* refers to the *speed* of compressions, not the actual number of compressions delivered per minute. Note that this compression rate will actually result in provision of <100 compressions

per minute, because you will pause to allow a second rescuer to provide 1 ventilation after every fifth compression. The actual number of compressions delivered per minute will vary from rescuer to rescuer and will be influenced by the compression rate and the speed with which the second rescuer can position the head, open the airway, and deliver ventilation.[136,232]

5. After 5 compressions, pause briefly for the second rescuer to open the airway with a head tilt–chin lift (or, if trauma is suspected, with a jaw thrust) and give 1 effective breath (the chest should rise with the breath). Compressions and ventilations should be coordinated to avoid simultaneous delivery and ensure adequate ventilation and chest expansion, especially when the airway is unprotected.[233]

Continue compressions and breaths in a ratio of 5:1 (for 1 or 2 rescuers). Note that this differs from the recommended ratio of 3:1 (compressions to ventilations) for the newly born or premature infant in the neonatal ICU (see "Part 11: Neonatal Resuscitation"). This difference is based on ease of teaching and skills retention for specific trained providers in the delivery room setting, with increased emphasis on effective and frequent ventilation needed for resuscitation of the newly born.

The 2 thumb–encircling hands technique may generate higher peak systolic and coronary perfusion pressure than the 2-finger technique, and healthcare providers prefer this technique to the alternative.[21,234–238] For this reason the 2 thumb–encircling hands chest compression technique is the preferred technique for *2 healthcare providers* to use in newly born infants and infants of appropriate size (Class IIb). This technique is *not* taught to the lay rescuer and is not practical for the healthcare provider working alone, who must alternate compression and ventilation.

Chest Compression Technique in the Child (Approximately 1 to 8 Years of Age) (Figure 15)

1. Place the heel of one hand over the lower half of the sternum, ensuring that you do not compress on or near the xiphoid process. Lift your fingers to avoid pressing on the child's ribs.

2. Position yourself vertically above the victim's chest and, with your arm straight, depress the sternum approximately one third to one half the depth of the child's chest. This corresponds to a compression depth of approximately 1 to 1½ inches, but these measurements are not precise. After the compression, release the pressure on the sternum, allowing it to return to normal position, but do not remove your hand from the surface of the chest.

3. Compress the sternum *at a rate of approximately 100 times per minute* (this corresponds to a rate that is slightly less than 2 compressions per second during the groups of 5 compressions). The compression *rate* refers to the *speed* of compressions, not the actual number of compressions delivered per minute. Note that this compression rate will actually result in provision of <100 compressions per minute because you will pause to provide 1 ventilation after every fifth compression. The actual number of compressions delivered per minute will vary from rescuer to rescuer and will be influenced

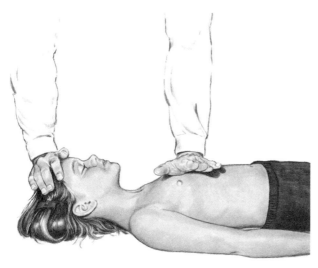

Figure 15. One-hand chest compression technique in child.

by the compression rate and the speed with which you can position the head, open the airway, and deliver ventilations.[136,232]

4. After 5 compressions, open the airway and give 1 effective rescue breath. Be sure the chest rises with the breath.
5. Return your hand immediately to the correct position on the sternum and give 5 chest compressions.
6. Continue compressions and breaths in a ratio of 5:1 (for 1 or 2 rescuers).

Note that many reasonable techniques are available to teach proper hand position for chest compression. The technique used should emphasize the importance of locating the lower half of the sternum, avoiding force on or near the xiphoid process and asymmetric force on the ribs. Emphasis should be placed on optimizing mechanics to depress the chest rhythmically approximately one third to one half the depth of the chest at a rate of approximately 100 times per minute and coordinating with rescue breaths to ensure delivery of adequate ventilation in between compressions without delay.

In large children and children ≥*8 years* of age, the adult 2-handed method of chest compression should be used to achieve an adequate depth of compression as follows (see "Part 3: Adult BLS"):

1. Place the heel of one hand on the lower half of the sternum. Place the heel of your other hand on top of the back of the first hand.
2. Interlock the fingers of both hands and lift the fingers to avoid pressure on the child's ribs.
3. Position yourself vertically above the victim's chest and, with your arm straight, press down on the sternum to depress it approximately 1½ to 2 inches. Release the pressure completely after each compression, allowing the sternum to return to its normal position, but do not remove your hands from the surface of the chest.
4. Compress the sternum *at a rate of approximately 100 times per minute* (this corresponds to a rate of slightly <2 compressions per second during the groups of 15 compressions). The compression *rate* refers to the *speed* of compressions, not the actual number of compressions

delivered per minute. Note that this compression rate will actually result in provision of <100 compressions each minute because you will pause to provide 2 ventilations after every group of 15 compressions. The actual number of compressions delivered per minute will vary from rescuer to rescuer and will be influenced by the compression rate and the speed with which you can position the head, open the airway, and deliver ventilation.[136,232]

5. After 15 compressions, open the airway with the head tilt–chin lift (if trauma to the head and neck is suspected, use the jaw-thrust maneuver to open the airway) and give 2 effective breaths.
6. Return your hands immediately to the correct position on the sternum and give 15 chest compressions.
7. Continue compressions and breaths in a ratio of 15:2 for 1 or 2 rescuers until the airway is secure (see "Part 3: Adult BLS").

Until the airway is secured, the compression-ventilation ratio of 15:2 is recommended for 1 or 2 rescuers for adult victims and victims ≥8 years of age. Once the airway is secured, 2 rescuers should use a 5:1 ratio of compressions and ventilations.

Coordination of Compressions and Rescue Breathing

External chest compressions for infants and children should always be accompanied by rescue breathing. In the infant and child, a compression-ventilation ratio of 5:1 is maintained for both 1 and 2 rescuers. The 2-rescuer technique should be taught to healthcare providers. For infants in the special resuscitation circumstances of the delivery room and neonatal intensive care setting, even more emphasis is placed on ventilation during resuscitation, and a 3:1 compression-ventilation ratio is recommended (see "Part 11: Neonatal Resuscitation").

When 2 rescuers are providing CPR for an infant or child with an unsecured airway, the rescuer providing the compressions should pause after every fifth compression to allow the second rescuer to provide 1 effective ventilation. This pause is necessary until the airway is secure (intubated). Once the airway is secure (the trachea is intubated), the pause is no longer necessary. However, coordination of compressions and ventilation may facilitate adequate ventilation even after tracheal intubation and is emphasized in the newly born (see "Part 11: Neonatal Resuscitation"). Compressions may be initiated after chest inflation and may augment active exhalation during CPR. Although the technique of simultaneous compression and ventilation may augment coronary perfusion pressure in some settings,[239–242] it may produce barotrauma and decrease ventilation and is not recommended. Priority is given to assuring adequate ventilation and avoidance of potentially harmful excessive barotrauma in children.[241]

Reassess the victim after 20 cycles of compressions and ventilations (slightly longer than 1 minute) and every few minutes thereafter for any sign of resumption of spontaneous breathing or signs of circulation. The number 20 is easy to remember, so it is used to provide a guideline interval for reassessment rather than an indication of the absolute number of cycles delivered in exactly 1 minute. In the delivery room setting, more frequent assessments of heart rate—approximately every 30 seconds—are recommended for the newly born (see "Part 11: Neonatal Resuscitation").

In infants, coordination of rapid compressions and ventilations by a single rescuer in a 5:1 ratio may be difficult.[232,243,244] To minimize delays, if no trauma is present, the rescuer can maintain airway patency during compressions by using the hand that is not performing compressions to maintain a head tilt (refer to Figure 15). Effective chest expansion should be visible with each breath you provide. If the chest does not rise, use the hand performing chest compressions to perform a chin lift (or jaw thrust) to open the airway when rescue breaths are delivered. Then return the hand to the sternum compression position to resume compressions after the breath is delivered. If trauma is present, the hand that is not performing compressions should maintain head stability during chest compressions.

In children, head tilt alone is often inadequate to maintain airway patency. Often both hands are needed to perform the head tilt–chin lift maneuver (or jaw thrust) with each ventilation. The time needed to position the hands for each breath, locate landmarks, and reposition the hand to perform compressions may reduce the total number of compressions provided in a minute. Therefore, when moving the hand performing the compressions back to the sternum, visualize and return your hand to the approximate location used for the previous sequence of compressions.

Compression-Ventilation Ratio
Ideal compression-ventilation ratios for infants and children are unknown. From an educational standpoint, a single universal compression-ventilation ratio for victims of all ages and all rescuers providing BLS and ALS interventions would be desirable. Studies of monitored rescuers have demonstrated that the 15:2 compression-ventilation ratio delivers more compressions per minute, and the 5:1 compression-ventilation ratio delivers more ventilations per minute.[136,232]

There is consensus among resuscitation councils that pediatric guidelines should recommend a compression-ventilation ratio of 3:1 for newly born infants (see "Part 11: Neonatal Resuscitation") and 5:1 for infants and children up to 8 years of age. A 15:2 compression-ventilation ratio is now recommended for older children (≥8 years of age) and adults for 1- or 2-rescuer CPR until the airway is secure. The rationale for maintaining age-specific differences in compression-ventilation ratios during resuscitation includes the following:

1. Respiratory problems are the most common cause of pediatric arrest, and most victims of pediatric cardiopulmonary arrest are hypoxic and hypercarbic. Therefore, effective ventilation should be emphasized.
2. Physiological respiratory rates in infants and children are faster than in adults.
3. Current providers are trained in and accustomed to these ratios. Any change from the current guidelines in a fundamental aspect of resuscitation steps should be supported by a high level of scientific evidence.

The actual number of delivered interventions (compressions and ventilations) per minute will vary from rescuer to rescuer and will depend on the compression rate, amount of

time the rescuer spends opening the airway and providing ventilation, and rescuer fatigue.[232,245,246] At present there is insufficient evidence to justify changing the current recommendations for compression-ventilation ratios in infants and children to a universal ratio (Class Indeterminate).

Emerging evidence in *adult* victims of cardiac arrest suggests that the provision of longer sequences of uninterrupted chest compressions (a compression-ventilation ratio >5:1) may be easier to teach and retain.[61,133] In addition, animal data suggests that longer sequences of uninterrupted chest compressions may improve coronary perfusion.[247,248] Finally, longer sequences of compressions may allow more efficient second-rescuer interventions in the out-of-hospital EMS setting.[243] These observations have led to a Class IIb recommendation for a 15:2 compression-ventilation ratio for 1- and 2-rescuer CPR in older children (≥8 years) and adults.

Compression-Only CPR
Clinical studies have established that outcomes are dismal when the pediatric victim of cardiac arrest remains in cardiac arrest until the arrival of EMS personnel. By comparison, excellent outcomes are typical when the child is successfully resuscitated before the arrival of EMS personnel.[9,15,16,40,46,249–252] Some of these patients were apparently resuscitated with "partial CPR," consisting of chest compressions or rescue breathing only. In some published surveys, healthcare providers have expressed reluctance to perform mouth-to-mouth ventilation for unknown victims of cardiopulmonary arrest.[253–255] This reluctance has also been expressed by some surveyed potential lay rescuers,[40,256] although reluctance has not been expressed about resuscitation of infants and children.

The effectiveness of "compression-only" or "no ventilation" CPR has been studied in animal models of *acute VF* sudden cardiac arrest and in some clinical trials of *adult* out-of-hospital cardiac arrest. Some evidence in adult animal models and limited adult clinical trials suggests that positive-pressure ventilation may not be essential during the initial 6 to 12 minutes of an *acute VF* cardiac arrest.[33,257–263] Spontaneous gasping and passive chest recoil may provide some ventilation during that time without the need for active rescue breathing.[259,260,262] In addition, cardiac output during chest compression is only approximately 25% of normal, so the ventilation necessary to maintain optimal ventilation-perfusion relationships may be minimal.[264,265] However, it does not appear that these observations can be applied to resuscitation of infants and children.

Well-controlled animal studies have established that simulated bystander CPR with chest compressions plus rescue breathing is superior to chest compressions alone or rescue breathing alone for asphyxial cardiac arrest and severe asphyxial hypoxic-ischemic shock (pulseless cardiac arrests). However, chest compression–only CPR and rescue breathing–only CPR have been shown to be effective early in animal models of pulseless arrest, and the application of either of these forms of "partial CPR" was found to be superior to no bystander CPR.

Preliminary evidence suggests that *both* chest compressions and active rescue breathing are necessary for optimal resuscitation of the asphyxial arrests most commonly encountered in children.[223,224] For pediatric cardiac arrest, the lay rescuer should provide immediate chest compressions and rescue breathing. If the lay rescuer is unwilling or unable to provide rescue breathing or chest compressions, it is better to provide either chest compressions or rescue breathing than no bystander CPR (Class IIb).

Circulatory Adjuncts and Mechanical Devices for Chest Compression

The use of mechanical devices to provide chest compressions during CPR is not recommended for children. These devices have been designed and tested for use in adults, and their safety and efficacy in children have not been studied. Active compression-decompression CPR (ACD-CPR) has been shown to increase cardiac output compared with standard CPR in adult animal models.[266,267] ACD-CPR maintains coronary perfusion during compression and decompression in humans[268,269] and provides ventilation if the airway is patent.[268,270] In clinical trials ACD-CPR has produced variable results, including improved short-term outcome (eg, return of spontaneous circulation and survival for 24 hours).[271–274] However, these improved outcomes are not consistent,[275] and no long-term survival benefits of ACD-CPR have been reported in most trials. On the basis of these variable clinical results, ACD-CPR is considered an optional technique for adult CPR (Class IIa). This technique cannot be recommended for use in children because it has not been studied in this age group (Class Indeterminate).

Interposed abdominal compression CPR (IAC-CPR) has been shown to increase blood flow in laboratory and computer models[276–278] of adult CPR. IAC-CPR has been shown to improve hemodynamics of CPR and return of spontaneous circulation for adult patients in some clinical in-hospital settings,[279,280] with no evidence of excessive harm. The technique is slightly more complex than standard CPR, however, and it does require an additional rescuer. IAC-CPR has been recommended as an alternative technique (Class IIb in-hospital) for trained adult healthcare providers. This technique cannot be recommended for use in children because it has not been studied in this age group.

Recovery Position

Although many recovery positions are used in the management of children, particularly in those emerging from anesthesia, no specific optimal recovery position can be universally endorsed on the basis of scientific study in children. There is consensus that an ideal recovery position should provide overall stability and considers the following: etiology of the arrest and stability of the cervical spine, risk for aspiration, attention to pressure points, ability to monitor adequacy of ventilation and perfusion, maintenance of a patent airway, and access to the patient for interventions.

Relief of Foreign-Body Airway Obstruction

BLS providers should be able to recognize and relieve complete FBAO. Three maneuvers to remove foreign bodies are suggested: back blows, chest thrusts, and abdominal thrusts. There are some differences between resuscitation councils as to the sequence of actions used to relieve FBAO, but the published data does not support the effectiveness of one sequence over another. There is consensus that lack of protection of the upper abdominal organs by the rib cage renders infants and young children at risk for iatrogenic trauma from abdominal thrusts.[281] Therefore, the use of abdominal thrusts is not recommended for relief of FBAO in infants (Class III).

Epidemiology and Recognition of FBAO

Most reported cases of FBAO in adults are caused by impacted food and occur while the victim is eating. Most reported episodes of choking in infants and children occur during eating or play, when parents or child care providers are present. The choking event is therefore commonly witnessed, and the rescuer usually intervenes when the victim is conscious.

Signs of FBAO in infants and children include the *sudden* onset of respiratory distress associated with coughing, gagging, or stridor (a high-pitched, noisy sound or wheezing). These signs and symptoms of airway obstruction may also be caused by infections such as epiglottitis and croup, which result in airway edema. However, signs of FBAO typically develop very abruptly, with no other signs of illness or infection. Infectious airway obstruction is often accompanied by fever, with other signs of congestion, hoarseness, drooling, lethargy, or limpness. If the child has an infectious cause of airway obstruction, the Heimlich maneuver and back blows and chest thrusts will not relieve the airway obstruction. The child must be taken immediately to an emergency facility.

Priorities for Teaching Relief of Complete FBAO

When FBAO produces signs of *complete* airway obstruction, act quickly to relieve the obstruction. If partial obstruction is present and the child is coughing forcefully, do not interfere with the child's spontaneous coughing and breathing efforts. Attempt to relieve the obstruction only if the cough is or becomes ineffective (loss of sound), respiratory difficulty increases and is accompanied by stridor, or the victim becomes unresponsive. Activate the EMS system as quickly as possible if the child is having difficulty breathing. If >1 rescuer is present, the second rescuer activates the EMS system while the first rescuer attends to the child.

If a *responsive infant* demonstrates signs of complete FBAO, deliver a combination of back blows and chest thrusts until the object is expelled or the victim becomes unresponsive. Although the data in this age group is limited, Heimlich thrusts are not recommended because abdominal thrusts may damage the relatively large and unprotected liver.[62,282]

If a responsive child (1 to 8 years of age) demonstrates signs of complete FBAO, provide a series of Heimlich subdiaphragmatic abdominal thrusts.[283,284] These thrusts increase intrathoracic pressure, creating artificial "coughs" that force air and the foreign body out of the airway.

Epidemiological data[13,285] does not distinguish between FBAO fatalities in which the victims are responsive when first encountered from those in which the victims are unresponsive when initially encountered. Anecdotal evidence, however, suggests that the lay rescuer is more likely to encounter a victim of FBAO who is conscious initially.

The likelihood that a cardiac arrest or unresponsiveness will be caused by an unsuspected FBAO is thought to be low.[13,285] However, the impact of averting a cardiac arrest in a responsive victim with complete airway obstruction would be significant.

The 1992 guidelines[1] recommendations for treatment of FBAO in the unconscious/unresponsive victim were time consuming to teach and perform and were often confusing to students. Training programs that attempt to teach large amounts of material to lay rescuers may fail to achieve core educational objectives (eg, the psychomotor skills of CPR), resulting in poor skills retention and performance.[60] Focused skills training results in superior levels of student performance compared with traditional CPR courses.[61,286–288] This data indicates a need to simplify CPR training for laypersons, including skills in relief of FBAO.

Expert panelists at the Second AHA International Evidence Evaluation Conference held in 1999 and at the International Guidelines 2000 Conference on CPR and ECC agreed that lay rescuer BLS courses should focus on teaching a small number of essential skills. These essential skills were identified as relief of FBAO in the responsive/conscious victim and the skills of CPR. Teaching of the complex skills set of relief of FBAO in the *unresponsive/unconscious victim* to *lay rescuers* is no longer recommended (Class IIb).

If the infant or child choking victim becomes unresponsive/unconscious during attempts to relieve FBAO, provide CPR for approximately 1 minute and then activate the EMS system. Several studies[289–293] indicate that chest compressions identical to those performed during CPR may generate sufficient pressure to remove a foreign body. If the lay rescuer appears to encounter an airway obstruction in the unresponsive victim during the sequence of CPR after attempting and reattempting ventilation, the rescuer should look for and remove the object if seen in the airway when the mouth is opened for rescue breathing. Then the rescuer continues CPR, including chest compressions and cycles of compressions and ventilation.

Healthcare providers should continue to perform abdominal thrusts for responsive adults and children with complete FBAO and alternating back blows and chest thrusts for responsive infants with complete FBAO. Healthcare providers should also be taught the sequences of action appropriate for relief of FBAO in *unresponsive* infants, children, and adults. These sequences of actions for healthcare providers are unchanged from the 1992 guidelines.

Relief of FBAO in the Responsive Infant: Back Blows and Chest Thrusts

The following sequence is used to clear a foreign-body obstruction from the airway of an infant. Back blows (Figure 16) are delivered while the infant is supported in the prone position, straddling the rescuer's forearm, with the head lower than the trunk. After 5 back blows, if the object has not been expelled, give up to 5 chest thrusts. These chest thrusts consist of chest compressions over the lower half of the sternum, 1 finger's breath below the intermammary line. This

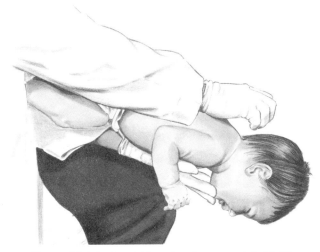

Figure 16. Infant back blows to relieve complete FBAO.

landmark is the same location used to provide chest compressions during CPR. Chest thrusts are delivered while the infant is supine, held on the rescuer's forearm, with the infant's head lower than the body.

Perform the following steps to relieve airway obstruction (the rescuer is usually seated or kneeling with the infant on the rescuer's lap):

1. Hold the infant prone with the head slightly lower than the chest, resting on your forearm. Support the infant's head by firmly supporting the jaw. Take care to avoid compressing the soft tissues of the infant's throat. Rest your forearm on the your thigh to support the infant.
2. Deliver up to 5 back blows forcefully in the middle of the back between the infant's shoulder blades, using the heel of the hand. Each blow should be delivered with sufficient force to attempt to dislodge the foreign body.
3. After delivering up to 5 back blows, place your free hand on the infant's back, supporting the occiput of the infant's head with the palm of your hand. The infant will be effectively cradled between your 2 forearms, with the palm of one hand supporting the face and jaw, while the palm of the other hand supports the occiput.
4. Turn the infant as a unit while carefully supporting the head and neck. Hold the infant in the supine position, with your forearm resting on your thigh. Keep the infant's head lower than the trunk.
5. Provide up to 5 quick downward chest thrusts in the same location as chest compressions—lower third of the sternum, approximately 1 finger's breadth below the intermammary line. Chest thrusts are delivered at a rate of approximately 1 per second, each with the intention of creating enough of an "artificial cough" to dislodge the foreign body.
6. If the airway remains obstructed, repeat the sequence of up to 5 back blows and up to 5 chest thrusts until the object is removed or the victim becomes unresponsive.

Relief of FBAO in the Responsive Child: Abdominal Thrusts (Heimlich Maneuver)

Note: Three maneuvers are suggested to relieve FBAO in the child: back blows, chest thrusts, and abdominal thrusts. Back blows and chest thrusts may be alternative interventions for

FBAO in children, and international training programs should train providers on the basis of ease of teaching and retention in their community.

Abdominal Thrusts With Victim Standing or Sitting

The rescuer should perform the following steps to relieve complete airway obstruction:

1. Stand or kneel behind the victim, arms directly under the victim's axillae, encircling the victim's torso.
2. Place the flat, thumb side of 1 fist against the victim's abdomen in the midline slightly above the navel and well below the tip of the xiphoid process.
3. Grasp the fist with the other hand and exert a series of up to 5 quick inward and upward thrusts (Figure 17). Do not touch the xiphoid process or the lower margins of the rib cage, because force applied to these structures may damage internal organs.[281,294,295]
4. Each thrust should be a separate, distinct movement, delivered with the intent to relieve the obstruction. Continue the series of up to 5 thrusts until the foreign body is expelled or the victim becomes unresponsive.

Relief of FBAO in the Unresponsive Infant or Child

Lay Rescuer Actions

If the infant or child becomes unresponsive, attempt CPR with a single addition—each time the airway is opened, look for the obstructing object in the back of the throat. *If you see an object*, remove it. This recommendation is designed to simplify layperson CPR training and ensure the acquisition of the core skills of rescue breathing and compression while still providing treatment to the FBAO victim.

Healthcare Provider Actions

Blind finger sweeps should not be performed in infants and children because the foreign body may be pushed back into the airway, causing further obstruction or injury to the supraglottic area.[296,297] When abdominal thrusts or chest thrusts are provided to the unresponsive/unconscious, non-breathing victim, open the victim's mouth by grasping both the tongue and lower jaw between the thumb and finger and lifting (tongue-jaw lift).[144] This action draws the tongue away from the back of the throat and may itself partially relieve the obstruction. If the foreign body is seen, carefully remove it.

If the *infant* victim becomes unresponsive, perform the following sequence:

1. Open the victim's airway using a tongue-jaw lift and look for an object in the pharynx. If an object is visible, remove it with a finger sweep. Do not perform a blind finger sweep.
2. Open the airway with a head tilt–chin lift and attempt to provide rescue breaths. If the breaths are not effective, reposition the head and reattempt ventilation.
3. If the breaths are still not effective, perform the sequence of up to 5 back blows and up to 5 chest thrusts.
4. Repeat steps 1 through 3 until the object is dislodged and the airway is patent or for approximately 1 minute. If the infant remains unresponsive after approximately 1 minute, activate the EMS system.

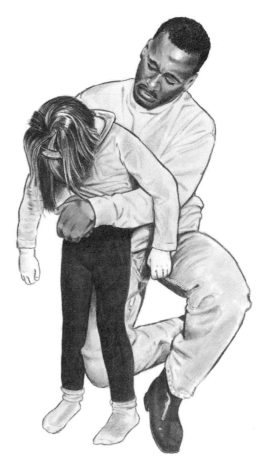

Figure 17. Abdominal thrusts performed for a responsive child with FBAO.

5. If breaths are effective, check for signs of circulation and continue CPR as needed, or place the infant in a recovery position if the infant demonstrates adequate breathing and signs of circulation.

If the *child* victim becomes unresponsive, place the victim in the supine position and perform the following sequence:

1. Open the victim's airway using a tongue-jaw lift and look for an object in the pharynx. If an object is visible, remove it with a finger sweep. However, do not perform a blind finger sweep.
2. Open the airway with a head tilt–chin lift, and attempt to provide rescue breaths. If breaths are not effective, reposition the head and reattempt ventilation.
3. If the breaths are still not effective, kneel beside the victim or straddle the victim's hips and prepare to perform the Heimlich maneuver abdominal thrusts as follows:
   a. Place the heel of one hand on the child's abdomen in the midline slightly above the navel and well below the rib cage and xiphoid process. Place the other hand on top of the first.
   b. Press both hands onto the abdomen with a quick inward and upward thrust (Figure 18). Direct each thrust upward in the midline and not to either side of the abdomen. If necessary, perform a series of up to 5 thrusts. Each thrust should be a separate and distinct movement of sufficient force to attempt to dislodge the airway obstruction.

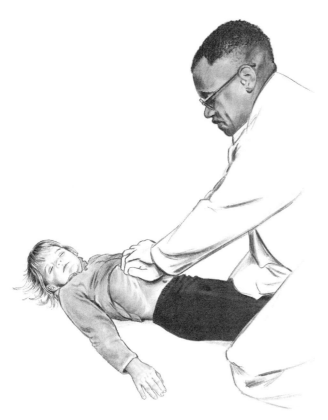

Figure 18. Abdominal thrusts performed for supine, unresponsive child.

4. Repeat steps 1 through 3 until the object is retrieved or rescuer breaths are effective.
5. Once effective breaths are delivered, assess for signs of circulation and provide additional CPR as needed or place the child in a recovery position if the child demonstrates adequate breathing and signs of circulation.

BLS in Special Situations

BLS for the Trauma Victim

The principles of resuscitation of the seriously injured child are the same as those for any pediatric patient. However, some aspects of pediatric trauma care require emphasis because improper resuscitation is a major cause of preventable pediatric trauma death.[298–300] Common errors in pediatric trauma resuscitation include failure to open and maintain the airway with cervical spine protection, inadequate or overzealous fluid resuscitation, and failure to recognize and treat internal bleeding. Ideally, a qualified surgeon should be involved early in the course of resuscitation. In regions with developed EMS systems, children with multisystem trauma should be transported rapidly to trauma centers with pediatric expertise. The relative value of aeromedical transport compared with ground transport of children with multiple trauma is unclear and should be evaluated by individual EMS systems.[301–303] It is likely that mode of transport preference will depend on EMS system characteristics.

BLS support requires meticulous attention to airway, breathing, and circulation from the moment of injury. The airway may become obstructed by soft tissues, blood, or

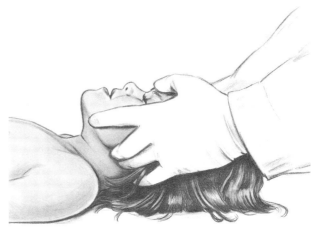

Figure 19. Spine immobilization with airway opening in child with potential head and neck trauma.

dental fragments. These causes of airway obstruction should be anticipated and treated. Airway control includes spinal immobilization, which is continued during transport and stabilization in an ALS facility. This is best accomplished by a combined jaw-thrust and spinal stabilization maneuver, using only the amount of manual control necessary to prevent cranial-cervical motion (Figure 19). The head tilt–chin lift is contraindicated because it may worsen existing cervical spinal injury. Rescuers should ensure that the neck is maintained in a neutral position because the prominent occiput of the child predisposes the neck to slight flexion when the child is placed on a flat surface.[226,304]

It may be difficult to immobilize the cervical spine of an infant or young child in a neutral position. When a young child is placed supine on a firm surface, the large occiput tends to encourage neck flexion.[305] Spinal immobilization of young children with a backboard with a recess for the head is recommended. If such a board is unavailable, the effect of a head recess can be simulated by placing a layer of towels or sheets ½ to 1 inch high on the board so that it elevates the torso (from shoulders to buttocks) and maintains the neck in neutral alignment.[225,226,306,307] The neck and airway should be in neutral position when the head rests on the backboard. Semirigid cervical collars are available in a wide range of sizes to help immobilize children of various sizes. The child's head and neck should be further immobilized with linen rolls and tape, with secondary immobilization of the child on a spine board.

If 2 rescuers are present, the first rescuer opens the airway with a jaw-thrust maneuver while the second rescuer ensures that the cervical spine is absolutely stabilized in a neutral position. Avoid traction on or movement of the neck because it may result in converting a partial to a complete spinal cord injury. Once the airway is controlled, immobilize the cervical spine with a semirigid cervical collar and a spine board, linen rolls, and tape. Throughout immobilization and during transport, support oxygenation and ventilation.[308]

BLS for the Submersion Victim

Submersion is a leading cause of death in children worldwide. The duration and severity of hypoxia sustained as the result of submersion is the single most important determinant of outcome. CPR, particularly rescue breathing, should be attempted as soon as the unresponsive submersion victim is pulled from the water. If possible, rescue breathing should be provided even while the victim is still in the water, if the rescuer's safety is ensured.

Many infants and children submerged for brief periods of time will respond to stimulation or rescue breathing alone.[15] If the child does not have signs of circulation (normal breathing, coughing, or movement) after initial rescue breaths are provided, begin chest compressions.

In 1994 the Institute of Medicine reviewed the recommendations of the AHA regarding resuscitation of submersion victims and supported the emphasis on initial establishment of effective ventilation.[62] There is no evidence that water acts as an obstructive foreign body, and time should not be wasted in attempting to remove water from the victim. Such maneuvers can cause injury but—more importantly—will delay CPR, particularly support of airway and ventilation.[62]

Additional special resuscitation situations are addressed in "Part 3, Adult BLS: Special Resuscitation Circumstances" and in "Part 11: Neonatal Resuscitation."

Family Presence During Resuscitation

Most family members would like to be present during the attempted resuscitation of a loved one, according to surveys in the United States and the United Kingdom.[309–314] Parents and those who care for chronically ill children are often knowledgeable about and comfortable with medical equipment and emergency procedures. Family members with no medical background report that being at the side of a loved one and saying goodbye during the final moments of life is extremely comforting.[309,315,316] Parents or family members often fail to ask if they can be present, but healthcare providers should offer the opportunity whenever possible.[312,315,317,318]

Family members present during resuscitation report that their presence helped them adjust to the death of their loved one,[309,311] and most indicate they would do so again.[309] Standardized psychological examinations suggest that family members present during resuscitation demonstrate less anxiety and depression and more constructive grief behavior than family members not present during resuscitation.[313]

When family members are present during resuscitative efforts, resuscitation team members should be sensitive to their presence. If possible, 1 member of the healthcare team should remain with the family to answer questions, clarify information, and offer comfort.[319]

In the prehospital setting, family members are typically present during resuscitation of a loved one. Prehospital care providers are often too busy to give undivided attention to the needs of family members. However, brief explanations and the opportunity to remain with the loved one can be comforting. Some EMS systems provide follow-up visits to family members after unsuccessful resuscitation attempts.

Termination of Resuscitative Efforts

Despite the best efforts of healthcare providers, most children who experience a cardiac arrest do not survive and never demonstrate return of spontaneous circulation. Return of spontaneous circulation is unlikely if the child fails to respond to effective BLS and ALS and ≥2 doses of epinephrine.[4,40,55] Special resuscitation circumstances, local resources, and underlying conditions and prognoses create a complex decision matrix for the resuscitation team. In general, in the absence of recurring or refractory VF or ventricular tachycardia, history of a toxic drug exposure or electrolyte imbalance, or a primary hypothermic injury, the resuscitation team should discontinue resuscitation efforts after 30 minutes, especially if there is no return of spontaneous circulation (Class IIa). For further discussion, see "Part 2: Ethical Aspects of CPR and ECC."

Maximizing the Effectiveness of Pediatric Basic Life Support Training

CPR is the critical link in the Chain of Survival, particularly for infants and children. For many years the AHA and members of ILCOR have promoted the goal of appropriate bystander (lay rescuer) response to every witnessed cardiopulmonary emergency, such as a choking child, a child in respiratory distress, or an infant or child in cardiac arrest. Although immediate bystander CPR can result in resuscitation even before the arrival of emergency personnel,[15,16] bystander CPR is not provided for a majority of victims of cardiac arrest.[4,40] Witnesses may fail to initiate resuscitation for several reasons; the most obvious is that they have not learned CPR.

CPR courses have evolved into instructor-based, classroom-based programs. Yet this approach is not effective in teaching the critical psychomotor skills of CPR. Several studies have documented the failure of lay rescuers to perform CPR after participating in these traditional courses.[286,320] In 1998 these findings led the AHA to convene the National ECC Educational Conference to discuss how to improve CPR skills performance and retention. The experts came to 2 major conclusions:

- Current CPR programs for lay rescuers contain too much cognitive material and provide insufficient "hands on" practice time.
- CPR programs for lay rescuers should focus on acquisition of specific psychomotor skills and retention of those skills over time.

Core Objectives

The core objectives for the Pediatric Basic Life Support course and modules are simple. After participation in a BLS course, the rescuer who assists an unresponsive victim will be able to

1. Recognize a situation in which resuscitation is appropriate.
2. Activate the EMS system when appropriate.
3. Retrieve and use an AED for the adult victim and the child victim ≥8 years old.
4. Provide effective ventilations (chest rises following use of mouth-to-mouth, mouth-to-mask, and mouth-to-barrier devices). Healthcare providers should be capable of providing bag-mask ventilation.

5. Provide effective chest compressions that generate a palpable pulse.
6. Perform all skills in a manner that is safe for the victim, rescuer, and bystanders.

The participant should remember how to perform these skills for ≥1 year after training.

If participants are to achieve core objectives, CPR programs must be simplified. They must focus on skills acquisition rather than cognitive knowledge. Training programs that attempt to teach large amounts of material fail to achieve core educational objectives (eg, the psychomotor skills of CPR), with poor participant skills retention and performance.[60] By comparison, focused training programs emphasizing skills acquisition result in superior levels of skills performance.[61,286-288]

This compelling data mandates consideration of the potential negative effects of science changes on teaching CPR. Consideration of these effects influenced debates about guidelines changes. Interventions that could produce even modest improvements in survival were more readily endorsed if they were easy to teach and would simplify CPR instruction. Conversely, interventions that would have a negative impact on CPR training (eg, complex instruction and extensive practice) had to be supported by higher levels of evidence of effectiveness to justify their introduction.

Course instructors should focus on ensuring participant mastery of core objectives. Skills practice time must be maximized and lecture time minimized. Resuscitation councils should evaluate skills acquisition by participants and use it to continuously improve resuscitation programs.

Audio and Visual CPR Performance Aids for BLS Interventions

CPR is a complex psychomotor task that is difficult to teach, learn, remember, and perform. Not surprisingly, observed CPR performance is often poor (inadequate compression depth, inadequate compression rate, etc). The use of audio and visual CPR performance aids during training can improve acquisition of CPR psychomotor skills (Class IIa). The use of audio prompts (eg, an audiotape with the appropriate cadence of "compress-compress-compress-breathe") improves CPR performance in both clinical and laboratory settings (Class IIb).[244,247,287,321,322] Use of these devices should be considered in areas where CPR is performed infrequently.

Areas of Overlap Within Guidelines for Pediatric BLS/ALS, Adult ACLS, and Newborn Resuscitation

Note that recommendations will overlap in areas where distinctions between age cutoffs and target audiences are blurred. Examples of overlapping areas between adult, pediatric, and neonatal recommendations include

- Compression-ventilation ratios of 15:2 versus 5:1 versus 3:1 and 2-finger versus 2 thumb–encircling hands versus 1-hand versus 2-hand compression technique
- When to "phone first" versus "phone fast"
- Chest-compression rate of approximately 120 events per minute for the newly born/neonate in the delivery room

versus at least 100 compressions per minute for BLS for infants beyond the newly born period and in the out-of-hospital setting versus approximately 100 compressions per minute for pediatric BLS
- Pulse check locations: carotid versus brachial versus femoral versus umbilical

Most of these overlapping areas are easily interpreted in the context of the training environment and target audience.

Areas of Controversy in International Guidelines 2000: Unresolved Issues and Need for Additional Research

There is great difficulty in creating advisory pediatric BLS statements for universal application. The ILCOR Pediatric Task Force reviewed the rationale for current internationally recognized guidelines in North America, South America, Europe, Australia, New Zealand, and southern Africa. The group identified several areas of controversy that require focused research. They are as follows:

- What is the prevalence and time course for presentation of VF during or after resuscitation?
- Should resuscitation sequences of interventions/algorithms be taught on the basis of the likelihood of presenting rhythm (eg, bradycardia-asystole most likely for children) or reversible etiology (eg, VF treated with defibrillation is most likely to be successfully resuscitated)?
- How many breaths should be initially attempted after opening the airway?
- At what heart rate should chest compressions be initiated?
- What is the optimal depth for chest compressions (one third to one half depth of chest versus specified number of inches or centimeters)?
- What sequence of interventions for the choking child is most appropriate: back blows versus abdominal thrusts versus chest thrusts?
- What defibrillation dose, type of waveform, and number of defibrillation shocks should be delivered after medication has been provided for VF in children?
- Should visual inspection of the mouth for a foreign body precede ventilation attempts in infants?
- What is an optimal recovery position for infants and children?
- Can a universal compression-ventilation ratio be adopted (5:1 versus 10:2 versus 15:2) that can accommodate all victims from infancy to adulthood?
- Is mouth-and-nose ventilation a better method than maternal mouth-to-infant-mouth-and-nose for ventilation of neonates and small infants?
- Can AEDs accurately and reliably be used in pediatric patients? Can AEDs provide a single optimal defibrillation "dose"?
- What are the frequency, etiology, and outcome of CPR provided by laypersons versus trained providers in a variety of home, out-of-hospital, and in-hospital settings?
- What is the impact of implementing universal resuscitation guidelines on arrest prevention, successful resuscitation,

and neurological performance outcomes from potential or actual cardiopulmonary arrest in infants and children?

Summary

The epidemiology and outcome of pediatric cardiopulmonary arrest and the priorities, techniques, and sequence of pediatric resuscitation assessments and interventions differ from those of adults. Current guidelines have been updated after extensive multinational evidence-based review and discussion over several years. Areas of controversy in current guidelines and recommendations made by consensus are detailed. A large degree of uniformity exists in the current guidelines advocated by the AHA, Council on Latin American Resuscitation, Heart and Stroke Foundation of Canada, European Resuscitation Council, Australian Resuscitation Council, and Resuscitation Council of Southern Africa. Differences are currently based on local and regional preferences, training networks, and customs rather than scientific controversy. Unresolved issues with potential for future universal application are highlighted.

Appendix

List of Pediatric BLS Classes of Recommendation

Phone first versus phone fast: Indeterminate

Provide chest compressions or rescue breathing as "better than nothing": Class IIb

Use of barrier devices in children: Indeterminate

Two versus 5 initial breaths: Indeterminate

Mouth-to-nose breathing: Class IIb

Healthcare providers should be trained to provide effective bag-mask ventilation: Class IIa

Goal of ventilation is "physiological" ventilation: Class IIa

Pulse check should not be taught to laypersons: Class IIa

Two thumb–encircling hands technique preferable to 2-finger technique for 2-rescuer healthcare provider CPR for infants: Class IIb

Universal compression-ventilation ratio: Indeterminate

ACD-CPR: Indeterminate

IAC-CPR: Indeterminate

Audio prompt for training: Class IIa

Audio prompt for CPR: Class IIb

Lay rescuers should not be taught complex relief of FBAO skills for unresponsive victim: Class IIb

Abdominal thrusts for infants: Class III

Termination of efforts after 30 minutes if no exceptional circumstances: Class IIa

Comparison Across Age Groups of Resuscitation Interventions

See the following Table.

TABLE. Comparison Across Age Groups of Resuscitation Interventions

CPR/Rescue Breathing	Adult and Older Child	Child (Approximately 1–8 Years of Age)	Infant (Less Than 1 Year of Age)	Neonate and Newly Born
Establish unresponsiveness, activate EMS				
Open airway (head tilt–chin lift or jaw thrust)	Head tilt–chin lift (if trauma is present, use jaw thrust)	Head tilt–chin lift (if trauma is present, use jaw thrust)	Head tilt–chin lift (if trauma is present, use jaw thrust)	Head tilt–chin lift (if trauma, use jaw thrust)
Check for breathing: (Look, Listen, Feel) If victim breathing: place in recovery position. If victim not breathing: give 2 effective slow breaths				
Initial	2 effective breaths at 2 seconds per breath	2 effective breaths at 1 to 1½ seconds per breath	2 effective breaths at 1 to 1½ seconds per breath	2 effective breaths at approximately 1 second per breath
Subsequent	12 breaths/min (approximate)	20 breaths/min (approximate)	20 breaths/min (approximate)	30–60 breaths/min (approximate)
Foreign-body airway obstruction	Abdominal thrusts or back blows or chest thrusts	Abdominal thrusts or back blows or chest thrusts	Back blows or chest thrusts (no abdominal thrusts)	Back blows or chest thrusts (no abdominal thrusts)
Signs of Circulation: Check for normal breathing, coughing or movement, pulse.* If signs of circulation present: provide airway and breathing support. If signs of circulation absent, begin chest compressions interposed with breaths	Pulse check (healthcare providers)* Carotid	(Healthcare providers)* Carotid	(Healthcare providers)* Brachial	(Healthcare providers)* Umbilical
Compression landmarks	Lower half of sternum	Lower half of sternum	Lower half of sternum (1 finger width below intermammary line)	Lower half of sternum (1 finger width below intermammary line)
Compression method	Heel of 1 hand, other hand on top	Heel of 1 hand	Two thumbs–encircling hands for 2-rescuer healthcare provider or 2 fingers	Two thumbs–encircling hands for 2-rescuer healthcare provider or 2 fingers
Compression depth	Approximately 1½ to 2 in	Approximately ⅓ to ½ the depth of the chest (1 to 1½ in)	Approximately ⅓ to ½ the depth of the chest (½ to 1 in)	Approximately ⅓ to ½ the depth of the chest
Compression rate	Approximately 100/min	Approximately 100/min	At least 100/min	Approximately 120 events/min (90 compressions/30 breaths)
Compression/ventilation ratio	15:2 (1 or 2 rescuers, unprotected airway) 5:1 (2 rescuers, protected airway)	5:1 (1 or 2 rescuers)	5:1 (1 or 2 rescuers)	3:1 (1 or 2 rescuers)

*Pulse check is performed as one of the "signs of circulation" assessed by healthcare providers. Lay rescuers check for other signs of circulation but do not check pulse.

References

1. Emergency Cardiac Care Committee and Subcommittees, American Heart Association. Guidelines for cardiopulmonary resuscitation and emergency cardiac care, VI: pediatric advanced life support [see comments]. *JAMA.* 1992;268:2262–2275.
2. Kaye W, Ornato JP, Peberdy M, Mancini ME, Nadkarni V, Truitt T. Factors associated with survival from in-hospital cardiac arrest: a pilot of the National Registry of Cardiopulmonary Resuscitation. *Circulation.* 1999;100:1–313. Abstract.
3. Zaritsky A, Nadkarni V, Hazinski MF, Foltin G, Quan L, Wright J, Fiser D, Zideman D, O'Malley P, Chameides L, Writing Group. Recommended guidelines for uniform reporting of pediatric advanced life support: the pediatric Utstein Style. A statement for healthcare professionals from a task force of the American Academy of Pediatrics, the American Heart Association, and the European Resuscitation Council. *Circulation.* 1995;92:2006–2020.
4. Young KD, Seidel JS. Pediatric cardiopulmonary resuscitation: a collective review [see comments]. *Ann Emerg Med.* 1999;33:195–205.

5. Hoyert DL, Kochanek KD, Murphy SL. Deaths: final data for 1997. *Natl Vital Stat Rep*. 1999;47:1–104.

6. Eisenberg M, Bergner L, Hallstrom A. Epidemiology of cardiac arrest and resuscitation in children. *Ann Emerg Med*. 1983;12:672–674.

7. Gausche M, Seidel JS, Henderson DP, Ness B, Ward PM, Wayland BW, Almeida B. Pediatric deaths and emergency medical services (EMS) in urban and rural areas. *Pediatr Emerg Care*. 1989;5:158–162.

8. Torphy DE, Minter MG, Thompson BM. Cardiorespiratory arrest and resuscitation of children. *Am J Dis Child*. 1984;138:1099–1102.

9. Friesen RM, Duncan P, Tweed WA, Bristow G. Appraisal of pediatric cardiopulmonary resuscitation. *Can Med Assoc J*. 1982;126:1055–1058.

10. Walsh CK, Krongrad E. Terminal cardiac electrical activity in pediatric patients. *Am J Cardiol*. 1983;51:557–561.

11. Zaritsky A. Cardiopulmonary resuscitation in children. *Clin Chest Med*. 1987;8:561–571.

12. National Safety Council. *1999 Injury Facts*. Itasca, Ill: National Safety Council; 1999.

13. Fingerhut LA, Cox CS, Warner M. International comparative analysis of injury mortality: findings from the ICE (International Collaborative Effort) on Injury Statistics, Vital and Health Statistics of the Centers for Disease Control and Prevention 1998.

14. Peters K, Kochanek K, Murphy S. Deaths: final data for 1996–1998. Hyattsville, Md: National Center for Health Statistics; National Vital Statistics Reports.

15. Kyriacou DN, Arcinue EL, Peek C, Kraus JF. Effect of immediate resuscitation on children with submersion injury. *Pediatrics*. 1994;94:137–142.

16. Hickey RW, Cohen DM, Strausbaugh S, Dietrich AM. Pediatric patients requiring CPR in the prehospital setting [see comments]. *Ann Emerg Med*. 1995;25:495–501.

17. Cummins RO, Hazinski MF, Kerber RE, Kudenchuk P, Becker L, Nichol G, Malanga B, Aufderheide TP, Stapleton EM, Kern K, Ornato JP, Sanders A, Valenzuela T, Eisenberg M. Low-energy biphasic waveform defibrillation: evidence-based review applied to emergency cardiovascular care guidelines: a statement for healthcare professionals from the American Heart Association Committee on Emergency Cardiovascular Care and the Subcommittees on Basic Life Support, Advanced Cardiac Life Support, and Pediatric Resuscitation. *Circulation*. 1998;97:1654–1667.

18. Nadkarni V, Hazinski MF, Zideman D, Kattwinkel J, Quan L, Bingham R, Zaritsky A, Bland J, Kramer E, Tiballs J. Pediatric resuscitation: an advisory statement from the Pediatric Working Group of the International Liaison Committee on Resuscitation. *Circulation*. 1997;95:2185–95.

19. Kattwinkel J, Niermeyer S, Nadkarni V, Tibballs J, Phillips B, Zideman D, Van Reempts P, Osmond M. An advisory statement from the Pediatric Working Group of the International Liaison Committee on Resuscitation. *Pediatrics*. 1999;103:e56.

20. Clements F, McGowan J. Finger position for chest compressions in cardiac arrest in infants. *Resuscitation* 2000;44:43–46.

21. Whitelaw CC, Slywka B, Goldsmith LJ. Comparison of a two-finger versus two-thumb method for chest compressions by healthcare providers in an infant mechanical model. *Resuscitation*. 2000;43:213–6.

22. Eckenhoff JE. Some anatomic considerations of the infant larynx influencing endotracheal anesthesia. *Anesthesiology*. 1951;12:401–410.

23. Coté CJ, et al, eds. *A Practice of Anesthesia for Infants and Children*. 2nd ed. Philadelphia, Pa: WB Saunders; 1993.

24. Nadkarni V. Ventricular fibrillation in the asphyxiated piglet model. In: Quan L, Franklin WH, eds. *Ventricular Fibrillation: a Pediatric Problem*. Armonk, NY: Futura Publishers; 2000:43–54.

25. Bayes de Luna A, Coumel P, Leclercq JF. Ambulatory sudden cardiac death: mechanisms of production of fatal arrhythmia on the basis of data from 157 cases. *Am Heart J*. 1989;117:151–9.

26. Cummins RO, Chamberlain DA, Abramson NS, Allen M, Baskett P, Becker L, Bossaert L, Delooz H, Dick W, Eisenberg M, et al. Recommended guidelines for uniform reporting of data from out-of-hospital cardiac arrest: the Utstein Style. Task Force of the American Heart Association, the European Resuscitation Council, the Heart and Stroke Foundation of Canada, and the Australian Resuscitation Council [see comments]. *Ann Emerg Med*. 1991;20:861–74.

27. Cummins RO. From concept to standard-of-care? Review of the clinical experience with automated external defibrillators. *Ann Emerg Med*. 1989;18:1269–1275.

28. Larsen MP, Eisenberg MS, Cummins RO, Hallstrom AP. Predicting survival from out-of-hospital cardiac arrest: a graphic model. *Ann Emerg Med*. 1993;22:1652–1658.

29. White RD, Vukov LF, Bugliosi TF. Early defibrillation by police: initial experience with measurement of critical time intervals and patient outcome. *Ann Emerg Med*. 1994;23:1009–1013.

30. Ladwig KH, Schoefinius A, Danner R, Gurtler R, Herman R, Koeppel A, Hauber P. Effects of early defibrillation by ambulance personnel on short- and long-term outcome of cardiac arrest survival: the Munich experiment. *Chest*. 1997;112:1584–1591.

31. Stiell IG, Wells GA, Field BJ, Spaite DW, De Maio VJ, Ward R, Munkley DP, Lyver MB, Luinstra LG, Campeau T, Maloney J, Dagnone E. Improved out-of-hospital cardiac arrest survival through the inexpensive optimization of an existing defibrillation program: OPALS study phase II. Ontario Prehospital Advanced Life Support [see comments]. *JAMA*. 1999;281:1175–1181.

32. White RD, Hankins DG, Bugliosi TF. Seven years' experience with early defibrillation by police and paramedics in an emergency medical services system. *Resuscitation*. 1998;39:145–151.

33. Van Hoeyweghen RJ, Bossaert LL, Mullie A, Calle P, Martens P, Buylaert WA, Delooz H, Belgian Cerebral Resuscitation Study Group. Quality and efficiency of bystander CPR. *Resuscitation*. 1993;26:47–52.

34. Bossaert L, Van Hoeyweghen R, the Cerebral Resuscitation Study Group. Bystander cardiopulmonary resuscitation (CPR) in out-of-hospital cardiac arrest. *Resuscitation*. 1989;17(suppl):S55–S69; discussion S199–S206.

35. Slonim AD, Patel KM, Ruttimann UE, Pollack MM. Cardiopulmonary resuscitation in pediatric intensive care units [see comments]. *Crit Care Med*. 1997;25:1951–1955.

36. Richman PB, Nashed AH. The etiology of cardiac arrest in children and young adults: special considerations for ED management. *Am J Emerg Med*. 1999;17:264–270.

37. Kuisma M, Suominen P, Korpela R. Paediatric out-of-hospital cardiac arrests: epidemiology and outcome. *Resuscitation*. 1995;30:141–150.

38. Kuisma M, Maatta T, Repo J. Cardiac arrests witnessed by EMS personnel in a multitiered system: epidemiology and outcome. *Am J Emerg Med*. 1998;16:12–16.

39. Finer NN, Horbar JD, Carpenter JH. Cardiopulmonary resuscitation in the very low birth weight infant: the Vermont Oxford Network experience. *Pediatrics*. 1999;104:428–434.

40. Sirbaugh PE, Pepe PE, Shook JE, Kimball KT, Goldman MJ, Ward MA, Mann DM. A prospective, population-based study of the demographics, epidemiology, management, and outcome of out-of-hospital pediatric cardiopulmonary arrest [see comments] [published erratum appears in *Ann Emerg Med*. 1999;33:358]. *Ann Emerg Med*. 1999;33:174–184.

41. Zaritsky A. Outcome following cardiopulmonary resuscitation in the pediatric intensive care unit [editorial; comment]. *Crit Care Med*. 1997;25:1937–1938.

42. Saugstad OD. Practical aspects of resuscitating asphyxiated newborn infants. *Eur J Pediatr*. 1998;157(suppl 1):S11–S15.

43. Palme-Kilander C. Methods of resuscitation in low-Apgar-score newborn infants: a national survey. *Acta Paediatr*. 1992;81:739–744.

44. World Health Organization. The World Health Report: *Report of the Director-General. 1995*. Geneva, Switzerland: World Health Organization; 1995.

45. Appleton GO, Cummins RO, Larson MP, Graves JR. CPR and the single rescuer: at what age should you "call first" rather than "call fast"? [see comments]. *Ann Emerg Med*. 1995;25:492–494.

46. Mogayzel C, Quan L, Graves JR, Tiedeman D, Fahrenbruch C, Herndon P. Out-of-hospital ventricular fibrillation in children and adolescents: causes and outcomes [see comments]. *Ann Emerg Med*. 1995;25:484–491.

47. Dieckmann RA, Vardis R. High-dose epinephrine in pediatric out-of-hospital cardiopulmonary arrest. *Pediatrics*. 1995;95:901–913.

48. Losek JD, Hennes H, Glaeser PW, Smith DS, Hendley G. Prehospital countershock treatment of pediatric asystole. *Am J Emerg Med*. 1989;7:7:571–575.

49. Safranek DJ, Eisenberg MS, Larsen MP. The epidemiology of cardiac arrest in young adults. *Ann Emerg Med*. 1992;21:1102–1106.

50. Schindler MB, Bohn D, Cox PN, McCrindle BW, Jarvis A, Edmonds J, Barker G. Outcome of out-of-hospital cardiac or respiratory arrest in children [see comments]. *N Engl J Med*. 1996;335:1473–1479.

51. Ronco R, King W, Donley DK, Tilden SJ. Outcome and cost at a children's hospital following resuscitation for out-of-hospital cardiopulmonary arrest. *Arch Pediatr Adolesc Med*. 1995;149:210–214.

52. Hazinski MF, Chahine AA, Holcomb GW III, Morris JA Jr. Outcome of cardiovascular collapse in pediatric blunt trauma. *Ann Emerg Med.* 1994;23:1229–1235.

53. Innes PA, Summers CA, Boyd IM, Molyneux EM. Audit of paediatric cardiopulmonary resuscitation. *Arch Dis Child.* 1993;68:487–491.

54. Losek JD, Hennes H, Glaeser P, Hendley G, Nelson DB. Prehospital care of the pulseless, nonbreathing pediatric patient. *Am J Emerg Med.* 1987;5:370–374.

55. Zaritsky A, Nadkarni V, Getson P, Kuehl K. CPR in children. *Ann Emerg Med.* 1987;16:1107–1111.

56. O'Rourke PP. Outcome of children who are apneic and pulseless in the emergency room. *Crit Care Med.* 1986;14:466–468.

57. Childhood injuries in the United States. Division of Injury Control, Center for Environmental Health and Injury Control, Centers for Disease Control [see comments]. *Am J Dis Child.* 1990;144:627–646.

58. Adgey AA, Johnston PW, McMechan S. Sudden cardiac death and substance abuse. *Resuscitation.* 1995;29:219–221.

59. Ackerman MJ. The long QT syndrome. *Pediatr Rev.* 1998;19:232–238.

60. Brennan RT, Braslow A. Skill mastery in cardiopulmonary resuscitation training classes. *Am J Emerg Med.* 1995;13:505–508.

61. Handley JA, Handley AJ. Four-step CPR: improving skill retention [published erratum appears in *Resuscitation.* 1998;37:199]. *Resuscitation.* 1998;36:3–8.

62. Rosen P, Stoto M, Harley J. The use of the Heimlich maneuver in near drowning: Institute of Medicine report. *J Emerg Med.* 1995;13:397–405.

63. Newacheck PW, Strickland B, Shonkoff JP, Perrin JM, McPherson M, McManus M, Lauver C, Fox H, Arango P. An epidemiologic profile of children with special health care needs [see comments]. *Pediatrics.* 1998;102:117–123.

64. McPherson M, Arango P, Fox H, Lauver C, McManus M, Newacheck PW, Perrin JM, Shonkoff JP, Strickland B. A new definition of children with special health care needs [comment]. *Pediatrics.* 1998;102:137–140.

65. Committee on Pediatric Emergency Medicine, American Academy of Pediatrics. Emergency preparedness for children with special health care needs. *Pediatrics.* 1999;104:e53.

66. Spaite DW, Conroy C, Tibbitts M, Karriker KJ, Seng M, Battaglia N, Criss EA, Valenzuela TD, Meislin HW. Use of emergency medical services by children with special health care needs. *Prehosp Emerg Care.* 2000;4:19–23.

67. Schultz-Grant LD, Young-Cureton V, Kataoka-Yahiro M. Advance directives and do not resuscitate orders: nurses' knowledge and the level of practice in school settings. *J Sch Nurs.* 1998;14:4–10, 12–13.

68. Seidel JS. Emergency medical services and the pediatric patient: are the needs being met? II: training and equipping emergency medical services providers for pediatric emergencies. *Pediatrics.* 1986;78:808–812.

69. Seidel JS. EMS-C in urban and rural areas: the California experience. In: *Emergency Medical Services for Children: Report of the 97th Ross Conference on Pediatric Research.* Columbus, Ohio: Ross Laboratories; 1989:808–812.

70. Applebaum D. Advanced prehospital care for pediatric emergencies. *Ann Emerg Med.* 1985;14:656–659.

71. Zaritsky A, French JP, Schafermeyer R, Morton D. A statewide evaluation of pediatric prehospital and hospital emergency services. *Arch Pediatr Adolesc Med.* 1994;148:76–81.

72. Graham CJ, Stuemky J, Lera TA. Emergency medical services preparedness for pediatric emergencies. *Pediatr Emerg Care.* 1993;9:329–331.

73. Cook RT Jr. The Institute of Medicine report on emergency medical services for children: thoughts for emergency medical technicians, paramedics, and emergency physicians. *Pediatrics.* 1995;96:199–206.

74. Makhmudova NM, Urinbaev MZ, Pak MA, Abukov MI, Faizieva NP. Organization of emergency medical services for the children in Tashkent [in Russian]. *Sov Zdravookhr.* 1990;55–59.

75. Foltin GL. Critical issues in urban emergency medical services for children. *Pediatrics.* 1995;96:174–179.

76. Brooks JG. Sudden infant death syndrome. *Pediatr Ann.* 1995;24:345–383.

77. American Academy of Pediatrics Task Force on Infant Positioning and SIDS. Positioning and sudden infant death syndrome (SIDS): update. *Pediatrics.* 1996;98:1216–1218.

78. American Academy of Pediatrics AAP Task Force on Infant Positioning and SIDS. Positioning and SIDS [published erratum appears in *Pediatrics.* 1992;90(2 pt 1):264] [see comments]. *Pediatrics.* 1992;89:1120–1126.

79. Willinger M, Hoffman HJ, Hartford RB. Infant sleep position and risk for sudden infant death syndrome: report of meeting held January 13 and 14, 1994, National Institutes of Health, Bethesda, MD [see comments]. *Pediatrics.* 1994;93:814–819.

80. Mitchell EA, Scragg R. Observations on ethnic differences in SIDS mortality in New Zealand. *Early Hum Dev.* 1994;38:151–157.

81. Blair PS, Fleming PJ, Bensley D, Smith I, Bacon C, Taylor E, Berry J, Golding J, Tripp J, Confidential Enquiry into Stillbirths and Deaths Regional Coordinators and Researchers. Smoking and the sudden infant death syndrome: results from 1993–5 case-control study for confidential inquiry into stillbirths and deaths in infancy [see comments]. *BMJ.* 1996;313:195–198.

82. Danesco E, Miller T, Spicer R. Incidence and costs of 1987–1994 childhood injuries: demographic breakdowns. *Pediatrics.* 2000;105:e27.

83. Guyer B, Ellers B. Childhood injuries in the United States: mortality, morbidity, and cost. *Am J Dis Child.* 1990;144:649–652.

84. Cushman R, James W, Waclawik H. Physicians promoting bicycle helmets for children: a randomized trial [see comments]. *Am J Public Health.* 1991;81:1044–1046.

85. Centers for Disease Control. Fatal injuries to children: United States, 1986. *JAMA.* 1990;264:952–953.

86. The National Committee for Injury Prevention and Control. Injury prevention: meeting the challenge. *Am J Prev Med.* 1989;5:1–303.

87. Giguere JF, St-Vil D, Turmel A, Di Lorenzo M, Pothel C, Manseau S, Mercier C. Airbags and children: a spectrum of C-spine injuries. *J Pediatr Surg.* 1998;33:811–816.

88. Bourke GJ. Airbags and fatal injuries to children. *Lancet.* 1996;347:560.

89. Hazinski MF, Eddy VA, Morris JA Jr. Children's traffic safety program: influence of early elementary school safety education on family seat belt use. *J Trauma.* 1995;39:1063–1068.

90. Patel DR, Greydanus DE, Rowlett JD. Romance with the automobile in the 20th century: implications for adolescents in a new millennium. *Adolesc Med.* 2000;11:127–139.

91. Harre N, Field J. Safe driving education programs at school: lessons from New Zealand. *Aust N Z J Public Health.* 1998;22:447–450.

92. Brown RC, Gains MJ, Greydanus DE, Schonberg SK. Driver education: position paper of the Society for Adolescent Medicine [see comments]. *J Adolesc Health.* 1997;21:416–418.

93. Robertson LS. Crash involvement of teenaged drivers when driver education is eliminated from high school. *Am J Public Health.* 1980;70:599–603.

94. Margolis LH, Kotch J, Lacey JH. Children in alcohol-related motor vehicle crashes. *Pediatrics.* 1986;77:870–872.

95. O'Malley PM, Johnston LD. Drinking and driving among US high school seniors, 1984–1997. *Am J Public Health.* 1999;89:678–684.

96. Lee JA, Jones-Webb RJ, Short BJ, Wagenaar AC. Drinking location and risk of alcohol-impaired driving among high school seniors. *Addict Behav.* 1997;22:387–393.

97. Quinlan KP, Brewer RD, Sleet DA, Dellinger AM. Characteristics of child passenger deaths and injuries involving drinking drivers [see comments]. *JAMA.* 2000;283:2249–2252.

98. Margolis LH, Foss RD, Tolbert WG. Alcohol and motor vehicle-related deaths of children as passengers, pedestrians, and bicyclists [see comments]. *JAMA.* 2000;283:2245–2248.

99. DiGuiseppi CG, Rivara FP, Koepsell TD, Polissar L. Bicycle helmet use by children: evaluation of a community-wide helmet campaign [see comments]. *JAMA.* 1989;262:2256–22561.

100. Thompson RS, Rivara FP, Thompson DC. A case-control study of the effectiveness of bicycle safety helmets [see comments]. *N Engl J Med.* 1989;320:1361–1367.

101. DiGuiseppi CG, Rivara FP, Koepsell TD. Attitudes toward bicycle helmet ownership and use by school-age children. *Am J Dis Child.* 1990;144:83–86.

102. Byard RW, Lipsett J. Drowning deaths in toddlers and preambulatory children in South Australia. *Am J Forensic Med Pathol.* 1999;20:328–332.

103. Sachdeva RC. Near drowning. *Crit Care Clin.* 1999;15:281–296.

104. Fergusson DM, Horwood LJ. Risks of drowning in fenced and unfenced domestic swimming pools. *N Z Med J.* 1984;97:777–779.

105. Forjuoh SN, Coben JH, Dearwater SR, Weiss HB. Identifying homes with inadequate smoke detector protection from residential fires in Pennsylvania. *J Burn Care Rehabil.* 1997;18:86–91.

106. Marshall SW, Runyan CW, Bangdiwala SI, Linzer MA, Sacks JJ, Butts JD. Fatal residential fires: who dies and who survives? *JAMA*. 1998; 279:1633–1637.

107. Rice DP, MacKenzie EJ, et al. *Cost of Injury in the United States: a Report to Congress*. Atlanta, Ga: Division of Injury, Epidemiology, and Control, Center for Environmental Health and Injury Control, Centers for Disease Control; 1989.

108. Hall J, Quincy M, Karter M. National Safety Council tabulations of National Center for Health Statistics mortality data. 1999.

109. An Evaluation of Residential Smoke Detector Performance Under Actual Field Conditions. Washington, DC: Federal Emergency Management Agency; 1980.

110. Fingerhut LA, Ingram DD, Feldman JJ. Firearm homicide among black teenage males in metropolitan counties: comparison of death rates in two periods, 1983 through 1985 and 1987 through 1989 [published erratum appears in *JAMA*. 1992;268:986]. *JAMA*. 1992;267:3054–3058.

111. Fingerhut LA. Firearm mortality among children, youth, and young adults 1–34 years of age, trends and current status: United States, 1985–90. *Adv Data*. 1993:1–20.

112. Beaman V, Annest JL, Mercy JA, Kresnow M, Pollock DA. Lethality of firearm-related injuries in the United States population. *Ann Emerg Med*. 2000;35:258–266.

113. Weil DS, Hemenway D. Loaded guns in the home: analysis of a national random survey of gun owners. *JAMA*. 1992;267:3033–3037.

114. Callahan CM, Rivara FP. Urban high school youth and handguns. A school-based survey. *JAMA*. 1992;267:3038–3042.

115. Cohen LR, Potter LB. Injuries and violence: risk factors and opportunities for prevention during adolescence. *Adolesc Med*. 1999;10: 125–135, vi.

116. Simon TR, Crosby AE, Dahlberg LL. Students who carry weapons to high school: comparison with other weapon-carriers. *J Adolesc Health*. 1999;24:340–348.

117. Brent DA, Perper JA, Allman CJ, Moritz GM, Wartella ME, Zelenak JP. The presence and accessibility of firearms in the homes of adolescent suicides: a case-control study [see comments]. *JAMA*. 1991;266: 2989–2995.

118. Svenson JE, Spurlock C, Nypaver M. Pediatric firearm-related fatalities: not just an urban problem. *Arch Pediatr Adolesc Med*. 1996;150: 583–587.

119. Wintemute GJ, Parham CA, Beaumont JJ, Wright M, Drake C. Mortality among recent purchasers of handguns [see comments]. *N Engl J Med*. 1999;341:1583–1589.

120. Kellermann AL, Rivara FP, Somes G, Reay DT, Francisco J, Banton JG, Prodzinski J, Fligner C, Hackman BB. Suicide in the home in relation to gun ownership [see comments]. *N Engl J Med*. 1992;327:467–472.

121. Kellermann AL, Rivara FP, Rushforth NB, Banton JG, Reay DT, Francisco JT, Locci AB, Prodzinski J, Hackman BB, Somes G. Gun ownership as a risk factor for homicide in the home [see comments]. *N Engl J Med*. 1993;329:1084–1091.

122. Christoffel KK. Toward reducing pediatric injuries from firearms: charting a legislative and regulatory course [see comments]. *Pediatrics*. 1991;88:294–305.

123. American Academy of Pediatrics Committee on Injury and Poison Prevention. Firearm injuries affecting the pediatric population. *Pediatrics*. 1992;89:788–790.

124. Christoffel KK. Pediatric firearm injuries: time to target a growing population. *Pediatr Ann*. 1992;21:430–436.

125. Rivara FP, Grossman DC, Cummings P. Injury prevention: second of two parts [see comments]. *N Engl J Med*. 1997;337:613–618.

126. Reilly JS. Prevention of aspiration in infants and young children: federal regulations. *Ann Otol Rhinol Laryngol*. 1990;99:273–276.

127. Harris CS, Baker SP, Smith GA, Harris RM. Childhood asphyxiation by food: a national analysis and overview. *JAMA*. 1984;251:2231–2315.

128. Rimell FL, Thome A Jr, Stool S, Reilly JS, Rider G, Stool D, Wilson CL. Characteristics of objects that cause choking in children [see comments]. *JAMA*. 1995;274:1763–1766.

129. Kuisma M, Alaspaa A. Out-of-hospital cardiac arrests of non-cardiac origin: epidemiology and outcome [see comments]. *Eur Heart J*. 1997; 18:1122–1128.

130. Mejicano GC, Maki DG. Infections acquired during cardiopulmonary resuscitation: estimating the risk and defining strategies for prevention. *Ann Intern Med*. 1998;129:813–828.

131. Dracup K, Moser DK, Doering LV, Guzy PM. Comparison of cardiopulmonary resuscitation training methods for parents of infants at high risk for cardiopulmonary arrest. *Ann Emerg Med*. 1998;32:170–177.

132. Eisenburger P, Safar P. Life supporting first aid training of the public: review and recommendations. *Resuscitation*. 1999;41:3–18.

133. Assar D, Chamberlain D, Colquhoun M, Donnelly P, Handley AJ, Leaves S, Kern KB, Mayor S. A rationale for staged teaching of basic life support. *Resuscitation*. 1998;39:137–143.

134. Amith G. Revising educational requirements: challenging four hours for both basic life support and automated external defibrillators. *New Horiz*. 1997;5:167–172.

135. Palmisano JM, Akingbola OA, Moler FW, Custer JR. Simulated pediatric cardiopulmonary resuscitation: initial events and response times of a hospital arrest team. *Respir Care*. 1994;39:725–729.

136. Whyte SD, Wyllie JP. Paediatric basic life support: a practical assessment. *Resuscitation*. 1999;41:153–157.

137. Whyte SD, Sinha AK, Wyllie JP. Neonatal resuscitation: a practical assessment. *Resuscitation*. 1999;40:21–25.

138. Ward P, Johnson LA, Mulligan NW, Ward MC, Jones DL. Improving cardiopulmonary resuscitation skills retention: effect of two checklists designed to prompt correct performance. *Resuscitation*. 1997;34: 221–225.

139. Hazinski MF. Is pediatric resuscitation unique? Relative merits of early CPR and ventilation versus early defibrillation for young victims of prehospital cardiac arrest [editorial; comment]. *Ann Emerg Med*. 1995; 25:540–543.

140. Ruben HM, Elam JO, Ruben AM, Greene DG. Investigation of upper airway problems in resuscitation, I: studies of pharyngeal x-rays and performance by laymen. *Anesthesiology*. 1961;22:271–279.

141. Safar P, Escarrage LA. Compliance in apneic anesthetized adults. *Anesthesiology*. 1959;20:283–289.

142. Elam JO, Greene DG, Schneider MA, et al. Head-tilt method of oral resuscitation. *JAMA*. 1960;172:812–815.

143. Guildner CW. Resuscitation: opening the airway: a comparative study of techniques for opening an airway obstructed by the tongue. *JACEP*. 1976;5:588–590.

144. Roth B, Magnusson J, Johansson I, Holmberg S, Westrin P. Jaw lift: a simple and effective method to open the airway in children. *Resuscitation*. 1998;39:171–174.

145. Baskett P, Nolan J, Parr M. Tidal volumes which are perceived to be adequate for resuscitation [see comments]. *Resuscitation*. 1996;31: 231–234.

146. Ruppert M, Reith MW, Widmann JH, Lackner CK, Kerkmann R, Schweiberer L, Peter K. Checking for breathing: evaluation of the diagnostic capability of emergency medical services personnel, physicians, medical students, and medical laypersons [see comments]. *Ann Emerg Med*. 1999;34:720–729.

147. Noc M, Weil MH, Sun S, Tang W, Bisera J. Spontaneous gasping during cardiopulmonary resuscitation without mechanical ventilation. *Am J Respir Crit Care Med*. 1994;150:861–864.

148. Poets CF, Meny RG, Chobanian MR, Bonofiglo RE. Gasping and other cardiorespiratory patterns during sudden infant deaths. *Pediatr Res*. 1999;45:350–354.

149. Handley AJ, Becker LB, Allen M, van Drenth A, Kramer EB, Montgomery WH. Single rescuer adult basic life support: an advisory statement from the Basic Life Support Working Group of the International Liaison Committee on Resuscitation (ILCOR). *Resuscitation*. 1997;34:101–108.

150. Fulstow R, Smith GB. The new recovery position, a cautionary tale [see comments]. *Resuscitation*. 1993;26:89–91.

151. Doxey J. Comparing Resuscitation Council (UK) recovery position with recovery position of 1992 European Resuscitation Council guidelines: a user's perspective. *Resuscitation*. 1998;39:161–169.

152. Turner S, Turner I, Chapman D, Howard P, Champion P, Hatfield J, James A, Marshall S, Barber S. A comparative study of the 1992 and 1997 recovery positions for use in the UK. *Resuscitation*. 1998;39: 153–160.

153. Wenzel V, Idris AH, Banner MJ, Fuerst RS, Tucker KJ. The composition of gas given by mouth-to-mouth ventilation during CPR [see comments]. *Chest*. 1994;106:1806–1810.

154. Htin KJ, Birenbaum DS, Idris AH, Banner MJ, Gravenstein N. Rescuer breathing pattern significantly affects O_2 and CO_2 received by patient during mouth-to-mouth ventilation. *Critical Care Med*. 1998;26:A56.

155. Zideman DA. Paediatric and neonatal life support. *Br J Anaesth*. 1997; 79:178–187.

156. Tonkin SL, Davis SL, Gunn TR. Nasal route for infant resuscitation by mothers [see comments]. *Lancet*. 1995;345:1353–1354.

157. Dembofsky CA, Gibson E, Nadkarni V, Rubin S, Greenspan JS. Assessment of infant cardiopulmonary resuscitation rescue breathing technique: relationship of infant and caregiver facial measurements. *Pediatrics.* 1999;103:E17.

158. Segedin E, Torrie J, Anderson B. Nasal airway versus oral route for infant resuscitation [letter; comment]. *Lancet.* 1995;346:382.

159. Wilson-Davis SL, Tonkin SL, Gunn TR. Air entry in infant resuscitation: oral or nasal routes? *J Appl Physiol.* 1997;82:152–155.

160. Miller MJ, Martin RJ, Carlo WA, Fouke JM, Strohl KP, Fanaroff AA. Oral breathing in newborn infants. *J Pediatr.* 1985;107:465–469.

161. Moss ML. The veloepiglottic sphincter and obligate nose breathing in the neonate. *J Pediatr.* 1965;67:330–331.

162. Nowak AJ, Casamassimo PS. Oral opening and other selected facial dimensions of children 6 weeks to 36 months of age. *J Oral Maxillofac Surg.* 1994;52:845–847; discussion 848.

163. Stocks J, Godfrey S. Nasal resistance during infancy. *Respir Physiol.* 1978;34:233–246.

164. Rodenstein DO, Perlmutter N, Stanescu DC. Infants are not obligatory nasal breathers. *Am Rev Respir Dis.* 1985;131:343–347.

165. Terndrup TE, Kanter RK, Cherry RA. A comparison of infant ventilation methods performed by prehospital personnel. *Ann Emerg Med.* 1989;18:607–611.

166. Berg MD, Idris AH, Berg RA. Severe ventilatory compromise due to gastric distention during pediatric cardiopulmonary resuscitation. *Resuscitation.* 1998;36:71–73.

167. Melker RJ. Asynchronous and other alternative methods of ventilation during CPR. *Ann Emerg Med.* 1984;13:758–761.

168. Melker RJ, Banner MJ. Ventilation during CPR: two-rescuer standards reappraised. *Ann Emerg Med.* 1985;14:397–402.

169. Goldman SL, McCann EM, Lloyd BW, Yup G. Inspiratory time and pulmonary function in mechanically ventilated babies with chronic lung disease. *Pediatr Pulmonol.* 1991;11:198–201.

170. Weiler N, Heinrichs W, Dick W. Assessment of pulmonary mechanics and gastric inflation pressure during mask ventilation. *Prehospital Disaster Med.* 1995;10:101–105.

171. Wenzel V, Idris AH, Banner MJ, Kubilis PS, Band R, Williams JL Jr, Lindner KH. Respiratory system compliance decreases after cardiopulmonary resuscitation and stomach inflation: impact of large and small tidal volumes on calculated peak airway pressure. *Resuscitation.* 1998;38:113–118.

172. Petito SP, Russell WJ. The prevention of gastric inflation: a neglected benefit of cricoid pressure. *Anaesth Intensive Care.* 1988;16:139–143.

173. Moynihan RJ, Brock-Utne JG, Archer JH, Feld LH, Kreitzman TR. The effect of cricoid pressure on preventing gastric insufflation in infants and children [see comments]. *Anesthesiology.* 1993;78:652–656.

174. US Agency for Health Care Policy and Research. Medical Treatment Effectiveness Research 1990.

175. Terndrup TE, Warner DA. Infant ventilation and oxygenation by basic life support providers: comparison of methods. *Prehospital Disaster Med.* 1992;7:35–40.

176. Hess D, Ness C, Oppel A, Rhoads K. Evaluation of mouth-to-mask ventilation devices. *Respir Care.* 1989;34:191–195.

177. Mondolfi AA, Grenier BM, Thompson JE, Bachur RG. Comparison of self-inflating bags with anesthesia bags for bag-mask ventilation in the pediatric emergency department. *Pediatr Emerg Care.* 1997;13:312–316.

178. Field D, Milner AD, Hopkin IE. Efficiency of manual resuscitators at birth. *Arch Dis Child.* 1986;61:300–302.

179. Milner AD. Resuscitation at birth. *Eur J Pediatr.* 1998;157:524–527.

180. Hirschman AM, Kravath RE. Venting vs ventilating: a danger of manual resuscitation bags. *Chest.* 1982;82:369–370.

181. Finer NN, Barrington KJ, Al-Fadley F, Peters KL. Limitations of self-inflating resuscitators. *Pediatrics.* 1986;77:417–420.

182. Jesudian MC, Harrison RR, Keenan RL, Maull KI. Bag-valve-mask ventilation: two rescuers are better than one: preliminary report. *Crit Care Med.* 1985;13:122–123.

183. Salem MR, Wong AY, Mani M, Sellick BA. Efficacy of cricoid pressure in preventing gastric inflation during bag-mask ventilation in pediatric patients. *Anesthesiology.* 1974;40:96–98.

184. Sellick BA. Cricoid pressure to control regurgitation of stomach contents during induction of anesthesia. *Lancet.* 1961;404–406.

185. Hartsilver EL, Vanner RG. Airway obstruction with cricoid pressure. *Anaesthesia.* 2000;55:208–211.

186. Palme C, Nystrom B, Tunell R. An evaluation of the efficiency of face masks in the resuscitation of newborn infants. *Lancet.* 1985;1:207–210.

187. Finer NN, Bates R, Tomat P. Low flow oxygen delivery via nasal cannula to neonates *Pediatr Pulmonol.* 1996;21:48–51.

188. Vain NE, Prudent LM, Stevens DP, Weeter MM, Maisels MJ. Regulation of oxygen concentration delivered to infants via nasal cannulas. *Am J Dis Child.* 1989;143:1458–1460.

189. Locke RG, Wolfson MR, Shaffer TH, Rubenstein SD, Greenspan JS. Inadvertent administration of positive end-distending pressure during nasal cannula flow. *Pediatrics.* 1993;91:135–138.

190. Mettey R, Masson G, Hoppeler A. Use of nasal cannula to induce positive expiratory pressure in neonatology [in French]. *Arch Fr Pediatr.* 1984;41:117–121.

191. Mather C, O'Kelly S. The palpation of pulses. *Anaesthesia.* 1996;51:189–191.

192. Cavallaro DL, Melker RJ. Comparison of two techniques for detecting cardiac activity in infants. *Crit Care Med.* 1983;11:189–190.

193. Brearley S, Shearman CP, Simms MH. Peripheral pulse palpation: an unreliable physical sign. *Ann R Coll Surg Engl.* 1992;74:169–171.

194. Bahr J, Klingler H, Panzer W, Rode H, Kettler D. Skills of lay people in checking the carotid pulse. *Resuscitation.* 1997;35:23–26.

195. Ochoa FJ, Ramalle-Gomara E, Carpintero JM, Garcia A, Saralegui I. Competence of health professionals to check the carotid pulse. *Resuscitation.* 1998;37:173–175.

196. Flesche CW, Zucker TP, Lorenz C, Nerudo B, Tarnow J. The carotid pulse check as a diagnostic tool to assess pulselessness during adult basic life support. *Euroanaesthesia.* 1995. Abstract.

197. Cummins RO, Hazinski MF. Cardiopulmonary resuscitation techniques and instruction: when does evidence justify revision? [editorial; comment]. *Ann Emerg Med.* 1999;34:780–784.

198. Flesche C, Neruda B, Breuer S, et al. Basic cardiopulmonary resuscitation skills: a comparison of ambulance staff and medical students in Germany. *Resuscitation.* 1994;28:s25. Abstract.

199. Flesche C, Neruda B, Neotages T, et al. Do cardiopulmonary skills among medical students meet current standards and patients' needs? *Resuscitation.* 1994;28:s25. Abstract.

200. Monsieurs KG, De Cauwer HG, Bossaert LL. Feeling for the carotid pulse: is five seconds enough? *Resuscitation.* 1996;31:S3. Abstract .

201. Flesche CW, Brewer S, Mandel LP, Brevik H, Tarnow J. The ability of health professional to check the carotid pulse. *Circulation.* 1994;90:288.

202. Eberle B, Dick WF, Schneider T, Wisser G, Doetsch S, Tzanova I. Checking the carotid pulse check: diagnostic accuracy of first responders in patients with and without a pulse. *Resuscitation.* 1996;33:107–116.

203. Whitelaw CC, Goldsmith LJ. Comparison of two techniques for determining the presence of a pulse in an infant [letter]. *Acad Emerg Med.* 1997;4:153–154.

204. Lundin M, Wiksten JP, Perakyla T, Lindfors O, Savolainen H, Skytta J, Lepantalo M. Distal pulse palpation: is it reliable? *World J Surg.* 1999;23:252–255.

205. Liberman M, Lavoie A, Mulder D, Sampalis J. Cardiopulmonary resuscitation: errors made by pre-hospital emergency medical personnel. *Resuscitation.* 1999;42:47–55.

206. Lcc CJ, Bullock LJ. Determining the pulse for infant CPR: time for a change? *Mil Med.* 1991;156:190–193.

207. Bush CM, Jones JS, Cohle SD, Johnson H. Pediatric injuries from cardiopulmonary resuscitation. *Ann Emerg Med.* 1996;28:40–44.

208. Spevak MR, Kleinman PK, Belanger PL, Primack C, Richmond JM. Cardiopulmonary resuscitation and rib fractures in infants: a postmortem radiologic-pathologic study. *JAMA.* 1994;272:617–618.

209. Kaplan JA, Fossum RM. Patterns of facial resuscitation injury in infancy. *Am J Forensic Med Pathol.* 1994;15:187–191.

210. Feldman KW, Brewer DK. Child abuse, cardiopulmonary resuscitation, and rib fractures. *Pediatrics.* 1984;73:339–342.

211. Nagel EL, Fine EG, Krischer JP, Davis JH. Complications of CPR. *Crit Care Med.* 1981;9:424.

212. Powner DJ, Holcombe PA, Mello LA. Cardiopulmonary resuscitation-related injuries. *Crit Care Med.* 1984;12:54–55.

213. Parke TR. Unexplained pneumoperitoneum in association with basic cardiopulmonary resuscitation efforts. *Resuscitation.* 1993;26:177–181.

214. Kramer K, Goldstein B. Retinal hemorrhages following cardiopulmonary resuscitation. *Clin Pediatr.* 1993;32:366–368.

215. Deleted in proof.

216. Theophilopoulos DT, Burchfield DJ. Accuracy of different methods for heart rate determination during simulated neonatal resuscitations. *J Perinatol.* 1998;18:65–67.

217. Connick M, Berg RA. Femoral venous pulsations during open-chest cardiac massage. *Ann Emerg Med.* 1994;24:1176–1179.

217a.Lubitz DS, Seidel JS, Chameides L, Luten RC, et al. A rapid method for estimating weight and resuscitation drug dosages from length in the pediatric age group. *Ann Emerg Med.* 1988;17:576–581.

218. Maier GW, Tyson GS Jr, Olsen CO, Kernstein KH, Davis JW, Conn EH, Sabiston DC Jr, Rankin JS. The physiology of external cardiac massage: high-impulse cardiopulmonary resuscitation. *Circulation.* 1984;70: 86–101.

219. Kouwenhoven WB, Jude JR, Knickerbocker GG. Closed-chest cardiac massage. *JAMA.* 1960;173:1064–1067.

220. Kern KB, Hilwig R, Ewy GA. Retrograde coronary blood flow during cardiopulmonary resuscitation in swine: intracoronary Doppler evaluation. *Am Heart J.* 1994;128:490–499.

221. Tucker KJ, Khan J, Idris A, Savitt MA. The biphasic mechanism of blood flow during cardiopulmonary resuscitation: a physiologic comparison of active compression-decompression and high-impulse manual external cardiac massage. *Ann Emerg Med.* 1994;24: 895–906.

222. Forney J, Ornato JP. Blood flow with ventilation alone in a child with cardiac arrest. *Ann Emerg Med.* 1980;9:624–626.

223. Berg RA, Hilwig RW, Kern KB, Babar I, Ewy GA. Simulated mouth-to-mouth ventilation and chest compressions (bystander cardiopulmonary resuscitation) improves outcome in a swine model of prehospital pediatric asphyxial cardiac arrest [see comments]. *Crit Care Med.* 1999;27:1893–1899.

224. Berg RA, Hilwig RW, Kern KB, Ewy GA. Bystander chest compression and assisted ventilation independently improve outcome from piglet asphyxial pulseless cardiac arrest. *Circulation.* 2000;101: 1743–1748.

225. Nypaver M, Treloar D. Neutral cervical spine positioning in children. *Ann Emerg Med.* 1994;23:208–211.

226. Herzenberg JE, Hensinger RN, Dedrick DK, Phillips WA. Emergency transport and positioning of young children who have an injury of the cervical spine: the standard backboard may be hazardous. *J Bone Joint Surg Am.* 1989;71:15–22.

227. Finholt DA, Kettrick RG, Wagner HR, Swedlow DB. The heart is under the lower third of the sternum: implications for external cardiac massage. *Am J Dis Child.* 1986;140:646–649.

228. Phillips GW, Zideman DA. Relation of infant heart to sternum: its significance in cardiopulmonary resuscitation. *Lancet.* 1986;1: 1024–1025.

229. Orlowski JP. Optimum position for external cardiac compression in infants and young children. *Ann Emerg Med.* 1986;15:667–673.

230. Shah NM, Gaur HK. Position of heart in relation to sternum and nipple line at various ages. *Indian Pediatr.* 1992;29:49–53.

231. Dean JM, Koehler RC, Schleien CL, Berkowitz I, Michael JR, Atchison D, Rogers MC, Traystman RJ. Age-related effects of compression rate and duration in cardiopulmonary resuscitation. *J Appl Physiol.* 1990;68:554–560.

232. Kinney SB, Tibballs J. An analysis of the efficacy of bag-valve-mask ventilation and chest compression during different compression-ventilation ratios in manikin-simulated paediatric resuscitation. *Resuscitation.* 2000;43:115–120.

233. Burchfield D, Erenberg A, Mullett MD, Keenan WJ, Denson SE, Kattwinkel J, Bloom R. Why change the compression and ventilation rates during CPR in neonates? Neonatal Resuscitation Steering Committee, American Heart Association and American Academy of Pediatrics [letter]. *Pediatrics.* 1994;93:1026–1027.

234. Thaler MM, Stobie GH. An improved technique of external cardiac compression in infants and young children. *N Engl J Med.* 1963;269: 606–610.

235. David R. Closed chest cardiac massage in the newborn infant. *Pediatrics.* 1988;81:552–554.

236. Todres ID, Rogers MC. Methods of external cardiac massage in the newborn infant. *J Pediatr.* 1975;86:781–782.

237. Ishimine P, Menegazzi J, Weinstein D. Evaluation of two-thumb chest compression with thoracic squeeze in a swine model of infant cardiac arrest. *Acad Emerg Med.* 1998;5.

238. Houri PK, Frank LR, Menegazzi JJ, Taylor R. A randomized, controlled trial of two-thumb vs two-finger chest compression in a swine infant model of cardiac arrest [see comment]. *Prehosp Emerg Care.* 1997;1:65–67.

239. Chandra N, Rudikoff M, Weisfeldt ML. Simultaneous chest compression and ventilation at high airway pressure during cardiopulmonary resuscitation. *Lancet.* 1980;1:175–8.

240. Babbs CF, Tacker WA, Paris RL, Murphy RJ, Davis RW. CPR with simultaneous compression and ventilation at high airway pressure in 4 animal models. *Crit Care Med.* 1982;10:501–504.

241. Hou SH, Lue HC, Chu SH. Comparison of conventional and simultaneous compression-ventilation cardiopulmonary resuscitation in piglets. *Jpn Circ J.* 1994;58:426–432.

242. Barranco F, Lesmes A, Irles JA, Blasco J, Leal J, Rodriguez J, Leon C. Cardiopulmonary resuscitation with simultaneous chest and abdominal compression: comparative study in humans. *Resuscitation.* 1990;20:67–77.

243. Wik L, Steen PA. The ventilation/compression ratio influences the effectiveness of two rescuer advanced cardiac life support on a manikin. *Resuscitation.* 1996;31:113–119.

244. Milander MM, Hiscok PS, Sanders AB, Kern KB, Berg RA, Ewy GA. Chest compression and ventilation rates during cardiopulmonary resuscitation: the effects of audible tone guidance [see comments]. *Acad Emerg Med.* 1995;2:708–713.

245. Nadkarni V, Tice L, Randall D, Corddry D. Metabolic effects on rescuer of varying compression-ventilation ratios during infant pediatric and adult CPR. *Crit Care Med.* 1999;27:A43.

246. Nadkarni V, Goodie B, Tice L, Cox T, Rose MJ. Evaluation of a universal compression/ventilation ratio for one-rescuer CPR in infant, pediatric and adult manikins *Crit Care Med.* 1997;25:A61.

247. Kern KB, Sanders AB, Raife J, Milander MM, Otto CW, Ewy GA. A study of chest compression rates during cardiopulmonary resuscitation in humans: the importance of rate-directed chest compressions. *Arch Intern Med.* 1992;152:145–149.

248. Kern KB, Hilwig RW, Berg RA, Ewy GA. Efficacy of chest compression-only BLS CPR in the presence of an occluded airway. *Resuscitation.* 1998;39:179–188.

249. Biggart MJ, Bohn DJ. Effect of hypothermia and cardiac arrest on outcome of near-drowning accidents in children. *J Pediatr.* 1990; 117:179–183.

250. Quan L, Gore EJ, Wentz K, Allen J, Novack AH. Ten-year study of pediatric drownings and near-drownings in King County, Washington: lessons in injury prevention. *Pediatrics.* 1989;83:1035–1040.

251. Fiser DH, Wrape V. Outcome of cardiopulmonary resuscitation in children. *Pediatr Emerg Care.* 1987;3:235–238.

252. Kemp AM, Sibert JR. Outcome in children who nearly drown: a British Isles study [see comments]. *BMJ.* 1991;302:931–933.

253. Ornato JP, Hallagan LF, McMahan SB, Peeples EH, Rostafinski AG. Attitudes of BCLS instructors about mouth-to-mouth resuscitation during the AIDS epidemic. *Ann Emerg Med.* 1990;19:151–156.

254. Brenner BE, Van DC, Cheng D, Lazar EJ. Determinants of reluctance to perform CPR among residents and applicants: the impact of experience on helping behavior. *Resuscitation.* 1997;35: 203–211.

255. Hew P, Brenner B, Kaufman J. Reluctance of paramedics and emergency medical technicians to perform mouth-to-mouth resuscitation. *J Emerg Med.* 1997;15:279–284.

256. Locke CJ, Berg RA, Sanders AB, Davis MF, Milander MM, Kern KB, Ewy GA. Bystander cardiopulmonary resuscitation: concerns about mouth-to-mouth contact. *Arch Intern Med.* 1995;155:938–943.

257. Berg RA, Kern KB, Sanders AB, Otto CW, Hilwig RW, Ewy GA. Bystander cardiopulmonary resuscitation: is ventilation necessary? *Circulation.* 1993;88:1907–1915.

258. Berg RA, Wilcoxson D, Hilwig RW, Kern KB, Sanders AB, Otto CW, Eklund DK, Ewy GA. The need for ventilatory support during bystander CPR. *Ann Emerg Med.* 1995;26:342–350.

259. Berg RA, Kern KB, Hilwig RW, Berg MD, Sanders AB, Otto CW, Ewy GA. Assisted ventilation does not improve outcome in a porcine model of single-rescuer bystander cardiopulmonary resuscitation. *Circulation.* 1997;95:1635–1641.

260. Berg RA, Kern KB, Hilwig RW, Ewy GA. Assisted ventilation during "bystander" CPR in a swine acute myocardial infarction model does not improve outcome. *Circulation.* 1997;96:4364–4371.

261. Chandra NC, Gruben KG, Tsitlik JE, Brower R, Guerci AD, Halperin HH, Weisfeldt ML, Permutt S. Observations of ventilation during resuscitation in a canine model. *Circulation.* 1994;90:3070–3075.

262. Tang W, Weil MH, Sun S, Kette D, Kette F, Gazmuri RJ, O'Connell F, Bisera J. Cardiopulmonary resuscitation by precordial com-

pression but without mechanical ventilation. *Am J Respir Crit Care Med.* 1994;150:1709–1713.

263. Noc M, Weil MH, Tang W, Turner T, Fukui M. Mechanical ventilation may not be essential for initial cardiopulmonary resuscitation. *Chest.* 1995;108:821–827.

264. Weil MH, Rackow EC, Trevino R, Grundler W, Falk JL, Griffel MI. Difference in acid-base state between venous and arterial blood during cardiopulmonary resuscitation. *N Engl J Med.* 1986;315: 153–156.

265. Sanders AB, Otto CW, Kern KB, Rogers JN, Perrault P, Ewy GA. Acid-base balance in a canine model of cardiac arrest. *Ann Emerg Med.* 1988;17:667–671.

266. Lindner KH, Pfenninger EG, Lurie KG, Schurmann W, Lindner IM, Ahnefeld FW. Effects of active compression-decompression resuscitation on myocardial and cerebral blood flow in pigs. *Circulation.* 1993;88:1254–1263.

267. Chang MW, Coffeen P, Lurie KG, Shultz J, Bache RJ, White CW. Active compression-decompression CPR improves vital organ perfusion in a dog model of ventricular fibrillation. *Chest.* 1994;106: 1250–1259.

268. Shultz JJ, Coffeen P, Sweeney M, Detloff B, Kehler C, Pineda E, Yakshe P, Adler SW, Chang M, Lurie KG. Evaluation of standard and active compression-decompression CPR in an acute human model of ventricular fibrillation. *Circulation.* 1994;89:684–693.

269. Baubin M, Haid C, Hamm P, Gilly H. Measuring forces and frequency during active compression decompression cardiopulmonary resuscitation: a device for training, research and real CPR. *Resuscitation.* 1999;43:17–24.

270. Cohen TJ, Tucker KJ, Lurie KG, Redberg RF, Dutton JP, Dwyer KA, Schwab TM, Chin MC, Gelb AM, Scheinman MM, et al, Cardiopulmonary Resuscitation Working Group. Active compression-decompression: a new method of cardiopulmonary resuscitation [see comments]. *JAMA.* 1992;267:2916–2923.

271. Plaisance P, Adnet F, Vicaut E, Hennequin B, Magne P, Prudhomme C, Lambert Y, Cantineau JP, Leopold C, Ferracci C, Gizzi M, Payen D. Benefit of active compression-decompression cardiopulmonary resuscitation as a prehospital advanced cardiac life support: a randomized multicenter study. *Circulation.* 1997;95:955–961.

272. Mauer D, Schneider T, Dick W, Withelm A, Elich D, Mauer M. Active compression-decompression resuscitation: a prospective, randomized study in a two-tiered EMS system with physicians in the field. *Resuscitation.* 1996;33:125–134.

273. Mauer DK, Nolan J, Plaisance P, Sitter H, Benoit H, Stiell IG, Sofianos E, Keiding N, Lurie KG. Effect of active compression-decompression resuscitation (ACD-CPR) on survival: a combined analysis using individual patient data. *Resuscitation.* 1999;41: 249–256.

274. Stiell IG, Hebert PC, Wells GA, Laupacis A, Vandemheen K, Dreyer JF, Eisenhauer MA, Gibson J, Higginson LA, Kirby AS, Mahon JL, Maloney JP, Weitzman BN. The Ontario trial of active compression-decompression cardiopulmonary resuscitation for in-hospital and prehospital cardiac arrest [see comments]. *JAMA.* 1996;275: 1417–1423.

275. Skogvoll E, Wik L. Active compression-decompression cardiopulmonary resuscitation: a population-based, prospective randomised clinical trial in out-of-hospital cardiac arrest. *Resuscitation.* 1999; 42:163–172.

276. Babbs CF. CPR techniques that combine chest and abdominal compression and decompression: hemodynamic insights from a spreadsheet model. *Circulation.* 1999;100:2146–2152.

277. Lurie KG. Recent advances in mechanical methods of cardiopulmonary resuscitation. *Acta Anaesthesiol Scand Suppl.* 1997;111:49–52.

278. Tang W, Weil MH, Schock RB, Sato Y, Lucas J, Sun S, Bisera J. Phased chest and abdominal compression-decompression: a new option for cardiopulmonary resuscitation. *Circulation.* 1997;95: 1335–1340.

279. Lindner KH, Wenzel V. [New mechanical methods for cardiopulmonary resuscitation (CPR): literature study and analysis of effectiveness]. *Anaesthesist.* 1997;46:220–230.

280. Sack JB, Kesselbrenner MB. Hemodynamics, survival benefits, and complications of interposed abdominal compression during cardiopulmonary resuscitation. *Acad Emerg Med.* 1994;1:490–497.

281. Majumdar A, Sedman PC. Gastric rupture secondary to successful Heimlich manoeuvre. *Postgrad Med J.* 1998;74:609–610.

282. Fink JA, Klein RL. Complications of the Heimlich maneuver. *J Pediatr Surg.* 1989;24:486–487.

283. Heimlich HJ. A life-saving maneuver to prevent food-choking. *JAMA.* 1975;234:398–401.

284. Day RL, Crelin ES, DuBois AB. Choking: the Heimlich abdominal thrust vs back blows: an approach to measurement of inertial and aerodynamic forces. *Pediatrics.* 1982;70:113–119.

285. National Center for Health Statistics and National Safety Council. *Data on Odds of Death Due to Choking.* 1998.

286. Braslow A, Brennan RT, Newman MM, Bircher NG, Batcheller AM, Kaye W. CPR training without an instructor: development and evaluation of a video self-instructional system for effective performance of cardiopulmonary resuscitation. *Resuscitation.* 1997;34:207–220.

287. Todd KH, Braslow A, Brennan RT, Lowery DW, Cox RJ, Lipscomb LE, Kellermann AL. Randomized, controlled trial of video self-instruction versus traditional CPR training. *Ann Emerg Med.* 1998; 31:364–369.

288. Todd KH, Heron SL, Thompson M, Dennis R, O'Connor J, Kellermann AL. Simple CPR: a randomized, controlled trial of video self-instructional cardiopulmonary resuscitation training in an African American church congregation [see comments]. *Ann Emerg Med.* 1999;34:730–737.

289. Langhelle A, Sunde K, Wik L, Steen PA. Airway pressure with chest compressions versus Heimlich manoeuvre in recently dead adults with complete airway obstruction. *Resuscitation.* 2000;44:105–108.

290. Sternbach G, Kiskaddon RT. Henry Heimlich: a life-saving maneuver for food choking. *J Emerg Med.* 1985;3:143–148.

291. Redding JS. The choking controversy: critique of evidence on the Heimlich maneuver. *Crit Care Med.* 1979;7:475–479.

292. Gordon AS, BMRP. Emergency management of foreign body obstruction. In: Safar P, Elam JO, eds. *Advances in Cardiopulmonary Resuscitation.* New York, NY; Springer-Verlag; 1977:39–50.

293. Guildner CW, Williams D, Subitch T. Airway obstructed by foreign material: the Heimlich maneuver. *JACEP.* 1976;5:675–677.

294. Bintz M, Cogbill TH. Gastric rupture after the Heimlich maneuver. *J Trauma.* 1996;40:159–160.

295. Cowan M, Bardole J, Dlesk A. Perforated stomach following the Heimlich maneuver. *Am J Emerg Med.* 1987;5:121–122.

296. Kabbani M, Goodwin SR. Traumatic epiglottis following blind finger sweep to remove a pharyngeal foreign body. *Clin Pediatr.* 1995;34:495–497.

297. Hartrey R, Bingham RM. Pharyngeal trauma as a result of blind finger sweeps in the choking child. *J Accid Emerg Med.* 1995;12: 52–54.

298. Dykes EH, Spence LJ, Young JG, Bohn DJ, Filler RM, Wesson DE. Preventable pediatric trauma deaths in a metropolitan region. *J Pediatr Surg.* 1989;24:107–110; discussion 110–111.

299. Esposito TJ, Sanddal ND, Dean JM, Hansen JD, Reynolds SA, Battan K. Analysis of preventable pediatric trauma deaths and inappropriate trauma care in Montana. *J Trauma.* 1999;47:243–251; discussion 251–253.

300. Suominen P, Rasanen J, Kivioja A. Efficacy of cardiopulmonary resuscitation in pulseless paediatric trauma patients. *Resuscitation.* 1998;36:9–13.

301. Koury SI, Moorer L, Stone CK, Stapczynski JS, Thomas SH. Air vs ground transport and outcome in trauma patients requiring urgent operative interventions. *Prehosp Emerg Care.* 1998;2:289–292.

302. Brathwaite CE, Rosko M, McDowell R, Gallagher J, Proenca J, Spott MA. A critical analysis of on-scene helicopter transport on survival in a statewide trauma system. *J Trauma.* 1998;45:140–144; discussion 144–146.

303. Moront ML, Gotschall CS, Eichelberger MR. Helicopter transport of injured children: system effectiveness and triage criteria. *J Pediatr Surg.* 1996;31:1183–1186; discussion 1187–1188.

304. Markenson D, Foltin G, Tunik M, Cooper A, Giordano L, Fitton A, Lanotte T. The Kendrick extrication device used for pediatric spinal immobilization. *Prehosp Emerg Care.* 1999;3:66–69.

305. Curran C, Dietrich AM, Bowman MJ, Ginn-Pease ME, King DR, Kosnik E. Pediatric cervical-spine immobilization: achieving neutral position? *J Trauma.* 1995;39:729–732.

306. Huerta C, Griffith R, Joyce SM. Cervical spine stabilization in pediatric patients: evaluation of current techniques [see comments]. *Ann Emerg Med.* 1987;16:1121–1126.

307. Treloar DJ, Nypaver M. Angulation of the pediatric cervical spine with and without cervical collar. *Pediatr Emerg Care.* 1997;13:5–8.

308. Soud T, Pieper P, Hazinski MF. Pediatric trauma. In: Hazinski MF. *Nursing Care of the Critically Ill Child*. St Louis, Mo: Mosby–Year Book; 1992:842–843.

309. Doyle CJ, Post H, Burney RE, Maino J, Keefe M, Rhee KJ. Family participation during resuscitation: an option. *Ann Emerg Med*. 1987; 16:673–675.

310. Hanson C, Strawser D. Family presence during cardiopulmonary resuscitation: Foote Hospital emergency department's nine-year perspective. *J Emerg Nurs*. 1992;18:104–106.

311. Barratt F, Wallis DN. Relatives in the resuscitation room: their point of view [see comments]. *J Accid Emerg Med*. 1998;15:109–111.

312. Meyers TA, Eichhorn DJ, Guzzetta CE. Do families want to be present during CPR? A retrospective survey. *J Emerg Nurs*. 1998; 24:400–405.

313. Robinson SM, Mackenzie-Ross S, Campbell Hewson GL, Egleston CV, Prevost AT. Psychological effect of witnessed resuscitation on bereaved relatives [see comments]. *Lancet*. 1998;352:614–617.

314. Boie ET, Moore GP, Brummett C, Nelson DR. Do parents want to be present during invasive procedures performed on their children in the emergency department? A survey of 400 parents. *Ann Emerg Med*. 1999;34:70–74.

315. Boyd R. Witnessed resuscitation by relatives. *Resuscitation*. 2000; 43:171–176.

316. Hampe SO. Needs of the grieving spouse in a hospital setting. *Nurs Res*. 1975;24:113–120.

317. Offord RJ. Should relatives of patients with cardiac arrest be invited to be present during cardiopulmonary resuscitation? *Intensive Crit Care Nurs*. 1998;14:288–293.

318. Shaner K, Eckle N. Implementing a program to support the option of family presence during resuscitation. *Assoc Care Child Health (ACCH) Advocate*. 1997;3:3–7.

319. Eichhorn DJ, Meyers TA, Mitchell TG, Guzzetta CE. Opening the doors: family presence during resuscitation. *J Cardiovasc Nurs*. 1996;10:59–70.

320. Moser DK, Coleman S. Recommendations for improving cardiopulmonary resuscitation skills retention. *Heart Lung*. 1992;21:372–380.

321. Doherty A, Damon S, Hein K, Cummins RO. Evaluation of CPR Prompt & Home Learning System for teaching CPR to lay rescuers. *Circulation*. 1998;98(suppl I):I-410. Abstract.

322. Starr LM. Electronic voice boosts CPR responses. *Occup Health Saf*. 1997;66:30–37.

Part 10: Pediatric Advanced Life Support

Major Guidelines Changes

International Terminology

In the preparation of these guidelines, we recognized that certain terms that are commonplace in the United States are uncommon internationally and vice versa. Because these are international guidelines, efforts were made to use terms consistently throughout. To avoid confusion, the reader should note the use of the following terms:

- *Tracheal tube*—commonly called an endotracheal tube. Note that a tracheal tube may be incorrectly placed in the esophagus, so the term does not mean a correctly positioned tube in the trachea. Moreover, a tracheostomy tube is not the same as a tracheal tube as used in these guidelines, even though both tubes are placed in the trachea. The procedure of placing a tracheal tube is still called *endotracheal intubation.*
- *Manual resuscitator*—refers to a bag-valve device used to provide mask, tracheal tube, or tracheostomy tube ventilation to a victim. A manual resuscitator may be self-inflating or flow-inflating (ie, an anesthesia manual resuscitator).
- *Exhaled CO_2 detection*—refers to detection of carbon dioxide in exhaled gas. End-tidal CO_2 monitors are a subset of exhaled CO_2 detectors, but they specifically detect and measure the quantity of CO_2 at the end of exhalation. Capnography graphically displays the change in exhaled CO_2 over time, whereas exhaled CO_2 detectors often are colorimetric systems designed to detect any CO_2 during exhalation and not just at the end of expiration.
- *Defibrillation*—although commonly used interchangeably with "shocks," defibrillation is the untimed (asynchronous) depolarization of the myocardium that *successfully* terminates ventricular fibrillation (VF) or pulseless ventricular tachycardia (VT). Thus, shocks are administered to victims in an attempt to achieve defibrillation.

Epidemiology and Recognition of Shock and Respiratory Failure

- We emphasize the need for better data regarding the epidemiology and treatment of pediatric cardiopulmonary arrest. There is a critical need for identification, tracking, and reporting of key resuscitation interventions and their relationship to various outcome measures, such as return of spontaneous circulation, survival, and neurological outcome. Published reports of resuscitation outcome are essential to provide data in future guideline reviews. Data collection efforts should use consistent terminology and record important time intervals. Critical elements for data collection have been described by an international consensus process called the Pediatric Utstein Guidelines for Reporting Outcome of Pediatric Cardiopulmonary Arrest.[1]
- An age-defined sequence of "phone fast" resuscitation is still appropriate for treatment of out-of-hospital arrest in infants and children, but a "phone first" approach to resuscitation from sudden collapse should be used for children at high risk for arrhythmias.

Support of Ventilation

- The method of advanced airway support (endotracheal intubation versus laryngeal mask versus bag-mask) provided to the patient should be selected on the basis of the training and skill level of providers in a given advanced life support (ALS) system and on the arrest characteristics and circumstances (eg, transport time and perhaps the cause of the arrest).
- Proficiency in the skill of bag-mask ventilation is mandatory for anyone providing ALS in prehospital and in-hospital settings (Class IIa).
- Secondary confirmation of proper tracheal tube placement is required for patients with a perfusing rhythm by capnography or exhaled CO_2 detection immediately after intubation and during transport (Class IIa). We strongly encourage the use of exhaled or end-tidal CO_2 detection. It is extremely reliable in a spontaneously perfusing victim (Class IIa), although it has lower specificity in the cardiac arrest victim (Class IIb). Adequate oxygenation should also be confirmed in a victim with a perfusing rhythm using pulse oximetry.

Fluid Therapy

- Rescuers should increase attention to early vascular access, including immediate intraosseous access for victims of cardiac arrest, and extend the use of intraosseous techniques to victims >6 years old.

Medications

- There is renewed emphasis on the need to identify and treat reversible causes of cardiac arrest and symptomatic arrhythmias, such as toxic drug overdose or electrolyte abnormalities.
- For cardiac arrest victims, we provide specific drug selection and dose recommendations but acknowledge the lack of adequate data to make such recommendations on the basis of firm evidence. For example, data supporting the use of high-dose epinephrine and the use of vasopressin in

Circulation. 2000;102(suppl I):I-291–I-342.
© 2000 American Heart Association, Inc.

Circulation is available at http://www.circulationaha.org

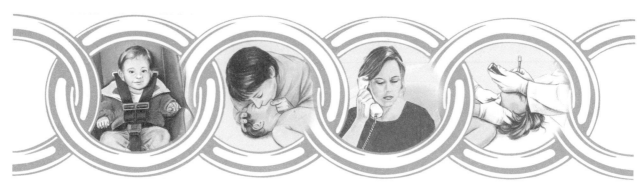

Figure 1. Pediatric Chain of Survival showing critical links of prevention, early CPR, early EMS activation, and early ALS. Additional links to definitive care and rehabilitation are also important after initial resuscitation and stabilization.

cardiac arrest is inadequate to allow firm recommendations (for further details, see the following section, "Drugs Used for Cardiac Arrest and Resuscitation").

Treatment of Arrhythmias

- We introduce vagal maneuvers into the treatment algorithm for supraventricular tachycardia.
- We introduce the drug amiodarone into the treatment algorithms for pediatric VT and shock-refractory VF.
- Automated external defibrillators (AEDs) may be used in the treatment of children ≥8 years of age (approximately >25 kg body weight) in cardiac arrest in the prehospital setting.

Postarrest Stabilization

- We place increased emphasis on postresuscitation interventions that may influence neurological survival, which include maintenance of normal ventilation rather than hyperventilation (Class IIa) in most victims, control of temperature (avoid hyperthermia), management of post-ischemic myocardial dysfunction, and glucose control.

Education and Training

- Simplification of education and reinforcement of skill acquisition and core competencies are essential in all American Heart Association courses. See also, in "Part 9: Pediatric Basic Life Support," Education and Training and Introduction.

Introduction

In contrast to cardiac arrest in adults, cardiopulmonary arrest in infants and children is rarely a sudden event and does not often result from a primary cardiac cause.[2] In adults, cardiopulmonary arrest is usually sudden and is primarily cardiac in origin; approximately 250 000 adults die annually of sudden cardiac arrest in the United States alone. Consequently, much of the research and training in adult cardiac resuscitation focuses on the identification and treatment of VF in the out-of-hospital setting, since this rhythm is the most amenable to effective therapy. Factors associated with increased survival after adult cardiopulmonary arrest include bystander CPR (relative odds of survival, 2.6; 95% confidence interval, 2.0 to 3.4)[3,4] and short interval to defibrillation.[5,6]

Cardiopulmonary (ie, cardiac) arrest in children is much less common than cardiac arrest in adults. When it does occur, pediatric cardiac arrest frequently represents the terminal event of progressive shock or respiratory failure. Causes of pediatric cardiac arrest are heterogeneous, including sudden infant death syndrome (SIDS), submersion/near-drowning, trauma, and sepsis. The progression from shock or respiratory failure to cardiac arrest associated with each of these causes may vary, making research or outcome reporting difficult, since there is not a "typical" type of cardiac arrest.

The cause of cardiac arrest also varies with age, the underlying health of the child, and the location of the event. In the out-of-hospital location, conditions such as trauma, SIDS, drowning, poisoning, choking, severe asthma, and pneumonia represent the most common causes of arrest. In the hospital, common causes of cardiac arrest include sepsis, respiratory failure, drug toxicity, metabolic disorders, and arrhythmias. These in-hospital causes often complicate an underlying condition. The Emergency Department represents a transition from the out-of-hospital to the hospital location. In the Emergency Department, cardiac arrest may be seen in children with underlying conditions typical for the hospital setting and in children with conditions seen more often in the out-of-hospital setting.

Throughout infancy and childhood, most out-of-hospital cardiac arrest occurs in or around the home. Beyond 6 months of age, trauma is the predominant cause of death.

Pediatric advanced life support (PALS) refers to the assessment and support of pulmonary and circulatory function in the period before an arrest and during and after an arrest. Consistent with the Chain of Survival (Figure 1), PALS should focus on prevention of the causes of arrest (SIDS, injury, and choking) and on early detection and rapid treatment of cardiopulmonary compromise and arrest in the critically ill or injured child. The components of PALS are similar in many respects to those of adult ACLS and include

- Basic life support
- Use of adjunctive equipment and special techniques to establish and maintain effective oxygenation, ventilation and perfusion
- Clinical and ECG monitoring and arrhythmia detection
- Establishment and maintenance of vascular access
- Identification and treatment of reversible causes of cardiopulmonary arrest

- Therapies for emergency treatment of patients with cardiac and respiratory arrest
- Treatment of patients with trauma, shock, respiratory failure, or other prearrest conditions

Because the etiology of cardiopulmonary emergencies and the available treatments and approaches may not be the same in out-of-hospital and hospital settings, these guidelines will highlight evaluation and treatment approaches that are recommended for each setting when appropriate.

These guidelines are based on clinical and experimental evidence of varying quality and quantity. Information on the strength of the scientific data leading to each new recommendation is provided. (For more information on the evidence evaluation process, see Reference 7.) Classes are defined fully in "Part 1: Introduction."

Ideally, treatments of choice are supported by excellent evidence and are Class I recommendations. Unfortunately the quality of published data on cardiac arrest and resuscitation, especially for children, usually dictates that consensus treatments included in the guidelines are Class IIa or IIb.

PALS for Children With Special Needs
Children with special healthcare needs have chronic physical, developmental, behavioral, or emotional conditions and also require health and related services of a type or amount not usually required by other children.[8–10] These children may require emergency care for acute, life-threatening complications that are unique to their chronic conditions, such as obstruction of a tracheostomy, failure of support technology (eg, ventilator failure), or progression of underlying respiratory failure or neurological disease. Approximately half of the EMS responses for children with special healthcare needs, however, are unrelated to those special needs.[11] Many involve traditional causes of EMS calls, such as trauma,[11] that require no treatment beyond the normal EMS standard of care.

Emergency care of children with special healthcare needs can be complicated by lack of specific medical information about the child's baseline condition, plan of medical care, current medications, and any "Do Not Attempt Resuscitation" orders. Certainly the best source of information about a chronically ill child is a concerned and compassionate person who cares for the child on a daily basis. If that person is unavailable or incapacitated (eg, after an automobile crash), some means is needed to access important information. A wide variety of methods have been developed to make this information immediately accessible, including the use of standard forms, containers kept in a standard place in the home (eg, the refrigerator), window stickers for the home, wallet cards, and medical alert bracelets. No one method of information communication has yet proved to be superior. A standardized form, the Emergency Information Form (EIF), was developed by the American Academy of Pediatrics and the American College of Emergency Physicians,[10] to be completed by the child's primary physician for use by EMS personnel and hospitals. This form is available electronically (http://www.pediatrics.org/cgi/content/full/104/4/e53). Parents and child-care providers should be encouraged to keep copies of essential medical information at home, with the

child, and at the child's school or child-care facility. School nurses should have copies of these forms and should be familiar with signs of deterioration in the child and any existing "Do Not Attempt Resuscitation" orders.[11,12]

If decisions are made by the physician, parents, and child (as appropriate) to limit resuscitative efforts or to withhold attempts at resuscitation, a physician order indicating the limits of resuscitative efforts must be written for use in the in-hospital setting, and in most countries a separate order must be written for the out-of-hospital setting. Legal issues and regulations vary from country to country and within the United States from state to state regarding requirements for these out-of-hospital "No CPR Directives." It is always important for a family to inform their local EMS system when such directives are established for out-of-hospital care. For further information about ethical issues of resuscitation, see also "Part 2: Ethical Aspects of CPR and ECC."

Whenever a child with a chronic or life-threatening condition is discharged from the hospital, parents, school nurses, and any home healthcare providers should be informed about possible causes of deterioration or complications that the child may experience and anticipated signs of deterioration. They should receive specific instructions about CPR and other interventions the child may require and instructions about whom to contact and why.[12]

If the child has a tracheostomy, anyone responsible for the child's care (including parents, school nurses, and home healthcare providers) should be taught to assess that the airway is patent, how to clear the airway, and how to provide CPR using the artificial airway. If CPR is required, rescue breathing and bag-mask ventilation are performed through the tracheostomy tube. As with any form of rescue breathing, the key sign of effective ventilation is adequate bilateral chest expansion. If the tracheostomy tube becomes obstructed and it is impossible to provide ventilation through it even after attempts to clear the tube with suctioning, remove and replace the tube. If a clean tube is unavailable, ventilation can be provided using mouth-to-stoma ventilation until an artificial airway can be placed through the stoma. Alternatively, if the upper airway is patent, it may be possible to provide effective conventional bag-mask ventilation through the nose and mouth while occluding the superficial tracheal stoma site.

International PALS Guidelines
Following the implementation of the 1992 guidelines,[13] the major international resuscitation councils (International Liaison Committee on Resuscitation [ILCOR]) participated in the development of advisory statements reflecting consensus recommendations based on existing resuscitation guidelines, practical experience, and informal interpretation and debate of an international resuscitation database.[14,15] A high degree of uniformity exists in current guidelines created by the major resuscitation councils for resuscitation of the newly born, neonates, infants, and young children. Controversies arise mostly from local and regional preferences or customs, training networks, and differences in availability of equipment and medication rather than from differences in interpretation of scientific evidence.

To develop this International Guidelines 2000 document on PALS, the Subcommittee on Pediatric Resuscitation of the AHA and other members of ILCOR identified issues or new developments worthy of further in-depth evaluation. From this list, areas of active research and evolving controversy were identified; evidence-based evaluation of each of these areas was conducted and debated, culminating in assignment of consensus-defined "levels of evidence" for specific guidelines questions. After identification and careful review of this evidence, the Pediatric Working Group of ILCOR updated the PALS guidelines, assigned classes of recommendations where possible, and objectively attempted to link the class of recommendation to the identified level of evidence. During these discussions the authors recognized the need to make recommendations for important interventions and treatment even when the only level of evidence was poor or absent. In the absence of specific pediatric data (outcome validity), recommendations were made or supported on the basis of common sense (face validity) or ease of teaching or skill retention (construct validity).

To reduce confusion and simplify education, whenever possible and appropriate, PALS recommendations are consistent with the adult BLS and ACLS algorithms and guidelines. Areas of departure from the adult algorithms and interventions are noted, and the rationale is explained in the text. Ultimately the practicality of implementing recommendations must be considered in the context of local resources (technology and personnel) and customs. No resuscitation protocol or guideline can be expected to appropriately anticipate all potential scenarios. Rather, these guidelines and treatment algorithms serve as a guiding template that will provide most critically ill children with appropriate support while thoughtful and appropriate etiology-based interventions are assembled and implemented.

Age Definitions: What Defines an Infant, Child, and Adult?

Definition of Newly Born, Neonate, Infant, and Child
The term "neonate" refers to infants in the first 28 days (month) of life.[16] In AHA ECC and ILCOR publications, the term "newly born" refers specifically to the *neonate* in the first minutes to hours following birth. This term is used to focus resuscitation knowledge and training on the time immediately after birth and during the first hours of life. *Newly born* is designed to emphasize those first hours of life, separate from the first month of life. The term "infant" includes the neonatal period and extends to the age of 1 year (12 months). For the purposes of these guidelines, the term "child" refers to the age group from 1 year to 8 years.

Pediatric BLS and ALS interventions tend to blur at the margins of age because there is no single anatomic, physiological, or management characteristic that is consistently different in the infant versus the child versus the adult victim of cardiac arrest. Furthermore, new technologies such as AEDs and the availability of airway and vascular access adjuncts that can be implemented with a minimum of advanced training create the need to reexamine previous recommendations for therapies based on age.

Anatomy
By consensus, the age cutoff for infants is 1 year. Note, however, that this definition is not based on specific anatomic or physiological differences between infants and children. For example, the differences between an 11-month-old "infant" and an 18-month-old "child" are smaller than the differences in anatomy and physiology between an 11-month-old and a 1-week-old infant. Historically the use of the term *child* was limited to ages 1 to 8 years for purposes of BLS education; cardiac compression can be done with 1 hand for victims up to the age of approximately 8 years. However, variability in the size of the victim or the size and strength of the rescuer can require use of the 2-handed adult compression technique for cardiac compression in younger children. For instance, a chronically ill 11-month-old infant may be sufficiently small to enable compression using the 2 thumb–encircling hands technique, and a 6- or 7-year-old may be too large for the 1-hand compression technique.

Further anatomic differences are noted in the airway of the child versus the adult. The narrowest portion of the airway in the child is at the level of the cricoid cartilage; in older children and adults the narrowest portion is at the level of the glottic opening. Moreover, the loose areolar tissue in the subglottic space allows for a natural seal without a cuffed tube in most children. Finally, attempting to squeeze a tube through the narrowed area of the cricoid cartilage increases the risk of subglottic stenosis. These anatomic differences and risk of complications led to the recommendation to use uncuffed tracheal tubes in children <8 years of age.[13]

Physiology
Respiratory and cardiac physiology evolves throughout infancy and childhood. In the newly born, for example, fluid-filled alveoli may require higher initial ventilation pressures than subsequent rescue breathing. In infants and children, lung inspiratory and expiratory time constants for alveolar filling and emptying may need to be adjusted according to both anatomic and physiological development. For example, the child with respiratory failure secondary to asthma clearly will require a different approach for mechanical ventilation support than a neonate with alveolar collapse caused by respiratory distress syndrome.

Epidemiology
Ideally the sequence of resuscitation should be tailored to the most likely cause of the arrest, but this increases the complexity of BLS and ALS education. For lay rescuers, CPR instruction must remain simple. Retention of current CPR skills and knowledge is now suboptimal, and more complex instruction is more difficult to teach, learn, remember, and perform. In the newly born infant, respiratory failure is the most common cause of cardiopulmonary deterioration and arrest. In the older infant and child, arrest may be related to progression of respiratory failure, shock, or neurological dysfunction. In general, pediatric out-of-hospital arrest is characterized by a progression from hypoxia and hypercarbia to respiratory arrest and bradycardia and then to asystolic cardiac arrest.[2,17,18] Therefore, a focus on immediate ventilation and compressions, rather than the "adult" approach of immediate EMS activation or defibrillation, appears to be

warranted. In this age group, early effective ventilation and oxygenation must be established as quickly as possible.

In some circumstances primary arrhythmic cardiac arrest is more likely than respiratory arrest, and the lay rescuer may be instructed to activate the EMS system first (eg, children with underlying cardiac disease or a history of arrhythmias). If a previously well child experiences a sudden witnessed collapse, this suggests a previously undetected cardiac disorder, and immediate activation of the EMS system may be beneficial. Children with sudden collapse may have a prolonged-QT syndrome, hypertrophic cardiomyopathy, or drug-induced cardiac arrest[19-21]; the latter is more likely in the adolescent age group, related to a drug overdose.

For optimal patient outcomes, all of the links of the Chain of Survival must be strong. Unfortunately the rate of bystander CPR is disappointing; bystander CPR is provided for only approximately 30% of out-of-hospital pediatric arrests.[2,17] A low rate of bystander CPR may mask improvements in the structure and function of the EMS system, since data in adults suggests a much worse outcome when bystander CPR is not provided.[3,5,6] Because all the links are connected, it is difficult to evaluate components of single links such as the optimal method of EMS system activation or the effect of specific EMS interventions.

In addition, local EMS response intervals, dispatcher training, and EMS protocols may dictate the most appropriate sequence of EMS activation and early life support interventions. For example, providing 1 minute of CPR is recommended in pediatric out-of-hospital arrest before activation of the EMS system.[13] Rather than using a uniform approach, however, perhaps the activation of the EMS system and the sequence of BLS support for out-of-hospital arrest should be based on the cause of arrest (ie, the cause of arrest could be separated into cardiac versus respiratory origin by lay rescuers). The increased educational complexity limits this approach, however. As noted above, if a cardiac cause is suspected on the basis of event circumstances, then immediate EMS activation may be more important than providing 1 minute of CPR. Once EMS providers arrive, early use of AEDs in children ≥8 years of age may help to better identify initial rhythms and rapidly treat children with a more favorable arrest rhythm (ie, VF or pulseless VT).[2]

Although recommending an etiology-based resuscitation sequence for lay rescuers may be more medically appropriate in certain circumstances, it is more complex and therefore harder to teach, learn, and remember. Consequently, after much deliberation and debate, we continue to recommend the same approach as stated in the 1992 guidelines[13]: phone first for adults and phone fast for children. Nevertheless, it is the responsibility of the healthcare provider to identify and train caretakers to call first when a child with a high risk of a primary cardiac event is identified. It is also appropriate to teach more knowledgeable providers to "call first" for a likely arrhythmic cardiac arrest (eg, sudden collapse at any age) and to "call fast" in other circumstances (eg, trauma, a submersion event, or an apparent choking event).

Recognition of Respiratory Failure and Shock

Survival after cardiac arrest in children averages 7% to 11%, with most survivors neurologically impaired. For this reason

we emphasize early recognition and treatment of respiratory failure and shock to prevent an arrest from occurring. To clarify terminology we use the following Pediatric Utstein Style[1] definitions: "respiratory arrest" is defined as the absence of respirations (ie, apnea) with detectable cardiac activity. This should be distinguished from *respiratory compromise leading to assisted ventilation*. In the latter, the patient may have respiratory distress with increased effort *or* inadequate respiratory effort with no distress. *Cardiac arrest* is the cessation of cardiac mechanical activity, determined by the inability to palpate a central pulse, unresponsiveness, and apnea (ie, no signs of circulation or life).

Deterioration in respiratory function or imminent respiratory arrest should be anticipated in infants or children who demonstrate any of the following signs: an increased respiratory rate, particularly if accompanied by signs of distress and increased respiratory effort; inadequate respiratory rate, effort, or chest excursion; diminished peripheral breath sounds; gasping or grunting respirations; decreased level of consciousness or response to pain; poor skeletal muscle tone; or cyanosis.

"Respiratory failure" is a clinical state characterized by inadequate oxygenation, ventilation, or both. Strict criteria for respiratory failure are difficult to define because the baseline oxygenation or ventilation of an individual infant or child may be abnormal. For example, an infant with cyanotic congenital heart disease would not be in respiratory failure on the basis of an oxygen saturation of 60%, whereas that would be an appropriate criterion in a child with normal cardiopulmonary physiology. Respiratory failure may be functionally characterized as a clinical state that requires intervention to prevent respiratory or cardiac arrest.

"Shock" is a clinical state in which blood flow and delivery of tissue nutrients do not meet tissue metabolic demand. Shock may occur with increased, normal, or decreased cardiac output or blood pressure. Since shock represents a continuum of severity, it is further characterized as being compensated or decompensated. "Decompensated shock" is defined as a clinical state of tissue perfusion that is inadequate to meet metabolic demand and hypotension (ie, a **systolic** blood pressure [SBP] less than the 5th percentile for age). The definition of hypotension in preterm neonates depends on the newborn's weight and gestational age.

For the PALS guidelines, *hypotension* is characterized by the following:

- For term neonates (0 to 28 days of age), SBP <60 mm Hg
- For infants from 1 month to 12 months, SBP <70 mm Hg
- For children >1 year to 10 years, SBP <70+(2×age in years)
- Beyond 10 years, hypotension is defined as an SBP <90 mm Hg

Note that these blood pressure thresholds will overlap with normal values, including the 5% of normal children who have an SBP lower than the 5th percentile for age.

Early (ie, *compensated*) shock is shock *without hypotension* (ie, shock with a "normal" blood pressure). Compensated shock is detected by evaluation of heart rate, presence and volume (strength) of peripheral pulses, and adequacy of end-organ perfusion. The latter includes assessment of mental status, capillary refill, skin temperature, and when available, monitoring urine output and determining the presence and magnitude of metabolic acidosis on laboratory evaluation.

Cardiac output is the product of heart rate and stroke volume. If stroke volume is compromised for any reason, tachycardia is a common physiological response in an attempt to maintain cardiac output. Therefore, sustained sinus tachycardia (ST) in the absence of known causes such as fever or pain may be an early sign of cardiovascular compromise. Bradycardia, on the other hand, may be a preterminal cardiac rhythm indicative of advanced shock, and it is often associated with hypotension. When cardiac output and systemic perfusion are compromised, the volume (strength or quality) of peripheral pulses is decreased, capillary refill time may be prolonged, and skin temperature is often cool despite a warm ambient temperature. In some children with shock, however, the pulses may be readily palpable and the skin temperature may be warm. The latter clinical picture, for example, is seen in children with early septic shock and represents inappropriate vasodilation of blood vessels in the skin and skeletal muscle.

Adjuncts for Airway and Ventilation

Standard Precautions

All fluids from patients should be treated as potentially infectious. Personnel should wear gloves and protective shields during procedures that are likely to expose them to droplets of blood, saliva, or other body fluids. Local precaution standards should be developed in the context of individual circumstances and available resources.

Out-of-Hospital Considerations

In the out-of-hospital setting, there is often a need to open the airway and to provide oxygen with or without ventilatory support. This requires the availability of a selection of face masks and a pediatric manual resuscitator (ventilation bag). The manual resuscitator may be used safely in infants and newborns by persons properly trained to avoid excess tidal volumes and pressure that can result in gastric inflation or overinflation of the lungs. Ventilation via a properly placed tracheal tube is the most effective and reliable method of assisted ventilation. However, this "gold standard" method requires mastery of the technical skill to successfully and safely place a tube in the trachea, and it may not always be appropriate in the out-of-hospital setting, depending on factors such as the experience and training of the healthcare provider and the transport time interval. In addition to the patient's condition, a wide variety of EMS system factors must be evaluated to identify the best method of securing the airway in a given setting. These factors include EMS provider training, the requirement for ongoing provider experience, the EMS indications for and techniques of pediatric endotracheal intubation, and the methods used to evaluate tube placement. In retrospective studies, increased accuracy and reduced complication rate are associated with increased training (including supervised time spent in the operating room as well as in the field),[17,22] the use of minimal requirements

ensuring adequate ongoing experience, and use of paralytic agents.[17,23,24]

In some EMS systems the success rate for pediatric intubation is relatively low and the complication rate is high.[25] This probably reflects the infrequent use of intubation skills by paramedics in a single-tiered system. In tiered EMS systems, the second tier of prehospital providers may have sufficient training and ongoing experience to perform intubation safely and effectively.[17] Dedicated critical care or interhospital transport personnel (including helicopter transport personnel) also may have a high success rate with endotracheal intubation.[24,26] Conversely, in the only prospective pediatric randomized, controlled trial comparing bag-mask ventilation with endotracheal intubation in the prehospital setting, bag-mask ventilation was generally as effective as endotracheal intubation; for the subgroup with respiratory failure, bag-mask ventilation was associated with improved survival.[25] It is important to note that the transport times were short for this EMS system, all providers received detailed training in bag-mask ventilation and endotracheal intubation, and individual ALS providers had infrequent opportunities to perform pediatric intubation. In summary, this study suggests that endotracheal intubation may not improve survival over bag-mask ventilation in all EMS systems, and endotracheal intubation appears to result in increased airway complications.[25]

On the basis of this data, anyone providing prehospital BLS care for infants and children should be trained to deliver effective oxygenation and ventilation using the bag-mask technique as the primary method of ventilatory support, particularly if transport time is short (Class IIa; level of evidence [LOE] 1, 2). Intubation of the seriously ill or injured pediatric patient in the out-of-hospital setting is a skill that requires both adequate initial training and ongoing experience plus outcome monitoring. If an EMS system chooses to provide out-of-hospital endotracheal intubation, the system should ensure proper initial training, monitoring of skill retention, and ongoing monitoring of the safety and effectiveness of this intervention.

When used by properly trained providers, medications can increase the success rate of endotracheal intubation[24,27] but may introduce additional risks. Because the risk from a misplaced tube is unacceptably high and clinical signs confirming tube placement in the trachea are not completely reliable,[28] use of a device to confirm tracheal tube placement in the field, in the transport vehicle, and on arrival to the hospital is desirable and strongly encouraged. Use of a device to confirm tube placement on arrival at the hospital is especially important because displacement of the tube is most likely to occur when the patient is moved into and out of the transport vehicle,[29] and animal data shows that detection of a displaced or obstructed tube using pulse oximetry or changes in heart rate or blood pressure may be delayed more than 3 minutes.[30] Secondary confirmation of tracheal tube position by use of exhaled CO_2 detection is strongly recommended in infants and children with a perfusing rhythm (Class IIa; LOE 3, 5, 7) and is recommended in patients in cardiac arrest (Class IIb; LOE 5, 7). Unfortunately these devices have been inadequately studied in children for use outside of the operating room (see "Noninvasive Respiratory Monitoring" later in this part), so additional data is needed before the use of these devices is made a Class I recommendation.

Oxygen Administration

Administer oxygen to all seriously ill or injured patients with respiratory insufficiency, shock, or trauma. In these patients inadequate pulmonary gas exchange and inadequate cardiac output resulting from conditions such as a low circulatory blood volume or disturbed cardiac function limit tissue oxygen delivery.

During cardiac arrest a number of factors contribute to severe progressive tissue hypoxia and the need for supplemental oxygen administration. At best, mouth-to-mouth ventilation provides 16% to 17% oxygen with a maximal alveolar oxygen tension of 80 mm Hg. Even optimal external chest compressions provide only a fraction of the normal cardiac output, so that blood flow and therefore delivery of oxygen to tissues are markedly diminished. In addition, CPR is associated with right-to-left pulmonary shunting caused by ventilation-perfusion mismatch, and respiratory conditions may further compromise oxygenation of the blood. The combination of low blood flow and usually low oxygenation leads to metabolic acidosis and organ failure. Oxygen should be administered to children demonstrating cardiopulmonary arrest or compromise to maximize arterial oxygen content even if measured arterial oxygen tension is high, because oxygen delivery to tissues may still be compromised by a low cardiac output. Whenever possible, humidify administered oxygen to prevent drying and thickening of pulmonary secretions; dried secretions may contribute to obstruction of natural or artificial airways.

Administer oxygen by nasal cannula, simple face masks, and nonrebreathing masks. The concentration of oxygen delivered depends on the oxygen flow rate and the patient's minute ventilation. As long as the flow of oxygen exceeds the maximal inspiratory flow rate, the prescribed concentration of oxygen will be delivered. If the inspiratory flow rate exceeds the oxygen flow rate, air is entrained, reducing the oxygen concentration delivered.

Masks

If the patient demonstrates effective spontaneous ventilation, use a simple face mask to provide oxygen at a concentration of 30% to 50%. If a higher concentration of oxygen is desired, it may be administered through a nonrebreathing mask, typically at a flow of 15 L/min. Masks should be available in a selection of sizes. To provide a consistent concentration of oxygen, the mask of appropriate size should provide an airtight seal without pressure on the eyes. A small under-mask volume is desirable to minimize rebreathing of exhaled gases. If the mask has an inflatable rim, the rim can mold to the contours of the child's face to minimize air leak.[31]

Nasal Cannulas

A nasal cannula is used to provide supplemental oxygen to a child who is breathing spontaneously. This low-flow device delivers varying inspired oxygen concentrations, depending on the child's respiratory rate and effort and the size of the child.[32] In young infants, nasal oxygen at 2 L/min can provide

an inspired oxygen concentration >50%. Nasal cannulas are often better tolerated than a face mask and are suitable to use in children who require modest oxygen supplementation. Nasal cannula flow rates >4 L/min for prolonged periods are often poorly tolerated because of the drying effect on the nasal mucosa.

Oropharyngeal and Nasopharyngeal Airways

An oropharyngeal airway is indicated for the unconscious infant or child if procedures to open the airway (eg, head tilt–chin lift or jaw thrust) fail to provide a clear, unobstructed airway. Do not use an oropharyngeal airway in the conscious child because it may induce vomiting.

Oropharyngeal airways are available for pediatric patients of all ages. Appropriate selection of airway size requires training and experience. An improperly sized oropharyngeal airway may fail to keep the tongue separated from the back of the pharynx or may actually cause airway obstruction. To select the proper size (length) of oropharyngeal airway from flange to distal tip, choose one equal to the distance from the central incisors to the angle of the jaw. To evaluate the size, place the airway next to the face.

Nasopharyngeal airways are soft rubber or plastic tubes that may be used in conscious patients requiring relief of upper airway obstruction. They may be useful in children with a diminished level of consciousness or in neurologically impaired children who have poor pharyngeal tone leading to upper airway obstruction. They are available in a selection of pediatric sizes. In very young patients, airway secretions and debris readily obstruct small nasopharyngeal airways, making them unreliable. Moreover, children may have large adenoids, which can lead to difficulty in placing the airway; trauma and bleeding may occur during placement. Large adenoids also may compress the nasopharyngeal airway after placement, leading to increased airway resistance and an ineffective airway.

Laryngeal Mask Airway

The laryngeal mask airway (LMA) is a device used to secure the airway in an unconscious patient. The LMA consists of a tube with a cuffed mask-like projection at the distal end. The LMA is introduced into the pharynx and advanced until resistance is felt as the tube locates in the hypopharynx. The balloon cuff is then inflated, which seals the hypopharynx, leaving the distal opening of the tube just above the glottic opening and providing a clear, secure airway. (See Figure 3 in "Part 6, Section 3: Adjuncts for Oxygenation, Ventilation, and Airway Control.")

LMAs are widely used in the operating room and provide an effective means of ventilation and oxygenation, but LMAs are contraindicated in an infant or child with an intact gag reflex. They may be useful in patients with difficult airways, and they have been used successfully in emergency airway control of adults in hospital and out-of-hospital settings.[33,34] They can be placed safely and reliably in infants and children,[35] although data suggests that proper training and supervision are needed to master the technique.[36,37] Data also suggests that mastering LMA insertion may be easier than mastering endotracheal intubation.[38] Indeed, nurses have been successfully trained to perform LMA insertion in adults in cardiac arrest,[39] and paramedics have been trained to insert an LMA with a higher success rate than endotracheal intubation.[40]

Although LMAs do not protect the airway from aspiration of refluxed gastric contents, a meta-analysis showed that aspiration is uncommon with LMA use in the operating room[41] and was less common than with bag-mask ventilation in adults undergoing in-hospital CPR.[42] Therefore, in the setting of cardiac or respiratory arrest, LMAs may be an effective alternative for establishing the airway when inserted by properly trained healthcare providers, but limited data comparing LMAs to bag-mask ventilation or endotracheal intubation in emergency pediatric resuscitation precludes a confident recommendation (Class Indeterminate; LOE 5, 7). Training for healthcare providers in the use of the LMA should not replace training to use bag-mask ventilation effectively.

An LMA may be more difficult to maintain during patient movement than a tracheal tube, making it problematic to use during transport. Careful attention is needed to ensure that the LMA position is maintained if the LMA is used in the out-of-hospital setting. Furthermore, the LMA is relatively expensive, and a number of sizes are needed to provide airway support to any child at risk. The cost of equipping out-of-hospital providers with LMA devices must be considered.

Ventilation Bags and Masks

Ventilation with a bag-mask device requires more skill than mouth-to-mouth or mouth-to-mask ventilation. A bag-mask device should be used only by personnel with proper training. Training should focus on selecting an appropriately sized mask and bag, opening the airway and securing the mask to the face, delivering adequate ventilation, and assessing the effectiveness of ventilation. We recommend periodic demonstration of proficiency.

Types of Ventilation Bags (Manual Resuscitators)

There are 2 basic types of manual resuscitators: self-inflating and flow-inflating. Ventilation bags used for resuscitation should be self-inflating and should be available in child and adult sizes, suitable for the entire pediatric age range.

Neonatal-size (250 mL) ventilation bags may be inadequate to support effective tidal volume and the longer inspiratory times required by full-term neonates and infants.[43] For this reason resuscitation bags used for ventilation of full-term newly borns, infants, and children should have a minimum volume of 450 to 500 mL. Studies using infant manikins showed that effective infant ventilation can be accomplished using pediatric (and larger) resuscitation bags.[44] *Regardless of the size of the manual resuscitator, take care to use only that force and tidal volume necessary to cause the chest to visibly rise.* Excessive ventilation volumes and airway pressures may compromise cardiac output by raising the intrathoracic pressure and by distending alveoli, increasing afterload on the right heart. In addition, excessive volumes may distend the stomach, impeding ventilation and increasing the risk of regurgitation and aspiration. In patients with small-airway obstruction (eg, asthma and bronchiolitis),

excessive tidal volumes and rate can result in air trapping, barotrauma, air leak, and severe compromise to cardiac output. In head-injured and postarrest patients, excessive ventilation volumes and rate may result in hyperventilation, with potentially adverse effects on neurological outcome. Therefore, the routine target in postarrest and head-injured patients should be physiological oxygenation and ventilation (Class IIa; LOE 5, 6; see "Postresuscitation Stabilization").

Ideally, manual resuscitators used for resuscitation should have either no pressure-relief valve or a pressure-relief valve with an override feature to permit use of high pressures to achieve visible chest expansion if necessary.[45] High pressures may be required during bag-mask ventilation of patients with upper or lower airway obstruction or poor lung compliance. In these patients a pressure-relief valve may prevent delivery of sufficient tidal volume.[32]

Self-Inflating Bags

The self-inflating bag delivers only room air (21% oxygen) unless supplemental oxygen is provided. At an oxygen inflow of 10 L/min, pediatric manual resuscitator devices without oxygen reservoirs deliver from 30% to 80% oxygen to the patient. The actual concentration of oxygen delivered is unpredictable because entrainment of variable quantities of room air occurs, depending on the tidal volume and peak inspiratory flow rate used. To deliver consistently higher oxygen concentrations (60% to 95%), all manual resuscitators used for resuscitation should be equipped with an oxygen reservoir. An oxygen flow of at least 10 to 15 L/min is necessary to maintain an adequate oxygen volume in the reservoir of a pediatric manual resuscitator; this should be considered the minimum flow rate.[32] The larger adult manual resuscitators require at least 15 L/min of oxygen to deliver high oxygen concentrations reliably.

To provide bag-mask ventilation, open the airway, seal the mask to the face, and deliver an adequate tidal volume. To open the airway and seal the mask to the face in the absence of suspected neck trauma, tilt the head back while 2 or 3 fingers are positioned under the angle of the mandible to lift it up and forward, moving the tongue off the posterior pharynx. Place the thumb and forefinger in a "C" shape over the mask and exert downward pressure on the mask while the other fingers maintain the jaw thrust to create a tight seal (Figure 2). This technique of opening the airway and sealing the mask to the face is called the "E-C clamp" technique. The third, fourth, and fifth fingers (forming an E) are positioned under the jaw to lift it forward; then the thumb and index finger (forming a C) hold the mask on the child's face. Determine appropriate mask size by the ability to seal it around the mouth and nose without covering the eyes or overlapping the chin. Once the mask is properly sealed, the other hand compresses the ventilation bag until the chest visibly rises.

Self-inflating bag-mask systems that contain a fish-mouth or leaf-flap outlet valve cannot be used to provide continuous supplemental oxygen to the child with spontaneous respirations. The valve in the self-inflating bag opens only if the bag is squeezed or the child's inspiratory effort is significant. If the bag is not squeezed, the valve usually remains closed, so

A

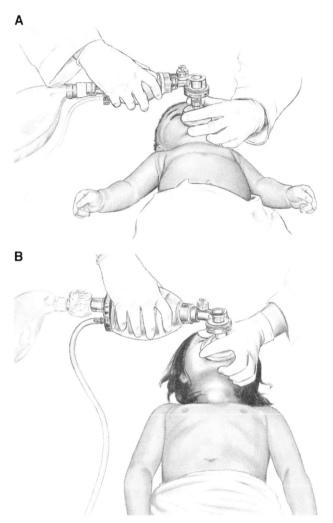

B

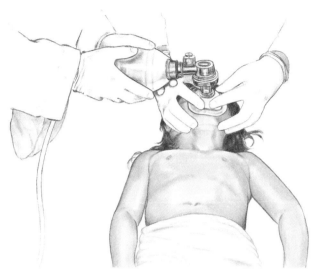

Figure 3. Two-rescuer bag-mask ventilation technique may provide superior ventilation when there is significant airway obstruction or poor lung compliance. One rescuer uses both hands to open the airway and maintain a tight mask-to-face seal while the other rescuer compresses the ventilation bag.

Figure 2. One-rescuer bag-mask ventilation demonstrating the "E-C clamp" technique of opening the airway. The thumb and forefinger form a "C" shape over the mask and exert downward pressure on the mask while the third, fourth, and fifth fingers (forming an E) are positioned along the jaw to maintain the jaw thrust. A, Infant; B, child.

Gastric Inflation and Cricoid Pressure
Gastric inflation in unconscious or obtunded patients can be minimized by increasing inspiratory time to deliver the necessary tidal volume at low peak inspiratory pressures. The rescuer must properly pace the rate of ventilation and ensure adequate time for exhalation.[25] To reduce gastric inflation, a second rescuer can apply cricoid pressure, but use this procedure only with an unconscious victim.[48] Cricoid pressure may also prevent regurgitation (and possible aspiration) of gastric contents.[49,50] Avoid excessive cricoid pressure because it may produce tracheal compression and obstruction or distortion of the upper airway anatomy.[51] Gastric inflation after prolonged bag-mask ventilation can limit effective ventilation[52]; inflation can be relieved by placement of a nasogastric or orogastric tube. If endotracheal intubation is performed, insertion of the gastric tube should follow the insertion of the tracheal tube.

Endotracheal Intubation
When used by properly trained providers, ventilation via a tracheal tube is the most effective and reliable method of assisted ventilation. Advantages of endotracheal intubation include the following:

- The airway is isolated to ensure adequate ventilation and delivery of oxygen without inflating the stomach.
- The risk of pulmonary aspiration of gastric contents is minimized.
- Inspiratory time and peak inspiratory pressures can be controlled.
- Secretions and other debris can be suctioned from the airways.
- Positive end-expiratory pressure can be delivered, if needed, through use of a positive end-expiratory pressure device on the exhalation port.

the child receives only a negligible amount of escaped oxygen and rebreathes the exhaled gases contained within the mask itself.

Flow-Inflating Bags
Flow-inflating bags (also called "anesthesia bags") refill only with oxygen inflow, and the inflow must be individually regulated. Since flow-inflating manual resuscitators are more difficult to use, they should be used by trained personnel only.[46] Flow-inflating bags permit the delivery of supplemental oxygen to a spontaneously breathing victim.

Two-Person Bag-Mask Ventilation
Superior bag-mask ventilation can be achieved with 2 persons, and this technique may be necessary when there is significant airway obstruction or poor lung compliance.[47] One rescuer uses both hands to open the airway and maintain a tight mask-to-face seal while the other rescuer compresses the ventilation bag (Figure 3). Both rescuers should observe the chest to ensure chest rise with each breath.

TABLE 1.   Pediatric Tracheal Tube and Suction Catheter Sizes*

Approximate Age/Size (Weight)	Internal Diameter of Tracheal Tube, mm	Suction Catheter Size, F
Premature infant (<1 kg)	2.5	5
Premature infant (1–2 kg)	3.0	5 or 6
Premature infant (2–3 kg)	3.0 to 3.5	6 or 8
0 month to 1 year/infant (3–10 kg)	3.5 to 4.0	8
1 year/small child (10–13 kg)	4.0	8
3 years/child (14–16 kg)	4.5	8 or 10
5 years/child (16–20 kg)	5.0	10
6 years/child (18–25 kg)	5.5	10
8 years/child to small adult (24–32 kg)	6.0 cuffed	10 or 12
12 years/adolescent (32–54 kg)	6.5 cuffed	12
16 years/adult (50+ kg)	7.0 cuffed	12
Adult female	7.0–8.0 cuffed	12 or 14
Adult male	7.0–8.0 cuffed	14

*These are approximations and should be adjusted on the basis of clinical experience. Tracheal tube selection for a child should be based on the child's size or age. One size larger and one size smaller should be allowed for individual variation. Color-coding based on length or size of the child may facilitate approximation of correct tracheal tube size.

Indications for endotracheal intubation include

- Inadequate central nervous system control of ventilation resulting in apnea or inadequate respiratory effort
- Functional or anatomic airway obstruction
- Excessive work of breathing leading to fatigue
- Need for high peak inspiratory pressures or positive end-expiratory pressures to maintain effective alveolar gas exchange
- Lack of airway protective reflexes
- Permitting paralysis or sedation for diagnostic studies while ensuring protection of the airway and control of ventilation

The airway of the child differs from that of the adult. The child's airway is more compliant, the tongue is relatively larger, the glottic opening is higher and more anterior in the neck, and the airway is proportionally smaller than in the adult. For these reasons, only highly trained medical providers who maintain their skill through experience or frequent retraining should attempt endotracheal intubation. If the provider lacks adequate training or experience, continued ventilation with a manual resuscitator and mask or an LMA may be appropriate until a more skilled provider is available.

The narrowest diameter of the child's airway is located below the vocal cords at the level of the cricoid cartilage. Since obstruction to passage of a tracheal tube may occur at a point just below the level of the glottic opening, uncuffed tubes typically are used for children <8 years old. However, cuffed tracheal tubes sized for younger children are available and may be appropriate under circumstances in which high inspiratory pressure is expected. For example, a child in respiratory failure from status asthmaticus or acute respiratory distress syndrome (ARDS) may benefit from a cuffed tracheal tube to permit use of higher ventilatory pressures.

Data suggests that using cuffed tracheal tubes in critically ill children results in complication rates that are no different from those for uncuffed tubes, provided that there is appropriate attention to monitoring cuff pressure.[53,54]

Suggested tracheal tubes and suction catheters for different ages (based on the average sizes of children at different ages) are listed in Table 1. For children older than 1 year, an estimate of tracheal tube size may also be made by use of the following equation:

Tracheal tube size (mm)=(age in years/4)+4.

If a cuffed tracheal tube is needed, a slight modification of this formula works well to predict the tracheal tube size[54]:

Tracheal tube size (mm)=(age in years/4)+3.

In general, tubes that are 0.5 mm smaller and 0.5 mm larger than estimated should be available. Because of the normal variation of body and airway size for a given age, appropriate tracheal tube selection is based more reliably on patient size than age.[55] Although the internal diameter of the tracheal tube may appear to be roughly equivalent to the size of the victim's little finger, estimation of tube size by this method may be difficult and unreliable.[56,57] An alternative method of tube size selection is based on a multicenter study that showed that a child's *body length* can predict correct tracheal tube size more accurately than the child's age.[55] Length-based resuscitation tapes may be helpful in identifying the correct tracheal tube size for children up to approximately 35 kg.[55]

Before attempting intubation, assemble the following equipment:

- A tonsil-tipped suction device or a large-bore suction catheter
- A suction catheter of appropriate size to fit into the tracheal tube
- A properly functioning manual resuscitator, oxygen source, and a face mask of appropriate size
- A stylet to provide rigidity to the tracheal tube and help guide it through and beyond the vocal cords. If a stylet is used, it is important to place the stylet tip 1 to 2 cm proximal to the distal end of the tracheal tube to prevent trauma to the trachea from the stylet. A sterile, water-soluble lubricant or sterile water may be helpful to moisten the stylet and aid its removal from the tracheal tube after successful placement.
- Three tracheal tubes, 1 tube of the estimated required size and tubes 0.5 mm smaller and 0.5 mm larger
- A laryngoscope blade and handle with a functioning bright light (and spare bulb and batteries if possible)
- An exhaled CO_2 detector (capnography or colorimetric) or, in older children and adolescents, an esophageal tube detector
- Tape to secure the tube and gauze to dry the face. An adhesive solution may also be used on the tube and face, or a tracheal tube holder may be considered. Assemble equipment to immobilize the child's head and shoulders, if appropriate.

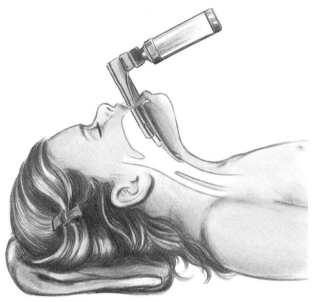

Figure 4. Position of laryngoscope with straight blade for pediatric intubation. The blade tip is usually passed over the epiglottis to rest above the glottic opening. Blade traction is used to lift the base of the tongue and directly elevate the epiglottis anteriorly, exposing the glottis.

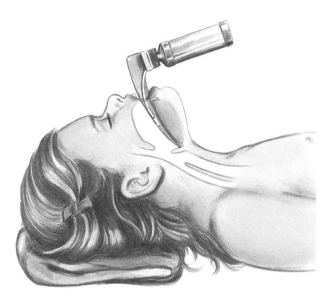

Figure 5. Position of laryngoscope with curved blade for pediatric intubation. The tip of the blade is usually passed into the vallecula (the space between the base of the tongue and the epiglottis) to displace the base of the tongue anteriorly, exposing the glottis.

The Intubation Procedure

In a child with a perfusing rhythm, endotracheal intubation should always be preceded by the administration of supplemental oxygen. Assist ventilation only if the patient's effort is inadequate. If a rapid sequence intubation (RSI) procedure is anticipated (see below), avoid assisted ventilation if possible because it often inflates the stomach and increases the risk of vomiting and aspiration. If trauma to the head and neck or multiple trauma is present, the cervical spine should be immobilized during intubation.

Since morbidity can occur from an improperly placed tracheal tube or from hypoxia created during prolonged intubation attempts, attempts should not exceed approximately 30 seconds, and the heart rate and pulse oximetry should be continuously monitored. Interrupt the intubation attempt for any of the following conditions: if bradycardia develops (ie, the heart rate drops precipitously or is <60 beats per minute [bpm]), the child's color or perfusion deteriorates, or the oxygen saturation by pulse oximetry falls to an unacceptable level. If any of these conditions develops, the intubation attempt generally should be interrupted and assisted ventilation provided with a ventilation bag-mask device and supplemental oxygen until the child's condition improves.

In some circumstances, such as in a child with ARDS, adequate oxygenation cannot be achieved with bag-mask ventilation. In this setting endotracheal intubation should be strongly considered despite the presence of cyanosis or bradycardia. Intubation is probably best performed by the most skilled provider present. In a child in cardiac arrest, do not delay intubation to apply a device to continuously monitor the rhythm. Furthermore, pulse oximetry will not function if the patient does not have detectable pulsatile perfusion.

Either a straight or a curved laryngoscope blade may be used. When a straight blade is used, the blade tip is usually passed over the epiglottis to rest above the glottic opening. Use the blade traction to lift the base of the tongue and directly elevate the epiglottis anteriorly, exposing the glottis (Figure 4). When using a curved blade, insert the tip of the blade into the vallecula (the space between the base of the tongue and the epiglottis) to displace the base of the tongue anteriorly. Do not use the laryngoscope blade and handle in a prying or levering motion, and do not place pressure directly on the teeth, lips, or gums (Figure 5).

Endotracheal intubation ideally should proceed when the glottic opening is visualized. Glottic visualization in infants and children requires that the head and neck be tipped (or angled) forward and the chin lifted into the "sniffing" position. Place the child's head on a small pillow (this flexes the neck slightly) to bring the larynx into optimal alignment for intubation.[58] In infants and children <2 years of age, use of a pillow to flex the neck is not necessary for oral intubation, and the head should be on a flat surface; often a small shoulder roll is used to elevate the shoulders.[58] As noted previously, if trauma to the head and neck or multiple trauma is present, attempt to immobilize the cervical spine during intubation.

The appropriate depth of insertion of a tracheal tube can be estimated from the following formula: Depth of insertion (cm)=internal tube diameter (in mm)×3. An alternative formula to estimate appropriate depth of insertion in children >2 years of age is this: Depth of insertion (cm)=(age in years/2)+12.

Verification of Proper Tube Placement

Once the tracheal tube is positioned, provide positive-pressure ventilation, observe chest wall movement, and listen for breath sounds over the peripheral lung fields. If the tube is properly positioned, there should be symmetrical, bilateral chest rise during positive-pressure ventilation, and breath sounds should be easily auscultated over both lung fields, especially in the axillary areas. Breath sounds should be absent over the upper abdomen.[28] The presence of water vapor in the tube is *not* a reliable indicator of proper tracheal tube position.[59] Tracheal tube placement should be confirmed by monitoring exhaled CO_2, *especially* in children with a perfusing rhythm (see "Noninvasive Respiratory Monitoring"). If there is any doubt about tracheal position of the tube, use the laryngoscope to verify tube position by seeing the tube pass through the glottic opening. In a patient monitored by continuous pulse oximetry, the oxygen saturation typically increases after successful intubation unless the child has severe alteration of oxygen diffusion across the alveolus or severe ventilation-perfusion mismatch (eg, ARDS or severe pneumonia).

After the tube is taped into place, confirm its position within the trachea clinically and by chest x-ray because transmitted breath sounds may be heard over the left hemithorax despite a right main bronchus intubation. In addition, the chest x-ray helps to identify and correct the position of a tube located high in the trachea, which is at high risk of displacement during movement.

Once the tracheal tube is placed and secured, maintain the head in a neutral position. Excessive movement of the head may displace the tracheal tube. Flexion of the head on the neck moves the tube farther into the airway, and extension of the head displaces the tube farther out of the airway.[60,61] In a responsive patient, consider placement of an oral airway adjacent to the tracheal tube, but not deeply enough into the oropharynx to stimulate a gag reflex, to prevent the child from biting down on the tube and obstructing the airway.

Rapid Sequence Intubation

RSI uses pharmacological agents to facilitate emergent endotracheal intubation while reducing adverse effects in responsive patients, including pain, arrhythmias, rise in systemic and intracranial pressures, airway trauma, gastric regurgitation and aspiration, hypoxemia, psychological trauma, and death. The term *rapid sequence intubation* is preferred over *rapid sequence induction* because the latter denotes the technique used by anesthesiologists for rapid airway control coincident with the initiation of anesthesia. In emergency settings, RSI should be seen not "as the initiation of anesthesia but rather as the use of deep sedation and paralysis to facilitate endotracheal intubation."[62]

In the United States, RSI is used frequently in Emergency Departments and intensive care units and to a lesser extent in the out-of-hospital setting. In many other countries, RSI is limited to trained anesthesiologists to minimize risks from the use of potent drugs to facilitate intubation. Regardless of where RSI is performed, only properly trained persons familiar with its indications and contraindications should use RSI. These persons must be proficient in the evaluation and management of the pediatric airway and must understand the medications (sedatives, neuromuscular blocking agents, and adjunctive agents) used during this procedure. The indications for RSI are the same as outlined above for endotracheal intubation. RSI is *not* indicated for patients in cardiac arrest or for those who are deeply comatose and require immediate intubation without delay. Relative contraindications to RSI include provider concern that intubation or mask ventilation may be unsuccessful; significant facial or laryngeal edema, trauma, or distortion; or a spontaneously breathing, adequately ventilated patient whose airway maintenance depends on his own upper airway muscle tone and positioning (eg, upper-airway obstruction or epiglottitis).[62]

An evidence-based analysis of RSI agents and procedures was not conducted at the evidence evaluation conferences leading to these guidelines. In addition, different pharmacological agents are used by protocol in different hospital and out-of-hospital settings. For these reasons, we cannot recommend uniform guidelines for RSI at this time. The inclusion of this information as an optional module in the PALS course is not an endorsement of RSI. To provide objective information on the value of RSI in various settings for future guidelines, healthcare systems using RSI should monitor the success rate and occurrence of complications.

Noninvasive Respiratory Monitoring

Pulse Oximetry

Pulse oximetry is an important noninvasive monitor of the child with respiratory insufficiency because it enables continuous evaluation of the arterial oxygen saturation. This monitoring technique is useful in both out-of-hospital and in-hospital settings.[63,64] It may provide early indication of respiratory deterioration causing hypoxemia (eg, from the loss of an artificial airway, disconnection of the oxygen supply, or impending or actual respiratory failure) and ideally should be used during stabilization and transport, because clinical recognition of hypoxemia is not reliable.[65] If peripheral perfusion is inadequate (eg, shock is present or the child is in cardiac arrest), pulse oximetry is unreliable and often unobtainable because accurate readings require the presence of pulsatile blood flow. In addition, if a patient is hyperoxygenated before intubation, incorrect tube position may not be recognized by pulse oximetry for a variable period depending on the rate of oxygen consumption.[30,66]

Exhaled or End-Tidal CO_2 Monitoring

Because clinical confirmation of tracheal tube placement may be unreliable, exhaled CO_2 detection using a colorimetric device or continuous capnography is recommended to confirm tube placement in infants (>2 kg) and in children (Class IIa; LOE 5, 6, 7). A positive color change or the presence of a capnography waveform showing exhaled CO_2 confirms tube position in the trachea when assessed after 6 ventilations.[67,68] Six ventilations are recommended to wash out CO_2 that may be present in the stomach and esophagus after bag-mask ventilation. After 6 ventilations, detected CO_2 can be presumed to be from the trachea rather than from a misplaced tube in the esophagus. Note that exhaled CO_2 may be detected with right main bronchus intubation, so exhaled CO_2 detection does not replace the need to document proper tube position in the trachea by chest x-ray and clinical examination.

Although detection of exhaled CO_2 in patients with a perfusing rhythm is both specific and sensitive for tube placement in the trachea, exhaled CO_2 detection is not as useful for patients in cardiac arrest. The presence of a color change or an exhaled CO_2 waveform reliably confirms tracheal tube placement, but the absence of detectable CO_2 does *not* confirm esophageal tube placement in the cardiac arrest patient. Infants, children, and adolescents in cardiac arrest may have limited pulmonary blood flow and therefore undetectable exhaled CO_2 despite proper placement of the tube in the trachea.[67,69] The low specificity of exhaled CO_2 monitoring in cardiac arrest limits the strength of recommendation of this test following intubation of a patient in cardiac arrest (Class IIb; LOE 3, 5, 6, 7).[69,70] In cardiac arrest the absence of a color change or detectable exhaled CO_2 by capnography may indicate either esophageal or tracheal tube placement.[69–71] If placement is uncertain, tube position must be confirmed by clinical examination and direct laryngeal examination.

In addition to cardiac arrest, other conditions leading to very low exhaled CO_2 may also produce misleading results. Clinical experience in adults, for example, suggests that severe airway obstruction (eg, status asthmaticus) and pulmonary edema may impair CO_2 elimination sufficiently to cause a false-negative test result.[70,72] If the detector is contaminated with acidic gastric contents or acidic drugs, such as tracheally administered epinephrine, the colorimetric detector may not be reliable. These problems cause a color change consistent with exhaled CO_2, but the detector remains a constant color throughout the respiratory cycle. Finally, intravenous bolus epinephrine administration may transiently reduce pulmonary blood flow and thus reduce the exhaled CO_2 below the limits of detection in cardiac arrest patients.[73]

Even though correct tracheal tube placement may not be confirmed by exhaled CO_2 detection in cardiac arrest, the absence of exhaled CO_2 may provide prognostic information in this setting. When correct tracheal tube position is confirmed, experience in animals[74] and adults[75–77] shows that absent or low detectable exhaled CO_2 correlates with poor outcome. In addition, efforts that improve closed-chest compression produce increases in exhaled CO_2.[78,79] This is consistent with data correlating cardiac output to exhaled CO_2 concentration.[80,81] There is only limited data relating exhaled CO_2 to outcome in pediatric cardiac arrest,[69] and animal data emphasizes the need to evaluate the exhaled CO_2 after providing several minutes of adequate ventilation in asphyxial arrests, since the initial values will be elevated.[82,83] On the basis of the limited data, no definite recommendation can be made about the use of exhaled CO_2 to predict outcome in children with cardiac arrest (Class Indeterminate; LOE 5, 6, 7), but we encourage the collection of outcome data correlated with exhaled CO_2 measurement.

Esophageal Detector Devices

Esophageal detector devices are based on the ability to readily aspirate air from the cartilage-supported trachea by drawing from gas in the lower airways. If the tracheal tube is placed in the esophagus, the walls of the esophagus collapse when aspiration is attempted by an esophageal detector device, preventing filling of a syringe or self-inflating rubber bulb.[71] In adults the esophageal detector device is very sensitive in identifying an esophageal tube placement when used in emergency intubations in patients with a perfusing rhythm.[84,85] In adults in cardiac arrest the esophageal detector device is useful to identify esophageal intubation, and it therefore can be used to supplement the potentially misleading information from exhaled CO_2 detection to confirm tracheal placement.[86] Although an esophageal detector device has been used successfully in children,[87] it appears to be unreliable in children <1 year of age,[88] in morbidly obese patients,[89] and in patients in late pregnancy.[90] In summary, there is insufficient data in emergency intubations in infants and children to recommend the routine use of an esophageal detector device (Class Indeterminate; LOE 5, 6, 7).

Verification of Tracheal Tube Position

Several points about the use of supplemental respiratory monitoring devices after intubation deserve emphasis.[91]

- No single confirmation technique is 100% reliable under all circumstances.
- Devices to confirm tracheal tube placement should always be used in the perfusing patient and are highly recommended in the cardiac arrest patient to supplement the physical examination because physical examination alone is unreliable.
- If the infant or child has a perfusing rhythm, exhaled CO_2 detection is the best method (most sensitive and specific) for verification of tube placement.
- Once placement is confirmed, the tube (and head, if appropriate) should be secured and the tube position at the level of the lip or teeth recorded.
- Repeated confirmation or continuous monitoring of tracheal tube position is highly recommended during stabilization and transport in the out-of-hospital or in-hospital setting.

If the condition of an intubated patient deteriorates, consider several possibilities that can be recalled by the mnemonic **DOPE**: **D**isplacement of the tube from the trachea, **O**bstruction of the tube, **P**neumothorax, and **E**quipment failure.

Miscellaneous Adjuncts to Airway and Ventilation

Suction devices (either portable or installed) should be available for emergency resuscitation. The portable unit should provide sufficient vacuum and flow for pharyngeal and tracheal suctioning. The installed unit should provide an airflow of >30 L/min at the end of the delivery tube and a vacuum of >300 mm Hg when the tube is clamped at full suction. Each device should have an adjustable suction regulator for use in children and intubated patients. Generally a maximum suction force of 80 to 120 mm Hg is used for suctioning the airway of the infant or child.[92] Large-bore, noncollapsible suction tubing should always be joined to the suction units, and semirigid pharyngeal tips (tonsil suction tips) and appropriate sizes of catheters should be available.

Pharyngeal and sterile tracheal suction catheters should be available in a variety of sizes (Table 1) and should be readily accessible. Tracheal suction catheters should have a Y-piece, T-piece, or lateral opening between the suction tube and the suction power control to regulate when suction is applied. The suction apparatus must be designed for easy cleaning and decontamination.

When it is impossible to oxygenate or ventilate the victim with a manual resuscitator or when intubation cannot be accomplished (eg, following severe facial trauma) and standard resuscitative measures to clear the airway fail, transtracheal catheter ventilation may be attempted.[93] Percutaneous needle cricothyrotomy provides effective ventilation and oxygenation in children during anesthesia if a jet ventilator is used,[94,95] although there is a risk of barotrauma.[94] There are only anecdotal reports of emergency oxygenation and ventilation using a transtracheal catheter in children, so further evaluation is required. Performance of needle cricothyrotomy requires specialized training. A large-bore (eg, 14-gauge) over-the-needle catheter is used to puncture the cricothyroid membrane percutaneously. The needle is then removed, and the catheter is joined with a standard (3-mm) tracheal tube adapter to an oxygen source and hand resuscitator bag or a high-pressure oxygen source.[96] This technique allows effective support of oxygenation, although CO_2 elimination may be suboptimal. Alternatively, emergency cricothyroidotomy may be performed using a modified Seldinger technique, whereby a small-bore needle is used to puncture the cricothyroid membrane.[97] A flexible wire is then inserted, followed by a dilator and finally a tracheostomy-like tube, permitting adequate oxygenation and ventilation. In an infant the small size of the cricothyroid membrane limits the feasibility of both techniques.

Circulatory Adjuncts

Bedboard
CPR should be performed where the victim is found. If cardiac arrest occurs in a hospital bed, place a firm support beneath the patient's back. A bedboard that extends from the shoulders to the waist and across the full width of the bed provides optimal support. The width of the board is especially important in larger children to avoid losing the force of compression by the mattress sinking down when the chest is compressed. Spine boards, preferably with head wells, should be used in ambulances and mobile life support units.[98,99] They provide a firm surface for CPR in the emergency vehicle or on a wheeled stretcher and also may be useful for extricating and immobilizing victims. In infants a firm surface should also be used under the back. The 2 thumb–encircling hands technique provides support by positioning the fingers behind the infant's back (see "Part 9: Pediatric Basic Life Support").

Mechanical Devices for Chest Compression
Mechanical devices to compress the sternum are not recommended for pediatric patients because they were designed and tested for use in adults, and data on pediatric safety and effectiveness is absent. Active compression-decompression CPR increases cardiac output compared with standard CPR in various animal models,[100,101] maintains coronary perfusion during compression and decompression CPR in humans,[102] and provides ventilation if the airway is open.[102] Clinical

trials report variable results with some benefit on short-term outcome measures (eg, return of spontaneous circulation and survival for 24 hours)[103–105] but no long-term survival benefits in most trials. On the basis of these variable clinical results, active compression-decompression CPR is considered an optional technique in adults (Class IIb; LOE 2, 5, 7). No recommendation can be made for children given the absence of clinical data (Class Indeterminate; LOE 7).

Interposed Abdominal Compression CPR
The technique of interposed abdominal compression CPR (IAC-CPR) does not use an adjunct piece of equipment but does require a third rescuer. This form of chest compression has been shown to increase blood flow in laboratory and computer models of adult CPR and in some in-hospital clinical settings. IAC-CPR has been recommended as an alternative technique (Class IIb) for in-hospital CPR in adult victims, but it cannot be recommended for use in children at this time.[106]

Medical Antishock Trousers
The effects of medical antishock trousers (MAST) during resuscitation of pediatric cardiac arrest are unknown, and the use of MAST cannot be recommended (Class III). The efficacy of MAST in the treatment of pediatric circulatory failure is controversial. Although MAST therapy was thought to be helpful in the treatment of hemorrhagic shock, randomized trials show either no benefit of MAST[107] or an increased mortality with their use.[108] One case series suggests that MAST may be useful in children with pelvic hemorrhage.[109] Potential complications of MAST include lower-extremity compartment syndrome and ischemia[110] and compromised ventilation.[111] If MAST are used, healthcare providers must be familiar with the proper indications, hazards, and complications of this therapy.

Open-Chest Cardiac Compression
Internal (open-chest) cardiac compression generates better cardiac output and cerebral and myocardial blood flow in animals[112] and adults[113] than closed-chest compressions, but comparable improvement in cardiac output may not be observed in infants and children because the chest wall is extremely compliant in this age group.[114,115] The use of open thoracotomy and direct cardiac compression does not appear to be beneficial in the treatment of blunt traumatic pediatric arrest and may increase the cost for short-term survivors,[116] although it is usually attempted relatively late in the course. Limited data suggests that early open-chest CPR may be useful in adults with nontraumatic arrest,[117] but this technique has not been evaluated in nontraumatic pediatric arrest. In the absence of adequate clinical data showing a beneficial effect, internal cardiac compression for children in cardiac arrest cannot be routinely recommended at this time (Class Indeterminate).

Extracorporeal Membrane Oxygenation
There is limited clinical experience with the use of extracorporeal membrane oxygenation (ECMO) to support the circulation after cardiac arrest. Most of the reported experience is

in children after cardiac surgery or in the cardiac catheterization laboratory.[118–120] Even with standard CPR for >50 minutes, long-term survival is possible with the use of ECMO in selected pediatric cardiac surgical patients,[118–120] although application of this technique requires specialized expensive equipment and a readily available experienced team. Emergency cardiopulmonary bypass also has been used, but it is difficult to achieve rapidly and may be associated with significant complications.[121] Nevertheless, occasional patients have attained neurologically intact survival despite intervals from arrest to cardiopulmonary bypass longer than 30 minutes.[122] Late application of cardiopulmonary bypass, however, was uniformly unsuccessful for 10 adults in an Emergency Department after prolonged arrest before bypass.[123] ECMO and emergency cardiopulmonary bypass should be considered optional techniques for selected patients when used by properly trained personnel in experienced specialty centers (Class IIb; LOE 5).

Establishing and Maintaining Vascular Access

Selection of Site and Priorities of Vascular Access

Vascular access is vital for drug and fluid administration but may be difficult to achieve in the pediatric patient.[124] During CPR the preferred access site is the largest, most accessible vein that does not require interruption of resuscitation.

Although central venous drug administration results in more rapid onset of action and higher peak drug levels than peripheral venous administration in adult resuscitation models,[125] these differences were not shown in a pediatric resuscitation model[126] and may not be important during pediatric CPR. Central venous lines provide more secure access to the circulation and permit administration of agents that might cause tissue injury if they infiltrate peripheral sites, such as vasopressors, hypertonic sodium bicarbonate, and calcium. For this reason, if a central venous catheter is in place at the time of arrest, it should be used (Class IIa; LOE 6, 7). Experienced providers may attempt central venous access, using the femoral, internal jugular, external jugular, or (in older children) subclavian vein. The femoral vein is probably the safest and easiest to cannulate. For rapid fluid resuscitation, a single-lumen, wide-bore, relatively short catheter is preferred because this results in lower resistance to flow. Catheter lengths of 5 cm in an infant, 8 cm in a young child, and 12 cm in an older child are usually suitable. If central venous pressure monitoring is desired from a femoral catheter, the catheter tip does not need to be inserted to a point above the diaphragm, provided that there is an unobstructed vena cava.[127,128]

Peripheral venous access provides a satisfactory route for administration of drugs or fluid if it can be achieved rapidly. Peripheral venipuncture can be performed in the veins of the arm, hand, leg, or foot. Drugs administered via peripheral vein during CPR should be followed by a rapid isotonic crystalloid flush (5 to 10 mL) to move the drugs into the central circulation.

The resuscitation team should use a protocol to establish vascular access during CPR. Such a protocol limits the time devoted to attempts at peripheral and central venous catheterization.[129] In infants and children requiring emergent access for severe shock or for prearrest conditions, establish intraosseous vascular access if reliable venous access cannot be achieved rapidly. The clinical hallmarks of decompensated shock or the prearrest state typically include at least several of the following signs: depressed level of consciousness, prolonged capillary refill, decreased or absent peripheral pulses, tachycardia, and a narrow pulse pressure. Because establishing vascular access in pediatric cardiac arrest victims is difficult, it may be preferable to attempt intraosseous access immediately.

If vascular access is not achieved rapidly in cardiac arrest patients and the airway is secured, lipid-soluble resuscitation drugs such as epinephrine may be administered through the tracheal route. Whenever a vascular route is available, however, it is preferable to tracheal drug administration (see below).

Intraosseous Access

An intraosseous cannula provides access to a noncollapsible marrow venous plexus, which serves as a rapid, safe, and reliable route for administration of drugs, crystalloids, colloids, and blood during resuscitation (Class IIa; LOE 3, 5).[130,131] Intraosseous vascular access often can be achieved in 30 to 60 seconds.[131,132] This technique uses a rigid needle, preferably a specially designed intraosseous or Jamshidi-type bone marrow needle. Although a styleted intraosseous needle is preferred to prevent obstruction of the needle with cortical bone, an 18-gauge butterfly needle has been used successfully to provide fluid resuscitation of children with severe dehydration[133] and may be considered but is not routinely recommended.

The intraosseous needle typically is inserted into the anterior tibial bone marrow; alternative sites include the distal femur, medial malleolus, or anterior superior iliac spine. In older children and adults, intraosseous cannulas were successfully inserted into the distal radius and ulna in addition to the proximal tibia.[134–136] The success rate for intraosseous cannulation tends to be lower in the prehospital setting in older children, but it still represents a reasonable alternative when vascular access cannot be achieved rapidly (Class IIa; LOE 5).[134,135]

Resuscitation drugs including epinephrine and adenosine, fluids, and blood products can be safely administered by the intraosseous route.[130,135] Potent catecholamine solutions also can be infused by the intraosseous route.[137] Onset of action and drug levels following intraosseous drug administration during CPR are comparable to those achieved following vascular administration, and drug concentrations similar to those from central venous administration have been documented.[138] To overcome the resistance of emissary veins, fluid for rapid volume resuscitation and viscous drugs and solutions may require administration under pressure via an infusion pump or forceful manual pressure.[139,140] Despite concerns that high-pressure infusion of blood may induce hemolysis and increase fat emboli to the lung, this was not observed in an experimental animal model.[141]

On the basis of animal studies the intraosseous route also may be used to obtain blood specimens for chemical and blood gas analysis and type and crossmatch, even during cardiac arrest.[142,143] Administration of sodium bicarbonate through an intraosseous cannula, however, eliminates the close correlation of intraosseous blood gases with mixed venous blood gases.[143] Complications were reported in <1% of patients after intraosseous infusion.[144,145] Complications include tibial fracture,[146] lower-extremity compartment syndrome or severe extravasation of drugs,[147,148] and osteomyelitis.[144,149] Some of these complications may be avoided by careful technique. Animal data[150,151] and one human follow-up study[152] showed that local effects of intraosseous infusion on the bone marrow and bone growth are minimal. Although microscopic pulmonary fat and bone marrow emboli have been reported,[153] they have never been reported clinically and appear to occur just as frequently during cardiac arrest without use of intraosseous drug administration.[153,154]

Tracheal Drug Administration

Until vascular access is obtained, the tracheal route may be used for administration of lipid-soluble drugs, including lidocaine, epinephrine, atropine, and naloxone (remembered with the mnemonic "LEAN").[155,156] Drugs that are not lipid soluble (eg, sodium bicarbonate and calcium) should *not* be administered by this route because they will injure the airways. Optimal drug dosages for administration by the tracheal route are unknown because drug absorption across the alveolar and bronchiolar epithelium during cardiac arrest may vary widely. Data from animal models,[157] including a neonatal piglet model[158] and one adult human study,[159] suggests, however, that a standard intravenous dose of epinephrine administered via the tracheal route produces serum concentrations that are only approximately 10% or less than those of an equivalent dose administered by the intravenous route. For this reason the recommended tracheal dose of epinephrine during pediatric resuscitation is approximately 10 times the dose given via an intravascular route (Class IIb; LOE 5, 6). It is logical to assume that doses of other resuscitation drugs administered tracheally should be increased compared with the intravenous dose.

When drugs are administered by the tracheal route, animal data suggests that dilution of the drug in up to 5 mL of normal saline followed by 5 manual ventilations results in equivalent absorption and pharmacological effect compared with administration through a catheter or feeding tube inserted into the tracheal tube.[160] Therefore, administration of drugs by the tracheal route is preferred, because administration via catheter or feeding tube is often cumbersome and depends on finding the correct-size catheter to place through the tracheal tube.

Fluid and Drug Therapy

Estimating Patient Weight in an Emergency

Pharmacotherapy in children is complicated by the need to adjust dosages to a wide variety of body weights. Unfortunately, during an emergency, particularly in the out-of-hospital and Emergency Department settings, the child's weight often is unknown. Skilled personnel may not accurately estimate a child's weight on the basis of appearance.[161]

Use of a growth chart to estimate weight from age is also impractical because a growth chart may not be readily available and the child's age may not be known. Moreover, there is a wide distribution of normal weight for a given age.

Length is easily measured and enables reliable calculation of emergency medication dosages. Tapes to determine weight from length are available with precalculated doses printed at various lengths. These tapes, based on normative data relating body length to weight, have been clinically validated.[55,161] Such tapes may be extremely helpful during management of pediatric emergencies. For hospitalized children, weight should be recorded and emergency drug doses precalculated, and this information should be easy to locate in case of an emergency.

Intravascular Fluids

Expansion of circulating blood volume is a critical component of PALS in children who have sustained trauma with acute blood loss. It may also be lifesaving in the treatment of nontraumatic shock, such as severe dehydration or septic shock.[162] Early restitution of circulating blood volume is important to prevent progression to refractory shock or cardiac arrest.[162] Volume expansion is best achieved with isotonic crystalloid solutions, such as Ringer's lactate or normal saline. Meta-analyses of studies comparing crystalloid to colloid administration in various types of shock or hypoalbuminemia suggests that albumin administration may be associated with increased mortality,[163,164] but few children were included in these studies and no firm recommendation can be made against the use of colloid solutions (eg, 5% albumin) in fluid resuscitation of infants and children.

Infusion of hypertonic saline solutions appears to be beneficial in studies of head-injured adult patients[165,166] and hypovolemic shock,[167] but there is insufficient data in children[168] to recommend the widespread use of these solutions at this time. Consistent with adult trauma life support guidelines, blood replacement is indicated in children with severe acute hemorrhage if the child remains in shock after infusion of 40 to 60 mL/kg of crystalloid.

Dextrose solutions (ie, 5% dextrose in water) should *not* be used for initial fluid resuscitation of children (Class III; LOE 6) because large volumes of glucose-containing intravenous solutions do not effectively expand the intravascular compartment and may result in hyperglycemia and a secondary osmotic diuresis. Hyperglycemia *before* cerebral ischemia worsens neurological outcome.[169] Hyperglycemia detected after traumatic or nontraumatic cardiac arrest is also associated with worse neurological outcome.[170,171] This data suggests that the presence of postarrest or postresuscitation hyperglycemia may reflect multiorgan system injury with impaired use of glucose (ie, postischemic hyperglycemia may be an epiphenomenon and not a cause of the poor neurological outcome).

If hypoglycemia is suspected or confirmed, it is readily treated with intravenous glucose (see "Glucose," below). During cardiac arrest, intravenous fluids are used to keep an intravenous line patent for drug administration and to flush drugs from the catheter toward the central venous circulation. In general, for children in cardiac arrest or receiving PALS,

Ringer's lactate or normal saline should be used because some drugs are incompatible in dextrose. Moreover, if the patient requires subsequent fluid resuscitation, use of these isotonic fluids avoids inadvertent bolus administration of dextrose-containing solutions.

Drugs Used for Cardiac Arrest and Resuscitation

Epinephrine

Epinephrine is an endogenous catecholamine with potent α- and β-adrenergic–stimulating properties. In cardiac arrest, α-adrenergic–mediated vasoconstriction is the most important pharmacological action; vasoconstriction increases aortic diastolic pressure and thus the coronary perfusion pressure, which is a critical determinant of success or failure of resuscitation.[172,173] Epinephrine-induced elevation of coronary perfusion pressure during chest compression enhances delivery of oxygen to the heart. Epinephrine also enhances the contractile state of the heart, stimulates spontaneous contractions, and increases the vigor and intensity of VF, increasing the success of defibrillation.[174]

The most commonly observed rhythms in the pediatric patient with cardiac arrest are asystole and bradyarrhythmia[2,175,176]; epinephrine may generate a perfusing rhythm in children with these rhythms. In a child with symptomatic bradycardia that is unresponsive to effective assisted ventilation and supplemental oxygenation, epinephrine may be given in a dose of 0.01 mg/kg (0.1 mL/kg of 1:10 000 solution) by the intravenous or intraosseous route or 0.1 mg/kg (0.1 mL/mg of 1:1000 solution) by the tracheal route. Because the action of catecholamines may be depressed by acidosis and hypoxemia,[177,178] attention to ventilation, oxygenation, and circulation is essential. Continuous epinephrine infusion (0.1 to 0.2 μg/kg per minute, titrated to effect) may be considered for refractory bradycardia.

High doses of epinephrine (10 to 20 times the routine dose) improve myocardial and cerebral blood flow in animals with cardiac arrest.[179,180] High rescue doses of epinephrine (0.2 mg/kg) were associated with improved survival and neurological outcome compared with that in a historic cohort in a single, nonblinded clinical trial of 20 children with witnessed cardiac arrest.[181] Enthusiasm was replaced by disappointment, however, after large multi-institutional adult studies,[182–186] well-controlled animal outcome studies,[187,188] and uncontrolled retrospective pediatric data[189,190] failed to show any benefit from high-dose epinephrine. Moreover, high-dose epinephrine can have adverse effects, including increased myocardial oxygen consumption during CPR, a postarrest hyperadrenergic state with tachycardia, hypertension and ventricular ectopy, myocardial necrosis, and worse postarrest myocardial dysfunction.[187,188,191,192] Finally, since great interpatient variability in catecholamine response is well established in the nonarrest state,[193,194] it is possible that a dangerous dose in one patient may be lifesaving in another.

The recommended initial resuscitation dose of epinephrine for cardiac arrest is 0.01 mg/kg (0.1 mL/kg of 1:10 000 solution) given by the intravenous or intraosseous route or 0.1 mg/kg (0.1 mL/kg of 1:1000 solution) by the tracheal route

(Table 2 and Figure 2); repeated doses are recommended every 3 to 5 minutes for ongoing arrest. The same dose of epinephrine is recommended for second and subsequent doses for unresponsive asystolic and pulseless arrest, but higher doses of epinephrine (0.1 to 0.2 mg/kg; 0.1 to 0.2 mL/kg of 1:1000 solution) by any intravascular route may be considered (Class IIb; LOE 6). If the initial dose of epinephrine is not effective, administer subsequent doses within 3 to 5 minutes and repeat every 3 to 5 minutes during resuscitation. If high-dose epinephrine is used, note that 2 different dilutions of epinephrine are needed; take care to avoid errors in selecting the correct concentration and dose. If the patient has continuous intra-arterial pressure monitoring during CPR, subsequent epinephrine doses can be titrated to effect. For example, standard epinephrine doses are rational if the aortic diastolic pressure is greater than approximately 20 mm Hg, whereas higher epinephrine doses are rational if the diastolic pressure is lower.

Epinephrine is absorbed when administered by the tracheal route, although absorption and resulting plasma concentrations are unpredictable.[158,195] The recommended tracheal dose is 0.1 mg/kg (0.1 mL/kg of a 1:1000 solution) (Class IIb; LOE 6). Once vascular access is obtained, administer epinephrine intravascularly, beginning with a dose of 0.01 mg/kg, if the victim remains in cardiac arrest.

A continuous infusion of epinephrine may be useful once spontaneous circulation is restored. The hemodynamic effects are dose related: low-dose infusions (<0.3 μg/kg per minute) generally produce prominent β-adrenergic action, and higher-dose infusions (>0.3 μg/kg per minute) result in β- and α-adrenergic–mediated vasoconstriction.[196] Since there is great interpatient variability in catecholamine pharmacology,[194,197] the infused dose should be titrated to the desired effect.

Administer epinephrine through a secure intravascular line, preferably into the central circulation. If the drug infiltrates into tissues, it may cause local ischemia, leading to tissue injury and ulceration. Epinephrine (and other catecholamines) are inactivated in alkaline solutions and should never be mixed with sodium bicarbonate. In patients with a perfusing rhythm, epinephrine causes tachycardia and often a wide pulse pressure and may produce ventricular ectopy. High infusion doses may produce excessive vasoconstriction, compromising extremity, mesenteric, and renal blood flow and resulting in severe hypertension and tachyarrhythmias.[187]

Atropine

Atropine is discussed in "Treatment of Bradyarrhythmias," below.

Vasopressin

Vasopressin is an endogenous hormone that acts at specific receptors to mediate systemic vasoconstriction (V_1 receptor) and reabsorption of water in the renal tubule (V_2 receptor). Marked secretion of vasopressin occurs in circulatory shock states and causes relatively selective vasoconstriction of blood vessels in the skin, skeletal muscle, intestine, and fat with relatively less vasoconstriction of the coronary, cerebral, and renal vascular beds. This hemodynamic action produces

TABLE 2.   PALS Medications for Cardiac Arrest and Symptomatic Arrhythmias

Drug	Dosage (Pediatric)	Remarks
Adenosine	0.1 mg/kg	Rapid IV/IO bolus
	Repeat dose: 0.2 mg/kg	Rapid flush to central circulation
	Maximum single dose: 12 mg	Monitor ECG during dose.
Amiodarone for pulseless VF/VT	5 mg/kg IV/IO	Rapid IV bolus
Amiodarone for perfusing tachycardias	Loading dose: 5 mg/kg IV/IO	IV over 20 to 60 minutes
	Maximum dose: 15 mg/kg per day	Routine use in combination with drugs prolonging QT interval is *not* recommended. Hypotension is most frequent side effect.
Atropine sulfate*	0.02 mg/kg	May give IV, IO or ET.
	Minimum dose: 0.1 mg	Tachycardia and pupil dilation may occur but *not* fixed dilated pupils.
	Maximum single dose: 0.5 mg in child, 1.0 mg in adolescent. May repeat once.	
Calcium chloride 10%=100 mg/mL (=27.2 mg/mL elemental Ca)	20 mg/kg (0.2 mL/kg) IV/IO	Give slow IV push for hypocalcemia, hypermagnesemia, calcium channel blocker toxicity, preferably via central vein. Monitor heart rate; bradycardia may occur.
Calcium gluconate 10%=100 mg/mL (=9 mg/mL elemental Ca)	60–100 mg/kg (0.6–1.0 mL/kg) IV/IO	Give slow IV push for hypocalcemia, hypermagnesemia, calcium channel blocker toxicity, preferably via central vein.
Epinephrine for symptomatic bradycardia*	IV/IO: 0.01 mg/kg (1:10 000, 0.1 mL/kg) ET: 0.1 mg/kg (1:1000, 0.1 mL/kg)	Tachyarrhythmias, hypertension may occur.
Epinephrine for pulseless arrest*	First dose:	
	IV/IO: 0.01 mg/kg (1:10 000, 0.1 mL/kg)	
	ET: 0.1 mg/kg (1:1000, 0.1 mL/kg)	
	Subsequent doses: Repeat initial dose or may increase up to 10 times (0.1 mg/kg, 1:1000, 0.1 mL/kg)	
	Administer epinephrine every 3 to 5 minutes.	
	IV/IO/ET doses as high as 0.2 mg/kg of 1:1000 may be effective.	
Glucose (10% or 25% or 50%)	IV/IO: 0.5–1.0 g/kg	For suspected hypoglycemia; avoid hyperglycemia.
	• 1–2 mL/kg 50%	
	• 2–4 mL/kg 25%	
	• 5–10 mL/kg 10%	
Lidocaine*	IV/IO/ET: 1 mg/kg	Rapid bolus
Lidocaine infusion (start after a bolus)	IV/IO: 20–50 μg/kg per minute	1 to 2.5 mL/kg per hour of 120 mg/100 mL solution or use "Rule of 6" (see Table 3)
Magnesium sulfate (500 mg/mL)	IV/IO: 25–50 mg/kg, Maximum dose: 2 g per dose	Rapid IV infusion for torsades or suspected hypomagnesemia; 10- to 20-minute infusion for asthma that responds poorly to β-adrenergic agonists.
Naloxone*	≤5 years or ≤20 kg: 0.1 mg/kg	For total reversal of narcotic effect. Use small repeated doses (0.01 to 0.03 mg/kg) titrated to desired effect.
	>5 years or >20 kg: 2.0 mg	
Procainamide for perfusing tachycardias (100 mg/mL and 500 mg/mL)	Loading dose: 15 mg/kg IV/IO	Infusion over 30 to 60 minutes; routine use in combination with drugs prolonging QT interval is *not* recommended.
Sodium bicarbonate (1 mEq/mL and 0.5 mEq/mL)	IV/IO: 1 mEq/kg per dose	Infuse slowly and only if ventilation is adequate.

IV indicates intravenous; IO, intraosseous; and ET, endotracheal.

*For endotracheal administration use higher doses (2 to 10 times the IV dose); dilute medication with normal saline to a volume of 3 to 5 mL and follow with several positive-pressure ventilations.

favorable increases in blood flow to the heart and brain in experimental models of cardiac arrest[198,199] and improved long-term survival compared with epinephrine.[200] Although adverse effects on splanchnic blood flow are a theoretical concern following large doses of vasopressin, modest declines in adrenal and renal blood flow are seen in experimental animals with no effect on intestinal or hepatic perfusion,[201] even after repeated doses.[202]

A small study in adults with VF resistant to defibrillation randomized subjects to receive epinephrine or vasopressin plus epinephrine.[203] The patients receiving vasopressin plus epinephrine were significantly more likely to survive to hospital admission and for 24 hours. Even low-dose vasopressin infusions demonstrated significant pressor effect in critically ill adults[204,205] and critically ill infants and children during evaluation for brain death and organ recovery.[206] Despite promising animal and limited clinical data,[207] there is no data on the use of vasopressin in pediatric cardiac arrest. Moreover, in a piglet model of prolonged asphyxial cardiac arrest, vasopressin was less effective than epinephrine.[208] Even though vasopressin is an alternative vasopressor in the treatment of adult shock-refractory VF, there is inadequate data to evaluate its efficacy and safety in infants and children at this time (Class Indeterminate; LOE 2, 6).

Calcium

Calcium is essential in myocardial excitation-contraction coupling. However, routine calcium administration does not improve outcome of cardiac arrest.[209] In addition, several studies implicated cytoplasmic calcium accumulation in the final common pathway of cell death.[210] Calcium accumulation results from calcium entering cells after ischemia and during reperfusion of ischemic organs; increased cytoplasmic calcium concentration activates intracellular enzyme systems, resulting in cellular necrosis.

Although calcium has been recommended in the treatment of electromechanical dissociation and asystole, experimental evidence for efficacy in either setting is lacking.[209,211] Therefore, routine administration of calcium in resuscitation of asystolic patients cannot be recommended. Calcium is indicated for treatment of documented hypocalcemia and hyperkalemia,[212] particularly in hemodynamically compromised patients. Ionized hypocalcemia is relatively common in critically ill children, particularly those with sepsis.[213,214] Calcium also should be considered for treatment of hypermagnesemia[215] and calcium channel blocker overdose[216] (Class IIa; LOE 5, 6).

There is little information about the optimal emergency dose of calcium. The currently recommended dose of 5 to 7 mg/kg of elemental calcium is based on extrapolation from adult data and limited pediatric data.[217] Calcium chloride 10% (100 mg/mL) is the calcium preparation of choice in children because it provides greater bioavailability of calcium than calcium gluconate.[217] A dose of 0.2 mL/kg of 10% calcium chloride will provide 20 mg/kg of the salt and 5.4 mg/kg of elemental calcium. The dose should be infused by slow intravenous push over 10 to 20 seconds during cardiac arrest or over 5 to 10 minutes in perfusing patients. In cardiac arrest, the dose may be repeated in 10 minutes if required.

Further doses should be based on measured deficits of ionized calcium.

Magnesium

Magnesium is a major intracellular cation and serves as a cofactor in >300 enzymatic reactions. The plasma magnesium concentration is composed of bound and unbound fractions in a manner that is similar to that of calcium; approximately 50% of the circulating magnesium is free (ie, ionized). In critically ill patients the total magnesium concentration may poorly reflect the physiological (ionized) concentration[218,219]; the latter can be measured with ion-selective electrodes. Particularly in pharmacological concentrations,[220] magnesium can inhibit calcium channels, which represents some of the potentially therapeutic effects of magnesium. Through inhibition of calcium channels and the subsequent reduction of intracellular calcium concentration, magnesium causes smooth muscle relaxation, which has been used in the treatment of acute severe asthma.[221] In addition, the effects of magnesium on calcium channels, and perhaps other membrane effects, have been useful in the treatment of torsades de pointes VT.[222]

The beneficial effect of magnesium in acute asthma is debated; studies report conflicting results.[221,223,224] In a randomized, prospective, double-blind pediatric trial, children who continued to have poor respiratory function (peak expiratory flow rate <60% of predicted) after 3 nebulized albuterol treatments were randomized to receive magnesium sulfate (25 mg/kg up to 2 g) or placebo.[221] The children in the magnesium group had significantly greater improvement in pulmonary function and were less likely to be admitted for treatment than the placebo group. The entry criteria for this study may explain why earlier studies failed to show a beneficial effect: the study population was composed of those children who failed routine management with 3 nebulized albuterol treatments before study entry. This observation is consistent with a similarly designed randomized, blinded trial in children[225] and a randomized, blinded clinical trial in adults showing that magnesium infusion (2 g over 20 minutes) produced a beneficial effect only in the most severely ill patients.[226] Thus, data does not support the routine use of magnesium in asthma therapy but shows that it may be beneficial in children with severe asthma despite routine medical therapy. A dose of 25 to 50 mg/kg (up to 2 g) may be given safely over 10 to 20 minutes by intravenous infusion.[225,227] Blood pressure and heart rate should be monitored during infusion. Although some evidence suggests that a threshold serum concentration is needed to produce a beneficial effect,[228,229] there is insufficient data to recommend trying to achieve a specific serum concentration.

Magnesium has been used in the treatment of a wide range of arrhythmias and was used in post–myocardial infarction patients to reduce ventricular arrhythmias. Data, however, supports only the routine use of magnesium sulfate in patients with documented hypomagnesemia or with torsades de pointes VT.[222,230] This is a unique polymorphic VT characterized by an ECG appearance of QRS complexes changing in amplitude and polarity so that they appear to rotate around an isoelectric line. It is seen in conditions distinguished by a long QT interval. Prolongation of the QT interval may occur in congenital conditions (eg, Romano-Ward and Jervell and Lange-Nielsen) or following drug toxicity. Type I_A anti-arrhythmics (eg, quinidine and disopyramide), type III (eg, sotalol and amiodarone), tricyclic antidepressants (see discussion below), and digitalis are all reported causes. In addition, unanticipated pharmacokinetic interactions may cause torsades de pointes; the interaction between cisapride and inhibitors of the cytochrome P450 system (eg, clarithromycin or erythromycin) is a recently recognized problem.[231] Regardless of the cause, magnesium sulfate in a rapid intravenous infusion (several minutes) of 25 to 50 mg/kg (up to 2 g) is recommended in the setting of torsades de pointes VT.

Glucose

Infants have high glucose requirements and low glycogen stores. As a result, during periods of increased energy requirements, such as shock, the infant may become hypoglycemic. For this reason, monitor blood glucose concentrations closely using rapid bedside tests during coma, shock, or respiratory failure. Documented hypoglycemia should be treated with an infusion of a glucose-containing solution. A dose of 2 to 4 mL/kg of 25% glucose (250 mg/mL) will provide 0.5 to 1.0 g/kg; 10% glucose (100 mg/mL) may be used at a dose of 5 to 10 mL/kg to deliver a similar quantity of glucose.

If possible, treat hypoglycemia with a continuous glucose infusion; bolus therapy with hypertonic glucose should be limited if possible because it may contribute to a sharp rise in serum osmolality and may result in an osmotic diuresis. Furthermore, hyperglycemia before cerebral ischemia worsens neurological outcome,[169,232] although the effect of hyperglycemia occurring *after* cerebral ischemia on neurological function is unknown. Combined administration of glucose, insulin, and potassium after an ischemic insult may be beneficial, based on data in adults showing that this infusion improves outcome and reduces complications after myocardial infarction.[233] In the absence of convincing data showing benefit or harm of hyperglycemia *after* arrest, the current recommendation is to ensure that the blood glucose concentration is at least normal during resuscitation and that hypoglycemia is avoided after resuscitation.

Sodium Bicarbonate

Although sodium bicarbonate previously was recommended for the treatment of severe metabolic acidosis in cardiac arrest, in most but not all[234] studies routine sodium bicarbonate administration failed to improve the outcome of cardiac arrest.[235] In children, respiratory failure is the major cause of cardiac arrest. Because sodium bicarbonate therapy transiently elevates CO_2 tension, administration of this drug to the pediatric patient during resuscitation may worsen existing respiratory acidosis. For these reasons treatment priorities for the infant or child in cardiac arrest should include assisting ventilation, supplementing oxygen, and restoring effective systemic perfusion (to correct tissue ischemia). Once effective ventilation is ensured and epinephrine plus chest compressions are provided to maximize circulation, use of sodium

bicarbonate may be considered for the patient with prolonged cardiac arrest (Class IIb; LOE 6, 7).

Administration of this drug also may be considered when shock is associated with documented severe metabolic acidosis (Class IIb), although clinical trials in acidotic critically ill adults failed to show a beneficial effect of sodium bicarbonate on hemodynamics despite improvements in metabolic acidosis.[236,237] There is no specific level of acidosis that requires treatment; the decision to administer sodium bicarbonate is determined by the acuity and severity of the acidosis and the child's circulatory state, among other factors. For example, a child with shock and marked metabolic acidosis from dehydration due to diabetic ketoacidosis does not require sodium bicarbonate in most circumstances and will respond well to fluid resuscitation and insulin administration alone.

Sodium bicarbonate is recommended in the treatment of symptomatic patients with hyperkalemia[238] (Class IIa; LOE 6, 7), hypermagnesemia, tricyclic antidepressant overdose, or overdose from other sodium channel blocking agents[239] (see "Special Resuscitation Situations" below; Class IIb; LOE 6, 7). Often patients with these metabolic or toxicological disorders will exhibit ECG abnormalities secondary to adverse effects on the heart.

When indicated, the initial dose of sodium bicarbonate is 1 mEq/kg (1 mL/kg of 8.4% solution) intravenously or via the intraosseous route (Table 2). A dilute solution (0.5 mEq/mL; 4.2% solution) may be used in neonates to limit the osmotic load, but there is no evidence that the dilute solution is beneficial in older infants or children. Further doses of sodium bicarbonate may be based on blood gas analyses. If such measurements are unavailable, subsequent doses of sodium bicarbonate may be considered after every 10 minutes of continued arrest. Even if available, arterial blood gas analysis may not accurately reflect tissue and venous pH during cardiac arrest or severe shock.[240,241] The role of sodium bicarbonate remains unclear in children who have documented postarrest metabolic acidosis.

Excessive sodium bicarbonate administration may have several adverse effects. Resulting metabolic alkalosis produces leftward displacement of the oxyhemoglobin dissociation curve with impaired delivery of oxygen to tissues,[242] acute intracellular shift of potassium, decreased plasma ionized calcium concentration, decreased VF threshold,[243] and impaired cardiac function. Hypernatremia and hyperosmolality may also result from excessive sodium bicarbonate administration.[244,245] Catecholamines are inactivated by bicarbonate and calcium precipitates when mixed with bicarbonate, so the intravenous tubing must be carefully irrigated with a 5- to 10-mL normal saline bolus after administration of sodium bicarbonate. A normal saline bolus (5 to 10 mL) should be given routinely between infusions of any resuscitation drugs.

Rhythm Disturbances

Although primary cardiac events are uncommon in the pediatric age group, the ECGs of all critically ill or injured children should be continuously monitored. In addition to

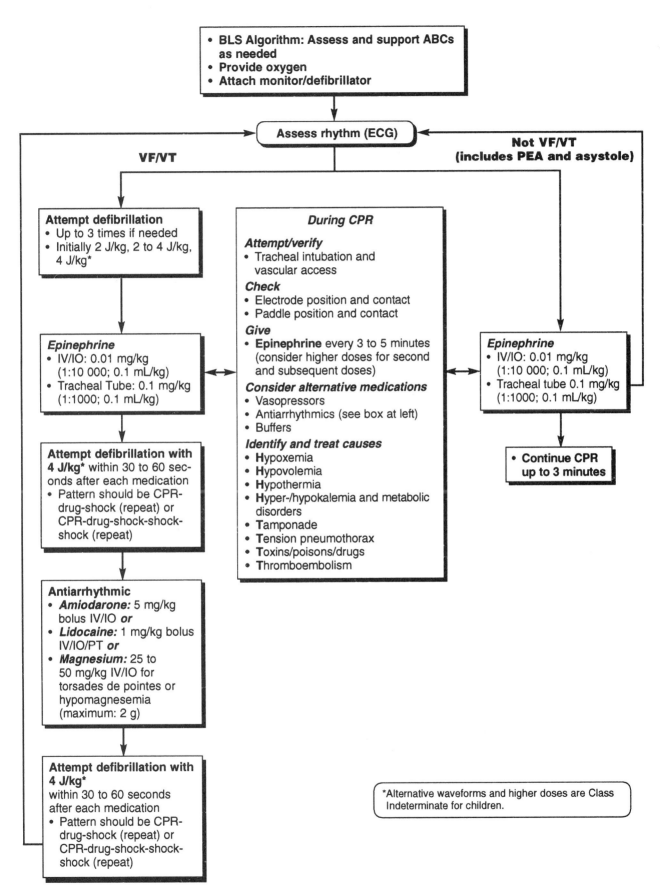

Figure 6. PALS pulseless arrest algorithm.

detecting cardiac arrhythmias, it is worthwhile to monitor changes in the heart rate in response to therapy. Most pediatric arrhythmias are the consequence of hypoxemia, acidosis, and hypotension rather than the cause of these clinical states, but children with myocarditis or cardiomyopathy are at increased risk of primary arrhythmias, as are children after heart surgery. In addition, a number of drugs taken in therapeutic or toxic amounts may cause arrhythmias. When rhythm is recorded in pediatric cardiac arrest victims in the out-of-hospital, Emergency Department, and hospital settings, the majority have asystole or some form of bradyarrhythmia, often with a wide QRS complex.[2,17]

Approximately 10% of reported pediatric cardiac arrest patients had VF or pulseless VT.[2] In a relatively large retrospective out-of-hospital pediatric study, VF was observed in approximately 20% of out-of-hospital cardiac arrest victims after exclusion of SIDS patients.[175]

The likelihood of VF increases with age, based on an analysis of out-of-hospital data. In children with nontraumatic arrest, VF was reported in only 3% of children from 0 to 8 years of age but was observed in 17% of victims from 8 to 30 years of age.[246] In the previously noted out-of-hospital study,[175] VF/VT was much more likely in children >9 years of age through adolescence (20%) than in those <4 years old (6.1% incidence if SIDS cases were included). In other out-of-hospital arrest studies, VF or VT occurred in 9% to 15% of children.[190,247]

The likelihood of detecting a ventricular arrhythmia may depend on the response time or other characteristics of the EMS system, since only 4% of 300 children experiencing an out-of-hospital arrest in the Houston metropolitan area had a ventricular arrhythmia identified on EMS arrival.[17] It is important to recognize and treat ventricular arrhythmias early, since the outcome is significantly better when these arrhythmias are promptly defibrillated than the reported outcome of children with asystole or other nonperfusing rhythms.[175,190,247]

The following sections will review rhythm disturbances moving from slow rhythms to fast rhythms then to VF. Although not technically a specific rhythm disturbance, pulseless electrical activity (PEA) will also be discussed (Figure 6). For each rhythm we review the epidemiology, etiology, and treatment.

Bradyarrhythmias

Hypoxemia, hypothermia, acidosis, hypotension, and hypoglycemia may depress normal sinus node function and slow conduction through the myocardium. In addition, excessive vagal stimulation (eg, induced by suctioning or during endotracheal intubation) may produce bradycardia. Finally, central nervous system insults such as increased intracranial pressure or brain stem compression can result in prominent bradycardia. Sinus bradycardia, sinus node arrest with a slow junctional or idioventricular rhythm, and atrioventricular (AV) block are the most common preterminal rhythms observed in infants and children. When bradycardia is due to heart block, consider drug-induced causes, such as digoxin toxicity, and acute inflammatory injury from myocarditis. In addition, infants and children

with a history of heart surgery are at increased risk of sick sinus syndrome or heart block secondary to injury to the AV node or conduction system. All slow rhythms that result in hemodynamic instability require immediate treatment (Figure 7).

Treatment of Bradyarrhythmias

In the small infant (<6 months), cardiac output is more dependent on heart rate than in the older infant and child; bradycardia is therefore more likely to cause symptoms in young infants. Clinically significant bradycardia is defined as a heart rate <60 bpm or a rapidly dropping heart rate despite adequate oxygenation and ventilation associated with poor systemic perfusion. Clinically significant bradycardia should be treated in a child of any age. Initial treatment should be directed to ensuring that the infant or child is breathing adequately and to providing supplemental oxygen. If a pharmacological agent is needed, epinephrine is the most useful drug in the treatment of symptomatic bradycardia in an infant or child, except for bradycardia caused by heart block or increased vagal tone (Figure 7; Class IIa; LOE 7, 8). For suspected vagally mediated bradycardia, atropine is the initial drug of choice. If the bradycardia persists after adequate oxygenation and ventilation and responds only transiently or not at all to bolus epinephrine or atropine administration, consider a continuous infusion of epinephrine or dopamine (Figure 7).

Atropine sulfate, a parasympatholytic drug, accelerates sinus or atrial pacemakers and increases AV conduction. Atropine is recommended in the treatment of symptomatic bradycardia caused by AV block or increased vagal activity (Class I), such as vagally mediated bradycardia during attempts at intubation. Although atropine may be used to treat bradycardia accompanied by poor perfusion or hypotension (Class IIb), epinephrine may be more effective in treating bradycardia accompanied by hypotension. When indicated, give atropine to treat bradycardia only after ensuring adequate oxygenation and ventilation and temperature (rule out hypothermia).

Small doses of atropine may produce paradoxical bradycardia[248]; the recommended dose is 0.02 mg/kg, with a minimum dose of 0.1 mg and a maximum single dose of 0.5 mg in a child and 1.0 mg in an adolescent.[248] The dose may be repeated in 5 minutes, to a maximum total dose of 1.0 mg in a child and 2.0 mg in an adolescent. Larger intravascular doses may be required in special resuscitation circumstances (eg, organophosphate poisoning).[249] If intravenous access is not readily available, atropine (0.02 mg/kg) may be administered tracheally,[250] although absorption into the circulation may be unreliable.[251]

Tachycardia may follow administration of atropine, but the agent is generally well tolerated in the pediatric patient. Atropine used to block vagally mediated bradycardia during intubation may have the undesirable effect of masking hypoxemia-induced bradycardia. Therefore, during attempts at intubation, monitor oxygen saturation with pulse oximetry and avoid prolonged attempts at intubation.

In selected cases of bradycardia caused by complete heart block or abnormal function of the sinus node, emergency

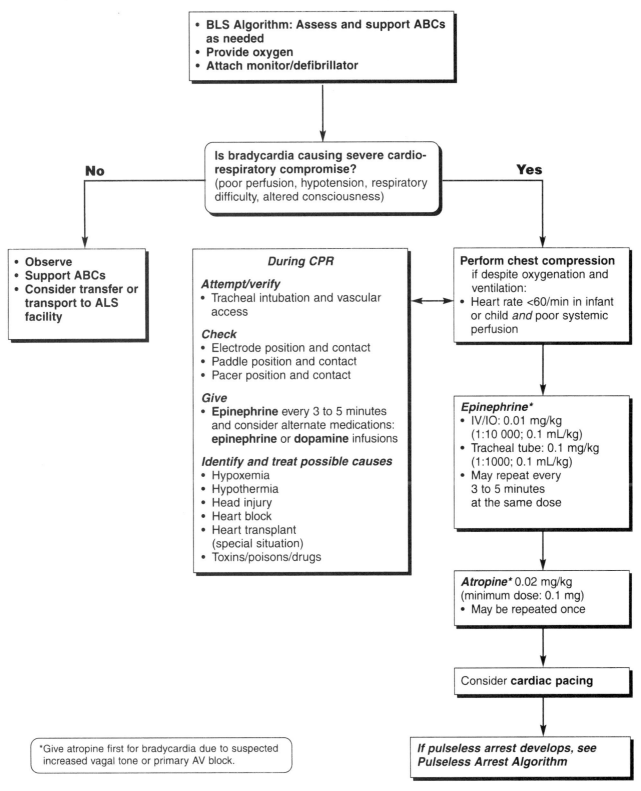

Figure 7. PALS bradycardia algorithm.

transthoracic pacing may be lifesaving.[252] Pacing is not helpful in children with bradycardia secondary to a postarrest hypoxic/ischemic myocardial insult or respiratory failure.[253] Pacing also was not shown to be effective in the treatment of asystole in children.[252,253]

Pulseless Electrical Activity

PEA is a clinical state characterized by organized electrical activity observed on a monitor or ECG in the absence of detectable cardiac output (ie, pulses). This clinical state often represents a preterminal condition that immediately precedes asystole. It frequently represents the final organized electrical state of a severely hypoxic, acidotic myocardium and is usually characterized on the monitor by a slow, wide-complex rhythm in a child who has experienced a prolonged period of hypoxia, ischemia, or hypercarbia. In this setting treat PEA in the same manner as asystole.

Occasionally PEA is due to a reversible cause that often occurs rapidly and represents a sudden impairment of cardiac output. When seen shortly after onset, the ECG rhythm may appear normal and the heart rate may be increased or be rapidly decreasing, but pulses or other evidence of detectable cardiac output are absent and the child appears lifeless. This subcategory of PEA is often called electromechanical dissociation (EMD). Causes of EMD are seen in Figure 6 (earlier in this segment) and can be recalled as the 4 H's and 4 T's. The 4 H's are severe **h**ypovolemia (eg, in trauma), **h**ypoxemia, **h**ypothermia, and **h**yperkalemia (and other metabolic imbalances). The 4 T's are **t**ension pneumothorax, pericardial **t**amponade, **t**oxins, and pulmonary **t**hromboembolus. If EMD is observed, search for evidence of these reversible causes and correct them if identified.

Treatment of PEA

Treat PEA in the same manner as asystole (Figure 6, pulseless arrest algorithm), with the caveat that reversible causes should be identified and corrected. If the patient remains pulseless after you have established an airway, ventilated the lungs, provided supplemental oxygen, and delivered chest compressions, give epinephrine (0.01 mg/kg initial dose). Several of the reversible causes of PEA (ie, hypovolemia, tension pneumothorax, and pericardial tamponade) may be at least partially corrected by the administration of a fluid bolus of normal saline or lactated Ringer's solution. Tension pneumothorax and pericardial tamponade, however, will also require more definitive therapy with needle aspiration or rapid drainage catheter placement. Check the child's temperature and perform immediate (ideally bedside) testing of glucose, electrolytes, and acid-base status. In the out-of-hospital setting, early recognition and effective treatment of PEA (and other rhythm disturbances associated with cardiac arrest) are emphasized on the basis of data reporting that a return of spontaneous circulation before arrival in the Emergency Department is associated with improved survival.[176,247,254]

Supraventricular Tachycardia

Supraventricular tachycardia (SVT) is the most common nonarrest arrhythmia during childhood and is the most common arrhythmia that produces cardiovascular instability during infancy. Usually caused by a reentrant mechanism, SVT in infants generally produces a heart rate >220 bpm and sometimes as high as 300 bpm. Lower heart rates may be observed in children during SVT. The QRS complex is narrow (ie, ≤0.08 seconds) in >90% of involved children,[255,256] making differentiation between marked sinus tachycardia (ST) due to shock and SVT somewhat difficult, particularly because either rhythm may be associated with poor systemic perfusion.

The following characteristics may aid differentiation between ST and SVT (Figure 8):

- A history consistent with shock (eg, dehydration or hemorrhage) is usually present with ST, whereas the history is often vague and nondescript with SVT.
- The heart rate is usually <220 bpm in infants and <180 bpm in children with ST, whereas infants with SVT typically have a heart rate >220 bpm, and children with SVT will typically have a heart rate >180 bpm.
- P waves may be difficult to identify in both ST and SVT once the ventricular rate exceeds 200 bpm, but they are usually present in infants and children with ST. If P waves are identifiable in ST, they are usually upright in leads I and aVF, whereas in SVT they are negative in leads II, III, and aVF.
- In ST the heart rate varies from beat to beat (variable R-R interval) and is often responsive to stimulation, but there is no beat-to-beat variability in SVT. Termination of SVT is abrupt, whereas the heart rate slows gradually in ST.

Cardiopulmonary stability during episodes of SVT is affected by the child's age, duration of SVT, prior ventricular function, and ventricular rate. Older children will typically complain of lightheadedness, dizziness, or chest discomfort, or simply note the fast heart rate. In infants, however, very rapid rates may be undetected for long periods until low cardiac output and shock develop. This deterioration in cardiac function occurs secondary to the combination of increased myocardial oxygen demand and limitation in myocardial oxygen delivery during the short diastolic phase associated with very rapid heart rates. If baseline myocardial function is impaired (eg, in a child with a cardiomyopathy), SVT can produce signs of shock in a relatively short time.

Wide-QRS SVT

Wide-QRS SVT (ie, SVT with aberrant conduction) is uncommon in infants and children. Correct diagnosis and differentiation from VT depends on careful analysis of at least a 12-lead ECG that may be supplemented by information from an esophageal lead. Obtain a patient and family history to help identify the presence of an underlying condition predisposing to stable VT. Because either SVT or VT can cause hemodynamic instability, do not base assumptions about the mechanism (ie, ventricular versus supraventricular) solely on the hemodynamic status of the patient. In most circumstances, wide-complex tachycardias should be treated as if they are VT (Figure 9).

Treatment of SVT

Vagal Maneuvers

In children with milder symptoms who are hemodynamically stable or during preparation for cardioversion or drug therapy, vagal maneuvers may be tried (Class IIa; LOE 4, 5, 7, 8). Success rates with these maneuvers are variable and depend on the presence of underlying conditions in the patient, the patient's level of cooperation, and the patient's age. Ice water applied to the face is most effective in infants and young children.[257,258] One method uses crushed ice mixed with water in a plastic bag or glove. Use care to apply the ice water mixture to the infant's face without obstructing ventilation. Other vagal maneuvers (ie,

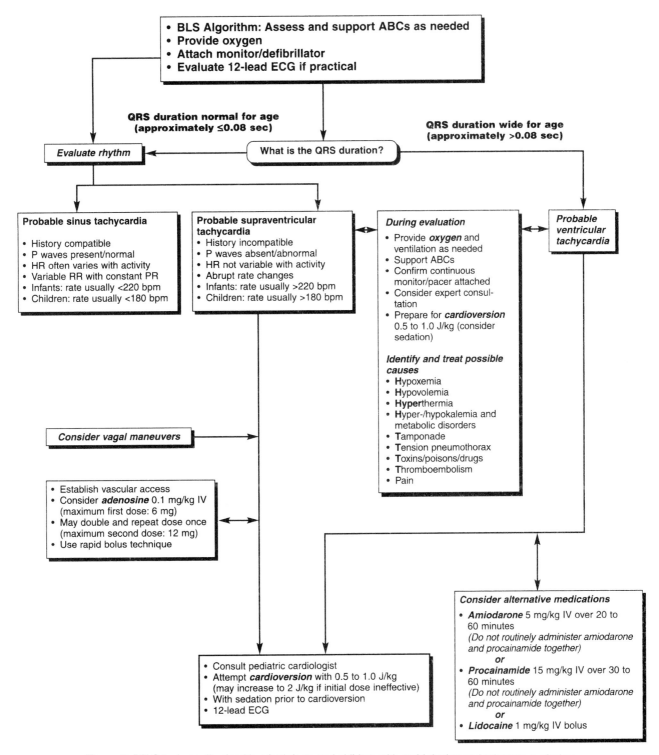

Figure 8. PALS tachycardia algorithm for infants and children with rapid rhythm and adequate perfusion.

carotid sinus massage or Valsalva) may be effective (Class IIb; LOE 5, 7) and appear to be safe on the basis of data obtained largely in older children, adolescents, and adults.[259–261] In children one technique for performing a Valsalva maneuver is to have the child blow through a straw.[260] Regardless of which vagal maneuver is attempted, obtain a 12-lead ECG before and after the vagal maneuver and monitor the ECG continuously during application of the ice water or vagal maneuver. Note that

application of external ocular pressure may be dangerous and should *not* be used to induce a vagal response.

Cardioversion
SVT that causes circulatory instability (eg, congestive heart failure with diminished peripheral perfusion, increased work of breathing and altered level of consciousness, or hypotension) is most expeditiously treated with electrical or chemical cardioversion. Synchronized electrical cardioversion is rec-

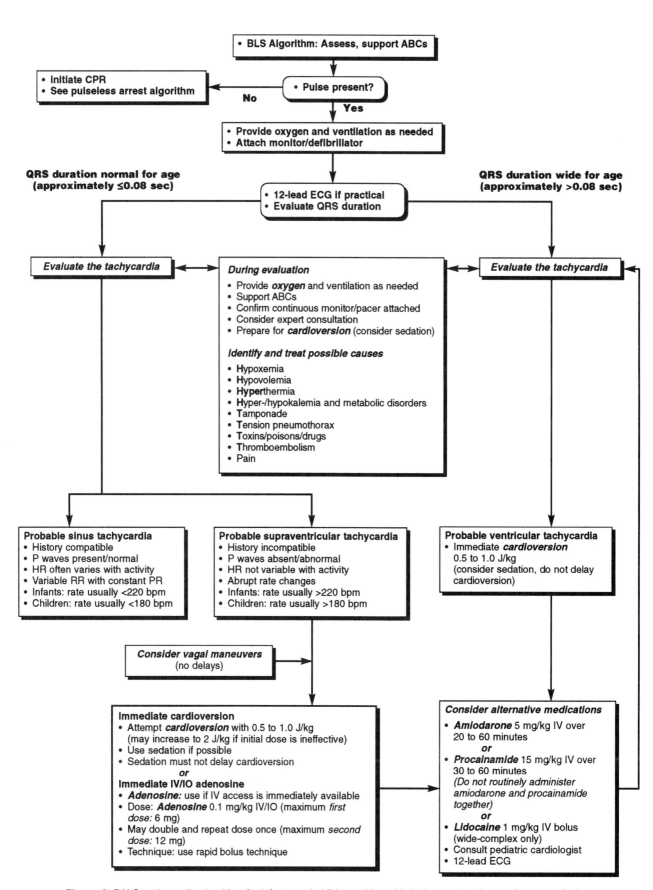

Figure 9. PALS tachycardia algorithm for infants and children with rapid rhythm and evidence of poor perfusion.

ommended at a starting dose of 0.5 to 1 J/kg. If vascular access is already available, adenosine may be administered before electrical cardioversion, but do not delay cardioversion if establishment of vascular access (intravenous or intraosseous) will require >20 to 30 seconds.

Adenosine

When medications are indicated, adenosine is the drug of choice for SVT in children (Class IIa; LOE 2, 3, 7).[256,262] If the patient is unstable, do not delay cardioversion to secure vascular access and deliver adenosine. Adenosine is an endogenous nucleoside that acts at specific receptors to cause a temporary block of conduction through the AV node; it interrupts the reentry circuits that involve the AV node. These reentry circuits are the underlying mechanism for the vast majority of SVT episodes in infants and children. Adenosine is very effective; side effects are minimal because its half-life is only 10 seconds. With continuous ECG monitoring, administer 0.1 mg/kg as a rapid intravenous bolus (Table 2). To enhance delivery of the drug to its site of action in the heart, the injection site should be as close to the heart as possible. A 2-syringe technique is recommended, 1 syringe containing the drug and 1 containing a saline flush of at least 5 mL. Because adenosine is metabolized by an enzyme on the surface of red blood cells (adenosine deaminase), a higher dose may be required for peripheral venous administration than if the drug is administered into a central vein.[256,262] If there is no effect, the dose may be doubled (0.2 mg/kg). The maximum recommended initial adult dose is 6 mg, and 12 mg is the maximum second dose. A single dose of adenosine should not exceed 12 mg.[256,262] Based on experimental data and a case report, adenosine may also be given by the intraosseous route.[263,264]

Verapamil Caution and Alternative Agents

Verapamil should *not* be used to treat SVT in infants because refractory hypotension and cardiac arrest have been reported following its administration (Class III; LOE 5),[265,266] and we discourage its use in children because it may cause hypotension and myocardial depression.[267] When used in children older than 1 year, verapamil is infused in a dose of 0.1 mg/kg. Procainamide and amiodarone are alternative agents for use in children with SVT and stable hemodynamics (Class IIb),[268,269] but they should not be used concurrently with agents that may prolong the QT interval. Therefore, amiodarone and procainamide generally should not be administered together because they both prolong the QT interval (Figure 9).

Treatment of Wide-QRS Tachycardia

The decision to initiate treatment is based on whether the patient is hemodynamically stable. In the absence of a mitigating history, wide-complex tachycardia associated with hemodynamic instability requires urgent treatment, based on the assumption that the rhythm is ventricular in origin (see "Treatment of VT and VF" below). Urgent treatment of a wide-complex tachycardia includes synchronized cardioversion if pulses are present and defibrillation shocks if pulses are lost. Signs of hemodynamic instability include evidence of compromised tissue perfusion and impaired level of consciousness. If the child is hemodynamically stable (ie, has

normal perfusion and level of consciousness), treatment can await further diagnostic studies. Early consultation with a pediatric cardiologist or other physician with appropriate expertise is recommended.

Ventricular Tachycardia and Ventricular Fibrillation

VT and VF are uncommon in children. When seen, consider congenital heart disease, cardiomyopathies, or acute inflammatory injury to the heart (eg, myocarditis). In addition, identify and treat reversible causes, including drug toxicity (eg, recreational drugs, tricyclic antidepressants, digoxin overdose, or toxicity from the combination of cisapride and macrolide antibiotics[231]), metabolic causes (eg, hyperkalemia, hypermagnesemia, hypocalcemia, or hypoglycemia), or hypothermia (see pulseless arrest algorithm, Figure 6).

Treatment of VT and VF

Hemodynamically Stable VT

If the child with VT is hemodynamically stable (ie, is alert with palpable distal pulses), careful evaluation and early consultation with a cardiologist are indicated before any therapy is given. Focus initial efforts on determining the origin of the tachycardia based on analysis of the 12-lead ECG and a carefully obtained history, including family history for ventricular arrhythmias or sudden death. If pharmacological therapy is undertaken, amiodarone (5 mg/kg over 20 to 60 minutes) should be considered (Class IIb; LOE 7). Procainamide (15 mg/kg over 30 to 60 minutes) or lidocaine (1 mg/kg over approximately 2 to 4 minutes) may be considered as alternative agents. A cautious approach is appropriate in children who are hemodynamically stable, because all of these drugs have intrinsic risks. Amiodarone and procainamide can cause hypotension, and procainamide is a potent negative inotrope. Close hemodynamic and ECG monitoring are required during and after the infusion of either agent. As noted previously, amiodarone and procainamide generally should not be administered together because both prolong the QT interval.

Cardioversion for VT With Pulses

In the infant or child with VT and palpable pulses associated with signs of shock (ie, low cardiac output, poor perfusion), immediate synchronized cardioversion is indicated (Figure 9). Depending on the severity of hemodynamic compromise and the patient's level of consciousness, cardioversion may be provided before vascular access is obtained. If the child is appropriately responsive and not in distress, there is often time to consult a cardiologist, obtain vascular access, and consider administration of sedation before cardioversion. In addition, it is important to consider drug or metabolic causes of the VT, especially in a child without a known predisposing cause for the arrhythmia. The rhythm should be examined for a torsades de pointes appearance. If torsades de pointes is suspected, administer 25 mg/kg of magnesium by a slow intravenous bolus over 10 to 20 minutes.

Pulseless VT/VF

Delivering shocks to produce defibrillation is the definitive therapy (Figure 2) for *pulseless* VT and VF. In this setting, deliver shocks immediately. Ventilation, oxygenation, and chest compressions should be delivered and vascular access may be attempted until the defibrillator arrives and is charged, but these interventions should not delay shocks. If the patient fails to defibrillate after 3 shocks (refer to Figure 6), administer intravenous epinephrine in a dose of 0.01 mg/kg (or 0.1 mg/kg for the tracheal route) and attempt defibrillation again within 30 to 60 seconds. If VF or pulseless VT continues after this epinephrine dose plus shock(s) or if VF/pulseless VT recurs, *amiodarone* (5 mg/kg by rapid intravenous bolus) may be used (Class Indeterminate; LOE 7) followed by another defibrillation attempt within 30 to 60 seconds after closed-chest compression to deliver the drug to its site of action. (Note that the pattern of treatment after the initial 3 shocks is "CPR-drug-shock, CPR-drug-shock." We recommend no more than 30 to 60 seconds of artificial circulation before the next shock.) The use of amiodarone is based on adult data of "shock-resistant VT/VF"[270] and experience with the use of amiodarone in children in the intensive care unit[268,269] (see Figures 6, 8, and 9 and Table 2). "Shock resistance" of a ventricular arrhythmia is defined as continued VF or pulseless VT (ie, requiring epinephrine and a fourth precordial shock) or the recurrence of VF/pulseless VT after initial shock(s) caused defibrillation. Amiodarone will not terminate VF, but it can prevent the recurrence of VF after a successful shock.[270] In summary, amiodarone administration in children with VT with a pulse is a Class IIb recommendation, whereas it is Class Indeterminate in VF and pulseless VT.

In the ACLS algorithm for treatment of pulseless VT and VF, shocks may be delivered in clusters of 3, separated by 1 minute of CPR and drug administration. This "CPR-drug-shock-shock-shock, CPR-drug-shock-shock-shock" pattern is an acceptable alternative to the "CPR-drug-shock, CPR-drug-shock" pattern of resuscitation.

Bretylium is no longer considered an appropriate agent because of the risk of hypotension,[271] the lack of demonstrable effectiveness in VT,[272] and the absence of published studies of its use in children (Class III; LOE 7). Because it cannot be administered rapidly, *procainamide* also is not considered an appropriate agent in VF or pulseless VT therapy. Although sotalol is not available in the United States as an intravenous preparation, intravenous sotalol may be considered in other countries and subsequently may be approved in the United States (Class IIb; LOE 7).

Amiodarone. Amiodarone is a highly lipid-soluble antiarrhythmic with complex pharmacology, making it difficult to classify. The oral form of the drug is poorly absorbed, which makes acute therapy by the oral route largely impractical. However, an intravenous preparation was approved in 1995, and amiodarone increasingly is used for a wide range of both atrial and ventricular arrhythmias in adults and children.[268,273] Amiodarone is a noncompetitive inhibitor of both α- and β-adrenergic receptors.[274] Secondary to this sympathetic block, intravenous administration of amiodarone produces vasodilation[275] and AV nodal suppression; the latter results from prolonging the AV nodal refractory period and slowing AV nodal conduction.[276] Amiodarone inhibits the outward

potassium current, which prolongs the QT interval.[277] This effect is thought to be its major action in acutely controlling arrhythmias, but it may also increase the propensity for polymorphic ventricular arrhythmias (ie, torsades de pointes tachycardia).[278] Fortunately this appears to be an uncommon complication.[279] Amiodarone also inhibits sodium channels, which slows conduction in the ventricular myocardium and prolongs QRS duration.[279,280] Amiodarone-induced sodium channel blockade is use dependent,[280] meaning that the drug is more effective at faster heart rates, which probably represents an important mechanism of its effectiveness in SVT and VT. Intravenous dosing recommendations in children are derived from a number of case series.[268,269,281] Amiodarone has been used most commonly in children to treat ectopic atrial tachycardia or junctional ectopic tachycardia after cardiac surgery[268,281,282] and VT in postoperative patients or children with underlying cardiac disease.[268,269,283] For both supraventricular and ventricular arrhythmias, a loading infusion of 5 mg/kg is recommended over several minutes to 1 hour, depending on the need to achieve a rapid drug effect. Repeated doses of 5 mg/kg up to a maximum of 15 mg/kg per day may be used as needed. Because of the high lipid solubility of amiodarone, measurement of drug levels correlates poorly with drug effect. The main acute side effect from intravenous administration is hypotension.[268,284] Terminal elimination of amiodarone is very prolonged, with a half-life lasting up to 40 days,[285] but this is relatively unimportant with acute loading. Elimination is not dependent on normal renal or hepatic function. Because of its complex pharmacology, poor oral absorption, and potential for long-term adverse effects, a pediatric cardiologist or similarly experienced provider should direct chronic amiodarone therapy. Potential long-term complications include interference with thyroid hormone metabolism leading to hypothyroidism or hyperthyroidism,[286] interstitial pneumonitis, corneal microdeposits, blue-gray skin discoloration, and elevated liver enzyme levels.[287] ARDS is an unusual but potentially life-threatening complication seen in patients receiving chronic amiodarone therapy who undergo a surgical procedure, especially a cardiac or pulmonary procedure.[288] Fortunately this has not been reported in children, but pulmonary fibrosis was reported in an infant receiving chronic therapy.[289] As use of amiodarone becomes more frequent, we encourage reporting the occurrence of this and other complications.

Lidocaine. Lidocaine is a sodium channel blocker that reduces the slope of phase 4 diastolic repolarization, which decreases automaticity and therefore suppresses ventricular arrhythmias.[290] Therapeutic concentrations raise the VF threshold[291] and therefore may protect against refibrillation after successful defibrillation. Although lidocaine has long been recommended for the treatment of ventricular arrhythmias in infants and children, data suggests that it is not very effective unless the arrhythmia is associated with focal myocardial ischemia.[292,293] Lidocaine may be considered in children with shock-resistant VF or pulseless VT (Class Indeterminate; LOE 5, 6, 7). The recommended dose is 1 mg/kg by rapid intravenous injection followed by an infusion, because the drug is rapidly redistributed, lowering the plasma concentration below the therapeutic range. Infusions are given at a rate of 20 to 50 μg/kg per minute. If there is more than a 15-minute delay between the bolus dose and start of an infusion, a second bolus dose of 0.5 to 1 mg/kg lidocaine may be given to rapidly restore therapeutic concentrations. Lidocaine toxicity from excessive plasma concentrations may be seen in patients with persistently poor cardiac output and hepatic or renal failure.[294] Excessive plasma concentrations may cause myocardial and circulatory depression and possible central nervous system symptoms, including drowsiness, disorientation, muscle twitching, or seizures. If reduced lidocaine clearance is expected or suspected, the infusion rate generally should not exceed 20 μg/kg per minute.

Procainamide. Procainamide is a sodium channel blocking antiarrhythmic agent that prolongs the effective refractory period of atria and ventricles and depresses the conduction velocity within the conduction system. This typically produces prolongation of conduction and refractoriness of accessory pathways, but somewhat paradoxically it shortens the effective refractory period of the AV node and increases AV nodal conduction. This may lead to increased heart rates when used to treat ectopic atrial tachycardia.[295] By slowing intraventricular conduction, procainamide prolongs the QT and PR intervals. Procainamide is effective in the treatment of atrial fibrillation, flutter, and SVT,[296,297] and it may be useful in the treatment of postoperative junctional ectopic tachycardia.[298] It also has been used to treat or suppress VT.[299] Despite a long history of use, there is little data on the effectiveness of procainamide compared with other antiarrhythmic agents in children.[300,301] Since procainamide must be given by a slow infusion to avoid toxicity from heart block, myocardial depression, and prolongation of the QT interval (which predisposes to torsades de pointes tachycardia), procainamide is not indicated in the treatment of VF or pulseless VT. In children with a perfusing rhythm associated with VT, procainamide may be considered (Class IIb; LOE 5, 6, 7; see Figures 6 and 9). Infuse the loading dose of 15 mg/kg over 30 to 60 minutes with continuous monitoring of the ECG and frequent blood pressure monitoring. If the QRS widens to >50% of baseline or hypotension occurs, stop the infusion. Since procainamide increases the likelihood of polymorphous VT developing, it generally should not be used in combination with another agent that prolongs the QT interval, such as amiodarone.

Epinephrine and Vasopressin. A vasoconstrictor regimen may be considered in shock-resistant VT/VF, since if systemic vasoconstriction is inadequate with routine therapy, coronary perfusion is limited and the myocardium is unlikely to respond to shocks. For these reasons high-dose epinephrine (0.1 to 0.2 mg/kg) may be considered in shock-resistant VF/pulseless VT (Class IIb; LOE 5, 6, 7). Data in animals and limited data in adults suggest that *vasopressin* may be helpful in VF and pulseless VT, but data is insufficient to allow recommendation for use in children (see previous discussion; Class Indeterminate).

Defibrillation, Cardioversion, and External Pacing

Defibrillation

Defibrillation is the untimed (asynchronous) depolarization of the myocardium that successfully terminates VF or pulseless VT. Electric shocks are used to achieve defibrillation; shocks produce a simultaneous depolarization of a critical mass of myocardial cells, which may then allow resumption of spontaneous depolarization, especially if the myocardium is oxygenated and normothermic and acidosis is not excessive. When VF occurs suddenly, an immediate shock is usually effective. If the arrest is prolonged or the child does not respond to the initial attempts at defibrillation, then ventilation, oxygenation, chest compressions, and pharmacological therapy may be needed to improve the metabolic environment of the myocardium (Figure 2).[302,303] Defibrillation is not effective in the treatment of asystolic arrest.[304]

The defibrillator paddle size is one determinant of transthoracic impedance, which in turn determines the current flow through the chest. The larger adult paddles, generally 8 to 10 cm in diameter, are recommended for children weighing over approximately 10 kg (approximately 1 year of age). The larger paddles reduce impedance and maximize current flow.[305,306] The selection of paddle size is based on providing the largest surface area of paddle or self-adhering electrode contact with the chest wall without contact between the paddles or electrodes. Since the electrical current will follow the path of least resistance, the electrode gel or gel pads from one electrode must not touch the gel or pads of the other electrode. If bridging occurs, a short circuit will be created and insufficient current will traverse the heart.[307] To meet these goals, infant paddles generally are recommended for infants weighing <10 kg, but larger paddles may be used as long as contact between the paddles is avoided.

The electrode–chest wall interface can be an electrode cream or paste or self-adhesive monitoring-defibrillation pads. Saline-soaked pads may cause arcing and are discouraged. Ultrasound gel is a poor conductor and should not be used. Bare paddles should not be used because they result in very high impedance,[308] and alcohol pads should not be used because they are poor conductors. Repeated shocks may also cause skin burns.[309]

The paddles are applied to the chest with firm pressure. Typically one paddle is placed over the right side of the upper chest and the other over the apex of the heart (to the left of the nipple over the left lower ribs). Alternatively, paddles or self-adhesive monitoring-defibrillation pads may be placed in an anterior-posterior position with one placed just to the left of the sternum and the other placed over the back.[310]

The optimum electrical energy dose for pediatric shocks to produce defibrillation is not conclusively established, but the available data suggests an initial dose of approximately 2 J/kg.[311,312] If this dose is unsuccessful, the energy dose should be doubled and repeated. If this dose is still unsuccessful, the victim should be shocked again with 4 J/kg. The first 3 defibrillation attempts should occur in rapid succession, with pauses long enough to confirm whether VF persists.

Newer defibrillators use biphasic waveforms; this waveform appears to be effective at lower energy doses.[7] Although there is no published data in young children, biphasic AEDs may be used in children ≥8 years (approximately >25 kg body weight) in the out-of-hospital setting (see "AEDs in Children" below). Manual biphasic defibrillators have also been developed. As information on energy dosing becomes available, these defibrillators may be used appropriately in young children.

If the initial 3 defibrillation attempts are unsuccessful, correct acidosis, hypoxemia, or hypothermia if present and administer epinephrine, perform CPR, and attempt defibrillation. If the repeat (fourth) shock is ineffective, administration of amiodarone (Class Indeterminate) is recommended, and lidocaine or high-dose epinephrine (Class IIb) may be considered. Defibrillation should be repeated with 4 J/kg (Figure 2) within 30 to 60 seconds after each drug (CPR-drug-shock, CPR-drug-shock) if VT/VF persists. An alternative therapeutic approach in shock-resistant VF or pulseless VT is CPR, drug administration, and then 3 shocks in succession.

The recommended energy dose of 2 J/kg is appropriate for children up to at least 8 years of age. As discussed below in the section on AEDs in children, the age or size at which a fixed-energy-dose "adult" defibrillator can be used is unknown. In the out-of-hospital setting, it may be reasonable to use adult defibrillation algorithms in children ≥8 years, and it certainly is reasonable to use adult energy doses in children who weigh at least 50 kg.

Increasing the shock energy dose is not indicated when defibrillation is initially successful but the rhythm deteriorates back to VF. In this situation, adjunctive medications (eg, amiodarone, lidocaine, or sotalol) may improve the success of subsequent defibrillation at the previously effective dose and prevent further recurrences. In addition, reversible causes of VF/VT should be sought and treated in patients with refractory VF/VT (ie, the 4 H's and 4 T's; see Figure 6).

AEDs in Children

In the prehospital setting, AEDs are commonly used in adults to assess cardiac rhythm and to deliver shocks to produce defibrillation. Data suggests that AEDs can accurately detect VF in children of all ages,[313–315] but there is inadequate data regarding the ability of AEDs to correctly identify tachycardic rhythms in infants.[315] Based on available data, AEDs may be considered for *rhythm identification* (Class IIb; LOE 3, 5) in children ≥8 years old but are not recommended for younger children or infants. The energy dose delivered by currently available monophasic and biphasic AEDs exceeds the recommended dose of 2 to 4 J/kg for most children <8 years of age. The median weight of children ≥8 years typically exceeds 25 kg (a weight of 25 kg corresponds to a body length of approximately 50 inches or 128 cm[161]). Thus, the delivered initial dose from an AED (150 to 200 J) will be <10 J/kg for most children ≥8 years. Animal data suggests that this may be a safe dose, so attempted defibrillation of VF/pulseless VT detected by an AED may be considered in these older children (Class Indeterminate; LOE 6), particularly in the out-of-hospital setting.[316] Locations that routinely care for children at risk for arrhythmias and cardiac arrest (eg, in-hospital settings) should continue to use defibrillators capable of appropriate energy adjustment. Attempted defibrillation of children younger than approximately 8 years with energy doses typical of AEDs cannot be recommended at this time. Biphasic waveform transthoracic defibrillation requires lower energy and appears to be effective in adults,[7] but there is inadequate data to recommend a biphasic energy dose for treatment of VF/pulseless VT in children (Class Indeterminate).

Synchronized Cardioversion

Synchronized cardioversion is the timed depolarization of myocardial cells that successfully restores a stable rhythm. It is used to treat the symptomatic patient with SVT or VT (with pulses) accompanied by poor perfusion, hypotension, or heart failure. It also may be used electively in children with stable VT or SVT at the direction of an appropriate cardiology specialist.

The synchronizer circuit on the defibrillator must be activated before each cardioversion attempt. The initial energy dose is approximately 0.5 to 1 J/kg. The dose is increased up to 2 J/kg with subsequent attempts if necessary. If a second shock is unsuccessful or the tachycardia recurs quickly, consider antiarrhythmic therapy before a third shock. Hypoxemia, acidosis, hypoglycemia, or hypothermia should be corrected if the patient fails to respond to attempts at cardioversion.

Noninvasive (Transcutaneous) Pacing

Noninvasive transcutaneous pacing has been used to treat adults with bradycardia or asystole.[317,318] Experience with children, however, is limited and does not support a beneficial effect of pacing on outcome of children with cardiac arrest.[252,253] Since this form of pacing is very uncomfortable, its use is reserved for children with profound symptomatic bradycardia refractory to BLS and ALS (Class IIb; LOE 5, 7), particularly when caused by underlying congenital or acquired heart disease producing complete heart block or sinus node dysfunction.[252]

Noninvasive pacing requires the use of an external pacing unit and 2 large adhesive-backed electrodes. If the child weighs <15 kg, pediatric (small or medium) electrodes are recommended.[252] The negative electrode is placed over the heart on the anterior chest and the positive electrode behind the heart on the back. If the back cannot be used, the positive electrode is placed on the right side of the anterior chest under the clavicle and the negative electrode on the left side of the chest over the fourth intercostal space, in the midaxillary area. Precise placement of electrodes does not appear to be necessary provided that the negative electrode is placed near the apex of the heart.[319,320]

Either asynchronous ventricular fixed-rate or ventricular-inhibited pacing may be provided; the latter is preferred. It will usually be necessary to adjust pacemaker output to ensure that every pacer impulse results in ventricular depolarization (capture). In general, if smaller electrodes are used, the pacer output required to produce capture will be higher.[252] If ventricular-inhibited pacing is performed, the sensitivity of

A

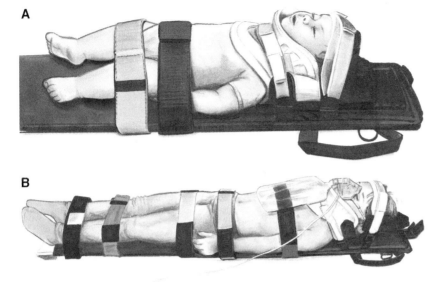

B

Figure 10. Example of spinal immobilization in trauma for infant (A) and child (B). Immobilization of an infant's or young child's cervical spine in a neutral position with specific care to avoid compromise of airway, breathing, and circulation and to maintain adequate visual and auscultory windows for monitoring.

the pacer's ECG detection must be adjusted so that intrinsic ventricular electric activity is appropriately sensed. To limit discomfort and to ensure a more reliable method of ongoing cardiac pacing, cardiology consultation is indicated if transcutaneous pacing is successful.

PALS for the Pediatric Trauma Victim

The principles of resuscitation of the seriously injured child are the same as those for any pediatric patient requiring PALS. Some aspects of pediatric trauma care, however, require emphasis, because improper resuscitation may be a major cause of preventable pediatric trauma death.[321] Common errors in pediatric trauma resuscitation include failure to open and maintain the airway, failure to provide appropriate fluid resuscitation for children (including those with head injury), and failure to recognize and treat internal bleeding. A qualified surgeon should be involved early in the course of the resuscitation. If possible, children with multisystem trauma should be transported rapidly to trauma centers with pediatric expertise. The relative value of aeromedical transport compared with ground transport of children with multiple trauma is unclear and should be evaluated by individual EMS systems.[322,323] Depending on the characteristics of each EMS system, it is likely that one mode of transport will be favored over the other.

Initial stabilization of the trauma victim involves 2 surveys: the Primary Survey and the Secondary Survey. Each focuses on assessment and treatment of life-threatening conditions. The Primary Survey includes the ABCs of BLS—including meticulous attention to **A**irway, **B**reathing, and **C**irculation—plus a "D" for **D**isability to evaluate neurological condition and an "E" for **E**xposure to keep the child warm and expose the skin to look for hidden injuries.

Airway control includes cervical spine immobilization, which must be continued during transport and stabilization in an ALS facility. Immobilization of an infant's or young child's cervical spine in a neutral position is challenging

because the occiput is large in young children.[99,324] Immobilization can best be achieved by using a backboard with a recess for the head or using a roll under the back from the shoulders to the buttocks.[98,99] Semirigid cervical collars are available in a wide variety of sizes. They can help maintain immobilization in children of various sizes. The head and neck should be further immobilized with towel rolls and tape, with secondary immobilization of the child on a spine board (Figure 10).

Breathing support is provided as needed. In the out-of-hospital setting, bag-mask ventilation may enable adequate support of oxygenation and ventilation, particularly when the transport time is short. Endotracheal intubation is indicated if the trauma victim's respiratory effort is inadequate, airway patency is compromised, or coma is present. Orotracheal intubation in the out-of-hospital setting should be performed only by properly trained and experienced providers. Regardless of the performance site, cervical spine immobilization

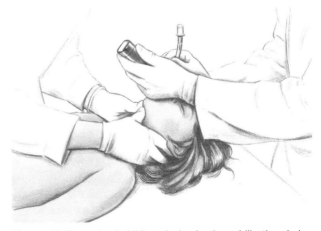

Figure 11. Example of child cervical spine immobilization during intubation in trauma. One provider maintains neutral position of neck and spine with care not to compromise airway while second provider performs endotracheal intubation.

should be addressed during the entire intubation procedure (Figure 11). Cricoid pressure may facilitate intubation when movement of the neck must be avoided. We particularly encourage confirmation of proper tracheal tube placement by use of capnography or exhaled CO_2 detection both after intubation and throughout transport (Class IIa), because hypoxemia and hypercarbia will complicate intracranial injury and are associated with poor outcome.

Although initial hyperventilation for patients with head trauma was previously recommended,[13] routine hyperventilation is not associated with an improved outcome in these patients[325] and may increase intrathoracic pressures, adversely affecting venous return and cardiac output. In addition, hyperventilation may adversely affect cerebral perfusion in areas of the brain still responsive to changes in PCO_2, leading to local or global brain ischemia.[326,327] Hyperventilation is no longer routinely recommended (Class III; LOE 3, 5, 6) and should be reserved for situations in which the victim has signs of increased intracranial pressure, such as transtentorial herniation. After intubation of the trauma patient, the goal of ventilatory support is to restore or maintain normal ventilation and good oxygenation.

In the traumatized victim, ventilation may be impaired by tension pneumothorax, open pneumothorax, hemothorax, or flail chest. Major thoracic injuries may be present in the absence of external evidence of chest trauma because the child's chest is extremely compliant. Even severe blunt chest trauma may fail to produce rib fractures. Thoracic injuries must be suspected, identified, and treated if there is a history of thoracoabdominal trauma or difficulty in providing effective ventilation.

After the airway is secured, a nasogastric or an orogastric tube should be inserted to prevent or relieve gastric inflation. Maxillofacial trauma and suspicion or confirmation of a basilar skull fracture are contraindications to blind nasogastric tube insertion because intracranial tube migration may result.[328]

Support of circulation in the trauma victim often requires treatment of hemorrhagic shock. Circulatory support of the pediatric trauma victim requires simultaneous control of external hemorrhage, assessment and support of systemic perfusion, and restoration and maintenance of blood volume. Control of external hemorrhage is best accomplished with direct pressure. Blind application of hemostatic clamps and use of tourniquets are contraindicated, except in traumatic amputation associated with bleeding from a major vessel.

If systemic perfusion is inadequate, provide rapid volume replacement with a bolus of 20 mL/kg of an isotonic crystalloid (eg, normal saline or lactated Ringer's solution) even if blood pressure is normal. Administer a second bolus (20 mL/kg) rapidly if heart rate, level of consciousness, capillary refill, and other signs of systemic perfusion fail to improve. The presence of hypotension traditionally was assumed to indicate a blood volume loss of $\geq 20\%$ and the need for urgent volume replacement and blood transfusion; however, minimal data supports this assumption. It is important to note that hypotension also may occur secondary to reversible causes such as a tension pneumothorax or pericardial tamponade, and hypotension may result from a neuro-

logical insult (eg, spinal cord injury or massive brain or brain stem injury resulting in loss of sympathetic nervous system control of peripheral vascular tone).

If the poorly perfused victim fails to respond to administration of 40 to 60 mL/kg of crystalloid, transfusion of 10 to 15 mL/kg of blood is indicated. Although type-specific crossmatched blood is preferred, O-negative blood may be used under urgent conditions. The blood should be warmed before transfusion; otherwise, rapid administration may result in significant hypothermia and can result in transient ionized hypocalcemia.[329,330] Consider intra-abdominal hemorrhage as a cause of continued hemodynamic instability despite adequate oxygenation, ventilation, and fluid resuscitation; surgical exploration may be needed. Undetected hemorrhage, particularly intra-abdominal hemorrhage, is a cause of preventable pediatric trauma mortality.[331,332]

Evaluation of neurological function (the "D" of Disability) requires application of a rapid neurological assessment, including a Glasgow Coma Scale (GCS) score. This scoring system evaluates eye opening, verbalization, and movement in response to stimulation. Serial assessments with the GCS allow rapid identification of any deterioration in the child's neurological status.

The "E" portion of the Primary Survey, Exposure, involves maintenance of a neutral thermal environment—keeping the child warm. A second meaning of exposure is to completely examine the child for hidden injuries.

The Secondary ABCD Trauma Survey involves more detailed evaluation and definitive therapy. This includes a head-to-toe assessment that is beyond the scope of these guidelines.

Special Resuscitation Situations

The principles of PALS introduced earlier in these guidelines are applicable in a wide variety of life-threatening circumstances. There are special situations, however, that require specific interventions that may differ from the routine PALS approach. Often these conditions are suggested by the history surrounding the event, knowledge of the common causes of arrest in various age groups, or rapidly obtained diagnostic tests. The special resuscitation situations covered in this section include toxicological emergencies and submersion/drowning. "Part 8: Advanced Challenges in Resuscitation" presents information on hypothermia, submersion/drowning/near-drowning, electrical injuries, and anaphylactic emergencies. The management principles of these emergencies are similar in adults and children.

Toxicological Emergencies

Based on data from the National Center for Health Statistics, drug-induced causes of death (eg, poisoning and overdose) are uncommon in younger children but become an important cause of death in the 15- to 24-year-old age group.[16] Similarly, a review of cardiac arrest in children and young adults suggests that toxicological causes are important in the adolescent age group.[19] The most important agents associated with cardiac arrest or requiring PALS are cocaine, narcotics, tricyclic antidepressants, calcium channel blockers, and β-adrenergic blockers.

The initial approach in toxicological emergencies uses basic PALS principles: assess and rapidly ensure adequate oxygenation, ventilation, and circulation. Subsequent priorities include reversing the adverse effects of the toxin, if possible, and preventing further absorption of the agent. Knowledge of the potential agent or recognition of characteristic clinical signs (toxidromes) for a particular toxin can be key to successful resuscitation. Unfortunately, since there are few well-controlled randomized trials of treatments for acute ingestions, most of the following recommendations are based on animal data and case series.

Cocaine

Cocaine has complex pharmacological effects, which are made more complex clinically by the varying onset, duration, and magnitude of these effects related to the route of administration and form of cocaine used.[333,334] Cocaine binds to the reuptake pump in presynaptic nerves, blocking the uptake of norepinephrine, dopamine, epinephrine, and serotonin from the synaptic cleft. This action leads to the local accumulation of these neurotransmitters, which produces both peripheral and central nervous system effects, depending on the receptors being activated. Accumulation of norepinephrine and epinephrine at β-adrenergic receptors leads to tachycardia, tremor, diaphoresis, and mydriasis. The tachycardia increases myocardial oxygen demand while reducing the time for diastolic coronary perfusion. Vasoconstriction and resultant hypertension develop from the accumulation of neurotransmitters at peripheral α-adrenergic receptors. Centrally mediated dopaminergic effects include mood elevation and movement disorders. Centrally mediated stimulation of serotonin (ie, 5-hydroxytryptamine; 5-HT) receptors results in exhilaration, hallucinations, and hyperthermia. Peripheral 5-HT–receptor stimulation results in coronary artery vasospasm.

The most frequent complication of cocaine use leading to hospitalization is acute coronary syndrome producing chest pain and various types of cardiac rhythm disturbances.[334,335] Acute coronary syndrome results from the combined effects of cocaine: stimulation of β-adrenergic myocardial receptors increases myocardial oxygen demand, and its α-adrenergic and 5-HT agonist actions cause coronary artery constriction, leading to ischemia. In addition, cocaine stimulates platelet aggregation,[336] perhaps through a secondary effect from cocaine-induced increases in circulating epinephrine.[337] Besides blocking reuptake of various amines, cocaine is a fast (ie, voltage-dependent) sodium channel inhibitor.[333] Sodium channel blockade prolongs the action potential propagation and therefore prolongs the QRS duration and impairs myocardial contractility.[333,338] Through the combination of adrenergic and sodium channel effects, cocaine use may cause various tachyarrhythmias, including VT and VF.

Initial treatment of the acute coronary syndrome consists of oxygen administration, continuous ECG monitoring, administration of a benzodiazepine (eg, diazepam or lorazepam; Class IIb; LOE 5, 6), and administration of aspirin and heparin.[339] Administration of aspirin and heparin has not been evaluated in clinical trials and is based on the concept of attempting to reverse the platelet-activating effects of cocaine

and biochemical manifestations of a procoagulant state. Substantial animal data shows that benzodiazepine administration is important,[340,341] probably because these drugs have anticonvulsant and central nervous system–depressant effects. There is no benefit and possible harm from the use of phenothiazines and butyrophenones (eg, haloperidol). Because animal experiments also show that hyperthermia is associated with a significant increase in toxicity,[341] aggressive cooling is indicated.

Although β-adrenergic blockers are a recommended treatment after myocardial ischemia in adults,[342] they are contraindicated in the setting of cocaine intoxication (Class III; LOE 5, 6, 7). In both animal[343] and human studies,[344,345] the addition of a β-adrenergic blocker results in increased blood pressure and coronary artery constriction. These adverse pharmacological effects are produced by antagonizing cocaine-induced β-adrenergic receptor stimulation, which normally causes vasodilation and counteracts the cocaine-induced increased stimulation of vasoconstricting α-adrenergic receptors. Although labetalol has mixed α- and β-adrenergic blocking actions, the latter dominates. This agent is not useful in the treatment of cocaine-induced acute coronary syndrome.[346]

To reverse coronary vasoconstriction, administration of the α-adrenergic blocker phentolamine may be considered but should follow oxygen, benzodiazepines, and nitroglycerin[339,347] (Class IIb; LOE 5, 6). The optimal dose of phentolamine is not known, and there is a risk of significant hypotension and tachycardia if excessive doses are used, so doses should be titrated to effect beginning with small intravenous infusions. Additional doses are infused after documenting ongoing hypertension or evidence of myocardial ischemia. Suggested doses for hypertension are 0.05 to 0.1 mg/kg intramuscularly or intravenously in a child up to a maximum of 2.5 to 5 mg, as recommended in adults.[348] The dose may be repeated every 5 to 10 minutes until blood pressure is controlled. Coronary vasospasm may also respond to nitroglycerin (Class IIa; LOE 5, 6).[349,350]

Because cocaine is a sodium channel blocker, consider administration of sodium bicarbonate in a dose of 1 to 2 mEq/kg in the treatment of ventricular arrhythmias. Although controlled human data is lacking, theoretical considerations and animal data[351,352] support this recommendation (Class IIb; LOE 5, 6, 7). Conversely, lidocaine, a local anesthetic that inhibits fast sodium channels, potentiates cocaine toxicity in animals.[353] Nevertheless, limited clinical experience has not documented adverse effects from lidocaine administration.[354] Therefore, lidocaine may be considered in the setting of cocaine-induced myocardial infarction (Class IIb; LOE 5, 6).

Although epinephrine may exacerbate cocaine-induced arrhythmias[355,356] and is contraindicated in ventricular arrhythmias if VF or pulseless VT occurs (Class III; LOE 6), epinephrine may be considered to increase coronary perfusion pressure during CPR (Class Indeterminate).

Tricyclic Antidepressants and Other Sodium Channel Blocking Agents

Tricyclic antidepressants continue to be a leading cause of morbidity and mortality despite the increasing availability of safer selective serotonin reuptake inhibitors for the treatment of depression. The toxic effects of tricyclic antidepressant agents result from their inhibition of fast (voltage-dependent) sodium channels in the brain and myocardium. This action is similar to that of other "membrane-stabilizing" agents (also called "quinidine-like" or "local anesthetics"). Besides tricyclic antidepressants, other sodium channel blockers include β-adrenergic blockers (particularly propranolol and sotalol), procainamide, quinidine, local anesthetics (eg, lidocaine), carbamazepine, type I$_C$ antiarrhythmics (eg, flecainide and encainide), and cocaine (see above).[338]

With serious intoxication, rhythm disturbances are due to prolongation of the action potential produced by inhibition of phase 0 of the action potential, resulting in delayed conduction. This intraventricular conduction delay results in QRS prolongation (particularly the terminal 40 milliseconds[357]) and a QRS duration ≥100 milliseconds.[358] The presence of these ECG abnormalities may be predictive of seizures and ventricular arrhythmia,[359] but this predictive effect is not confirmed by all investigators.[358,360] More recently an R wave in lead aVR ≥3 mm or an R wave–to–S wave ratio in lead aVR ≥0.7 was reported to be a superior predictor of serious toxicity.[361,362] Tricyclic antidepressants also inhibit potassium channels, leading to prolongation of the QT interval. Through blockade of both sodium and potassium channels, high concentrations of tricyclic antidepressants (and other sodium channel blockers) may result in preterminal sinus bradycardia and heart block with junctional or ventricular wide-complex escape beats.[338]

Treatment of sodium channel blocker toxicity includes protecting the airway, ensuring adequate oxygenation and ventilation, continuous monitoring of the ECG, and administering sodium bicarbonate (Class IIa; LOE 5, 6, 7). Infuse sodium bicarbonate only after the airway is opened and ventilation is ensured. Sodium bicarbonate narrows the QRS complex, shortens the QT interval, and increases myocardial contractility. These actions often suppress ventricular arrhythmias and reverse hypotension.[239,363] Experimental data suggests that the antiarrhythmic effect of sodium bicarbonate results from overcoming sodium channel blockade with hypertonic sodium, although the production of alkalosis per se may be important for some of these agents.[363,364] Regardless of the exact mechanism, the goal is to raise the sodium concentration and arterial pH. This can be achieved by administering 1- to 2-mEq/kg bolus infusions of sodium bicarbonate until the arterial pH is at least >7.45. After bolus administration, sodium bicarbonate may be infused as a solution of 150 mEq NaHCO$_3$ per liter in D$_5$W titrated to maintain alkalosis. In severe intoxications, consensus recommendations are to increase the pH to a level between 7.50 and 7.55; higher pH values are not recommended because of the risk of adverse effects.[338,365] The role of hyperventilation-induced alkalosis is not clear,[363,366] and its benefit may be related to the specific agent ingested[364]; therefore, maintenance of at least normal ventilation is recommended.

If hypotension is present, administer normal saline boluses (10 mL/kg each) in addition to sodium bicarbonate. Because tricyclic antidepressants block reuptake of norepinephrine at the neuromuscular junction, leading to catecholamine deple-

tion, a vasopressor may be necessary to maintain adequate vascular tone and blood pressure. Norepinephrine or epinephrine can be effective; anecdotal data supports treatment with norepinephrine rather than dopamine.[367,368] The superiority of norepinephrine over dopamine presumably is due to depletion of catecholamines, which will reduce the hemodynamic actions of dopamine because it is partly dependent on releasable stores of norepinephrine.[196] Pure β-adrenergic agonists are contraindicated (eg, dobutamine and isoproterenol) because they may worsen hypotension by causing vasodilation. If vasopressors are insufficient to maintain blood pressure, ECMO and cardiopulmonary bypass may be effective,[369,370] but they require the rapid availability of equipment and trained personnel. Early identification of at-risk patients and referral to a center capable of providing this therapy should be considered.

If ventricular arrhythmias do not respond to sodium bicarbonate, lidocaine may be considered, although some investigators argue against its use, because it is also a sodium channel blocker[353] (Class IIb; LOE 6, 7). Other Class I$_A$ (quinidine, procainamide) and Class I$_C$ (flecainide, propafenone) antiarrhythmic agents are contraindicated because they may exacerbate the cardiac toxicity (Class III; LOE 6, 8). Class III antiarrhythmics (eg, amiodarone and sotalol) prolong the QT interval and thus also are not indicated.[365]

Calcium Channel Blocker Toxicity

The increasing use of calcium channel blockers for the treatment of hypertension and congestive heart failure makes them available for accidental or intentional overdose. Although there are 3 different classes of these agents, based on their relative effects on the myocardium and vascular smooth muscle, in the overdosed patient these selective properties are inconsequential.[216] All of these agents bind to calcium channels, thereby inhibiting the influx of calcium into cells. The clinical manifestations of toxicity include bradyarrhythmias (due to inhibition of pacemaker cells and AV block) and hypotension (due to vasodilation and impaired cardiac contractility).[216] Altered mental status, including syncope, seizures, and coma, may occur because of cerebral hypoperfusion.

The initial approach to therapy is to provide oxygenation and ventilation, continuously monitor the ECG, and perform frequent clinical assessments, including close monitoring of blood pressure and hemodynamic status. Consider continuous intra-arterial blood pressure monitoring in symptomatic patients. If hypotension occurs, it may respond to normal saline bolus administration in milder cases, but with more severe intoxication it is often unresponsive to fluid administration. To avoid pulmonary edema, limit fluid boluses to 5 to 10 mL/kg, with careful reassessment after each bolus because of the high frequency of myocardial dysfunction in such patients. Calcium is often infused in calcium channel blocker overdose in an attempt to overcome the channel blockade, but case reports suggest only variable effectiveness (Class IIb; LOE 5, 6, 8).[216,371] The optimal dose of calcium is unclear. If used, calcium chloride is the generally recommended salt, because it results in greater elevation of the ionized calcium concentration.[217] Doses of 20 mg/kg (0.2 mL/kg) of 10% calcium chloride infused over 5 to 10 minutes may be provided, followed by infusions of 20 to 50 mg/kg per hour if a beneficial effect is observed. Ionized calcium concentrations should be monitored to limit toxicity from hypercalcemia.

High-dose vasopressor therapy (norepinephrine or epinephrine) may be considered on the basis of successful treatment of bradycardia and hypotension associated with severe calcium channel blocker toxicity (Class IIb; LOE 5).[372] High-dose vasopressor infusions require careful monitoring of the patient and titration of the infusion rate to the desired hemodynamic effect. Animal data[373,374] and a recent small case series[375] suggest that insulin plus glucose may be beneficial in calcium channel blocker toxicity (Class Indeterminate; LOE 5, 6). Precise dosage recommendations are unavailable. A loading dose of glucose (0.5 g/kg) may be followed by an infusion at 0.5 g/kg per hour. Following the glucose bolus, an insulin bolus of 0.5 to 1.0 U/kg is suggested, followed by 0.5 U/kg per hour. The goal is to maintain the glucose concentration between 100 and 200 mg/dL by titrating the rate of glucose administration. Presumably the beneficial effect of combined insulin-glucose therapy results from better myocardial use of glucose by activation of pyruvate dehydrogenase, which stimulates ATP production through aerobic metabolism. Careful monitoring of glucose concentration is needed to avoid hypoglycemia, the main adverse effect of this therapy. Because insulin and glucose stimulate movement of potassium from the extracellular to the intracellular space, potassium concentrations should be monitored closely, and exogenous potassium infusions are often needed.

β-Adrenergic Blocker Toxicity

β-Adrenergic blockers compete with norepinephrine and epinephrine at the β-adrenergic receptor, resulting in bradycardia and decreased cardiac contractility. In severe intoxication, some β-adrenergic blockers have sodium channel blocking effects as well (eg, propranolol and sotalol), leading to prolongation of the QRS and QT interval. Hypotension, usually with bradycardia, and varying degrees of heart block are common clinical manifestations of β-blocker toxicity.[376] Altered mental status, including seizures and coma, may occur, particularly with propranolol.[376,377]

The initial approach to treatment includes providing adequate oxygenation and ventilation, assessing perfusion, and establishing vascular access and treating shock if present. Continuous ECG monitoring and frequent clinical reassessment are also important. To overcome the β-adrenergic blockade, epinephrine infusions may be effective,[378] although very high infusion doses may be needed[379] (Class Indeterminate; LOE 5, 6). On the basis of animal data[376,380] and case reports,[378] glucagon also may be considered in the treatment of β-adrenergic blocker overdose (Class IIb; LOE 5, 6). In adults and adolescents, 5 to 10 mg of glucagon may be slowly infused over several minutes, followed by an intravenous infusion of 1 to 5 mg per hour. Bolus doses of 1 mg have been used in younger children. The diluent supplied by the manufacturer contains phenol and should not be used when these large bolus doses and subsequent continuous infusions are given, because phenol may cause hypotension, seizures, or arrhythmias.[381] If a dose ≥2 mg is needed, reconstitute the glucagon in sterile water at a final concentration <1 mg/mL.

As with calcium channel blocker overdose, glucose plus insulin also may be useful, with 1 animal study showing that it was superior to glucagon (Class Indeterminate; LOE 6).[374] When an intraventricular conduction delay is observed (ie, prolonged QRS interval), sodium bicarbonate may be used, as previously discussed.

β-Adrenergic blockade reduces cytoplasmic calcium concentration and thus reduces inotropy and chronotropy (ie, heart rate). Limited animal data[382] and a few small clinical uncontrolled case series[371,383] suggest that calcium administration may be beneficial, although other clinical reports suggest that it has no beneficial effect.[384,385] Calcium may be considered if administration of glucagon and catecholamine is not effective (Class IIb; LOE 5, 6).

Opioid Toxicity

Narcotics produce central nervous system depression and may cause hypoventilation, apnea, and respiratory failure requiring PALS. Naloxone is an effective opioid receptor antagonist that has been used in >20 years of clinical experience, and it remains the treatment of choice to reverse narcotic toxicity (Class IIa; LOE 4, 5, 6, 7).[14,386] Although naloxone administration is generally well tolerated,[387,388] both animal[389] and clinical data suggest that adverse events may occur, such as ventricular arrhythmias, acute pulmonary edema,[390] asystole, or seizures.[391] The opioid system and adrenergic system are interrelated; opioid antagonists stimulate sympathetic nervous system activity.[392] Moreover, hypercapnia stimulates the sympathetic nervous system. Animal data suggests that if ventilation is provided to normalize the partial pressure of arterial CO_2 before naloxone administration, the sudden rise in epinephrine concentration and its attendant toxic effects are blunted.[389] Thus, ventilation is recommended before the administration of naloxone (Class IIb; LOE 5, 6). The recommended dose of naloxone is 0.1 mg/kg administered intravenously, up to 2 mg in a single dose.[393] Alternatively, to avoid sudden hemodynamic effects from opioid reversal, repeated doses of 0.01 to 0.03 mg/kg may be used. Naloxone may be administered intramuscularly,[387] subcutaneously,[394] or through the tracheal tube, but its onset of action via these alternative routes may be delayed, particularly if the patient is poorly perfused.

Drowning/Submersion

Treatment of the submersion victim requires no particular alteration from the PBLS/PALS approach. Resuscitation, particularly rescue breathing, should begin when the child is in the water. The Heimlich maneuver is *not* indicated before rescue breathing is begun, and it should not be performed unless foreign-body airway obstruction is suspected.[395] The provision of prompt BLS has been linked with improved outcome following resuscitation in children.[254,396] Poor prognostic indicators after submersion include a prolonged submersion interval in non-icy water, VF on initial rhythm,[396] and absence of perfusing rhythm on arrival in the local

Emergency Department.[2,396] Signs of increased intracranial pressure that develop subsequent to a submersion injury are consistent with devastating neurological insult, but there is no evidence that invasive monitoring or aggressive treatment of the increased intracranial pressure alters outcome.[397–399]

Postresuscitation Stabilization

The postresuscitation phase begins after initial stabilization of the patient with shock or respiratory failure or after return of spontaneous circulation in a patient who was in cardiac arrest. This phase may include transport to a pediatric tertiary-care facility or intrahospital transport from the Emergency Department or ward and ongoing care in a pediatric intensive care unit. The goals of postresuscitation care are to preserve brain function, avoid secondary organ injury, seek and correct the cause of illness, and enable the patient to arrive at a tertiary-care setting in the best possible physiological state.

Care of the critically ill or injured child is complex, requiring knowledge and experience in the evaluation of all organ systems, assessment and monitoring of physiological functions, and management of multiple organ failure. Postresuscitation stabilization continues assessment and support of the ABCs (airway, breathing, and circulation) and adds attention to preservation of neurological function and avoidance of multisystem organ failure. Frequent reassessment of the patient is necessary because the patient's hemodynamic status often deteriorates after a brief period of stability.

After stabilization of the airway and support of oxygenation, ventilation, and perfusion, a secondary survey is performed that includes the patient's bones, joints, and skin. This survey carefully examines the patient for evidence of trauma and assesses the patient's neurological status. The medical history (allergies, illnesses, medications, and immunizations) and serious but not life-threatening conditions (such as renal and hepatic dysfunction) are then evaluated. Details on the postresuscitation evaluation and preservation of several organ systems are reviewed below.

Respiratory System

After resuscitation all children should receive supplemental oxygen until adequate oxygenation is confirmed by direct PaO_2 measurement or use of pulse oximetry and until adequate oxygen-carrying capacity (ie, hemoglobin concentration) is confirmed. In the postarrest setting, ongoing evidence of significant respiratory distress with agitation, poor air exchange, cyanosis, or hypoxemia requires support of oxygenation and ventilation, which is usually achieved by elective intubation and mechanical ventilation. To achieve airway control so that diagnostic studies such as a CT scan can be safely performed, elective endotracheal intubation using appropriate sedation and paralysis (see "Rapid Sequence Intubation") is sometimes used. After endotracheal intubation, tube position is assessed by clinical examination combined with a confirmatory test such as detection of exhaled CO_2 (Class IIb). Ongoing confirmation of tube placement using intermittent or continuous monitoring of exhaled CO_2 is also recommended (Class IIb), especially if the patient undergoes interhospital or intrahospital transport. Before patient transport, secure the tracheal tube and confirm the tube position

within the trachea by clinical examination and chest x-ray if available. In both hospital and out-of-hospital settings, oxygen saturation and the cardiac rhythm and rate should be continuously monitored, and blood pressure, breath sounds, perfusion, and color should be assessed frequently in intubated patients with a perfusing rhythm.

Reevaluate tracheal tube position and patency in patients who remain agitated despite effective mechanical ventilatory support and each time the patient is moved, such as into or out of a transport vehicle. If the condition of an intubated patient deteriorates, consider several possibilities that can be recalled by the mnemonic **DOPE: D**isplacement of the tube from the trachea, **O**bstruction of the tube, **P**neumothorax, and **E**quipment failure. If tracheal tube position and patency are confirmed and mechanical ventilation failure and pneumothorax are ruled out, the presence of agitation may require analgesia for pain control (eg, fentanyl or morphine) and/or sedation for confusion, anxiety, or agitation (eg, lorazepam, midazolam, or ketamine). Occasionally, neuromuscular blocking agents (eg, vecuronium or pancuronium) combined with analgesia or sedation are needed to optimize ventilation and minimize the risk of barotrauma or accidental tube dislodgment. In the hospital, continuous capnography is helpful in mechanically ventilated patients to avoid hypoventilation or hyperventilation, which may occur inadvertently during transport and diagnostic procedures.[400] Gastric distention may also cause discomfort and interfere with ventilation; if distention develops, an orogastric or nasogastric tube should be inserted.

Initial mechanical or manual ventilation of an intubated patient should provide 100% oxygen at a typical rate of 20 to 30 breaths per minute for infants and 12 to 20 breaths per minute for older children. Provision of effective ventilation depends on the respiratory rate and tidal volume. In general, the delivered tidal volume should be just sufficient to cause the chest to rise. Occasionally, higher rates or tidal volumes may be needed if intrinsic pulmonary disease or intracranial hypertension is present. Conversely, patients with conditions involving air trapping (eg, asthma and bronchiolitis) often require lower respiratory rates to allow prolonged expiratory time. If a mechanical ventilator is being used, initial delivered tidal volumes should be 7 to 10 mL/kg, sufficient to cause visible chest expansion and audible breath sounds over the distal lung fields.

Ventilator peak inspiratory pressure should begin at 20 to 25 cm H_2O and should be gradually increased until chest expansion is observed and breath sounds are adequate bilaterally. Higher inspiratory pressures may be needed in the presence of some lung diseases, but avoid peak pressures in excess of 35 cm H_2O if possible. To avoid high peak pressure during volume ventilation (ie, delivering a preset volume of gas rather than a preset inspiratory pressure), inspiratory time should be at least 0.6 to 1.0 second; longer times are often useful in conditions characterized by lower-airway obstruction (such as asthma or bronchiolitis) or poor lung compliance (eg, ARDS). A positive end-expiratory pressure of 2 to 5 cm H_2O is routinely provided; higher positive end-expiratory pressure may be necessary if diffuse alveolar disease or marked ventilation-perfusion mismatch associated with hypoxemia is present. Obtain an arterial blood gas analysis after 10 to 15 minutes on the initial ventilatory settings, and make adjustments in ventilatory support accordingly. Correlating the arterial P_{CO_2} with end-tidal CO_2 and correlating arterial oxygen saturation with pulse oximetry are useful procedures to permit continuous monitoring of ventilation and oxygenation. Perform frequent clinical assessment of the effectiveness of ventilation by observing for agitation, cyanosis, decreased breath sounds, chest wall movement, tachycardia, and spontaneous respiratory efforts that are asynchronous with mechanical ventilation. All intubated patients should be monitored with continuous pulse oximetry.

Transcutaneous oxygen and CO_2 sensors are used in children, particularly neonates and infants,[401,402] but changes in oxygenation or ventilation are not rapidly detected with these techniques. Conversely, transcutaneous monitors correlate more accurately with arterial blood P_{CO_2} than end-tidal detectors.[401,403] Repeated clinical evaluation is crucial also because transcutaneous monitors may be inaccurate or may not function reliably, especially in the presence of hypothermia or poor perfusion.

Cardiovascular System

Persistent circulatory dysfunction is observed frequently after resuscitation from cardiac arrest.[404,405] Frequent or continuous clinical evaluation is needed to detect evidence of inadequate cardiac output and shock. Maintaining adequate cardiac output and oxygen delivery to tissues is the key to preserving multiorgan function. Clinical signs of inadequate systemic perfusion include decreased capillary refill, absent or decreased intensity of distal pulses, altered mental status, cool extremities, tachycardia, decreased urine output, and hypotension. Decreased cardiac output or shock may be secondary to insufficient volume resuscitation, loss of peripheral vascular tone, and/or myocardial dysfunction. Treatment of altered perfusion includes fluid resuscitation, vasoactive agents to increase or decrease vascular resistance, inotropic agents, and/or correction of hypoxia and metabolic disorders. Heart rate, blood pressure, and oximetry monitoring should be continuous, and clinical evaluation should be repeated at least every 5 minutes. Cuff blood pressure measurements may be inaccurate in the child who remains hemodynamically unstable; consider direct arterial monitoring as soon as feasible in patients with continued cardiovascular compromise. Urine output is an important indicator of splanchnic organ perfusion; peripheral perfusion, heart rate, and mental status are nonspecific indicators that may be affected by ambient temperature, pain, fear, or neurological function. Blood pressure may be normal despite the presence of shock. For hemodynamically compromised patients, urine output generally should be monitored with an indwelling catheter.

Laboratory evaluation of the patient's circulatory state includes arterial blood gas analysis and evaluation of serum electrolytes, glucose, and calcium levels. The presence of metabolic (lactic) acidosis suggests the presence of tissue hypoxia caused by hypoxemia or ischemia. If cardiac output is adequate, a repeated arterial blood gas or lactic acid measurement typically shows improved acidosis and a reduced lactate concentration. A chest x-ray may help evaluate intravascular volume; a small heart is consistent with hypovolemia and a large heart is consistent with volume overload or myocardial dysfunction. Similarly, clear lung fields are inconsistent with cardiogenic shock, whereas pulmonary edema suggests heart failure, volume overload, ARDS, or diffuse pneumonia.

Drugs Used to Maintain Cardiac Output

The following section provides general information on the use of vasoactive and inotropic agents to maintain cardiac output and blood pressure in the postarrest period or in children with compromised hemodynamics at risk of cardiac arrest (Table 3). Note that although these agents are widely used, there is no clinical data comparing agents in the postarrest period that documents an advantage for outcome of one or more agents. In addition, the pharmacokinetics and pharmacodynamics (ie, clinical response to a given infusion rate) of these agents vary from patient to patient and even from hour to hour in the same patient. Factors that influence the effects of these agents include the child's age and maturity, underlying disease process (which influences receptor density and response), metabolic state, acid-base balance, autonomic and endocrine responses, and hepatic and renal function. Therefore, the recommended infusion doses listed below are starting points; the infusions must be adjusted according to measured patient response to achieve the desired effect.

After cardiac arrest or resuscitation from shock, the victim may have ongoing hemodynamic compromise secondary to a combination of inadequate cardiac pumping function, excessively increased systemic or pulmonary vascular resistance, or very low systemic vascular resistance. The last is most common in the patient with septic shock, although recent data shows that most children with *fluid-refractory* septic shock have high rather than low systemic vascular resistance and poor myocardial pumping function.[406] Children with cardiogenic shock typically have poor myocardial function and a compensatory increase in systemic and pulmonary vascular resistance as the body attempts to maintain an adequate blood pressure.

The classes of agents used to maintain circulatory function can be divided into inotropes, vasopressors, and vasodilators. Inotropes increase cardiac pumping function and often increase heart rate as well. Vasopressors increase systemic and pulmonary vascular resistance; they are most commonly used in children with inappropriately low systemic vascular resistance. Vasodilators are designed to reduce systemic and pulmonary vascular resistance. Although they do not directly increase pumping function, vasodilators reduce ventricular afterload, which often improves stroke volume and therefore cardiac output. They are the only class of agents that can increase cardiac output and simultaneously reduce myocardial oxygen demand.

Optimal use of these agents requires knowledge of the patient's cardiovascular physiology, which is not always clearly discerned from the clinical examination. Invasive hemodynamic monitoring, including measurement of central venous pressure, pulmonary capillary wedge pressure, and cardiac output, may be needed.[406] Furthermore, a number of the vasoactive agents have different hemodynamic effects at different infusion rates. For example, at low infusion rates,

TABLE 3.   PALS Medications to Maintain Cardiac Output and for Postresuscitation Stabilization

Medication	Dose Range	Comment	Preparation*
Amrinone	IV/IO loading dose: 0.75–1.0 mg/kg IV over 5 minutes; may repeat 2 times IV/IO infusion: 5–10 μg/kg per minute	Inodilator	6 × body weight (in kg) = No. of mg diluted to total 100 mL; then 1 mL/h delivers 1 μg/kg per minute
Dobutamine	IV/IO infusion: 2–20 μg/kg per minute	Inotrope; vasodilator	6 × body weight (in kg) = No. of mg diluted to total 100 mL; then 1 mL/h delivers 1 μg/kg per minute
Dopamine	IV/IO infusion: 2–20 μg/kg per minute	Inotrope; chronotrope; renal and splanchnic vasodilator in lower doses; pressor in higher doses	6 × body weight (in kg) = No. of mg diluted to total 100 mL; then 1 mL/h delivers 1 μg/kg per minute
Epinephrine	IV/IO infusion: 0.1–1.0 μg/kg per minute	Inotrope; chronotrope; vasodilator in lower doses and pressor in higher doses	0.6 × body weight (in kg) = No. of mg diluted to total 100 mL; then 1 mL/h delivers 0.1 μg/kg per minute
Lidocaine	IV/IO loading dose: 1 mg/kg IV/IO infusion: 20–50 μg/kg per minute	Antiarrhythmic, mild negative inotrope. Use lower infusion rate if poor cardiac output or poor hepatic function.	60 × body weight (in kg) = No. of mg diluted to total 100 mL; then 1 mL/h delivers 10 μg/kg per minute *or* **alternative premix** 120 mg/100 mL at 1 to 2.5 mL/kg per hour
Milrinone	IV/IO loading dose: 50–75 μg/kg IV/IO infusion: 0.5–0.75 μg/kg per minute	Inodilator	0.6 × body weight (in kg) = No. of mg diluted to total 100 mL; then 1 mL/h delivers 0.1 μg/kg per minute
Norepinephrine	IV/IO infusion: 0.1–2.0 μg/kg per minute	Vasopressor	0.6 × body weight (in kg) = No. of mg diluted to total 100 mL; then 1 mL/h delivers 0.1 μg/kg per minute
Prostaglandin E$_1$	IV/IO infusion: 0.05–0.1 μg/kg per minute	Maintains patency of ductus arteriosus in cyanotic congenital heart disease. Monitor for apnea, hypotension, and hypoglycemia.	0.3 × body weight (in kg) = No. of mg diluted to total 50 mL; then 1 mL/h delivers 0.1 μg/kg per minute
Sodium nitroprusside	IV/IO infusion: 1–8 μg/kg per minute	Vasodilator Prepare only in dextrose in water	6 × body weight (in kg) = No. of mg diluted to total 100 mL; then 1 mL/h delivers 1 μg/kg per minute

IV indicates intravenous; IO, intraosseous.

*Most infusions may be calculated on the basis of the "Rule of 6" as illustrated in the table. Alternatively, a standard concentration may be used to provide more dilute or more concentrated drug solution, but then an individual dose must be calculated for each patient and each infusion rate as follows: Infusion rate (mL/h) = [weight (kg) × dose (μg/kg per minute) × 60 min/h]/concentration (μg/mL). Diluent may be 5% dextrose in water, 5% dextrose in half-normal saline, normal saline, or Ringer's lactate unless noted otherwise.

epinephrine is a potent inotrope and lowers systemic vascular resistance through a prominent action on vascular β-adrenergic receptors. At higher infusion rates, epinephrine remains a potent inotrope and increases systemic vascular resistance by activating vascular α-adrenergic receptors. Since the pharmacokinetic and pharmacodynamic responses are not uniform across ages and across different diseases, careful monitoring of the patient's response to vasoactive agents is needed for optimal use.

Epinephrine

An epinephrine infusion is indicated in the treatment of shock with diminished systemic perfusion from any cause that is unresponsive to fluid resuscitation. Epinephrine is a potent inotrope and typically is infused at a rate sufficient to increase systemic vascular resistance and therefore blood pressure. Epinephrine is also a potent chronotrope (ie, it increases heart rate). It may be useful in patients with hemodynamically significant bradycardia that is unresponsive to oxygenation and ventilation. Epinephrine may be preferable to dopamine in patients with *marked* circulatory instability, particularly in infants (see "Dopamine," below). Infusions are prepared as listed in Table 3. The infusion is generally initiated at 0.1 to

0.3 μg/kg per minute and is titrated up to 1 μg/kg per minute based on the observed hemodynamic effects (see also Table 2). Epinephrine should be infused only into a secure intravenous line because tissue infiltration may cause local ischemia and ulceration. Epinephrine also may cause atrial or ventricular tachyarrhythmias, severe hypertension, and metabolic changes. Metabolic changes consist of hyperglycemia, increased lactate concentration,[407] and hypokalemia.

Dopamine

Dopamine is an endogenous catecholamine with complex cardiovascular effects. At low infusion rates (0.5 to 2 μg/kg per minute), dopamine typically increases renal and splanchnic blood flow with little effect on systemic hemodynamics, although increases in blood pressure and cardiac output were observed in neonates after infusions as low as 0.5 to 1.0 μg/kg per minute.[408] At infusion rates >5 μg/kg per minute, dopamine can result in both direct stimulation of cardiac β-adrenergic receptors and indirect stimulation through the release of norepinephrine stored in cardiac sympathetic nerves.[196] Myocardial norepinephrine stores are depleted in chronic congestive heart failure and also may be diminished in infants because sympathetic nervous system myocardial innervation is incomplete during the first months of life. In either condition the inotropic action of dopamine may be reduced.[196] Consistent with observations in animals,[409] dopamine tends to increase pulmonary vascular resistance in children after cardiac surgery, particularly if their pulmonary vascular resistance was elevated at baseline.[196,410]

Since it possesses inotropic and vasopressor effects, dopamine is used in the treatment of circulatory shock following resuscitation or when shock is unresponsive to fluid administration and is characterized by a low systemic vascular resistance[406,411] (Class IIb; LOE 5, 6, 7). Dopamine must be infused through a secure intravenous line. Infusions (Table 3) are usually begun at 2 to 5 μg/kg per minute and may be increased to 10 to 20 μg/kg per minute in an effort to improve blood pressure, perfusion, and urine output. Infusion rates exceeding 20 μg/kg per minute may result in excessive vasoconstriction and a loss of renal vasodilating effects,[196] although as previously noted there is substantial interpatient variability in kinetics and response. If further inotropic support is needed, either epinephrine or dobutamine may be preferable to a dopamine infusion of >20 μg/kg per minute. If further vasopressor support is needed to maintain blood pressure despite high-dose dopamine infusion, norepinephrine or epinephrine is generally preferred. Although not a concern after short-term use, if dopamine infusions are used for several days it may adversely affect thyroid function by inhibiting thyrotropin-stimulating hormone release from the pituitary gland.[412]

Dopamine infusions may produce tachycardia, vasoconstriction, and ventricular ectopy. Infiltration of dopamine into tissues can produce local tissue necrosis. Dopamine and other catecholamines are partially inactivated in alkaline solutions and therefore should not be mixed with sodium bicarbonate.

Dobutamine Hydrochloride
Dobutamine hydrochloride is a synthetic catecholamine with a relatively selective effect on β_1-adrenergic receptors and a lesser effect on β_2-adrenergic receptors. Thus, dobutamine is a relatively selective inotrope, increasing myocardial contractility and usually decreasing peripheral vascular tone. It is effective in improving cardiac output and blood pressure in neonates and children.[193,413] Dobutamine may be particularly useful in the treatment of low cardiac output secondary to poor myocardial function,[414] such as following cardiac arrest.[405] Dobutamine is usually infused in a dose range of 2 to 20 μg/kg per minute (Tables 2 and 3). Higher infusion rates may produce tachycardia or ventricular ectopy. Pharmacokinetics and clinical responses to specific dobutamine doses vary widely among pediatric patients,[193,413,414] so the drug must be titrated according to individual patient response.

Norepinephrine
Norepinephrine is the neurotransmitter released from sympathetic nerves; it is therefore a potent inotropic agent that also activates peripheral α- and β-adrenergic receptors. At the infusion rates used clinically, α-adrenergic effects predominate and result in both the beneficial and adverse effects of norepinephrine. Since it is a potent vasoconstricting agent, norepinephrine is reserved for children with low systemic vascular resistance that is unresponsive to fluid resuscitation. This is most commonly seen in children with septic shock but also may be seen in spinal shock and anaphylaxis. Although

intuitive reasoning would suggest that norepinephrine will worsen renal and splanchnic perfusion secondary to its vasoconstrictive actions, clinical data in adults shows that it improves splanchnic perfusion and renal function in hypotensive patients with septic shock,[415,416] particularly if combined with dobutamine.[407] Furthermore, infusing low doses of dopamine with norepinephrine appears to increase splanchnic blood flow and urine output, providing some degree of protection from excessive vasoconstriction.[417,418] Certainly urine output and the magnitude of metabolic acidosis should be monitored carefully during a norepinephrine infusion.

Prepare norepinephrine infusions as noted in Table 3 and infuse at rates of 0.1 to 2 μg/kg per minute. Adjust the infusion rate to achieve the desired change in blood pressure and perfusion. Since norepinephrine increases systemic vascular resistance and blood pressure, its expected chronotropic effect on heart rate is reduced and the heart rate may actually decrease despite β-adrenergic stimulation. The main toxicities are hypertension, organ ischemia (including distal extremity vascular beds), and arrhythmias. Norepinephrine should be infused through a secure vascular line, preferably one that is placed centrally.

Sodium Nitroprusside
Sodium nitroprusside is a vasodilator that reduces tone in all vascular beds by stimulating local nitric oxide production. It has no direct effect on the myocardium when infused at therapeutic doses, but cardiac output often increases following nitroprusside administration because systemic and pulmonary vascular resistance (ie, ventricular afterload) fall. Sodium nitroprusside is indicated in the treatment of shock or low cardiac output states characterized by high vascular resistance. It is also used in the treatment of severe hypertension. Although its vasodilating action may seem to contraindicate its use in patients with low blood pressure, in cardiogenic shock the ability of sodium nitroprusside to increase stroke volume usually more than offsets the decrease in systemic vascular resistance so that blood pressure is stabilized or increased. This is seen in the following equation describing the relationship between these hemodynamic parameters: BP=CO×SVR, where BP is blood pressure, CO is cardiac output, and SVR is systemic vascular resistance. If the increase in cardiac output is proportionately larger than the fall in systemic vascular resistance induced by sodium nitroprusside (or other vasodilators), blood pressure will increase rather than decrease. If the patient is volume depleted, sodium nitroprusside is contraindicated, because hypotension is likely.

Since sodium nitroprusside is rapidly metabolized, it must be infused continuously. The drug must be prepared in dextrose in water and cannot be infused with a saline-containing solution. This may create the need for a separate infusion site. Infusions are typically started at 1 μg/kg per minute and adjusted as needed up to 8 μg/kg per minute. Nitroprusside undergoes metabolism by endothelial cells and red blood cells, releasing nitric oxide and cyanide. The latter is rapidly metabolized in the liver to thiocyanate, provided that hepatic function is adequate. High infusion rates or diminished hepatic function may exceed the ability of the liver to metabolize cyanide, resulting in clinical toxicity.[419] Furthermore, the hepatic metabolite thiocyanate must be renally excreted. In patients with poor renal function, thiocyanate may accumulate, leading to central nervous system dysfunction that ranges from irritability to seizures, abdominal pain, nausea, and vomiting. Thiocyanate levels should be measured in patients receiving prolonged sodium nitroprusside infusions, particularly if the infusion rate exceeds 2 μg/kg per minute.

Inodilators

This class of agents combines inotropic stimulation of the heart with vasodilation of the systemic and pulmonary vascular beds. The agents currently available are *amrinone* and *milrinone*. Unlike catecholamines, inodilators do not depend on activation of receptors. Instead, these agents inhibit phosphodiesterase type III, which results in an increase in the intracellular concentration of cAMP. In the myocardium, cAMP acts as a second messenger increasing cardiac contractility; heart rate is increased to a lesser extent because phosphodiesterase type III is more prevalent in myocytes and vascular smooth muscle than it is in the pacemaker cells of the heart. Indeed, the action of inodilators is most notable in vascular smooth muscle, so this class of agents acts much like a combination of sodium nitroprusside and a selective inotrope such as dobutamine.

Inodilators are used to treat children with myocardial dysfunction and increased systemic or pulmonary vascular resistance. They are used for conditions such as congestive heart failure in postoperative cardiac surgical patients or patients with dilated cardiomyopathy and even in selected children with septic shock and myocardial dysfunction with a high systemic vascular resistance.[420,421] Like vasodilators, inodilators have the ability to augment cardiac output with little effect on myocardial oxygen demand and often with little change in heart rate. Blood pressure is generally well maintained, provided that the patient has adequate intravascular volume. In the presence of hypovolemia, the potent vasodilating action will result in hypotension.

The major disadvantage of this class of agents is that they have relatively long elimination half-lives. They must be administered with a loading dose followed by an infusion. The latter may lead to a false sense that a change in infusion rate results in a rapid change in hemodynamic effect. Hemodynamic changes will occur when the change in infusion rate produces significant changes in the plasma concentration. Since 3 half-lives are needed to reach approximately 90% of the steady-state concentration at a given infusion rate, and assuming a 6-hour half-life, approximately 18 hours is needed to achieve the ultimate hemodynamic effect following a change in the amrinone infusion rate. Milrinone has a half-life of approximately 1.5 hours,[422] so a new steady-state concentration will occur approximately 4.5 hours after a change in infusion rate. Similarly, if toxicity occurs, stopping the infusion will not eliminate the adverse effect. Instead, you will need to wait until the drug is metabolized over several hours.

Amrinone is given as a loading dose of approximately 0.75 to 1 mg/kg over 5 minutes. If the patient tolerates this load, it may be repeated up to 2 times to a total load of 3 mg/kg followed by an infusion of 5 to 10 μg/kg per minute. There is a 6-fold variation in amrinone pharmacokinetics in children,

making it difficult to predict the optimal infusion rate.[423] In infants <4 weeks of age and in patients with renal dysfunction,[424] amrinone clearance will be low, leading to a greater risk of toxicity. If hypotension occurs during the loading dose, give 5 to 10 mL/kg of normal saline or other appropriate fluid and position the patient flat or head down if the patient can tolerate this position. If the patient remains hypotensive despite fluid loading, then a vasopressor agent needs to be used, and no further loading of amrinone should be given. For short-term stabilization, the patient may be treated with just a loading dose without an infusion. If the patient's renal function is more severely affected than recognized initially, the amrinone concentration will accumulate during an infusion, resulting in excessive vasodilation and hypotension that may not present until ≥12 to 24 hours after the initiation of an amrinone infusion. The other major side effect of amrinone is increased platelet destruction,[425] so the platelet count should be checked every 12 to 24 hours when starting an amrinone infusion.

Milrinone is a newer inodilator agent that is also cleared by the kidney, but because it has a shorter half-life than amrinone,[421,422] it is often preferred. Milrinone also has less effect on platelets. Milrinone has been used in children to increase cardiac output and decrease systemic vascular resistance in septic shock[420,422]; these effects require that the patient is adequately fluid resuscitated and has an elevated systemic vascular resistance. Based on pharmacokinetic data, milrinone initially is given as a bolus of 50 to 75 μg/kg followed by an infusion of 0.5 to 0.75 μg/kg per minute.[421,422]

Neurological Preservation

Central nervous system dysfunction may either contribute to or result from a cardiac arrest. The key to preserving neurological function is the rapid restoration and maintenance of adequate oxygen delivery to the brain and avoidance of secondary injury to the neurons. Therefore, if there is evidence of significant central nervous system depression that may prevent adequate airway protection or respiratory drive, intubation and controlled ventilation are recommended. Data does not support the routine use of hyperventilation in brain-injured patients. Indeed, data suggests that hyperventilation may impair neurological outcome, most likely because of a combination of adverse effects on cardiac output, cerebral venous return, and cerebral vascular tone.[325]

Recent data suggests that postarrest or postischemia hypothermia (core temperatures of 33°C to 36°C) may have beneficial effects on neurological function.[426,427] There is insufficient data, however, to recommend the routine application of hypothermia (Class Indeterminate), but postarrest patients with core temperatures <37.5°C should not be actively rewarmed (Class IIb) unless the core temperature is <33°C, in which case they should be rewarmed to 34°C (Class IIb). Conversely, increased core temperature increases metabolic demand by 10% to 13% for each degree Celsius increase in temperature above normal. Since increasing metabolic demand may worsen neurological injury, it is not surprising that the presence of fever following brain injury is associated with worsened neurological outcome in adults with cerebral ischemia.[428] In the brain-injured patient or in the postarrest patient with compromised cardiac output, correct hyperthermia with active cooling to achieve a normal core temperature (Class IIa; LOE 5, 6, 7). Prevent shivering because it will increase metabolic demand. Sedation may be adequate to control shivering, but neuromuscular blockade may be needed.

Seizures may occur at any time after a significant hypoxic-ischemic insult to the brain, such as that following a cardiac arrest. If seizures occur, search for a correctable metabolic cause such as hypoglycemia or an electrolyte disturbance. Because seizures greatly increase cerebral metabolic demand at a time when cerebral blood flow may be compromised, aggressive treatment of these postischemia seizures is indicated. Initial control of the seizures is typically best achieved with the use of a benzodiazepine such as lorazepam, diazepam, or midazolam. Although the concept seems rational, there is no clinical data supporting the routine administration of an antiepileptic to prevent postarrest seizures. Conversely, if the postarrest or head-injured patient requires neuromuscular blockade, a cerebral function monitor is needed to detect seizure activity. If a cerebral function monitor is unavailable, the patient may be loaded with an anticonvulsant such as phenytoin, fosphenytoin, or phenobarbital in an attempt to prevent unrecognized seizures and further brain injury.

Renal System

Decreased urine output (<1.0 mL/kg per hour in infants and children or <30 mL per hour in adolescents) in the postresuscitation period may result from prerenal causes (such as dehydration and inadequate systemic perfusion), renal ischemic damage, or a combination of these conditions. Determine baseline serum urea nitrogen and creatinine values as soon as possible. Volume depletion may be treated with additional fluid administration (see "Intravascular Fluids"). Treat myocardial dysfunction with vasoactive drug therapy as described in the drug section. Nephrotoxic and renally excreted medications should be avoided or administered cautiously until renal status is determined. For example, pancuronium administration may result in very prolonged neuromuscular blockade, because it is renally excreted.

Gastrointestinal System

If bowel sounds are absent, abdominal distention is present, or the patient requires mechanical ventilation, an orogastric or nasogastric tube should be inserted to prevent or treat gastric distention. Blind nasogastric tube placement is contraindicated in the patient with serious facial trauma or basilar skull fracture because intracranial tube migration may result.[328]

General Postresuscitation Care

Once the patient's cardiopulmonary status is stable, change intraosseous lines to intravenous ones and secure all intravenous lines. Splint any apparent fractures. The underlying cause of the arrest (infection, ingestion, etc) should be treated if known. Because hypoglycemia and hypothermia are frequently observed, monitor serum glucose level and core body temperature frequently and take corrective measures as needed. Recommended guidelines for treatment (Table 4) and equipment (Table 5) for stabilization of seriously ill or injured children may be consulted.[429]

TABLE 4.   Summary of Postresuscitation Care

	Intervention
Airway	Tracheal intubation with confirmation of tube position and repeat confirmation on movement/transport
	Secure tube before transport
	Gastric decompression
Breathing	100% inspired oxygen
	Provide mechanical ventilation targeting normal ventilation goals (P_{CO_2} 35 to 40 mm Hg)
	Monitor continuous pulse oximetry and exhaled CO_2 (or capnography) if available
Circulation	Ensure adequate intravascular volume (volume titration)
	Optimize myocardial function and systemic perfusion (inotropes, vasopressors, vasodilators)
	Monitor capillary refill, blood pressure, continuous ECG, urine output; measure arterial blood gas and lactate to assess degree of acidosis, if available
	Ideally maintain 2 routes of functional vascular access
Disability	Perform rapid secondary survey including brief neurological assessment
	Avoid hyperglycemia, treat hypoglycemia (monitor glucose)
	If seizures are observed, medicate with anticonvulsant agents
	Obtain laboratory studies (if available): arterial blood gases, glucose, electrolytes, hematocrit, chest radiograph
Exposure	Avoid and correct hyperthermia (monitor temperature)
	Avoid profound hypothermia <33°C

Be sure to communicate interventions and status of the patient to family and to transport and receiving providers.

Interhospital Transport

Ideally, postresuscitation care is provided by trained medical personnel in specialized pediatric intensive care units. Transportation to these units should be coordinated with the receiving unit to ensure that the child is safely delivered to a pediatric tertiary-care facility in stable or improved condition.[430] To reduce the likelihood of complications during transport, the transport team members preferably should receive training and experience in the care of critically ill and injured children[29,431] and should be supervised by a physician with experience and training in pediatric emergency medicine or pediatric critical care. The mode of transport as well as the composition of the team should be established for each EMS system, based on the care required by an individual patient.[432] In general, if a pediatric and adult team are available within the same time frame, the pediatric team is preferred. The weather, distance, and the patient's condition will determine the selection of surface ambulance, fixed-wing aircraft, or helicopter. Equipment that should be available for transport of children is listed in Table 6.

Family Presence During Resuscitation

According to surveys in the United States and the United Kingdom,[433–438] most family members would like to be present during the attempted resuscitation of a loved one. Parents and providers of care for chronically ill children are often knowledgeable about and comfortable with medical equipment and emergency procedures. Family members with

TABLE 5.   Suggested Equipment, Supplies, and Drugs for EMS ALS Responders

Equipment	
Backboard and spine board (preferably with head well)	Suction catheters (5F, 6F, 8F, 10F, 12F, 14F, and tonsil tip)
Blood pressure cuffs in newborn, infant, child, and adult sizes	Obstetric pack
Exhaled CO_2 monitor	Thermal blanket
Semirigid cervical collars in several pediatric sizes	Water-soluble lubricant
*Laryngoscope with straight blades, Nos. 0, 1, 2, and 3 (curved blades may be used in size 2 and 3)	**Drugs**
Monitor/defibrillator (including small paddles/electrodes optional)	Albuterol in 2.5-mg unit doses, or equivalent bronchodilator for inhalation
External pacemaker	Adenosine
Oxygen source	Amiodarone
Pediatric self-inflating bag-mask resuscitator with newborn, infant, and child masks	Atropine sulfate
Pediatric femur splint	Benzodiazepine (for seizure control; eg, diazepam, lorazepam, midazolam)
Pulse oximeter	Calcium chloride or calcium gluconate
Stethoscope	Dopamine
Stiff cervical collars in infant and child sizes	Diphenhydramine
Tracheal tube placement confirmation devices	Epinephrine 1 mg/mL (1:1000)
Standard precautions equipment	Epinephrine 1 mg/10 mL (1:10 000)
Portable suction capability	Flumazenil (benzodiazepine antagonist) (optional)
Supplies	Glucose 50% and/or 25% and/or 10%
Arm boards (6, 8, and 15 in)	Glucagon
*Tracheal tubes, cuffed (6.0, 6.5, 7.0, 7.5, and 8.0 mm)	Insulin
*Tracheal tubes, uncuffed (2.5, 3.0, 3.5, 4.0, 4.5, 5.0, 5.5 mm)	Lidocaine
Intraosseous infusion needles	Magnesium sulfate
Minidrip intravenous burettes	Narcotic analgesic (eg, morphine sulfate)
Nasal cannulas in infant and child sizes	Naloxone
Normal saline or lactated Ringer's solution	Procainamide
Oral airways, 0–5	Prostaglandin E_1 (optional)
Over-the-needle catheters (24-, 22-, 20-, 18-, 16-, 14-gauge)	Sodium bicarbonate
Pediatric nonrebreathing mask	Steroid (eg, dexamethasone, methylprednisolone)
Simple oxygen masks in infant and child sizes	

*If tracheal intubation is within the scope of the provider's practice.

no medical background report that being at the side of a loved one and saying goodbye during the final moments of life are extremely comforting.[435,439] Parents or family members often fail to ask if they can be present, but healthcare providers should offer the opportunity whenever possible.[437,439,440]

Family members present during resuscitation report that it helped their adjustment to the death of the loved one,[433,435] and most indicate they would participate again.[435] Standardized psychological examinations suggest that family members present during resuscitation show less anxiety and depression and more constructive grieving behavior than family members not present during the resuscitation.[438]

When family members are present during resuscitative efforts, resuscitation team members should be sensitive to the presence of the family member. When family members are present during an in-hospital resuscitation, if possible one person should remain with the family member to answer questions, clarify information, and provide comfort.[441]

Termination of Resuscitative Efforts

Despite the best efforts of healthcare providers, most children experiencing a cardiac arrest will not survive. There may be transient return of spontaneous circulation, with death occurring subsequently in the intensive care unit. Alternatively, some children will not respond to prolonged efforts. If a child fails to respond to at least 2 doses of epinephrine with a return of spontaneous circulation, the child is unlikely to survive.[2,17,442] In the absence of recurring or refractory VF or VT, history of a toxic drug exposure, or a primary hypothermic insult, resuscitative efforts may be discontinued if there is no return of spontaneous circulation despite ALS interventions. In general, this requires no more than 30 minutes. Further discussion on the ethics of resuscitation is contained in Part 2.

TABLE 6. Suggested Equipment for Pediatric Transport

ALS	BLS	Pediatric Kit
x	x	Standard precaution equipment
x	x	Oxygen source
x	x	Neonatal-infant masks
x	x	Pediatric self-inflating bag-mask resuscitator
x	x	Pediatric masks in 3 sizes
x	x	Nasal cannulas, infant and child
x	x	Oral airways, 00-5
x		*Tracheal tubes, uncuffed 2.5 to 5.5 mm and cuffed 6.0 to 8.0 mm
x		Intubating stylet, 6F
x	x	Bulb syringe
x		Suction catheters (6F, 8F, 10F, 12F, and 14F)
x		*Laryngoscope blades, straight Nos. 0, 1, 2, and 3 and curved Nos. 2, 3, and 4 (optional)
x	x	Blood pressure cuffs, infant and child
x		Buretrol (Metriset)
x		Over-the-needle catheters, 24- to 16-gauge
x		Butterfly cannulas, 23- to 19-gauge
x		Tourniquets, infant and child
x		Intraosseous needles, 18- to 15-gauge
x		Pediatric Magill forceps
x		Pediatric defibrillator paddles/electrodes
x		Pediatric ECG electrodes
x	x	Pediatric traction splint
x	x	Cervical immobilization devices (eg, semirigid collars, wedge)
x	x	Extrication device short board
x	x	Swaddler or immobilization device
x	x	Cord clamps
x		Point-of-care glucose analysis capability
x		Gastric decompression tube, 8F to 16F
x		Meconium aspirator
x		Pulse oximeter and transport ECG monitor
x		Tracheal tube placement confirmation equipment (CO_2 detection/esophageal detector)
x	x	Stethoscope
x	x	Portable suction device
x	x	Obstetric pack
x	x	Thermal blanket
x	x	Water-soluble lubricant
x	x	Infant car seat
x	x	Nasopharyngeal airways (18F to 34F)
x	x	Glasgow Coma Scale score reference
x	x	Pediatric trauma score reference
x		Hand-held nebulizer
x		Length/weight-based drug dosing reference
x		Resuscitation drugs and IV fluids that meet local standards of care

*If within the scope of trained providers practice.

Future Directions

These guidelines more clearly indicate the quality of evidence for our recommendations than heretofore. There are few recommendations that have sufficient evidence to merit a Class IIa status, much less a Class I status. This observation represents an opportunity and a call to action to obtain better information to guide future guideline developers. Since the rate of cardiac arrest in infants and children is relatively low, a single center is unlikely to gather sufficient data to answer some of the important questions. Instead, a multi-institutional effort is needed to collect data using a consistent set of definitions.[1] The AHA is sponsoring the development of a National Registry for Cardiopulmonary Resuscitation (NRCPR) that should help address this need for data. We encourage widespread participation, which will lead to improved evidence-based guidelines.

References

1. Zaritsky A, Nadkarni V, Hazinski MF, Foltin G, Quan L, Wright J, Fiser D, Zideman D, O'Malley P, Chameides L, et al. Recommended guidelines for uniform reporting of pediatric advanced life support: the pediatric Utstein style: a statement for healthcare professionals from a task force of the American Academy of Pediatrics, the American Heart Association, and the European Resuscitation Council. *Pediatrics*. 1995; 96:765–779.
2. Young KD, Seidel JS. Pediatric cardiopulmonary resuscitation: a collective review. *Ann Emerg Med*. 1999;33:195–205.
3. Van Hoeyweghen RJ, Bossaert LL, Mullie A, Calle P, Martens P, Buylaert WA, Delooz H, Belgian Cerebral Resuscitation Group. Quality and efficiency of bystander CPR. *Resuscitation*. 1993;26:47–52.
4. Bossaert L, Van Hoeyweghen R, the Cerebral Resuscitation Study Group. Bystander cardiopulmonary resuscitation (CPR) in out-of-hospital cardiac arrest. *Ann Emerg Med*. 1989;17(suppl):S55–S69.
5. Nichol G, Stiell IG, Laupacis A, Pham B, De Maio VJ, Wells GA. A cumulative meta-analysis of the effectiveness of defibrillator-capable emergency medical services for victims of out-of-hospital cardiac arrest. *Ann Emerg Med*. 1999;34:517–525.
6. Stiell IG, Wells GA, DeMaio VJ, Spaite DW, Field BJ III, Munkley DP, Lyver MB, Luinstra LG, Ward R. Modifiable factors associated with improved cardiac arrest survival in a multicenter basic life support/ defibrillation system: OPALS Study phase I results. Ontario Prehospital Advanced Life Support. *Ann Emerg Med*. 1999;33:44–50.
7. Cummins RO, Hazinski MF, Kerber RE, Kudenchuk P, Becker L, Nichol G, Malanga B, Aufderheide TP, Stapleton EM, Kern K, Ornato JP, Sanders A, Valenzuela T, Eisenberg M. Low-energy biphasic waveform defibrillation: evidence-based review applied to emergency cardiovascular care guidelines: a statement for healthcare professionals from the American Heart Association Committee on Emergency Cardiovascular Care and the Subcommittees on Basic Life Support, Advanced Cardiac Life Support, and Pediatric Resuscitation. *Circulation*. 1998;97:1654–1667.
8. McPherson M, Arango P, Fox H, Lauver C, McManus M, Newacheck PW, Perrin JM, Shonkoff JP, Strickland B. A new definition of children with special health care needs. *Pediatrics*. 1998;102:137–140.
9. Newacheck PW, Strickland B, Shonkoff JP, Perrin JM, McPherson M, McManus M, Lauver C, Fox H, Arango P. An epidemiologic profile of children with special health care needs. *Pediatrics*. 1998;102:117–123.
10. Committee on Pediatric Emergency Medicine, American Academy of Pediatrics. Emergency preparedness for children with special health care needs. *Pediatrics*. 1999;104:e53.
11. Spaite DW, Conroy C, Tibbitts M, Karriker KJ, Seng M, Battaglia N, Criss EA, Valenzuela TD, Meislin HW. Use of emergency medical services by children with special health care needs. *Prehosp Emerg Care*. 2000;4:19–23.
12. Schultz-Grant LD, Young-Cureton V, Kataoka-Yahiro M. Advance directives and do not resuscitate orders: nurses' knowledge and the level of practice in school settings. *J Sch Nurs*. 1998;14:4–10, 12–13.
13. Subcommittee on Pediatric Resuscitation AHA. Guidelines for cardiopulmonary resuscitation and emergency cardiac care, VI: pediatric advanced life support. *JAMA*. 1992;268:2262–2275.

14. Kattwinkel J, Niermeyer S, Nadkarni V, Tibballs J, Phillips B, Zideman D, Van Reempts P, Osmond M. An advisory statement from the Pediatric Working Group of the International Liaison Committee on Resuscitation. *Pediatrics.* 1999;103:e56.

15. Nadkarni V, Hazinski MF, Zideman D, Kattwinkel J, Quan L, Bingham R, Zaritsky A, Bland J, Kramer E, Tibballs J. Pediatric resuscitation: an advisory statement from the Pediatric Working Group of the International Liaison Committee on Resuscitation. *Circulation.* 1997;95: 2185–2195.

16. Hoyert DL, Kochanek KD, Murphy SL. Deaths: final data for 1997. *National Vital Statistics Report.* 1999;47:1–105.

17. Sirbaugh PE, Pepe PE, Shook JE, Kimball KT, Goldman MJ, Ward MA, Mann DM. A prospective, population-based study of the demographics, epidemiology, management, and outcome of out-of-hospital pediatric cardiopulmonary arrest. *Ann Emerg Med.* 1999;33:174–184.

18. Kuisma M, Suominen P, Korpela R. Paediatric out-of-hospital cardiac arrests: epidemiology and outcome. *Resuscitation.* 1995;30:141–150.

19. Richman PB, Nashed AH. The etiology of cardiac arrest in children and young adults: special considerations for ED management. *Am J Emerg Med.* 1999;17:264–270.

20. Adgey AAJ, Johnston PW, McMechan S. Sudden cardiac death and substance abuse. *Resuscitation.* 1995;29:219–221.

21. Ackerman MJ. The long QT syndrome. *Pediatr Rev.* 1998;19:232–238.

22. Brownstein DR, Quan L, Orr R, Wentz KR, Copass MK. Paramedic intubation training in a pediatric operating room. *Am J Emerg Med.* 1992;10:418–420.

23. Ma OJ, Atchley RB, Hatley T, Green M, Young J, Brady W. Intubation success rates improve for an air medical program after implementing the use of neuromuscular blocking agents. *Am J Emerg Med.* 1998;16: 125–127.

24. Sing RF, Rotondo MF, Zonies DH, Schwab CW, Kauder DR, Ross SE, Brathwaite CC. Rapid sequence induction for intubation by an aeromedical transport team: a critical analysis. *Am J Emerg Med.* 1998;16: 598–602.

25. Gausche M, Lewis RJ, Stratton SJ, Haynes BE, Gunter CS, Godrich SM, Poore PD, McCollough MD, Henderson DP, Pratt FD, Seidel JS. A prospective randomized study of the effect of out-of-hospital pediatric endotracheal intubation on survival and neurological outcome. *JAMA.* 2000;283:783–790.

26. Thomas SH, Harrison T, Wedel SK. Flight crew airway management in four settings: a six-year review. *Prehosp Emerg Care.* 1999;3:310–315.

27. Ma MH, Hwang JJ, Lai LP, Wang SM, Huang GT, Shyu KG, Ko YL, Lin JL, Chen WJ, Hsu KL, et al. Transesophageal echocardiographic assessment of mitral valve position and pulmonary venous flow during cardiopulmonary resuscitation in humans. *Circulation.* 1995;92: 854–61.

28. Andersen KH, Schultz-Lebahn T. Oesophageal intubation can be undetected by auscultation of the chest. *Acta Anaesthesiol Scand.* 1994;38: 580–582.

29. Beyer AJ III, Land G, Zaritsky A. Nonphysician transport of intubated pediatric patients: a system evaluation. *Crit Care Med.* 1992;20: 961–966.

30. Poirier MP, Gonzalez Del-Rey JA, McAneney CM, DiGiulio GA. Utility of monitoring capnography, pulse oximetry, and vital signs in the detection of airway mishaps: a hyperoxemic animal model. *Am J Emerg Med.* 1998;16:350–352.

31. Palme C, Nystrom B, Tunell R. An evaluation of the efficiency of face masks in the resuscitation of newborn infants. *Lancet.* 1985;1:207–210.

32. Finer NN, Barrington KJ, Al-Fadley F, Peters KL. Limitations of self-inflating resuscitators. *Pediatrics.* 1986;77:417–420.

33. Rumball CJ, MacDonald D. The PTL, Combitube, laryngeal mask, and oral airway: a randomized prehospital comparative study of ventilatory device effectiveness and cost-effectiveness in 470 cases of cardiorespiratory arrest. *Prehosp Emerg Care.* 1997;1:1–10.

34. Martin SE, Ochsner MG, Jarman RH, Agudelo WE, Davis FE. Use of the laryngeal mask airway in air transport when intubation fails. *J Trauma.* 1999;47:352–357.

35. Berry AM, Brimacombe JR, Verghese C. The laryngeal mask airway in emergency medicine, neonatal resuscitation, and intensive care medicine. *Int Anesthesiol Clin.* 1998;36:91–109.

36. Lopez-Gil M, Brimacombe J, Cebrian J, Arranz J. Laryngeal mask airway in pediatric practice: a prospective study of skill acquisition by anesthesia residents. *Anesthesiology.* 1996;84:807–811.

37. Lopez-Gil M, Brimacombe J, Alvarez M. Safety and efficacy of the laryngeal mask airway: a prospective survey of 1400 children. *Anaesthesia.* 1996;51:969–972.

38. Brimacombe J. The advantages of the LMA over the tracheal tube or facemask: a meta- analysis. *Can J Anaesth.* 1995;42:1017–1023.

39. Baskett PJF (coordinator). The use of the laryngeal mask airway by nurses during cardiopulmonary resuscitation: results of a multicentre trial. *Anaesthesia.* 1994;49:3–7.

40. Pennant JH, Walker MB. Comparison of the endotracheal tube and laryngeal mask in airway management by paramedical personnel. *Anesth Analg.* 1992;74:531–534.

41. Brimacombe JR, Berry A. The incidence of aspiration associated with the laryngeal mask airway: a meta-analysis of published literature. *J Clin Anesth.* 1995;7:297–305.

42. Stone BJ, Chantler PJ, Baskett PJ. The incidence of regurgitation during cardiopulmonary resuscitation: a comparison between the bag valve mask and laryngeal mask airway. *Resuscitation.* 1998;38:3–6.

43. Field D, Milner AD, Hopkin IE. Efficiency of manual resuscitators at birth. *Arch Dis Child.* 1986;61:300–302.

44. Terndrup TE, Kanter RK, Cherry RA. A comparison of infant ventilation methods performed by prehospital personnel. *Ann Emerg Med.* 1989;18:607–611.

45. Hirschman AM, Kravath RE. Venting vs ventilating: a danger of manual resuscitation bags. *Chest.* 1982;82:369–370.

46. Mondolfi AA, Grenier BM, Thompson JE, Bachur RG. Comparison of self-inflating bags with anesthesia bags for bag-mask ventilation in the pediatric emergency department. *Pediatr Emerg Care.* 1997;13: 312–316.

47. Jesudian MC, Harrison RR, Keenan RL, Maull KI. Bag-valve-mask ventilation: two rescuers are better than one: preliminary report. *Crit Care Med.* 1985;13:122–123.

48. Moynihan RJ, Brock-Utne JG, Archer JH, Feld LH, Kreitzman TR. The effect of cricoid pressure on preventing gastric insufflation in infants and children. *Anesthesiology.* 1993;78:652–656.

49. Salem MR, Wong AY, Mani M, Sellick BA. Efficacy of cricoid pressure in preventing gastric inflation during bag-mask ventilation in pediatric patients. *Anesthesiology.* 1974;40:96–98.

50. Sellick BA. Cricoid pressure to control regurgitation of stomach contents during induction of anesthesia. *Lancet.* 1961;2:404–406.

51. Hartsilver EL, Vanner RG. Airway obstruction with cricoid pressure. *Anaesthesia.* 2000;55:208–211.

52. Berg MD, Idris AH, Berg RA. Severe ventilatory compromise due to gastric distention during pediatric cardiopulmonary resuscitation. *Resuscitation.* 1998;36:71–73.

53. Deakers TW, Reynolds G, Stretton M, Newth CJ. Cuffed endotracheal tubes in pediatric intensive care. *J Pediatr.* 1994;125:57–62.

54. Khine HH, Corddry DH, Kettrick RG, Martin TM, McCloskey JJ, Rose JB, Theroux MC, Zagnoev M. Comparison of cuffed and uncuffed endotracheal tubes in young children during general anesthesia. *Anesthesiology.* 1997;86:627–631.

55. Luten RC, Wears RL, Broselow J, Zaritsky A, Barnett TM, Lee T, Bailey A, Valley R, Brown R, Rosenthal B. Length-based endotracheal tube and emergency equipment in pediatrics. *Ann Emerg Med.* 1992;21: 900–904.

56. King BR, Baker MD, Braitman LE, Seidl-Friedman J, Schreiner MS. Endotracheal tube selection in children: a comparison of four methods. *Ann Emerg Med.* 1993;22:530–534.

57. van den Berg AA, Mphanza T. Choice of tracheal tube size for children: finger size or age-related formula? *Anaesthesia.* 1997;52:701–703.

58. Westhorpe RN. The position of the larynx in children and its relationship to the ease of intubation. *Anaesth Intensive Care.* 1987;15:384–388.

59. Kelly JJ, Eynon CA, Kaplan JL, de Garavilla L, Dalsey WC. Use of tube condensation as an indicator of endotracheal tube placement. *Ann Emerg Med.* 1998;31:575–578.

60. Donn SM, Kuhns LR. Mechanism of endotracheal tube movement with change of head position in the neonate. *Pediatr Radiol.* 1980;9:37–40.

61. Hartrey R, Kestin IG. Movement of oral and nasal tracheal tubes as a result of changes in head and neck position. *Anaesthesia.* 1995;50: 682–687.

62. Gerardi MJ, Sacchetti AD, Cantor RM, Santamaria JP, Gausche M, Lucid W, Foltin GL. Rapid-sequence intubation of the pediatric patient. Pediatric Emergency Medicine Committee of the American College of Emergency Physicians [see comments]. *Ann Emerg Med.* 1996;28: 55–74.

63. Bota GW, Rowe BH. Continuous monitoring of oxygen saturation in prehospital patients with severe illness: the problem of unrecognized hypoxemia. *J Emerg Med.* 1995;13:305–311.

64. Aughey K, Hess D, Eitel D, Bleecher K, Cooley M, Ogden C, Sabulsky N. An evaluation of pulse oximetry in prehospital care. *Ann Emerg Med.* 1991;20:887–891.

65. Brown LH, Manring EA, Kornegay HB, Prasad NH. Can prehospital personnel detect hypoxemia without the aid of pulse oximeters? *Am J Emerg Med.* 1996;14:43–44.

66. Birmingham PK, Cheney FW, Ward RJ. Esophageal intubation: a review of detection techniques. *Anesth Analg.* 1986;65:886–891.

67. Bhende MS, Thompson AE, Orr RA. Utility of an end-tidal carbon dioxide detector during stabilization and transport of critically ill children. *Pediatrics.* 1992;89:1042–1044.

68. Bhende MS, Thompson AE, Cook DR, Saville AL. Validity of a disposable end-tidal CO_2 detector in verifying endotracheal tube placement in infants and children. *Ann Emerg Med.* 1992;21:142–145.

69. Bhende MS, Thompson AE. Evaluation of an end-tidal CO_2 detector during pediatric cardiopulmonary resuscitation. *Pediatrics.* 1995;95:395–399.

70. Ornato JP, Shipley JB, Racht EM, Slovis CM, Wrenn KD, Pepe PE, Almeida SL, Ginger VF, Fotre TV. Multicenter study of a portable, hand-size, colorimetric end-tidal carbon dioxide detection device. *Ann Emerg Med.* 1992;21:518–523.

71. Cardoso MM, Banner MJ, Melker RJ, Bjoraker DG. Portable devices used to detect endotracheal intubation during emergency situations: a review. *Crit Care Med.* 1998;26:957–964.

72. Ward KR, Yealy DM. End-tidal carbon dioxide monitoring in emergency medicine, 2: clinical applications. *Acad Emerg Med.* 1998;5:637–646.

73. Cantineau JP, Merckx P, Lambert Y, Sorkine M, Bertrand C, Duvaldestin P. Effect of epinephrine on end-tidal carbon dioxide pressure during prehospital cardiopulmonary resuscitation. *Am J Emerg Med.* 1994;12:267–270.

74. Kern KB, Sanders AB, Voorhees WD, Babbs CF, Tacker WA, Ewy GA. Changes in expired end-tidal carbon dioxide during cardiopulmonary resuscitation in dogs: A prognostic guide for resuscitation efforts. *J Am Coll Cardiol.* 1989;13:1184–1189.

75. Callaham M, Barton C. Prediction of outcome of cardiopulmonary resuscitation from end-tidal carbon dioxide concentration. *Crit Care Med.* 1990;18:358–362.

76. Levine RL, Wayne MA, Miller CC. End-tidal carbon dioxide and outcome of out-of-hospital cardiac arrest. *N Engl J Med.* 1997;337:301–306.

77. Varon AJ, Morrina J, Civetta JM. Clinical utility of a colorimetric end-tidal CO_2 detector in cardiopulmonary resuscitation and emergency intubation. *J Clin Monit.* 1991;7:289–293.

78. Ward K, Sullivan JR, Zelenak RR, et al. A comparison of interposed abdominal compression CPR and standard CPR by monitoring end-tidal Pco_2. *Ann Emerg Med.* 1989;18:831–837.

79. Ward KR, Menegazzi JJ, Zelenak RR, Sullivan RJ, McSwain N Jr. A comparison of chest compressions between mechanical and manual CPR by monitoring end-tidal PCO_2 during human cardiac arrest. *Ann Emerg Med.* 1993;22:669–674.

80. Weil MH, Bisera J, Trevino RP, Rackow EC. Cardiac output and end-tidal carbon dioxide. *Crit Care Med.* 1985;13:907–909.

81. Ornato JP, Garnett AR, Glauser FL. Relationship between cardiac output and the end-tidal carbon dioxide tension. *Ann Emerg Med.* 1990;19:1104–1106.

82. Bhende MS, Karasic DG, Karasic RB. End-tidal carbon dioxide changes during cardiopulmonary resuscitation after experimental asphyxial cardiac arrest. *Am J Emerg Med.* 1996;14:349–350.

83. Berg RA, Henry C, Otto CW, Sanders AB, Kern KB, Hilwig RW, Ewy GA. Initial end-tidal CO_2 is markedly elevated during cardiopulmonary resuscitation after asphyxial cardiac arrest. *Pediatr Emerg Care.* 1996;12:245–248.

84. Kasper CL, Deem S. The self-inflating bulb to detect esophageal intubation during emergency airway management. *Anesthesiology.* 1998;88:898–902.

85. Zaleski L, Abello D, Gold MI. The esophageal detector device: does it work? *Anesthesiology.* 1993;79:244–247.

86. Bozeman WP, Hexter D, Liang HK, Kelen GD. Esophageal detector device versus detection of end-tidal carbon dioxide level in emergency intubation. *Ann Emerg Med.* 1996;27:595–599.

87. Wee MY, Walker AK. The oesophageal detector device: an assessment with uncuffed tubes in children. *Anaesthesia.* 1991;46:869–871.

88. Haynes SR, Morton NS. Use of the oesophageal detector device in children under one year of age. *Anaesthesia.* 1990;45:1067–1069.

89. Lang DJ, Wafai Y, Salem MR, Czinn EA, Halim AA, Baraka A. Efficacy of the self-inflating bulb in confirming tracheal intubation in the morbidly obese. *Anesthesiology.* 1996;85:246–253.

90. Baraka A, Khoury PJ, Siddik SS, Salem MR, Joseph NJ. Efficacy of the self-inflating bulb in differentiating esophageal from tracheal intubation in the parturient undergoing cesarean section. *Anesth Analg.* 1997;84:533–537.

91. O'Connor R, Swor RA. National Association of EMS Physicians position paper: verification of endotracheal tube placement following intubation. *Prehosp Emerg Care.* 1999;3:248–250.

92. Zander J, Hazinski MF. Pulmonary disorders: airway obstruction. In: Hazinski MF, ed. *Nursing Care of the Critically Ill Child.* St Louis, Mo: Mosby-Year Book; 1992.

93. Klain M, Keszler H, Brader E. High frequency jet ventilation in CPR. *Crit Care Med.* 1981;9:421–422.

94. Depierraz B, Ravussin P, Brossard E, Monnier P. Percutaneous transtracheal jet ventilation for paediatric endoscopic laser treatment of laryngeal and subglottic lesions. *Can J Anaesth.* 1994;41:1200–1207.

95. Ravussin P, Bayer-Berger M, Monnier P, Savary M, Freeman J. Percutaneous transtracheal ventilation for laser endoscopic procedures in infants and small children with laryngeal obstruction: report of two cases. *Can J Anaesth.* 1987;34:83–86.

96. Peak DA, Roy S. Needle cricothyroidotomy revisited. *Pediatr Emerg Care.* 1999;15:224–226.

97. Barrachina F, Guardiola JJ, Ano T, Ochagavia A, Marine J. Percutaneous dilatational cricothyroidotomy: outcome with 44 consecutive patients. *Intensive Care Med.* 1996;22:937–940.

98. Nypaver M, Treloar D. Neutral cervical spine positioning in children. *Ann Emerg Med.* 1994;23:208–211.

99. Herzenberg JE, Hensinger RN, Dedrick DK, Phillips WA. Emergency transport and positioning of young children who have an injury of the cervical spine: the standard backboard may be hazardous. *J Bone Joint Surg Am.* 1989;71:15–22.

100. Lindner KH, Pfenninger EG, Lurie KG, Schurmann W, Lindner IM, Ahnefeld FW. Effects of active compression-decompression resuscitation on myocardial and cerebral blood flow in pigs. *Circulation.* 1993;88:1254–1263.

101. Chang MW, Coffeen P, Lurie KG, Shultz J, Bache RJ, White CW. Active compression-decompression CPR improves vital organ perfusion in a dog model of ventricular fibrillation. *Chest.* 1994;106:1250–1259.

102. Shultz JJ, Coffeen P, Sweeney M, Detloff B, Kehler C, Pineda E, Yakshe P, Adler SW, Chang M, Lurie KG. Evaluation of standard and active compression-decompression CPR in an acute human model of ventricular fibrillation. *Circulation.* 1994;89:684–693.

103. Plaisance P, Adnet F, Vicaut E, Hennequin B, Magne P, Prudhomme C, Lambert Y, Cantineau JP, Leopold C, Ferracci C, Gizzi M, Payen D. Benefit of active compression-decompression cardiopulmonary resuscitation as a prehospital advanced cardiac life support: a randomized multicenter study. *Circulation.* 1997;95:955–961.

104. Mauer D, Schneider T, Dick W, Withelm A, Elich D, Mauer M. Active compression-decompression resuscitation: a prospective, randomized study in a two-tiered EMS system with physicians in the field. *Resuscitation.* 1996;33:125–134.

105. Stiell IG, Hebert PC, Wells GA, Laupacis A, Vandemheen K, Dreyer JF, Eisenhauer MA, Gibson J, Higginson LA, Kirby AS, Mahon JL, Maloney JP, Weitzman BN. The Ontario trial of active compression-decompression cardiopulmonary resuscitation for in-hospital and prehospital cardiac arrest. *JAMA.* 1996;275:1417–1423.

106. Waldman PJ, Walters BL, Grunau CFV. Pancreatic injury associated with interposed abdominal compressions in pediatric cardiopulmonary resuscitation. *Am J Emerg Med.* 1984;2:510–512.

107. Chang FC, Harrison PB, Beech RR, Helmer SD. PASG: does it help in the management of traumatic shock? *J Trauma.* 1995;39:453–456.

108. Mattox KL, Bickell W, Pepe PE, Burch J, Feliciano D. Prospective MAST study in 911 patients. *J Trauma.* 1989;29:1104–1111.

109. Brunette DD, Fifield G, Ruiz E. Use of pneumatic antishock trousers in the management of pediatric pelvic hemorrhage. *Pediatr Emerg Care.* 1987;3:86–90.

110. Aprahamian C, Gessert G, Bandyk DF, Sell L, Stiehl J, Olson DW. MAST-associated compartment syndrome (MACS): a review. *J Trauma.* 1989;29:549–555.

111. Blomquist S, Aberg T, Solem JO, Steen S. Lung mechanics, gas exchange and central circulation during treatment of intra-abdominal hemorrhage with pneumatic anti-shock garment and intra-aortic balloon occlusion: an experimental study in pigs. *Eur Surg Res.* 1994;26: 240–247.

112. Bircher N, Safar P. Manual open-chest cardiopulmonary resuscitation. *Ann Emerg Med.* 1984;13:770–773.

113. Boczar ME, Howard MA, Rivers EP, Martin GB, Horst HM, Lewandowski C, Tomlanovich MC, Nowak RM. A technique revisited: hemodynamic comparison of closed- and open-chest cardiac massage during human cardiopulmonary resuscitation. *Crit Care Med.* 1995;23:498–503.

114. Beaver BL, Colombani PM, Buck JR, Dudgeon DL, Bohrer SL, Haller JA Jr. Efficacy of emergency room thoracotomy in pediatric trauma. *J Pediatr Surg.* 1987;22:19–23.

115. Redding JS, Cozine RA. A comparison of open-chest and closed-chest cardiac massage in dogs. *Anesthesiology.* 1961;22:280–285.

116. Sheikh A, Brogan T. Outcome and cost of open- and closed-chest cardiopulmonary resuscitation in pediatric cardiac arrests. *Pediatrics.* 1994;93:392–398.

117. Takino M, Okada Y. The optimum timing of resuscitative thoracotomy for non-traumatic out-of-hospital cardiac arrest. *Resuscitation.* 1993;26: 69–74.

118. Duncan BW, Ibrahim AE, Hraska V, del Nido PJ, Laussen PC, Wessel DL, Mayer JE Jr, Bower LK, Jonas RA. Use of rapid-deployment extracorporeal membrane oxygenation for the resuscitation of pediatric patients with heart disease after cardiac arrest. *J Thorac Cardiovasc Surg.* 1998;116:305–311.

119. del-Nido PJ, Dalton HJ, Thompson AE, Siewers RD. Extracorporeal membrane oxygenator rescue in children during cardiac arrest after cardiac surgery. *Circulation.* 1992;86(suppl II):II-300–II-304.

120. Dalton HJ, Siewers RD, Fuhrman BP, Del Nido P, Thompson AE, Shaver MG, Dowhy M. Extracorporeal membrane oxygenation for cardiac rescue in children with severe myocardial dysfunction. *Crit Care Med.* 1993;21:1020–1028.

121. Mair P, Hoermann C, Moertl M, Bonatti J, Falbesoner C, Balogh D. Percutaneous venoarterial extracorporeal membrane oxygenation for emergency mechanical circulatory support. *Resuscitation.* 1996;33: 29–34.

122. Cochran JB, Tecklenburg FW, Lau YR, Habib DM. Emergency cardiopulmonary bypass for cardiac arrest refractory to pediatric advanced life support. *Pediatr Emerg Care.* 1999;15:30–32.

123. Martin GB, Rivers EP, Paradis NA, Goetting MG, Morris DC, Nowak RM. Emergency department cardiopulmonary bypass in the treatment of human cardiac arrest. *Chest.* 1998;113:743–751.

124. Rosetti V, Thompson B, Aprahamian C, Darin J, Mateer J. Difficulty and delay in intravascular access in pediatric arrests. *Ann Emerg Med.* 1984;13:406.

125. Hedges JR, Barsan WB, Doan LA, Joyce SM, Lukes SJ, Dalsey WC, Nishiyama H. Central versus peripheral intravenous routes in cardiopulmonary resuscitation. *Am J Emerg Med.* 1984;2:385–390.

126. Fleisher G, Caputo G, Baskin M. Comparison of external jugular and peripheral venous administration of sodium bicarbonate in puppies. *Crit Care Med.* 1989;17:251–254.

127. Lloyd TR, Donnerstein RL, Berg RA. Accuracy of central venous pressure measurement from the abdominal inferior vena cava. *Pediatrics.* 1992;89:506–508.

128. Berg RA, Lloyd TR, Donnerstein RL. Accuracy of central venous pressure monitoring in the intraabdominal inferior vena cava: a canine study. *J Pediatr.* 1992;120:67–71.

129. Kanter RK, Zimmerman JJ, Strauss RH, Stoeckel KA. Pediatric emergency intravenous access: evaluation of a protocol. *Am J Dis Child.* 1986;140:132–134.

130. Fiser D. Intraosseous infusion. *N Engl J Med.* 1990;322:1579–1581.

131. Banerjee S, Singhi SC, Singh S, Singh M. The intraosseous route is a suitable alternative to intravenous route for fluid resuscitation in severely dehydrated children. *Indian Pediatr.* 1994;31:1511–1520.

132. Glaeser P, Losek J, Nelson D, et al. Pediatric intraosseous infusions: impact on vascular access time. *Am J Emerg Med.* 1988;6:330–332.

133. Daga SR, Gosavi DV, Verma B. Intraosseous access using butterfly needle. *Trop Doct.* 1999;29:142–144.

134. Glaeser PW, Hellmich TR, Szewczuga D, Losek JD, Smith DS. Five-year experience in prehospital intraosseous infusion in children and adults. *Ann Emerg Med.* 1993;22:1119–1124.

135. Guy J, Haley K, Zuspan SJ. Use of intraosseous infusion in the pediatric trauma patient. *J Pediatr Surg.* 1993;28:158–161.

136. Waisman M, Waisman D. Bone marrow infusion in adults. *J Trauma.* 1997;42:288–293.

137. Berg R. Emergency infusion of catecholamines into bone marrow. *Am J Dis Child.* 1984;138:810–811.

138. Andropoulos DB, Soifer SJ, Schrieber MD. Plasma epinephrine concentrations after intraosseous and central venous injection during cardiopulmonary resuscitation in the lamb. *J Pediatr.* 1990;116:312–315.

139. Orlowski JP, Porembka DT, Gallagher JM, Lockrem JD, VanLente F. Comparison study of intraosseous, central intravenous, and peripheral intravenous infusions of emergency drugs. *Am J Dis Child.* 1990;144: 112–117.

140. Warren DW, Kissoon N, Sommerauer JF, Rieder MJ. Comparison of fluid infusion rates among peripheral intravenous and humerus, femur, malleolus, and tibial intraosseous sites in normovolemic and hypovolemic piglets. *Ann Emerg Med.* 1993;22:183–186.

141. Plewa MC, King RW, Fenn-Buderer N, Gretzinger K, Renuart D, Cruz R. Hematologic safety of intraosseous blood transfusion in a swine model of pediatric hemorrhagic hypovolemia. *Acad Emerg Med.* 1995; 2:799–809.

142. Johnson L, Kissoon N, Fiallos M, Abdelmoneim T, Murphy S. Use of intraosseous blood to assess blood chemistries and hemoglobin during cardiopulmonary resuscitation with drug infusions. *Crit Care Med.* 1999;27:1147–1152.

143. Abdelmoneim T, Kissoon N, Johnson L, Fiallos M, Murphy S. Acid-base status of blood from intraosseous and mixed venous sites during prolonged cardiopulmonary resuscitation and drug infusions. *Crit Care Med.* 1999;27:1923–1928.

144. Heinild S, Sodergaard T, Tudvad F. Bone marrow infusions in childhood: experiences from 1000 infusions. *J Pediatr.* 1974;30: 400–412.

145. Rosetti VA, Thompson BM, Miller J, Mateer JR, Aprahamian C. Intraosseous infusion: an alternative route of pediatric intravascular access. *Ann Emerg Med.* 1985;14:885–888.

146. La Fleche FR, Slepin MJ, Vargas J, Milzman DP. Iatrogenic bilateral tibial fractures after intraosseous infusion attempts in a 3 month old infant. *Ann Emerg Med.* 1989;18:1099–1101.

147. Vidal R, Kissoon N, Gayle M. Compartment syndrome following intraosseous infusion. *Pediatrics.* 1993;91:1201–1202.

148. Simmons CM, Johnson NE, Perkin RM, van Stralen D. Intraosseous extravasation complication reports. *Ann Emerg Med.* 1994;23:363–366.

149. Rosovsky M, FitzPatrick M, Goldfarb CR, Finestone H. Bilateral osteomyelitis due to intraosseous infusion: case report and review of the English-language literature. *Pediatr Radiol.* 1994;24:72–73.

150. Pollack CV Jr, Pender ES, Woodall BN, Tubbs RC, Iyer RV, Miller HW. Long-term local effects of intraosseous infusion on tibial bone marrow in the weanling pig model. *Am J Emerg Med.* 1992;10:27–31.

151. Brickman KR, Rega P, Schoolfield L, Harkins K, Weisbrode SE, Reynolds G. Investigation of bone developmental and histopathologic changes from intraosseous infusion. *Ann Emerg Med.* 1996;28: 430–435.

152. Fiser RT, Walker WM, Seibert JJ, McCarthy R, Fiser DH. Tibial length following intraosseous infusion: a prospective, radiographic analysis. *Pediatr Emerg Care.* 1997;13:186–188.

153. Orlowski JP, Julius CJ, Petras RE, Porembka DT, Gallagher JM. The safety of intraosseous infusions: risks of fat and bone marrow emboli to the lungs. *Ann Emerg Med.* 1989;18:1062–1067.

154. Fiallos M, Kissoon N, Abdelmoneim T, Johnson L, Murphy S, Lu L, Masood S, Idris A. Fat embolism with the use of intraosseous infusion during cardiopulmonary resuscitation. *Am J Med Sci.* 1997;314:73–79.

155. Ward J Jr. Endotracheal drug therapy. *Am J Emerg Med.* 1983;1:71–82.

156. Johnston C. Endotracheal drug delivery. *Pediatr Emerg Care.* 1992;8: 94–97.

157. Ralston SH, Tacher WA, Showen L, Carter A, Babbs CF. Endotracheal versus intravenous epinephrine during electromechanical dissociation with CPR in dogs. *Ann Emerg Med.* 1985;14:1044–1048.

158. Kleinman ME, Oh W, Stonestreet BS. Comparison of intravenous and endotracheal epinephrine during cardiopulmonary resuscitation in newborn piglets. *Crit Care Med.* 1999;27:2748–2754.

159. Quinton DN, O'Byrne G, Aitkenhead AR. Comparison of endotracheal and peripheral intravenous adrenaline in cardiac arrest: is the endotracheal route reliable? *Lancet.* 1987;1:828–829.

160. Jasani MS, Nadkarni VM, Finkelstein MS, Mandell GA, Salzman SK, Norman ME. Endotracheal epinephrine administration technique effects in pediatric porcine hypoxic-hypercarbic arrest. *Crit Care Med.* 1994; 22:1174–1180.

161. Lubitz DS, Seidel JS, Chameides L, Luten RC, Zaritsky AL, Campbell FW. A rapid method for estimating weight and resuscitation drug dosages from length in the pediatric age group. *Ann Emerg Med.* 1988; 17:576–581.

162. Carcillo J, Davis A, Zaritsky A. Role of early fluid resuscitation in pediatric septic shock. *JAMA.* 1991;266:1242–1245.

163. Schierhout G, Roberts I. Fluid resuscitation with colloid or crystalloid solutions in critically ill patients: a systematic review of randomised trials. *BMJ.* 1998;316:961–964.

164. Cochrane Injuries Group Albumin Reviewers. Human albumin administration in critically ill patients: systematic review of randomised controlled trials. *BMJ.* 1998;317:235–240.

165. Qureshi AI, Suarez JI, Bhardwaj A, Mirski M, Schnitzer MS, Hanley DF, Ulatowski JA. Use of hypertonic (3%) saline/acetate infusion in the treatment of cerebral edema: effect on intracranial pressure and lateral displacement of the brain. *Crit Care Med.* 1998;26:440–446.

166. Schwarz S, Schwab S, Bertram M, Aschoff A, Hacke W. Effects of hypertonic saline hydroxyethyl starch solution and mannitol in patients with increased intracranial pressure after stroke. *Stroke.* 1998;29: 1550–1555.

167. Rocha e Silva M. Hypertonic saline resuscitation. *Medicina.* 1998;58: 393–402.

168. Simma B, Burger R, Falk M, Sacher P, Fanconi S. A prospective, randomized, and controlled study of fluid management in children with severe head injury: lactated Ringer's solution versus hypertonic saline [see comments]. *Crit Care Med.* 1998;26:1265–1270.

169. Cherian L, Goodman JC, Robertson CS. Hyperglycemia increases brain injury caused by secondary ischemia after cortical impact injury in rats [see comments]. *Crit Care Med.* 1997;25:1378–1383.

170. Ashwal S, Schneider S, Tomasi L, Thompson J. Prognostic implications of hyperglycemia and reduced cerebral blood flow in childhood near-drowning. *Neurology.* 1990;40:820–823.

171. Longstreth WT Jr, Copass MK, Dennis LK, Rauch-Matthews ME, Stark MS, Cobb LA. Intravenous glucose after out-of-hospital cardiopulmonary arrest: a community-based randomized trial. *Neurology.* 1993;43: 2534–2541.

172. Niemann JT, Criley JM, Rosborough JP, Niskanen RA, Alferness C. Predictive indices of successful cardiac resuscitation after prolonged arrest and experimental cardiopulmonary resuscitation. *Ann Emerg Med.* 1985;14:521–528.

173. Sanders AB, Ewy GA, Taft TV. The prognostic and therapeutic importance of the aortic diastolic pressure in resuscitation from cardiac arrest. *Crit Care Med.* 1984;12:871–873.

174. Otto C, Yakaitis R, Blitt C. Mechanism of action of epinephrine in resuscitation from asphyxial arrest. *Crit Care Med.* 1981;9:321–324.

175. Mogayzel C, Quan L, Graves JR, Tiedeman D, Fahrenbruch C, Herndon P. Out-of-hospital ventricular fibrillation in children and adolescents: causes and outcomes. *Ann Emerg Med.* 1995;25:484–491.

176. Hickey RW, Cohen DM, Strausbaugh S, Dietrich AM. Pediatric patients requiring CPR in the prehospital setting. *Ann Emerg Med.* 1995;25: 495–501.

177. Huang YG, Wong KC, Yip WH, McJames SW, Pace NL. Cardiovascular responses to graded doses of three catecholamines during lactic and hydrochloric acidosis in dogs. *Br J Anaesth.* 1995;74:583–590.

178. Preziosi MP, Roig JC, Hargrove N, Burchfield DJ. Metabolic acidemia with hypoxia attenuates the hemodynamic responses to epinephrine during resuscitation in lambs. *Crit Care Med.* 1993;21:1901–1907.

179. Brown CG, Werman HA. Adrenergic agonists during cardiopulmonary resuscitation. *Resuscitation.* 1990;19:1–16.

180. Gonzales ER, Ornato JP, Garnett AR, Levine RL, Young DS, Racht EM. Dose-dependent vasopressor response to epinephrine during CPR in human beings. *Ann Emerg Med.* 1989;18:920–926.

181. Goetting MG, Paradis NA. High-dose epinephrine improves outcome from pediatric cardiac arrest. *Ann Emerg Med.* 1991;20:22–26.

182. Brown CG, Martin DR, Pepe PE, Stueven H, Cummins RO, Gonzalez E, Jastremski M, the Multicenter High-Dose Epinephrine Study Group. A comparison of standard-dose and high-dose epinephrine in cardiac arrest outside the hospital. *N Engl J Med.* 1992;327:1051–1055.

183. Callaham M, Madsen CD, Barton CW, Saunders CE, Daley M, Pointer J. A randomized trial of high-dose epinephrine and norepinephrine versus standard dose epinephrine in prehospital cardiac arrest. *JAMA.* 1992;268:2667–2672.

184. Lipman J, Wilson W, Kobilski S, Scribante J, Lee C, Kraus P, Cooper J, Barr J, Moyes D. High-dose adrenaline in adult in-hospital asystolic

185. Lindner KH, Ahnefeld FW, Prengel AW. Comparison of standard and high-dose adrenaline in the resuscitation of asystole and electromechanical dissociation. *Acta Anaesthesiol Scand.* 1991;35:253–256.

186. Sherman BW, Munger MA, Foulke GE, Rutherford WF, Panacek EA. High-dose versus standard-dose epinephrine treatment of cardiac arrest after failure of standard therapy. *Pharmacotherapy.* 1997;17:242–7.

187. Berg RA, Otto CW, Kern KB, Sanders AB, Hilwig RW, Hansen KK, Ewy GA. High-dose epinephrine results in greater early mortality after resuscitation from prolonged cardiac arrest in pigs: a prospective, randomized study. *Crit Care Med.* 1994;22:282–290.

188. Berg RA, Otto CW, Kern KB, Hilwig RW, Sanders AB, Henry CP, Ewy GA. A randomized, blinded trial of high-dose epinephrine versus standard-dose epinephrine in a swine model of pediatric asphyxial cardiac arrest. *Crit Care Med.* 1996;24:1695–1700.

189. Carpenter TC, Stenmark KR. High-dose epinephrine is not superior to standard-dose epinephrine in pediatric in-hospital cardiopulmonary arrest. *Pediatrics.* 1997;99:403–408.

190. Dieckmann RA, Vardis R. High-dose epinephrine in pediatric out-of-hospital cardiopulmonary arrest. *Pediatrics.* 1995;95:901–913.

191. Rivers EP, Wortsman J, Rady MY, Blake HC, McGeorge FT, Buderer NM. The effect of the total cumulative epinephrine dose administered during human CPR on hemodynamic, oxygen transport, and utilization variables in the postresuscitation period. *Chest.* 1994;106:1499–1507.

192. Tang W, Weil MH, Sun S, Noc M, Yang L, Gazmuri RJ. Epinephrine increases the severity of postresuscitation myocardial dysfunction. *Circulation.* 1995;92:3089–93.

193. Berg RA, Donnerstein RL, Padbury JF. Dobutamine infusions in stable, critically ill children: pharmacokinetics and hemodynamic actions. *Crit Care Med.* 1993;21:678–86.

194. Berg RA, Padbury JF. Sulfoconjugation and renal excretion contribute to the interpatient variation of exogenous catecholamine clearance in critically ill children. *Crit Care Med.* 1997;25:1247–51.

195. Chernow B, Holbrook P, D'Angona DS Jr, Zaritsky A, Casey LC, Fletcher JR, Lake CR. Epinephrine absorption after intratracheal administration. *Anesth Analg.* 1984;63:829–832.

196. Zaritsky AL. Catecholamines, inotropic medications, and vasopressor agents. In: Chernow B, ed. *The Pharmacologic Approach to the Critically Ill Patient.* Ed 3. Baltimore, Md: Williams & Wilkins; 1994: 387–404.

197. Fisher DG, Schwartz PH, Davis AL. Pharmacokinetics of exogenous epinephrine in critically ill children. *Crit Care Med.* 1993;21:111–117.

198. Lindner KH, Prengel AW, Pfenninger EG, Lindner IM, Strohmenger HU, Georgieff M, Lurie KG. Vasopressin improves vital organ blood flow during closed-chest cardiopulmonary resuscitation in pigs. *Circulation.* 1995;91:215–221.

199. Prengel AW, Lindner KH, Keller A. Cerebral oxygenation during cardiopulmonary resuscitation with epinephrine and vasopressin in pigs. *Stroke.* 1996;27:1241–1248.

200. Wenzel V, Lindner KH, Krismer AC, Voelckel WG, Schocke MF, Hund W, Witkiewicz M, Miller EA, Klima G, Wissel J, Lingnau W, Aichner FT. Survival with full neurologic recovery and no cerebral pathology after prolonged cardiopulmonary resuscitation with vasopressin in pigs. *J Am Coll Cardiol.* 2000;35:527–533.

201. Prengel AW, Lindner KH, Wenzel V, Tugtekin I, Anhaupl T. Splanchnic and renal blood flow after cardiopulmonary resuscitation with epinephrine and vasopressin in pigs. *Resuscitation.* 1998;38:19–24.

202. Wenzel V, Lindner KH, Krismer AC, Miller EA, Voelckel WG, Lingnau W. Repeated administration of vasopressin but not epinephrine maintains coronary perfusion pressure after early and late administration during prolonged cardiopulmonary resuscitation in pigs. *Circulation.* 1999;99:1379–1384.

203. Lindner KH, Dirks B, Strohmenger HU, Prengel AW, Lindner IM. Randomised comparison of epinephrine and vasopressin in patients. *Lancet.* 1997;349:535–537.

204. Rozenfeld V, Cheng JW. The role of vasopressin in the treatment of vasodilation in shock states. *Ann Pharmacother.* 2000;34:250–254.

205. Morales DL, Gregg D, Helman DN, Williams MR, Naka Y, Landry DW, Oz MC. Arginine vasopressin in the treatment of 50 patients with postcardiotomy vasodilatory shock. *Ann Thorac Surg.* 2000;69: 102–106.

206. Katz K, Lawler J, Wax J, O'Connor R, Nadkarni V. Vasopressin pressor effect in critically ill children during evaluation for brain death and organ recovery. *Resuscitation.* In press.

207. Rosenzweig EB, Starc TJ, Chen JM, Cullinane S, Timchak DM, Gersony WM, Landry DW, Galantowicz ME. Intravenous arginine-vasopressin in children with vasodilatory shock after cardiac surgery. *Circulation.* 1999;100(suppl II):II-182–II-186.

208. Voeckel WG, Lurie KG, Lindner KH, McKnite S, Zielinski T, Lindstrom P, Wenzel V. Comparison of epinephrine and vasopressin in a pediatric porcine model of asphyxial cardiac arrest. *Circulation.* 1999; 100(suppl I):I-316. Abstract.

209. Stueven H, Thompson B, Aprahamian C, Tonsfeldt D, Kastenson E. Lack of effectiveness of calcium chloride in refractory asystole. *Ann Emerg Med.* 1985;14:630–632.

210. Katz A, Reuter H. Cellular calcium and cardiac cell death. *Am J Cardiol.* 1979;44:188–190.

211. Stueven H, Thompson B, Aprahamian C, Tonsfeldt D, Kastenson E. The effectiveness of calcium chloride in refractory electromechanical dissociation. *Ann Emerg Med.* 1985;14:626–629.

212. Bisogno JL, Langley A, Von Dreele MM. Effect of calcium to reverse the electrocardiographic effects of hyperkalemia in the isolated rat heart: a prospective, dose-response study. *Crit Care Med.* 1994;22:697–704.

213. Cardenas-Rivero N, Chernow B, Stoiko MA, Nussbaum SR, Todres ID. Hypocalcemia in critically ill children. *J Pediatr.* 1989;114:946–951.

214. Zaritsky A. Cardiopulmonary resuscitation in children. *Clin Chest Med.* 1987;8:561–571.

215. Bohman VR, Cotton DB. Supralethal magnesemia with patient survival. *Obstet Gynecol.* 1990;76:984–986.

216. Ramoska EA, Spiller HA, Winter M, Borys D. A one-year evaluation of calcium channel blocker overdoses: toxicity and treatment. *Ann Emerg Med.* 1993;22:196–200.

217. Broner CW, Stidham GL, Westenkirchner DF, Watson DC. A prospective, randomized, double-blind comparison of calcium chloride and calcium gluconate therapies for hypocalcemia in critically ill children. *J Pediatr.* 1990;117:986–989.

218. Fiser RT, Torres A Jr, Butch AW, Valentine JL. Ionized magnesium concentrations in critically ill children. *Crit Care Med.* 1998;26:2048–2052.

219. Maggioni A, Orzalesi M, Mimouni FB. Intravenous correction of neonatal hypomagnesemia: effect on ionized magnesium. *J Pediatr.* 1998;132:652–655.

220. Hirota K, Sato T, Hashimoto Y, Yoshioka H, Ohtomo N, Ishihara H, Matsuki A. Relaxant effect of magnesium and zinc on histamine-induced bronchoconstriction in dogs. *Crit Care Med.* 1999;27:1159–63.

221. Ciarallo L, Sauer AH, Shannon MW. Intravenous magnesium therapy for moderate to severe pediatric asthma: results of a randomized, placebo-controlled trial. *J Pediatr.* 1996;129:809–814.

222. Banai S, Tzivoni D. Drug therapy for torsade de pointes. *J Cardiovasc Electrophysiol.* 1993;4:206–210.

223. Green SM, Rothrock SG. Intravenous magnesium for acute asthma: failure to decrease emergency treatment duration or need for hospitalization. *Ann Emerg Med.* 1992;21:260–265.

224. Tiffany BR, Berk WA, Todd IK, White SR. Magnesium bolus or infusion fails to improve expiratory flow in acute asthma exacerbations. *Chest.* 1993;104:831–834.

225. Gurkan F, Haspolat K, Bosnak M, Dikici B, Derman O, Ece A. Intravenous magnesium sulphate in the management of moderate to severe acute asthmatic children nonresponding to conventional therapy. *Eur J Emerg Med.* 1999;6:201–205.

226. Bloch H, Silverman R, Mancherje N, Grant S, Jagminas L, Scharf SM. Intravenous magnesium sulfate as an adjunct in the treatment of acute asthma. *Chest.* 1995;107:1576–1581.

227. Pabon H, Monem G, Kissoon N. Safety and efficacy of magnesium sulfate infusions in children with status asthmaticus. *Pediatr Emerg Care.* 1994;10:200–203.

228. Rolla G, Bucca C, Brussino L, Colagrande P. Effect of intravenous magnesium infusion on salbutamol-induced bronchodilatation in patients with asthma. *Magnes Res.* 1994;7:129–33.

229. Okayama H, Aikawa T, Okayama M, Sasaki H, Mue S, Takishima T. Bronchodilating effect of intravenous magnesium sulfate in bronchial asthma. *JAMA.* 1987;257:1076–1078.

230. Fazekas T, Scherlag BJ, Vos M, Wellens HJ, Lazzara R. Magnesium and the heart: antiarrhythmic therapy with magnesium. *Clin Cardiol.* 1993; 16:768–74.

231. van Haarst AD, van 't Klooster GA, van Gerven JM, Schoemaker RC, van Oene JC, Burggraaf J, Coene MC, Cohen AF. The influence of cisapride and clarithromycin on QT intervals in healthy volunteers. *Clin Pharmacol Ther.* 1998;64:542–6.

232. Sieber FE, Traystman RJ. Special issues: glucose and the brain. *Crit Care Med.* 1992;20:104–114.

233. Díaz R, Paolasso EA, Piegas LS, Tajer CD, Moreno MG, Corvalan R, Isea JE, Romero G. Metabolic modulation of acute myocardial infarction. The ECLA (Estudios Cardiologicos Latinoamerica) Collaborative Group. *Circulation.* 1998;98:2227–2234.

234. Vukmir RB, Bircher N, Radovsky A, Safar P. Sodium bicarbonate may improve outcome in dogs with brief or prolonged cardiac arrest. *Crit Care Med.* 1995;23:515–522.

235. Levy MM. An evidence-based evaluation of the use of sodium bicarbonate during cardiopulmonary resuscitation. *Crit Care Clin.* 1998;14:457–483.

236. Cooper DJ, Walley KR, Wiggs BR, Russell JA. Bicarbonate does not improve hemodynamics in critically ill patients who have a lactic acidosis: a prospective, controlled clinical study. *Ann Intern Med.* 1990; 112:492–498.

237. Mathieu D, Neviere R, Billard V, Fleyfel M, Wattel F. Effects of bicarbonate therapy on hemodynamics and tissue oxygenation in patients with lactic acidosis: a prospective, controlled clinical study. *Crit Care Med.* 1991;19:1352–1356.

238. Ettinger PO, Regan TJ, Olderwurtel HA. Hyperkalemia, cardiac conduction and the electrocardiogram: a review. *Am Heart J.* 1974;88:360–71.

239. Hoffman JR, Votey SR, Bayer M, Silver L. Effect of hypertonic sodium bicarbonate in the treatment of moderate-to-severe cyclic antidepressant overdose. *Am J Emerg Med.* 1993;11:336–341.

240. Weil M, Rackow E, Trevino R, Grundler W, Falk J, Griffel M. Difference in acid-base state between venous and arterial blood during cardiopulmonary resuscitation. *N Engl J Med.* 1986;315:153–156.

241. Steedman DJ, Robertson CE. Acid base changes in arterial and central venous blood during cardiopulmonary resuscitation. *Arch Emerg Med.* 1992;9:169–176.

242. Bellingham AJ, Detter JC, Lenfant C. Regulatory mechanisms of hemoglobin oxygen affinity in acidosis and alkalosis. *J Clin Invest.* 1971;50:700–706.

243. Bishop RL, Weisfeldt ML. Sodium bicarbonate administration during cardiac arrest: effect on arterial pH, PCO_2, and osmolality. *JAMA.* 1976;235:506–509.

244. Mattar JA, Neil MH, Shubin H, Stein L. Cardiac arrest in the critically ill, II: hyperosmolal states following cardiac arrest. *Am J Med.* 1974; 56:162–168.

245. Aufderheide TP, Martin DR, Olson DW, Aprahamian C, Woo JW, Hendley GE, Hargarten KM, Thompson B. Prehospital bicarbonate use in cardiac arrest: a 3-year experience. *Am J Emerg Med.* 1992;10:4–7.

246. Appleton GO, Cummins RO, Larson MP, Graves JR. CPR and the single rescuer: at what age should you "call first" rather than "call fast"? *Ann Emerg Med.* 1995;25:492–494.

247. Losek JD, Hennes H, Glaeser P, Hendley G, Nelson DB. Prehospital care of the pulseless, nonbreathing pediatric patient. *Am J Emerg Med.* 1987;5:370–374.

248. Dauchot P, Gravenstein JS. Effects of atropine on the electrocardiogram in different age groups. *Clin Pharmacol Ther.* 1971;12:274–280.

249. Zwiener RJ, Ginsburg CM. Organophosphate and carbamate poisoning in infants and children. *Pediatrics.* 1988;81:121–126.

250. Howard RF, Bingham RM. Endotracheal compared with intravenous administration of atropine. *Arch Dis Child.* 1990;65:449–450.

251. Lee PL, Chung YT, Lee BY, Yeh CY, Lin SY, Chao CC. The optimal dose of atropine via the endotracheal route. *Ma Tsui Hsueh Tsa Chi.* 1989;27:35–38.

252. Beland MJ, Hesslein PS, Finlay CD, Faerron-Angel JE, Williams WG, Rowe RD. Noninvasive transcutaneous cardiac pacing in children. *PACE Pacing Clin Electrophysiol.* 1987;10:1262–1270.

253. Quan L, Graves JR, Kinder DR, Horan S, Cummins RO. Transcutaneous cardiac pacing in the treatment of out-of-hospital pediatric cardiac arrests. *Ann Emerg Med.* 1992;21:905–909.

254. Kyriacou DN, Arcinue EL, Peek C, Krauss JF. Effect of immediate resuscitation on children with submersion injury. *Pediatrics.* 1994;94:137–142.

255. Kugler JD, Danford DA. Management of infants, children, and adolescents with paroxysmal supraventricular tachycardia. *J Pediatr.* 1996; 129:324–338.

256. Losek JD, Endom E, Dietrich A, Stewart G, Zempsky W, Smith K. Adenosine and pediatric supraventricular tachycardia in the emergency department: multicenter study and review. *Ann Emerg Med.* 1999;33:185–191.

257. Sreeram N, Wren C. Supraventricular tachycardia in infants: response to initial treatment. *Arch Dis Child.* 1990;65:127–129.

258. Aydin M, Baysal K, Kucukoduk S, Cetinkaya F, Yaman S. Application of ice water to the face in initial treatment of supraventricular tachycardia. *Turk J Pediatr.* 1995;37:15–17.

259. Ornato JP, Hallagan LF, Reese WA, Clark RF, Tayal VS, Garnett AR, Gonzalez ER. Treatment of paroxysmal supraventricular tachycardia in the emergency department by clinical decision analysis. *Am J Emerg Med.* 1988;6:555–560.

260. Lim SH, Anantharaman V, Teo WS, Goh PP, Tan AT. Comparison of treatment of supraventricular tachycardia by Valsalva maneuver and carotid sinus massage. *Ann Emerg Med.* 1998;31:30–35.

261. Waxman MB, Wald RW, Sharma AD, Huerta F, Cameron DA. Vagal techniques for termination of paroxysmal supraventricular tachycardia. *Am J Cardiol.* 1980;46:655–664.

262. Overholt E, Rheuban K, Gutgesell H, Lerman B, Dimarco J. Usefulness of adenosine for arrhythmias in infants and children. *Am J Cardiol.* 1988;61:336–340.

263. Getschman SJ, Dietrich AM, Franklin WH, Allen HD. Intraosseous adenosine: as effective as peripheral or central venous administration? *Arch Pediatr Adolesc Med.* 1994;148:616–619.

264. Friedman FD. Intraosseous adenosine for the termination of supraventricular tachycardia in an infant. *Ann Emerg Med.* 1996;28:356–358.

265. Epstein ML, Kiel EA, Victorica BE. Cardiac decompensation following verapamil in infants with supraventricular tachycardia. *Pediatrics.* 1985;75:737–740.

266. Kirk CR, Gibbs JL, Thomas R, Radley-Smith R, Qureshi SA. Cardiovascular collapse after verapamil in supraventricular tachycardia. *Arch Dis Child.* 1987;62:1265–1266.

267. Rankin AC, Rae AP, Oldroyd KG, Cobbe SM. Verapamil or adenosine for the immediate treatment of supraventricular tachycardia. *Q J Med.* 1990;74:203–208.

268. Perry JC, Fenrich AL, Hulse JE, Triedman JK, Friedman RA, Lamberti JJ. Pediatric use of intravenous amiodarone: efficacy and safety in critically ill patients from a multicenter protocol. *J Am Coll Cardiol.* 1996;27:1246–1250.

269. Perry JC, Knilans TK, Marlow D, Denfield SW, Fenrich AL, Friedman RA. Intravenous amiodarone for life-threatening tachyarrhythmias in children and young adults. *J Am Coll Cardiol.* 1993;22:95–98.

270. Kudenchuk PJ, Cobb LA, Copass MK, Cummins RO, Doherty AM, Fahrenbruch CE, Hallstrom AP, Murray WA, Olsufka M, Walsh T. Amiodarone for resuscitation after out-of-hospital cardiac arrest due to ventricular fibrillation. *N Engl J Med.* 1999;341:871–878.

271. Kowey PR, Levine JH, Herre JM, Pacifico A, Lindsay BD, Plumb VJ, Janosik DL, Kopelman HA, Scheinman MM, the Intravenous Amiodarone Multicenter Investigators Group. Randomized, double-blind comparison of intravenous amiodarone and bretylium in the treatment of patients with recurrent, hemodynamically destabilizing ventricular tachycardia or fibrillation. *Circulation.* 1995;92:3255–3263.

272. Chandrasekaran S, Steinberg JS. Efficacy of bretylium tosylate for ventricular tachycardia. *Am J Cardiol.* 1999;83:115–117.

273. Naccarelli GV, Wolbrette DL, Patel HM, Luck JC. Amiodarone: clinical trials. *Curr Opin Cardiol.* 2000;15:64–72.

274. Bauthier J, Broekhuysen J, Charlier R, Richard J. Nature of the inhibition by amiodarone of isoproterenol-induced tachycardia in the dog. *Arch Int Pharmacodyn Ther.* 1976;219:45–51.

275. Kosinski EJ, Albin JB, Young E, Lewis SM, LeLand OS Jr. Hemodynamic effects of intravenous amiodarone. *J Am Coll Cardiol.* 1984;4:565–570.

276. Singh BN. Amiodarone: historical development and pharmacologic profile. *Am Heart J.* 1983;106:788–797.

277. Yabek SM, Kato R, Singh BN. Effects of amiodarone and its metabolite, desethylamiodarone, on the electrophysiologic properties of isolated cardiac muscle. *J Cardiovasc Pharmacol.* 1986;8:197–207.

278. Mattioni TA, Zheutlin TA, Dunnington C, Kehoe RF. The proarrhythmic effects of amiodarone. *Prog Cardiovasc Dis.* 1989;31:439–446.

279. Mason JW. Amiodarone. *N Engl J Med.* 1987;316:455–466.

280. Mason JW, Hondeghem LM, Katzung BG. Block of inactivated sodium channels and of depolarization-induced automaticity in guinea pig papillary muscle by amiodarone. *Circ Res.* 1984;55:278–285.

281. Raja P, Hawker RE, Chaikitpinyo A, Cooper SG, Lau KC, Nunn GR, Cartmill TB, Sholler GF. Amiodarone management of junctional ectopic tachycardia after cardiac surgery in children. *Br Heart J.* 1994;72:261–265.

282. Figa FH, Gow RM, Hamilton RM, Freedom RM. Clinical efficacy and safety of intravenous amiodarone in infants and children. *Am J Cardiol.* 1994;74:573–7.

283. Pongiglione G, Strasburger JF, Deal BJ, Benson DW Jr. Use of amiodarone for short-term and adjuvant therapy in young patients. *Am J Cardiol.* 1991;68:603–8.

284. Scheinman MM, Levine JH, Cannom DS, Friehling T, Kopelman HA, Chilson DA, Platia EV, Wilber DJ, Kowey PR, The Intravenous Amiodarone Multicenter Investigators Group. Dose-ranging study of intravenous amiodarone in patients with life-threatening ventricular tachyarrhythmias. *Circulation.* 1995;92:3264–3272.

285. Holt DW, Tucker GT, Jackson PR, Storey GC. Amiodarone pharmacokinetics. *Am Heart J.* 1983;106:840–847.

286. Nademanee K, Piwonka RW, Singh BN, Hershman JM. Amiodarone and thyroid function. *Prog Cardiovasc Dis.* 1989;31:427–437.

287. Raeder EA, Podrid PJ, Lown B. Side effects and complications of amiodarone therapy. *Am Heart J.* 1985;109:975–983.

288. Donaldson L, Grant IS, Naysmith MR, Thomas JS. Acute amiodarone-induced lung toxicity. *Intensive Care Med.* 1998;24:626–630.

289. Bowers PN, Fields J, Schwartz D, Rosenfeld LE, Nehgme R. Amiodarone induced pulmonary fibrosis in infancy. *Pacing Clin Electrophysiol.* 1998;21:1665–1667.

290. Bigger JT Jr, Mandel WJ. Effect of lidocaine on the electrophysiologic properties of ventricular muscle and Purkinje fibers. *J Clin Invest.* 1970;49:63–77.

291. Chow MSS, Kluger J, DiPersio DM, Lawrence R, Fieldman A. Antifibrillatory effects of lidocaine and bretylium immediately post CPR. *Am Heart J.* 1985;110:938–943.

292. Wesley RC Jr, Resh W, Zimmerman D. Reconsiderations of the routine and preferential use of lidocaine in the emergent treatment of ventricular arrhythmias. *Crit Care Med.* 1991;19:1439–1444.

293. Armengol RE, Graff J, Baerman JM, Swiryn S. Lack of effectiveness of lidocaine for sustained, wide complex QRS complex tachycardia. *Ann Emerg Med.* 1989;18:254–257.

294. Thompson PD, Melmon KL, Richardson JA, Cohn D, Steinbrunn W, Cudihee R, Rowland M. Lidocaine pharmacokinetics in advanced heart failure, liver disease, and renal failure in humans. *Ann Intern Med.* 1973;78:499–508.

295. Mehta AV, Sanchez GR, Sacks EJ, Casta A, Dunn JM, Donner RM. Ectopic automatic atrial tachycardia in children: clinical characteristics, management and follow-up. *J Am Coll Cardiol.* 1988;11:379–385.

296. Hjelms E. Procainamide conversion of acute atrial fibrillation after open-heart surgery compared with digoxin treatment. *Scand J Thorac Cardiovasc Surg.* 1992;26:193–196.

297. Boahene KA, Klein GJ, Yee R, Sharma AD, Fujimura O. Termination of acute atrial fibrillation in the Wolff-Parkinson-White syndrome by procainamide and propafenone: importance of atrial fibrillatory cycle length. *J Am Coll Cardiol.* 1990;16:1408–1414.

298. Walsh EP, Saul JP, Sholler GF, Triedman JK, Jonas RA, Mayer JE, Wessel DL. Evaluation of a staged treatment protocol for rapid automatic junctional tachycardia after operation for congenital heart disease. *J Am Coll Cardiol.* 1997;29:1046–1053.

299. Singh BN, Kehoe R, Woosley RL, Scheinman M, Quart B. Multicenter trial of sotalol compared with procainamide in the suppression of inducible ventricular tachycardia: a double-blind, randomized parallel evaluation. Sotalol Multicenter Study Group. *Am Heart J.* 1995;129:87–97.

300. Luedtke SA, Kuhn RJ, McCaffrey FM. Pharmacologic management of supraventricular tachycardias in children, 1: Wolff-Parkinson-White and atrioventricular nodal reentry. *Ann Pharmacother.* 1997;31:1227–1243.

301. Luedtke SA, Kuhn RJ, McCaffrey FM. Pharmacologic management of supraventricular tachycardias in children, 2: atrial flutter, atrial fibrillation, and junctional and atrial ectopic tachycardia. *Ann Pharmacother.* 1997;31:1347–1359.

302. Cobb LA, Fahrenbruch CE, Walsh TR, Copass MK, Olsufka M, Breskin M, Hallstrom AP. Influence of cardiopulmonary resuscitation prior to defibrillation in patients with out-of-hospital ventricular fibrillation. *JAMA.* 1999;281:1182–1188.

303. Yakaitis RW, Ewy GA, Otto CW, Taren DL, Moon TE. Influence of time and therapy on ventricular defibrillation in dogs. *Crit Care Med.* 1980;8:157–163.

304. Losek JD, Hennes H, Glaeser PW, Smith DS, Hendley G. Prehospital countershock treatment of pediatric asystole. *Am J Emerg Med.* 1989;7:571–575.

305. Atkins DL, Sirna S, Kieso R, Charbonnier F, Kerber RE. Pediatric defibrillation: importance of paddle size in determining transthoracic impedance. *Pediatrics*. 1988;82:914–918.

306. Atkins DL, Kerber RE. Pediatric defibrillation: current flow is improved by using "adult" electrode paddles. *Pediatrics*. 1994;94:90–93.

307. Caterine MR, Yoerger DM, Spencer KT, Miller SG, Kerber RE. Effect of electrode position and gel-application technique on predicted transcardiac current during transthoracic defibrillation. *Ann Emerg Med*. 1997;29:588 595.

308. Sirna SJ, Ferguson DW, Charbonnier F, Kerber RE. Factors affecting transthoracic impedance during electrical cardioversion. *Am J Cardiol*. 1988;62:1048–1052.

309. McNaughton GW, Wyatt JP, Byrne JC. Defibrillation: a burning issue in coronary care units! *Scott Med J*. 1996;41:47–48.

310. Garcia LA, Kerber RE. Transthoracic defibrillation: does electrode adhesive pad position alter transthoracic impedance? *Resuscitation*. 1998;37:139–143.

311. Gutgesell HP, Tacker WA, Geddes LA, Davis S, Lie JT, McNamara DG. Energy dose for ventricular defibrillation of children. *Pediatrics*. 1976;58:898–901.

312. Chameides L, Brown GE, Raye JR, Todres DI, Viles PH. Guidelines for defibrillation in infants and children: report of the American Heart Association target activity group: cardiopulmonary resuscitation in the young. *Circulation*. 1977;56:502A–503A.

313. Atkins DL, Hartley LL, York DK. Accurate recognition and effective treatment of ventricular fibrillation by automated external defibrillators in adolescents. *Pediatrics*. 1998;101:393–397.

314. Cecchin F, Perry JC, Berul CI, Jorgenson DB, Brian DW, Lyster T, Snider DE, Zimmerman AA, Lupinetti FM, Rosenthal GL, Rule D, Atkins DL. Accuracy of automatic external defibrillator analysis algorithm in young children. *Circulation*. 1999;100(suppl I):I-663. Abstract.

315. Hazinski MF, Walker C, Smith H, Deshpande J. Specificity of automatic external defibrillator rhythm analysis in pediatric tachyarrhythmias. *Circulation*. 1997;96(suppl I):I-561.

316. Babbs CF, Tacker WA, VanVleet JF, Bourland JD, Geddes LA. Therapeutic indices for transchest defibrillator shocks: effective, damaging, and lethal electrical doses. *Am Heart J*. 1980;99:734–738.

317. Zoll PM, Zoll RH, Falk RH, Clinton JE, Eitel DR, Antman EM. External noninvasive temporary cardiac pacing: clinical trials. *Circulation*. 1985; 71:937–944.

318. Niemann JT, Haynes KS, Garner D, Rennie CJ III, Jagels G, Stormo O. Post countershock pulseless rhythms: response to CPR, artificial cardiac pacing and adrenergic agonists. *Ann Emerg Med*. 1985;15:112–120.

319. Falk RH, Ngai ST. External cardiac pacing: influence of electrode placement on pacing threshold. *Crit Care Med*. 1986;14:931–932.

320. Oral H, Brinkman K, Pelosi F, Flemming M, Tse HF, Kim MH, Michaud GF, Knight BP, Goyal R, Strickberger SA, Morady F. Effect of electrode polarity on the energy required for transthoracic atrial defibrillation. *Am J Cardiol*. 1999;84:228–230, A8.

321. Dykes EH, Spence LJ, Young JG, Bohn DJ, Filler RM, Wesson DE. Preventable pediatric trauma deaths in a metropolitan region. *J Pediatr Surg*. 1989;24:107–110.

322. Koury SI, Moorer L, Stone CK, Stapczynski JS, Thomas SH. Air vs ground transport and outcome in trauma patients requiring urgent operative interventions. *Prehosp Emerg Care*. 1998;2:289–292.

323. Moront ML, Gotschall CS, Eichelberger MR. Helicopter transport of injured children: system effectiveness and triage criteria. *J Pediatr Surg*. 1996;31:1183–1186; discussion 1187–8.

324. Curran C, Dietrich AM, Bowman MJ, Ginn-Pease ME, King DR, Kosnik E. Pediatric cervical-spine immobilization: achieving neutral position? *J Trauma*. 1995;39:729–732.

325. Muizelaar JP, Marmarou A, Ward JD, Kontos HA, Choi SC, Becker DP, Gruemer H, Young HF. Adverse effects of prolonged hyperventilation in patients with severe head injury: a randomized clinical trial. *J Neurosurg*. 1991;75:731–739.

326. Robertson CS, Valadka AB, Hannay HJ, Contant CF, Gopinath SP, Cormio M, Uzura M, Grossman RG. Prevention of secondary ischemic insults after severe head injury. *Crit Care Med*. 1999;27:2086–2095.

327. Schneider GH, Sarrafzadeh AS, Kiening KL, Bardt TF, Unterberg AW, Lanksch WR. Influence of hyperventilation on brain tissue-PO_2, PCO_2, and pH in patients with intracranial hypertension. *Acta Neurochir Suppl*. 1998;71:62–65.

328. Baskaya MK. Inadvertent intracranial placement of a nasogastric tube in patients with head injuries. *Surg Neurol*. 1999;52:426–427.

329. Rutledge R, Sheldon GF, Collins ML. Massive transfusion. *Crit Care Clin*. 1986;2:791–805.

330. Niven MJ, Zohar M, Shimoni Z, Glick J. Symptomatic hypocalcemia precipitated by small-volume blood transfusion. *Ann Emerg Med*. 1998; 32:498–501.

331. Ramenofsky ML, Luterman A, Quindlen E, Riddick L, Curreri PW. Maximum survival in pediatric trauma: the ideal system. *J Trauma*. 1984;24:818–823.

332. Luterman A, Ramenofsky M, Berryman C, Talley MA, Curreri PW. Evaluation of prehospital emergency medical service (EMS): defining areas for improvement. *J Trauma*. 1983;23:702–707.

333. Bauman JL, Grawe JJ, Winecoff AP, Hariman RJ. Cocaine-related sudden cardiac death: a hypothesis correlating basic science and clinical observations. *J Clin Pharmacol*. 1994;34:902–911.

334. Hollander JE, Hoffman RS, Gennis P, Fairweather P, DiSano MJ, Schumb DA, Feldman JA, Fish SS, Dyer S, Wax P, et al. Prospective multicenter evaluation of cocaine-associated chest pain. Cocaine Associated Chest Pain (COCHPA) Study Group. *Acad Emerg Med*. 1994;1: 330–339.

335. Brody SL, Slovis CM, Wrenn KD. Cocaine-related medical problems: consecutive series of 233 patients. *Am J Med*. 1990;88:325–331.

336. Zurbano MJ, Heras M, Rigol M, Roig E, Epelde F, Miranda F, Sanz G, Escolar G, Ordinas A. Cocaine administration enhances platelet reactivity to subendothelial components: studies in a pig model. *Eur J Clin Invest*. 1997;27:116–120.

337. Karch SB. Cardiac arrest in cocaine users. *Am J Emerg Med*. 1996;14: 79–81.

338. Kolecki PF, Curry SC. Poisoning by sodium channel blocking agents. *Crit Care Clin*. 1997;13:829–848.

339. Hoffman RS, Hollander JE. Evaluation of patients with chest pain after cocaine use. *Crit Care Clin*. 1997;13:809–828.

340. Derlet RW, Albertson TE. Diazepam in the prevention of seizures and death in cocaine-intoxicated rats. *Ann Emerg Med*. 1989;18:542–546.

341. Catravas JD, Waters IW, Walz MA, Davis WM. Acute cocaine intoxication in the conscious dog: pathophysiologic profile of acute lethality. *Arch Int Pharmacodyn Ther*. 1978;235:328–340.

342. Freemantle N, Cleland J, Young P, Mason J, Harrison J. β-Blockade after myocardial infarction: systematic review and meta regression analysis. *BMJ*. 1999;318:1730–1737.

343. Kenny D, Pagel PS, Warltier DC. Attenuation of the systemic and coronary hemodynamic effects of cocaine in conscious dogs: propranolol versus labetalol. *Basic Res Cardiol*. 1992;87:465–477.

344. Lange RA, Cigarroa RG, Flores ED, McBride W, Kim AS, Wells PJ, Bedotto JB, Danziger RS, Hillis LD. Potentiation of cocaine-induced coronary vasoconstriction by beta- adrenergic blockade. *Ann Intern Med*. 1990;112:897–903.

345. Sand IC, Brody SL, Wrenn KD, Slovis CM. Experience with esmolol for the treatment of cocaine-associated cardiovascular complications. *Am J Emerg Med*. 1991;9:161–163.

346. Boehrer JD, Moliterno DJ, Willard JE, Hillis LD, Lange RA. Influence of labetalol on cocaine-induced coronary vasoconstriction in humans. *Am J Med*. 1993;94:608–610.

347. Lange RA, Cigarroa RG, Yancy CW Jr, Willard JE, Popma JJ, Sills MN, McBride W, Kim AS, Hillis LD. Cocaine-induced coronary-artery vasoconstriction. *N Engl J Med*. 1989;321:1557–1562.

348. Benitz WE, Tatro DS. *The Pediatric Drug Handbook*. St Louis, Mo: Mosby-Year Book; 1995.

349. Brogan WC III, Lange RA, Kim AS, Moliterno DJ, Hillis LD. Alleviation of cocaine-induced coronary vasoconstriction by nitroglycerin. *J Am Coll Cardiol*. 1991;18:581–586.

350. Hollander JE, Hoffman RS, Gennis P, Fairweather P, DiSano MJ, Schumb DA, Feldman JA, Fish SS, Dyer S, Wax P, et al. Nitroglycerin in the treatment of cocaine associated chest pain: clinical safety and efficacy. *J Toxicol Clin Toxicol*. 1994;32:243–256.

351. Kerns W II, Garvey L, Owens J. Cocaine-induced wide complex dysrhythmia. *J Emerg Med*. 1997;15:321–329.

352. Beckman KJ, Parker RB, Hariman RJ, Gallastegui JL, Javaid JI, Bauman JL. Hemodynamic and electrophysiological actions of cocaine: effects of sodium bicarbonate as an antidote in dogs. *Circulation*. 1991; 83:1799–1807.

353. Derlet RW, Albertson TE, Tharratt RS. Lidocaine potentiation of cocaine toxicity. *Ann Emerg Med*. 1991;20:135–138.

354. Shih RD, Hollander JE, Burstein JL, Nelson LS, Hoffman RS, Quick AM. Clinical safety of lidocaine in patients with cocaine-associated myocardial infarction. *Ann Emerg Med*. 1995;26:702–706.

355. Keller DJ, Todd GL. Acute cardiotoxic effects of cocaine and a hyperadrenergic state in anesthetized dogs. *Int J Cardiol.* 1994;44:19–28.

356. Gillis RA, Hernandez YM, Erzouki HK, Raczkowski VF, Mandal AK, Kuhn FE, Dretchen KL. Sympathetic nervous system mediated cardiovascular effects of cocaine are primarily due to a peripheral site of action of the drug. *Drug Alcohol Depend.* 1995;37:217–30.

357. Wolfe TR, Caravati EM, Rollins DE. Terminal 40-ms frontal plane QRS axis as a marker for tricyclic antidepressant overdose. *Ann Emerg Med.* 1989;18:348–351.

358. Harrigan RA, Brady WJ. ECG abnormalities in tricyclic antidepressant ingestion. *Am J Emerg Med.* 1999;17:387–393.

359. Boehnert MT, Lovejoy FH Jr. Value of the QRS duration versus the serum drug level in predicting seizures and ventricular arrhythmias after an acute overdose of tricyclic antidepressants. *N Engl J Med.* 1985;313:474–479.

360. Foulke GE. Identifying toxicity risk early after antidepressant overdose. *Am J Emerg Med.* 1995;13:123–126.

361. Liebelt EL, Francis PD, Woolf AD. ECG lead aVR versus QRS interval in predicting seizures and arrhythmias in acute tricyclic antidepressant toxicity. *Ann Emerg Med.* 1995;26:195–201.

362. Liebelt EL, Ulrich A, Francis PD, Woolf A. Serial electrocardiogram changes in acute tricyclic antidepressant overdoses. *Crit Care Med.* 1997;25:1721–1726.

363. McCabe JL, Cobaugh DJ, Menegazzi JJ, Fata J. Experimental tricyclic antidepressant toxicity: a randomized, controlled comparison of hypertonic saline solution, sodium bicarbonate, and hyperventilation. *Ann Emerg Med.* 1998;32:329–333.

364. Bou-Abboud E, Nattel S. Relative role of alkalosis and sodium ions in reversal of class I antiarrhythmic drug-induced sodium channel blockade by sodium bicarbonate. *Circulation.* 1996;94:1954–1961.

365. Shanon M, Liebelt E. Targeted management strategies for cardiovascular toxicity from tricyclic antidepressant overdose: the pivotal role for alkalinization and sodium loading. *Pediatr Emerg Care.* 1998;14:293–298.

366. Bessen HA, Niemann JT. Improvement of cardiac conduction after hyperventilation in tricyclic antidepressant overdose. *J Toxicol Clin Toxicol.* 1985;23:537–546.

367. Teba L, Schiebel F, Dedhia HV, Lazzell VA. Beneficial effect of norepinephrine in the treatment of circulatory shock caused by tricyclic antidepressant overdose. *Am J Emerg Med.* 1988;6:566–568.

368. Tran TP, Panacek EA, Rhee KJ, Foulke GE. Response to dopamine vs norepinephrine in tricyclic antidepressant-induced hypotension. *Acad Emerg Med.* 1997;4:864–868.

369. Williams JM, Hollingshed MJ, Vasilakis A, Morales M, Prescott JE, Graeber GM. Extracorporeal circulation in the management of severe tricyclic antidepressant overdose. *Am J Emerg Med.* 1994;12:456–458.

370. Larkin GL, Graeber GM, Hollingshed MJ. Experimental amitriptyline poisoning: treatment of severe cardiovascular toxicity with cardiopulmonary bypass. *Ann Emerg Med.* 1994;23:480–486.

371. Henry M, Kay MM, Viccellio P. Cardiogenic shock associated with calcium-channel and beta blockers: reversal with intravenous calcium chloride. *Am J Emerg Med.* 1985;3:334–336.

372. Lewis M, Kallenbach J, Germond C, Zaltzman M, Muller F, Steyn J, Zwi S. Survival following massive overdose of adrenergic blocking agents (acebutolol and labetalol). *Eur Heart J.* 1983;4:328–332.

373. Kline JA, Tomaszewski CA, Schroeder JD, Raymond RM. Insulin is a superior antidote for cardiovascular toxicity induced by verapamil in the anesthetized canine. *J Pharmacol Exp Ther.* 1993;267:744–750.

374. Kerns W II, Schroeder D, Williams C, Tomaszewski C, Raymond R. Insulin improves survival in a canine model of acute beta-blocker toxicity. *Ann Emerg Med.* 1997;29:748–757.

375. Yuan TH, Kerns WP II, Tomaszewski CA, Ford MD, Kline JA. Insulin-glucose as adjunctive therapy for severe calcium channel antagonist poisoning. *J Toxicol Clin Toxicol.* 1999;37:463–474.

376. Kerns W II, Kline J, Ford MD. Beta-blocker and calcium channel blocker toxicity. *Emerg Med Clin North Am.* 1994;12:365–390.

377. Cruickshank JM, Neil-Dwyer G, Cameron MM, McAinsh J. Beta-adrenoreceptor-blocking agents and the blood-brain barrier. *Clin Sci.* 1980; 59(suppl 6):453s–455s.

378. Weinstein RS. Recognition and management of poisoning with beta-adrenergic blocking agents. *Ann Emerg Med.* 1984;13:1123.

379. Avery GJ II, Spotnitz HM, Rose EA, Malm JR, Hoffman BF. Pharmacologic antagonism of beta-adrenergic blockade in dogs, I: hemodynamic effects of isoproterenol, dopamine, and epinephrine in acute propranolol administration. *J Thorac Cardiovasc Surg.* 1979;77:267–276.

380. Zaritsky AL, Horowitz M, Chernow B. Glucagon antagonism of calcium channel blocker-induced myocardial dysfunction. *Crit Care Med.* 1988; 16:246–251.

381. Mofenson HC, Caraccio TR, Laudano J. Glucagon for propranolol overdose. *JAMA.* 1986;255:2025–2026. Letter.

382. Love JN, Hanfling D, Howell JM. Hemodynamic effects of calcium chloride in a canine model of acute propranolol intoxication. *Ann Emerg Med.* 1996;28:1–6.

383. Haddad LM. Resuscitation after nifedipine overdose exclusively with intravenous calcium chloride. *Am J Emerg Med.* 1996;14:602–603.

384. Horowitz BZ, Rhee KJ. Massive verapamil ingestion: a report of two cases and a review of the literature. *Am J Emerg Med.* 1989;7:624–631.

385. Watling SM, Crain JL, Edwards TD, Stiller RA. Verapamil overdose: case report and review of the literature. *Ann Pharmacother.* 1992;26: 1373–1378.

386. American Academy of Pediatrics Committee on Drugs. Naloxone dosage and route of administration for infants and children: addendum to emergency drug doses for infants and children. *Pediatrics.* 1990;86:484–485.

387. Sporer KA, Firestone J, Isaacs SM. Out-of-hospital treatment of opioid overdoses in an urban setting. *Acad Emerg Med.* 1996;3:660–667.

388. Yealy DM, Paris PM, Kaplan RM, Heller MB, Marini SE. The safety of prehospital naloxone administration by paramedics. *Ann Emerg Med.* 1990;19:902–905.

389. Mills CA, Flacke JW, Flacke WE, Bloor BC, Liu MD. Narcotic reversal in hypercapnic dogs: comparison of naloxone and nalbuphine. *Can J Anaesth.* 1990;37:238–244.

390. Prough DS, Roy R, Bumgarner J, Shannon G. Acute pulmonary edema in healthy teenagers following conservative doses of intravenous naloxone. *Anesthesiology.* 1984;60:485–486.

391. Osterwalder JJ. Naloxone: for intoxications with intravenous heroin and heroin mixtures: harmless or hazardous? A prospective clinical study. *J Toxicol Clin Toxicol.* 1996;34:409–416.

392. Kienbaum P, Thurauf N, Michel MC, Scherbaum N, Gastpar M, Peters J. Profound increase in epinephrine concentration in plasma and cardiovascular stimulation after mu-opioid receptor blockade in opioid-addicted patients during barbiturate-induced anesthesia for acute detoxification [see comments]. *Anesthesiology.* 1998;88:1154–1161.

393. American Academy of Pediatrics Committee on Drugs. Emergency drug doses for infants and children with naloxone in newborns: clarification. *Pediatrics.* 1989;83:803.

394. Wanger K, Brough L, Macmillan I, Goulding J, MacPhail I, Christenson JM. Intravenous vs subcutaneous naloxone for out-of-hospital management of presumed opioid overdose. *Acad Emerg Med.* 1998;5:293–299.

395. Rosen P, Stoto M, Harley J. The use of the Heimlich maneuver in near drowning: Institute of Medicine report. *J Emerg Med.* 1995;13:397–405.

396. Quan L, Wentz KR, Gore EJ, Copass MK. Outcome and predictors of outcome in pediatric submersion victims receiving prehospital care in King County, Washington. *Pediatrics.* 1990;86:586–593.

397. Spack L, Gedeit R, Splaingard M, Havens PL. Failure of aggressive therapy to alter outcome in pediatric near-drowning. *Pediatr Emerg Care.* 1997;13:98–102.

398. Lavelle JM, Shaw KN. Near drowning: is emergency department cardiopulmonary resuscitation or intensive care unit cerebral resuscitation indicated? *Crit Care Med.* 1993;21:368–373.

399. Bohn DJ, Biggar WD, Smith CR, Conn AW, Barker GA. Influence of hypothermia, barbiturate therapy, and intracranial pressure monitoring on morbidity and mortality after near drowning. *Crit Care Med.* 1986; 14:529–534.

400. Tobias JD, Lynch A, Garrett J. Alterations of end-tidal carbon dioxide during the intrahospital transport of children. *Pediatr Emerg Care.* 1996;12:249–251.

401. Tobias JD, Meyer DJ. Noninvasive monitoring of carbon dioxide during respiratory failure in toddlers and infants: end-tidal versus transcutaneous carbon dioxide. *Anesth Analg.* 1997;85:55–58.

402. O'Connor TA, Grueber R. Transcutaneous measurement of carbon dioxide tension during long-distance transport of neonates receiving mechanical ventilation. *J Perinatol.* 1998;18:189–192.

403. Hand IL, Shepard EK, Krauss AN, Auld PA. Discrepancies between transcutaneous and end-tidal carbon dioxide monitoring in the critically ill neonate with respiratory distress syndrome. *Crit Care Med.* 1989;17:556–559.

404. Lucking SE, Pollack MM, Fields AI. Shock following generalized hypoxic-ischemic injury in previously healthy infants and children. *J Pediatr.* 1986;108:359–364.

405. Kern KB, Hilwig RW, Berg RA, Rhee KH, Sanders AB, Otto CW, Ewy GA. Postresuscitation left ventricular systolic and diastolic dysfunction: treatment with dobutamine. *Circulation*. 1997;95:2610–2613.

406. Ceneviva G, Paschall JA, Maffei F, Carcillo JA. Hemodynamic support in fluid-refractory pediatric septic shock. *Pediatrics*. 1998;102:e19.

407. Levy B, Bollaert PE, Charpentier C, Nace L, Audibert G, Bauer P, Nabet P, Larcan A. Comparison of norepinephrine and dobutamine to epinephrine for hemodynamics, lactate metabolism, and gastric tonometric variables in septic shock: a prospective, randomized study. *Intensive Care Med*. 1997;23:282–287.

408. Padbury JF, Agata Y, Baylen BG, Ludlow JK, Polk DH, Goldblatt E, Pescetti J. Dopamine pharmacokinetics in critically ill newborn infants. *J Pediatr*. 1987;110:293–8.

409. Mentzer RM Jr, Alegre CA, Nolan SP. The effects of dopamine and isoproterenol on the pulmonary circulation. *J Thorac Cardiovasc Surg*. 1976;71:807–814.

410. Booker PD, Evans C, Franks R. Comparison of the haemodynamic effects of dopamine and dobutamine in young children undergoing cardiac surgery. *Br J Anaesth*. 1995;74:419–423.

411. Ushay HM, Notterman DA. Pharmacology of pediatric resuscitation. *Pediatr Clin North Am*. 1997;44:207–33.

412. Van den Berghe G, de Zegher F, Lauwers P. Dopamine suppresses pituitary function in infants and children. *Crit Care Med*. 1994;22:1747–1753.

413. Habib DM, Padbury JF, Anas NG, Perkin RM, Minegar C. Dobutamine pharmacokinetics and pharmacodynamics in pediatric intensive care patients. *Crit Care Med*. 1992;20:601–608.

414. Martinez AM, Padbury JF, Thio S. Dobutamine pharmacokinetics and cardiovascular responses in critically ill neonates. *Pediatrics*. 1992;89:47–51.

415. Martin C, Papazian L, Perrin G, Saux P, Gouin F. Norepinephrine or dopamine for the treatment of hyperdynamic septic shock? *Chest*. 1993;103:1826–1831.

416. Redl-Wenzl EM, Armbruster C, Edelmann G, Fischl E, Kolacny M, Wechsler-Fordos A, Sporn P. The effects of norepinephrine on hemodynamics and renal function in severe septic shock states. *Intensive Care Med*. 1993;19:151–154.

417. Hoogenberg K, Smit AJ, Girbes AR. Effects of low-dose dopamine on renal and systemic hemodynamics during incremental norepinephrine infusion in healthy volunteers. *Crit Care Med*. 1998;26:260–265.

418. Juste RN, Panikkar K, Soni N. The effects of low-dose dopamine infusions on haemodynamic and renal parameters in patients with septic shock requiring treatment with noradrenaline. *Intensive Care Med*. 1998;24:564–568.

419. Rindone JP, Sloane EP. Cyanide toxicity from sodium nitroprusside: risks and management. *Ann Pharmacother*. 1992;26:515–519.

420. Barton P, Garcia J, Kouatli A, Kitchen L, Zorka A, Lindsay C, Lawless S, Giroir B. Hemodynamic effects of i.v. milrinone lactate in pediatric patients with septic shock: a prospective, double-blinded, randomized, placebo-controlled, interventional study. *Chest*. 1996;109:1302–1312.

421. Bailey JM, Miller BE, Lu W, Tosone SR, Kanter KR, Tam VK. The pharmacokinetics of milrinone in pediatric patients after cardiac surgery. *Anesthesiology*. 1999;90:1012–1018.

422. Lindsay CA, Barton P, Lawless S, Kitchen L, Zorka A, Garcia J, Kouatli A, Giroir B. Pharmacokinetics and pharmacodynamics of milrinone lactate in pediatric patients with septic shock. *J Pediatr*. 1998;132:329–334.

423. Allen-Webb EM, Ross MP, Pappas JB, McGough EC, Banner W Jr. Age-related amrinone pharmacokinetics in a pediatric population. *Crit Care Med*. 1994;22:1016–1024.

424. Lawless ST, Zaritsky A, Miles M. The acute pharmacokinetics and pharmacodynamics of amrinone in pediatric patients. *J Clin Pharmacol*. 1991;31:800–803.

425. Ross MP, Allen-Webb EM, Pappas JB, McGough EC. Amrinone-associated thrombocytopenia: pharmacokinetic analysis. *Clin Pharmacol Ther*. 1993;53:661–667.

426. Bernard SA, Jones BM, Horne MK. Clinical trial of induced hypothermia in comatose survivors of out-of-hospital cardiac arrest. *Ann Emerg Med*. 1997;30:146–153.

427. Marion DW, Leonov Y, Ginsberg M, Katz LM, Kochanek PM, Lechleuthner A, Nemoto EM, Obrist W, Safar P, Sterz F, Tisherman SA, White RJ, Xiao F, Zar H. Resuscitative hypothermia. *Crit Care Med*. 1996;24:S81–S89.

428. Ginsberg MD, Busto R. Combating hyperthermia in acute stroke: a significant clinical concern. *Stroke*. 1998;29:529–534.

429. Seidel J, Tittle S, Hodge D III, Garcia V, Sabato K, Gausche M, Scherer LR, Gerardi M, Baker MD, Weber S, Iakahashi I, Boechler E, Jalalon S. Guidelines for pediatric equipment and supplies for emergency departments. Committee on Pediatric Equipment and Supplies for Emergency Departments. National Emergency Medical Services for Children Resource Alliance. *J Emerg Nurs*. 1998;24:45–48.

430. Henning R. Emergency transport of critically ill children: stabilisation before departure. *Med J Aust*. 1992;156:117–24.

431. Edge WE, Kanter RK, Weigle CGM, Walsh RF. Reduction of morbidity in interhospital transport by specialized pediatric staff. *Crit Care Med*. 1994;22:1186–1191.

432. Guidelines Committee of the American College of Critical Care Medicine, Society of Critical Care Medicine and American Association of Critical-Care Nurses Transfer Guidelines Task Force. Guidelines for the transfer of critically ill patients. *Crit Care Med*. 1993;21:931–937.

433. Barratt F, Wallis DN. Relatives in the resuscitation room: their point of view. *J Accid Emerg Med*. 1998;15:109–11.

434. Boie ET, Moore GP, Brummett C, Nelson DR. Do parents want to be present during invasive procedures performed on their children in the emergency department? A survey of 400 parents. *Ann Emerg Med*. 1999;34:70–4.

435. Doyle CJ, Post H, Burney RE, Maino J, Keefe M, Rhee KJ. Family participation during resuscitation: an option. *Ann Emerg Med*. 1987;16:673–675.

436. Hanson C, Strawser D. Family presence during cardiopulmonary resuscitation: Foote Hospital emergency department's nine-year perspective. *J Emerg Nurs*. 1992;18:104–106.

437. Meyers TA, Eichhorn DJ, Guzzetta CE. Do families want to be present during CPR? A retrospective survey. *J Emerg Nurs*. 1998;24:400–405.

438. Robinson SM, Mackenzie-Ross S, Campbell Hewson GL, Egleston CV, Prevost AT. Psychological effect of witnessed resuscitation on bereaved relatives. *Lancet*. 1998;352:614–617.

439. Boyd R. Witnessed resuscitation by relatives. *Resuscitation*. 2000;43:171–176.

440. Offert RJ. Should relatives of patients with cardiac arrest be invited to be present during CPR? *Intensive Crit Care Nursing*. 1998;14:288–293.

441. Eichhorn DJ, Meyers TA, Mitchell TG, Guzzetta CE. Opening the doors: family presence during resuscitation. *J Cardiovasc Nurs*. 1996;10:59–70.

442. Zaritsky A, Nadkarni V, Getson P, Kuehl K. CPR in children. *Ann Emerg Med*. 1987;16:1107–1110.

Part 11: Neonatal Resuscitation

Major Guidelines Changes

The Pediatric Working Group of the International Liaison Committee on Resuscitation (ILCOR) developed an advisory statement published in 1999. This statement listed the following principles of resuscitation of the newly born:

- Personnel capable of initiating resuscitation should attend every delivery. A minority (fewer than 10%) of newly born infants require active resuscitative interventions to establish a vigorous cry or regular respirations, maintain a heart rate >100 beats per minute (bpm), and achieve good color and tone.
- When meconium is observed in the amniotic fluid, deliver the head, and suction meconium from the hypopharynx on delivery of the head. If the newly born infant has absent or depressed respirations, heart rate <100 bpm, or poor muscle tone, carry out direct tracheal suctioning to remove meconium from the airway.
- Establishment of adequate ventilation should be of primary concern. Provide assisted ventilation with attention to oxygen delivery, inspiratory time, and effectiveness as judged by chest rise if stimulation does not achieve prompt onset of spontaneous respirations or the heart rate is <100 bpm.
- Provide chest compressions if the heart rate is absent or remains <60 bpm despite adequate assisted ventilation for 30 seconds. Coordinate chest compressions with ventilations at a ratio of 3:1 and a rate of 120 events per minute to achieve approximately 90 compressions and 30 breaths per minute.
- Administer epinephrine if the heart rate remains <60 bpm despite 30 seconds of effective assisted ventilation and circulation (chest compressions).

At the Guidelines 2000 Conference, we made the following recommendations:

Temperature

- Cerebral hypothermia; avoidance of perinatal hyperthermia
  —Avoid hyperthermia (Class III).
  —Although several recent animal and human studies have suggested that selective cerebral hypothermia may protect against brain injury in the asphyxiated infant, we cannot recommend routine implementation of this therapy until appropriate controlled human studies have been performed (Class Indeterminate).

Oxygenation and Ventilation

- Room air versus 100% oxygen during positive-pressure ventilation

—100% oxygen has been used traditionally for rapid reversal of hypoxia. Although biochemical and preliminary clinical evidence suggests that lower inspired oxygen concentrations may be useful in some settings, data is insufficient to justify a change from the recommendation that 100% oxygen be used if assisted ventilation is required.
  —If supplemental oxygen is unavailable and positive-pressure ventilation is required, use room air (Class Indeterminate).

- Laryngeal mask as an alternative method of establishing an airway
  —When used by appropriately trained providers, the laryngeal mask airway may be an effective alternative for establishing an airway during resuscitation of the newly born infant, particularly if bag-mask ventilation is ineffective or attempts at tracheal intubation have failed (Class Indeterminate).
- Confirmation of tracheal tube placement by exhaled CO_2 detection
  —Exhaled CO_2 detection can be useful in the secondary confirmation of tracheal intubation in the newly born, particularly when clinical assessment is equivocal (Class Indeterminate).

Chest Compressions

- Preferred technique for chest compressions
  —Two thumb–encircling hands chest compression is the preferred technique for chest compressions in newly born infants and older infants when size permits (Class IIb).
  —For chest compressions, we recommend a relative depth of compression (one third of the anterior-posterior diameter of the chest) rather than an absolute depth. Chest compressions should be sufficiently deep to generate a palpable pulse.

Medications, Volume Expansion, and Vascular Access

- Epinephrine dose
  —Administer epinephrine if the heart rate remains <60 bpm after a minimum of 30 seconds of adequate ventilation and chest compressions (Class I).
  —Epinephrine administration is particularly indicated in the presence of asystole.

Circulation. 2000;102(suppl I):I-343–I-357.
© 2000 American Heart Association, Inc.

Circulation is available at http://www.circulationaha.org

- Choice of fluid for acute volume expansion
  —Emergency volume expansion may be accomplished by an isotonic crystalloid solution such as normal saline or Ringer's lactate. O-negative red blood cells may be used if the need for blood replacement is anticipated before birth (Class IIb).
  —Albumin-containing solutions are no longer the fluid of choice for initial for initial volume expansion because their availability is limited, they introduce a risk of infectious disease, and an association with increased mortality has been observed.

- Alternative routes for vascular access
  —Intraosseous access can be used as an alternative route for medications/volume expansion if umbilical or other direct venous access is not readily available (Class IIb).

Ethics

- Noninitiation and discontinuation of resuscitation
  —There are circumstances (relating to gestational age, birth weight, known underlying condition, lack of response to interventions) in which noninitiation or discontinuation of resuscitation in the delivery room may be appropriate (Class IIb).

Introduction

Resuscitation of the newly born infant presents a different set of challenges than resuscitation of the adult or even the older infant or child. The transition from placental gas exchange in a liquid-filled intrauterine environment to spontaneous breathing of air requires dramatic physiological changes in the infant within the first minutes to hours after birth.

Approximately 5% to 10% of the newly born population require some degree of active resuscitation at birth (eg, stimulation to breathe),[1] and approximately 1% to 10% born in the hospital are reported to require assisted ventilation.[2] More than 5 million neonatal deaths occur worldwide each year. It has been estimated that birth asphyxia accounts for 19% of these deaths, suggesting that the outcome might be improved for more than 1 million infants per year through implementation of simple resuscitative techniques.[3] Although the need for resuscitation of the newly born infant often can be predicted, such circumstances may arise suddenly and may occur in facilities that do not routinely provide neonatal intensive care. Thus, it is essential that the knowledge and skills required for resuscitation be taught to all providers of neonatal care.

With adequate anticipation, it is possible to optimize the delivery setting with appropriately prepared equipment and trained personnel who are capable of functioning as a team during neonatal resuscitation. At least 1 person skilled in initiating neonatal resuscitation should be present at every delivery. An additional skilled person capable of performing a complete resuscitation should be immediately available.

Neonatal resuscitation can be divided into 4 categories of action:

- Basic steps, including rapid assessment and initial steps in stabilization

- Ventilation, including bag-mask or bag-tube ventilation
- Chest compressions
- Administration of medications or fluids

Tracheal intubation may be required during any of these steps. All newly born infants require rapid assessment, including examination for the presence of meconium in the amniotic fluid or on the skin; evaluation of breathing, muscle tone, and color; and classification of gestational age as term or preterm. Newly born infants with a normal rapid assessment require only routine care (warmth, clearing the airway, drying). All others receive the initial steps, including warmth, clearing the airway, drying, positioning, stimulation to initiate or improve respirations, and oxygen as necessary.

Subsequent evaluation and intervention are based on a triad of characteristics: (1) respirations, (2) heart rate, and (3) color. Most newly born infants require only the basic steps, but for those who require further intervention, the most crucial action is establishment of adequate ventilation. Only a very small percentage will need chest compressions and medications.[4]

Certain special circumstances have unique implications for resuscitation of the newly born infant. Care of the infant after resuscitation includes not only supportive care but also ongoing monitoring and appropriate diagnostic evaluation. In certain clinical circumstances, noninitiation or discontinuation of resuscitation in the delivery room may be appropriate. Finally, it is important to document resuscitation interventions and responses in order to understand an individual infant's pathophysiology as well as to improve resuscitation performance and study resuscitation outcomes.[5–8]

Background

Changes in Neonatal Resuscitation Guidelines, 1992 to 2000

The ILCOR Pediatric Working Group consists of representatives from the American Heart Association (AHA), European Resuscitation Council (ERC), Heart and Stroke Foundation of Canada (HSFC), Australian Resuscitation Council (ARC), New Zealand Resuscitation Council (NZRC), Resuscitation Council of Southern Africa (RCSA), and Council of Latin America for Resuscitation (CLAR). Members of the Neonatal Resuscitation Program (NRP) Steering Committee of the American Academy of Pediatrics (AAP) and representatives of the World Health Organization (WHO) joined the ILCOR Pediatric Working Group to extend existing advisory recommendations for pediatric and neonatal basic life support[9] to comprehensive basic and advanced resuscitation for the newly born.[10] Careful review of the guidelines of constituent organizations[11–17] and current international literature formed the basis for the 1999 ILCOR advisory statement.[10] We have included consensus recommendations from that statement at the beginning of this document.

Using questions and controversies identified during the ILCOR process, the Neonatal Resuscitation Program Steering Committee (AAP), the Pediatric Working Group (ILCOR), and the Pediatric Resuscitation Subcommittee of the Emergency Cardiovascular Care Committee (AHA) carried out further evidence evaluation. At the Evidence Evaluation

Conference and International Guidelines 2000 Conference on CPR and ECC, these groups and panels of international experts and participants developed additional recommendations. The International Guidelines 2000 recommendations form the basis of this document.

Definition of "Newly Born," "Neonate," and "Infant"

Although the guidelines for neonatal resuscitation focus on newly born infants, most of the principles are applicable throughout the neonatal period and early infancy. The term "newly born" refers specifically to the infant in *the first minutes to hours after birth*. The term "neonate" is generally defined as an infant during the first 28 days of life. Infancy includes the neonatal period and extends through 12 months of age.

Unique Physiology of the Newly Born

The transition from fetal to extrauterine life is characterized by a series of unique physiological events: the lungs change from fluid-filled to air-filled, pulmonary blood flow increases dramatically, and intracardiac and extracardiac shunts (foramen ovale and ductus arteriosus) initially reverse direction and subsequently close. Such physiological considerations affect resuscitative interventions in the newly born.

For initial lung expansion, fluid-filled alveoli may require higher ventilation pressures than are commonly used in rescue breathing during infancy.[18,19] Physical expansion of the lungs, with establishment of functional residual capacity and increase in alveolar oxygen tension, both mediate the critical decrease in pulmonary vascular resistance and result in an increase in pulmonary blood flow after birth. Failure to normalize pulmonary vascular resistance may result in persistence of right-to-left intracardiac and extracardiac shunts (persistent pulmonary hypertension). Failure to adequately expand alveolar spaces may result in intrapulmonary shunting of blood with resultant hypoxemia. In addition to disordered cardiopulmonary transition, disruption of the fetoplacental circulation also may render the newly born at risk for resuscitation because of acute blood loss.

Developmental considerations at various gestational ages also influence pulmonary pathology and resuscitation physiology in the newly born. Surfactant deficiency in the premature infant alters lung compliance and resistance.[20] Meconium passed into the amniotic fluid may be aspirated, leading to airway obstruction. Complications of meconium aspiration are particularly likely in infants small for gestational age and those born post term or with significant perinatal compromise.[21]

Although certain physiological features are unique to the newly born, others pertain to infants throughout the neonatal period and into the first months of life. Severe illness due to a wide variety of conditions continues to manifest as disturbances in respiratory function (cyanosis, apnea, respiratory failure). Convalescing preterm infants with chronic lung disease often require significant ventilatory support regardless of the etiology of their need for resuscitation. Persistent pulmonary hypertension, persistent patency of the ductus arteriosus, and intracardiac shunts may produce symptoms

during the neonatal period or even into infancy. Thus, many of the considerations and interventions that apply to the newly born may remain important for days, weeks, or months after birth.

The point at which neonatal resuscitation guidelines should be replaced by pediatric resuscitation protocols varies for individual patients. Objective data is lacking on optimal compression-ventilation ratios by age and disease state. However, infants with acute or chronic lung disease may benefit from a lower compression-ventilation ratio well into infancy. For these infants, continued use of some aspects of the neonatal guidelines is reasonable. Conversely, a neonate with a cardiac arrhythmia resulting in poor perfusion requires use of protocols more fully detailed in pediatric advanced life support. Factors of age, pathophysiology, and caregiver training should be evaluated for each patient and the most appropriate resuscitation routines and care setting identified.

Anticipation of Resuscitation Need

Anticipation, adequate preparation, accurate evaluation, and prompt initiation of support are the critical steps to successful neonatal resuscitation.

Communication

Appropriate preparation for an anticipated high-risk delivery requires communication between the person(s) caring for the mother and those responsible for resuscitation of the newly born. Communication among caregivers should include details of antepartum and intrapartum maternal medical conditions and treatment as well as specific indicators of fetal condition (fetal heart rate monitoring, lung maturity, ultrasonography). Table 1 lists examples of the antepartum and intrapartum circumstances that place the newly born infant at risk.

Preparation for Delivery

Personnel

Personnel capable of initiating resuscitation should attend every delivery. At least 1 such person should be responsible solely for care of the infant. A person capable of carrying out a complete resuscitation should be immediately available for normal low-risk deliveries and in attendance for all deliveries considered high risk. More than 1 experienced person should attend an anticipated high-risk delivery. Resuscitation of a severely depressed newly born infant requires at least 2 persons, 1 to ventilate and intubate if necessary and another to monitor heart rate and perform chest compressions if required. A team of 3 or more persons with designated roles is highly desirable during an extensive resuscitation including medication administration. A separate team should be present for each infant of a multiple gestation. Each resuscitation team should have an identified leader, and all team members should have specifically defined roles.

Equipment

Although the need for resuscitation at birth often can be predicted by risk factors, for many infants resuscitation cannot be anticipated.[22] Therefore, a clean and warm environment with a complete inventory of resuscitation equip-

TABLE 1. Conditions Associated With Risk to Newborns

Antepartum risk factors

  Maternal diabetes

  Pregnancy-induced hypertension

  Chronic hypertension

  Chronic maternal illness

    Cardiovascular

    Thyroid

    Neurological

    Pulmonary

    Renal

  Anemia or isoimmunization

  Previous fetal or neonatal death

  Bleeding in second or third trimester

  Maternal infection

  Polyhydramnios

  Oligohydramnios

  Premature rupture of membranes

  Post-term gestation

  Multiple gestation

  Size-dates discrepancy

  Drug therapy, eg,

    Lithium carbonate

    Magnesium

    Adrenergic-blocking drugs

  Maternal substance abuse

  Fetal malformation

  Diminished fetal activity

  No prenatal care

  Age <16 or >35 years

Intrapartum risk factors

  Emergency cesarean section

  Forceps or vacuum-assisted delivery

  Breech or other abnormal presentation

  Premature labor

  Precipitous labor

  Chorioamnionitis

  Prolonged rupture of membranes (>18 hours before delivery)

  Prolonged labor (>24 hours)

  Prolonged second stage of labor (>2 hours)

  Fetal bradycardia

  Non-reassuring fetal heart rate patterns

  Use of general anesthesia

  Uterine tetany

  Narcotics administered to mother within 4 hours of delivery

  Meconium-stained amniotic fluid

  Prolapsed cord

  Abruptio placentae

  Placenta previa

ment and drugs should be maintained at hand and in fully operational condition wherever deliveries occur. Table 2 presents a list of suggested neonatal supplies, medications, and equipment.

Standard precautions should be followed carefully in delivery areas, where exposure to blood and body fluids is likely. All fluids from patients should be treated as potentially infectious. Personnel should wear gloves and other appropriate protective barriers when handling newly born infants or contaminated equipment. Techniques involving mouth suction by the healthcare provider should not be used.

Evaluation

Determination of the need for resuscitative efforts should begin immediately after birth and proceed throughout the resuscitation process. An initial complex of signs (meconium in the amniotic fluid or on the skin, cry or respirations, muscle tone, color, term or preterm gestation) should be evaluated rapidly and simultaneously by visual inspection. Actions are dictated by integrated evaluation rather than by evaluation of a single vital sign, followed by action on the result, and then evaluation of the next sign (sequential action). Evaluation and intervention for the newly born are often simultaneous processes, especially when >1 trained provider is present. To enhance educational retention, this process is often taught as a sequence of distinct steps. The appropriate response to abnormal findings also depends on the time elapsed since birth and how the infant has responded to previous resuscitative interventions.

Response to Extrauterine Environment

Most newly born infants will respond to the stimulation of the extrauterine environment with strong inspiratory efforts, a vigorous cry, and movement of all extremities. If these responses are intact, color improves steadily from cyanotic or dusky to pink, and heart rate can be assumed to be adequate. The infant who responds vigorously to the extrauterine environment and who is term can remain with the mother to receive routine care (warmth, clearing the airway, drying). Indications for further assessment under a radiant warmer and possible intervention include

- Meconium in the amniotic fluid or on the skin
- Absent or weak responses
- Persistent cyanosis
- Preterm birth

Further assessment of the newly born infant is based on the triad of respiration, heart rate, and color.

Respiration

After initial respiratory efforts, the newly born infant should be able to establish regular respirations sufficient to improve color and maintain a heart rate >100 bpm. Gasping and apnea are signs that indicate the need for assisted ventilation.[23]

Heart Rate

Heart rate is determined by listening to the precordium with a stethoscope or feeling pulsations at the base of the umbilical cord. Central and peripheral pulses in the neck and extremities

TABLE 2.   Neonatal Resuscitation Supplies and Equipment

Suction equipment

   Bulb syringe

   Mechanical suction and tubing

   Suction catheters, 5F or 6F, 8F, and 10F or 12F

   8F feeding tube and 20-mL syringe

   Meconium aspiration device

Bag-and-mask equipment

   Neonatal resuscitation bag with a pressure-release valve or pressure manometer (the bag must be capable of delivering 90% to 100% oxygen)

   Face masks, newborn and premature sizes (masks with cushioned rim preferred)

   Oxygen with flowmeter (flow rate up to 10 L/min) and tubing (including portable oxygen cylinders)

Intubation equipment

   Laryngoscope with straight blades, No. 0 (preterm) and No. 1 (term)

   Extra bulbs and batteries for laryngoscope

   Tracheal tubes, 2.5, 3.0, 3.5, and 4.0 mm ID

   Stylet (optional)

   Scissors

   Tape or securing device for tracheal tube

   Alcohol sponges

   CO_2 detector (optional)

   Laryngeal mask airway (optional)

Medications

   Epinephrine 1:10 000 (0.1 mg/mL)—3-mL or 10-mL ampules

   Isotonic crystalloid (normal saline or Ringer's lactate) for volume expansion—100 or 250 mL

   Sodium bicarbonate 4.2% (5 mEq/10 mL)—10-mL ampules

   Naloxone hydrochloride 0.4 mg/mL—1-mL ampules; or 1.0 mg/mL—2-mL ampules

   Normal saline, 30 mL

   Dextrose 10%, 250 mL

   Normal saline "fish" or "bullet" (optional)

   Feeding tube, 5F (optional)

   Umbilical vessel catheterization supplies

      Sterile gloves

      Scalpel or scissors

      Povidone-iodine solution

      Umbilical tape

      Umbilical catheters, 3.5F, 5F

      Three-way stopcock

   Syringes, 1, 3, 5, 10, 20, and 50 mL

   Needles, 25-, 21-, and 18-gauge or puncture device for needleless system

Miscellaneous

   Gloves and appropriate personal protection

   Radiant warmer or other heat source

   Firm, padded resuscitation surface

   Clock (timer optional)

   Warmed linens

   Stethoscope

   Tape, ½ or ¾ inch

   Cardiac monitor and electrodes and/or pulse oximeter with probe (optional for delivery room)

   Oropharyngeal airways

are often difficult to feel in infants,[24,25] but the umbilical pulse is readily accessible in the newly born and permits assessment of heart rate without interruption of ventilation for auscultation. If pulsations cannot be felt at the base of the cord, auscultation of the precordium should be performed. Heart rate should be consistently >100 bpm in an uncompromised newly born infant. An increasing or decreasing heart rate also can provide evidence of improvement or deterioration.

Color

An uncompromised newly born infant will be able to maintain a pink color of the mucous membranes without supplemental oxygen. Central cyanosis is determined by examining the face, trunk, and mucous membranes. Acrocyanosis is usually a normal finding at birth and is not a reliable indicator of hypoxemia, but it may indicate other conditions, such as cold stress. Pallor may be a sign of decreased cardiac output, severe anemia, hypovolemia, hypothermia, or acidosis.

Techniques of Resuscitation

The techniques of neonatal resuscitation are discussed below and are outlined in the algorithm (see Figure).

Basic Steps

Warmth

Preventing heat loss in the newly born is vital because cold stress can increase oxygen consumption and impede effective resuscitation.[26,27] Hyperthermia should be avoided, however, because it is associated with perinatal respiratory depression[28,29] (Class III, level of evidence [LOE] 3). Whenever possible, deliver the infant in a warm, draft-free area. Placing the infant under a radiant warmer, rapidly drying the skin, removing wet linen immediately, and wrapping the infant in prewarmed blankets will reduce heat loss. Another strategy for reducing heat loss is placing the dried infant skin-to-skin on the mother's chest or abdomen to use her body as a heat source.

Recent animal and human studies have suggested that selective (cerebral) hypothermia of the asphyxiated infant may protect against brain injury.[30–32] Although this is a promising area of research, we cannot recommend routine implementation until appropriate controlled studies in humans have been performed (Class Indeterminate, LOE 2).

Clearing the Airway

The infant's airway is cleared by positioning of the infant and removal of secretions if needed.

Positioning

The newly born infant should be placed supine or lying on its side, with the head in a neutral or slightly extended position. If respiratory efforts are present but not producing effective tidal ventilation, often the airway is obstructed; immediate efforts must be made to correct overextension or flexion or to remove secretions. A blanket or towel placed under the shoulders may be helpful in maintaining proper head position.

Suctioning

If time permits, the person assisting delivery of the infant should suction the infant's nose and mouth with a bulb syringe after delivery of the shoulders but before delivery of the chest. Healthy, vigorous, newly born infants generally do not require suctioning after delivery.[33] Secretions may be wiped from the nose and mouth with gauze or a towel. If suctioning is necessary, clear secretions first from the mouth and then the nose with a bulb syringe or suction catheter (8F or 10F). Aggressive pharyngeal suction can cause laryngeal spasm and vagal bradycardia[34] and delay the onset of spontaneous breathing. In the absence of meconium or blood, limit mechanical suction with a catheter in depth and duration. Negative pressure of the suction apparatus should not exceed 100 mm Hg (13.3 kPa or 136 cm H_2O). If copious secretions are present, the infant's head may be turned to the side, and suctioning may help clear the airway.

Clearing the Airway of Meconium

Approximately 12% of deliveries are complicated by the presence of meconium in the amniotic fluid.[35] When the amniotic fluid is meconium-stained, suction the mouth, pharynx, and nose as soon as the head is delivered (intrapartum suctioning) regardless of whether the meconium is thin or thick.[36] Either a large-bore suction catheter (12F to 14F) or bulb syringe can be used.[37] Thorough suctioning of the nose, mouth, and posterior pharynx before delivery of the body appears to decrease the risk of meconium-aspiration syndrome.[36] Nevertheless, a significant number (20% to 30%) of meconium-stained infants will have meconium in the trachea despite such suctioning and in the absence of spontaneous respirations.[38,39] This suggests the occurrence of in utero aspiration and the need for tracheal suctioning after delivery in *depressed* infants.

If the fluid contains meconium and the infant has absent or depressed respirations, decreased muscle tone, or heart rate <100 bpm, perform direct laryngoscopy immediately after birth for suctioning of residual meconium from the hypopharynx (under direct vision) and intubation/suction of the trachea.[40,41] There is evidence that tracheal suctioning of the vigorous infant with meconium-stained fluid does not improve outcome and may cause complications (Class I, LOE 1).[42,43] Warmth can be provided by a radiant heater; however, drying and stimulation generally should be delayed in such infants. Accomplish tracheal suctioning by applying suction directly to a tracheal tube as it is withdrawn from the airway. Repeat intubation and suctioning until little additional meconium is recovered or until the heart rate indicates that resuscitation must proceed without delay. If the infant's heart rate or respiration is severely depressed, it may be necessary to institute positive-pressure ventilation despite the presence of some meconium in the airway. Suction catheters inserted through the tracheal tube may be too small to accomplish initial removal of particulate meconium; subsequent use of suction catheters inserted through a tracheal tube may be adequate to continue removal of meconium. Delay gastric suctioning to prevent aspiration of swallowed meconium until initial resuscitation is complete. Meconium-stained infants who develop apnea or respiratory distress should receive tracheal suctioning before positive-pressure ventilation, even if they are initially vigorous.

Tactile Stimulation

Drying and suctioning produce enough stimulation to initiate effective respirations in most newly born infants. If

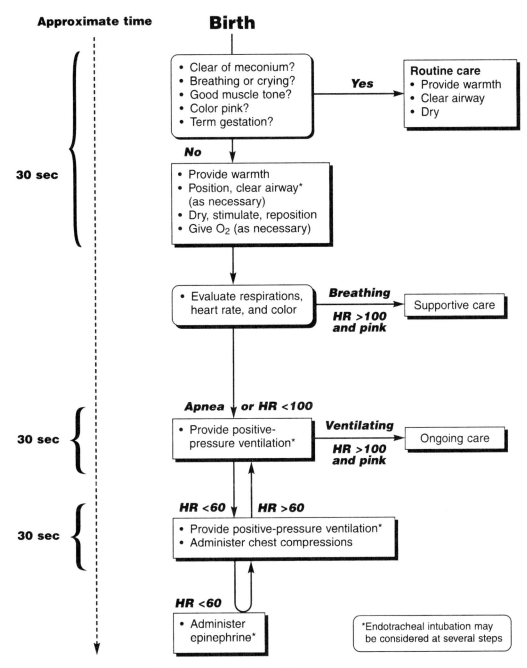

Algorithm for resuscitation of the newly born infant.

an infant fails to establish spontaneous and effective respirations after drying with a towel or gentle rubbing of the back, flicking the soles of the feet may initiate spontaneous respirations. Avoid more vigorous methods of stimulation. Tactile stimulation may initiate spontaneous respirations in newly born infants who are experiencing primary apnea. If these efforts do not result in prompt onset of effective ventilation, discontinue them because the infant is in secondary apnea and positive-pressure ventilation will be required.[23]

Oxygen Administration
Hypoxia is nearly always present in a newly born infant who requires resuscitation. Therefore, if cyanosis, bradycardia, or other signs of distress are noted in a breathing newborn during stabilization, administration of 100% oxygen is indicated while determining the need for additional intervention. Free-flow oxygen can be delivered through a face mask and flow-inflating bag, an oxygen mask, or a hand cupped around oxygen tubing. The oxygen source should deliver at least 5 L/min, and the oxygen should be held close to the face to maximize the inhaled concentration. Many self-inflating bags will not passively deliver sufficient oxygen flow (ie, when not being squeezed). The goal of supplemental oxygen use should be normoxia; sufficient oxygen should be administered to achieve pink color in the mucous membranes. If cyanosis returns when supplemental oxygen is withdrawn, post-

resuscitation care should include monitoring of administered oxygen concentration and arterial oxygen saturation.

Ventilation

Most newly born infants who require positive-pressure ventilation can be adequately ventilated with a bag and mask. Indications for positive-pressure ventilation include apnea or gasping respirations, heart rate <100 bpm, and persistent central cyanosis despite 100% oxygen.

Although the pressure required for establishment of air breathing is variable and unpredictable, higher inflation pressures (30 to 40 cm H_2O or higher) and longer inflation times may be required for the first several breaths than for subsequent breaths.[18,19] Visible chest expansion is a more reliable sign of appropriate inflation pressures than any specific manometer reading. The assisted ventilation rate should be 40 to 60 breaths per minute (30 breaths per minute when chest compressions are also being delivered). Signs of adequate ventilation include bilateral expansion of the lungs, as assessed by chest wall movement and breath sounds, and improvement in heart rate and color. If ventilation is inadequate, check the seal between mask and face, clear any airway obstruction (adjust head position, clear secretions, open the infant's mouth), and finally increase inflation pressure. Prolonged bag-mask ventilation may produce gastric inflation; this should be relieved by insertion of an 8F orogastric tube that is aspirated with a syringe and left open to air. If such maneuvers do not result in adequate ventilation, endotracheal intubation should follow.

After 30 seconds of adequate ventilation with 100% oxygen, spontaneous breathing and heart rate should be checked. If spontaneous respirations are present and the heart rate is ≥100 bpm, positive-pressure ventilation may be gradually reduced and discontinued. Gentle tactile stimulation may help maintain and improve spontaneous respirations while free-flow oxygen is administered. If spontaneous respirations are inadequate or if heart rate remains below 100 bpm, assisted ventilation must continue with bag and mask or tracheal tube. If the heart rate is <60 bpm, continue assisted ventilation, begin chest compressions, and consider endotracheal intubation.

The key to successful neonatal resuscitation is establishment of adequate ventilation. Reversal of hypoxia, acidosis, and bradycardia depends on adequate inflation of fluid-filled lungs with air or oxygen.[44,45] Although 100% oxygen has been used traditionally for rapid reversal of hypoxia, there is biochemical evidence and preliminary clinical evidence to argue for resuscitation with lower oxygen concentrations.[46-48] Current clinical data, however, is insufficient to justify adopting this as routine practice. If assisted ventilation is required, deliver 100% oxygen by positive-pressure ventilation. If supplemental oxygen is unavailable, initiate resuscitation of the newly born infant with positive-pressure ventilation and room air (Class Indeterminate, LOE 2).

Ventilation Bags

Resuscitation bags used for neonates should be no larger than 750 mL; larger bag volumes make it difficult to judge delivery of the small tidal volumes (5 to 8 mL/kg) that newly born infants require. Bags for neonatal resuscitation can be either self-inflating or flow-inflating.

Self-Inflating Bags

The self-inflating bag refills independently of gas flow because of the recoil of the bag. To permit rapid reinflation, most bags of this type have an intake valve at one end that pulls in room air, diluting the oxygen flowing into the bag at a fixed rate. Delivery of high concentrations of oxygen (90% to 100%) with a self-inflating bag requires an attached oxygen reservoir.

To maintain inflation pressure for at least 1 second, a minimum bag volume of 450 to 500 mL may be necessary. If the device contains a pressure-release valve, it should release at approximately 30 to 35 cm H_2O pressure and should have an override feature to permit delivery of higher pressures if necessary to achieve good chest expansion. Self-inflating bags that are not pressure limited or that have a device to bypass the pressure-release valve should be equipped with an in-line manometer. Do not use self-inflating bags to deliver oxygen passively through the mask because the flow of oxygen is unreliable unless the bag is being squeezed.

Flow-Inflating Bags

The flow-inflating (anesthesia) bag inflates only when compressed gas is flowing into it and the patient outlet is at least partially occluded. Proper use requires adjustment of the flow of gas into the gas inlet, adjustment of the flow of gas out through the flow-control valve, and creation of a tight seal between the mask and face. Because a flow-inflating bag is capable of delivering very high pressures, a manometer should be connected to the bag to monitor peak and end-expiratory pressures. More training is required for proper use of the flow-inflating bag than the self-inflating bag,[49] but the flow-inflating bag can provide a greater range of peak inspiratory pressures and more reliable control of oxygen concentration. High concentrations of oxygen may be delivered passively through the mask of a flow-inflating bag.

Face Masks

Masks should be of appropriate size to seal around the mouth and nose but not cover the eyes or overlap the chin. A range of sizes should be available. A round mask can seal effectively on the face of a small infant; anatomically shaped masks better fit the contours of a large term infant's face. Masks should be designed to have low dead space (<5 mL). A mask with a cushioned rim is preferable to one without because the cushioned rim facilitates creation of a tight seal without exerting excessive pressure on the face.[50]

Laryngeal Mask Airway Ventilation

Masks that fit over the laryngeal inlet have been shown to be effective for ventilating newly born full-term infants.[51] There is limited data on the use of these devices in small preterm infants,[52] however, and their use in the setting of meconium-stained amniotic fluid has not been studied. The laryngeal mask airway, when used by appropriately trained providers, may be an effective alternative for establishing an airway in resuscitation of the newly born infant, especially in the case of ineffective bag-mask ventilation or failed endotracheal intubation (Class Indeterminate, LOE 5). However, we cannot recommend routine use of the laryngeal mask airway at

TABLE 3. Suggested Tracheal Tube Size and Depth of Insertion According to Weight and Gestational Age

Weight, g	Gestational Age, wk	Tube Size, mm (ID)	Depth of Insertion From Upper Lip, cm
<1000	<28	2.5	6.5–7
1000–2000	28–34	3.0	7–8
2000–3000	34–38	3.5	8–9
>3000	>38	3.5–4.0	>9

ID indicates inner diameter.

this time, and the device cannot replace endotracheal intubation for meconium suctioning.

Endotracheal Intubation

Endotracheal intubation may be indicated at several points during neonatal resuscitation:

- When tracheal suctioning for meconium is required
- If bag-mask ventilation is ineffective or prolonged
- When chest compressions are performed
- When tracheal administration of medications is desired
- Special resuscitation circumstances, such as congenital diaphragmatic hernia or extremely low birth weight

The timing of endotracheal intubation may also depend on the skill and experience of the resuscitator.

Keep the supplies and equipment for endotracheal intubation together and readily available in each delivery room, nursery, and Emergency Department. Preferred tracheal tubes have a uniform diameter (without a shoulder) and have a natural curve, a radiopaque indicator line, and markings to indicate the appropriate depth of insertion. If a stylet is used, it must not protrude beyond the tip of the tube. Table 3 provides a guideline for selection of tracheal tube sizes and depths of insertion. Positioning the vocal cord guide (a line proximal to the tip of the tube) at the level of the vocal cords should position the tip of the tube above the carina. Proper depth of insertion can also be estimated by calculating the depth at the lips according to the following formula:

weight in kilograms + 6 cm = insertion depth at lip in cm

Perform endotracheal intubation orally, using a laryngoscope with a straight blade (size 0 for premature infants, size 1 for term infants). Insert the tip of the laryngoscope into the vallecula or onto the epiglottis and elevate gently to reveal the vocal cords. Cricoid pressure may be helpful. Insert the tube to an appropriate depth through the vocal cords as indicated by the vocal cord guide line and check its position by the centimeter marking at the upper lip. Record and maintain this depth of insertion. Variation in head position will alter the depth of insertion and may predispose to unintentional extubation or endobronchial intubation.[53,54]

After endotracheal intubation, confirm the position of the tube by the following:

- Observing symmetrical chest-wall motion
- Listening for equal breath sounds, especially in the axillae, and for absence of breath sounds over the stomach
- Confirming absence of gastric inflation

- Watching for a fog of moisture in the tube during exhalation
- Noting improvement in heart rate, color, and activity of the infant

An exhaled-CO_2 monitor may be used to verify tracheal tube placement.[55] These devices are associated with some false-negative but few false-positive results.[56] Monitoring of exhaled CO_2 can be useful in the secondary confirmation of tracheal intubation in the newly born, particularly when clinical assessment is equivocal (Class Indeterminate, LOE 5). Data about sensitivity and specificity of exhaled CO_2 detectors in reflecting tracheal tube position is limited in newly born infants. Extrapolation of data from other age groups is problematic because conditions common to the newborn period, including inadequate pulmonary expansion, decreased pulmonary blood flow, and small tidal volumes, may influence the interpretation of the exhaled CO_2 concentration.

Chest Compressions

Asphyxia causes peripheral vasoconstriction, tissue hypoxia, acidosis, poor myocardial contractility, bradycardia, and eventually cardiac arrest. Establishment of adequate ventilation and oxygenation will restore vital signs in the vast majority of newly born infants. In deciding when to initiate chest compressions, consider the heart rate, the change of heart rate, and the time elapsed after initiation of resuscitative measures. Because chest compressions may diminish the effectiveness of ventilation, do not initiate them until lung inflation and ventilation have been established.

The general indication for initiation of chest compressions is a heart rate <60 bpm despite adequate ventilation with 100% oxygen for 30 seconds. Although it has been common practice to give compressions if the heart rate is 60 to 80 bpm and the heart rate is not rising, ventilation should be the priority in resuscitation of the newly born. Provision of chest compressions is likely to compete with provision of effective ventilation. Because no scientific data suggests an evidence-based resolution, the ILCOR Working Group recommends that compressions be initiated for a heart rate of <60 bpm based on construct validity (ease of teaching and skill retention).

Compression Technique

Compressions should be delivered on the lower third of the sternum.[57,58] Acceptable techniques are (1) 2 thumbs on the sternum, superimposed or adjacent to each other according to the size of the infant, with fingers encircling the chest and supporting the back (the 2 thumb–encircling hands technique), and (2) 2 fingers placed on the sternum at right angles to the chest with the other hand supporting the back.[59–61] Data suggests that the 2 thumb–encircling hands technique may offer some advantages in generating peak systolic and coronary perfusion pressure and that providers prefer this technique to the 2-finger technique.[59–63] For this reason, we prefer the 2 thumb–encircling hands technique for healthcare providers performing chest compressions in newly born infants and older infants whose size permits its use (Class IIb, LOE 5).

Consensus of the ILCOR Working Group supports a relative rather than absolute depth of compression (ie, compress to approximately one third of the anterior-posterior diameter of the chest) to generate a palpable pulse. The pediatric basic life support guidelines recommend a relative compression depth of one third to one half of the anterior-posterior dimension of the chest. In the absence of specific data about ideal compression depth, these guidelines recommend compression to approximately one third the depth of the chest, but the compression depth must be adequate to produce a palpable pulse. Deliver compressions smoothly. A compression to relaxation ratio with a slightly shorter compression than relaxation phase offers theoretical advantages for blood flow in the very young infant.[64] Keep the thumbs or fingers on the sternum during the relaxation phase.

Coordinate compressions and ventilations to avoid simultaneous delivery.[65] There should be a 3:1 ratio of compressions to ventilations, with 90 compressions and 30 breaths to achieve approximately 120 events per minute. Thus, each event will be allotted approximately 1/2 second, with exhalation occurring during the first compression following each ventilation. Reassess the heart rate approximately every 30 seconds. Continue chest compressions until the spontaneous heart rate is ≥60 bpm.

Medications

Drugs are rarely indicated in resuscitation of the newly born infant.[66] Bradycardia in the newly born infant is usually the result of inadequate lung inflation or profound hypoxia, and adequate ventilation is the most important step in correcting bradycardia. Administer medications if, despite adequate ventilation with 100% oxygen and chest compressions, the heart rate remains <60 bpm.

Medications and Volume Expansion

Epinephrine

Administration of epinephrine is indicated when the heart rate remains <60 bpm after a minimum of 30 seconds of adequate ventilation and chest compressions (Class I). Epinephrine is particularly indicated in the presence of asystole.

Epinephrine has both α- and β-adrenergic–stimulating properties; however, in cardiac arrest, α-adrenergic–mediated vasoconstriction may be the more important action.[67] Vasoconstriction elevates the perfusion pressure during chest compression, enhancing delivery of oxygen to the heart and brain.[68] Epinephrine also enhances the contractile state of the heart, stimulates spontaneous contractions, and increases heart rate.

The recommended intravenous or endotracheal dose is 0.1 to 0.3 mL/kg of a 1:10 000 solution (0.01 to 0.03 mg/kg), repeated every 3 to 5 minutes as indicated. The data regarding effects of high-dose epinephrine for resuscitation of newly born infants is inadequate to support routine use of higher doses of epinephrine (Class Indeterminate, LOE 4). Higher doses have been associated with exaggerated hypertension but lower cardiac output in animals.[69,70] The sequence of hypotension followed by hypertension likely increases the risk of intracranial hemorrhage, especially in preterm infants.[71]

Volume Expanders

Volume expanders may be necessary to resuscitate a newly born infant who is hypovolemic. Suspect hypovolemia in any infant who fails to respond to resuscitation. Consider volume expansion when there has been suspected blood loss or the infant appears to be in shock (pale, poor perfusion, weak pulse) and has not responded adequately to other resuscitative measures (Class I). The fluid of choice for volume expansion is an isotonic crystalloid solution such as normal saline or Ringer's lactate (Class IIb, LOE 7). Administration of O-negative red blood cells may be indicated for replacement of large-volume blood loss (Class IIb, LOE 7). Albumin-containing solutions are less frequently used for initial volume expansion because of limited availability, risk of infectious disease, and an observed association with increased mortality.[72]

The initial dose of volume expander is 10 mL/kg given by slow intravenous push over 5 to 10 minutes. The dose may be repeated after further clinical assessment and observation of response. Higher bolus volumes have been recommended for resuscitation of older infants. However, volume overload or complications such as intracranial hemorrhage may result from inappropriate intravascular volume expansion in asphyxiated newly born infants as well as in preterm infants.[73,74]

Bicarbonate

There is insufficient data to recommend routine use of bicarbonate in resuscitation of the newly born. In fact, the hyperosmolarity and CO_2-generating properties of sodium bicarbonate may be detrimental to myocardial or cerebral function.[75–77] Use of sodium bicarbonate is discouraged during brief CPR. If it is used during prolonged arrests unresponsive to other therapy, it should be given only after establishment of adequate ventilation and circulation.[78] Later use of bicarbonate for treatment of persistent metabolic acidosis or hyperkalemia should be directed by arterial blood gas levels or serum chemistries, among other evaluations. A dose of 1 to 2 mEq/kg of a 0.5 mEq/mL solution may be given by slow intravenous push (over at least 2 minutes) after adequate ventilation and perfusion have been established.

Naloxone

Naloxone hydrochloride is a narcotic antagonist without respiratory-depressant activity. It is specifically indicated for reversal of respiratory depression in a newly born infant whose mother received narcotics within 4 hours of delivery. Always establish and maintain adequate ventilation before administration of naloxone. Do not administer naloxone to newly born infants whose mothers are suspected of having recently abused narcotic drugs because it may precipitate abrupt withdrawal signs in such infants.

The recommended dose of naloxone is 0.1 mg/kg of a 0.4 mg/mL or 1.0 mg/mL solution given intravenously, endotracheally, or—if perfusion is adequate—intramuscularly or subcutaneously. Because the duration of action of narcotics may exceed that of naloxone, continued monitoring of respiratory function is essential, and repeated naloxone doses may be necessary to prevent recurrent apnea.

TABLE 4. Special Circumstances in Resuscitation of the Newly Born Infant

Condition	History/Clinical Signs	Actions
Mechanical blockage of the airway		
Meconium or mucus blockage	Meconium-stained amniotic fluid	Intubation for suctioning/ventilation
	Poor chest wall movement	
Choanal atresia	Pink when crying, cyanotic when quiet	Oral airway
		Endotracheal intubation
Pharyngeal airway malformation	Persistent retractions, poor air entry	Prone positioning, posterior nasopharyngeal tube
Impaired lung function		
Pneumothorax	Asymmetrical breath sounds	Needle thoracentesis
	Persistent cyanosis/bradycardia	
Pleural effusions/ascites	Diminished air movement	Immediate intubation
	Persistent cyanosis/bradycardia	Needle thoracentesis, paracentesis
		Possible volume expansion
Congenital diaphragmatic hernia	Asymmetrical breath sounds	Endotracheal intubation
	Persistent cyanosis/bradycardia	Placement of orogastric catheter
	Scaphoid abdomen	
Pneumonia/sepsis	Diminished air movement	Endotracheal intubation
	Persistent cyanosis/bradycardia	Possible volume expansion
Impaired cardiac function		
Congenital heart disease	Persistent cyanosis/bradycardia	Diagnostic evaluation
Fetal/maternal hemorrhage	Pallor; poor response to resuscitation	Volume expansion, possibly including red blood cells

Routes of Medication Administration

The tracheal route is generally the most rapidly accessible route for drug administration during resuscitation. It may be used for administration of epinephrine and naloxone, but it should not be used during resuscitation for administration of caustic agents such as sodium bicarbonate. The tracheal route of administration may result in a more variable response to epinephrine than the intravenous route[79–81]; however, neonatal data is insufficient to recommend a higher dose of epinephrine for tracheal administration.

Attempt to establish intravenous access in neonates who fail to respond to tracheally administered epinephrine. The umbilical vein is the most rapidly accessible venous route; it may be used for epinephrine or naloxone administration as well as for administration of volume expanders and bicarbonate. Insert a 3.5F or 5F radiopaque catheter so that the tip is just below skin level and a free flow of blood returns on aspiration. Deep insertion poses the risk of infusion of hypertonic and vasoactive medications into the liver. Take care to avoid introduction of air emboli into the umbilical vein.

Peripheral sites for venous access (scalp or peripheral vein) may be adequate but are usually more difficult to cannulate. Naloxone may be given intramuscularly or subcutaneously but only after effective assisted ventilation has been established and only if the infant's peripheral circulation is adequate. We do not recommend administration of resuscitation drugs through the umbilical artery because the artery is often not rapidly accessible and complications may result if vasoactive or hypertonic drugs (eg, epinephrine or bicarbonate) are given by this route.

Intraosseous lines are not commonly used in newly born infants because the umbilical vein is more accessible, the small bones are fragile, and the intraosseous space is small in a premature infant. Intraosseous access has been shown to be useful in the neonate and older infant when vascular access is difficult to achieve.[82] Intraosseous access can be used as an alternative route for medication/volume expansion if umbilical or other direct venous access is not readily attainable (Class IIb, LOE 5).

Special Resuscitation Circumstances

Several circumstances have unique implications for resuscitation of the newly born infant. Prenatal diagnosis and certain features of the perinatal history and clinical course may alert the resuscitation team to these special circumstances. Meconium aspiration (see above), multiple birth, and prematurity are common conditions with immediate implications for the resuscitation team at delivery. Other circumstances that may affect opening of the airway, timing of endotracheal intubation, and selection and administration of volume expanders are presented in Table 4.

Prematurity

The incidence of perinatal depression is markedly increased among preterm neonates because of the complications associated with preterm labor and the physiological immaturity and lability of the preterm infant.[83] Diminished lung compliance, respiratory musculature, and respiratory drive may contribute to the need for assisted ventilation.

Some experts recommend early elective intubation of extremely preterm infants (eg, <28 weeks of gestation) to help establish an air-fluid interface,[84] while others recommend that this be accomplished with oxygen administration via mask or nasal prongs.[85] Many infants younger than 30 to

TABLE 5. Apgar Scoring

Sign	Score		
	0	1	2
Heart rate	Absent	Slow (<100 bpm)	≥100 bpm
Respirations	Absent	Slow, irregular	Good, crying
Muscle tone	Limp	Some flexion	Active motion
Reflex irritability (catheter in nares, tactile stimulation)	No response	Grimace	Cough, sneeze, cry
Color	Blue or pale	Pink body, blue extremities	Completely pink

bpm indicates beats per minute.

31 weeks will undergo intubation for surfactant administration after the initial stages of resuscitation have been successful.[86]

A number of factors can complicate resuscitation of the premature infant. Because premature infants have low body fat and a high ratio of surface area to body mass, they are also more difficult to keep warm. Their immature brains and the presence of a fragile germinal matrix predispose them to development of intracranial hemorrhage after episodes of hypoxia or rapid changes in vascular pressure and osmolarity.[77,87,88] For this reason, avoid rapid boluses of volume expanders or hyperosmolar solutions.

Multiple Births

Multiple births are more frequently associated with a need for resuscitation because of abnormalities of placentation, compromise of cord blood flow, or mechanical complications during delivery. Monozygotic multiple fetuses may also have abnormalities of blood volume resulting from interfetal vascular anastomoses.

Postresuscitation Issues

Continuing Care of the Newly Born Infant After Resuscitation

Supportive or ongoing care, monitoring, and appropriate diagnostic evaluation are required after resuscitation. Once adequate ventilation and circulation have been established, the infant is still at risk and should be maintained in or transferred to an environment in which close monitoring and anticipatory care can be provided. Postresuscitation monitoring should include monitoring of heart rate, respiratory rate, administered oxygen concentration, and arterial oxygen saturation, with blood gas analysis as indicated. Document blood pressure and check the blood glucose level during stabilization after resuscitation. Consider ongoing blood glucose screening and documentation of calcium. A chest radiograph may help elucidate underlying causes of the arrest or detect complications, such as pneumothorax. Additional postresuscitation care may include treatment of hypotension with volume expanders or pressors, treatment of possible infection or seizures, initiation of appropriate fluid therapy, and documentation of observations and actions.

Documentation of Resuscitation

Thorough documentation of assessments and resuscitative actions is essential for good clinical care, for communication, and for medicolegal concerns. The Apgar scores quantify and summarize the response of the newly born infant to the extrauterine environment and to resuscitation (Table 5).[89,90] Assign Apgar scores at 1 and 5 minutes after birth and then sequentially every 5 minutes until vital signs have stabilized. The Apgar scores should not dictate appropriate resuscitative actions, nor should interventions for depressed infants be delayed until the 1-minute assessment. Complete documentation must also include a narrative description of interventions performed and their timing.

Continuing Care of the Family

When time permits, the team responsible for care of the newly born should introduce themselves to the mother and family before delivery. They should outline the proposed plan of care and solicit the family's questions. Especially in cases of potentially lethal fetal malformations or extreme prematurity, the family should be asked to articulate their beliefs and desires about the extent of resuscitation, and the team should outline its planned approach (see below).

After delivery the mother continues to be a patient herself, with physical and emotional needs. The team caring for the newly born infant should inform the parents of the infant's condition at the earliest opportunity. If resuscitation is necessary, inform the parents of the procedures undertaken and their indications. Encourage the parents to ask questions, and answer their questions as frankly and honestly as possible. Make every effort to enable the parents to have contact with the newly born infant.

Ethics

There are circumstances in which noninitiation or discontinuation of resuscitation in the delivery room may be appropriate. However, national and local protocols should dictate the procedures to be followed. Changes in resuscitation and intensive care practices and neonatal outcome make it imperative that all such protocols be reviewed regularly and modified as necessary.

Noninitiation of Resuscitation

The delivery of extremely immature infants and infants with severe congenital anomalies raises questions about initiation of resuscitation.[91–93] Noninitiation of resuscitation in the delivery room is appropriate for infants with confirmed gestation <23 weeks or birth weight <400 g, anencephaly, or confirmed trisomy 13 or 18. Current data suggests that resuscitation of these newly born infants is very unlikely to result in survival or survival without severe disability[94] (Class IIb, LOE 5).[95] However, antenatal information may be incomplete or unreliable. In cases of uncertain prognosis, including uncertain gestational age, resuscitation options include a trial of therapy and noninitiation or discontinuation of resuscitation after assessment of the infant. In such cases, initiation of resuscitation at delivery does not mandate continued support.

Noninitiation of support and later withdrawal of support are generally considered to be ethically equivalent; however, the latter approach allows time to gather more complete clinical information and to provide counseling to the family. Ongoing evaluation and discussion with the parents and the healthcare team should guide continuation versus withdrawal of support. In general, there is no advantage to delayed, graded, or partial support; if the infant survives, outcome may be worsened as a result of this approach.

Discontinuation of Resuscitation

Discontinuation of resuscitative efforts may be appropriate if resuscitation of an infant with cardiorespiratory arrest does not result in spontaneous circulation in 15 minutes. Resuscitation of newly born infants after 10 minutes of asystole is very unlikely to result in survival or survival without severe disability (Class IIb, LOE 5).[96–99] We recommend local discussions to formulate guidelines consistent with local resources and outcome data.

References

1. Saugstad OD. Practical aspects of resuscitating asphyxiated newborn infants. *Eur J Pediatr.* 1998;157(suppl 1):S11–S15.
2. Palme-Kilander C. Methods of resuscitation in low-Apgar-score newborn infants: a national survey. *Acta Paediatr.* 1992;81:739–744.
3. *World Health Report.* Geneva, Switzerland: World Health Organization; 1995.
4. Perlman JM, Risser R. Cardiopulmonary resuscitation in the delivery room: associated clinical events. *Arch Pediatr Adolesc Med.* 1995;149: 20–25.
5. Cummins RO, Chamberlain DA, Abramson NS, et al. Recommended guidelines for uniform reporting of data from out-of-hospital cardiac arrest: the Utstein style. *Circulation.* 1991;84:960–975.
6. Cummins RO, Chamberlain DA, Hazinski MF, et al. Recommended guidelines for reviewing, reporting, and conducting research on in-hospital resuscitation: the in-hospital "Utstein style." *Circulation.* 1997;95:2213–2239.
7. Zaritsky A, Nadkarni V, Hazinski MF, Foltin G, Quan L, Wright J, Fiser D, Zideman D, O'Malley P, Chameides L, Writing Group. Recommended guidelines for uniform reporting of pediatric advanced life support: the pediatric Utstein style: a statement for healthcare professionals from a task force of the American Academy of Pediatrics, the American Heart Association, and the European Resuscitation Council. *Circulation.* 1995; 92:2006–2020.
8. Idris AH, Becker LB, Ornato JP, Hedges JR, Bircher NG, Chandra NC, Cummins RO, Dick W, Ebmeyer U, Halperin HR, Hazinski MF, Kerber RE, Kern KB, Safar P, Steen PA, Swindle MM, Tsitlik JE, von Planta I, von Planta M, Wears RL, Weil MH, Writing Group. Utstein-style guidelines for uniform reporting of laboratory CPR research: a statement for healthcare professionals from a task force of the American Heart Association, the American College of Emergency Physicians, the American College of Cardiology, the European Resuscitation Council, the Heart and Stroke Foundation of Canada, the Institute of Critical Care Medicine, the Safar Center for Resuscitation Research, and the Society for Academic Emergency Medicine. *Circulation.* 1996;94:2324–2336.
9. Nadkarni V, Hazinski MF, Zideman D, Kattwinkel J, Quan L, Bingham R, Zaritsky A, Bland J, Kramer E, Tiballs J. Paediatric life support: an advisory statement by the Paediatric Life Support Working Group of the International Liaison Committee on Resuscitation. *Resuscitation.* 1997; 34:115–127.
10. Kattwinkel J, Niermeyer S, Nadkarni V, Tiballs J, Phillips B, Zideman D, Van Reempts P, Osmond M. ILCOR advisory statement: resuscitation of the newly born infant: an advisory statement from the pediatric working group of the International Liaison Committee on Resuscitation. *Circulation.* 1999;99:1927–1938.
11. Guidelines for cardiopulmonary resuscitation and emergency cardiac care: Emergency Cardiac Care Committee and Subcommittees, American Heart Association, part V: pediatric basic life support [see comments]. *JAMA.* 1992;268:2251–2261.
12. Bloom RS, Cropley C, AHA/AAP Neonatal Resuscitation Program Steering Committee, American Heart Association. American Academy of Pediatrics. Textbook of Neonatal Resuscitation/Ronald S. Bloom, Catherine Cropley, and the AHA/AAP Neonatal Resuscitation Program Steering Committee [Rev. ed.];1 v. (various pagings): ill.; 28 cm. Elk Grove Village, IL: American Academy of Pediatrics: American Heart Association; 1994.
13. Kloeck WGJ, Kramer E. Resuscitation Council of Southern Africa: new recommendations for BLS in adults, children and infants. *Trauma Emerg Med.* 1997;14:13–32.
14. Advanced Life Support Committee of the Australian Resuscitation Council. Paediatric advanced life support: Australian Resuscitation Council guidelines: Advanced Life Support Committee of the Australian Resuscitation Council. *Med J Aust.* 1996;165:199–201, 204–206.
15. European Resuscitation Council. Pediatric basic life support: to be read in conjunction with the International Liaison Committee on Resuscitation Pediatric Working Group Advisory Statement (April 1997). *Resuscitation.* 1998;37:97–100.
16. European Resuscitation Council. Pediatric advanced life support: to be read in conjunction with the International Liaison Committee on Resuscitation Pediatric Working Group Advisory Statement (April 1997). *Resuscitation.* 1998;37:101–102.
17. European Resuscitation Council. Recommendations on resuscitation of babies at birth: to be read in conjunction with the International Liaison Committee on Resuscitation Pediatric Working Group Advisory Statement (April 1997). *Resuscitation.* 1998;37:103–110.
18. Vyas H, Milner AD, Hopkin IE, Boon AW. Physiologic responses to prolonged slow-rise inflation in the resuscitation of the asphyxiated newborn infant. *J Pediatr.* 1981;99:635–639.
19. Vyas H, Field D, Milner AD, Hopkin IE. Determinants of the first inspiratory volume and functional residual capacity at birth. *Pediatr Pulmonol.* 1986;2:189–193.
20. Jobe A. The respiratory system. In: Fanaroff AA, Martin RJ, et al, eds. *Neonatal Perinatal Medicine.* St Louis, Mo: CV Mosby; 1997:991–1018.
21. Gregory GA, Gooding CA, Phibbs RH, Tooley WH. Meconium aspiration in infants: a prospective study. *J Pediatr.* 1974;85:848–852.
22. Peliowski A, Finer NN. Birth asphyxia in the term infant. In: Sinclair JC, Bracken MB, et al, eds. *Effective Care of the Newborn Infant.* Oxford, UK: Oxford University Press; 1992:249–273.
23. Dawes GF. *Fetal and Neonatal Physiology: A Comparative Study of the Changes at Birth.* Chicago, Ill: Year Book Medical Publishers; 1968: 149–151.
24. Whitelaw CC, Goldsmith LJ. Comparison of two techniques for determining the presence of a pulse in an infant [letter]. *Acad Emerg Med.* 1997;4:153–154.
25. Theophilopoulos DT, Burchfield DJ. Accuracy of different methods for heart rate determination during simulated neonatal resuscitations. *J Perinatol.* 1998;18:65–67.
26. Gandy GM, Adamson SK Jr, Cunningham N, Silverman WA, James LS. Thermal environment and acid-base homeostasis in human infants during the first few hours of life. *J Clin Invest.* 1964;43:751–758.
27. Dahm LS, James LS. Newborn temperature and calculated heat loss in the delivery room. *Pediatrics.* 1972;49:504–513.
28. Perlman JM. Maternal fever and neonatal depression: preliminary observations. *Clin Pediatr.* 1999;38:287–291.
29. Lieberman E, Lang J, Richardson DK, Frigoletto FD, Heffner LJ, Cohen A. Intrapartum maternal fever and neonatal outcome. *Pediatrics.* 2000; 105:8–13.
30. Vannucci RC, Perlman JM. Interventions for perinatal hypoxic-ischemic encephalopathy [see comments]. *Pediatrics.* 1997;100:1004–1014.
31. Edwards AD, Wyatt JS, Thoreson M. Treatment of hypoxic-ischemic brain damage by moderate hypothermia. *Arch Dis Child Fetal Neonatal Ed.* 1998;78:F85–F88.

32. Gunn AJ, Gluckman PD, Gunn TR. Selective head cooling in newborn infants after perinatal asphyxia: a safety study [see comments]. *Pediatrics.* 1998;102:885–892.

33. Estol PC, Piriz H, Basalo S, Simini F, Grela C. Oro-naso-pharyngeal suction at birth: effects on respiratory adaptation of normal term vaginally born infants. *J Perinatal Med.* 1992;20:297–305.

34. Cordero L Jr, Hon EH. Neonatal bradycardia following nasopharyngeal stimulation. *J Pediatr.* 1971;78:78:441–447.

35. Wiswell TE, Tuggle JM, Turner BS. Meconium aspiration syndrome: have we made a difference? [see comments]. *Pediatrics.* 1990;85:85:715–721.

36. Carson BS, Losey RW, Bowes WA Jr, Simmons MA. Combined obstetric and pediatric approach to prevent meconium aspiration syndrome. *Am J Obstet Gynecol.* 1976;126:126:712–715.

37. Locus P, Yeomans E, Crosby U. Efficacy of bulb versus DeLee suction at deliveries complicated by meconium stained amniotic fluid [see comments]. *Am J Perinatol.* 1990;7:87–91.

38. Rossi EM, Philipson EH, Williams TG, Kalhan SC. Meconium aspiration syndrome: intrapartum and neonatal attributes [see comments]. *Am J Obstet Gynecol.* 1989;161:1106–1110.

39. Falciglia HS. Failure to prevent meconium aspiration syndrome. *Obstet Gynecol.* 1988;71:71:349–353.

40. Greenough A. Meconium aspiration syndrome: prevention and treatment. *Early Hum Dev.* 1995;40:955–981.

41. Wiswell TE, Bent RC. Meconium staining and the meconium aspiration syndrome: unresolved issues. *Pediatr Clin North Am.* 1993;40:955–981.

42. Wiswell TE. Meconium in the Delivery Room Trial Group: delivery room management of the apparently vigorous meconium-stained neonate: results of the multicenter collaborative trial. *Pediatrics.* 2000;105:1–7.

43. Linder N, Aranda JV, Tsur M, et al. Need for endotracheal intubation and suction in meconium-stained neonates. *J Pediatr.* 1988;112:613–615.

44. de Burgh Daly M, Angell-James JE, Elsner R. Role of carotid-body chemoreceptors and their reflex interactions in bradycardia and cardiac arrest. *Lancet.* 1979;1:764–767.

45. de Burgh Daly M. Interactions between respiration and circulation. In: Cherniack NS, Widdicombe JG, eds. *Handbook of Physiology, Section 3, The Respiratory System.* Bethesda, Md: American Physiological Society; 1986:529–595.

46. Rootwelt T, Odden J, Hall C, Ganes T, Saugstad OD. Cerebral blood flow and evoked potentials during reoxygenation with 21 or 100% O_2 in newborn pigs. *J Appl Physiol.* 1993;75:2054–2060.

47. Ramji S, Ahuja S, Thirupuram S, Rootwelt T, Rooth G, Saugstad OD. Resuscitation of asphyxic newborn infants with room air or 100% oxygen. *Pediatr Res.* 1993;34:809–812.

48. Saugstad OD, Rootwellt T, Aalen O. Resuscitation of asphyxiated newborn infants with room air or oxygen: an international controlled trial: the Resair 2 Study. *Pediatrics.* 1998;102:e1.

49. Kanter RK. Evaluation of mask-bag ventilation in resuscitation of infants. *Am J Dis Child.* 1987;141:761–763.

50. Palme C, Nystrom B, Tunell R. An evaluation of the efficiency of face masks in the resuscitation of newborn infants. *Lancet.* 1985;1:207–210.

51. Paterson SJ, Byrne PJ, Molesky MG, Seal RF, Finucane BT. Neonatal resuscitation using the laryngeal mask airway [see comments]. *Anesthesiology.* 1994;80:1248–1253, discussion 27A.

52. Gandini D, Brimacombe JR. Neonatal resuscitation with the laryngeal mask airway in normal and low birth weight infants. *Anesth Analg.* 1999;89:642–643.

53. Todres ID, deBros F, Kramer SS, Moylan FM, Shannon DC. Endotracheal tube displacement in the newborn infant. *J Pediatr.* 1976;89:126–127.

54. Rotschild A, Chitayat D, Puterman ML, Phang MS, Ling E, Baldwin V. Optimal positioning of endotracheal tubes for ventilation of preterm infants. *Am J Dis Child.* 1991;145:1007–1012.

55. Aziz HF, Martin JB, Moore JJ. The pediatric end-tidal carbon dioxide detector role in endotracheal intubation in newborns. *J Perinatol.* 1999;19:110–113.

56. Bhende MS, Thompson AE, Orr RA. Utility of an end-tidal carbon dioxide detector during stabilization and transport of critically ill children. *Pediatrics.* 1992;89:1042–1044.

57. Orlowski JP. Optimum position for external cardiac compression in infants and young children. *Ann Emerg Med.* 1986;15:667–673.

58. Phillips GW, Zideman DA. Relation of infant heart to sternum: its significance in cardiopulmonary resuscitation. *Lancet.* 1986;1:1:1024–1025.

59. Thaler MM, Stobie GHC. An improved technique of external cardiac compression in infants and young children. *N Engl J Med.* 1963;269:606–610.

60. David R. Closed chest cardiac massage in the newborn infant. *Pediatrics.* 1988;81:552–554.

61. Todres ID, Rogers MC. Methods of external cardiac massage in the newborn infant. *J Pediatr.* 1975;86:781–782.

62. Menegazzi JJ, Auble TE, Nicklas KA, Hosack GM, Rack L, Goode JS. Two-thumb versus two-finger chest compression during CPR in a swine infant model of cardiac arrest [see comments]. *Ann Emerg Med.* 1993;22:240–243.

63. Houri PK, Frank LR, Menegazzi JJ, Taylor R. A randomized, controlled trial of two-thumb vs two-finger chest compression in a swine infant model of cardiac arrest [see comment]. *Prehosp Emerg Care.* 1997;1:65–67.

64. Dean JM, Koehler RC, Schleien CL, Berkowitz I, Michael JR, Atchison D, Rogers MC, Traystman RJ. Age-related effects of compression rate and duration in cardiopulmonary resuscitation. *J Appl Physiol.* 1990;68:554–560.

65. Berkowitz ID, Chantarojanasiri T, Koehler RC, Schleien CL, Dean JM, Michael JR, Rogers MC, Traystman RJ. Blood flow during cardiopulmonary resuscitation with simultaneous compression and ventilation in infant pigs. *Pediatr Res.* 1989;26:558–564.

66. Burchfield DJ. Medication use in neonatal resuscitation. *Clin Perinatol.* 1999;26:683–691.

67. Zaritsky A, Chernow B. Use of catecholamines in pediatrics. *J Pediatr.* 1984;105:341–350.

68. Berkowitz ID, Gervais H, Schleien CL, Koehler RC, Dean JM, Traystman RJ. Epinephrine dosage effects on cerebral and myocardial blood flow in an infant swine model of cardiopulmonary resuscitation. *Anesthesiology.* 1991;75:1041–1050.

69. Berg RA, Otto CW, Kern KB, Hilwig RW, Sanders AB, Henry CP, Ewy GA. A randomized, blinded trial of high-dose epinephrine versus standard-dose epinephrine in a swine model of pediatric asphyxial cardiac arrest. *Crit Care Med.* 1996;24:1695–1700.

70. Burchfield DJ, Preziosi MP, Lucas VW, Fan J. Effect of graded doses of epinephrine during asphyxia-induced bradycardia in newborn lambs. *Resuscitation.* 1993;25:235–244.

71. Pasternak JF, Groothus DR, Fischer JM, Fischer DP. Regional cerebral blood flow in the beagle puppy model of neonatal intraventricular hemorrhage: studies during systemic hypertension. *Neurology.* 1983;33:559–566.

72. Cochrane Injuries Group Albumin Reviewers. Human albumin administration in critically ill patients: systematic review of randomised controlled trials. *BMJ.* 1998;317:235–240.

73. Usher R, Lind J. Blood volume of the newborn premature infant. *Acta Paediatr Scand.* 1965;54:419–431.

74. Funato M, Tamai H, Noma K, et al. Clinical events in association with timing of intraventricular hemorrhage in preterm infants. *J Pediatr.* 1992;121:614–619.

75. Kette F, Weil MH, von Planta M, Gazmuri RJ, Rackow EC. Buffer agents do not reverse intramyocardial acidosis during cardiac resuscitation. *Circulation.* 1990;81:1660–1666.

76. Kette F, Weil MH, Gazmuri RJ. Buffer solutions may compromise cardiac resuscitation by reducing coronary perfusion pressure [published correction appears in *JAMA.* 1991;266:3286] [see comments]. *JAMA.* 1991;266:2121–2126.

77. Papile LA, Burstein J, Burstein R, Koffler H, Koops B. Relationship of intravenous sodium bicarbonate infusions and cerebral intraventricular hemorrhage. *J Pediatr.* 1978;93:834–836.

78. Hein HA. The use of sodium bicarbonate in neonatal resuscitation: help or harm? *Pediatrics.* 1993;91:496–497.

79. Lindemann R. Resuscitation of the newborn: endotracheal administration of epinephrine. *Acta Paediatr Scand.* 1984;73:210–212.

80. Lucas VW, Preziosi MP, Burchfield DJ. Epinephrine absorption following endotracheal administration: effects of hypoxia-induced low pulmonary blood flow. *Resuscitation.* 1994;27:31–34.

81. Mullett CJ, Kong JQ, Romano JT, Polak MJ. Age-related changes in pulmonary venous epinephrine concentration and pulmonary vascular response after intratracheal epinephrine. *Pediatr Res.* 1992;31:458–461.

82. Ellemunter H, Simma B, Trawoger R, Maurer H. Intraosseous lines in preterm and full term neonates. *Arch Dis Child Fetal Neonatal Ed.* 1999;80:F74–75.

83. MacDonald HM, Mulligan JC, Allen AC, Taylor PM. Neonatal asphyxia, I: relationship of obstetric and neonatal complications to

neonatal mortality in 38,405 consecutive deliveries. *J Pediatr.* 1980; 96:898–902.

84. Poets CF, Sens B. Changes in intubation rates and outcome of very low birth weight infants: a population study. *Pediatrics.* 1996;98:24–27.

85. Avery ME, Tooley WH, Keller JB, et al. Is chronic lung disease in low birth weight infants preventable? a survey of eight centers. *Pediatrics.* 1987;79:26–30.

86. Kattwinkel J. Surfactant: evolving issues. *Clin Perinatol.* 1998;25:17–32.

87. Simmons MA, Adcock EW III, Bard H, Battaglia FC. Hypernatremia and intracranial hemorrhage in neonates. *N Engl J Med.* 1974;291:6–10.

88. Hambleton G, Wigglesworth JS. Origin of intraventricular haemorrhage in the preterm infant. *Arch Dis Child.* 1976;51:651–659.

89. Apgar V, James LS. Further observations of the newborn scoring system. *Am J Dis Child.* 1962;104:419–428.

90. Chamberlain G, Banks J. Assessment of the Apgar score. *Lancet.* 1974; 2:1225–1228.

91. Byrne PJ, Tyebkhan JM, Laing LM. Ethical decision-making and neonatal resuscitation. *Semin Perinatol.* 1994;18:36–41.

92. Davies JM, Reynolds BM. The ethics of cardiopulmonary resuscitation, I: background to decision making. *Arch Dis Child.* 1992;67:1498–1501.

93. Landwirth J. Ethical issues in pediatric and neonatal resuscitation. *Ann Emerg Med.* 1993;22:502–507.

94. Tyson JE, Younes N, Verter J, Wright LL. Viability, morbidity, and resource use among newborns of 501- to 800-g birth weight: National Institute of Child Health and Human Development Neonatal Research Network. *JAMA.* 1996;276:1645–1651.

95. Finer NN, Horbar JD, Carpenter JH. Cardiopulmonary resuscitation in the very low birth weight infant: the Vermont Oxford Network experience. *Pediatrics.* 1999;104:428–434.

96. Davis DJ. How aggressive should delivery room cardiopulmonary resuscitation be for extremely low birth weight neonates? [see comments]. *Pediatrics.* 1993;92:447–450.

97. Jain L, Ferre C, Vidyasagar D, Nath S, Sheftel D. Cardiopulmonary resuscitation of apparently stillborn infants: survival and long-term outcome [see comments]. *J Pediatr.* 1991;118:778–782.

98. Yeo CL, Tudehope DI. Outcome of resuscitated apparently stillborn infants: a ten year review. *J Paediatr Child Health.* 1994;30:129–133.

99. Casalaz DM, Marlow N, Speidel BD. Outcome of resuscitation following unexpected apparent stillbirth. *Arch Dis Child Fetal Neonatal Ed.* 1998; 78:F112–F115.

Part 12: From Science to Survival
Strengthening the Chain of Survival in Every Community

ECC in the Community: How to Ensure Effectiveness

Many clinicians, administrators, and researchers have recognized the need to improve community systems of ECC to optimize patient survival. In 1992 this section of the guidelines described in detail the structural components of a "Chain of Survival." Eight years later the same systematic, organized, coordinated effort in a community remains the strongest recommendation we can make to save more people from out-of-hospital cardiac arrest.[1] The metaphor of links of a chain[1a] has proved successful across many aspects of resuscitation and ECC. For example, the Utstein guidelines for evaluating outcomes from in-hospital cardiac arrest[2] and examining pediatric cardiopulmonary emergencies[3] were developed from the Chain of Survival perspective. As originally formulated, the out-of-hospital Utstein guidelines were intended to provide a structure to evaluate an emergency system. The usefulness of the Utstein template has been confirmed by the many communities that have identified weaknesses in the "links" of their ECC system. Communities continue to implement modifications and optimize treatment for their critical out-of-hospital patients.[4]

The central question to be answered is whether a community's ECC system provides optimal patient survival. Achieving the optimal survival rate for out-of-hospital cardiac arrest in every community is the challenge now and in the future. What is optimal in one community, however, may not be possible in all communities. Early reports of high survival in mid-sized cities provided the EMS prototype adopted by most communities.[5,6] Obstacles to providing care in rural and large metropolitan areas create different challenges for EMS systems.[7] Each community will need to examine and devise its own mechanisms to achieve the goal of optimal patient survival. Traditionally, quality assurance in ECC has measured process variables, but the emphasis of quality assurance for cardiac arrest care should be expanded to examine outcome variables in the entire ECC system.[8,9] The shift in emphasis on system evaluation is necessary because the Chain of Survival is necessary for optimal outcome.[10]

The Chain of Survival

The 1992 guidelines[11] described early access, early CPR, early defibrillation, and early advanced care as essential components of a series of actions designed to reduce the mortality associated with cardiac arrest (Figure 1). These vital links were echoed by the International Liaison Committee on Resuscitation (ILCOR) advisory statements in 1997.[12]

Survival from cardiac arrest depends on a series of critical interventions. If one of these critical actions is neglected or delayed, survival is unlikely. The American Heart Association has used the term "Chain of Survival" to describe this sequence. This chain has 4 interdependent links: early access, early basic CPR, early defibrillation, and early ACLS. The Chain of Survival concept underscores several important principles:

1. If any link in the chain is inadequate, survival rates will be poor. Weakness in system components is the major explanation for variability in survival rates reported over the past 20 years.[4,5]
2. Although all links must be strong, the inevitable question always arises: Which link is the most important? Certainly, recognition of the emergency and initiation of the Chain is essential—if no one recognizes the emergency and begins to act, survival will be poor.[4] Because rapid defibrillation is the only "sufficient" intervention (ie, defibrillation and only defibrillation can reverse a ventricular fibrillation [VF] arrest), it is often proclaimed to be "the single most important factor in determining survival from adult sudden cardiac arrest." The truth, however, is even more satisfying and more in keeping with the concept of a "Chain of Survival." Each link in the Chain of Survival is important (see below).
3. The effectiveness of an ECC system cannot be identified by examining an individual link—the whole system must be evaluated. The survival rate to hospital discharge has emerged as the "gold standard" for determining the effectiveness of treatment of cardiac arrest. Recently, considerable progress has been made in providing clear methodological guidelines for study design, uniform terminology, and reporting of results.[5,13,14] This progress should facilitate future research on CPR and implementation of the Chain of Survival in each community. (See Table 1 for definitions of terms.)

At least 2 large-scale studies have investigated which patient variables and which emergency system variables were significantly related to survival to hospital discharge.[15,16] A number of variables (male sex, age, witnessed arrest, etc) had at least some significant relationship with survival. The investigators tried to identify the fewest variables that could explain the greatest differences in survival rates. Surprisingly, most of the differences in survival were explained by just 2 performance variables: the intervals *collapse to CPR* and

Circulation. 2000;102(suppl I):I-358–I-370.
© 2000 American Heart Association, Inc.

Circulation is available at http://www.circulationaha.org

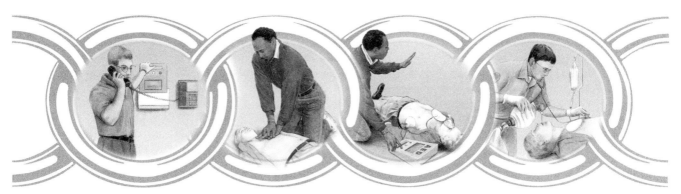

Figure 1. The ECC systems concept is displayed schematically by the "Chain of Survival" metaphor.

collapse to defibrillation. These results provided even more support for the Chain of Survival concept when investigators observed that it was the *interaction* of early CPR with early defibrillation that was most powerful: without *both factors,* (1) CPR starting within 5 minutes and (2) defibrillation occurring within 10 minutes, the value of early defibrillation or early CPR was lost. This interaction becomes dramatically clear in a simple 2×2 table (Table 2).

TABLE 1. Definitions and Terminology in ECC[67]

Cardiac arrest—Cardiac arrest is the cessation of cardiac mechanical activity. It is a clinical diagnosis, confirmed by unresponsiveness, absence of detectable pulse, and apnea (or agonal respirations).

Cardiopulmonary resuscitation (CPR)—CPR is an attempt to restore spontaneous circulation through any of a broad range of maneuvers and techniques.

Basic CPR—Basic CPR is the attempt to restore spontaneous circulation by using chest wall compressions and pulmonary ventilation.

Bystander CPR, layperson CPR, or citizen CPR—These terms are synonymous; however, *bystander CPR* is preferred. Bystander CPR is an attempt to provide basic CPR by a person not at that moment part of the organized emergency response system.

Basic life support (BLS)—BLS is the phase of ECC that includes recognition of cardiac arrest, access to the EMS system, and basic CPR. It may also refer to the educational program in these subjects.

Advanced CPR or advanced cardiovascular life support (ACLS)—These terms refer to attempts to restore spontaneous circulation with basic CPR plus advanced airway management, tracheal intubation, defibrillation, and intravenous medications. ACLS may also refer to the educational program that provides guidelines for these techniques.

Emergency medical services (EMS) or emergency personnel—Persons who respond to medical emergencies in an official capacity are emergency (or EMS) personnel. The EMS system has 2 major divisions: EMS dispatchers and EMS responders.

    EMS dispatchers—EMS personnel responsible for dispatching EMS responders to the scene of medical emergencies and providing telephone instructions to bystanders at the scene while professionals are en route.

    EMS responders—EMS personnel who respond to medical emergencies by going to the scene in an emergency vehicle. They may be first-, second-, or third-tier responders, depending on the EMS system. They may be trained in ACLS or BLS. All should be capable of performing defibrillation. *Emergency medical technician (EMT)* usually denotes BLS training. *Paramedic* or *EMT-P* usually denotes ACLS training.

ECC system—The ECC system refers to all aspects of ECC, including that rendered by emergency personnel. The extended ECC system also includes bystander CPR, rapid activation of the EMS system, emergency departments, intensive care units, cardiac rehabilitation, cardiac prevention programs, BLS and ACLS training programs, and citizen defibrillation.

Chain of Survival—The Chain of Survival is a metaphor to communicate the interdependence of a community's emergency response to cardiac arrest. This response is composed of 4 links: early access, early CPR, early defibrillation, and early ACLS. If a link is weak or missing, the result will be poor survival despite excellence in the rest of the ECC system.

Presumed cardiac cause—Cardiac arrest due to presumed cardiac cause is the major focus of ECC. When reporting cardiac outcome data, studies of cardiac arrest should exclude arrests due to obvious noncardiac causes. Because of practical considerations (lack of autopsy information, cost), all arrests are considered to be of cardiac cause unless an obvious noncardiac cause can be identified. Common noncardiac diagnoses that should be separated during analysis of cardiac arrest outcome include sudden infant death syndrome, drug overdose, suicide, drowning, trauma, exsanguination, and terminal illness.

Time intervals—The Utstein recommendations have provided a rational nomenclature for important time intervals. Time intervals should be reported as the A-to-B interval, which represents the period that begins at time point A and ends at time point B. These are more informative than imprecise terms like *downtime* or *response time.* The following terms, for example, are suggested:

    911-call–to-dispatch interval—The interval from the time the call for help is first received by the 911 center until the time the emergency vehicle leaves for the scene.

    Vehicle-dispatch–to-scene interval—The interval beginning when the emergency vehicle departs for the scene and ending when EMS responders indicate that the vehicle has stopped at the scene or address. This does not include the time interval until emergency personnel arrive at the patient's side or the interval until defibrillation occurs.

    Vehicle-at-scene–to–patient-access interval—The interval from when the emergency response vehicle stops moving at the scene or address until EMS responders are at the patient's side.

    Call-to-defibrillation interval—The interval from receipt of the call at the emergency response system center until the patient receives the first shock.

TABLE 2. Influence of Early CPR and Early Defibrillation on Percent of Survival to Hospital Discharge[34]

Collapse to CPR	Collapse to Defibrillation	
	<10 min	>10 min
<5 min	37%	7%
>5 min	20%	0%

The First Link: Early Access

Early access encompasses the events initiated after the patient's collapse until the arrival of EMS personnel prepared to provide care. Recognition of early warning signs, such as chest pain and shortness of breath, that encourage patients to activate the emergency response system before collapse is a key component of this link. With a cardiac arrest the following events must occur rapidly:

- Early identification of the patient's collapse by someone who activates the system
- Rapid notification (usually by telephone) of EMS response team
- Rapid recognition by dispatchers of a potential cardiac arrest
- Rapid dispatch instructions to available EMS responders (first-, second-, and third-tier EMS personnel) to guide them to the patient
- Rapid arrival of EMS responders at the scene
- Arrival of an EMS responder with all necessary equipment at the patient's side
- Identification of the cardiac arrest

All of these events must take place before defibrillation or advanced care can occur; each of these events is a vital part of the early access link. In most communities responsibility for these events rests with the EMS telephone system, dispatcher, and responders.

The Telephone Call to Activate the Emergency Response System: Key Role of an Area-Wide Dedicated Emergency Telephone Number

Widespread use of a 2- or 3-digit dedicated emergency telephone number has simplified and shortened access to emergency assistance. Many countries have established area-wide emergency telephone numbers. Table 3 displays the emergency telephone number used in many countries throughout the world.[17] International travelers can access a website for the emergency numbers of more than 200 countries: http://ambulance.ie.eu.org.

Unfortunately, many communities do not have the service of a single EMS telephone number. Providing emergency response service through a dedicated unique number should be a top priority for all communities. Enhanced EMS phone service is preferable.

The increasing sophistication of telecommunication systems now makes it possible for emergency medical dispatchers (EMDs) to identify the location and telephone number of the incoming telephone call. This invaluable feature (called "enhanced 911" in the United States) requires a costly software and hardware upgrade. Cellular telephone calls to

TABLE 3. Emergency Response System Numbers

Country	Emergency Telephone Number
Albania	17
Argentina	101
Australia	000
Austria	144
Belarus	03
Belgium	100
Bosnia	94
Brazil	192
Bulgaria	155
Canada	911
Chile	131
China	120
Croatia	94
Cypress	112
Czechia/Czech Republic	155
Denmark	122
Dominican Republic	911
Finland	0112
France	15
Germany	112
Greece	166
Guatemala	123
Hong Kong	999
Hungary	104
Iceland	112
India	102
Indonesia	118
Ireland	112/999
Israel	101
Italy	118
Jamaica	110
Japan	119
Kenya	999
Korea	119
Malaysia	999
Mexico	080
Monaco	112
Netherlands	112
New Zealand	111
Norway	113
Philippines	166
Poland	999
Portugal	115
Romania	06
Russia	03
Slovakia	115
Slovenia	94
South Africa	10177
Spain	061
Sweden	112
Switzerland	114
Taiwan	119
Thailand	191
Turkey	118
United Kingdom	999
United States	911
Yugoslavia	94
Zimbabwe	994

emergency medical dispatchers cannot be included in such "enhanced services" because only the location of the connecting cell is identified. The amazing growth in the use of cellular phones, however, demands a solution to this problem. Features may be added to cellular telephones and cellular networks to enable tracking of emergency calls from cellular phones. Such features should be mandatory and widely implemented.

Emergency Medical Dispatchers and the Emergency Medical Dispatch System
Rapid emergency medical dispatch has emerged as a critical component of the early access link.[18–22] Traditionally, however, the dispatchers who answer the emergency calls were simply that—"dispatchers"—identifying the nature of the call ("fire, police, emergency medical"), the location, and then switching to the appropriate service to receive details. All EMS dispatch systems must be able to immediately answer all emergency medical calls, quickly determine the nature of the emergency, identify the nearest appropriate EMS responder unit(s), dispatch the unit to the scene in <1 minute on average, and provide critical information to EMS responders about the type of emergency.

In the late 1980s EMS leaders began to explore whether EMDs could actually stay on the telephone with the callers and offer medical advice to the caller. (See also "Part 3: Adult Basic Life Support.") This led to the highly successful concept of "prearrival instructions,"[21,22] in which the EMD quickly interviews the caller to learn more about the emergency. The EMD then offers to give the caller advice or instructions on what to do while waiting for the EMS responders to arrive. Internationally, EMDs now give prearrival instructions, and there is widespread acknowledgment that these instructions have improved outcomes.

Simultaneously with the development of protocols for prearrival instructions, Eisenberg and colleagues, in Seattle–King County, Washington, developed and validated CPR instructions for the dispatcher to offer to the caller.[23,24] These dispatcher-assisted CPR instructions are now standard practice for dispatch centers all over the globe. The "template" instructions first developed in King County have been translated into >10 languages. Dispatcher-directed CPR requires only 2 to 4 hours of additional dispatcher training, and it has been shown in controlled trials to be feasible and effective.[24,25,25a]

An article in the *New England Journal of Medicine* in 2000 by Hallstrom and colleagues used EMDs to conduct a prospective, randomized, controlled trial of chest compression–only CPR.[25a] This work was an indirect confirmation of the success of some of the more controversial instructions in telephone CPR, namely, elimination of the pulse check (too difficult for lay rescuers to perform) and replacing the complicated directions on locating the sternal compression point to a simple "press right between the nipples." These "controversial" shortcuts in CPR instructions were actually put into service >12 years ago, with no problems resulting from their implementation.

The growth of interest in public access defibrillation (PAD) and the growing use of automated external defibrilla-

tors (AEDs) by family members of high-risk cardiac patients led to the inevitable question of EMD-assisted defibrillation. Early work by Doherty and colleagues[26] in Seattle–King County, Washington, confirmed the ease with which this could be achieved and implemented across large EMS systems. The caller is instructed to place both the AED and the telephone next to the victim. The dispatcher simply listens with the rescuer to the voice prompts of the AED, and together they work through the directions.

The EMS Responder System
The EMS responder system is usually composed of responders trained in BLS, ACLS, or both.[19] The system may provide either a single-tier or multi-tier level of response.[27] Most 1-tier systems use ACLS-trained responders (paramedics), although some provide only BLS. Two-tier systems generally provide first-responder units staffed with emergency medical technicians or firefighters close to the scene,[19] followed by the second tier of ACLS responders. Two-tier systems in which first responders are trained in early defibrillation are most effective in providing rapid ACLS.[6,28]

Once dispatched, EMS responders must quickly reach the site of the cardiac arrest, locate the patient, and arrive at the patient's side with all necessary equipment. The following are important considerations:

1. *EMS travel interval*—The interval it takes an EMS responder to reach the scene is critical for survival of the cardiac arrest victim. Communities have learned to shorten this interval by adding response vehicles, placing response vehicles strategically, and improving traffic paths. Multi-tiered systems appear to have the fastest response intervals because they have more first-responder units. Many communities report an EMS transit interval of approximately 5 minutes for first responders. This interval is too long when the goal is to provide CPR and defibrillation within 4 minutes of an EMS emergency call. Providing rapid EMS response in rural areas with smaller populations remains a challenge.
2. *Locating the patient*—Few studies have actually noted the time interval from arrival of EMS responders at the scene address until their arrival at the patient's side.[29] This interval, previously assumed to be negligible, is difficult to document because most systems have no means of recording this time.
3. *Carrying the correct equipment*—The first EMS responders dispatched to treat a patient with cardiac arrest must carry a defibrillator, oxygen, and airway management equipment.[30] They must also arrive at the patient's side in <4 to 5 minutes if defibrillation is to be performed within 5 minutes of the call.

The Second Link: Early CPR

Bystander CPR is the second link in the Chain of Survival. CPR is most effective when started immediately after the victim's collapse. Many studies have confirmed the value of early CPR by lay rescuers.[15,16,31–35] The probability of survival approximately doubles when bystanders initiate CPR before the arrival of EMS personnel.[15] The contribution of bystander CPR to survival appears particularly significant for infants and children; the best survival from out-of-hospital collapse has been documented among infants resuscitated by parents,[36] near-drowning victims who receive immediate CPR,[37] and children resuscitated by bystanders.[38]

The 1992 conference recommended the development of community-wide CPR programs in as many locations as possible, including schools, military bases, housing complexes, work sites, and public buildings. Communities need to remove barriers that discourage citizens from learning and performing CPR. Creating community-wide change, however, can be challenging. Several randomized community intervention trials, including one in which a short CPR training video was distributed to various households, failed to show an increased likelihood of either CPR being performed or EMS being called.[39–42] Targeting relatives of high-risk persons also failed to show an increased likelihood of CPR being performed in an emergency.[43] In contrast, parents of high-risk infants who learn CPR appear to perform it willingly and successfully.[36]

One significant barrier to CPR performance is the complexity of the CPR skills set as commonly taught. Multiple studies have documented poor skills retention by participants in traditional didactic CPR courses.[44,45] New approaches to teaching CPR, including a simplified curriculum and practice-while-watching and practice-after-watching videos, have been more successful in teaching core skills to participants than traditional courses.[46] Computerized prompt devices or web-based instruction may offer benefit for teaching or reviewing the skills of CPR. Innovative approaches are necessary to focus on participant skill acquisition.

The Third Link: Early Defibrillation

Early defibrillation is the link in the Chain of Survival that is most likely to improve survival.[1,47–51] The placement of AEDs in the hands of large numbers of people trained in their use may be the key intervention to increase the chances of survival of patients with out-of-hospital cardiac arrest.[51] AEDs are computerized, low-maintenance, user-friendly defibrillators that analyze the victim's rhythm to determine whether a shockable rhythm is present. When the AED detects a shockable rhythm, it charges, then prompts the rescuer to press a shock button to deliver a shock. These devices are highly accurate (sensitivity for VF and specificity for non-VF >95% for virtually all AEDs) and can significantly reduce the time to defibrillation (see "Part 4: The Automated External Defibrillator").

Early Defibrillation

The AHA, ERC, and ILCOR recommend that every emergency vehicle that may transport cardiac arrest patients be equipped with a defibrillator and that emergency personnel be equipped with, trained to use, and permitted to operate this device.[30,52] To achieve this goal, the International Association of Fire Chiefs has endorsed equipping fire-suppression units with AEDs.[51]

Several options for rapid defibrillation exist. Although AEDs dominate the BLS level of the EMS market, defibrillation also can be performed with manual or semiautomated external defibrillators. Manual defibrillation requires interpretation of a monitor or rhythm strip and is usually performed by responders trained in ACLS. Even so, manual defibrillation by emergency medical technicians trained to recognize VF improves survival.[47,53]

The widespread effectiveness and demonstrated safety of the AED have made it acceptable for use by nonprofessional responders. Lay responders must still be trained in CPR and use of the defibrillators. PAD programs, in which AEDs are placed in the hands of trained rescuers, have had initial success in police departments,[54–58] airplanes,[59,60] and casinos.[61] For early defibrillation programs to be successful, defibrillators must be placed in the hands of rescuers who will arrive *before* traditional EMS personnel. If time to defibrillation is not shortened, survival will not increase.[62]

With limited EMS resources, defibrillators should be given priority over many other medical devices, such as automatic transport ventilators. The cost of defibrillators has steadily declined, making purchase of these devices more attractive. Participants in the 1992 Guidelines Conference recommended that

- AEDs be widely available for use by persons who have been appropriately trained
- All firefighting personnel who perform CPR and first aid be equipped with and trained to operate AEDs
- AEDs be placed in gathering places of >10 000 people
- In those states in which it is necessary, legislation be enacted to allow all EMS personnel to perform early defibrillation

Participants in the international Guidelines 2000 Conference expressed the opinion that PAD may prove to be the decade's most effective and successful improvement in ECC (See Public Access Defibrillation in "Part 4: The Automated External Defibrillator"). PAD programs should include the following:

1. Preparation and planning
2. Establishment of pre-event training and program
3. Post–clinical event monitoring of quality improvement and critical incident stress debriefing

The Fourth Link: Early ACLS

Early ACLS provided by paramedics at the scene is another critical link in the management of cardiac arrest. EMS systems should have sufficient staff to provide a minimum of 2 responders trained in ACLS. Because of the difficulties in treating cardiac arrest in the field, additional responders should be present. In systems with survival rates of >20% for patients with VF, response teams have at a minimum 2 ACLS providers plus 2 BLS personnel at the scene.[63] Most experts agree that 4 responders (2 trained in ACLS and 2 trained in BLS) provide the most effective team in resuscitation of cardiac arrest victims. Although not every EMS system can attain this level of response, every system should actively pursue this goal.

Research Challenges for the Future

The best way to evaluate the Chain of Survival in a community is to assess survival to hospital discharge and

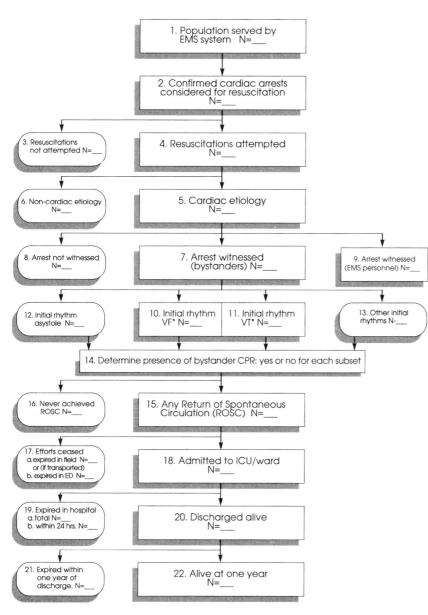

Figure 2. Recommended Utstein-style template for reporting data on cardiac arrest. VF and ventricular tachycardia (VT) should be reported separately through the template. Reproduced with permission from Reference 14.

*VF and VT should be reported separately through template

identify delays in activation of the chain. The best way to improve the Chain of Survival is to develop high levels of evidence needed to refine resuscitation guidelines. To meet these goals, clinical research is essential. This research should use common definitions and terminology to allow comparisons and sharing of information across regions and internationally. The Utstein templates (Figures 2 through 4) should be used.[3,64,65]

The best way to evaluate the strength of the community Chain of Survival is to assess the survival rates achieved by the ECC system. The cost of data collection for a system may be significant, but only through evaluation can systems routinely improve their services. Thus, conference participants strongly endorsed the position that all ECC systems should assess their performance through ongoing evaluation. For evaluation data to be meaningful, it is necessary to compare EMS systems. This in turn requires

standardized definitions and terms of reference. Until recently, uniform terminology was not available, producing a cardiac arrest Tower of Babel.[5] Survival rates reported in the literature range from 2% to 44%. It is not yet understood whether these profound variations are due to differences in population, treatment protocol, system organization, rescuer skills, or reporting practices.

There is now international consensus on the importance of using standard terminology and methods to evaluate survival and the Chain of Survival. Considerable effort has been directed to create clear, unambiguous terminology, establish a uniform method of reporting outcome data, and improve methods of research in cardiac arrest.[2,3,64] Improving the ECC system, however, first requires an accurate measurement of the survival rate for each community. This can be achieved by implementing the following recommendations:

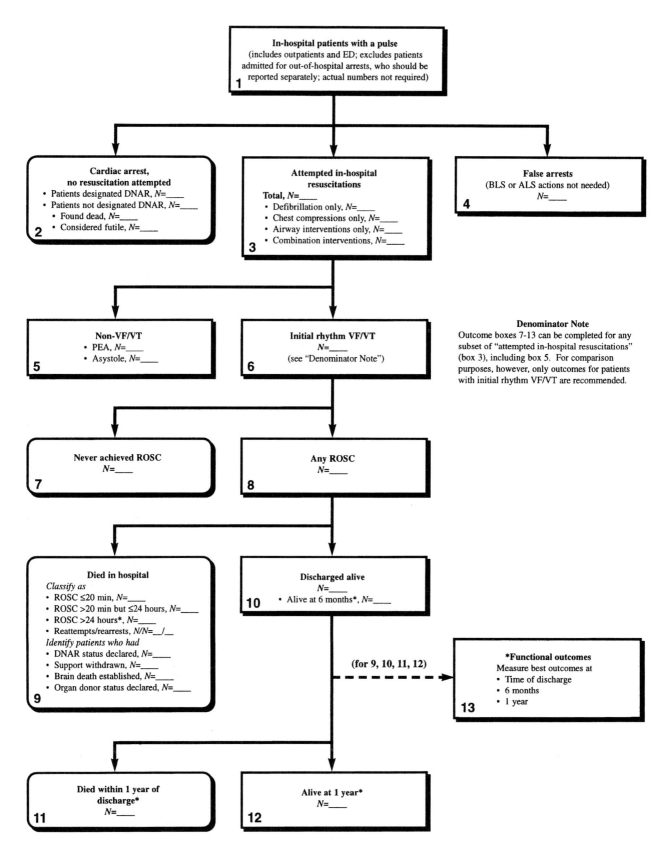

Figure 3. Template for reporting results of in-hospital resuscitation. Reproduced with permission from Reference 2.

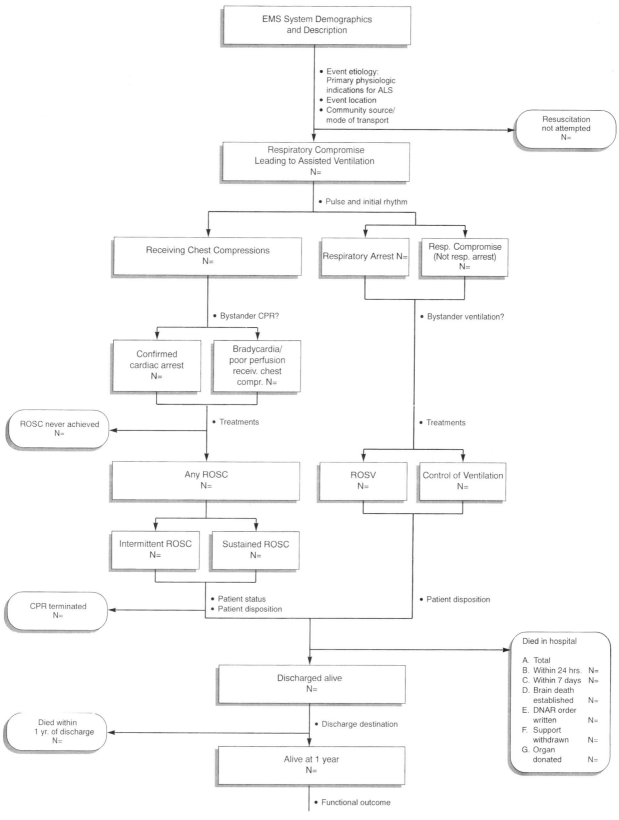

Figure 4. Template for reporting results of pediatric resuscitation. Reproduced with permission from Reference 3.

TABLE 4. Recommended Clinical Data to Collect*[67]

Location and time of cardiac arrest
Any precipitating event/obvious noncardiac cause
Time of receipt of call for help
Time of dispatch of emergency vehicle
Time first-response vehicle stops at scene
Confirmed cardiac arrest, witnessed or unwitnessed
Bystander CPR performed and time initiated
Arrest after arrival of emergency response personnel
Time of first CPR efforts
Initial ECG rhythm
Treatment provided and corresponding times
Time of first defibrillation
Return of spontaneous circulation and time
Final patient status at scene
Patient status on arrival in Emergency Department
Status after Emergency Department treatment
Status at hospital admission
Status at hospital discharge
Time of death
Discharged alive
Alive at 1 year (if possible)
Neurological assessment (if possible)

*Describe the method by which each data point is obtained (estimated or measured).

1. Develop an evaluation process for the ECC system.
2. Include an accurate assessment of survival rate by using standardized terminology and reporting methods. This focus on quality improvement should identify practical goals, given the structure and demographic characteristics of the local system; identify current performance, including survival rate; identify gaps between goals and current performance; identify strategies to improve system performance; and evaluate whether performance improves with these modifications.
3. Design the evaluation specifically to benefit the local community. As a secondary interest, information should be shared regionally and nationally to help other communities develop optimal systems.
4. In assessing survival, integrate evolving concepts of consensus terminology, data collection, system description, and CPR research methods into EMS systems.

Consensus Terminology

The terms and definitions listed in Table 1, referred to as the Utstein style,[2,3,64] were developed by a joint task force of the American Heart Association, the European Resuscitation Council, the Heart and Stroke Foundation of Canada, the Resuscitation Council of Southern Africa, the Australian Resuscitation Council, and the New Zealand Resuscitation Council. These terms are intended as a starting point for achieving uniform terminology. Collectively they represent a major improvement over past practice. The emphasis has been to develop terms that will have universal applicability and replace the imprecise terms previously used in the cardiac arrest literature. The terms and definitions in Table 1 should

be used whenever possible to reduce confusion in reporting cardiac arrest data.

Data Collection

Hundreds of potentially important events start and then stop during the course of a cardiac arrest. Events do not always occur in the same order, nor will all patients experience all events. Despite the complexity of cardiac arrest data, certain minimal data must be gathered (Table 4).

Population Served

It is important to report accurately the size of the population served by the EMS system so that the incidence of cardiac arrest within a community can be calculated (incidence equals number of cardiac arrests per population served per unit of time). Incidence of cardiac arrest may reflect the overall health of a community, which may in turn affect the survival rate. Reporting gender, education, socioeconomic factors, and age allows collection of important epidemiological data and identification of high-risk groups. The level of CPR training in the community also should be reported.

Confirmed Cardiac Arrests Considered for Resuscitation, Resuscitations Attempted, and Resuscitations Not Attempted

The number of unresponsive, pulseless, and breathless persons for whom emergency response personnel are called should be documented. This is the maximum number of cardiac arrest patients to use for analysis. Some patients will be excluded in subsequent analyses (eg, those with traumatic arrests, those "dead on arrival," or those in whom resuscitation was not attempted). After these exclusions the total number of cardiac arrests should be categorized as "resuscitation attempted" and "resuscitation not attempted," and the criteria or rationale for nonattempted resuscitations should be reported.

Arrest After Arrival of Emergency Personnel

Approximately 10% of cardiac arrest patients collapse after the arrival of emergency personnel.[7,66,67] During data analysis these cases should be considered separately from unwitnessed and bystander-witnessed arrests, for 2 reasons. First, the presence or absence of bystander CPR and the call-to-arrival interval do not apply to these patients. Inclusion of arrests witnessed by paramedics with other cases would distort tabulation of the percentage of bystander CPR and measurements of the call-to-arrival interval. Second, patients in this category provide important clinical information that deserves separate analysis.

The arrest-after-arrival subgroup may provide one of the best measures of EMS responder performance. Because other symptoms precipitated the call for help, however, the pathophysiological explanation for arrest after arrival may differ from that of sudden, unexpected arrests.

Stopping CPR Efforts in the Field

Many studies have shown the futility of transporting patients to the Accident and Emergency Department if return of spontaneous circulation is not achieved with adequate ACLS in the field.[68-70] Some EMS systems routinely terminate unsuccessful CPR efforts in the field, whereas others transport every patient in whom resuscitation is attempted. No one disputes that the survival rate among these patients is dismally low, at <1%. A dilemma remains over how to determine which patients may benefit from additional care. Reported data should include the number of patients for whom efforts were discontinued at the scene and in the Emergency Department and specific criteria for termination of efforts.

Cardiac Rhythms

Analysis of cardiac rhythms is complicated because of the many different abnormal ECG patterns and because most patients experience changing rhythms during a cardiac arrest.[71] The distinction between asystole and fine VF should be made for all patients. Deflections on the surface ECG of <1 mm (calibrated at 10 mm/mV) are defined as asystole, whereas ≥1 mm is VF. "Pulseless electrical activity" is a term that includes electromechanical dissociation, pseudo-electromechanical dissociation, idioventricular rhythms, pulseless ventricular escape rhythms, postdefibrillation idioventricular rhythms, and bradyasystolic rhythms. For purposes of uniform reporting, all pulseless rhythms with electrical activity should be included as "other rhythms." For all cases of cardiac arrest, emergency personnel should report the initial rhythm noted. When a patient arrests after emergency responders arrive, personnel should report the initial rhythm immediately. They should also classify ECG rhythms into 1 of 4 categories: VF, ventricular tachycardia, asystole, and other (all pulseless electrical activity should be included in "other").

Outcomes

In a review of 36 communities,[5] 11 different working definitions of *survivor* were reported. Four outcomes that provide the most useful information are (1) return of spontaneous circulation, (2) successful hospital admission, (3) successful hospital discharge, and (4) long-term survival with some assessment of neurological function. This data should be reported.

Time Points and Intervals

A great deal of confusion has resulted from the use of imprecise terms for the timing of cardiac arrest events. For example, *response time*, *downtime*, and *time to definitive care* have all had a variety of meanings. For clarity, the times at which an event starts and stops should be referred to as *time points*. The interval from *time point A* to *time point B* should be referred to as the *A-to-B interval*.

Lack of accuracy in documenting time is still a problem. Most communities depend on EMS personnel to accurately document the timing of cardiac arrest events. In reality these times are usually estimated by EMS personnel after the patient has arrived in the Emergency Department. This method is inaccurate. Newer defibrillator/monitors with audio event recorders, notebook computers, bar code readers, and other technologies are available to allow EMS responders to document each event. If these devices can be synchronized with emergency response system clocks, they will help provide answers to the many questions posed by researchers and ECC systems in future analyses. The ideal documentation

system should be hands-free and should automatically record the time a device is turned on or used. Conference participants recommended the following:

- Recording the best available time points for patient collapse, initiation of CPR, receipt of emergency response system call, rescue vehicle dispatch, rescue vehicle arrival, first CPR by emergency response personnel, first defibrillatory shock, return of spontaneous circulation, and abandonment of CPR (death)
- Describing how time data was documented
- Developing mechanisms to synchronize all emergency response system clocks (those of EMS dispatch centers, dispatchers, and responders)
- Striving to make data collection hands-free and automated

In-Hospital Data

The outcome of patients with in-hospital cardiac arrest has not been analyzed extensively. Researchers have noted a number of methodological problems in studying the in-hospital arrest population. The analysis is confounded with comorbid variables, such as terminal diseases and serious underlying illnesses. It has been thought that this would lead to a disproportionate number of deaths. The claim has been that out-of-hospital cardiac arrests represent a more homogeneous population and cannot be compared with in-hospital cardiac arrests.

The facts do not support these concerns, however. Not all in-hospital cardiac arrest patients die, and many out-of-hospital patients also have a terminal disease or underlying illness. In 7 recent in-hospital studies the aggregate survival rate was 11% (of 1804 arrests, 199 hospital discharges), a rate better than the rates achieved in some out-of-hospital studies.[14] Although there may be important differences in the pathophysiological bases of some in-hospital cardiac arrests (a higher percentage of pulmonary embolism, hyperkalemia, etc), the outcomes of in-hospital cardiac arrests appear to be similar to out-of-hospital arrests (see Figure 3).

There are advantages to studying in-hospital patients. Documentation is improved, and arrest-to-defibrillation intervals are shorter. Research protocols and data collection techniques requiring advanced or invasive monitoring are more feasible and can be rapidly implemented in the hospital. Most hospitals have resuscitation teams that respond to all arrests. This consistency in response increases consistency in treatment protocols and documentation. The patient's medical history and condition leading to the arrest are often documented in medical records. Patients with no-CPR status are clearly identified, eliminating prehospital situations in which emergency personnel are called to attend to a patient who should not receive resuscitative efforts. The complete cardiac arrest history is in the hospital medical record, eliminating the need to merge multiple data sources. A single clock (the hospital clock) runs during the arrest reducing the likelihood of lack of synchronization between time points. In addition, autopsies are performed after many unsuccessful resuscitations. These may provide important additional data. Participants in the national conference recommended encouraging research on in-hospital cardiac arrests and applying the prehospital Chain of Survival model to in-hospital cardiac arrest, including activities such as in-hospital early defibrillation programs using AEDs.

A Systematic Approach to Resuscitation Data Collection: The Utstein Template for Out-of-Hospital Cardiac Arrest

The original Utstein template (Figure 2) provides cardiac arrest researchers with a uniform format for data reporting. This is important because of confusion and inconsistencies in survival rate statistics in the past. Some researchers have reported analysis of only favorable subgroups (ie, patients with witnessed VF). Others have excluded from analysis patients pronounced dead at the scene. This variability in reporting practices has produced different denominators for the survival rate and made comparisons impossible. The template approach should facilitate comparisons between communities and reduce confusion about calculation of survival rates. The template provides a uniform method of calculating an overall survival rate and defines a subgroup stratification that can be used for further analysis.

Emergency Medical Dispatch, Emergency Medical Systems, and the Accident and Emergency Department

The 1985 national conference made recommendations for both prehospital and in-hospital ECC units. These guidelines, however, have been implemented in a variety of ways. There are major differences among EMS systems in how they fulfill their responsibilities with dispatching, staffing, training level, equipment, skills (such as defibrillation, tracheal intubation, venous access), communication technologies, administration, and ratio of rescue personnel to population.[72] Of even more importance are the variations in how the EMS components coordinate and fit together.

With such wide variation in EMS systems, it is difficult to make comparisons. Investigators have not agreed on the optimal EMS system configuration, but research data has now identified those features common to consistently successful out-of-hospital ECC systems. Analysis of some systems with high survival rates for out-of-hospital cardiac arrest reveals these common effective practices:

- Two-tiered EMS systems have improved survival rates over 1-tiered systems.
- Any system in which the first-responding personnel can use AEDs has better outcomes than systems that do not have first-responder defibrillation.
- Multi-tiered systems using deployment rules based on concepts of priority dispatching are effective.
- Cross-training of personnel in dual-service systems (fire and emergency medical) allows aggressive use of fire department personnel and equipment for emergency medical responses.
- EMS systems with active medical control and supervision (medical supervisors at the scene, in the field) have better outcomes than those with passive medical control (retrospective chart reviews).
- The system has actively involved citizenry, defined as having

—High incidence of citizens trained in CPR
—Training in lay responder defibrillation
—Emergency phone calls made and completed as soon as possible after the witnessed emergency
—On arrival, EMS personnel observe lay responders attempting acceptable CPR on a high percentage of all witnessed arrests

These preliminary findings need confirmation by assorted communities. These communities should possess enough variability and population to identify critical factors leading to the high survival rates. Each part of the system—dispatch and first-, second-, and third-tier responders—must be clearly defined so that we can learn the strengths and weaknesses of different structures.

Analysis will be facilitated by describing the EMS dispatch system in terms of type of communication (eg, 911, enhanced 911, or computer-aided dispatch) and method of dispatch, describing each EMS responder, specifying the number of tiers and the role each tier plays during a cardiac arrest, and listing the major interventions in cardiac arrest treatment and obstacles or delays encountered.

Performing the Outcome Assessment: The Chain of Providers

The Chain of Survival model suggests an important dynamic to consider when performing an evaluation of an EMS system. It implies a chain of providers to treat victims of cardiac arrest. This chain of providers should perform the system evaluation. The long-term goal is not merely to collect data but to improve the ECC system. All members of the chain of providers must be represented in the outcome assessment team because the assessment will naturally evolve into the improvement process.

The outcome assessment team may benefit from having representatives of various health departments, EMS systems, police departments, hospitals, universities, industry, and organizations active in BLS and ACLS training. Often a nonpartisan organization such as a resuscitation council or association can facilitate the genesis of this diverse team and serve as an umbrella over the work to be done. A representative team should assess the Chain of Survival, including all interested providers in the process, and identify (1) current performance, (2) community-specific goals, (3) gaps between current performance and goals, (4) ways to improve the ECC system, and (5) whether performance improves after modifications. This process should be a long-term, ongoing effort in every community.

Design of Cardiac Arrest Studies

In the development of a Chain of Survival assessment, the process of working together may be as important as scientific results. For example, EMS personnel may feel threatened by the review process. ACLS-level providers may question why administrators wish to collect information on how long it takes to defibrillate, or dispatchers may feel that they are being singled out for scrutiny. Hospitals provide much of the outcome data, but they also are reluctant to undergo outside scrutiny. In reality local politics cannot be separated from the assessment. Most concerns can be addressed, however, and the effort can move forward if the team represents all providers. Each community must develop its own assessment process to evaluate its Chain of Survival.

The National Registry of Cardiopulmonary Resuscitation

The National Registry of Cardiopulmonary Resuscitation (NRCPR) is a national database for collection of information on in-hospital resuscitation interventions. Sponsored by the American Heart Association, the NRCPR, using modified Utstein templates, gathers the information collected by subscribers. Each participating hospital receives quarterly reports comparing its outcome data with that of an appropriate peer group. This information will undoubtedly be of great value for quality-assurance monitoring within participating medical centers. In addition, the registry will yield valuable information about large groups of inpatients, with analysis within subgroups.[73]

For information about subscribing to the NRCPR, contact www.info@nrcpr.org.

Summary

Cardiac arrest treatment continues to evolve. Adequate treatment of the individual patient requires that the whole ECC system function smoothly, consistently, and rapidly. To maximize community-wide survival rates, a careful evaluation of the entire Chain of Survival is necessary, using standard measurements of performance. The challenge for the next decade is to establish this infrastructure and conduct multicenter, prospective, controlled clinical trials to better define the key factors that will improve survival from cardiac arrest in every community.

References

1. Cummins RO, Ornato JP, Thies WH, Pepe PE. Improving survival from sudden cardiac arrest: the "chain of survival" concept. A statement for health professionals from the Advanced Cardiac Life Support Subcommittee and the Emergency Cardiac Care Committee, American Heart Association. *Circulation*. 1991;83:1832–1847.

1a. Ahnefekt FW. Die Wiederbelebung bei Kreislaufstillstand. *Verh Dtsch Ges Inn Med*. 1968;74:279–287.

2. Cummins RO, Chamberlain D, Hazinski MF, Nadkarni V, Kloeck W, Kramer E, Becker L, Robertson C, Koster R, Zaritsky A, Bossaert L, Ornato JP, Callanan V, Allen M, Steen P, Connolly B, Sanders A, Idris A, Cobbe S. Recommended guidelines for reviewing, reporting, and conducting research on in-hospital resuscitation: the in-hospital "Utstein style." A statement for healthcare professionals from the American Heart Association, the European Resuscitation Council, the Heart and Stroke Foundation of Canada, the Australian Resuscitation Council, and the Resuscitation Councils of Southern Africa. *Resuscitation*. 1997;34:151–183.

3. Zaritsky A, Nadkarni V, Hazinski MF, Foltin G, Quan L, Wright J, Fiser D, Zideman D, O'Malley P, Chameides L, Writing Group. Recommended guidelines for uniform reporting of pediatric advanced life support: the pediatric Utstein Style. A statement for healthcare professionals from a task force of the American Academy of Pediatrics, the American Heart Association, and the European Resuscitation Council. *Circulation*. 1995;92:2006–2020.

4. Cummins RO, Chamberlain DA, Abramson NS, Allen M, Baskett P, Becker L, Bossaert L, Delooz H, Dick W, Eisenberg M, et al. Recommended guidelines for uniform reporting of data from out-of-hospital cardiac arrest: the Utstein Style. Task Force of the American Heart Association, the European Resuscitation Council, the Heart and Stroke Foundation of Canada, and the Australian Resuscitation Council [see comments]. *Ann Emerg Med*. 1991;20:861–874.

5. Eisenberg MS, Cummins RO, Damon S, Larsen MP, Hearne TR. Survival rates from out-of-hospital cardiac arrest: recommendations for uniform definitions and data to report. *Ann Emerg Med*. 1990;19:1249–1259.

6. Eisenberg MS, Horwood BT, Cummins RO, Reynolds-Haertle R, Hearne TR. Cardiac arrest and resuscitation: a tale of 29 cities. *Ann Emerg Med*. 1990;19:179–186.

7. Becker LB, Ostrander MP, Barrett J, Kondos GT. Outcome of CPR in a large metropolitan area: where are the survivors? [see comments]. *Ann Emerg Med*. 1991;20:355–361.

8. Johnson JC. Quality assurance in EMS. In: Roush WR, Aranosian RD, Blair TMH, Handal, KA, Kellow RC, Steward RD, eds. *Principles of EMS Systems: A Comprehensive Text for Physicians*. Dallas, Tex: American College of Emergency Physicians; 1989.

9. US Agency for Health Care Policy and Research. *Medical Treatment Effectiveness Research*. Bethesda, Md: National Institutes of Health; 1990.

10. Cummins RO. The "chain of survival" concept: how it can save lives. *Heart Dis Stroke*. 1992;1:43–45.

11. Emergency Cardiac Care Committee and Subcommittees, American Heart Association. Guidelines for cardiopulmonary resuscitation and emergency cardiac care, I: introduction [see comments]. *JAMA*. 1992;268:2171–2183.

12. Cummins RO, Chamberlain DA. Advisory statements of the International Liaison Committee on Resuscitation. *Circulation*. 1997;95:2172–2210.

13. Jastremski MS. In-hospital cardiac arrest. *Ann Emerg Med*. 1993;22:113–117.

14. Weaver WD, Cobb LA, Hallstrom AP, Copass MK, Ray R, Emery M, Fahrenbruch C. Considerations for improving survival from out-of-hospital cardiac arrest. *Ann Emerg Med*. 1986;15:1181–1186.

15. Larsen MP, Eisenberg MS, Cummins RO, Hallstrom AP. Predicting survival from out-of-hospital cardiac arrest: a graphic model. *Ann Emerg Med*. 1993;22:1652–1658.

16. Valenzuela TD, Roe DJ, Cretin S, Spaite DW, Larsen MP. Estimating effectiveness of cardiac arrest interventions: a logistic regression survival model. *Circulation*. 1997;96:3308–3313.

17. Bossaert L, ed. The prehospital management of acute heart attacks: recommendations of a task force of the European Society of Cardiology and the European Resuscitation Council. *European Resuscitation Council Guidelines for Resuscitation*. Amsterdam, Netherlands: Elsevier; 1998.

18. Clawson JJ. Emergency medical dispatching. In: *Principles of EMS Systems*. Roush WR, Aranosian RD, Blair TMH, Handal KA, Kellow RC, Steward RD, eds. Dallas, Tex: American College of Emergency Physicians; 1989:119–133.

19. Pepe PE, Almaguer DR. Emergency medical services personnel and ground transport vehicles. *Probl Crit Care*. 1990;4:470–476.

20. Curka PA, Pepe PE, Ginger VF, Sherrard RC. Computer-aided EMS priority dispatch: ability of a computed triage system to safely spare paramedics from responses not requiring advanced life support. *Ann Emerg Med*. 1991;20:446. Abstract.

21. Clawson JJ. Emergency medical dispatch. In: Kuehl AE, ed. *EMS Medical Directors' Handbook*. St Louis, Mo: Mosby Year Book; 1989:59–90.

22. National Association of EMS Physicians. Emergency medical dispatching: a position paper. *Prehospital Disaster Med*. 1989;19:536–546.

23. Carter WB, Eisenberg MS, Hallstrom AP, Schaeffer S. Development and implementation of emergency CPR instruction via telephone. *Ann Emerg Med*. 1984;13:695–700.

24. Eisenberg MS, Hallstrom AP, Carter WB, Cummins RO, Bergner L, Pierce J. Emergency CPR instruction via telephone. *Am J Public Health*. 1985;75:47–50.

25. Kellermann AL, Hackman BB, Somes G. Dispatcher-assisted cardiopulmonary resuscitation: validation of efficacy. *Circulation*. 1989;80:1231–1239.

25a. Hallstrom A, Cobb L, Johnson E, Copass M. Cardiopulmonary resuscitation by chest compression alone or with mouth-to-mouth ventilation. *N Engl J Med*. 2000;342:1546–1553.

26. Doherty A, Cummins R, Damon S. Evaluation of CPR Prompt & Home Learning System for teaching CPR to lay rescuers. *Circulation*. 1998;98(suppl I):I-410.

27. Braun O, McCallion R, Fazackerley J. Characteristics of midsized urban EMS systems. *Ann Emerg Med*. 1990;19:536–546.

28. Pepe PE, Bonnin MJ, Almaguer DR. The effect of tiered system implementation on sudden death survival rates. *Prehospital Disaster Med*. 1989;4:71. Abstract.

29. Campbell JC, Gratton MC, Robinson WA. Meaningful response time interval: is it an elusive dream? *Ann Emerg Med*. 1991;83:433.

30. Kerber RE. Statement on early defibrillation from the Emergency Cardiac Care Committee, American Heart Association. *Circulation*. 1991; 83:2233.

31. Cummins RO, Eisenberg MS. Prehospital cardiopulmonary resuscitation: is it effective? *JAMA*. 1985;253:2408–2412.

32. Ritter G, Wolfe RA, Goldstein S, Landis JR, Vasu CM, Acheson A, Leighton R, Medendrop SV. The effect of bystander CPR on survival of out-of-hospital cardiac arrest victims. *Am Heart J*. 1985;110:932–937.

33. Bossaert L, Van Hoeyweghen R, the Cerebral Resuscitation Study Group. Bystander cardiopulmonary resuscitation (CPR) in out-of-hospital cardiac arrest. *Resuscitation*. 1989;17(suppl):S55–S69; discussion S199–S206.

34. Cummins RO, Eisenberg MS, Hallstrom AP, Litwin PE. Survival of out-of-hospital cardiac arrest with early initiation of cardiopulmonary resuscitation. *Am J Emerg Med*. 1985;3:114–119.

35. Cummins RO, Graves JR. Clinical results of standard CPR: prehospital and inhospital resuscitation. In Kaye W, Bircher NG, eds. *Cardiopulmonary Resuscitation*. New York, NY: Churchill-Livingston; 1989.

36. Dracup K, Moser DK, Doering LV, Guzy PM. Comparison of cardiopulmonary resuscitation training methods for parents of infants at high risk for cardiopulmonary arrest. *Ann Emerg Med*. 1998;32:170–177.

37. Kyriacou DN, Arcinue EL, Peek C, Kraus JF. Effect of immediate resuscitation on children with submersion injury. *Pediatrics*. 1994;94: 137–142.

38. Hickey RW, Cohen DM, Strausbaugh S, Dietrich AM. Pediatric patients requiring CPR in the prehospital setting [see comments]. *Ann Emerg Med*. 1995;25:495–501.

39. Bilger MC, Giesen BC, Wollan PC, White RD. Improved retention of the EMS activation component (EMSAC) in adult CPR education. *Resuscitation*. 1997;35:219–224.

40. Meischke H, Dulberg EM, Schaeffer SS, Henwood DK, Larsen MP, Eisenberg MS. "Call fast, Call 911": a direct mail campaign to reduce patient delay in acute myocardial infarction. *Am J Public Health*. 1997; 87:1705–1709.

41. Simons-Morton DG, Goff DC, Osganian S, Goldberg RJ, Raczynski JM, Finnegan JR, Zapka J, Eisenberg MS, Proschan MA, Feldman HA, Hedges JR, Luepker RV, REACT Research Group. Rapid early action for coronary treatment: rationale, design, and baseline characteristics [see comments]. *Acad Emerg Med*. 1998;5:726–738.

42. Eisenberg M, Damon S, Mandel L, Tewodros A, Meischke H, Beaupied E, Bennett J, Guildner C, Ewell C, Gordon M. CPR instruction by videotape: results of a community project. *Ann Emerg Med*. 1995;25: 198–202.

43. Dracup K, Moser DK, Taylor SE, Guzy PM. The psychological consequences of cardiopulmonary resuscitation training for family members of patients at risk for sudden death. *Am J Public Health*. 1997;87: 1434–1439.

44. Kaye W, Rallis SF, Mancini ME, Linhares KC, Angell ML, Donovan DS, Zajano NC, Finger JA. The problem of poor retention of cardiopulmonary resuscitation skills may lie with the instructor, not the learner or the curriculum. *Resuscitation*. 1991;21:67–87.

45. Brennan RT, Braslow A. Skill mastery in cardiopulmonary resuscitation training classes. *Am J Emerg Med*. 1995;13:505–508.

46. Braslow A, Brennan RT, Newman MM, Bircher NG, Batcheller AM, Kaye W. CPR training without an instructor: development and evaluation of a video self-instructional system for effective performance of cardiopulmonary resuscitation. *Resuscitation*. 1997;34:207–220.

47. Stults KR, Brown DD, Kerber RE. Efficacy of an automated external defibrillator in the management of out-of-hospital cardiac arrest: validation of the diagnostic algorithm and initial clinical experience in a rural environment. *Circulation*. 1986;73:701–709.

48. Wright D, James C, Marsden AK, Mackintosh AF. Defibrillation by ambulance staff who have had extended training [see comments]. *BMJ*. 1989;299:96–97.

49. Paris PM. EMT-defibrillation: a recipe for saving lives. *Am J Emerg Med*. 1988;6:282–287.

50. Cummins RO, Thies W. Encouraging early defibrillation: the American Heart Association and automated external defibrillators. *Ann Emerg Med*. 1990;19:1245–1248.

51. Cobb LA, Eliastam M, Kerber RE, Melker R, Moss AJ, Newell L, Paraskos JA, Weaver WD, Weil M, Weisfeldt ML. Report of the American Heart Association Task Force on the Future of Cardiopulmonary Resuscitation. *Circulation*. 1992;85:2346–23455.

52. Kloeck W, Cummins RO, Chamberlain D, Bossaert L, Callanan V, Carli P, Christenson J, Connolly B, Ornato JP, Sanders A, Steen P. Early defibrillation: an advisory statement from the Advanced Life Support Working Group of the International Liaison Committee on Resuscitation. *Circulation*. 1997;95:2183–2184.

53. Cummins RO. From concept to standard-of-care? Review of the clinical experience with automated external defibrillators. *Ann Emerg Med*. 1989; 18:1269–1275.

54. Kellermann AL, Hackman BB, Somes G, Kreth TK, Nail L, Dobyns P. Impact of first-responder defibrillation in an urban emergency medical services system [see comments]. *JAMA*. 1993;270:1708–1713.

55. White RD, Vukov LF, Bugliosi TF. Early defibrillation by police: initial experience with measurement of critical time intervals and patient outcome. *Ann Emerg Med*. 1994;23:1009–1013.

56. White RD, Asplin BR, Bugliosi TF, Hankins DG. High discharge survival rate after out-of-hospital ventricular fibrillation with rapid defibrillation by police and paramedics. *Ann Emerg Med*. 1996;28:480–485.

57. Davis EA, Mosesso VN Jr. Performance of police first responders in utilizing automated external defibrillation on victims of sudden cardiac arrest. *Prehosp Emerg Care*. 1998;2:101–107.

58. Mosesso VN Jr, Davis EA, Auble TE, Paris PM, Yealy DM. Use of automated external defibrillators by police officers for treatment of out-of-hospital cardiac arrest. *Ann Emerg Med*. 1998;32:200–207.

59. O'Rourke MF, Donaldson E, Geddes JS. An airline cardiac arrest program [see comments]. *Circulation*. 1997;96:2849–2853.

60. Page RL, Hamdan MH, McKenas DK. Defibrillation aboard a commercial aircraft. *Circulation*. 1998;97:1429–1430.

61. Valenzuela TD, Bjerke HS, Clark LL, et al. Rapid defibrillation by nontraditional responders: the Casino Project. *Acad Emerg Med*. 1998;5:414–415.

62. Sweeney TA, Runge JW, Gibbs MA, Raymond JM, Schafermeyer RW, Norton HJ, Boyle-Whitesel MJ. EMT defibrillation does not increase survival from sudden cardiac death in a two-tiered urban-suburban EMS system. *Ann Emerg Med*. 1998;31:234–240.

63. Pepe PE, Bonnin MJ, Mattox KL. Regulating the scope of EMS. *Prehospital Disaster Med*. 1990;5:59–63.

64. Cummins RO, Chamberlain DA, Abramson NS, et al. Recommended guidelines for uniform reporting of data from out-of-hospital cardiac arrest: the Utstein style. *Circulation*. 1991;84:960–975.

65. Cummins RO, Chamberlain D, Hazinski MF, et al. Recommended guidelines for reviewing, reporting, and conducting research on in-hospital resuscitation: the in-hospital "Utstein style." *Circulation*. 1997;95:2213–2239.

66. Eisenberg MS, Cummins RO, Litwin PE, Hallstrom AP. Out-of-hospital cardiac arrest: significance of symptoms in patients collapsing before and after arrival of paramedics. *Am J Emerg Med*. 1986;4:116–120.

67. Pepe PE, Bonnin MJ, Clark PS. Clinical predictors of survival in paramedic-witnessed cardiac arrest. *Prehospital Disaster Med*. 1989;4:71. Abstract.

68. Kellermann AL, Staves DR, Hackman BB. In-hospital resuscitation following unsuccessful prehospital advanced cardiac life support: "heroic efforts" or an exercise in futility? *Ann Emerg Med*. 1988;17:589–594.

69. Gray WA, Capone RJ, Most AS. Unsuccessful emergency medical resuscitation: are continued efforts in the emergency department justified? [see comments]. *N Engl J Med*. 1991;325:1393–1398.

70. Bonnin MJ, Pepe PE, Clark PS. Key role of prehospital resuscitation in survival from out-of-hospital cardiac arrest. *Ann Emerg Med*. 1990; 19:466. Abstract.

71. Brown C. Physiologic measurement of the ventricular fibrillation ECG signal: estimating the duration of ventricular fibrillation. *Ann Emerg Med*. 1993;22:70–74.

72. Stout J. System status management. *J Emerg Med Serv*. 1989;14:65–67.

73. Kaye W, Ornato JP, Peberdy M, Mancini ME, Nadkarni V, Truitt T. Factors associated with survival from in-hospital cardiac arrest: a pilot of the National Registry of Cardiopulmonary Resuscitation. *Circulation*. 1999;100(suppl I):I-313. Abstract.

The Most Important Changes in the International ECC and CPR Guidelines 2000

Richard O. Cummins, MD; Mary Fran Hazinski, RN, MSN*

Background

The release of new resuscitation guidelines has a profound effect on clinical practice and on resuscitation teaching. New guidelines produce changes in the marketing and sales of resuscitation products. New guidelines stimulate discussions and debates surrounding the evidence and the rationale. We recognize the strong possibility that many people will concentrate on just a small number of specific details and will overlook the major conceptual changes in how we developed the guidelines and in the basic principles that provide the foundation for these new guidelines. In the following sections we summarize what we consider significant revisions and innovations in resuscitation concepts and principles.

1. Resuscitation Guidelines Now Internationally Developed, Science-Based, and Evidence-Based

The Guidelines 2000 Conference was a fulfillment of important changes that have been under way since 1992.[1–3] The most important changes are expressed in the subtitle of the conference name: "an international consensus on science." The conference was part of an international process, culminating in an international scientific collaboration, fulfilling a mission to produce international guidelines. In addition, for the conference to succeed as a consensus on science, participants had to be strongly committed to the principles of evidence-based guideline development.

At the 1992 guidelines conference, an international panel of experts on resuscitation set a goal to make international resuscitation guidelines as consistent as possible by the year 2000.[1–3] If all scientists review the same science and evaluate it using the same criteria, they reasoned, we should come to the same conclusions and recommendations about how to resuscitate patients. This goal of a single international version of evidence-based, scientific resuscitation guidelines is now a reality with the publication of this document. These international guidelines have grown from several years of planning and review of evidence, reaching a pinnacle at the Guidelines 2000 Conference, the forum for the final presentation and discussion of the draft recommendations.

The 1999 Evidence Evaluation Conference and the Guidelines 2000 Conference were not just new versions of the ECC and CPR conference of the American Heart Association with some invited guests from non-AHA organizations. The participating international leaders ignored parochial issues of meeting venue, financing, and numbers of participants. Instead, the international leadership took the only step that could give us truly international guidelines: both AHA and non-AHA experts and consultants occupied every decision-making position that could influence the final conclusions. These positions included panel chairs, expert presenters, expert reviewers, first draft authors, discussion group leaders, peer reviewers, and editorial board members. Regional and national differences seemed to vanish as participants concentrated on review of evidence, critical appraisal, and debate about conclusions.

We can develop valid resuscitation guidelines only by review of *all* the science and *all* the evidence published internationally, including non–English-language sources. Because good research is being performed and published around the world, guideline developers must have a mechanism to capture this international evidence. The need to capture the world's scientific conclusions created a daunting task that required international planning and consultation. The emphasis on international participation came not from a sense of hospitality but from a sense of quality improvement.

Because of concern that some participants and experts would be unfamiliar with the principles of critical appraisal and evidence-based guideline development, a Research Task Force, with international liaisons, was appointed by ILCOR and the ECC Committee/Subcommittees. The objectives of the Task Force were to specify how to perform critical appraisal of scientific literature and, in particular, how to develop evidence-based scientific guidelines. The Task Force produced a consensus document to explain evidence-based guideline processes to all participants. This document was pilot-tested multiple times with appropriate revisions and modifications after each of 3 evaluation meetings: the Mini Evidence Evaluation Conference, March 1999; the Evidence Evaluation Conference, September 1999; and the Guidelines 2000 Conference, February 2000. This statement, titled "How

*With contributions from the representatives of the resuscitation councils of ILCOR, including the Resuscitation Council of Southern Africa, the New Zealand Resuscitation Council, the Heart and Stroke Foundation of Canada, the European Resuscitation Council, the Australian Resuscitation Council, and the American Heart Association; the Members of the Emergency Cardiovascular Care (ECC) Committee and ECC Subcommittees; and the Editors of the Science Product Development Panel, ECC Programs, American Heart Association. R.O. Cummins and M.F. Hazinski are Senior Science Editors, American Heart Association ECC Programs.

Circulation. 2000;102(suppl I):I-371–I-376.

© 2000 American Heart Association, Inc.

Circulation is available at http://www.circulationaha.org

to Develop Evidence-Based Resuscitation Guidelines," supplied the rationale and template for ECC guideline development.[4] An appendix provided a fill-in-the-blanks worksheet that paralleled the steps recommended in the statement. To gain experience and further develop this evidence-based approach, we applied the recommendations to a proposed guideline for an automated external defibrillator (AED) that used an impedance-compensated biphasic waveform.[5]

The template worksheet was then made available on diskette and online. All topic experts for the Evidence Evaluation Conference completed or contributed to a worksheet. Anyone, whether a participant in the conference or not, could propose a new guideline. We asked only that proposers share with us the evidence they had identified and on which they based their proposals. Anyone who wanted to propose a new guideline could obtain a file from the AHA with directions and a template worksheet. (This worksheet can be downloaded from http://www.americanheart.org/ECC/index.html. Interested persons can also download the statement "How to Develop Evidence-Based Resuscitation Guidelines" from this web site.)

2. Expanded Scope of ECC: From Before the Heart Stops Beating to After the Pulse Returns

During the 1990s resuscitation leaders and experts realized that the range of topics discussed in the ECC and CPR guidelines needed to expand. ILCOR, along with the AHA, recognized that there were dangers associated with limiting the guidelines to patients who have lost their pulse and are in full cardiac arrest. Frequently rescuers and clinicians encounter patients "on their way to a cardiac arrest." Proper interventions at this point may stabilize a patient and keep him or her from further deterioration.

In the United States the AHA ECC programs have added a new course called ACLS for Experienced Providers. This course was designed to address a growing list of prearrest conditions that if treated effectively before the heart stopped would not deteriorate to the point of needing resuscitation. Furthermore, these prearrest conditions would still affect the therapeutic approach if the victim continued to deteriorate despite the prearrest treatments. Life-threatening hyperkalemia provides an example of such a prearrest-to-arrest continuum, as does a lethal overdose of a tricyclic antidepressant. Obviously knowledge of the problem of high potassium or a tricyclic antidepressant overdose will drive the therapeutic approach used after the arrest. The well-trained provider would not simply look at the display of a PEA arrhythmia on the monitor and follow the PEA algorithm.

Included in this expanded list of arrest etiologies are a number of conditions that require specific guidelines but until now have not had precise recommendations, eg, asthma, anaphylaxis, electrolyte disturbances, and toxin-induced disturbances in rhythm and blood pressure. Although these were evidence-based and reviewed in a consensus fashion by many international participants, these special resuscitation conditions did not receive full, face-to-face, international, evidence-based review. Complete international, evidence-

based review and consensus for these topics is planned for the near future and will be provided in supplemental materials.

3. First Aid, CPR, and Defibrillation in the Workplace

The International Guidelines 2000 present a new section on first aid in the workplace. In the United States and most other countries involved in resuscitation research, workplace injuries are a leading cause of death and disability. Deaths from fatal injuries, however, are still only about one third of all workplace deaths. The remaining two thirds are due to sudden cardiac arrest from ventricular fibrillation or other urgent cardiovascular emergencies. In US workplaces, subject to specific federal regulations, trained lay rescuers are expected to respond to all emergencies. Workplace responders need evidence-based guidelines for the response to these emergencies. Because the ECC and CPR guidelines already provide protocols to manage more than two thirds of life-threatening worksite events, it was natural to add evidence-based first aid guidelines to the existing CPR and early defibrillation protocols.[6] The published research for most first aid topics, however, is insufficient to support higher-level classes of recommendations for all actions. Most first aid guidelines merited only a IIb or an Indeterminate class (classes of recommendation are discussed in Part 1). However, we expect the need for evidence-based first aid recommendations to foster additional research on these topics.

4. Elimination of Pulse Check by Lay Rescuers

Since 1992 many published studies have documented the inability of lay rescuers (and usually healthcare professionals as well) to determine accurately the presence or absence of a carotid pulse.[7–16]

When laypersons assess for a pulse, they take too long and are often wrong in their assessment. The large number of errors made in assessing the pulse in simulations is alarming. In actual witnessed arrests, responders may fail to provide chest compressions and fail to apply an AED to people who they mistakenly think have a pulse. This result is called a false-negative (or type II) error—an error that denies a victim an opportunity to be resuscitated. [This topic is discussed in more detail in the editorial titled "Guidelines Based on Fear of Type II (False-Negative) Errors."] By extrapolation from existing data we estimate that this false-negative error will occur in approximately 10% of all of witnessed cardiac arrest victims.

To increase the number of victims who receive appropriate resuscitation, these guidelines recommend elimination of the pulse check for lay rescuers. The training will substitute a simple step: *evaluate for signs of circulation* (normal breathing, coughing, or movement in response to rescue breaths).

5. Revision and Simplification of Adult BLS Compression Rate and Compression-Ventilation Ratio

The compression rate for adult victims (≥8 years of age) has been changed to a specific target (approximately 100 compressions per minute) rather than a broad range (80 to 100 compressions per minute). This change should simplify training and retention by making the compression rate for adults and children (1 to 8 years of age) the same. This recommendation is based on the observation that every time compressions are stopped, multiple compressions are required to reestablish adequate blood flow. In addition, many rescuers compress at a rate much lower than the recommended rate. A recommendation to aim for a 25% higher rate should help bring the average rate into an acceptable range.

The adult compression-ventilation ratio has been simplified to a 15:2 ratio for both 1- and 2-rescuer CPR until the airway is secure (then a 5:1 compression-ventilation ratio can be used for 2-rescuer CPR). Again, this recommendation was prompted by the observation that multiple compressions are required before adequate blood flow resumes after each time the rescuer interrupts compressions to deliver a rescue breath. This change will reduce the number of times per minute that chest compressions are interrupted and will increase the number of chest compressions per minute.

6. Changes in the Foundations of Education, Training, and Evaluation: Skills-Based, Video-Mediated Instruction for Lay Rescuers

For several years educators have criticized the lecture-based approach to teaching and learning CPR. Education experts have rightly criticized loosely scheduled courses packed with information about diverse topics and focused on lectures rather than on acquisition of a small number of critical skills.[17–19] To acquire CPR skills, participants need hands-on practice; excessive lecture time reduces skills practice time. Principles of adult education and evidence documenting the success of video-based learning have led to endorsement and acceptance of video-based teaching techniques.[20–23] These "practice-as-you-watch" and "watch-then-practice" techniques promote acquisition of skills in skills-based educational programs for lay rescuers.

All innovative educational programs should be pilot-tested and evaluated on objective criteria. The program's success at teaching is measured by the percentage of participants who can demonstrate satisfactory critical skills.[24] The AHA has adopted a "watch-then-practice" video-based medium, having documented that as the most effective didactic method for skills acquisition.[25] This focus on skills acquisition represents a dramatic shift in the approach to teaching CPR. By the next iteration of these guidelines research should be able to document whether this shift in teaching techniques makes lay rescuers more likely to learn and perform CPR. The more important outcome should be whether this approach increases the frequency of bystander CPR for out-of-hospital cardiac arrest.

7. Outcome-Driven Education and Evaluation

CPR educators should be able to identify the core learning objectives of any CPR course for any participant.[26] CPR education should emphasize these core objectives and should evaluate whether the participants meet these objectives. Regardless of whether a CPR course teaches a lay rescuer or a healthcare provider, the course should be structured to eliminate extraneous material and focus the participant on acquisition of core information and skills. A course that uses skills or written evaluations should also focus on the core objectives. If the participant then fails to achieve the core objectives, the course (including the instructor) may be at fault.[19] This represents a dramatic departure from the old "pass-fail" philosophy that failure was the fault of the participant. It is now clear that when participants fail to learn it may be that instructors fail to teach.

8. Teaching ACLS: The Primary and Secondary ABCD Surveys as a Unifying Approach to Assessment and Management

ACLS training since 1994 has reformulated cardiac arrest treatment away from a rhythm-based treatment approach to a unifying approach based on reviewing the Primary and Secondary ABCD Surveys.[27–29] All ACLS algorithms in 2000 are oriented around this system, taking the same generic approach to all problems (the primary and secondary ABCD approach), with specific modifications introduced at the second D (differential diagnosis).

The new ACLS for Experienced Providers Course became available in the United States in 1999.[30] The topics addressed in the course were developed to appeal to experienced people who have already taken an ACLS Provider Course. Nevertheless, the ACLS Course for Experienced Providers adopted the primary and secondary ABCD model, noting it to be a logical, uniform, and easily memorized approach.

9. Acute Coronary Syndromes and Acute Ischemic Stroke: Increased Efforts to Achieve Rapid Identification, Rapid Transport, Prearrival Treatment, and Prearrival Notification of the Emergency Department

With the availability and reported success of fibrinolytic therapy for acute coronary syndromes and ischemic stroke, more emphasis must be placed on what appears to be the major obstacle to early fibrinolytic therapy: patient delay.[31] Patients who may be eligible for fibrinolytic treatment must reach a treatment center and be evaluated within the narrow therapeutic window for administration of these drugs. Although patient delays are addressed in other programs, prehospital providers and Emergency Departments must be organized so that they occupy as little of the therapeutic window as possible. To achieve this goal, prehospital care providers must be able to do the following:

- Screen for patients with a high likelihood of an acute coronary syndrome or a potential stroke; immediately transport these patients to appropriate treatment centers.
- Contact and alert emergency facilities that a candidate for fibrinolytic therapy is en route (prearrival notification).
- Initiate diagnostic (eg, 12-lead ECGs or stroke screening exams) and therapeutic actions when indicated. (Where locally appropriate and authorized, this can include field fibrinolytic protocols and antihypertensive protocols.)

To achieve the goal of treatment within the therapeutic window, Emergency Departments and specialists in emergency medicine must be able to do the following:

- Meet the recommended stroke evaluation targets for patients who are potential fibrinolytic candidates. These targets include multiple steps from arrival to disposition, including door-to-physician evaluation, to CT scan obtained, to CT scan interpreted and fibrinolytic decision made.
- Meet the recommended acute coronary syndrome evaluation targets for patients who are potential candidates for fibrinolytic therapy or percutaneous coronary interventions.

10. Devices for Secondary Confirmation of Proper Tracheal Tube Placement: Techniques to Prevent Dislodgment of Tracheal Tubes

For the first time, the ECC guidelines for PALS and ACLS include 2 new recommendations to use devices and techniques for secondary confirmation of tracheal tube placement and to prevent tracheal tube dislodgment after it has been placed:

- Use a validated secondary confirmation technique to confirm tracheal tube placement, in addition to primary confirmation through physical examination.
- Use a specific, validated technique or device to prevent tracheal tube dislodgment, especially in the prehospital setting or whenever transport of the patient is necessary.

The rationale for these important new recommendations is presented in a companion editorial, "Guidelines Based on the Principle 'First, Do No Harm.'" The rationale for this step is based less on hard, definitive evidence and more on a *philosophy of care* (ie, do no harm). These recommendations were driven by an imperative to prevent harm rather than to initiate an intervention because of support from powerful and compelling evidence.

11. Comparable Effectiveness: Competent Ventilation Using Bag-Mask Device May Be as Effective as Compromised Ventilation Using Tracheal Tube

The recent publication of a prospective, randomized trial compared the effectiveness of out-of-hospital ventilations via tracheal tube placement versus ventilations via bag-mask for pediatric emergencies.[32] The results, which confirmed the 2 interventions as equivalent, challenged the concept that ventilation via a properly placed tracheal tube was resuscitation's "gold standard." The choice of ventilatory support (bag-mask ventilation or tracheal intubation) should be based on the clinical condition of the patient, transport time to Emergency Department care, and the experience, training, and expertise of the rescuers. Proficiency in bag-mask ventilation is mandatory for anyone providing BLS or ACLS in the prehospital setting and is of higher priority than skill in tracheal intubation. In locations where prehospital intubation is preferred, quality assurance monitoring must be in place to document rates of successful intubation and rates and severity of complications. Secondary confirmation of tracheal tube placement (see point 10) should be performed immediately after intubation, during transport, and during any movement of the patient.

12. Pharmacological Therapy for Adult and Pediatric Cardiac Arrest and for Pediatric Arrhythmias With Poor Perfusion

Whenever possible, the pediatric guidelines for drug therapy for cardiac arrest and significant arrhythmias have been made consistent with the pharmacological guidelines for adult resuscitation. The adult evidence-based recommendations, however, may not be the best model on which to base pediatric recommendations. On review of the evidence supporting the effectiveness of antiarrhythmics for adult VF or pulseless VT, only amiodarone received an acceptable, effective classification (IIb).[33] Other traditional agents such as lidocaine, bretylium, and procainamide received an indeterminate rating because valid, prospective, randomized trials confirming effectiveness were absent. Similarly, there is insufficient data in the pediatric population to support any agent beyond a Class IIb recommendation. Most PALS recommendations are classed Indeterminate. A major objective of the Subcommittee on Pediatric Resuscitation is to obtain definitive evidence to answer these clinical questions in time for the next iteration of the guidelines.

13. Support for Family Presence at Resuscitation Attempts

When questioned, most family members state that they would like to be present during the attempted resuscitation of a loved one, especially when the resuscitation attempt involves a child. A number of studies have confirmed the desire of family members to be present either at the last minutes of a loved one's life or at the recovery of an effective heartbeat.[5,34–36a] Whenever possible, family members should be given this option, but they will require support and specific attention during the resuscitation. Furthermore, such initiatives require advance planning, discussions among all the staff, and general commitment to work through initial problems. If at all possible, a member of the resuscitation team should remain with the family members while they are in the resuscitation suite. This team member can answer their questions, provide support, and recognize when the family members might need to leave.

14. Honoring Out-of-Hospital No-CPR Advance Directives

In the United States, since 1992 more and more states have instituted regulations that permit EMS personnel to honor advance directives or no-CPR documents/bracelets when they arrive on the scene. For many years the principle followed was *"if called, EMS personnel institute all clinically indicated emergency procedures."* On arrival of EMS personnel at the location of a pulseless person, the protocols required initiation of resuscitative efforts regardless of futility or the prearrest wishes of the victim. The International Guidelines 2000 strongly encourage all US EMS systems to address this issue and follow the lead of our colleagues from Europe and other countries. Those systems place much emphasis on the important role of EMS responders to support the survivors.

15. Death Pronouncement in the Field, Survivor Support Plans, the Futility of Transport of Patients Needing Continued CPR

There has been little evidence that EMS systems and Medical Control Emergency Departments in the United States have reacted to the large and consistently negative experience with transporting pulseless patients from the field to the Emergency Department.[37–44] The survival rate of patients who fail to respond to effective ALS care in the field has never been improved by high-speed, potentially dangerous transportation to an Emergency Department. Researchers in Europe report the same dismal outcomes.[45,46] Unless patients are suffering from rare, specific pathological conditions (eg, hypothermia, drug overdose), there are no in-hospital interventions that will successfully resuscitate patients who fail out-of-hospital efforts.[47] High-speed transport of pulseless patients persists to a large extent because EMS personnel are uncomfortable with having to stop efforts in a victim's home and, in effect, making such a public acknowledgment of failure.[48] In addition, both family and personnel experience discomfort with leaving a body at the scene. The indignity, futility, and danger involved with these transports, however, must end, as it has in many countries.

The solution requires thoughtful planning for the steps to follow when resuscitative efforts stop in the field. Answers to the following questions require reflection, but the answers are available: what are the legal requirements for death certification? for disposition of the body? for post-event survivor support? This is not a new guideline in the United States. Mature EMS systems such as in Seattle–King County, Washington, USA, have implemented protocols for certification of death in the out-of-hospital setting for >20 years.[49] A recent statement from the National Association of EMS Physicians provides an excellent review of this topic, including a thorough list of recommendations almost identical to the guidelines included in the International Guidelines 2000.[48] These futile transports must stop; a little planning and work are all that is necessary.

Summary

Many people involved with resuscitation have specific interests and enthusiasm. They will review the new guidelines to see how their favorite interventions fared. This essay lists a number of the new guidelines that merit special attention: support for family presence at resuscitations, pronouncing death at the scene rather than after futile transport efforts, honoring advance directives, comparable effectiveness of bag-mask ventilation versus tracheal intubation, revision of compression rates and compression-ventilation ratios, and devices to confirm tracheal intubation and prevent tube dislodgment.

Even more important are the new principles and concepts that the International Guidelines 2000 endorse: international guideline science, international guideline development, evidence-based guidelines, training by objectives, expanded scope of ECC to first aid and periarrest conditions, avoidance of false-negative (type II) errors, video-mediated instruction, and a philosophy to "do no harm."

The number and magnitude of these new guidelines reflect the dynamic nature of resuscitation at the start of the 21st century. There is great optimism that these new and revised guidelines will help achieve our ultimate objective. This objective is to be ready when fate brings some lives to a premature end. If we are, we can restore more of these people to a high-quality life, ready for many more years of living.

References

1. Cummins RO, Chamberlain DA. Advisory statements of the International Liaison Committee on Resuscitation. *Circulation.* 1997;95:2172–2173.
2. Chamberlain D, Cummins RO. International emergency cardiac care: support, science, and universal guidelines. *Ann Emerg Med.* 1993;22(2 pt 2):508–511.
3. Cummins RO, Eisenberg MS. Cardiopulmonary resuscitation: American style. *BMJ.* 1985;291:1401–1403.
4. Cummins RO, Hazinski MF, Billi J, Babbs C, Kerber R, Ornato J. How to develop evidence-based ECC and CPR guidelines. Syllabus for the International Guidelines Conference on CPR and ECC, February 6–8, 2000. Dallas, Tex: American Heart Association.
5. Cummins RO, Hazinski MF, Kerber RE, Kudenchuk P, Becker L, Nichol G, Malanga B, Aufderheide TP, Stapleton EM, Kern K, Ornato JP, Sanders A, Valenzuela T, Eisenberg M. Low-energy biphasic waveform defibrillation: evidence-based review applied to emergency cardiovascular care guidelines: a statement for healthcare professionals from the American Heart Association Committee on Emergency Cardiovascular Care and the Subcommittees on Basic Life Support, Advanced Cardiac Life Support, and Pediatric Resuscitation. *Circulation.* 1998;97:1654–1667.
6. Eisenburger P, Safar P. Life supporting first aid training of the public: review and recommendations. *Resuscitation.* 1999;41:3–18.
7. Handley AJ, Becker LB, Allen M, van Drenth A, Kramer EB, Montgomery WH. Single rescuer adult basic life support: an advisory statement from the Basic Life Support Working Group of the International Liaison Committee on Resuscitation (ILCOR). *Resuscitation.* 1997;34:101–108.
8. Handley AJ, Becker LB, Allen M, van Drenth A, Kramer EB, Montgomery WH. Single-rescuer adult basic life support: an advisory statement from the Basic Life Support Working Group of the International Liaison Committee on Resuscitation. *Circulation.* 1997;95:2174–2179.
9. Flesche CW, Breuer S, Mandel LP, Brevik H, Tarnow J. The ability of health professionals to check the carotid pulse. *Circulation.* 1994;90(suppl I):I-288. Abstract.
10. Flesche CW, Zucker TP, Lorenz C, Neruda B, Tarnow J. The carotid pulse check as a diagnostic tool to assess pulselessness during adult basic life support. *Euroanesthesia.* 1995;95:72. Abstract.
11. Bahr J, Klingler H, Panzer W, Rode H, Kettler D. Skills of lay people in checking the carotid pulse. *Resuscitation.* 1997;35:23–26.
12. Monsieurs KG, De Cauwer HG, Bossaert LL. Feeling for the carotid pulse: is five seconds enough? *Resuscitation.* 1996;31:S3.
13. Cummins RO, Hazinski MF. Cardiopulmonary resuscitation techniques and instruction: when does evidence justify revision? [editorial; comment]. *Ann Emerg Med.* 1999;34:780–784.
14. Ochoa FJ, Ramalle-Gomara E, Lisa V, Saralegui I. The effect of rescuer fatigue on the quality of chest compressions. *Resuscitation.* 1998;37:149–152.
15. Flesche C, Neruda B, Breuer S, Tarnow J. Basic cardiopulmonary resuscitation skills: a comparison of ambulance staff and medical students in Germany. *Resuscitation.* 1994;28:S25. Abstract.
16. Flesche C, Neruda B, Noetages P, Tarnow J. Do cardiopulmonary skills among medical students meet current standards and patients' needs? *Resuscitation* 1994;28:S25. Abstract.
17. Kaye W, Mancini ME. Teaching adult resuscitation in the United States: time for a rethink. *Resuscitation.* 1998;37:177–187.
18. Kaye W, Wynne G, Marteau T, et al. An advanced resuscitation training course for preregistration house officers. *J R Coll Physicians Lond.* 1990;24:51–54.
19. Kaye W, Rallis SF, Mancini ME, et al. The problem of poor retention of cardiopulmonary resuscitation skills may lie with the instructor, not the learner or the curriculum. *Resuscitation.* 1991;21:67–87.

20. Brennan RT, Braslow A. Skill mastery in cardiopulmonary resuscitation training classes. *Am J Emerg Med.* 1995;13:505–508.

21. Braslow A, Brennan RT, Newman MM, Bircher NG, Batcheller AM, Kaye W. CPR training without an instructor: development and evaluation of a video self-instructional system for effective performance of cardiopulmonary resuscitation. *Resuscitation.* 1997;34:207–220.

22. Todd KH, Heron SL, Thompson M, Dennis R, O'Connor J, Kellermann AL. Simple CPR: a randomized, controlled trial of video self-instructional cardiopulmonary resuscitation training in an African American church congregation. *Ann Emerg Med.* 1999;34:730–737.

23. Todd KH, Braslow A, Brennan RT, et al. A randomized, controlled trial of video self-instruction versus traditional CPR training. *Ann Emerg Med.* 1998;31:364–369.

24. Aufderheide T, Stapleton E, Hazinski MF, Cummins RO. *Heartsaver AED for the Lay Rescuer and First Responder.* Dallas, Tex: American Heart Association; 1998.

25. Deleted in proof.

26. Deleted in proof.

27. Montgomery WH, Brown DD, Hazinski MF, Clawsen J, Newell LD, Flint L. Citizen response to cardiopulmonary emergencies. *Ann Emerg Med.* 1993;22(2 pt 2):428–434.

28. Billi JE, Membrino GE. Education in adult advanced cardiac life support training programs: changing the paradigm. *Ann Emerg Med.* 1993;22: 475–483.

29. Billi JE. The educational direction of the ACLS training program. *Ann Emerg Med.* 1993;22:484–488.

30. Cummins RO, Hazinski MF. *Instructor's Manual: Advanced Cardiac Life Support for Experienced Providers.* Dallas, Tex: American Heart Association; 1999.

31. Katzan IL, Furlan AJ, Lloyd LE, Frank JI, Harper DL, Hinchey JA. Use of tissue-type plasminogen activator for acute ischemic stroke: the Cleveland area experience. *JAMA.* 2000;283:1151–1158.

32. Gausche M, Lewis RJ, Stratton SJ, Haynes BE, Gunter CS, Goodrich SM, Poore PD, McCollough MD, Henderson DP, Pratt FD, Seidel JS. Effect of out-of-hospital pediatric endotracheal intubation on survival and neurological outcome: a controlled clinical trial. *JAMA.* 2000;283:783–790.

33. Kudenchuk PJ, Cobb LA, Copass MK, et al. Amiodarone for resuscitation after out-of-hospital cardiac arrest due to ventricular fibrillation *N Engl J Med.* 1999;341:871–879.

34. Boie ET, Moore GO, Brummett C, Nelson DR. Do parents want to be present during invasive procedures performed on their children in the emergency department? A survey of 400 parents. *Ann Emerg Med.* 1999;34:70–74.

35. Boyd R. Witnessed resuscitation by relatives. *Resuscitation.* 2000;43: 171–176.

36. Adams S, Whitlock M, Bloomfield P, Baskett PJF. Should relatives be allowed to watch resuscitation? *BMJ.* 1994;308:1687–1689.

36a. Robinson SM, Mackenzie Ross S, Campbell Hewson GL, et al. Psychological effect of witnessed resuscitation on bereaved relatives. *Lancet.* 1998;352:614–617.

37. Bonnin M, Swor R. Outcomes in unsuccessful field resuscitation attempts. *Ann Emerg Med.* 1989;18:507–512.

38. Bonnin M, Pepe P, Kimball K, Clark P. Distinct criteria for termination of resuscitation in the out-of-hospital setting. *JAMA.* 1993;270: 1457–1462.

39. Gray W, Capone R, Most A. Unsuccessful emergency medical resuscitation: are continued efforts in the emergency department justified? *N Engl J Med.* 1991;325:1393–1398.

40. Gray W. Prehospital resuscitation: the good the bad and the futile. *JAMA.* 1993;270:1471–1472.

41. Kellerman A, Staves D, Hackman B. In-hospital resuscitation following unsuccessful prehospital advanced cardiac life support: "heroic efforts" or an exercise in futility? *Ann Emerg Med.* 1988;17:589–594.

42. Kellermann A, Hackman B. Terminating unsuccessful advanced cardiac life support in the field. *Am J Emerg Med.* 1987;5:548–549.

43. Kellermann AL. Criteria for dead-on-arrivals, prehospital termination of CPR, and do-not-resuscitate orders [see comments]. *Ann Emerg Med.* 1993;22:47–51.

44. Kellermann A, Hackman B, Somes G. Predicting the outcome of unsuccessful prehospital advanced cardiac life support. *JAMA.* 1993;270: 1433–1436.

45. Herlitz J, Ekstrom L, Axelson A, et al. Continuation of CPR on admission to Emergency Department after out-of-hospital cardiac arrest: occurrence, characteristics and outcome. *Resuscitation.* 1997;33:223–231.

46. Naess A-C, Steen E, Steen PA. Ethics in treatment decisions during out-of-hospital resuscitation. *Resuscitation.* 1997;33:245–256.

47. Eisenberg MS, Cummins RO. Termination of CPR in the prehospital arena [editorial]. *Ann Emerg Med.* 1985;14:1106–1107.

48. Bailey ED, Wydro GC, Cone DC, and the National Association of EMS Physicians (NAEMSP) Standards and Clinical Practice Committee. Termination of resuscitation in the prehospital setting for adult patients suffering nontraumatic cardiac arrest: a position statement from the NAEMSP. *Prehosp Emerg Care.* 2000;4:190–195.

49. Dull SM, Graves JR, Larsen MP, Cummins RO. Expected death and unwanted resuscitation in the prehospital setting. *Ann Emerg Med.* 1994; 23:997–1002.

Guidelines Based on Fear of Type II (False-Negative) Errors
Why We Dropped the Pulse Check for Lay Rescuers

Richard O. Cummins, MD; Mary Fran Hazinski, RN, MSN

The new guidelines for CPR and ECC strongly emphasize evidence as the basis for all new clinical recommendations. The *level* of evidence may range from a high of Level 1 (one or more randomized, controlled clinical trials) to a low of Level 8 (rational conjecture, common sense, or accepted historically as standard practice). Nonevidence factors can influence the selection of the final class of recommendation, such as the expense of interventions, the ease of teaching, and the consequences of error. A technique that might improve resuscitation outcomes based on animal evidence, eg, open-chest CPR, turns out to be complex, difficult to learn, and difficult to implement. Such a technique would not merit as strong a recommendation as a technique that produced more modest improvements in survival but did so with superior ease of teaching, learning, and implementing.

Two principles that were less familiar to the International Guidelines 2000 experts came into play in several of the debates over the final class of recommendation:

- Avoid "false-negative" (type II) errors in patient assessment.
- Keep any risks from the interventions as close to zero as possible.

We have followed these principles in developing 3 new guidelines recommendations:

- Elimination of the pulse check for lay rescuers.
- Secondary confirmation techniques for tracheal tube placement. These are additions to current overreliance on physical examination as the best confirmation technique.
- More specific methods to prevent tracheal tube dislodgment.

As a general rule clinicians develop a strong imperative always to avoid what are called type II errors or the error of accepting false-negatives.[1–6] This imperative has been a clinical heuristic (decision-making principle) for many decades. Simply stated, whenever a clinician ponders a differential diagnosis, he or she makes 1 of 2 diagnoses: either the disease is *present* or the disease is *absent*. This diagnosis of a disease can be in error in either of 2 ways:

- The clinician's diagnosis is "no disease" when in fact the disease is present (a false-negative, or type II, error).

- The clinician's diagnosis is "disease present," when in truth the disease is not present (a false-positive, or type I, error).

Epidemiologists and statisticians have used the classic 2×2 table to express these relationships between "truth"—disease present or disease absent—and the physician's clinical diagnosis—disease present or disease absent (see Table 1).[3,7]

The classic 2×2 matrix has many uses in clinical epidemiology and diagnostic decision making. Clinicians, researchers, and epidemiologists use the 2×2 matrix to calculate the sensitivity, specificity, and accuracy of diagnostic tests as well as probability, odds ratios, and likelihood for positive or negative treatment outcomes. In statistics the 2×2 matrix enters into calculations for testing the "null" hypothesis, sample size, study *power*, and probability value related to the probability of α and β errors.[7] (Statisticians and others will recognize that a type II or false-negative error rate is the same dilemma statisticians face when they calculate probability value: the probability of accepting the "null hypothesis" when, in fact, the null hypothesis is wrong. The use of double negatives ["yes, the null hypothesis is of no benefit"] can make this a confusing topic.)

No clinician, however, considers false-negative and false-positive (type I and type II) errors to be equivalent in importance or concern. If a clinician has the misfortune to make a wrong clinical diagnosis, which of the following would be a more grievous error: (a) to tell a patient that he or she is *well* when in truth the patient has a serious illness (false-negative or type II error) or (b) to tell the patient that he or she is *ill* with a serious condition when in reality the patient is in glowing health (false-positive or type 1 error)?

The false-negative (type II) error causes an opportunity for a "cure" to be missed. Most clinicians would contend that this is a much more severe mistake than a false-positive (type I) error, ie, thinking a disease is present when it is not. False-positive mistakes have the negative consequences of producing worry, concern, and unnecessary treatment. If the treatment itself lacks serious side effects and poses no harm to the patient, retracting a negative diagnosis and replacing it with a clean bill of health would have few if any negative consequences.

The Pulse Check: A Diagnostic Test
The pulse check, under scrutiny by a number of researchers in the 1990s, is in reality a *diagnostic test*.[8–23]

Circulation. 2000;102(suppl I):I-377–I-379.
© 2000 American Heart Association, Inc.

Circulation is available at http://www.circulationaha.org

TABLE 1. 2×2 Table That Compares the Results of a Diagnostic Test With the "True" Status of the Patient

		"TRUTH" → Status of the Patient		
		Disease Present	Disease Absent	N
Diagnostic test	Test positive: disease present	A Correct diagnosis: disease present	B Type I error: false positive	A+B
	Test negative: disease absent	C Type II error: false negative	D Correct diagnosis: disease absent	C+D
		A+C	B+D	Total Number

The palpation of the carotid artery "tests" for the "diagnosis" of cardiac arrest. If this "disease" is present and the rescuer correctly diagnoses "no pulse," the rescuer starts CPR and (frequently) attaches an AED and delivers shocks.

If the pulseless state is present and the rescuer, in error, states that he or she feels a pulse (false-negative), then the rescuer fails to provide CPR and neglects to check for VF with an AED. This type of false-negative error yields considerable negative consequences, the most telling being the loss of a chance to save a life.

One of the more important pulse check studies was first presented in 1994 at the Scientific Congress of the European Resuscitation Council, in Mainz, Germany.[8] This simple but elegant study alerted resuscitation experts to the danger of false-positive errors. The authors noted that when rescuers thought a pulse was absent, they were correct most of the time (60%) and started their CPR and AED protocols. For the other 40% of patients about whom the rescuers were in error and the model victims really had a pulse, the rescuers started CPR unnecessarily. Table 2 includes the actual numbers from this study by Eberle and colleagues.

From the occasions when the rescuers thought that *disease was present* (n=53) and the *disease really was present* (n=59), we can calculate the sensitivity (53/59=90%). This meant, however, that 10% of the time (100% minus 90%) the victim was falsely diagnosed as having a pulse (n=6) when in fact the pulse was absent (n=59).

If we make several assumptions, we can see the consequences of this 10% type II error rate for the pulse check. Consider a person who suddenly collapses in a cardiac arrest. The nearest witness is a CPR-trained family friend or relative. After checking unresponsiveness and calling the emergency response system, the rescuer would perform steps "A" and "B" and arrive at the "C" of the ABCs. The rescuer needs to check for a pulse. With a false-negative error rate of 10%, the person doing the pulse check will state the equivalent of *"I feel a pulse: we do not need chest compressions"* approximately 1 out of every 10 witnessed arrests. The consequence for that victim is that the rescuer will withhold CPR and AED application inappropriately.

If we consider a hypothetical population of 100 people who experience a sudden, witnessed collapse, 70 to 80 people will be in VF. We know that with early defibrillation, the rate of survival to hospital discharge for the VF victims could be 50% to 70%. A range of 35 to 56 people (50% of 70 to 70% of 80) should have been discharged alive. With the 10% false-negative rate, however, approximately 4 to 6 potential survivors will not survive because CPR and early defibrillation have been withheld.

This possibility for such a severe problem arises because healthcare providers assume that lay rescuers can attend a basic life support course and leave with the ability to accurately detect both the *absence* of a pulse and the *presence* of a pulse. The positive consequences of the plan to drop the pulse check for the lay rescuer is that now the rescuer will start CPR on the basis of unresponsiveness and the absence of any signs of life. All of our hypothetical 100 people in cardiac arrest will receive the positive benefits of early CPR. This avoids having CPR omitted for 10 out of 100 people in need of the intervention.

What are the major consequences of dropping the pulse check for lay responders? What benefits are being sacrificed? What harm may ensue? Elimination of the pulse check should simplify CPR training because rescuers must learn fewer action steps and because the pulse check is the most difficult CPR action to master. Simple training for a simple skill

TABLE 2. 2×2 Table That Compares the Results of a Diagnostic Test of Carotid Pulse Check With the "True" Status of the Patient

		"TRUE" Status of the Patient		
		Disease Present ("No Pulse: Cardiac Arrest!")	Disease Absent ("Good Pulse!")	N
Diagnostic test	Rescuer thinks DISEASE PRESENT ("no pulse: cardiac arrest!")	53 Sensitivity: number of times rescuer thinks no pulse/number of times there is no pulse: 53/59=90%	66 Type I error: number of times rescuer thinks there is no pulse/number of times there is pulse	119
	Rescuer thinks DISEASE ABSENT ("good pulse: no CPR, no AED")	6 Type II error (false negative): a cardiac arrest but rescuer thinks pulse present	81 Specificity: times rescuer thinks disease absent/times disease really is absent	87
		59	147	206

Modified from Reference 24. Based on data from Reference 8.

increases the probability that a lay responder will perform successfully some time in the future.

In addition, the data suggests that of 100 people who collapse but still maintain a pulse, lay responders will "diagnose" the disease of "no pulse" up to 40 times. Thus, a rather high number of people will receive unnecessary ventilations and chest compressions. We must remember, however, that the guidelines still direct the lay rescuer to "check for signs of life" and avoid depending on just the pulse check. Experts speculate that these people diagnosed falsely as "cardiac arrest: begin chest compression" will begin to display other signs of life when the mouth-to-mask ventilations and the forceful chest compressions begin. Attempts to perform unnecessary CPR on people who do not need it probably will not continue for more than 1 or 2 cycles.

The widespread expectation that public access defibrillation (PAD) will continue to expand over the next decade led to a final concern expressed at the Guidelines 2000 Conference. Will dropping the pulse check for lay rescuers produce a conflict with currently accepted indications for attaching and activating an AED? AED instructions provided by AED manufacturers state that AEDs should be attached and placed in assess-and-treat mode only for people in cardiac arrest. The pulse check is necessary to determine cardiac arrest and be consistent with the labeling from AED manufacturers. Does dropping the pulse check for lay responders mean they will be unable to participate in PAD programs? Participation could be denied because lay responders will not be trained to perform the essential step required for AED attachment. This sounds like speculation on a conundrum based on semantics. Eliminating the pulse check should not develop into an obstacle to PAD expansion. The FDA and the AED manufacturers have begun very reasonable dialogue on this issue, which should be resolved in a short time.

In conclusion, the International Guidelines 2000 recommend elimination of the pulse check for lay rescuers as a Class IIa recommendation. When the question of the accuracy and validity of the pulse check was raised, we had to adjust our perspective in two ways. First, it was critical to begin to evaluate the pulse check as exactly what it is—a diagnostic test. Once analyzed in this way the shortcomings of the pulse check became glaringly apparent. The pulse check performs poorly when used as a diagnostic tool by lay responders.

The most significant error that could result from continued use of the pulse check would be a type II error—belief in a false-negative result. Such an error will lead at once to failure to diagnose cardiac arrest, failure to start CPR, and failure to assess the arrest rhythm for VF for approximately 10% of victims of cardiac arrest. A diagnostic test with life or death consequences that has an overall accuracy of only 75% (90% sensibility; 60% specificity) is unacceptable and must be discontinued. This new guideline should eliminate an inaccurate test and increase the number of victims of cardiac arrest who receive chest compressions and early defibrillation.

Finally, we must add the benefits that come from simplifying CPR teaching. Elimination of the pulse check will reduce the number of CPR steps and the skills that the rescuer must learn, remember, and do. Such simplification will increase the likelihood that lay rescuers will learn CPR, perform CPR, and save more lives.

References

1. Sackett DL. Evidence-based medicine and treatment choices. *Lancet*. 1997;349:570–573.
2. Sackett D. Rules of evidence and clinical recommendations on the use of antithrombotic agents. *Chest*. 1989;95:2S–3S.
3. Sackett D, Richard W, Rosenberg W, et al. *Evidence-Based Medicine: How to Practice and Teach EBM*. New York, NY: Churchill Livingstone; 1997.
4. Sackett D, Haynes R, Guyatt G, Tugwell P. *Clinical Epidemiology: A Basic Science for Clinical Medicine*. 2nd ed. Boston, Mass: Little, Brown & Co; 1991.
5. Sackett D, Haynes R, Tugwell P. *Clinical Epidemiology: A Basic Science for Clinical Epidemiology*. Boston, Mass: Little, Brown & Co; 1985.
6. Sackett DL, Rosenberg WM, Gray JA, Haynes RB, Richardson WS. Evidence based medicine: what it is and what it isn't. *BMJ*. 1996;312:71–72.
7. Lang T, Secic M. *How To Report Statistics in Medicine: Annotated Guidelines for Authors, Editors, and Reviewers*. Philadelphia, Pa: American College of Physicians; 1997.
8. Eberle B, Dick WF, Schneider T, Wisser G, Doetsch S, Tzanova I. Checking the carotid pulse check: diagnostic accuracy of first responders in patients with and without a pulse. *Resuscitation*. 1996;33:107–116.
9. Brennan R, Braslow A. Skill mastery in cardiopulmonary resuscitation training classes. *Am J Emerg Med*. 1995;13:505–508.
10. Brennan R, Braslow A, Batcheller A, Kaye W. A reliable and valid method for evaluating cardiopulmonary resuscitation training outcomes. *Resuscitation*. 1996;32:85–93.
11. Bahr J, Klinger H, Panzer W, Rode H, Kettler D. Skills of lay people in checking the carotid pulse. *Resuscitation*. 1997;35:23–26.
12. Bahr J. CPR education in the community. *Eur J Emerg Med*. 1994;1:190–192.
13. Flesche C, Neruda B, Breuer S, Tarnow J. Basic cardiopulmonary resuscitation skills: a comparison of ambulance staff and medical students in Germany. *Resuscitation*. 1994;28:S25. Abstract.
14. Flesche C, Neruda B, Noetages P, Tarnow J. Do cardiopulmonary skills among medical students meet current standards and patients' needs? *Resuscitation*. 1994;28:S25. Abstract.
15. Mather C, O'Kelly S. The palpation of pulses. *Anaesthesia*. 1996;51:189–191.
16. McConnell EA. Assessing a carotid pulse. *Nursing*. 1994;24:22.
17. Gough JE, Kerr MK, Henderson RA, Brown LH, Dunn KA. Do pulse checks cause a significant delay in the initial defibrillation sequence? *Resuscitation*. 1997;34:23–25.
18. Montgomery WH, Brown DD, Hazinski MF, Clawsen J, Newell LD, Flint L. Citizen response to cardiopulmonary emergencies. *Ann Emerg Med*. 1993;22(2 pt 2):428–434.
19. Flesche CW, Breuer S, Mandel LP, Brevik H, Tarnow J. The ability of health professionals to check the carotid pulse. *Circulation*. 1994;90(suppl I):I-288. Abstract.
20. Flesche CW, Zucker TP, Lorenz C, Neruda B, Tarnow J. The carotid pulse check as a diagnostic tool to assess pulselessness during adult basic life support. *Euroanaesthesia*. 1995;95:72. Abstract.
21. Monsieurs KG, De Cauwer HG, Bossaert LL. Feeling for the carotid pulse: is five seconds enough? *Resuscitation*. 1996;31:S3.
22. Becker LB, Berg RA, Pepe PE et al. A reappraisal of mouth-to-mouth ventilation during bystander-initiated cardiopulmonary resuscitation. *Circulation*. 1997;96:2012–2112.
23. Basic Life Support Working Party of the European Resuscitation Council. Guidelines for basic life support. *Resuscitation*. 1992;24:103–110.
24. Cummins RO, Hazinski MF. Cardiopulmonary resuscitation techniques and instruction: when does evidence justify revision? *Ann Emerg Med*. 1999;34:780–784.

Guidelines Based on the Principle "First, Do No Harm"

New Guidelines on Tracheal Tube Confirmation and Prevention of Dislodgment

Richard O. Cummins, MD; Mary Fran Hazinski, RN, MSN

In 1992 ECC experts thought the "gold standard" to confirm correct tracheal tube placement was the multiple, time-honored physical examination criteria:

- See the tube passing through the cords.
- Hear proper sounds when checking 5-point auscultation.
- See the chest expand with each ventilation.
- Note improvement in the level of oxygen saturation.
- See vapor condense in the tube with ventilations.

The experts and clinicians working on recommendations in 1992 rejected several proposals to add secondary confirmation techniques to the resuscitation guidelines. They did not recommend qualitative single-use devices that measured expired CO_2, largely because of expense. They did not accept the inexpensive esophageal detector device (EDD), in large part because the evidence revealed that errors still occurred with them. Continuous quantitative expired CO_2 measurements as a method to detect tube dislodgment were not even mentioned 8 years ago.

The original goals of secondary confirmation techniques were to

- Always identify and remove all esophageal intubations (100% sensitivity to failed intubations)
- Never remove a tracheal tube that is in the trachea (100% specificity to successful intubations).

In 1992 no secondary detection technique performed at this level, and none do now (2000). The evidence the experts used to support the decision to not recommend secondary confirmation devices was their strong confidence in a flawed assumption: the hallowed *confirmation by physical examination criteria* simply could not be improved (Level 8 evidence). In addition, no one asked the question, Does discovery of a tracheal tube in the esophagus in the Accident and Emergency Department or the postanesthesia recovery area indicate an original esophageal tube placement, or an unrecognized tracheal tube displacement that took place after proper tracheal intubation? Guidelines on how to prevent tracheal tube dislodgment were nonexistent. The 1994 ACLS textbook contained only a 2-word recommendation: "secure tube."

Between 1992 and 2000, however, an increasing body of information about high rates of errors in medicine began to accumulate.[1-3] Resuscitation leaders became concerned that patients under their care were experiencing undetected esophageal intubation and undetected tracheal tube dislodgment at a frequency far higher than commonly recognized. The "evidence" that raised these suspicions was indirect and retrospective. Esophageal intubation and tube dislodgment are perceived to be uncommon events. This frequency is so low that a single practitioner may never be involved personally with such an event. In many locations quality assurance committees review these episodes if they learn about them. Quality assurance records, however, are sealed and not available for discovery.

Teachers and practitioners in residency training programs in anesthesiology, emergency medicine, and paramedic programs at academic medical centers hear about and know of these problems locally, often because they were the professionals who discovered the out-of-place tube.[4] This experience in teaching and training programs leads to widespread suspicion that the true rate of misplaced or dislodged tracheal tubes is much higher than ever suspected.[5-10] These complications are extremely serious—if unrecognized they inevitably result in death or severe neurological injury. Most importantly, these are preventable tragedies that devastate families and friends and cut short many young lives.

Recent studies on errors in medicine contend that an accepted tenet of the culture of healthcare providers is to cover up or obscure errors like unrecognized esophageal intubations.[2,11] In terms of open, candid discussions oriented toward remedies, the medical culture lags far behind other professional groups who must maintain life or death skills.[14,15] Aviation pilots have been the most common comparison group with doctors.[14,15]

In the United States any discovered esophageal intubation or tracheal tube dislodgment often results in the filing of a wrongful death or injury lawsuit against the responsible physicians, institutions, or other healthcare providers. Reviews of databases of legal cases and filed lawsuits are one way of getting a sense of how often these events might be occurring. Informal reviews of some of these private databases by the authors confirm the existence of many lawsuits

Circulation. 2000;102(suppl I):I-380–I-384.
© 2000 American Heart Association, Inc.

Circulation is available at http://www.circulationaha.org

filed because tracheal tubes are misplaced originally or dislodged after initial proper placement.

One subspecialty society in the United States has established a unique and highly valuable source of information on malpractice claims against anesthesiologists, called the *American Society of Anesthesiology (ASA) Closed Claims Project*, established by Professor Fred Cheney of the University of Washington in the mid 1980s. The cases in this database are serious misadventures that occur even in the rigidly controlled environment of the operating room or in preoperative or postoperative locations.[12] The cases involve a myriad of problems: teeth and jaw injuries, nerve injuries, problems in gas delivery, equipment failures, eye injuries, and even cases in which operations have been performed during persistent "awareness/awake states." The ASA reports the most damaging events, such as unrecognized esophageal intubations or unrecognized tube dislodgment during the operation, transfer, or movement by the patient.[13]

One of the most admirable features of this ASA project has been the willingness of departments of anesthesiology to identify, analyze, and report these errors. Each event is classified into preventable versus not preventable, and investigators make considerable efforts to determine what was the most likely cause of the event: operator use error, operator maintenance error, equipment design, equipment malfunction, and predictable and unpredictable component failures. This allows open discussion of corrective measures, redesigns, or even new devices. All actions attempt to move the specialty closer and closer to the zero-risk goal.

Of great help to anesthesiology have been evaluations and discussion of whether some new monitoring device or technique, if used in the adverse event cases, would have prevented the mishap. For example, as long ago as 1974 to 1988—4 years before the concept was rejected at the 1992 Guidelines Conference—the ASA examined 1097 claims and concluded that monitoring devices would have completely prevented 32% of the morbidity and mortality. Pulse oximetry and capnometry were the 2 monitoring techniques judged most useful; taken together they could have prevented 93% of the preventable mishaps.[13]

Historically the ASA has been the major leader in the movement to commit to the concept "first, do no harm." To use positive terminology, experts and advisors now speak of the need to "create a *zero-risk* environment" in which to conduct anesthesiology. Over the past 2 decades these principles have coalesced and blended with the principles of the human-engineering/human-factor design movements.[1] The principles include a rejection of the quality assurance model of "find the bad apple; eliminate the problem." Furthermore, we now have widespread acceptance of the concept that errors in medicine must not be attributed to "bad or unskilled or ignorant practitioners, who never learned and never remember."[2,14] Instead, we must view errors in medicine, as in the aviation industry[15] and other public safety organizations, more as system errors or defects in the practice culture and environment than as defects in the practitioners.[2]

The practitioner makes an error because the design of the equipment or the design of the immediate practice environ-

ment makes the error possible. The solutions proposed are to reduce the possibility of error to zero, not by focusing on the practitioner's lack of technique but by engineering around the physician and around the technique. Make errors impossible wherever feasible, so that errors become very difficult to commit. Examples abound in medical devices: fuses, circuit breakers, connector couplings, plugs, warning lights, and simplicity at all user-device interfaces.

There are many examples of harm occurring from errors in medication.[3] Anesthesiology has been deeply involved with hospital-wide efforts to reduce these errors. A medication that provides an excellent example is one that can cause a fatal anaphylactoid reaction, but this reaction is so rare that few clinicians have ever heard of it. The zero-risk approach, when applied to this problem, concluded that the best way to achieve this goal was to remove the medication completely from the hospital premises. With the drug totally unavailable in a facility, the risk of repeat reactions approached zero.

Despite the current trend to focus more on device and system design, it is not possible to remove the operator entirely from responsibility when things go wrong. A review of hundreds of reports of defibrillator failures in the 1980s revealed that the large majority of these failures were operator errors rather than defibrillator malfunctions.[16] In many cases the operators were failing because the devices had not been designed from the perspective of creating a zero risk. When manufacturers began designing automated external defibrillators for unsophisticated users, such as nontraditional responders, the need to create a zero-risk device became acute. Today AEDs provide, in general, good examples of design with a priority on eliminating all possible operator errors. Of interest in the operator-versus-device error debate is that the majority of the "operator failures" reported in the 1980s would be impossible to commit today if the operator were using a modern AED.

AED design continues to evolve especially in the user-device interface. The concept of user-critical steps was borrowed from military training for flying aircraft. A user-critical step is one that the user *must* perform or proper operation will not occur. Here are the 6 user-critical steps required by early AED models: (1) turn the device on, (2) attach pads to the patient, (3) attach cables to pads, (4) attach cables to the AED unit, (5) press the ANALYZE button, and (6) press the SHOCK button. Failure to perform any one of these steps means that a person in ventricular fibrillation will not be shocked. Every time an operator is expected to "do" is giving the operator a chance to "fail."

By the end of 1999, manufacturers had taken on this challenge to eliminate as many user-critical steps as possible. They have done a good job by taking the following actions to eliminate steps: (1) pads preattached to the cables, (2) cables preattached to the AED, (3) POWER ON to occur automatically when the lid is opened, and (4) analysis begins when the pads complete an impedance-measuring circuit across the chest. This leaves just 2 user-critical steps: attach the pads; press the SHOCK button. This is thoughtful design engineering demonstrating the zero-risk concept: 2-step AEDs will experience far fewer operator failures than 6-step devices.

Despite the imperative to make medical devices "operator-proof," it is impossible to take the operator or practitioner completely out of the picture. There always remain significant skill requirements in resuscitation, with the psychomotor skill of tracheal intubation looming as the highest challenge for most practitioners. How can responsible individuals make the practitioner error-proof or mold the individual into a zero-risk performer?

In March 2000 the *British Medical Journal* devoted parts of several issues to the topic of error in medicine. Leaders in this field place great hope on high-fidelity simulators that can train multiple responders to coordinate and work together as a team during resuscitative efforts. Many thoughtful innovations under way in training simulators are integrating sophisticated sensors and pressure gauges with interactive, virtual reality programs. The programs can now handle the problem of reacting not to predetermined instructions but to the actions and decisions of the trainee.

At the international Guidelines 2000 Conference these concepts and principles were ubiquitous. The experts, clinicians, and other participants encountered numerous areas in which objective evidence is weak or absent and fails to support evidence-based recommendations. The experts and resource people often invoked the basic principles of "first, do no harm," "accept only zero-risk interventions," and "never commit type II (false-negative) diagnostic errors."

The most dramatic example of this approach was provided by an excellent prospective study of out-of-hospital, paramedic-performed, pediatric tracheal intubation.[17] The study, led by Marianne Gausche and her colleagues in the Los Angeles County EMS system, California, USA, reached the surprising conclusion that in this particular system, with well-trained but inexperienced paramedics traveling short distances (5-minute transport interval) to receiving hospitals, intubation did not improve survival over bag-mask ventilation.

Other results in this study hit the supporters of out-of-hospital provision of advanced resuscitation care with stunning force. Out of 177 pediatric patients who were intubated and transported to the Emergency Department for further care, a total of 15, or 8% (15/177), were determined to have either esophageal intubation or unrecognized dislodgment of the tracheal tube sometime between the original intubation attempt and placement on the Emergency Department stretchers. Faced with this data, the Medical Director of the Los Angeles EMS system, Sam Stratton, took appropriate action, directing that all equipment for pediatric intubation be removed from the emergency vehicles. Authorization for the medics to attempt pediatric intubation was withdrawn. This incident provides an excellent example of taking the necessary, and highly controversial, actions needed to create a zero-risk intervention. Drs Gausche and Stratton merit our admiration.

How should this data on esophageal intubation be interpreted? Esophageal intubation and unrecognized dislodgment of a tracheal tube are mortal errors. In their conscientious

efforts to help their patients, some paramedics commit an act that contributes directly to the death of their patient. The advanced intervention of tracheal intubation combined with the diagnostic skills of the medics (to detect tube misplacement) is far from being a zero-risk action.

The chief investigators from the Los Angeles study first presented their results in May 1998 at the Scientific Assembly of the Society for Academic Emergency Medicine. At that same conference investigators from Orlando, Florida, presented an equally disturbing abstract of high rates of out-of-hospital paramedic esophageal intubations for adults and children.[6,8,18] For 8 months physicians evaluated all patients arriving at a regional trauma center with a tracheal tube inserted by out-of-hospital personnel. On arrival of patients at the Emergency Department, physicians discovered a stunning 25% of the patients (27 patients out of 108) to have improperly placed tracheal tubes. For 18 of the 27 the tube was in the esophagus; in 9 of the 27 the tube was above the vocal cords. The investigators considered this incidence of out-of-hospital, unrecognized, misplaced tracheal tubes excessively high. They started a reevaluation of their out-of-hospital training and protocols, but they have not yet published their complete results.

These 2 studies, reported in national newspapers, stimulated a strong sense of urgency at the Guidelines 2000 Conference. Here was an intervention that clinicians and practitioners regarded as definitive therapy for victims of cardiopulmonary emergencies, but it was beginning to appear to be a dangerous weapon in the hands of out-of-hospital ACLS personnel. Although tracheal intubation attempts always had the potential to harm the patient, this was the first indisputable evidence that these iatrogenic tragedies were taking a toll.

What Is the Solution?

The attendees at the Guidelines 2000 Conference shared the intense concern of many that ACLS providers may be inadvertently causing death from esophageal intubation or undetected tube dislodgment. Everyone was receptive to proposals to add recommendations to the guidelines to reduce these adverse events. The available techniques include the following:

- *Qualitative end-tidal CO_2 detectors* that undergo a color change when expired CO_2 passes across the detector surface
- *Quantitative end-tidal CO_2 measurement devices called capnometers.* These monitors digitally display a single numeric value for the highest level of expired CO_2 reached during expiration, a process called *capnometry.* Cutoff levels identify when the tube end is in the trachea versus the esophagus or hypopharyngeal area.
- *Quantitative capnographic waveform monitors* that provide, in a process called *capnography*, a continuous display of the amount of CO_2 expired over time. The waveform of patients with a pulse and with the tracheal tube in place shows a very distinct pattern of CO_2 level during expiration from dead space, the alveoli, and then inspiration. In patients with cardiac arrest, however, use of expired CO_2

detectors can lead to unnecessary removal of a properly placed tracheal tube. But devices that use *capnographic waveforms* are so sensitive that the devices can detect residual CO_2 when the tube is in the trachea.

- *Esophageal detector devices (EDDs).* EDDs work by having a care provider insert a tracheal tube and then attach an EDD to the distal end. A quick pull of the EDD plunger (or compression of the aspiration bulb) will produce an easy aspiration of air if the tracheal tube is in the trachea. If the tracheal tube is in the esophagus, the aspiration pulls the mucosal wall of the esophagus against the distal openings in the tracheal tube and either the bulb will not reexpand or the syringe plunger will not pull outward.

Endorsement of either of these devices was slow because the clinical expectation was for devices that were virtually 100% accurate with all uses. Each of these confirmation techniques, however, has significant accuracy problems. End-tidal CO_2 measurements, for instance, are relatively inaccurate in patients without blood flow or a beating heart. The CO_2 is simply not delivered to the lungs for exhalation. The more common error, therefore, is a false-positive error in which the operator is led to think the tube is in the esophagus. The operator's response should be to remove the tracheal tube unnecessarily, which is a type I or false-positive error.

The EDDs, however, are much better for the cardiac arrest patient, because the measurement does not depend on a beating heart. There are, however, a number of situations in which EDDs will indicate to the operator that the tube is in the trachea when it is not. This is the dreaded "type II or false-negative error," in which the diagnostic test looks for "disease," in this case an esophageal intubation. The accompanying editorial on the pulse check discusses the significance of committing a false-negative (consequence can be death) versus a false-positive (consequence can be unnecessary treatment) error. In people with marked obesity or chronic lung disease with chest hyperexpansion or in victims in whom the stomach was filled with air during CPR, EDDs will often rapidly reexpand, indicating tube placement in the trachea. This finding, however, is a false-negative result, leading the operator to think the tube is in the trachea and therefore safe to leave in place. In reality the tube is in the esophagus, often leading to severe consequences.

Obviously perfection in terms of secondary confirmation of endotracheal intubation is unlikely. Both types of devices have significant rates of false-positives and false-negatives. Capnographic waveform monitors are the method of choice, but the devices can run to hundreds of dollars, posing a distinct disadvantage in some settings. In general, an algorithmic approach using several techniques is being recommended for prehospital care.[6,19] Distinguishing clinical features are the presence or absence of a pulse.

- If a *pulse is present,* rely on the colorimetric, qualitative CO_2 techniques.
- If a *pulse is absent,* use the colorimetric CO_2 device. But if the device shows no color change, add the test of the EDD.

No air rush with positive suction indicates that the tracheal tube is in the esophagus—**therefore** reintubate. Air rush with no suction indicates that the tube is in the trachea—**therefore** secure the tube.

Evidence is just beginning to accumulate about securing the tube in place to prevent dislodgment. We lack high-level evidence because the problem is so difficult to study. Some work suggests a surprisingly large amount of tube movement with minimal head and neck flexion and extension. Anesthesiologists have been vocal and adamant about their traditional techniques of tape-and-string to secure the tube, contending an error-free history. A respected textbook of emergency medicine has only 1 illustration on this topic; it features line drawings of how to tear and split adhesive tape, with no mention of the many commercial tube holders available. At this time the Guidelines 2000 Conference can make only a Class IIB recommendation for the use of commercial tube holders, especially for intubations in the out-of-hospital setting. Despite the large number of manufacturers of tracheal tube holders, none supplies objective evidence comparing holder versus no holder or one brand of holder versus another. Recent legal and clinical trial data plus observational epidemiology, however, create a high level of suspicion that the problem of tracheal tube displacement may be devastatingly large.

Summary

In summary, this editorial and the one on pulse check point out another area in which a total reliance on evidence-based guidelines may do our patients a disservice. The debate over dropping the pulse check hinged less on the strength of the evidence and more on the widespread clinical principle of fear of false-negative errors. The discussion of secondary confirmation of tracheal tube placement also lacks a strong base of evidence that identifies the one best technique of tube confirmation for patients with a pulse versus those without a pulse. The principles of the zero-risk intervention and first, do no harm come into play in this situation. We must deal with the growing awareness of the fact that tracheal intubation is not only a potentially lethal intervention but now is also a confirmed lethal intervention, and at a much higher death rate than has ever been suspected. Factors that contribute to the transformation of the tracheal tube from a life-saving to a death-causing intervention are being identified by honest and open researchers. National societies in emergency medicine are responding appropriately. We strongly recommend shifting from making an evidence-based recommendation to instead making a principle-based recommendation—killing our patients is unacceptable; we must act on the widespread concept regarding errors in medicine. We must adopt zero-risk interventions in all possible situations.

References

1. Berwick DM, Leape LL. Reducing errors in medicine. *BMJ.* 1999;319: 136–137.
2. Bisset A, Libertiny G. Risks of medicine and air travel. *BMJ.* 1999;319: 1135–1136.

3. Brennan TA, Leape LL, Laird NM, Hebert L, Localio AR, et al. Incidence of adverse events and negligence in hospitalized patients: results of the Harvard Medical Practice Study I. *N Engl J Med*. 1991;324:370–376.

4. White SJ, Slovis CM. Inadvertent esophageal intubation in the field: reliance on a fool's "gold standard." *Acad Emerg Med*. 1997;4:89–91.

5. Falk J, Rackow E, Weil M. End-tidal carbon dioxide concentration during cardiopulmonary resuscitation. *N Engl J Med*. 1988;318:607–611.

6. Falk JL, Sayre MR. Confirmation of airway placement. *Prehosp Emerg Care*. 1999;2:273–278.

7. Wayne MA, Slovis CM, Pirallo RG. Management of difficult airways in the field. *Prehosp Emerg Care*. 1999;2:290–296.

8. Falk JL. Misplaced tubes. *Prehosp Emerg Care*. 2000;4:202–203. Letter.

9. Ho J. Misplaced tubes. *Prehosp Emerg Care*. 2000;4:202–203. Letter.

10. Wayne M, Levine R, Miller C. Use of end-tidal carbon dioxide to predict outcome in prehospital cardiac arrest. *Ann Emerg Med*. 1995;25:762–767.

11. Helmreich RL. Error, stress, and teamwork in medicine and aviation: cross sectional surveys. *BMJ*. 2000;320:745–749.

12. Cheney FW, Posner K, Caplan RA, Ward RJ. Standard of care and anesthesia liability. *JAMA*. 1989;261:1599–1603.

13. Tinker JH, Dull DL, Caplan RA, Ward RJ, Cheney FW. Role of monitoring devices in prevention of anesthetic mishaps: a closed claims analysis. *Anesthesiology*. 1989;71:541–546.

14. Vincent C. Research into medical accidents: a case of negligence? *BMJ*. 1989;299:1150–1153.

15. Sexton JB, Thomas EJ, Helmreich RL. Error, stress, and teamwork in medicine and aviation: cross sectional surveys. *BMJ*. 2000;320:745–9.

16. Cummins R, Chesemore K, White R. Defibrillator failures: causes of problems and recommendations for improvement. *JAMA*. 1990;264:1019–1025.

17. Gausche M, Henderson D, Brownstein D, Foltin G. The education of out-of-hospital emergency medical personnel in pediatrics: report of a national task force. *Prehosp Emerg Care*. 1998;2:56–61.

18. Katz S, Falk J, Wash M. Misplaced endotracheal tubes by paramedics in an urban emergency medical services system. *Acad Emerg Med*. 1998; 5:429. Abstract.

19. O'Connor RE, Swor RA, Standards and Clinical Practice Committee, National Association of EMS Physicians. Verification of endotracheal tube placement following intubation. *Prehosp Emerg Care*. 1999;3:248–250.

Electrical Treatments in ECC
Moderators: Leo L. Bossaert, MD, Sergio Timerman, MD, Roger D. White, MD
Panel Members: Dianne L. Atkins, MD, Richard E. Kerber, MD, Joseph P. Ornato, MD

Education and Training: How Best to Achieve Our Objectives?
Moderators: Walter G.J. Kloeck, MD, BCh, Thomas E. Terndrup, MD
Panel Members: John E. Billi, MD, Peggy Chehardy, EdD, CHES, Anthony J. Handley, MD, Edward R. Stapleton, EMT-P

Education and Training: Innovations to Improve Learning and Performance
Moderator: Mary Beth Mancini, RN, MSN
Panel Members: John E. Billi, MD, Alidene Doherty, RN, CCRN, Teresa C. Juarbe, RN, PhD, Thomas E. Terndrup, MD

Ethical/Legal Issues in Resuscitation
Moderators: Nisha C. Chandra-Strobos, MD, Petter A. Steen, MD
Panel Members: Norman S. Abramson, MD, Rein DeVos, PhD, Mary E. Fallat, MD, Thomas Finucane, MD, John Kattwinkel, MD, Paul E. Pepe, MD, MPH

Community Approaches to ECC
Moderators: Graham Nichol, MD, MPH, Edward R. Stapleton, EMT-P
Panel Members: Lisa A. Carlson, RN, MS, CPNP, Alidene Doherty, RN, CCRN, Carlos Reyes, MD

Postresuscitation Care
Moderators: Terry Vanden Hoek, MD, Charles L. Schleien, MD, Fritz R. Sterz, MD
Panel Members: Ivor S. Douglas, MD, Hendrik W. Gervais, MD, Robert W. Hickey, MD

Circulatory Adjuncts and Alternative CPR Techniques
Moderators: Karl B. Kern, MD, Peter T. Morley, MD
Panel Members: Charles F. Babbs, MD, PhD, Henry R. Halperin, MD, MA, Norman A. Paradis, MD, Lars Wik, MD

Pharmacologic Control of Heart Rate and Rhythm
Moderators: Paul Dorian, MD, Saul Drajer, MD, Peter J. Kudenchuk, MD
Panel Members: Edgar R. Gonzalez, PharmD, Keith G. Lurie, MD, Peter T. Morley, MD, Ricardo Samson, MD

Toxicology: When Drugs/Toxins Affect Resuscitation Protocols
Moderators: Thomas G. Martin, MD, MPH, Mitchell P. Ross, MD, Francisco de la Torre, MD
Panel Member: Judd E. Hollander, MD

Challenging Resuscitation Problems: Special Situations for Experienced Providers
Moderators: Richard O. Cummins, MD, MPH, MSc, Walter G.J. Kloeck, MD, BCh
Panel Members: John Field, MD, Anthony J. Handley, MD, David G.C. McCann, MD, Petter A. Steen, MD

Research — The Future of Resuscitation
Moderators: Peter J.F. Baskett, MD, Gordon A. Ewy, MD
Panel Members: Douglas Chamberlain, MD, Leon Chameides, MD, Leonard A. Cobb, MD, Janice Jones, MD, Karl H. Lindner, MD, John Kattwinkel, MD, Richard E. Kerber, MD, Rose Marie Robertson, MD, Peter Safar, MD, Charles L. Schleien, MD, Petter A. Steen, MD, Max Harry Weil, MD, PhD

Guidelines 2000 Conference Moderators and Panelists

Norman S. Abramson, MD, University of Pittsburgh, Pittsburgh, PA
Dianne L. Atkins, MD, University of Iowa, Iowa City, IA
Tom P. Aufderheide, MD, Medical College of Wisconsin, Milwaukee, WI
Charles F. Babbs, MD, PhD, Purdue University, West Lafayette, IN
Thomas A. Barnes, EdD, RRT, Northeastern University, Boston, MA
William Barsan, MD, University of Michigan, Ann Arbor, MI
Peter J.F. Baskett, MD, Stanton Court, Wiltshire, England
Lance B. Becker, MD, University of Chicago Hospital, Chicago, IL
Robert A. Berg, MD, University of Arizona, Tucson, AZ
Paul A. Berlin, MS, NREMT-P, Gig Harbor, WA
John E. Billi, MD, University of Michigan, Ann Arbor, MI
Nicholas G. Bircher, MD, Montefiore University Hospital, Pittsburgh, PA
Leo L. Bossaert, MD, University of Antwerp, Antwerp, Belgium
Vic Callanan, MD, Townsville General Hospital, Townsville, Queensland, Australia
Pierre Carli, MD, SAMU de Paris, Paris, France
Lisa A. Carlson, RN, MS, CPNP, Primary Children's Medical Center, Salt Lake City, UT
Douglas Chamberlain, MD, Brighton, England
Leon Chameides, MD, Hartford, CT
Nisha C. Chandra-Strobos, MD, Johns Hopkins University School of Medicine, Baltimore, MD
Peggy Chehardy, PhD, CHES, Tulane University, New Orleans, LA
Leonard A. Cobb, MD, Harborview Medical Center, Seattle, WA
Richard O. Cummins, MD, MPH, MSc, University of Washington Medical Center, Seattle, WA
Rein DeVos, PhD, Academic Medicine Center, Amsterdam, Netherlands
Alidene Doherty, BSN, CCRN, Issaquah Fire Department, Issaquah, WA
Paul Dorian, MD, St Michael's Hospital, Toronto, Ontario, Canada
Ivor S. Douglas, MD, New York Presbyterian Medical Center, New York, NY
Saul Drajer, MD, Argentina Cardiology Foundation, Buenos Aires, Argentina
Mickey S. Eisenberg, MD, PhD, University of Washington Medical Center, Seattle, WA

Gordon A. Ewy, MD, University of Arizona, Tucson, AZ
Mary E. Fallat, MD, University of Louisville, Louisville, KY
John Field, MD, Pennsylvania State University College of Medicine, Hershey, PA
Tom G. Finucane, MD, Johns Hopkins University School of Medicine, Baltimore, MD
Marianne Gausche, MD, Harbor-UCLA Medical Center, Torrance, CA
Michael J. Gerardi, MD, Morristown Memorial Hospital, Morristown, NJ
Hendrik W. Gervais, MD, PhD, Johannes Gutenberg University, Mainz, Germany
Louis Gonzales, BS, NREMT-P, Temple College, Temple, TX
Edgar R. Gonzalez, PharmD, Mechanicsville, VA
Judy Goodman, Iowa-Illinois Safety Council, Des Moines, IA
Henry R. Halperin, MD, MA, Johns Hopkins University School of Medicine, Baltimore, MD
Anthony J. Handley, MD, Colchester, Essex, England
Mary Fran Hazinski, RN, MSN, Vanderbilt University, Nashville, TN
Mark C. Henry, MD, State University of New York at Stony Brook, Stony Brook, NY
Johan Herlitz, MD, Sahlgrenska University, Goteborg, Sweden
Robert W. Hickey, MD, University of Pittsburgh, Pittsburgh, PA
Judd E. Hollander, MD, University of Pennsylvania, Philadelphia, PA
Ahamed H. Idris, MD, University of Florida, Gainesville, FL
Janice Jones, PhD, Georgetown University, Washington, DC
Teresa C. Juarbe, RN, PhD, University of California at San Francisco, San Francisco, CA
John Kattwinkel, MD, University of Virginia, Charlottesville, VA
Richard E. Kerber, MD, University of Iowa, Iowa City, IA
Karl B. Kern, MD, University of Arizona, Tucson, AZ
Walter G.J. Kloeck, MD, BCh, Johannesburg, South Africa
Rashmi U. Kothari, MD, Borgess Research Institute, Kalamazoo, MI
Peter J. Kudenchuk, MD, University of Washington Medical Center, Seattle, WA
Alain Leizorovicz, MD, University of Lyon, Lyon, France
Karl H. Lindner, MD, The Leopold-Franzens-University of Innsbruck, Innsbruck, Austria
Katherine A. Littrell, RN, PhD, Genentech Inc, South San Francisco, CA
Keith G. Lurie, MD, University of Minnesota Medical School, Minneapolis, MN
David G.C. McCann, MD, Donaldsonville, GA
Mary Beth Mancini, RN, MSN, Parkland Health and Hospital System, Dallas, TX
Thomas G. Martin, MD, MPH, University of Washington Medical Center, Seattle, WA
William H. Montgomery, MD, Straub Clinic and Hospital, Honolulu, HI

Peter T. Morley, MD, Royal Melbourne Hospital, Victoria, Australia

Vinay M. Nadkarni, MD, A. I. duPont Hospital for Children, Wilmington, DE

Graham Nichol, MD, MPH, University of Ottawa, Ottawa, Ontario, Canada

Susan Niermeyer, MD, The Children's Hospital, Denver, CO

Jerry P. Nolan, MD, Bath, England

Joseph P. Ornato, MD, Medical College of Virginia, Richmond, VA

Martin H. Osmond, MDCM, Children's Hospital of Eastern Ontario, Ottawa, Ontario, Canada

Charles W. Otto, MD, PhD, University of Arizona, Tucson, AZ

Norman A. Paradis, MD, University of Colorado Health Science Center, Denver, CO

Michael J. Parr, MD, University of New South Wales, Liverpool, Australia

Mary Ann Peberdy, MD, Medical College of Virginia, Richmond, VA

Paul E. Pepe, MD, MPH, The University of Texas Southwestern Medical Center, Dallas, TX

Barbara Phillips, MD, Royal Liverpool Children's Hospital, Liverpool, England

Carlos Reyes, MD, Ministerio de Salva, Santiago, Chile

Flavio Ribichini, MD, Laboratorio di Emodinamica Divisione di Cardiologia, Cuneo, Italy

Colin Robertson, MD, The Royal Infirmary of Edinburgh, Scotland

Rose Marie Robertson, MD, Vanderbilt University Medical Center, Nashville, TN

Mitchell P. Ross, MD, University of Louisville, Louisville, KY

Peter Safar, MD, Safar Center for Resuscitation, University of Pittsburgh, Pittsburgh, PA

Ricardo A. Samson, MD, University of Arizona, Tucson, AZ

Arthur B. Sanders, MD, MHA, University of Arizona, Tucson, AZ

Charles L. Schleien, MD, Columbia University, New York, NY

Donna L. Seger, MD, Vanderbilt University Medical Center, Nashville, TN

Michael Shuster, MD, Heart and Stroke Foundation of Canada, Ottawa, Ontario, Canada

Michael J. Silka, MD, University of Southern California, Los Angeles, CA

Adam J. Singer, MD, State University at Stony Brook, Stony Brook, NY

Lynn A. Smaha, MD, Guthrie Clinic, Sayre, PA

Edward R. Stapleton, EMT-P, State University at Stony Brook, Stony Brook, NY

Petter A. Steen, MD, Ullevaal University Hospital, Oslo, Norway

Fritz R. Sterz, MD, Universitatsklinik fur Notfallmedizin, Wien, Austria

Wanchun Tang, MD, Institute of Critical Care Medicine, Palm Springs, CA

Thomas E. Terndrup, MD, University of Alabama at Birmingham, Birmingham, AL

James Tibballs, MD, Royal Children's Hospital, Melbourne, Australia

Sergio Timerman, MD, National Committee on Resuscitation FUNCOR, Sao Paulo, Brazil

Francisco de la Torre, MD, Universitario Val d'Hebron, Barcelona, Spain

Patrick Van Reempts, MD, PhD, University Hospital Antwerp, Antwerp, Belgium

Terry Vanden Hoek, MD, University of Chicago, Chicago, IL

Max Harry Weil, MD, PhD, Institute of Critical Care Medicine, Palm Springs, CA

Volker Wenzel, MD, University of Innsbruck, Innsbruck, Austria

Roger D. White, MD, Mayo Clinic, Rochester, MN

Lars Wik, MD, National Hospital of Norway, Oslo, Norway

Arno Zaritsky, MD, Children's Hospital of The King's Daughters, Norfolk, VA

Evidence Evaluation Conference (September 1999)

Panels

Ventilation
Moderators: Volker Wenzel, MD, Ahamed H. Idris, MD
Panel Members: William H. Montgomery, MD, Jerry P. Nolan, MD, Michael J. Parr, MD, Gail E. Rasmussen, MD, Wanchun Tang, MD, James Tibballs, MD, Lars Wik, MD

Newly Born
Moderators: John Kattwinkel, MD, Patrick Van Reempts, MD, PhD
Panel Members: David Azzopardi, MD, David Burchfield, MD, Alistair Gunn, MD, Anthony Milner, MD, Susan Niermeyer, MD, Jeffrey Perlman, MD, Ola Didrik Saugstad, MD, Alfonso J. Solimano, MD, Tom Wiswell, MD

Pharmacology – Antiarrhythmics
Moderators: Paul Dorian, MD, Peter J. Kudenchuk, MD
Panel Members: Dianne L. Atkins, MD, Edgar R. Gonzalez, PharmD, Anton P.M. Gorgels, MD, Peter T. Morley, MD, Colin Robertson, MD, Ricardo A. Samson, MD, Michael J. Silka, MD, Bramah N. Singh, MD

Airway Devices
Moderators: Thomas A. Barnes, EdD, RRT, Jerry Nolan, MD
Panel Members: David Macdonald, BSc, ALS, Charles W. Otto, MD, Paul E. Pepe, MD, MPH, Michael R. Sayre, MD, Michael Shuster, MD, Arno Zaritsky, MD

Education
Moderators: Walter G.J. Kloeck, MD, BCh, Thomas E. Terndrup, MD
Panel Members: Anthony J. Handley, MD, Harriet Hawkins, RN, CCRN, Teresa C. Juarbe, RN, PhD, Mary Beth Mancini, RN, MSN, Pip Mason, RN, Edward R. Stapleton, EMT-P, Elinor Wilson, RN, PhD

Acute Coronary Syndromes
Moderators: Leo L. Bossaert, MD, John Field, MD
Panel Members: Tom P. Aufderheide, MD, Johan Herlitz, MD, PhD, Alain

Leizorovicz, MD, Katherine A. Littrell, RN, PhD, Joseph P. Ornato, MD, Mary Ann Peberdy, MD, Flavio Ribichini, MD

AEDs and PAD
Moderators: Sergio Timerman, MD, Roger D. White, MD
Panel Members: Dianne L. Atkins, MD, Leo L. Bossaert, MD, Mary Fran Hazinski, RN, MSN, Richard E. Kerber, MD, Mary Beth Mancini, RN, Joseph P. Ornato, MD, Mary Ann Peberdy, MD, Linda Quan, MD, Wanchun Tang, MD

Pharmacology – Pressors
Moderators: Karl H. Lindner, MD, Vinay M. Nadkarni, MD
Panel Members: Robert A. Berg, MD, Walter G.J. Kloeck, MD, BCh, Peter T. Morley, MD, Charles W. Otto, MD, Norman A. Paradis, MD, Jeffrey Perlman, MD, Ian Stiell, MD, MSc

International Chain of Survival
Moderator: Ian Jacobs, PhD
Panel Members: Vic Callanan, MD, Allen Jaffe, MD, William Landau, MD, Pip Mason, RN, Terence Valenzuela, MD, Norman Vetter, MD, Richard D. Wetzel, MD

Action Sequences for the Lay Rescuer
Moderators: Marc Gay, EMT-P, Paul E. Pepe, MD, MPH
Panel Members: Robert A. Berg, MD, Nicholas Bircher, MD, Leonard A. Cobb, MD, Vic Callanan, MD, Rein de Vos, MD, Alfred Hallstrom, PhD, Anthony J. Handley, MD, Robert W. Hickey, MD, Ian Jacobs, PhD, Arno Zaritsky, MD, David A. Zideman, MD

Pediatric Applications
Moderators: Leon Chameides, MD, Mary Fran Hazinski, RN, MSN
Panel Members: Dianne L. Atkins, MD, Mary E. Fallat, MD, Barbara Phillips, MD, Linda Quan, MD, Charles L. Schleien, MD, Thomas E. Terndrup, MD, James Tibballs, MD, David A. Zideman, MD

Toxicology
Moderators: Francisco de Latorre, MD, Thomas G. Martin, MD, MPH
Panel Members: Andrew Dawson, MD, Robert S. Hoffman, MD, Judd E. Hollander, MD, Albert Jaeger, MD, William Kerns II, MD, Mitchell P. Ross, MD

Chest Compressions and BLS-D
Moderators: Robert A. Berg, MD, Barbara Phillips, MD
Panel Members: Leonard A. Cobb, MD, Alidene Doherty, BSN, CCRN, Gordon A. Ewy, MD, Michael J. Gerardi, MD, Anthony J. Handley, MD, Sharon Kinney, RN, Arthur B. Sanders, MD, MHA, Jonathan Wyllie, MD

Adjuncts for CPR and Compressions
Moderators: Karl B. Kern, MD, Peter T. Morley, MD
Panel Members: Charles F. Babbs, MD, PhD, Francisco De Latorre, MD, Henry R. Halperin, MD, MA, Keith G. Lurie, MD, Joseph P. Ornato, MD, Edison F. Paiva, MD, Norman A. Paradis, MD

Pediatric Airway
Moderators: Arno Zaritsky, MD, David A. Zideman, MD
Panel Members: Waldemar Carlo, MD, Marianne Gausche, MD, Mary Fran Hazinski, RN, MSN, Vinay M. Nadkarni, MD, Martin H. Osmond, MDCM, Gail Rasmussen, RN

Stroke
Moderators: Werner Hacke, MD, Rashmi U. Kothari, MD
Panel Members: Thomas Brott, MD, Elco H. Dykstra, MD, Anthony Furlan, MD, Jerome R. Hoffman, MD, Robert Hoffman, MD, Walter Koroshetz, MD, John Marler, MD, Michael R. Sayre, MD

Post-Resuscitation Therapy
Moderators: Martin H. Osmond, MDCM, Charles L. Schleien, MD
Panel Members: Gerba Buunk, MD, Ivor Douglas, MD, Hendrik Gervais, MD, Robert W. Hickey, MD, Jamie Hutchinson, MD, Volker Wenzel, MD

Ethics
Moderators: Nisha C. Chandra-Strobos, MD, Petter A. Steen, MD
Panel Members: Norman S. Abramson, MD, Rein de Vos, PhD, Dietrich Kettler, MD, Paul E. Pepe, MD, MPH

Evidence Evaluation Conference Moderators and Panelists

Norman S. Abramson, MD, University of Pittsburgh, Pittsburgh, PA

Dianne L. Atkins, MD, University of Iowa, Iowa City, IA

Tom P. Aufderheide, MD, Medical College of Wisconsin, Milwaukee, WI

Dennis Azzopardi, MD, Hammersmith Hospital, London, England

Charles F. Babbs, MD, PhD, Purdue University, West Lafayette, IN

Thomas A. Barnes, EdD, RRT, Northeastern University, Boston, MA

Robert A. Berg, MD, University of Arizona, Tucson, AZ

Nicholas G. Bircher, MD, Montefiore University Hospital, Pittsburgh, PA

Leo L. Bossaert, MD, University of Antwerp, Antwerp, Belgium

Thomas Brott, MD, Mayo Clinic Jacksonville, Jacksonville, FL

David Burchfield, MD, University of Florida, Gainsville, FL

Gerba Buunk, MD, Franciscus Hospital, Roosendaal, Netherlands

Vic Callanan, MD, Townsville General Hospital, Townsville, Queensland, Australia

Waldemar Carlo, MD, FAAP, University of Alabama-Birmingham, Birmingham, AL

Leon Chameides, MD, Hartford, CT

Nisha C. Chandra-Strobos, MD, Johns Hopkins University School of Medicine, Baltimore, MD

Leonard A. Cobb, MD, Harborview Medical Center, Seattle, WA

Richard O. Cummins, MD, MPH, MSc, University of Washington Medical Center, Seattle, WA

Andrew Dawson, MD, Newcastle Master Misericordiae Hospital, Newcastle, Australia

Edison F. de Pavia, MD, FUNCOR, Sao Paulo, Brazil

Rein DeVos, PhD, Academic Medicine Center, Amsterdam, Netherlands

Alidene Doherty, BSN, CCRN, Issaquah Fire Department, Issaquah, WA

Paul Dorian, MD, St Michael's Hospital, Toronto, Ontario, Canada

Ivor S. Douglas, MD, New York Presbyterian Medical Center, New York, NY

Eelco H. Dykstra, MD, PECEMMS Foundation, Apeldoorn, Netherlands

Gordon A. Ewy, MD, University of Arizona, Tucson, AZ

Mary E. Fallat, MD, University of Louisville, Louisville, KY

John Field, MD, Pennsylvania State University College of Medicine, Hershey, PA

Anthony Furlan, MD, Cleveland Clinic Foundation, Cleveland, OH

Marianne Gausche, MD, Harbor-UCLA Medical Center, Torrance, CA

Mark Gay, EMT-P, Heart and Stroke Foundation of Canada, Longueuil, Canada

Michael J. Gerardi, MD, Morristown Memorial Hospital, Morristown, NJ

Hendrik W. Gervais, MD, PhD, Johannes Gutenberg University, Mainz, Germany

Louis Gonzales, BS, NREMT-P, Temple College, Temple, TX

Edgar R. Gonzalez, PharmD, Mechanicsville, VA

Anton P.M. Gorgels, MD, Amsterdam, Netherlands

Alistair Gunn, MD, Auckland School of Medicine, Auckland, New Zealand

Werner Hacke, MD, University of Heidelberg, Heidelberg, Germany

Alfred P. Hallstrom, PhD, University of Washington, Seattle, WA

Henry R. Halperin, MD, MA, Johns Hopkins University School of Medicine, Baltimore, MD

Anthony J. Handley, MD, Colchester, Essex, England

Mary Fran Hazinski, RN, MSN, Vanderbilt University, Nashville, TN

Mark C. Henry, MD, State University of New York at Stony Brook, Stony Brook, NY

Johan Herlitz, MD, Sahlgrenska University, Goteborg, Sweden

Robert W. Hickey, MD, University of Pittsburgh, Pittsburgh, PA

Jerome Hoffman, MD, New York Poison Center, New York, NY

Robert Hoffman, MD University of Pennsylvania, Philadelphia, PA

Judd E. Hollander, MD, University of Pennsylvania, Philadelphia, PA

Jamie Hutchinson, MD, University of Ottawa, Ottawa, Canada

Ahamed H. Idris, MD, University of Florida, Gainesville, FL

Ian Jacobs, MD, University of Southern Australia, Nedlands, Australia

Albert Jaeger, MD, PhD, Hospitaux Universitaires de Strasbourg, Strasbourg, France

Teresa C. Juarbe, RN, PhD, University of California at San Francisco, San Francisco, CA

John Kattwinkel, MD, University of Virginia, Charlottesville, VA

Richard E. Kerber, MD, University of Iowa, Iowa City, IA

Karl B. Kern, MD, University of Arizona, Tucson, AZ

William Kerns II, MD, Carolinas Medical Center, Charlotte, NC

Dietrich Ketter, MD, George-August-University Goettingen, Goettingen, Germany

Sharon Kinney, RN, The University of Melbourne, Melbourne, Australia

Walter G.J. Kloeck, MD, BCh, Johannesburg, South Africa

Walter Koroshetz, MD, Massachusetts General Hospital, Boston, MA

Rashmi U. Kothari, MD, University of Cincinnati, Cincinnati, OH

Peter J. Kudenchuk, MD, University of Washington Medical Center, Seattle, WA

William Landau, University of Washington, Seattle, WA

Alain Leizorovicz, MD, University of Lyon, Lyon, France

Karl H. Lindner, MD, The Leopold-Franzens-University of Innsbruck, Innsbruck, Austria

Katherine A. Littrell, RN, PhD, Genentech Inc, South San Francisco, CA

Keith G. Lurie, MD, University of Minnesota Medical School, Minneapolis, MN

Mary Beth Mancini, RN, MSN, Parkland Health and Hospital System, Dallas, TX

David MacDonald, BSc, ALS, Vancouver, Canada

John Marler, MD, National Institutes of Health, Bethesda, MD

Thomas G. Martin, MD, MPH, University of Washington Medical Center, Seattle, WA

Anthony Milner, MD, St Thomas Hospital, London, England

William H. Montgomery, MD, Straub Clinic and Hospital, Honolulu, HI

Peter T. Morley, MD, Royal Melbourne Hospital, Victoria, Australia

Vinay M. Nadkarni, MD, A. I. duPont Hospital for Children, Wilmington, DE

Susan Niermeyer, MD, The Children's Hospital, Denver, CO

Jerry P. Nolan, MD, Bath, England

Joseph P. Ornato, MD, Medical College of Virginia, Richmond, VA

Martin H. Osmond, MDCM, Children's Hospital of Eastern Ontario, Ottawa, Ontario, Canada

Charles W. Otto, MD, PhD, University of Arizona, Tucson, AZ

Norman A. Paradis, MD, University of Colorado Health Science Center, Denver, CO

Michael J. Parr, MD, University of New South Wales, Liverpool, Australia

Mary Ann Peberdy, MD, Medical College of Virginia, Richmond, VA

Paul E. Pepe, MD, MPH, Allegheny University, Pittsburgh, PA

Jeffrey Perlman, MD, University of Texas, Southwestern Medical School, Dallas, TX

Barbara Phillips, MD, Royal Liverpool Children's Hospital, Liverpool, England

Flavio Ribichini, MD, Laboratorio di Emodinamica Divisione di Cardiologia, Cuneo, Italy

Linda Quan, MD, Children's Regional Medical Center, Seattle, WA

Gail Rasmussen, MD, St Jude's Children's Hospital, Memphis, TN

Colin Robertson, MD, The Royal Infirmary of Edinburgh, Scotland

Mitchell P. Ross, MD, University of Louisville, Louisville, KY

Ricardo A. Samson, MD, University of Arizona, Tucson, AZ

Arthur B. Sanders, MD, MHA, University of Arizona, Tucson, AZ

Ola Didrik Saugstad, MD, The National Hospital, Oslo, Norway

Michael R. Sayre, MD, University of Cincinnati, Cincinnati, OH

Charles L. Schleien, MD, Columbia University, New York, NY

Michael W. Shannon, MD, MPH, Children's Hospital of Boston, Boston, MA

Michael Shuster, MD, Heart and Stroke Foundation of Canada, Ottawa, Ontario, Canada

Michael J. Silka, MD, University of Southern California, Los Angeles, CA

Bramah N. Singh, MD, University of California, Los Angeles, CA

Edward R. Stapleton, EMT-P, State University at Stony Brook, Stony Brook, NY

Ian Stiell, MD, MSc, Loeb Research Institute, Ottawa, Canada

Wanchun Tang, MD, Institute of Critical Care Medicine, Palm Springs, CA

Thomas E. Terndrup, MD, University of Alabama at Birmingham, Birmingham, AL

James Tibballs, MD, Royal Children's Hospital, Melbourne, Australia

Sergio Timerman, MD, National Committee on Resuscitation FUNCOR, Sao Paulo, Brazil

Francisco de la Torre, MD, Universitario Val d'Hebron, Barcelona, Spain

Terence Valenzuela, MD, University of Arizona, Tucson, AZ

Patrick Van Reempts, MD, PhD, University Hospital Antwerp, Antwerp, Belgium

Norman Vetter, MD, UWCM, Cardiff, UK

Volker Wenzel, MD, University of Innsbruck, Innsbruck, Austria

Roger D. White, MD, Mayo Clinic, Rochester, MN

Lars Wik, MD, National Hospital of Norway, Oslo, Norway

Elinor Wilson, MD, Heart and Stroke Foundation of Canada

Thomas Wiswell, Discovery Laboratories, Doylestown, PA

Jonathan Wyllie, MD, South Cleveland Hospital, Cleveland, England

Arno Zaritsky, MD, Children's Hospital of The King's Daughters, Norfolk, VA

David A. Zideman, MD, Hammersmith Hospital, London, England